THIRTEENTH EDITION

Health & Wellness

Gordon Edlin, PhD

Emeritus Professor of Genetics
University of California, Davis

Eric Golanty, PhD

Emeritus Professor of Health, Wellness,
and Physical Education
Las Positas College

JONES & BARTLETT
LEARNING

World Headquarters
Jones & Bartlett Learning
5 Wall Street
Burlington, MA 01803
978-443-5000
info@jblearning.com
www.jblearning.com

Jones & Bartlett Learning books and products are available through most bookstores and online booksellers. To contact Jones & Bartlett Learning directly, call 800-832-0034, fax 978-443-8000, or visit our website, www.jblearning.com.

Substantial discounts on bulk quantities of Jones & Bartlett Learning publications are available to corporations, professional associations, and other qualified organizations. For details and specific discount information, contact the special sales department at Jones & Bartlett Learning via the above contact information or send an email to specialsales@jblearning.com.

16030-7

Production Credits
VP, Product Management: David D. Cella
Director of Product Management: Cathy L. Esperti
Product Assistant: Rachael Souza
Director of Production: Jenny L. Corriveau
Senior Production Editor: Nancy Hitchcock
Director of Marketing: Andrea DeFronzo
Production Services Manager: Colleen Lamy
VP, Manufacturing and Inventory Control: Therese Connell
Composition: Exela Technologies, Inc.

Cover Design: Kristin E. Parker
Director of Rights & Media: Joanna Gallant
Rights & Media Specialist: Merideth Tumasz
Media Development Editor: Shannon Sheehan/Troy Liston
Cover Image (Title Page, Part Opener): © yurok/Getty Images
Printing and Binding: LSC Communications
Cover Printing: LSC Communications

Library of Congress Cataloging-in-Publication Data

Names: Edlin, Gordon, 1932- author. | Golanty, Eric, author.
Title: Health & wellness / Gordon Edlin, PhD, Emeritus Professor of Genetics,
    University of California, Davis Eric Golanty, PhD, Emeritus Professor of
    Health, Wellness, and Physical Education, Las Positas College.
Other titles: Health and wellness
Description: Thirteenth [edition]. | Burlington, Massachusetts: Jones &
    Bartlett Learning, [2019] | Includes bibliographical references and index.
Identifiers: LCCN 2018022619 | ISBN 9781284144130 (paperback)
Subjects: LCSH: Health. | Holistic medicine. | BISAC: HEALTH & FITNESS /
    General.
Classification: LCC RA776 .E24 2019 | DDC 613—dc23
LC record available at https://lccn.loc.gov/2018022619

6048

Printed in the United States of America
22 21 20 19 18   10 9 8 7 6 5 4 3 2

BRIEF CONTENTS

CONTENTS

FEATURES

Health Tips

Managing Stress

Wellness Guide

Global Wellness

Dollars & Health Sense

PREFACE

It is with particular pride that we present the 13th edition of *Health and Wellness*. Publication of this edition in 2018 represents 36 years of continuous use of this textbook by students and instructors since the first edition appeared in 1982. A lot has happened to us (the authors), to book publishing, and to the world since then. We are much older, books are available online in digital format, and the world has changed in ways too numerous to mention. However, the visions we had of health and how to achieve it are as true today as they were 30 years ago. When we conceived of writing a textbook that instructors could use to teach health, we chose to present the rationale and scientific evidence for prevention of disease and illness and for individual self-responsibility for fostering and maintaining one's health. The idea of self-responsibility is now accepted as fundamental in health education. Your behaviors, lifestyle, mental attitudes, and physical activities are what lead to overall health and wellness. Medical science is making truly remarkable advances in curing or alleviating serious conditions such as hepatitis C infections, some cases of cystic fibrosis, and a number of previously untreatable cancers. However, it is even more important today to take charge of your own health. As the pandemics of heart disease, obesity, and diabetes spread around the world, as pollution threatens the livability of the environment and climate change threatens the health of the entire planet, everyone must understand how their behaviors and attitudes contribute to their personal health or illness and the living things that share the Earth with them. The information and guidelines that we set out in previous editions of this book are no less applicable in today's world.

How to Use This Text

We have developed a number of features to help you learn about health and wellness in this book.

Each chapter of the book begins with a list of *Learning Objectives* to help you focus on the most important concepts in that chapter.

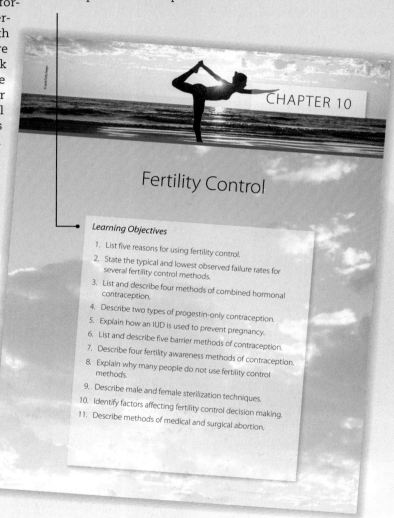

CHAPTER 10

Fertility Control

Learning Objectives

1. List five reasons for using fertility control.
2. State the typical and lowest observed failure rates for several fertility control methods.
3. List and describe four methods of combined hormonal contraception.
4. Describe two types of progestin-only contraception.
5. Explain how an IUD is used to prevent pregnancy.
6. List and describe five barrier methods of contraception.
7. Describe four fertility awareness methods of contraception.
8. Explain why many people do not use fertility control methods.
9. Describe male and female sterilization techniques.
10. Identify factors affecting fertility control decision making.
11. Describe methods of medical and surgical abortion.

school, often rushing to and from work and home, and hence are at risk for automobile accidents.

Alcohol-using students are at risk for auto and other kinds of accidents. Athletically active students are at risk for sports injuries.

Also, a variety of environmental and social forces present barriers to healthful living. For example, someone may want to become more physically active to manage stress or weight and to reduce the risks of heart disease and cancer. However, that person may live in a car-dependent community where work, school, and services are located miles apart and where there are no sidewalks, bike lanes, or nearby parks.

TERMS

Foundation Health Status: seven categories of health goals that represent the major public health concerns in the United States

Leading Health Indicators (LHIs): a set of high-priority Healthy People 2020 objectives and ways to achieve them

self-esteem: the judgment one places on one's self-worth

Key Terms are defined on or near the page on which they are introduced, as well as in the glossary at the end of the book.

(planets and stars). Our planet is aging in the sense that its resources are being used up and the environment is changing. The nuclear reactions that fuel the sun will eventually slow down, and the sun is expected to explode about 5 billion years from now.

Many people associate aging with sickness, disability, loneliness, and increased inactivity. However, such negative views of aging are exaggerated; many older persons today are mentally, sexually, and physically active and continue to work well into their 80s or even 90s.

In America, negative views about aging are still prominent in movies, television, and, especially, advertising.

> I don't want to achieve immortality through my work.
> I want to achieve immortality by not dying.
>
> *Woody Allen*

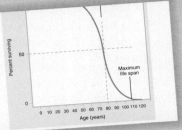

Epigrams enliven each chapter with thought-provoking (and often humorous) quotations about health.

locked or blocked. Hundreds of people were trapped in the buildings and died from burns or suffocation; hundreds more were seriously burned or injured.

About 360,000 residential fires occur in the United States each year. Those fires are responsible for about 13,000 injuries and 2,500 deaths and a loss of $7 billion. Fires in the home may be attributed to many factors: fireplaces, wood stoves, kerosene or space heaters, improper placement of appliances, faulty wiring of the house or appliances, grease fires in the kitchen (loose sleeves dangling over open flames), improper storage of combustible materials, or a careless smoker in the house.

Death rates from fires or burns have markedly decreased since the 1950s. Smoke detectors, portable ladders, and fire extinguishers have helped reduce fatalities. Also, many elementary school students are receiving annual training from local fire departments concerning fire safety. Prevention and education are, once again, the best strategies to eliminate unintentional injuries from fires and burns. Each household should have a planned escape route, smoke detectors placed at key locations throughout the home, and posted emergency phone numbers. Everyone should know how to operate a fire extinguisher and know exactly where it is kept, and in two-story houses, a portable ladder should be readily accessible.

Fire Retardants Fire retardants are chemicals added to clothing, drapes, furniture, bedding, and other fabrics to help prevent the spread of a fire should one start. Most fire retardant chemicals are toxic—they usually are carcinogenic when tested on laboratory animals, and they can pollute land and water and harm the environment. The amount of fire retardant chemicals added to fabrics and furniture is considerable—up to 5% of the fabric's weight. In the 1970s, two fire retardants (called *brominated tris* and *chlorinated tris*) that had been added to children's sleepwear for years were finally banned. These chemicals are carcinogenic and are absorbed into the body from pajamas and other bedding containing fire retardant chemicals. These substances are still added to the foam and fabrics used in furniture. The risk to health and to the environment far outweighs the risk of a fire in a home spreading from furniture. This is especially true now that most homes have smoke detectors. Also, all states, the District of Columbia, and Canada require that all cigarettes be fire-safe.

Firearms

Many Americans view ownership of guns as a constitutional right; others believe that it is a privilege and that ownership should be restricted and regulated. One aspect of firearms is incontrovertible—they cause thousands of deaths and injuries each year.

Firearm-related deaths fall into three categories: unintentional, intentional,

> The hour of departure has arrived and we go our separate ways—I to die and you to live. Which is better, God only knows.
>
> *Socrates*

Kids and Guns: Sometimes a Fatal Mix

Car accidents are the leading cause of unintentional death among children under age 18. The second leading cause of death in that age group is accidental or deliberate discharge of a firearm. Among all high-income countries in the world, 91% of firearm deaths of children younger than 14 years occur in the United States.

Every week about 50 American children die from a bullet wound (see table). Add nearly 5,800 nonfatal gun injuries in this age group annually, and it becomes clear that guns present a serious health risk to American children.

Gun-Related Deaths Among American Children by Age Group, 2012–2014

Age Group	Total	Homicide	Suicide	Unintentional
0–12 years	403	229	150	24
13–17 years	2,080	1,068	543	469

Source: Fowler, K. A. (2017). Childhood firearm injuries in the United States. *Pediatrics,* 140, doi: 10.1542/peds.2017-2298

The vast majority of young children are killed in their homes, often unintentionally as a result playing with loaded guns or involvement in family violence and homicide among adults. Teens are just as likely to be killed by a firearm in a home or on the streets. Suicide by gun is almost always at home. The majority of children are killed with a handgun.

Protecting Kids from Firearm Death

Parents can take the following steps to help protect their children from death by firearm (University of Michigan Mott Children's Hospital, 2017):

• Parents who keep firearms at home should keep the guns locked and unloaded, with the ammunition locked in a separate location.

• Before a child goes to a friend's house, parents should ask the friend's parent whether the family has firearms in the house, and how they are stored. This can be part of all the usual things you would discuss before a visit, like allergies, snacks, sunscreen, etc.

• Parents of teenagers should store guns safely to lessen the risk of gun suicide attempt, even if their children have been educated about guns.

Data from Fowler, K.A. (2017). Childhood firearm injuries in the United States. Pediatrics, 140, XXX–XXX; University of Michigan Mott Children's Hospital, Gun safety for children and youth (www.med.umich.edu/yourchild/topics/guns.htm)

and undetermined. Studies show that having access to a firearm increases the risk of a firearm-related injury or death. If you keep one or more firearms in your home, you should be trained in their use and take all possible safeguards to prevent intentional or unintentional injury or death. All firearms should be locked away. Guns should never be stored loaded. Ammunition should be kept locked in a separate location.

Health Tips in every chapter enable students to make immediate changes to their behavior.

Global Wellness boxes explore health and wellness topics as they impact different countries and cultures.

After Childhood and Adulthood There's Oldhood

We're all familiar with the periods of childhood and adulthood. But you don't hear much about "oldhood." Childhood is the time of considerable physical, emotional, and social development, for which there are expectations, guidelines, rules, teachers, mentors, and laws. Most cultures have a marker for when childhood ends and adulthood begins, such as turning 18 or getting married. Unlike childhood, adulthood is given over to meeting the demands of work/career, marriage, parenthood, and other responsibilities, and their attendant stresses and strains. Oldhood, which also has markers, such as turning 65 or retiring from an occupation, is often seen as a time of diminishing capacity and opportunity. However, as with any other time in the life span, if one has one's health and financial and social support, oldhood can present an enormous diversity of opportunities for new experiences, work, creativity, and joy. There are fewer responsibilities and stress, and more time for exercise, sleep, and indulging one's intellect, and even engaging in a long-put-off passion. Oldhood may be the final epoch of life, but it does not have to be the least rewarding.

Persons surviving to age 55 today can expect to live, on average, another 25 years; those surviving to age 75 can expect to live another 10 to 12 years. Many of these older people are relatively healthy and the length of time that they will be disabled before death is short. In general, people who live to the oldest ages without disabilities are those who have practiced good nutrition, were physically and mentally active, and did not use tobacco or drink alcohol excessively.

More and more attention is being paid to the role of nutrition in healthy aging. Increased consumption of fresh fruits and vegetables is thought to slow the aging processes; those containing antioxidant chemicals are regarded as particularly potent antiaging foods. These include avocado, berries, broccoli, cabbage, carrots, citrus, grapes, onions, tomatoes, and spinach. Coffee and tea also contain significant amounts of antioxidants. But according to believers in the antioxidant theory of aging, supplements still are needed to ensure that you are getting sufficient amounts of antioxidant vitamins and minerals.

Every age of life provides opportunities for growth and satisfaction. Even though we have no way of knowing when serious illness or death will confront us, we do have control of how we live each day and the satisfactions we find in life. The way we choose to live when we are young will greatly affect our health later. For example, smoking while young increases the likelihood of developing cancer and heart disease later. Drinking alcohol to excess and taking unnecessary chances invite accidents that can cause death or permanent disability. Although each person's life span is partly determined by genes, environmental factors, such as nutrition, exercise, and lifestyle, are also important in determining not only how long we live but how well we live.

challenge. Generally, increasing age is associated with increasing disability and functional impairments, such as loss of mobility, sight, or hearing. One goal of gerontology is to find ways to minimize or postpone the disabilities that accompany aging so that quality of life extends to, or close to, the end of life.

The scientific evidence is now quite overwhelming that most of the disability and long-term medical care in elderly persons results from major chronic diseases that were already present in midlife. The most significant predictors of a healthy old age are low blood pressure and low serum glucose levels, not being obese, and not smoking cigarettes while young. These factors are also important in predicting such diseases as cardiovascular disease, cancer, and diabetes. Thus, the evidence points to the importance of developing healthy habits while young if the "golden years" are going to be enjoyed with one's physical and mental abilities intact.

TERMS

hospice: a place for terminally ill patients to spend the time before death in an environment that attends to their physical, emotional, and spiritual needs but does not administer any further treatments; hospice care also can be given in a patient's home

---

Wellness Guides offer tips, techniques, and steps toward a healthy lifestyle and self-responsibility.

Financial Incentives to Get Healthy

Imagine the following scenario. Your employer wants the staff to be healthier by becoming more physically active, so the company is going to pay employees to walk 7,000 steps a day. Steps are counted via a smartphone app, and the total number of steps is transmitted to the program's exercise central database for recording. Participants receive $25 to enroll. In their monthly paychecks, they receive $20 for each month of participation in the program and any earnings from walking. Your employer is offering three incentive options. Which option would you choose?

Pay4play	Double winner	Take the money (and run)
Receive $2 for each day you walk 7,000 steps.	Receive a lottery number between 00 and 99 on each day you walk 7,000 steps. One winning number is drawn each day. You receive $5 for a one-digit match and $50 for a two-digit match (and a bump in your health for walking even if you don't win any money).	Receive a $60 credit at the first of each month. Deduct $2 a day for each day you do not meet the 7,000-step requirement.

Behavioral economists and health professionals are experimenting with ways to incentivize health behavior changes. The fictitious program described here is derived from an actual experiment of similar design conducted by researchers at the

University of Pennsylvania Perelman School of Medicine (Patel, et al., 2016). The results are depicted in the accompanying graph. From the data in the graph, which incentive is the most powerful? Was that the one you chose? Can you explain the results?

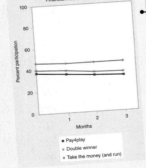

Financial incentives to get healthy

■ Pay4play
× Double winner
＋ Take the money (and run)

• Employees receive company-supplied training and time at work to engage in various types of physical activities.
• New housing developments are required to include inviting public spaces, parks, walking and biking paths, and close access to public transportation and shopping to minimize driving.
• Walking during work hours is encouraged by placing parking lots some distance from buildings, giving employees pedometers or fitness apps, resetting elevators to run slowly to encourage walking stairs, and making staircases wide, carpeted, brightly painted, and with music and picture windows.
• Communities designate and maintain "safe walking" routes for schoolchildren and adult walkers.
• Colleges, universities, churches, and other organizations offer programs that encourage walking and other types of physical activity.

The Definition of Physical Activity

Physical activity is anything you do when you are not sitting or lying down, from clicking your computer's mouse to running a marathon. Among Americans and residents of developed countries, physical activity occurs in the following contexts (Table 7.2):

• *Doing household tasks,* such as washing the floor, being with and taking care of children, and gardening
• *Work-related movement,* for example, walking from a desk to the elevator, being a server in a restaurant, or working in construction
• *Leisure-time activities,* such as taking a walk or engaging in recreational exercise such as dancing, running, swimming, or tennis
• *Skill-based performance activities,* for example, exercising the body (or specific body regions) in order to excel at a particular activity or sport

Physical activity is scientifically defined in terms of the amount of energy expended to produce movement. Movement occurs when energy derived from food

TERMS

sedentary behavior: a pattern of living that lacks sufficient physical activity for good health

---

Most people usually think of health as the absence of disease. But what about someone who has a relatively harmless genetic disorder, such as an extra toe? Is this individual less healthy than a person with the usual number of toes? Different perhaps, but not necessarily less healthy.

It is true that not feeling sick is one important aspect of health. Just as important, however, is having a sense of optimum well-being—a state of physical, mental, emotional, social, and spiritual wellness. In this view, health is defined not only by being unencumbered by disease and disability but also by living in harmony with yourself and with your social and physical environments. You foster your own health and well-being when you take responsibility for avoiding harmful behaviors (e.g., not smoking cigarettes), limiting your exposure to health risks (e.g., not drinking alcohol and driving; limiting the consumption of junk food), and undertaking healthy behaviors and practices such as consuming nutritious food, exercising regularly, attending to your mental well-being, and supporting actions that contribute to the health and well-being of your community (e.g., limiting pollution and reducing violence).

> The health of a people is really the foundation upon which all their happiness and all their powers as a state depend.
>
> *Benjamin Disraeli*

In this chapter, we discuss the definition of health, how modern lifestyles contribute to an enormous degree of chronic illness throughout the world, and how adopting healthy living habits can help people maintain wellness. Throughout this text, we show you ways to maximize your health by understanding how your mind and body function, how to limit exposure to pollution and toxic substances, how to make informed decisions about health and health care, how to be responsible for your actions and behaviors, and how social, economic, and political forces affect your ability to lead a healthy life. Learning to be responsible for the degree of health and vitality you want while you are young helps to ensure lifelong wellness and the capacity to cope with sickness when it does occur.

Models of Health

Scientists and health educators have developed two main ways to define health: the medical model and the wellness, or holistic, model.

The Medical Model of Health

The medical model of health's main tenet is that health is the absence of one or more of the "five Ds"—death, disease, discomfort, disability, and dissatisfaction. In other words,

Mind–Body Harmony

When you are well and healthy, your body systems function harmoniously. If one of your organs is not functioning properly, however, the other organs may not be able to function correctly either, and you may become ill. Thus, disease may be regarded as the disruption of physical and mental harmony of the whole person.

In traditional Western science and medicine, mind–body harmony is considered in terms of homeostasis, the tendency

The Yin–Yang Symbol
This symbol represents the harmonious balance of forces in nature and in people. The white and dark dots show that there is always some yin in a person's yang component and vice versa. The goal in life and nature, according to the traditional Asian view, is to maintain a harmonious balance between yin and yang forces.

for coordinated self-regulation among bodily processes that leads to optimum functioning and survival. Many Asian philosophies embody an idea of mind–body harmony. This idea is based on a universal energy called chi (qi), which must be distributed harmoniously throughout the mind–body to attain and maintain health. Harmony is expressed as a balance of forces called yin and yang. Yin and yang represent the opposing and complementary aspects of the universal chi that is present in everything, including our bodies. Yang forces are characterized as light, positive, creative, full of movement, and having the nature of heaven. Yin forces are characterized as dark, negative, quiet, receptive, and having the nature of earth.

In Asian philosophies and medicine, body and mind are regarded as inseparable. Yin and yang apply to both mental and physical processes. When yin and yang forces are in balance in an individual, a state of harmony exists and the person experiences health and wellness. However, if either yin or yang forces come to predominate in a person, a state of disharmony is produced and disease may result.

Treatment of disease is designed to reestablish harmony of the mind and body. The balance of yin and yang forces must be restored so that health returns.

T'ai chi chi'uan and *qigong* (pronounced jé-kung) are Chinese mind–body methods that are practiced by many North Americans to help maintain health and harmony. These exercises are especially useful for older persons whose bodies can no longer manage vigorous exercise. People who practice *qigong* experience lower blood pressure, improved circulation, and enhanced immune system functions.

Managing Stress boxes give you practical strategies for coping with stress.

Providing Chemical Constituents

Your body is made up of billions of atoms and molecules arranged in particular combinations and proportions. Most of the atoms and molecules that now make up your body were not part of you even a few weeks ago because living things continually exchange their chemical constituents with the environment. The food you consume provides your body with replacement chemicals, which are utilized to manufacture the biological substances that make you you. Your body can manufacture most of the chemicals it needs, but it cannot manufacture 40 of them. These are called the essential nutrients (Table 5.4). Failure to obtain adequate amounts of any essential nutrient can result in weakness, ill-health, or a deficiency disease such as goiter from lack of iodine. Inadequate intake of vitamin A is the most common cause of blindness in children worldwide (World Health Organization, 2016).

Researchers have determined the daily amount of the essential and other nutrients consistent with good health. Many countries and the World Health Organization have produced dietary recommendations based on this research. In the United States, these recommendations, called Dietary Reference Intakes, or DRIs, are issued by the Food and Nutrition Board of the National Academy of Science's Institute of Medicine (U.S. Department of Agriculture, 2017). DRIs are issued for men and women in reasonably good health, pregnant

Table 5.4

The Essential Nutrients*

Amino acids	Fats	Water	Vitamins	Minerals
Isoleucine	Linoleic acid		Ascorbic acid (vitamin C)	Calcium
Leucine	Linolenic acid		Biotin	Chlorine
Lysine			Cobalamin (vitamin B₁₂)	Chromium
Methionine			Folic acid	Cobalt
Phenylalanine			Niacin (vitamin B₃)	Copper
Threonine			Pantothenic acid	Iodine
Tryptophan			Pyridoxine (vitamin B₆)	Iron
Valine			Riboflavin (vitamin B₂)	Magnesium
Arginine†			Thiamine (vitamin B₁)	Manganese
Histidine†			Vitamin A	Molybdenum
			Vitamin D	Phosphorus
			Vitamin E	Potassium
			Vitamin K	Selenium
				Sodium
				Sulfur
				Zinc

*Must be obtained from food.
†Not essential for adults; needed for growth in children.

Ways to Reduce Food Waste

Plan
Make a weekly menu. Prepare a shopping list noting how many meals you'll make with each item and buy no more than what you expect to use. Keep a list of meals and their ingredients that you enjoy. Avoid buying foods you already have. Buying in bulk is thrifty only if you use the food before it spoils.

Store
Store fruits and vegetables for maximum freshness. Freeze, preserve, or can surplus fruits and vegetables. To slow ripening, store bananas, apples, and tomatoes by themselves, and store fruits and vegetables in different bins. Wash berries prior to eating to prevent mold.

Prep
Wash, dry, chop, dice, slice, and place fresh food items in clear storage containers soon after shopping for use later in the week. Prep and freeze meals ahead of time. Freeze bread, sliced fruit, or meat you know won't eat soon.

Save Money
Cook or eat what you already have at home before buying more (soups, casseroles, stir fries, sauces, baked goods, pancakes, or smoothies). Use the edible parts of food that you normally do not eat (stale bread for croutons, sautéed beet tops, vegetable scraps for stock). Have "eat the leftovers" night each week. At restaurants, order only what you can finish; be aware of side

dishes included with entrees; take home the leftovers for your next meal.

Divert from Landfills
Donate to food banks nutritious, safe, and untouched food. Compost food scraps rather than throw them away.

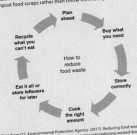

Data from U.S. Environmental Protection Agency. (2017). Reducing food waste at home. Retrieved from https://www.epa.gov/recycle/reducing-wasted-food-home.

Dollars & Health Sense boxes focus on the influence of economic forces on individual and community health; for example, the marketing of worthless and sometimes dangerous supplements and devices for weight management, fitness, and stress relief; direct-to-consumer advertising in the marketing of minimally effective and sometimes dangerous pharmaceuticals; and cigarette advertising to encourage youths to start smoking.

Chapters conclude with *Critical Thinking About Health*—a set of questions that present controversial or thought-provoking situations and ask you to examine your opinions and explore your biases.

End-of-chapter material includes *Chapter Summary and Highlights* (a brief review of the chapter), *For Your Health* (new self-evaluation exercises), *References*, *Suggested Readings*, and *Recommended Websites* where you can find additional health information.

Critical Thinking About Health

1. The accompanying graph shows the results of a test of a new drug. Four groups of patients were involved. Group 1 received a placebo; group 2, 20 mg of the drug; group 3, 40 mg; and group 4, 80 mg.
   a. Do the data support the hypothesis that the drug is effective? Why or why not?
   b. What percentage of people get well without the drug? What's a likely explanation?
   c. What's the maximum percentage of people that can be expected to get well from taking the drug?
   d. If 80 mg produces the desired effect in the largest number of people, why didn't the experimenters report the effects of 100 mg?
2. Bob Kozlo came home from work early one day. Upon hearing his dad's car pull up in the driveway, Jamie, Bob's 16-year-old son, quickly disposed of the joint he and his friend Max were sharing. Mr. Kozlo, who as a teenager also had experimented with marijuana, smelled the telltale odor and knew immediately what Jamie and Max had been up to.
   a. Should Mr. Kozlo ignore this situation or take some kind of action, and if so, what should he do?
   b. Should he tell Max's parents?

   c. What is your opinion of teenagers experimenting with marijuana or any other drugs, including alcohol and tobacco?
3. Why are some drugs illegal? What characteristics distinguish a legal drug from an illegal one? If you had unlimited power and resources, what would you do to solve the illegal drug problem in the United States?
4. In what ways has substance use and abuse touched your life?

Chapter Summary and Highlights

Chapter Summary

Before recorded human history, our ancestors accidentally left containers of ripe fruit or wet grains out in the open where microorganisms began the process of fermentation. When they drank the liquid, their thoughts and behaviors changed. They liked it. They had discovered alcohol. So began a systematic search for leaves, roots, flowers, or mushrooms that could alter thoughts, feelings, and sensations or cure various ailments. Human history and drugs became forever entwined. The shamans, witch doctors, and healers became powerful forces for new knowledge.

A drug is a chemical substance that can produce a change in human (and animal) physiology. The change can be beneficial or harmful, fast or slow acting, long lasting or temporary, addicting or nonaddicting. Many of the most effective drugs used today to treat physical and mental ailments are derived from substances originally discovered in nature. Alcohol, nicotine, opium derivatives, marijuana, and cocaine are still the most widely used drugs. Whether a drug is legal or illegal today has nothing to do with the drug's effectiveness, usefulness, or safety. Consumption of alcohol (and smoking tobacco) causes far more disease and death than all illegal drugs

combined. Prescription drugs do great good as well as great harm. To preserve your health, think carefully about what drugs you ingest or inhale.

Drug abuse is a major problem in today's societies. Drug abuse really means overuse of a drug to the point where a person cannot function and has lost control of his or her life. Addiction or dependence on alcohol, heroin, cocaine, prescription pain killers, tranquilizers, or "uppers and downers" is an example of drug abuse. A person also can become physically or mentally tolerant to a drug, which means that larger doses are needed to achieve the desired effect. All drugs, legal and illegal, have secondary effects that may be dangerous or undesirable. When using any drug, be aware of undesirable side effects or adverse reactions. There are many ways to cope with life's problems without immediately seeking a drug-related solution.

Highlights

- People have been ingesting drugs throughout recorded history for a variety of reasons, including altering thoughts and feelings, curing illness, and facilitating social interaction.

For Your Health

Communication is an integral part of healthy relationships. Do the Listening Exercise (in the Workbook, Chapter 8) to enhance your ability to communicate with important

References

American Academy of Pediatrics. (2012). Newborn male circumcision. Retrieved from https://www.aap.org /en-us/about-the-aap/aap-press-room/pages /newborn-male-circumcision.aspx

Dhejne, C., et al. (2016). Mental health and gender dysphoria: A review of the literature. *International Review of Psychiatry, 28*, 44–57.

Franco, O. H., et al. (2016). Use of plant-based therapies and menopausal symptoms: A systematic review and meta-analysis. *Journal of the American Medical Association, 315*, 2554–2563.

McMahon, C. G., et al. (2013). Standard operating procedures in the disorders of orgasm and ejaculation. *Journal of Sexual Medicine, 10*, 204–229.

Suggested Readings

The Boston Women's Health Book Collective. (2011). *Our bodies, ourselves: A book by and for women.* New York: Touchstone. This book reflects the vital health concerns of women of diverse ages, ethnic and racial backgrounds, and sexual orientation–a must-read for every woman. Companion website is https://www. ourbodiesourselves.org.

Golanty, E., & Edlin, G. (2011). *Human sexuality: The basics.* Sudbury, MA: Jones & Bartlett Learning. A basic college-level text.

Gottman, J. M. (2004). *The seven principles for making marriage work.* New York: Orion. A renowned couples researcher and professor of marital therapy shows how to maintain healthy intimate relationships.

Harvard Medical School. (2017). Men's sexual health. Retrieved from http://www.health.harvard.edu/topics /mens-sexual-health. Numerous authoritative articles on a range of physical, psychological, interpersonal, and social factors influence a man's sexual health.

Recommended Websites

Daily Reproductive Health Report
Daily news stories on human sexuality and reproduction, from the Kaiser Family Foundation.

Go Ask Alice!
A health (including sexuality, sexual health, and relationships) question-and-answer Internet service produced by the Columbia University Health Education Program.

MayoClinic.com
Sexual health basics by the Mayo Clinic staff.

Sex Information and Education Council of the United States (SIECUS)
Information and education about sexuality and responsible sexual choices.

Critical Thinking About Health

1. Set aside some time to reflect on (and write down) your earliest learning experiences about sexuality. Were they open and positive or shrouded with secrecy and shame? How have these experiences shaped your adult sexual attitudes and behaviors? What, if anything, would you like to change?
2. Make a list of situations and relationships in which sexual activity is permissible for you personally. Would your list be different for your son or daughter? Explain.
3. In the United States when a boy is born, the parents are faced with the decision of whether to have him circumcised. Proponents of circumcision cite a number of reasons for supporting it: religion, culture, health, or hygiene. Opponents of circumcision say that it is unnecessary surgery that brings with it unnecessary risk and pain to the child. What are your beliefs on circumcision? On what do you base your beliefs? Talk to someone who disagrees with you and see if your beliefs change or soften.

Chapter Summary and Highlights

Chapter Summary

Awareness of sex and sexuality arises in childhood when we become aware of our biological sex and that there are two sexes. Which one am I? Then we learn to establish a social sexual identity, the gender identity. Even as a child we develop our sexual orientation, the sense of the sex to which we are attracted. People display a spectrum of sexual orientations just as people have a range of intellectual abilities. If everyone realized that sexual orientation is a complex trait like intelligence, perhaps there would be much less prejudice and violence against people whose sexual orientation and preferences differ from their own. As we grow and mature both physically and emotionally, we feel the need to explore our sexuality with others of the opposite sex or with those of the same sex.

Intimacy is a basic human need. Infants bond with mothers (or a substitute caretaker) shortly after birth. As we grow older we share intimate thoughts and feelings with family and friends. Some thoughts and feelings are easily shared; others are not. Becoming physically intimate with another person for the first time can have a profound effect on one's sexual and psychological development, relationships should be entered into with trust and understanding the principles of a fast-paced world, taking time to develop relationships is often ignored. Today, people often seek immediate sexual gratification as a major goal of their social interaction. Learn to treasure your

The text also includes appendixes on relaxation exercises and stress management techniques (including guides for yoga and t'ai chi). A workbook has been included at the end of the text to provide you with self-assessments and activities to explore your own health.

What's New

The following are some examples of topics that are new to this edition or have been expanded upon from prior editions:

- 29 new and updated boxed features, including:
  - Health Tips: Tips for Meeting Basic Human Needs
  - Wellness Guide: What Do Indoor Tanning Beds and Cigarettes Have in Common?
  - Dollars & Health Sense: Plastic Microbeads and Microfibers Pollute Oceans and Seas
  - Global Wellness: After Childhood and Adulthood, There's Oldhood
- New and updated illustrations, photos, and tables highlighting important health information, such as Chapter 18, Table 18.6, "Alcohol-Related Illness, Worldwide," and Chapter 19, Figure 19.1, "Adult Health Insurance Coverage in U.S. by Percent"
- Extensive changes made to Chapter 8, Healthy Sexuality and Intimate Relationships, to expand on the LGBTQ community

- Chapter 19, Making Decisions About Health Care, has been updated to discuss changing healthcare policies
- References, Suggested Reading, and Recommended Websites have been updated for every chapter

Instructor Resources

Qualified Instructors will receive a full suite of Instructor Resources, including the following:

- 3,000 new and updated assessment items, including Practice Activities, Midterm, and Final Exam
- More than 250 slides in PowerPoint format
- An updated Instructor's Manual containing Discussion Questions and Model Answers
- Updated weblinks to relevant health-related sites, including myOptumHealth and the Center for Disease Control and Prevention (CDC)

Student Resources

- Interactive eBook
- Revised Student Workbook with various health-related activities, such as Can I Read a Food Label? and My Sexual Values
- New writable PDFs available online
- New and updated Practice Questions

REVIEWERS

Lawrence E. Acker, Harris-Stowe State University

Pat Alsader, Planned Parenthood of West Central Illinois

David Anspaugh, Memphis State University

Catherine G. Ansuini, Buffalo State College

Jennifer Austin, Colby-Sawyer College

Judy B. Baker, East Carolina University

Cynthia Bartok, Bastyr University

N. K. Bhagavan, University of Hawaii Medical School

Nancy J. Binkin, Centers for Disease Control and Prevention

David Birch, Indiana University

Barbara Brehm-Curtis, Smith College

Rita Buckley Connolly, St. Joseph's University

Tyrone R. Burkett, The Pennsylvania State University

Donald Calitri, Eastern Kentucky University

Barbara Coombs, San Francisco City College

Linda Chaput, W. H. Freeman Publishers

Dorothy Coltrin, De Anza College

Geoffrey Cooper, Harvard Medical School

Bernice Daugherty, Lander University

Nicholas J. DiCicco, Camden County College

Judy Drolet, Southern Illinois University at Carbondale

William E. Dunscombe, Union County College

Philip Duryea, University of New Mexico

Seymour Eiseman, California State University–Northridge

Carol Ellison, Berkeley, California

Marlene Henry Fletcher, Central Texas College

Marianne Frauenknecht, Western Michigan University

Laura Fox Fudacz, Ivy Tech Community College of Indiana

Nicole Gegel, Illinois State University

Katherine Gieg, Missouri Baptist University

Mai Goldsmith, Southern Illinois University at Edwardsville

Wretha G. Goodpaster, Morehead State University

Catherine M. Headley, Judson College

Allan C. Henderson, California State University–Long Beach

Meg Henning, Keene State

Sherry Hineman, University of California–San Diego

Leo Hollister, Stanford Medical Center

Stanley Inkelis, Harbor General Hospital

John Janowiak, Appalachian State University

William Kane, University of New Mexico

Mark Kittleson, Southern Illinois University at Carbondale

Tim Knickelbein, Normandale Community College

Dr. Jerome Kotecki, Ball State University

Dawn Larsen, Mankato State University

Pat Lefler, Bluegrass Community and Technical College

C. H. "Pete" LeRoy, New Mexico Highlands University

Karen M. Lew, University of Miami

Will Lotter, University of California–Davis

Beverly Saxton Mahoney, The Pennsylvania State University

Mary Martin, University of California–San Francisco

Sharon Mathis, Benedictine College

Patricia L. McDiarmid, Springfield College

Marion Micke, Illinois State University

Dr. Pardess Mitchell, William Rainey Harper College

Peter J. Morano, Central Connecticut State University

Richard P. Morris, Rollins College

Linda J. Mukina Felker, Edinboro University of Pennsylvania

Debra J. C. Murray, University of North Carolina at Chapel Hill

Anne Nadakavukaren, Illinois State University

Ann Neilson, College of Saint Rose

Marion Nestle, New York University

Roberta Ogletree, Southern Illinois University at Carbondale

Larry Olsen, The Pennsylvania State University

Elizabeth O'Neill, Central Connecticut State University

David Phelps, Oregon State University

Richard Plant, South Middlesex Community College

Bruce Ragon, Indiana University

Kerry J. Redican, Virginia Technical University

Dwayne Reed, Buck Institute for Research on Aging

Janet Reis, University of Illinois at Urbana–Champaign

Russell E. Robinson, Shippensburg University

Jennifer L Scheid, Daemen College

A NOTE OF THANKS

Throughout all of the editions of *Health and Wellness*, many people have contributed support and guidance. This book has benefited greatly from their comments, opinions, thoughtful critiques, expert knowledge, and constructive suggestions. We are most appreciative for their participation in this project. We would especially like to thank Brian Luke Seaward, Paramount Wellness Institute; James Walsh; Esther M. Weekes; Martin Schulz; Shae Bearden; Rocky Young; Bharti Temkin; and Laura Jones-Swann and Scott O. Roberts, Texas Tech University.

We also want to thank our editors (past and present), especially Art Bartlett and Julie Bolduc, and all of the people at Jones & Bartlett Learning for their unflagging support of this textbook over the years. This new edition could not have been published without the efforts of the staff at Jones & Bartlett Learning and the Health Science team: Cathy Esperti, Rachael Souza, Nancy Hitchcock, Merideth Tumasz, and Shannon Sheehan. To all, we express our appreciation.

PART ONE

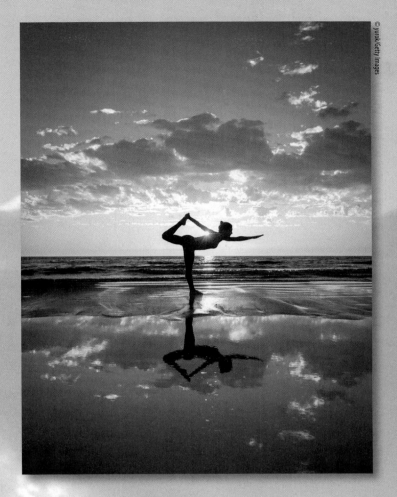

©yurok/Getty Images

Achieving Wellness

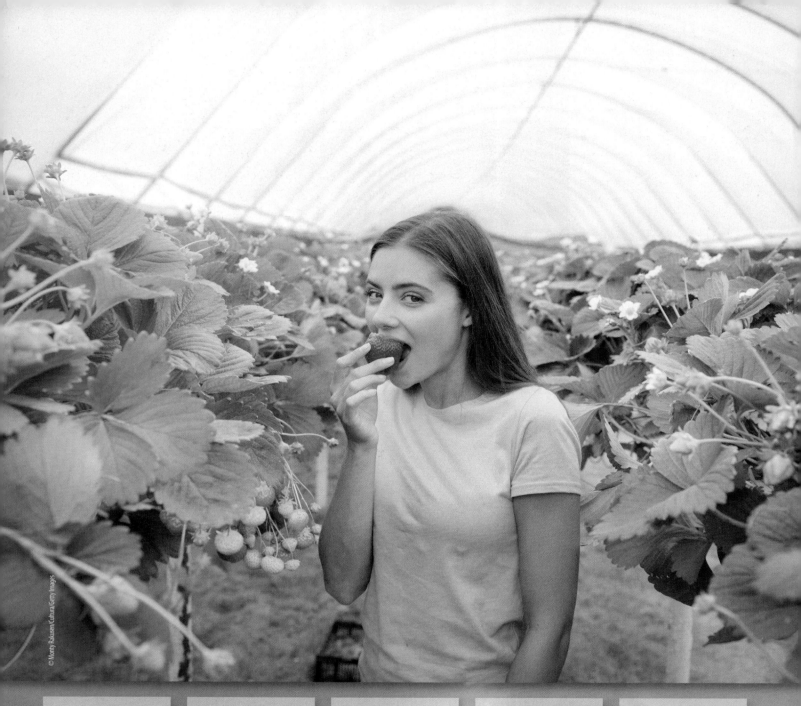

© Monty Rakusen/Cultura/Getty Images

Health Tips

The Two-Minute Stress Reducer

Reduce Stress When Sitting in Front of a Computer

Dollars & Health Sense

Profiting from Making People Sick

How Much Money Is a Life Worth?

Global Wellness

Chronic Diseases in Rich and Poor Countries: The Causes Differ

Managing Stress

Mind–Body Harmony

Wellness Guide

Spirituality, Religion, and Health

Social Determinants of Health

CHAPTER 1

The Definition of Health

Learning Objectives

1. Describe the medical and wellness models of health.

2. List the key points of the World Health Organization definition of health.

3. List and describe the six dimensions of wellness.

4. List the three health behaviors responsible for most of the actual causes of death.

5. Define *lifestyle disease*.

6. Identify the goals of Healthy People 2020.

7. List and describe the major health issues of college students.

8. Describe the Health Belief Model, Transtheoretical Model, and Theory of Reasoned Action/Theory of Planned Behavior.

Most people usually think of health as the absence of disease. But what about someone who has a relatively harmless genetic disorder, such as an extra toe? Is this individual less healthy than a person with the usual number of toes? Different perhaps, but not necessarily less healthy.

It is true that not feeling sick is one important aspect of health. Just as important, however, is having a sense of optimum well-being—a state of physical, mental, emotional, social, and spiritual wellness. In this view, health is defined not only by being unencumbered by disease and disability but also by living in harmony with yourself and with your social and physical environments. You foster your own health and well-being when you take responsibility for avoiding harmful behaviors (e.g., not smoking cigarettes), limiting your exposure to health risks (e.g., not drinking alcohol and driving; limiting the consumption of junk food), and undertaking healthy behaviors and practices such as consuming nutritious food, exercising regularly, attending to your mental well-being, and supporting actions that contribute to the health and well-being of your community (e.g., limiting pollution and reducing violence).

> The health of a people is really the foundation upon which all their happiness and all their powers as a state depend.
>
> *Benjamin Disraeli*

In this chapter, we discuss the definition of health, how modern lifestyles contribute to an enormous degree of chronic illness throughout the world, and how adopting healthy living habits can help people maintain wellness. Throughout this text, we show you ways to maximize your health by understanding how your mind and body function, how to limit exposure to pollution and toxic substances, how to make informed decisions about health and health care, how to be responsible for your actions and behaviors, and how social, economic, and political forces affect your ability to lead a healthy life. Learning to be responsible for the degree of health and vitality you want while you are young helps to ensure lifelong wellness and the capacity to cope with sickness when it does occur.

Models of Health

Scientists and health educators have developed two main ways to define health: the medical model and the wellness, or holistic, model.

The Medical Model of Health

The **medical model** of health's main tenet is that health is the absence of one or more of the "five Ds"—death, disease, discomfort, disability, and dissatisfaction. In other words,

Mind–Body Harmony

When you are well and healthy, your body systems function harmoniously. If one of your organs is not functioning properly, however, the other organs may not be able to function correctly either, and you may become ill. Thus, disease may be regarded as the disruption of physical and mental harmony of the whole person.

In traditional Western science and medicine, mind–body harmony is considered in terms of homeostasis, the tendency for coordinated self-regulation among bodily processes that leads to optimum functioning and survival. Many Asian philosophies embody an idea of mind–body harmony. This idea is based on a universal energy called **chi** (qi), which must be distributed harmoniously throughout the mind–body to attain and maintain health. Harmony is expressed as a balance of forces called yin and yang. Yin and yang represent the opposing and complementary aspects of the universal chi that is present in everything, including our bodies. Yang forces are characterized as light, positive, creative, full of movement, and having the nature of heaven. Yin forces are characterized as dark, negative, quiet, receptive, and having the nature of earth.

In Asian philosophies and medicine, body and mind are regarded as inseparable. Yin and yang apply to both mental and physical processes. When yin and yang forces are in balance in an individual, a state of harmony exists and the person experiences health and wellness. However, if either yin or yang forces come to predominate in a person, a state of disharmony is produced and disease may result.

Treatment of disease is designed to reestablish harmony of the mind and body. The balance of yin and yang forces must be restored so that health returns.

T'ai chi ch'uan and *qigong* (pronounced jê-kung) are Chinese mind–body methods that are practiced by many North Americans to help maintain health and harmony. These exercises are especially useful for older persons whose bodies can no longer manage vigorous exercise. People who practice *qigong* experience lower blood pressure, improved circulation, and enhanced immune system functions.

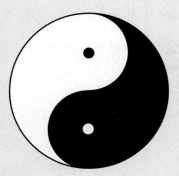

The Yin–Yang Symbol

This symbol represents the harmonious balance of forces in nature and in people. The white and dark dots show that there is always some yin in a person's yang component and vice versa. The goal in life and nature, according to the traditional Asian view, is to maintain a harmonious balance between yin and yang forces.

if you are not sick, disabled, or mentally unstable, or otherwise miserable, you are defined as healthy. The medical model relies almost exclusively on biological explanations of disease and illness and is interpreted in terms of malfunction of organs, cells, and other biological systems (e.g., liver disease, heart disease, or osteoporosis). In the medical model, the absence of health is determined by the presence of observable or measurable symptoms. In times of sickness, the restoration of health is accomplished by successfully treating the underlying cause of the disease. If that is not possible, then the goal is to alleviate symptoms.

Within the medical model, the health of a population can be measured in terms of **vital statistics**, which are data on the degree of illness (**morbidity**) and the numbers of deaths (**mortality**) in a given population. Vital statistics include the following:

Incidence: the number of new cases of disease or illness during a particular time period, generally expressed per 100,000 population. Example: The incidence of influenza in 2016 among Americans of all ages was 12.7 per 100,000 persons.

Prevalence: the total number of people in a community, country, or other group with a particular health status. Example: The prevalence of high blood pressure among U.S. adults is about 70 million.

These statistical measurements allow comparisons between populations and also within the same population over time.

The strength of the medical model is determining with reasonable biological precision the cause of many illnesses or their debilitating symptoms and providing treatments that cure a disease, ameliorate symptoms, or restore function to a damaged body part. Anyone who has been cured of a serious infection by taking antibiotics or undergone a lifesaving surgical procedure can attest to that. A weakness of the medical model is the tendency not to consider or deal with psychological and social factors that affect medical and health issues, nor has it been very successful in encouraging healthy lifestyles, reducing unhealthy behaviors, and fostering a healthy environment.

For example, overweight and obesity, which are a worldwide pandemic, are caused in most instances by overconsumption of low-nutrient food and by too little physical activity. Rather than addressing personal living habits and social conditions, the response of the medical model to overweight and obesity is to treat patients with drugs, surgery, or both to alter the biological aspects of the condition. In fact, surgically tying off most of the stomach in obese individuals is one of the fastest-growing surgical procedures in the United States.

The Wellness Model of Health

The **wellness model** emphasizes self-healing, the promotion of health, and the prevention of illness rather than solely the treatment of symptoms of disease. The World Health Organization (WHO) employs a wellness definition of health, as follows: **health** is "a state of complete physical, mental, and social well-being and not merely the absence of disease and infirmity." This definition is so broad and covers so much that some people find it meaningless. Its universality, however, is exactly right. People's lives, and therefore their health, are affected by every aspect of life: environmental influences such as climate; the availability of nutritious food, comfortable shelter, clean air to breathe, and pure water to drink; and other people, including family, lovers, employers, coworkers, friends, and associates of various kinds.

The WHO definition of health recognizes the interrelatedness of the physical, psychological, emotional, social, spiritual, and environmental factors that contribute to the overall quality of a person's life. All parts of

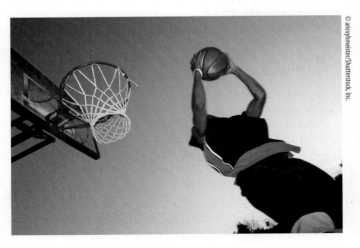

A healthy lifestyle depends on exercise.

© aricyhmeister/Shutterstock, Inc.

TERMS

chi: a Chinese term referring to the balance of energy in the body

health: state of sound physical, mental, and social well-being

incidence: the number of new cases of a particular disease

medical model: interprets health in terms of the absence of disease and disability

morbidity: the number of persons in a population who are ill

mortality: death rate; number of deaths per unit of population (e.g., per 100, 10,000, or 1,000,000) in a specific region, age range, or other group

prevalence: the number of people within a population with a particular disease

vital statistics: numerical data relating to birth, death, disease, marriage, and health

wellness model: encompasses the physiological, mental, emotional, social, spiritual, and environmental aspects of health

the mind, body, and environment are interdependent. The Old English root of our word health (*hal*, meaning well or whole) implies that there is more to health than freedom from sickness. Health means (1) being free from symptoms of disease and pain as much as possible; (2) being active, able to do what you want and what you must at the appropriate time; and (3) being in good spirits and feeling emotionally healthy most of the time.

Jesse Williams (1939), one of the founders of modern health education, echoes the WHO definition by describing health as

> that condition of the individual that makes possible the highest enjoyment of life, the greatest constructive work, and that shows itself in the best service to the world. . . . Health as freedom from disease is a standard of mediocrity; health as a quality of life is a standard of inspiration and increasing achievement.

Attaining health is a lifelong dynamic process that takes into account all the decisions we make daily, such as which foods we eat, the amount of exercise we get, whether we drink alcohol before driving, wear seat belts, or smoke cigarettes. Every choice we make potentially affects health and wellness. Sometimes the social and physical environments present obstacles to making healthful choices. For example, a person may know not to eat fatty, fast food every day, but this kind of food may be easier to obtain than healthier alternatives. Wellness includes recognizing that some social influences are not healthy and finding healthier alternatives. It also includes taking actions to make the social and physical environments healthier for all.

Health is not something suddenly achieved at a specific time, like getting a college degree. Rather, health is a process—indeed, a way of life—through which you develop and encourage every aspect of your body, mind, and spirit to interrelate harmoniously as much of the time as possible.

Consider how the wellness model views the headache. About 50% of American adults experience at least one headache each year. Although a headache can be the result of brain injury or the symptom of another illness, more often it is caused by emotional stress that produces a tightening of the muscles in the head and neck (tension headache). These contracting muscles increase the blood pressure in the head, thereby causing the pain of headache.

> You can observe a lot just by watching.
> *Yogi Berra*

The medical model advocates relieving a headache by taking acetaminophen, aspirin, or some other drug that can alter the physiological mechanisms that produce the pain. In contrast, the wellness approach advocates determining the source of the tensions—worry, anger, or frustration—and then attempting to reduce or eliminate it.

Identifying and eliminating the sources of tension and anxiety in your life is the surest way to prevent headaches. Some people have learned to use "having a headache" as a means of avoiding unpleasant situations, such as school or work obligations. As children they may have observed their parents coping with tension and stress by "getting a headache," and so they, too, learned that "having a headache" can be used to avoid anxiety-provoking experiences. Have you developed such an avoidance mechanism?

Dimensions of Health and Wellness

The wellness model of health has six dimensions of health and wellness: emotional, intellectual, spiritual, occupational, social, and physical:

1. **Emotional wellness** requires understanding emotions and coping with problems that arise in everyday life. A person with emotional wellness is able to maintain a sense of humor, recognize feelings and appropriately express them, strive to meet emotional needs, and take responsibility for his or her behavior.
2. **Intellectual wellness** involves having a mind open to new ideas and concepts. If you are intellectually

The Two-Minute Stress Reducer

Stressed out?
Be still.
And take a
D
E
E
P
Breath.

Center Yourself

Focus your attention inward. Allow thoughts, ideas, and sensations to pass through your mind without reacting to any of them. You will notice them pass out of your mind, only to be replaced by new thoughts and sensations. Continue to breathe deeply and slowly and watch the passing of the thoughts that stress you.

Empty Your Mind

Acknowledge that you have preconceived ideas and ingrained habits of perceiving. Know that you can empty your mind of distressing thoughts and replace them with ones that create inner harmony.

Ground Yourself

Feel the sensation of your body touching the earth. Place your feet (or your bottom if you are sitting, or your entire body if you are lying down) firmly on the earth. Let your awareness come to your point of contact with the earth, and feel gravity connecting you to Mother Earth and stabilizing you.

Connect

Allow yourself to feel your physical and spiritual connection with all living things. Remind yourself that with every breath you are reestablishing your connection with all of nature.

healthy, you seek new experiences and challenges. A person with intellectual wellness is able to communicate effectively in speaking and in writing, see more than one side of an issue, keep abreast of global issues, and exhibit good life- and time-management skills.

3. **Spiritual wellness** is the state of harmony with yourself and others. It is the ability to balance inner needs with the demands of the rest of the world. A person with spiritual wellness is able to examine personal values and beliefs, search for meanings that help explain the purpose of life, have a clear understanding of right and wrong, and appreciate natural forces in the universe.

4. **Occupational wellness** is being able to enjoy what you are doing to earn a living and contribute to society, whether it be going to college or working as an office assistant, food server, doctor, construction manager, or accountant. In a job, it means having skills such as critical thinking, problem solving, and communicating well. A person with occupational wellness is able to feel a sense of accomplishment in his or her work, balance work and other aspects of life, find satisfaction in being creative and innovative, and seek challenges at work.

5. **Social wellness** refers to the ability to perform social roles effectively, comfortably, and without harming others. A person with social wellness is able to develop positive relationships with loved ones, develop relationships with friends, enjoy being with others, and effectively communicate with others who may be different.

6. **Physical wellness** is a healthy body maintained by eating right, exercising regularly, avoiding harmful habits, making informed and responsible decisions about health, seeking medical care when needed, and participating in activities that help prevent illness. A person with physical wellness is able to exercise regularly and select a well-balanced diet; participate in safe, responsible sexual behavior; make informed choices about medicinal use and medical care; and maintain a positive, health-promoting lifestyle.

Because wellness is dynamic and continuous, no dimension of wellness functions in isolation. When you have a high level of wellness or optimal health, all dimensions are integrated and functioning together. The person's environment (including work, school, family, community) and his or her physical, emotional, intellectual, occupational, spiritual, and social dimensions of wellness are in tune with one another to produce harmony.

Spirituality, Religion, and Health

Many people believe that spirituality—finding meaning, hope, comfort, and inner peace through religion, a connection with Nature, or some force larger than oneself—plays a role in health and illness. Spiritual experiences tend to engender feelings of compassion and empathy; peace of mind; relatedness and communion with a force, power, or set of values larger than oneself; and harmony with the environment. These feelings are believed to be a cornerstone of health because they represent a balance between the inner and outer aspects of human experience. For some, the spiritual dimension of life is embodied in the practice of a specific religion. For others, the spiritual dimension is nonreligious yet part of a personal philosophy. Many practices can help people experience the spiritual realms of existence—prayer, meditation, yoga, musical and artistic endeavors, and helping others are but a few common ones.

Becoming more spiritually aware, regardless of the chosen path, can lead to a healthier life. Being in touch with your spiritual feelings helps you handle life's ups and downs with understanding and compassion for yourself and others. You become open to love in the highest sense of its meaning, which is acceptance and tolerance. You begin to love yourself despite your problems and hang-ups. You love your family and friends when relations are strained. You see beauty and harmony in more and more aspects of living. And occasionally—however fleetingly—you may experience the truly wondrous feeling of being completely and joyfully alive.

Measuring Health

Scientists use a variety of methods to measure health. Some methods count the number of individuals in a population in a particular health-related life situation, such as the number of adults who have had a heart attack or the number of children who die within 6 months of birth (infant mortality). Usually, these numbers are compared to similar measures for that population group from prior years or to other populations to determine if the frequency of the particular situation is increasing or decreasing. For example, the incidence of death from heart disease in the

TERMS

emotional wellness: understanding emotions and knowing how to cope with problems that arise in everyday life and how to manage stress

intellectual wellness: having a mind open to new ideas and concepts

occupational wellness: enjoyment of what you are doing to earn a living and contribute to society

physical wellness: maintaining a healthy body by eating right, exercising regularly, avoiding harmful habits, and making informed, responsible decisions about your health

social wellness: ability to perform social roles effectively, comfortably, and without harming others

spiritual wellness: state of balance and harmony with yourself and others

Social Determinants of Health

The interrelationships among biology, individual behavior, access to quality health services, social factors, and policies determine individual and population health. Because health is affected by nearly all aspects of a person's life, assessing health status requires evaluating not only facets of traditional medical care and public health, but also societal factors such as education, housing, transportation, agriculture, the physical environment, and social and economic forces. For example, increasing taxes on tobacco sales can improve individual and population health by reducing tobacco smoking. Federal automobile safety regulations reduce rates of injuries and deaths from motor vehicle accidents. Social factors and conditions of the environment affect health in a variety of ways; for example, millions of people in the United States live in places that have unhealthy levels of ozone or other air pollutants, thus increasing the risk of asthma and other respiratory diseases.

Social and Economic Determinants of Health

- Availability of resources to meet daily needs, such as educational and job opportunities, living wages, and healthful foods
- Social norms and attitudes, such as discrimination
- Exposure to crime, violence, and social disorder, such as the presence of trash
- Social support and social interactions
- Exposure to mass media and emerging technologies, such as the Internet or smartphones
- Socioeconomic conditions, such as concentrated poverty
- Quality schools
- Transportation options
- Public safety
- Residential segregation

Physical Determinants of Health

- Natural environment, such as plants, weather, or climate change
- Built environment, such as buildings or transportation
- Worksites, schools, and recreational settings
- Housing, homes, and neighborhoods
- Exposure to toxic substances and other physical hazards
- Physical barriers, especially for people with disabilities
- Aesthetic elements, such as good lighting, trees, or benches

HealthyPeople.gov. (n.d.). Determinants of health. Retrieved from https://www.healthypeople.gov/2020/about/foundation-health-measures/Determinants-of-Health.

United States as measured by the percentage of affected adults has been declining for over a hundred years. Or, the U.S. infant mortality rate, measured in deaths per 100,000 live births, is the highest among the 20 most economically developed countries.

Another measure of health is the Disability Adjusted Life Year, or DALY, which is an estimate of the number of years lost due to ill-health, disability, or early death. DALY is generally used to compare the health status of population groups, for example, between Ireland and South Africa. **Burden of disease** is a measure of population health that aims to quantify the gap between the ideal of living to old age in good health, and the current situation where healthy life is shortened by illness, injury, disability, and premature death.

The **health-related quality of life and well-being (HRQoL)** goes beyond direct measures of the degree of medical diagnoses, life expectancy, and causes of death to include nonmedical factors that affect a person's quality of life, including **well-being**, which consists of the qualities of positive emotions and life satisfaction. As such, health-related quality of life includes physical, mental, emotional, and social aspects of life. Scientists utilize several tools to measure health-related quality of life: self-reported assessments of physical and mental quality of life, fatigue, pain, emotional distress, social activities, and roles; scientific surveys that evaluate how frequently individuals feel very healthy and satisfied or content with life; individuals' personal assessments of the quality of their relationships, their positive emotions, their resilience, and the realization of their potential; and individuals' assessments of the impact of their health on their social participation, including education, employment, civic, social, and leisure activities, and to what degree, if any, a functional limitation (e.g., vision loss, mobility difficulty, or intellectual disability) affects living a long and satisfying life.

Lifestyle Diseases

In the early part of the twentieth century, infectious diseases—those caused by bacteria, viruses, and other parasites—were the leading causes of death, in large part because modern public health methods and modern drugs, such as antibiotics, were not available. In 1918, millions of people around the world died from influenza, the cause of which was unknown at that time, but is now known to be a virus.

Today, the leading causes of death in the United States and much of the industrialized world are not due to infections but to "lifestyle diseases" (**Table 1.1**). These diseases, such as heart disease and cancer, mostly result from people's behaviors and the ways in which they live.

Heart disease, for example, results primarily from poor diet, cigarette smoking, lack of exercise, high levels of stress, high blood pressure, and high levels of blood cholesterol. Cancer is associated with poor nutrition, smoking cigarettes, and exposure to hazardous substances in the environment. An unhealthy lifestyle is also at the root of many instances of lung disease (from cigarette smoking) and type 2 diabetes and kidney disease (from being

Table 1.1

Ten Leading Causes of Death in the United States for All Ages, All Races, and Both Sexes, 1900 and 2016

1900	2016
1. Tuberculosis	Heart disease
2. Pneumonia	Cancer
3. Diarrhea and enteritis	Chronic lower respiratory diseases (e.g., emphysema/bronchitis)
4. Liver disease	Accidents
5. Heart disease	Stroke/disease of brain blood vessels
6. Injuries	Alzheimer's disease
7. Stroke	Diabetes (mostly type 2)
8. Bronchitis	Flu and pneumonia
9. Cancer	Kidney disease
10. Diphtheria	Suicide

In 1900, five of the top causes of death were infectious illnesses. In 2016, only one of the top leading causes of death was from infection; all others were from lifestyle diseases.

Data from Centers for Disease Control and Prevention, National Center for Health Statistics. Retrieved from www.cdc.gov/nchs/data/fastats/leading-causes-of-death.htm and https://www.cdc.gov/nchs/data/hus/hus16.pdf#019

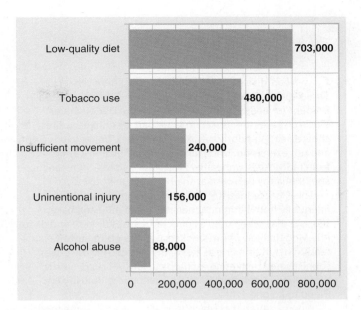

Low-quality diet — 703,000
Tobacco use — 480,000
Insufficient movement — 240,000
Uninentional injury — 156,000
Alcohol abuse — 88,000

(x-axis: 0   200,000   400,000   600,000   800,000)

■ **Figure 1.1**

Deaths Due to Preventable Causes, United States, 2017
Nearly half of the 2.7 million American deaths are caused by lifestyle factors such as poor diet, tobacco use, insufficient body movement, unintentional injuries (falls, motor vehicle accidents, poisoning and opiate overdose), and alcohol abuse.

Sources: Renata, M. et al. (2017). Association Between Dietary Factors and Mortality from Heart Disease, Stroke, and Type 2 Diabetes in the United States. *Journal of the American Medical Association, 317,* 912–924. U.S. Centers for Disease Control, National Center for Health Statistics, www.cdc.gov/nchs/index.htm.

overweight). In some instances, suicide and accidents are from stress or drug and alcohol use.

A major characteristic of many lifestyle diseases is that they are **chronic diseases**, meaning that they persist for years or life. Chronic diseases lower the quality of life of the affected persons and usually shorten the life span. A chronic disease also tends to affect a patient's family and is costly to the healthcare system. About 86% of total annual U.S. health expenditures of $2.7 trillion is for chronic and mental health conditions. About half that amount is spent on medical care for diseases that are largely preventable, such as heart disease, many cancers, high blood pressure, and type 2 diabetes (Centers for Disease Control and Prevention, 2017a).

When a person dies, the cause of death is generally identified in terms of the organ system(s) that failed and resulted in the person's death, for example, heart disease, cirrhosis of the liver, cancer of the lung. This may not, however, identify the root causes of that death. For example, saying someone died of lung cancer does not tell us that the actual cause of death was smoking. When deaths are examined for their actual causes and not simply what is reported on death certificates, the results show that approximately half of the 2.7 million deaths in the United States each year are due to lifestyle factors (**Figure 1.1**).

Leading the list of life-shortening behaviors is poor diet. Low consumption of fruits, vegetables, nuts, and seeds and high consumption of salt, meat, processed grains, and sugar contribute to 703,000 American deaths annually. Next to poor diet is tobacco use, which is responsible for more than 480,000 American deaths per year. Smoking cigarettes and cigars, chewing tobacco, and being exposed to secondhand smoke contribute substantially to deaths caused by cancer of all kinds, heart

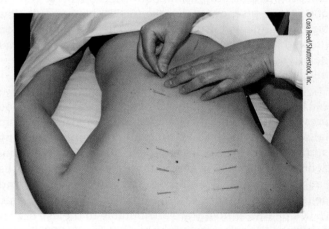

© Cora Reed/Shutterstock, Inc.

Many alternative medical practices, such as chiropractic, massage, and acupuncture, are now considered legitimate medical treatments and are often covered by insurance.

TERMS

burden of disease: the gap between the ideal of living to old age in good health and a current situation in which life is shortened by illness

chronic disease: a disease that persists for years or even a lifetime

health-related quality of life and well-being (HRQoL): a measure of health that includes non-medical factors

well-being: qualities of life that include positive emotions (e.g., happiness, contentment) and life satisfaction

Profiting from Making People Sick

Heart disease, stroke, lung cancer, colon cancer, type 2 diabetes, and chronic obstructive pulmonary disease account for nearly half of all deaths in the United States. These diseases are caused in large part by unhealthy lifestyle choices: eating poorly, smoking cigarettes, being overweight, and not exercising. Unfortunately, many businesses profit from individuals' unhealthy lifestyles—indeed, some encourage unhealthy behavior as the basis of their business.

The tobacco industry is the prime example of profiting financially from harming others. No other industry makes a product that, when used as directed, causes disease and death. Knowing that long-term smokers (i.e., their best customers) tend to begin smoking as teens, the tobacco industry uses sophisticated marketing methods to lure young people to smoke and to get them hooked. The tobacco industry is a friend to no one.

Whereas it is not as obvious as with tobacco, some food companies, for example, also profit from harming their customers. A typical serving of fast food (e.g., burger, fries, and a soft drink or shake) contains around 1,000 calories, about half or more of most individuals' energy requirement for one day. Approximately one-third to one-half of those calories are from saturated fat, a prime contributor to heart and blood vessel disease. Fast food also contains large amounts of salt, which also contributes to heart and blood vessel disease. This is why a steady diet of fast food can lead to weight problems and associated illnesses like type 2 diabetes.

Some of America's largest corporations are in the business of supplying consumers with less-than-healthy amounts of sugar. The sugar is contained in packaged foods (from ketchup to breakfast cereals), snack foods, fast food, and sugar-sweetened beverages, such as sodas, energy drinks, and sports drinks. Sugar-sweetened beverages alone deliver 36% of the added sugar that Americans consume, contributing to the risk of heart disease and type 2 diabetes. And, unlike other products to which sugar is added, sugar-sweetened beverages have no nutritional value; they can readily be replaced by healthy beverages such as water and low-fat milk. Efforts to limit the damage to health from added sugar in food include taxing sugar-sweetened beverages in order to lessen consumption, particularly among youth, and encouraging food companies to voluntarily reduce the amount of sugar added to their products.

You need not wait for the actions of government and industry to better your health. You can start today by resisting efforts of others to profit from distributing ill health and by adopting healthy living habits.

---

disease, high blood pressure, stroke, bronchitis, chronic obstructive pulmonary disease (COPD), pneumonia, low birth weight, and burns from fires. The enormous toll on life and health exacted by tobacco use is the reason that health agencies, doctors, and governments overwhelmingly recommend avoiding tobacco use.

Low-to-no physical activity is responsible for 240,000 deaths, principally from heart disease, high blood pressure, stroke, and diabetes. Unintentional injures from falls, motor vehicle accidents, and poisonings including opiate overdose are responsible for 156,000 annual deaths. Alcohol abuse accounts for nearly 88,000 deaths each year from alcohol toxicity, motor vehicle and pedestrian accidents, and homicides. In contrast, only 25,000 deaths annually are attributable to the use of illegal drugs. Unsafe sex is responsible for 20,000 deaths from AIDS and other diseases.

Type 2 Diabetes as a Lifestyle Disease

Diabetes is a disease in which the amount of sugar in the blood increases to unhealthy levels as a result of malfunctions in the body's sugar-regulating system. Diabetes can cause blindness, blood vessel problems, kidney failure, heart damage, and death. There are two forms of diabetes:

Type 1 (insulin-dependent). The pancreas (a digestive organ) is diseased and is unable to manufacture the hormone insulin, which regulates the level of sugar in the blood. Medical treatment involves frequent injections of insulin.

Type 2 (non-insulin-dependent). Too much fat in the blood (generally from being overweight) causes body cells to resist the actions of insulin. This is called *insulin resistance*; it causes blood levels of sugar to rise. Over time, insulin-producing cells in the pancreas become damaged and produce less insulin. Treatment includes increasing exercise, decreasing the consumption of calories to produce weight (fat) loss, and possibly injections of insulin or drugs that decrease insulin resistance.

That type 2 diabetes is a lifestyle disease is illustrated by the migration of Jews from Yemen to Israel in the late 1940s. At that time, the prevalence of type 2 diabetes among Yemenite Jews was less than 1 case per 1,000 individuals. Thirty years later, the same population, now adapted to a Western lifestyle in Israel, had a rate of almost 12 cases of type 2 diabetes per 1,000 individuals.

The Pima Indians who live in the southwestern United States offer another example of type 2 diabetes as a lifestyle disease. Traditionally, these Native Americans lived mostly on maize, beans, wild game, and vegetables. They were active, lean, and strong. Because forced relocation removed them from their traditional environment, today many Pimas have adopted living habits characteristic of most Americans, and hence many are overweight and about 40% have type 2 diabetes, the highest incidence in the world.

Currently, about 30 million adult Americans are diagnosed with type 2 diabetes. This is 12% of the

U.S. population and puts the United States first among developed nations in the prevalence of this disease. About 90 million American adults (about 37% of the adult population) have a condition called *prediabetes*. About 70% of people with prediabetes will develop type 2 diabetes within 10 years. Type 2 diabetes is strongly associated with being overweight: For every 20% increase in body weight, the chance of developing type 2 diabetes doubles. As a consequence of the epidemic of overweight and obesity in the United States, type 2 diabetes has become a major health problem.

Type 2 diabetes is a problem not only in the United States but also around the world. In 2000, the global number of people with diabetes was about 171 million (2.5% of the world's population). In 2014, about 442 million people worldwide had diabetes (about 8.5% of the world's population). By the year 2025, the number of people with diabetes is expected to be more than 550 million.

Research has conclusively shown that eating healthfully and regularly engaging in moderate physical activity can reverse and prevent type 2 diabetes (Centers for Disease Control and Prevention, 2017b). This is the reason everyone is encouraged to adopt healthy eating practices and engage in moderate physical activity.

Whereas each individual is responsible for her or his lifestyle decisions, scientists and health professionals know that many lifestyle diseases, including type 2 diabetes, require community-wide efforts to help individuals make healthy choices (Katz, 2009). For example, institutions can insist that vending machines contain healthy foods instead of junk food. Stairwells can be made visually attractive and have music or video to encourage walking instead of riding elevators. Municipalities can ensure that subdivisions have sidewalks and many parks. Rather than being at a centralized location, food service can be located at the periphery of large institutions to encourage walking.

Many health insurers and employers have begun to offer financial incentives to employees to make healthy changes in their lifestyles. Some companies give employees time off to exercise during work hours and financial rewards for losing weight. Some companies also penalize and even fire employees who violate no-smoking rules. In a 2008 poll, 91% of American employers believed that they could reduce their healthcare costs by getting employees to adopt healthier lifestyles (Mello & Rosenthal, 2008).

Nearsightedness

Another dramatic example of how modern lifestyles affect health concerns vision. Many children and a majority of adults in modern societies wear glasses or contact lenses to correct for nearsightedness (myopia). When our ancestors had to forage and hunt for food, acute vision was probably essential to survival and, of course, corrective lenses were unknown. During early development, a child's eye adapts to the visual information the eyes receive from the

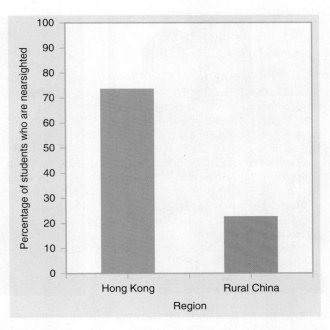

■ Figure 1.2

Comparison of visual acuity of 18- to 28-year-old students in Hong Kong with youths in rural areas of China. Most of the rural youths have normal vision, whereas most of the Hong Kong students are myopic.

Data from J. Wallman. (1994). Nature and nurture of myopia. *Nature, 371*, 201–202.

environment. Looking at distant objects tends to produce normal vision or eyes that are slightly farsighted. Today, almost all children watch TV and computer screens for many hours a day and also read books, magazines, and newspapers—all of which require close-up vision. These activities tend to cause myopia in many children.

The influence of modern lifestyles on vision was documented by measuring the vision of young people in rural China compared with the vision of Chinese students in Hong Kong (Seppa, 2013). Most of the young people in the rural environment had normal vision or were slightly farsighted (**Figure 1.2**). In contrast, most of the Chinese students in Hong Kong were nearsighted, many to a considerable degree. Thus, if one considers 20/20 vision desirable, our modern lifestyle, which involves much close-up vision, is likely to affect eye development and may produce myopia. Until we understand more about the environmental and genetic cues that affect visual development, children should be encouraged to spend time outdoors, where their eyes are more likely to focus on distant objects.

The U.S. Medical Care System

In the United States, the medical model of health has given rise to an enormous, complex, and expensive industry. Most of the resources of the medical industry are devoted to treating people who are already sick. Very little effort is made to prevent illness and disease or to

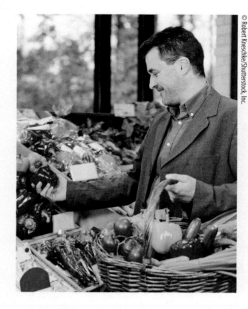
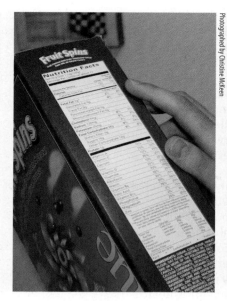
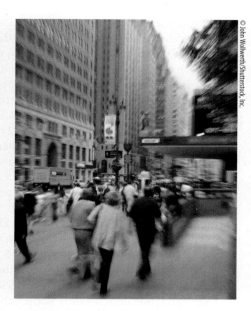

Simple behaviors in our everyday lives can positively affect health: Eat five servings of fruits and vegetables every day, read food labels to make wise choices, and walk instead of drive whenever possible.

encourage self-responsibility for health. Although, in reality, the system we all pay for and use is one of sickness care, it is called a healthcare system.

There is little doubt that the U.S. medical care system can deliver high-quality sickness care. However, it produces less health for Americans than do the analogous care systems in nearly all other high-income countries, including Canada, Australia, Japan, Sweden, France, and the United Kingdom. Compared to those countries, the United States has higher rates of chronic disease and early death among adults and higher rates of untimely death and injuries among adolescents and small children, and larger percentages of people with obesity, type 2 diabetes, heart disease, chronic lung disease, and arthritis (Woolf & Aron, 2013). Reasons for the United States' poor health rankings are lack of access to, and deficiencies in, the medical care system; high rates of unhealthy

behaviors, such as excess calorie consumption; high rates of poverty and other adverse social conditions; and an unhealthy environment.

One factor that does not explain why Americans are not as healthy as residents of other high-income countries is money spent on medical care. The United States spends twice as much per capita on medical care than do other economically developed countries (**Table 1.2**). In 2015, the total yearly cost of U.S. medical care was $3.2 trillion, nearly 20% of the country's wealth. Insurance companies, doctors, for-profit hospitals, and pharmaceutical and medical device companies compete vigorously for this vast treasure (see box "How Much Is a Life Worth?"). These entities have every incentive to maintain the current sickness system and little incentive to support disease prevention and self-responsibility for health. Consider that in the United States the medical management

How Much Money Is a Life Worth?

When U.S. federal agencies consider adopting new regulations intended to promote health or prevent injury or death, they try to figure out if the new regulations are cost-effective, that is, is gain in health worth the cost to attain it.

For example, let's assume that of the several thousand water systems in the United States, 2,000 would have to spend a combined total of $3 billion to modernize so that arsenic levels could be reduced to required (safe) levels. Let's also assume that spending this $3 billion would save the lives of 60 people per year who would otherwise die of arsenic toxicity. If the costs of modernizing the water systems were spread over 20 years, then the $3 billion would save 20 × 60 = 1,200 lives. That works out to $2.5 million per life saved.

Is the new regulation worth the cost? Most definitely, according to "value of a statistical life" (VSL) calculations used by most federal agencies. Although each agency has its own specific VSL, the values for early and middle-aged adults tend be between $6 million and $9 million per life; the VSL for someone over age 65 is about half that for someone in middle age. The VSL represents how much a person or employer is willing to pay to greatly reduce or eliminate a fatal risk. It is not based on earning power, an estimate of one's contribution to society, or how much someone is loved by family and friends.

It's been pointed out that $6 million to $9 million per life seems reasonable until you're talking about yourself or someone you care about. Then, the dollar value of a life is close to infinite.

Table 1.2

Per Capita Medical Care Spending in Developed Countries (2016)

Country	Per capita spending in U.S. Dollars
United States	9,882
Switzerland	7,919
Norway	6,647
Germany	5,551
Canada	4,753
Australia	4,708
France	4,704
Japan	4,519
United Kingdom	4,192
Italy	3,391
Israel	2,822
Russia	1,351
Mexico	1,040

Data from Organisation for Economic Co-operation and Development (OECD). (2017). *Health at a Glance: OECD Indicators*. Retrieved from http://dx.doi.org/10.1787/health_glance-2017-en.

of type 2 diabetes with drugs and surgery costs $14,000 a year per patient, whereas managing the disease with healthy nutrition and moderate physical activity costs almost nothing.

Recognizing that Americans are paying more for health and getting less, the U.S. Congress in 2010 passed the Affordable Care Act (ACA), the major provisions of which went into effect in 2013. The central feature of the ACA is to provide everyone access to medical care regardless of income, age, and health status ("preexisting conditions"). Because every dollar spent on disease prevention and support of a wellness lifestyle saves at least three dollars in sickness care costs, the act also calls for increased preventive services such as vaccinations, disease screening, and individual wellness/disease prevention, including smoking cessation and obesity and type 2 diabetes prevention. The law also helps employers and communities institute and strengthen wellness programs.

Healthy People 2020

Each decade, the U.S. government issues health objectives for the nation, the latest of which is Healthy People 2020 (HealthyPeople.gov, 2017). The main goals of Healthy People 2020 are (1) to help individuals of all ages live longer and improve their quality of life, and (2) to eliminate health disparities among segments of the U.S. population, including differences by gender, race or ethnicity, education or income, disability, geographic location, or sexual orientation.

Healthy People 2020 recognizes that families, schools, worksites, communities, states, and national organizations must help individuals live healthfully. This means that not only are individuals asked to make healthy lifestyle choices based on sound health knowledge but also that communities strive to provide quality education, housing, and transportation; health-promoting social and physical environments; and access to quality medical care. For example, informing people that it is healthy to consume five servings of fresh fruits and vegetables each day is insufficient if their community does not have stores or other sources of healthy food. Also, advising people to walk more is insufficient if their communities are not safe or lack parks or sidewalks.

Healthy People 2020 consists of nearly 1,200 specific health objectives grouped into 42 topic areas (**Figure 1.3**),

> The only way to keep your health is to eat what you don't want, drink what you don't like, and do what you'd rather not.
>
> *Mark Twain*

1. Access to Quality Health Service
2. Adolescent Health
3. Arthritis, Osteoporosis, and Chronic Back Conditions
4. Blood Disorders and Blood Safety
5. Cancer
6. Chronic Kidney Disease
7. Dementias, including Alzheimer's Disease
8. Diabetes
9. Disability and Secondary Conditions
10. Early and Middle Childhood
11. Educational and Community-Based Programs
12. Environmental Health
13. Family Planning and Sexual Health
14. Food Safety
15. Genomics
16. Global Health
17. Healthcare-Associated Infections
18. Health Communication
19. Health-Related Quality of Life and Well-Being
20. Hearing and Other Sensory Communication Disorders
21. Heart Disease and Stroke
22. HIV
23. Immunizations and Infectious Diseases
24. Injury and Violence Prevention
25. Lesbian, Gay, Bisexual, and Transgender Health
26. Maternal, Infant, and Child Health
27. Medical Product Safety
28. Mental Health and Mental Disorders
29. Nutrition and Weight Status
30. Occupational Safety and Health
31. Older Adults
32. Oral Health
33. Physical Activity and Fitness
34. Preparedness
35. Public Health Infrastructure
36. Respiratory Diseases
37. Sexually Transmitted Diseases
38. Sleep Health
39. Social Determinants of Health
40. Substance Abuse
41. Tobacco Use
42. Vision and Hearing

■ **Figure 1.3**

Topic Areas for Healthy People 2020
Modified from U.S. Department of Health and Human Services Office of Disease Prevention and Health Promotion. *Healthy People 2020*. Washington, DC. Retrieved from http://healthypeople.gov/2020/topicsobjectives2020/default.aspx.

© Skip Nall/Photodisc/Getty Images

each with a specific goal. Examples of specific goals are the following:

- *Cancer* (Topic Area #5): Reduce the number of new cancer cases as well as the illness, disability, and death caused by cancer.
- *Disability and Secondary Conditions* (Topic Area #9): Promote the health of people with disabilities, prevent secondary conditions, and eliminate disparities between people with and without disabilities in the U.S. population.
- *Food Safety* (Topic Area #14): Reduce foodborne illnesses.

A subset of Healthy People 2020 objectives, called **Leading Health Indicators (LHIs)**, have been selected to communicate high-priority health issues and actions that can be taken to address them.

Several of the goals in Healthy People 2020 are grouped into seven categories, called **Foundation Health Status**, which reflect the major health concerns in the United States (**Figure 1.4**). Foundation Health Status is intended to help everyone more easily understand the overall health of the U.S. population and the most important changes required to improve individual health and the health of families and communities. Each of the categories depends to some extent on the following factors:

- The information people have about their health and how to make improvements
- Choices people make (behavioral factors)
- Where and how people live (environmental, economic, and social conditions)
- The type, amount, and quality of health care people receive (access to health care and characteristics of the healthcare system)

The overarching goal of Healthy People 2020 is to help individuals be as healthy and well as possible. Healthy People 2020 encourages individuals, families, communities, schools, and places of employment to promote the health of everyone. As of 2014, 14 of the 26 Leading Health Indicators had shown improvement since 2010; 4 had met or exceeded their 2020 target goals. These include improvements in air quality, reductions in child exposure to secondhand smoke, more adults meeting guidelines for physical activity, increases in disease screening, and a reduction in tobacco smoking. Leading Health Indicators showing no improvement or worsening health outcomes included increases in rates of suicide, depression among youth, and childhood obesity and no change in fruit and vegetable consumption and diabetes control (Koh, 2014).

1. **Life Expectancy (with International Comparison).** The average number of years individual Americans would be expected to live, measured from birth and at age 65, compared to peer Organization for Economic Co-operation and Development (OECD) countries

2. **Healthy Life Expectancy.** The expected years of life in good or better health, years of life free of limitation of activity, and years of life free of selected chronic diseases

3. **Years of Potential Life Lost (with International Comparison).** The degree of premature death; that is, the total number of years not lived by people who die before reaching a given age, compared to 31 OECD countries and determined for both sexes by cause of death

4. **Physically and Mentally Unhealthy Days.** The number of days in the past 30 days that individuals rated their physical or mental health as not good

5. **Self-Assessed Health Status.** How an individual perceives his or her health, rating it as excellent, very good, good, fair, or poor

6. **Limitation of Activity.** The long-term reduction in a person's ability to do his or her usual activities caused by physical, mental, or emotional problems and assessed by asking people about their limitations in activities of daily living (such as bathing/showering, dressing, eating, getting into and out of bed, walking, using the toilet); instrumental activities of daily living (such as using the telephone, doing light housework, doing heavy housework, preparing meals, shopping for personal items, managing money); play, school, or work; and remembering

7. **Chronic Disease Prevalence.** The number of Americans with one or more of the following chronic diseases: cardiovascular disease, arthritis, diabetes, asthma, cancer, and chronic obstructive pulmonary disease (COPD)

■ **Figure 1.4**

Healthy People 2020 Foundation Health Status

Modified from U.S. Department of Health and Human Services. Office of Disease Prevention and Health Promotion. *Healthy People 2020*. Washington, DC. Retrieved from http://healthypeople.gov/2020/about/GenHealthAbout.aspx.

Health Issues of College Students

About 16 million people attend U.S. colleges and universities. About half are "traditional" students, those who enrolled in college directly from high school; others are "nontraditional students," those who enrolled in college after having devoted months or years to working, military service, traveling, and/or raising a family. A variety of health issues can affect college students' academic performance (**Table 1.3**). Some typical health issues for college students include the following:

Mental health. Students are exposed to a variety of stressors and pressures that can impair their mental health. Academic overload, tests, and competition can create feelings of insecurity, anxiety, inferiority, and depression. Traditional students may be lonely and have difficulty adjusting to early adulthood. Nontraditional students may feel isolated and without social support. Stress can impair sleep and lead to depression.

Food and weight. Time pressures and the easy availability of junk food induce many students to consume lots of sugar (candy, sodas) and fat (fast food) and insufficient amounts of fruits and vegetables. Students may use food to cope with stress and uncomfortable emotions. Many students are overly concerned about their body size and shape to meet social expectations of attractiveness, causing some

Table 1.3

Health Impediments to Academic Performance Reported by American College Students

Health Issue	Percentage Reporting
Stress	34
Sleep difficulties	21
Anxiety	24
Cold/flu/sore throat	16
Depression	17
Upper respiratory infection	6
Alcohol use	4
Allergies	3

Data from American College Health Association (2017). *American College Health Association-National College Health Assessment II: Reference Group Undergraduates Executive Summary Spring 2017*. Retrieved from: http://www.acha-ncha.org/docs/ACHA-NCHA-II_spring_2017_Reference_Group_Executive_summary.pdf.

to develop eating disorders. Many college students are among the two-thirds of North American adults who are overweight. Thus, weight control is an issue for many students.

Health care. A large proportion of U.S. college students has limited access to health care because their colleges do not have comprehensive services and they are without health insurance.

Substance use and abuse. Many students use tobacco, alcohol, and other drugs to cope with stress and unpleasant feelings or to fit in socially. Alcohol abuse is related to sexual assault and date rape, unintended pregnancies (from not using contraceptives properly or at all), and acquiring an STD (from not practicing safer sex).

Sexual and relationship health. Sexually active students of any age are at risk for acquiring an STD, becoming unintentionally pregnant, or becoming involved in sexual assault, especially acquaintance or date rape. Sexual activity to relieve academic stress, increase self-esteem, gain peer acceptance, or relieve loneliness can be mentally and spiritually damaging. Married students may find that the time and energy demands of college work create stress in their marital relationships.

Accidents and injuries. Many students commute to school, often rushing to and from work and home, and hence are at risk for automobile accidents. Alcohol-using students are at risk for auto and other kinds of accidents. Athletically active students are at risk for sports injuries.

Also, a variety of environmental and social forces present barriers to healthful living. For example, someone may want to become more physically active to manage stress or weight and to reduce the risks of heart disease and cancer. However, that person may live in a car-dependent community where work, school, and services are located miles apart and where there are no sidewalks, bike lanes, or nearby parks.

Making Healthy Lifestyle Changes

A major assumption of health education is that nearly everyone has a basic desire to be healthy and well but that many people acquire habits of thought and behavior that may make them less well rather than more. One goal of health education, therefore, is to provide knowledge and information so individuals can develop healthful attitudes and skills. With healthful attitudes and skills, it is reasoned, people will adopt healthy behaviors because they naturally want to do what is best for themselves.

It is said that knowledge is power, but with regard to living healthfully, that isn't always the case. Almost everyone knows that smoking cigarettes, driving after drinking alcohol, and eating junk food are unhealthy, but many people do those things anyway. Simply knowing what to do is no guarantee that a person will do it.

> If you find yourself in a hole, stop digging.
> *Will Rogers*

One must act. Living healthfully requires action based on accurate knowledge. Action has the components of goals, strategies for attaining goals including managing obstacles, and expectations of whether you will be successful (called outcome expectancies).

Goals A goal can be something you want or something you want to prevent or avoid. There are short-term goals ("I want to get a good night's sleep") and long-term goals ("I want to get my degree"). Goals can be clearly defined ("I'm going to study this Friday night instead of partying") or fuzzy ("I want to do better at school").

Goals reflect a person's or a culture's values, which are beliefs about what is important. Two values that affect health are valuing oneself (**self-esteem**) and valuing the physical and social environments in which one lives. When you value yourself, you are more likely to engage in healthful behaviors and have a high degree of psychological well-being (Adler & Stewart, 2004). When you value your physical and social environments, you are more likely to contribute to making them clean, healthy, and supportive, that is, to be helpful to others in attaining their goals.

Strategies for Action Strategies involve your ability to generate plans for attaining your goals and your attitudes about your ability to carry out those plans.

TERMS

Foundation Health Status: seven categories of health goals that represent the major public health concerns in the United States

Leading Health Indicators (LHIs): a set of high-priority Healthy People 2020 objectives and ways to achieve them

self-esteem: the judgment one places on one's self-worth

Generating plans involves research, critical thinking, and creativity. You want to seek the knowledge and experiences of others, and you want to evaluate it critically to be sure it is authoritative and authentic. For example, when using the Internet to obtain health information, you must determine the authoritativeness of the source of the information and ask yourself in whose interest is this information posted on the Web, yours or parties who want you to act on their behalf, such as advertisers and sellers of products. The creative aspect of planning involves generating a variety of possible paths (brainstorming) and evaluating the ones with the greatest likelihood for success.

Besides planning what to do, people assess whether they can carry out the actions required to accomplish a goal. This belief is called **self-efficacy**. Self-efficacy is associated with confident, encouraging inner self-talk, such as "I can do it," and "I won't give up."

Slogans like "Just do it," although seemingly encouraging self-efficacy, can undermine it because they ignore the fact that not every goal is realistic or attainable and no one can do everything no matter how hard he or she tries. Generating false hopes to accomplish the impossible damages one's sense of self-efficacy and self-esteem.

Agency is the belief that one can influence the nature and quality of one's life, rather than believing that one's fate is determined by reacting to circumstances not in one's control. People exhibit agency when they develop intentions and motivations for manifesting them, act on their own behalf in accordance with their values and goals, and evaluate the consequences of their actions in terms of their original goals and strategies. Agency means acknowledging that obstacles to accomplishing one's goals are ever present, and thus not a cause to become stressed. In the face of obstacles, one is flexible and is willing to change goals and strategies that are not working rather than letting discouragement engender defeat. Repeated success at accomplishing goals leads to confidence and vitality rather than insecurity and passivity. It also leads to strengthening hope, the general expectation that one will experience good outcomes in life.

Expectations for Success People pursue goals with expectations about the outcomes of their efforts. **Optimism**—imagining a high probability of attaining your goal—motivates, whereas **pessimism**—imagining a low probability of attaining your goal—stifles. Optimism is associated with perceiving negative events as specific, temporary obstacles to be overcome, whereas pessimism is associated with explaining negative events as self-caused (it's my fault), stable (it will last forever), and global (it's going to ruin everything). A pessimistic explanatory style is associated with a greater degree of illness and a shorter life expectancy (Rasmussen, 2009) because pessimists are more likely (1) to be anxious and depressed, (2) to believe that living healthfully or getting

help from others when ill won't make things better, and (3) to experience a state of chronic stress and its negative physiological and immune consequences.

Optimism also is associated with the tendency to perceive oneself as being able to move toward a desired goal and/or away from an undesirable goal. Optimism is associated with inner self-talk that is encouraging and hopeful ("I'll find a way to solve this problem"). On the other hand, the self-talk associated with pessimism is anxious ("I'm not sure what to do"; "I'm not sure it will work out") and self-critical ("I'm inept"). Optimism has been shown to be associated with successfully confronting health problems, lessening the risk of developing coronary heart disease and stroke, due to the adoption of healthy lifestyles, and greater ability to handle stress (Carver & Scheier, 2014).

One reason people resist making healthy lifestyle changes is that an unhealthy attitude or behavior is rewarding in some way, even if it is harmful in some other way (e.g., smoking cigarettes to relieve stress). To change a health behavior, a person must believe that the benefits of change outweigh the costs and that she or he is capable of making the desired change. Rituals such as New Year's resolutions and slogans such as "Just do it" offer unrealistic models of how habits are changed. Desire and willpower alone are insufficient; research, planning, and enlisting social support are required as well. Following are three models that describe the process of health behavior change.

The Health Belief Model

The Health Belief Model (HBM) was originally developed as a systematic method to explain and predict preventive health behavior, but it has been revised to include general health motivation for the purpose of distinguishing illness and sick-role behavior from healthy behavior. Key aspects of the model are described as follows:

- **Perceived susceptibility.** Each individual has his or her own perception of the likelihood of experiencing a condition that would adversely affect his or her health. Individuals vary widely in their perception of susceptibility to a disease or condition. Some deny the possibility of contracting an adverse condition. Others admit to a statistical possibility of disease susceptibility. And still others believe there is real danger that they will experience an adverse condition or contract a given disease.
- **Perceived seriousness.** Perceived seriousness refers to the beliefs a person holds concerning the effects of a given disease or condition on his or her life. These effects can be considered from the point of view of the differences that a disease would create—for instance, pain and discomfort, loss of work time, financial burdens, difficulties with family, problems with relationships, and susceptibility to future conditions. It is important to include these emotional and financial

burdens when considering the seriousness of a disease or condition.

- **Perceived benefits of taking action.** Taking action toward the prevention of disease or toward dealing with an illness is the next step after an individual has accepted the susceptibility to a disease and recognized its seriousness. The action a person chooses will be influenced by his or her beliefs regarding the benefits of the action, particularly if they outweigh the perceived costs.
- **Barriers to taking action.** Action may not take place even though an individual believes that the benefits to taking action are significant. This may be because of barriers, which can include inconvenience, cost, unpleasantness, pain, or upset. These characteristics may lead a person away from taking the desired action.
- **Cues to action.** An individual's perception of the levels of susceptibility and seriousness provides the force to act. Benefits, minus barriers, provide the path of action. However, "cues to action" may be required for the desired behavior to occur. These cues to action may be internal or external. An internal cue can be a sign, symptom, or feeling interpreted by someone as a health issue that needs attention, for example, noticing that one's clothes are too tight or that it's harder to walk up stairs. An external cue is a message or suggestion from someone such as a healthcare provider or a family member that it's a good idea to participate in some health-related behavior. Examples of external cues to action include a reminder email from a doctor to get screened for a disease or a friend or family member getting sick ("That could happen to me").

The Transtheoretical Model

One of the most influential models of health behavior change is the Transtheoretical Model, or Process of Change Model (Prochaska, DiClemente, & Norcross, 1992). This model recognizes that change occurs through the following stages:

- **Precontemplation.** The person is not considering changing a particular behavior in the foreseeable future. Many individuals in this stage are unaware or underaware of their problems. Information is important during this stage.
- **Contemplation.** The person becomes aware that change is desirable but has not committed to act. The person often focuses on why it would be difficult to change. Information on options on how to change the behavior can be helpful during this stage.
- **Preparation.** The person desires change and commits to making that change in the near future, usually within the next 30 days. Instead of thinking why he or she can't take action, the focus is on what can be done to begin. The person creates a realistic plan for making a change, including overcoming obstacles. This stage may include announcing the change to friends and family, researching how to make the

change, making a calendar, or setting up a diary or journal to record progress and obstacles to progress.

- **Action.** The person implements the plan. The old behavior and the environmental situations that reinforced that behavior are stopped and new behaviors and environmental supports are adopted. Obstacles are expected and noted, and strategies for overcoming them are implemented. Progress through this stage may take six months or more.
- **Maintenance.** The person strengthens the change, recognizing that lapses and even temptations to give up will occur. "Ebb and flow" are to be expected and are not to be seen as failures. The person can remind himself or herself of the many benefits of and gains from the behavior change to help combat relapse.
- **Termination.** The person is not tempted to return to the previous behavior.

The Theory of Reasoned Action/Theory of Planned Behavior

The Theory of Reasoned Action/Theory of Planned Behavior posits that changing a health behavior begins with an intention to adopt a new behavior (e.g., stop smoking). The intention is a combination of a positive attitude about performing the behavior (e.g., "not smoking is good") and the person's thoughts about how others will respond to the behavior (e.g., "my girlfriend will be happy if I stop"). Furthermore, change is affected by the person's perceptions of how much control he or she has over successfully bringing about the desired change (e.g., "I can do this if I get some support").

A Healthy Lifestyle Starts with You

Being healthy and well starts with you. The medical care system—doctors and other medical providers, pharmaceutical companies, hospitals, clinics, insurance companies, and to some degree the government—can help you when you are sick. However, only you can make life goals to be healthy and well; to take responsibility for the ways that your thoughts, feelings, and behaviors affect your life; to care for rather than harm yourself; to choose

TERMS

agency: the belief that one can influence the nature and quality of one's life, rather than believing that one's fate is determined by reacting to circumstances not in one's control

optimism: the thought process of imagining a high probability of attaining a goal

pessimism: the thought process of imagining a low probability of attaining a goal

self-efficacy: the belief that one can carry out the actions required to accomplish a goal

Chronic Diseases in Rich and Poor Countries: The Causes Differ

Chronic diseases are the leading causes of death throughout the world. Besides causing death, chronic diseases reduce the quality of life of affected individuals, often for many years. Four chronic diseases—heart disease, cancer, respiratory disease, and type 2 diabetes—account for over 40 million deaths per year worldwide (World Health Organization, 2017). By 2025, the number of deaths worldwide from those four chronic diseases is expected to increase to nearly 50 million annually.

In economically developed countries, such as Japan, the United States, Australia, and most of Europe, nearly 50% of the chronic disease burden is associated with five risk factors: tobacco use, high blood pressure, alcohol use, high cholesterol, and overweight (**Table 1.4**). On the other hand, in the least economically developed countries, deaths from chronic disease result from different risk factors: underweight, unsafe sex (causing HIV/AIDS), unsafe water and sanitation, and indoor smoke from cooking. As poor countries develop economically, the risk factors for chronic disease resemble those of developed countries.

Recognizing that heart disease, cancer, respiratory disease, and type 2 diabetes are largely preventable, international health organizations are searching for ways to stem the rising tide of chronic disease in developing countries. Not only is there a desire to offer people an improved quality of life but also there is the recognition that economic development is slowed or stalled when a country carries a large burden of disease. The more a poor country's meager financial resources are used to deal with an increasing number of people with chronic diseases, the less money there is to build schools, roads, electricity-generating plants, and other infrastructure. To the degree that disease retards economic advancement, it contributes to poverty and its discontents, including terrorism born of frustration.

To reduce the burden of chronic disease in developing countries, individuals must be encouraged and taught how to live more healthfully. Moreover, governments will need to regulate transnational economic activities that can negatively affect the public health. For example, to limit the damage caused by tobacco smoking, in 2003, the World Health Organization sponsored the Framework Treaty on Tobacco Control, agreed to by 168 countries, which includes a comprehensive ban on all tobacco advertising, promotion, and sponsorship; elimination of illicit trade in tobacco products; banning of tobacco sales to and by minors; agricultural diversification and the promotion of alternative livelihoods; and an increase in taxes on tobacco products to discourage consumption. Similar efforts will be required to limit consumption of sugar, fat, and cholesterol and thereby reduce the burdens of heart disease, high blood pressure, type 2 diabetes, and overweight (Yach et al., 2004).

Table 1.4

Percentage of Deaths from Chronic Disease Risk Factors in Developed and Developing Countries

Risk factor	Developed countries (1.4 billion people)	Developing countries (2.4 billion people)	Least developed countries (2.3 billion people)
Tobacco use	12.2	4.0	2.0
High blood pressure	10.9	5.0	2.5
Alcohol use	9.2	6.2	***
High cholesterol	7.6	2.1	1.9
Overweight	7.4	2.7	***
Low fruit and vegetable consumption	3.9	1.9	***
Physical inactivity	3.3	***	***
Underweight	***	3.1	14.9
Unsafe water, sanitation, hygiene	***	1.7	5.5
Unsafe sex	10.2	***	0.8
Indoor smoke	***	1.9	3.9

Developed countries include the United States, Japan, and Australia.
Developing countries include China, Brazil, and Thailand.
Least developed countries include India, Mali, and Nigeria.
***Indicates a low percentage of deaths.

Adapted from D. Yach et al. (2004). The global burden of chronic disease. *Journal of the American Medical Association, 291,* 2616–2622.

to learn and adopt health-promoting behaviors; and to contribute to the development and maintenance of a health-promoting society.

Scientists at the University of California at Berkeley undertook a multiyear study to determine, among other things, behaviors that contribute to health and longevity. Their findings include the following:

- No smoking
- Getting 7 to 8 hours of sleep per night
- Maintaining body weight not less than 10% and not more than 30% of recommended for height and body frame
- Regular exercise
- Little or no alcohol consumption
- Eating breakfast regularly
- Little between-meal snacking

Analyzing data from nearly 17,000 Americans, scientists at the U.S. Centers for Disease Control and Prevention determined that certain lifestyle practices can reduce the risk of chronic diseases and death (Ford et al., 2009; Ford et al., 2011). These practices include not smoking, maintaining body weight (body mass index of 30 or less), performing about 3.5 hours of physical activity per week (30 to 45 minutes per day), and consuming a diet containing at least five servings of fruits and vegetables per day, whole-grain bread, little meat, and zero to low consumption of alcohol, salt, and junk food. Unfortunately, fewer than 6% Americans engage in all of these lifestyle practices; 10% engage in none. The trend in the United States over the past 20 years has been toward living less healthfully rather than more.

It is clear from many kinds of health research that each one of us needs to do more to maintain and improve our health. When one is young, thinking about

Reduce Stress When Sitting in Front of a Computer

If you sit at a computer for more than 30 minutes at a time, remember to stand up and stretch the muscles of your neck, shoulders, and back. Do stretches for at least 5 minutes to avoid headaches, fatigue, and muscle cramps. Studies show that virtually everyone raises and hunches their shoulders as soon as they sit down at a computer. About one-third start breathing shallowly. The American Institute of Stress recommends practicing slow, deep breathing while using a computer.

health is the last thing one is interested in doing. We (the authors) certainly did not worry about our health when we were teenagers or even in college. Moreover, 50 years ago, eating as much meat as you could afford, smoking cigarettes, and getting drunk were generally accepted behaviors. When you are 20 years old, thinking about being 60 or 70 years old is unimaginable. Unlike 50 years ago, we now know that protecting health is something that has to begin while you are young. Making lifestyle changes when you already are old (and presumably wiser) is mostly too late.

Health is similar to retirement: It is something you have to plan for and pay attention to while you are young. For example, putting away just a few dollars every month adds up to an enormous sum in 50 years, but most of us never think about doing it. The same holds true for health. Making small, positive changes in your health and lifestyle now will pay enormous dividends in the future.

Critical Thinking About Health

1. As pointed out in this chapter, the major health issues of college students are sexual health, mental health, substance abuse, weight, accidents and injuries, and health care. Discuss which of these issues is of most concern to you personally. Explain your reasons and worries. How can you deal with your concerns in a way that will improve your health?

2. Describe one lifestyle behavior you routinely engage in that you regard as harmful to your health (smoking, for example). Discuss your reasons for continuing to engage in this unhealthy behavior. Consider what you might do to change this behavior and list the steps you would take to accomplish the healthy change. Do you believe that you can make the healthy change?

3. What is the significance to American society of the data in Figure 1.1?

4. Imagine that you are the Surgeon General of the United States, who formulates national health policy. (A former surgeon general, C. Everett Koop, formulated the crusade against tobacco smoking a generation ago.) Describe what you believe is the primary health problem in the United States today. Justify your choice with as many facts as you can. Describe the steps you believe should be taken by government, private companies, organizations, and individuals to eradicate this health problem.

Chapter Summary and Highlights

Chapter Summary

The word *health* can have many meanings. For some, being healthy simply means not being sick. For others, physical health and strength matter most, and emotional and mental health are of lesser concern. For others, emotional and spiritual well-being are paramount. If you are concerned with *all* aspects of your health, you think of health holistically. A holistic approach to health means that you strive for physical, mental, emotional, and spiritual well-being. You also try to live in harmony with your environment and with friends, family, and society.

Many people born in the past 20 years will live to 100 years of age or more. Adopting healthy lifestyles while young will help ensure a healthy old age. Most people are born healthy but become unwell because of unhealthy lifestyles. Chronic diseases such as heart disease, cancer, diabetes, and others are primarily due to unhealthy lifestyle choices such as smoking tobacco, drinking alcohol to excess, overeating and becoming overweight, and a lack of regular physical exercise. Maintaining a healthy body and mind will help you recover from occasional sickness and injuries that are inevitable parts of life.

The path to physical, mental, emotional, and spiritual health is to set health goals for yourself beginning now. Adopt healthy habits that feel right for you. Perhaps the most important word to remember in striving for a healthy lifestyle is *moderation*. Eat when hungry and do not eat more once you are full. Refrain from mindless snacking when bored or while engaged in sedentary recreational activities (watching TV, playing video games, using social media). Make movement a part of your daily life. Walk more, use stairs instead of elevators, ride a bike, dance, or do yoga. And be sure to take time to quiet your mind, especially when you are angry, stressed, or upset.

Health does not come from outside ourselves. The key to a healthy life has always been self-responsibility. Doctors, hospitals, drugs, and government rules cannot make you healthy. They can help prevent illness and injuries and often restore body and brain to a semblance of normal functioning. But you are always the one responsible for your moment-to-moment, day-to-day health.

Highlights

- Health is not only the absence of disease but also living in harmony with oneself, friends and relatives, and social and physical environments.
- Health means being responsible for preventing personal illness and injuries as well as knowing when to seek medical help.
- Three models used to describe health are medical, environmental, and holistic, or wellness.
- A holistic approach to health emphasizes prevention of disease and injury and self-responsibility for nutrition, exercise, and other aspects of lifestyle that promote wellness.
- The dimensions of wellness are emotional, intellectual, spiritual, occupational, social, and physical.

- Many illnesses (e.g., diabetes, heart disease, cancer) are "lifestyle diseases," that is, primarily attributable to unhealthy living habits. Taking responsibility for your health while you are young is the best way to reduce the risk of chronic disease later in life.
- Unhealthy lifestyles and behaviors are responsible for half of all deaths in the United States each year.

- Healthy People 2020 is a set of national health objectives characterized by enhancing the quality of life, reducing the incidence of preventable diseases and premature deaths, and reducing disparity in health status among different demographic groups.
- Changing health behaviors requires knowledge, planning, and social support.

For Your Health

Determine your level of wellness by completing the Health and Wellness Assessment (Exercise 1.1) in the Workbook. Do the other exercises for Chapter 1 to examine other aspects of your health.

References

Adler, N., & Stewart, J. (2004). Self-esteem. John D. and Catherine T. MacArthur Research Network on Socioeconomic Status and Health. Retrieved June 7, 2005, from http://www.macses.ucsf.edu/Research/Psychosocial/notebook/selfesteem.html

American Diabetes Association. (2013). Prevention. Retrieved from http://www.diabetes.org/diabetes-basics/prevention/

Carver, C. S., & Scheier, M. F. (2014). Dispositional optimism. *Trends in Cognitive Science*, 18, 293–399.

Centers for Disease Control and Prevention. (2017a). Chronic disease overview. Retrieved from https://www.cdc.gov/chronicdisease/overview/

Centers for Disease Control and Prevention. (2017b). National Diabetes Prevention Program. Retrieved from https://www.cdc.gov/diabetes/prevention/index.html

Ford, E. S., et al. (2011). Low-risk behaviors and all-cause mortality: Findings from the National Health and Nutrition Examination Survey III Mortality Study. *American Journal of Public Health*, 101(10), 1922–1929.

Ford, E. S., et al. (2009). Healthy living is the best revenge. *Archives of Internal Medicine, 169*, 1355–1362.

Healthy People.gov. (2017). Healthy People 2020. Retrieved from http://www.healthypeople.gov

Katz, M. H. (2009). Structural interventions for addressing chronic health problems. *Journal of the American Medical Association, 302*, 683–685.

Koh, H. K. (2014). Healthy People 2020: A report card on the health of the nation. *Journal of the American Medical Association, 311*, 2475–2476.

Mello, M. M., & Rosenthal, M. B. (2008). Wellness programs and lifestyle discrimination: The legal limits. *New England Journal of Medicine, 359*, 192–199.

Prochaska, J. O., DiClemente, C. C., & Norcross, J. C. (1992). In search of how people change. *American Psychologist, 47*, 1102–1104.

Rasmussen, H. N. (2009). Optimism and physical health: A meta-analytic review. *Annals of Behavioral Medicine, 37*, 239–256.

Seppa, N. (2013, February 9). Urban eyes, *Science News*, 22.

Williams, J. F. (1939). *Personal hygiene applied*. Philadelphia: W. B. Saunders.

Woolf, S. H., & Aron, L. Y. (Eds.). (2013). *U.S. Health in International Perspective: Shorter Lives, Poorer Health*. Washington, DC: National Academies Press.

World Health Organization. (2011). Global status report on noncommunicable diseases. Retrieved June 6, 2011, from http://www.who.int/chp/ncd_global_status_report/en/index.html

Yach, D., et al. (2004). The global burden of chronic diseases. *Journal of the American Medical Association, 291*, 2616–2622.

Suggested Readings

American Public Health Association. (2012). Public Health and Chronic Disease. Retrieved from http://www.apha.org/NR/rdonlyres/9A621245-FFB6-465F-8695-BD783EF2E040/0/ChronicDiseaseFact_FINAL.pdf. In 2010, the five most costly and preventable chronic conditions cost the United States nearly $347 billion—30% of total health spending.

Barondess, J. A. (2005). On the preservation of health. *Journal of the American Medical Association, 294,* 3024–3026. Presents the idea that health is best maintained by adopting healthy living habits early in life and practicing them consistently as one grows older.

Breslow, L. (1999). From disease prevention to health promotion. *Journal of the American Medical Association, 281,* 1030–1033. Discusses why health promotion is more important than disease prevention.

Centers for Disease Control and Prevention. (1999). Achievements in public health, 1900–1999: Control of infectious diseases. *Morbidity and Mortality Weekly Report, 48,* 621–629. Discusses the massive decline in deaths from infectious diseases in the United States during the twentieth century.

Cohen, J. T., et al. (2008). Does preventive care save money? *New England Journal of Medicine, 358,* 661–663. Quantifies the costs savings of many preventive health measures (e.g., smoking relapse, screening all 65-year-olds for diabetes).

Fineberg, H. V. (2013). The paradox of disease prevention: Celebrated in principle, resisted in practice. *Journal of the American Medical Association, 310,* 85–90. Identifies 12 obstacles in medical practice to preventing illness and disease and 6 strategies to overcome these obstacles.

King, D. E., et al. (2007). Turning back the clock: Adopting a healthy lifestyle in middle age. *American Journal of Medicine, 120,* 598–603. Shows that middle-aged Americans who newly adopt four healthy behaviors (consuming five or more servings of fruits and vegetables per day, exercising regularly, maintaining a normal body weight, and not smoking cigarettes) are healthier and live longer than those who do not.

Recommended Websites

American Holistic Health Association
Information on healthy lifestyle choices and enhancing your level of wellness.

Healthy People 2020 Goals
The U.S. government's national health objectives, which are designed to identify the most significant preventable threats to health and to establish national goals to reduce these health risks.

The Mayo Clinic
This site carries authoritative information on a variety of health topics.

MedlinePlus
The U.S. National Library of Medicine offers information and education on more than 600 health topics.

National Center for Health Statistics
Data on all aspects of health and disease in the United States, from the Centers for Disease Control and Prevention.

The Partnership to Fight Chronic Disease
A national coalition of patients, healthcare providers, community organizations, business and labor groups, and health policy experts committed to raising awareness of the number one cause of death, disability, and rising healthcare costs in the United States: rising rates of preventable and treatable chronic diseases.

World Health Organization Global Health Atlas
Standardized data and statistics for infectious diseases at country, regional, and global levels supported through information on demography, socioeconomic conditions, and environmental factors. Data can be accessed in the form of reports, charts, and interactive maps.

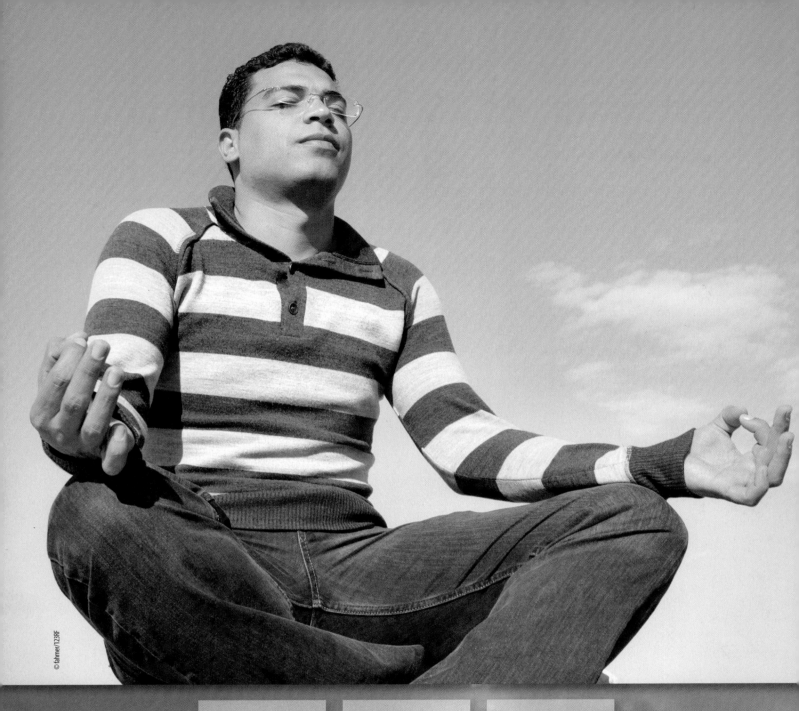

Health Tips

Repeating This Phrase May Improve Your Health

Make Up Your Own Mantra for Changing Behaviors

Image Visualization Reduces Stress

Managing Stress

Biofeedback

Focusing Attention

Relaxation with Music

Wellness Guide

Using Your Mind to Heal Your Body

Positive Thinking Has the Power to Improve Health

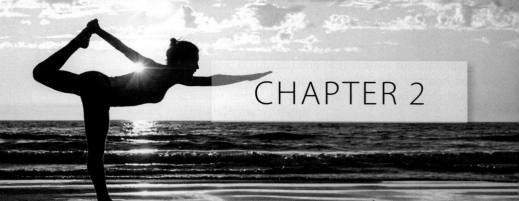

CHAPTER 2

Mind–Body Communications Maintain Wellness

Learning Objectives

1. Describe three ways the mind and body communicate biologically.

2. Define *psychosomatic illness*.

3. Describe and give examples of the placebo effect and the nocebo effect.

4. Describe how faith, religion, and spirituality affect health.

5. Explain hypnotherapy.

6. Describe meditation and image visualization.

Many people believe that good health is related primarily to healthy nutrition and near daily physical activity. Although both are vital to health, other important factors affecting health are your thoughts, feelings, beliefs, attitudes, and values. Positive thoughts about yourself and others and positive emotions such as happiness and love contribute to vitality, optimism, and joy, which can motivate living healthfully, aid healing and recovery from illness and injury, and increase longevity (Dockray & Steptoe, 2010). Negative thoughts and emotions can contribute to depression, pessimism, and decreased health and longevity.

> Life is not measured by the number of breaths we take, but by the moments that take our breath away.
>
> *George Carlin*

Many people think of health and healing in terms of drugs, medical treatments, and surgery. However, health and healing also are accomplished by mental processes such as faith, magic, and spiritual practices. Even in our culture we recognize that attitudes play an important role in promoting health and recovering from illness. Most physicians are aware that a person's attitude greatly affects the probability of recovery from illness. We've all heard of the patient's "will to live."

The mind affects health and well-being because the mind and body are parts of a unified whole. No body exists without a mind; no mind exists without a body. The mind and body communicate with each other by means of the nervous, endocrine (hormone), and immune systems, allowing thoughts, beliefs, and feelings to change body chemistry and physiology and vice versa.

Advances in identifying the biological mechanisms of mind–body communication confirm that the mind can affect health in powerful ways. Joy, creativity, and contentment lead to a state of mind–body harmony, which we experience as bodily health and subjective well-being. Fear, anxiety, stress, and depression contribute to mind–body disharmony, which increases risks for a variety of illnesses, impedes healing, and fosters a sense that life is difficult and unpleasant.

There are ways to focus the mind to promote health, prevent disease, and foster healing in times of illness. Among them are biofeedback, relaxation, hypnosis, guided imagery, autogenic training, and meditation (Table 2.1). Modern Western medicine has begun to utilize mind–body techniques, and researchers are elucidating the biological mechanisms that underlie mind–body communications and their effects on health and wellness. In this chapter, we discuss mind–body interactions and how they affect health and well-being.

Mechanisms of Mind–Body Communication

Nerve cells in the brain's thought and feeling centers connect to other nerve cells in the brain and body, hormone-producing tissues and organs, and immune

Table 2.1

Mind–Body Methods for Promoting Health and Preventing and Recovering from Illness

Method	Description
Autogenic training	Silent repetition of one of six autogenic phrases to produce a state of deep relaxation
Biofeedback	Using an electronic device to "feed back" information about the activity of a particular region of the body to alter that activity
Guided imagery	Using mental images suggested by a "guide" to produce relaxation and/or develop a skill
Hypnosis	Focusing attention and lessening awareness of surroundings to produce a relaxed state that is open to suggestion
Image visualization	Using self-generated mental images to produce relaxation and/or develop a skill
Meditation	Focusing awareness on a self-produced inner sound ("mantra") or an external sound, or image, or one's breathing to lessen attentiveness to external stimuli
Relaxation response	Mental method to produce relaxation
Virtual reality therapy	Using computer-generated environments to simulate an experience to treat psychological difficulties

cells throughout the body. In this way, mental activty is able to influence many of the body's physiological processes and thereby affect health.

The Autonomic Nervous System

A major pathway by which the mind and body communicate is through the **autonomic nervous system** (ANS), a group of nerves that regulate many of the body's physiological processes, such as heart rate, blood pressure, breathing, and the functioning of the gastrointestinal, urinary, and reproductive systems (**Figure 2.1**). Centers in the brain, principally in the brain stem and hypothalamus, receive information about the state of the body and/or environment and, in response, activate the nerve fibers of the ANS to maintain appropriate physiological balance. For example, when you exercise, the ANS stimulates the heart's pacemaker cells to increase your heart rate, thus increasing the amount of blood pumped to moving muscles.

The autonomic nervous system derives its name from the fact that its activities normally operate without conscious control. Thus, when jogging, you do not think about how fast your heart should beat or whether you should sweat to cool yourself when jogging. Even though the ANS functions without conscious control, the signals it sends to the body can be affected by thoughts and feelings. For example, nearly all students are familiar with the nervous stomach and sweaty palms that accompany the stress of

Sympathetic

Dilates pupils

Inhibits salivation

Dilates bronchi
(lungs)

Stimulates
heartbeat

Stimulates
adrenal gland

Inhibits digestion
(stomach, pancreas,
liver, spleen)

Dilates bladder

Parasympathetic

Constricts pupils

Stimulates salivation

Constricts bronchi
(lungs)

Slows heartbeat

Inhibits adrenal
gland

Stimulates digestion
(stomach, pancreas,
liver, spleen)

Contracts bladder

■ **Figure 2.1**

Functions Controlled by the Autonomic Nervous System
The autonomic nervous system has two parts or divisions. The sympathetic division and the parasympathetic division regulate functions that normally are not under conscious control, such as breathing, digestion, and heart rate.

taking an important exam. Realizing that it is possible to do poorly on an exam (a thought) leads to anxiety (an emotion), which activates the ANS to produce symptoms. Panic has an immediate effect on breathing and heart rate, and stress can constrict blood vessels, causing headaches or high blood pressure.

Many students live fast-paced, hectic lives that are full of time pressures and stress. Besides doing school assignments, many students work at jobs, and nearly all try to maintain harmonious social relationships with family and friends, which take time and attention. Moreover, the modern environment is filled with smartphones, computers, the Internet, TV, video games, and other stimuli that compete for one's attention. Trying to accommodate all of life's demands produces near continuous physiologic arousal mediated by the sympathetic nerves of the ANS, causing, among other things, sleep disturbances, muscle tension, gastrointestinal symptoms, and an increased risk for cardiovascular disease.

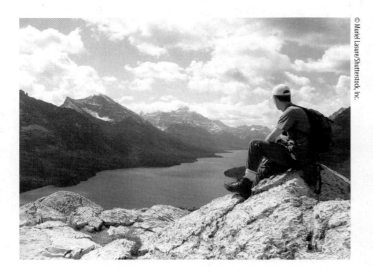

© Muriel Lasure/Shutterstock, Inc.

It is possible to counteract ANS-mediated arousal by putting 20 to 30 minutes or more of quiet time into your life each day. (If you must, schedule it in your day-planner.) You can employ any of a number of techniques designed to lessen ANS arousal and create a sense of mind—body harmony (see Table 2.1). Or you can find a quiet spot in a park or a room where you can comfortably and silently reflect on and be grateful for the good things in your life and let go, for a time, of the problems of the world and what you need to accomplish that day and in your life.

Hormones

Besides the autonomic nervous system, the mind can affect physiology via the endocrine (hormone) system. **Hormones** are chemicals produced by special organs and tissues in the body. Each hormone regulates specific biological functions (**Figure 2.2**). Hormones notify the body of changes outside and inside the body that must be responded to in order to maintain health.

Many hormones respond to changes in thoughts and feelings. For example, if the mind interprets a situation as threatening or frightening, regardless of whether the danger is real or imagined, centers in the brain responsible

TERMS

autonomic nervous system: the special group of nerves that control some of the body's organs and their functions

hormones: chemicals produced in the body that regulate body functions

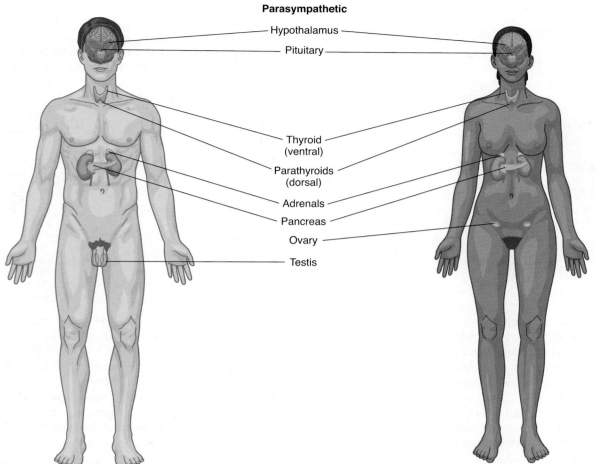

Parasympathetic

Hypothalamus
Pituitary
Thyroid (ventral)
Parathyroids (dorsal)
Adrenals
Pancreas
Ovary
Testis

■ **Figure 2.2**

Where Hormones Are Released
Hormones are released from different glands throughout the body. The synthesis and release of these hormones are regulated by the mind and autonomic nervous system. Hormones carry chemical messages that tell organs in the body how to respond to stimuli.

for emotions signal other parts of the brain and body to release hormones, such as adrenaline and cortisol, into the bloodstream. These hormones circulate to several of the body's organs and tissues to make the body alert and ready to deal with the danger.

Hormones manufactured in the brain can affect other areas of the brain; however, most hormones that originate in the brain are released into the circulatory system and travel throughout the body. Certain brain hormones have been associated with increases or decreases in particular feelings and behaviors (see **Table 2.2**). Thus, the environment, the brain (mind), and hormones (chemical messengers) are intricately interconnected and, ultimately, can determine health.

Using Your Mind to Heal Your Body

Have you ever cut or burned your hand? Perhaps you were cutting up food and the knife slipped, or perhaps you reached for a pan on the stove, forgetting that the handle was hot. The usual response to such accidents is anger at being careless or forgetful and anger at the sudden pain. We jump around and get upset, which generally exacerbates the injury and delays healing. A much better response to minor injuries that do not require immediate medical attention is the following.

In case of a cut, place a clean cloth over the wound and press gently to help stop the bleeding. Then sit or lie down. Close your eyes and allow yourself to become mentally and physically quiet. In your mind, visualize the injured part and see it as it was just before the accident. Then imagine the process of healing. See the skin coming back together. Feel the pain recede. Notice diminished bleeding. Continue doing this for 5 minutes or longer until you feel calm. If the accident caused a burn, place an ice bag or cool, wet cloth over the wound. Then lie down and visualize the skin becoming cooler and looking like the normal skin around the burn.

By immediately calming the mind after an injury, inflammation and other harmful physiological reactions in the area are reduced. Healing processes begin immediately when you send positive, calming thoughts and images to the injured area. Continue to visualize healing in the injured area.

Table 2.2

Hormone Levels Can Affect Moods, Thoughts, Feelings, and Behaviors

Hormone	Effects of high levels
Cortisol	High blood levels of cortisol increase stress and alertness, decrease sensitivity to pain, impair memory processing, and increase depression.
Dopamine	High blood levels of dopamine increase pleasure and motivation and decrease sadness.
Oxytocin	High blood levels of oxytocin increase trust and feelings of attachment and decrease fear.
Vasopressin	High blood levels of vasopressin increase sexual arousal and attention but decrease anxiety.
Serotonin	High blood levels of serotonin increase aggression and obsessive thoughts.

The Immune System

Besides the ANS and endocrine system, the mind and body communicate via the immune system. The immune system is responsible for combating infections and ridding the body of foreign organisms and toxic substances. Immune system cells, tissues, and organs are located throughout the body. The immune system can be influenced by the mind via the nervous and endocrine systems. Nerves of the sympathetic nervous system connect to certain immune tissues, such as bone marrow, lymph nodes, and spleen. Many immune cells respond to the presence of the hormone cortisol as part of the stress response. Moreover, the immune system releases special chemicals called *cytokines*, which can affect the nervous and endocrine systems.

Many studies have demonstrated that the mind can affect the workings of the immune system. It is well known that stress and negative mood states can weaken the immune system and that methods to reduce stress such as mindfulness meditation and t'ai chi can strengthen immune response (Antoni, 2012). Positive emotions, such as feeling calm and peaceful, happy, and optimistic about life, can enhance immune function (Pressman & Black, 2012).

The Mind Can Create Illness or Wellness

That thoughts and feelings can alter physiological processes means that individuals have the power to influence their health for ill or for well-being. For thousands of years, belief in the healing powers of a deity or special person, such as a king, priest, or shaman, or ascribing healing powers to a potion or elixir, have been employed to heal the sick by ridding the body and/or spirit of demons and evil spirits. Today's patients have faith in the knowledge of their physicians and the medicines they prescribe just as people of ancient civilizations believed in their priests

and herbs. Any improvement in a patient's condition is likely a combination of faith in the healer and the efficacy of the treatment.

Ancient Egyptian papyri show that although the priest–physicians of ancient Egypt prescribed herbs and performed surgeries, their treatments relied on the belief of the people in the healing power of the gods. Priests would put patients into a trance in a temple and tell them that when they awakened, they would be healed. And often they were.

The Greeks and Romans had gods, oracles, and temples of healing. Their priests also used trance and sleeplike mental states to impart healing suggestions to receptive minds. Sometimes "miraculous cures" resulted. Greek and Roman emperors and priests also healed by the

> Faith. You can do little with it and nothing without it.
>
> *Samuel Butler*

"laying on of hands"; people were healed because they believed that their rulers had divine powers. King Pyrrhus of Epirus is reputed to have cured sick patients solely by the touch of his big toe.

All religions teach that divine persons have the power to heal. The New Testament recounts many examples of the healing power of Jesus.

> Is any sick among you? Let him call for the Elders of the church and let them pray over him, anointing him with oil in the name of the Lord; and the prayer of faith shall save the sick.
>
> —James 5:14–15

> That evening they brought him many who were possessed with demons, and he cast out the spirits with a word, and healed all who were sick.
>
> —Matthew 8:14

> And he said to her, "Daughter, your faith has made you well; go in peace and be healed of your diseases."
>
> —Mark 5:34

Repeating This Phrase May Improve Your Health

In the early 1900s, a French pharmacist named Emile Coué (1857–1926) became famous for using autosuggestion to cure people of all kinds of ailments. His most famous autosuggestion, which millions of people recited to themselves, was: "Every day, in every way, I'm getting better and better."

Try this autosuggestion or make up one of your own to fit a particular situation you want to improve. Repeat the suggestion in your mind as often as feels comfortable. Do it without effort or expectation. Autosuggestion is a powerful tool for improving health and for healing.

Nearly 50% of Americans use prayer to help them cope with illness (Wachholtz & Sambamoorthi, 2011). People pray for their own health and the health of others; they pray individually and in prayer groups. People pray to God, a "guardian angel," or a deceased loved one for support and personal strength to cope with illness. Research shows that religiosity/spirituality is associated with reduced mortality among relatively healthy individuals, but not those who are ill (Chida et al., 2009). This finding may reflect that the social support offered by religious affiliation and the enhanced immune function from positive emotions such as security and confidence are associated with religious experience. Studies have been unable to find any therapeutic effects of intercessory prayer, in which groups pray for the health and recovery of patients either with or without the patients' knowledge (Roberts et al., 2009).

At times of serious illness or when death is a possibility, many individuals want their physicians to be aware of their spiritual or religious beliefs. On the other hand, for routine health matters most patients do not want their physicians to be directly involved in their health-related spiritual experiences. Most doctors believe that a patient's spiritual outlook is important to handling health difficulties and that physicians should ask patients about spiritual and religious issues, although few physicians believe that it is appropriate for them to recommend prayer and religious activities to patients (Sulmasy, 2009).

The Mind Can Create Illness

Psychosomatic Illnesses The power of the mind to cause illness is borne out by a long list of **psychosomatic illnesses** (**Figure 2.3**). These conditions are caused, in large measure, by mental states and attitudes such as persistent anxiety, depression, and stress that produce

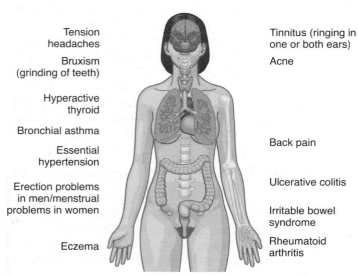

Tension headaches
Bruxism (grinding of teeth)
Hyperactive thyroid
Bronchial asthma
Essential hypertension
Erection problems in men/menstrual problems in women
Eczema

Tinnitus (ringing in one or both ears)
Acne
Back pain
Ulcerative colitis
Irritable bowel syndrome
Rheumatoid arthritis

■ **Figure 2.3**

Psychosomatic Illnesses
Many diseases and disorders of the body are partly caused by thoughts and feelings.

unhealthy physiological changes. That is why these illnesses are called psychosomatic, a term derived from the Greek (*psych*, mind; *soma*, body).

Many people believe that psychosomatic means imaginary, that "it's all in the head." This is not the case. The damage to the gastrointestinal tract in someone with stress-related irritable bowel syndrome is just as real as the damage caused by an infection or injury. Psychosomatic means that thoughts and feelings are at the root of the physiological abnormalities causing the symptoms.

Modern medicine tends not to treat psychosomatic illnesses directly. Physicians prefer to use drugs that suppress symptoms, but rarely do they address the underlying mental states that cause the illness. This is caused in part by their training, which focuses on biological causes of disease, and in part by doctors not having time to probe the lifestyle of a patient with a psychosomatic illness; also, the patient's health insurer is not likely to pay for the doctor to do so.

Somatic Symptom Disorder Somatic symptom disorder refers to the occurrence of physical symptoms usually, but not always, without the presence of detectable injury or disease. Psychological and social problems such as depression or anger may cause pain (especially low back pain), fatigue, nausea, diarrhea, and sexual problems. It is estimated that 25% to 75% of all patients who visit primary care physicians suffer from somatic symptoms. These are difficult to treat, time-consuming for physicians to diagnose, and expensive for the healthcare system. A common complaint is pain of long duration in several parts of the body that cannot be explained by any medical condition or injury.

The lives that many people choose to live or are forced to live by financial or family circumstances can cause mind–body disruption that eventually produces pain and sickness. People suffering from somatic symptom disorder are not feigning sickness; they have lost mind–body harmony to a serious degree. Health can be restored with knowledge of how the mind and body interact and the application of methods that produce insight to the particular issue. Compassionate professional help and guidance are also beneficial.

The Mind Can Create Wellness

The power of the mind to create wellness is illustrated by studies that show that positive emotions are associated with healthful biological changes. For example, a group of English civil service workers were asked to rate their state of happiness several times during a typical work day while researchers measured blood pressure, heart rate, and stress hormone (cortisol) levels. Those with the highest happiness ratings showed the lowest heart rate and stress hormone levels (there was no effect of happiness on blood pressure).

The role of humor in maintaining health has a long history. Plato advocated humor as a means to lighten the burdens of the soul and to improve one's health. From medieval court jesters to modern circus clowns, laughter has been used to help people forget their problems, to restore mind–body harmony, and to foster health and healing. In 1979, Norman Cousins, a well-known magazine editor, described how he had cured himself of a rare untreatable disease (ankylosing spondylitis) by watching humorous movies for months until he had laughed himself well (Cousins, 1979). Scientific studies have confirmed that humor has a positive effect on the immune system by increasing levels of natural killer cells that help prevent infections (Bennett & Lengacher, 2009). Humor elevates pain thresholds by activating endorphins (hormones released in the brain) that affect pain responses. Humor reduces stress and anxiety in cancer patients, becoming a powerful adjunct to medicines in the healing process (Roaldsen et al., 2015).

Dr. Madan Lal Kataria, an Indian physician who has been dubbed the Guru of Giggling, has developed a set of laughter exercises that are likened to yoga poses (Khatchadourian, 2010). Dr. Kataria recommends that people learn to laugh without jokes or funny videos on a regular schedule as a means to better health. He has established laughter clubs all over the world with an estimated 250,000 members. Perhaps, if more people laughed more often, many of the world's conflicts would be solved.

Mind–Body Healing

Placebo Effect

Another example of the mind contributing to wellness is the **placebo effect** (from the Latin "I shall please"), which refers to the lessening of symptoms or the curing of disease by a person's belief in the curative power of an inert medicine (called a *sugar pill* or *placebo*) or belief in the healing power of a person or special words or objects. Although placebo is often thought to be a fake medicine that tricks a patient into feeling better, in actuality a placebo produces identifiable biological changes; healing is not imagined or just "all in the head." Placebos work because the *expectation* of effectiveness brings about real physiological changes in the body that lead to healing.

For example, researchers used functional magnetic resonance imaging (fMRI) to map changes in blood flow in the brains of volunteers (Wager et al., 2004). The volunteers were subjected to harmless but occasionally painful electric shocks or heat. When they believed an antipain cream had been applied to their arm, they rated the pain as less intense. Moreover, placebo pain relief was related to decreased brain activity in pain-sensitive brain regions and was associated with increased activity during anticipation of pain in other brain regions, providing evidence that placebos alter the experience of pain.

Placebo-induced pain relief likely occurs because the expectation of relief increases the body's manufacture or release of its own internal pain-relieving chemicals, endorphins, and cannabinoids (Medoff & Colloca, 2015). For example, after having wisdom teeth removed, adults were given morphine or placebo for pain relief; about 33% of those receiving placebo experienced pain relief. Then, a chemical that blocks the effects of morphine and endorphins, called *naloxone*, was given to any patient who had experienced pain relief, either from morphine or placebo. All patients receiving naloxone experienced return of their pain. Thus, it was shown that the expectation of pain relief can stimulate the manufacture and release of endorphins.

The placebo effect is so common and powerful that the U.S. Food and Drug Administration requires that a new drug undergo a *double-blind, placebo-controlled* trial. This means comparing one group of patients' responses to a new drug with a different matched group's responses to a placebo (the control group). So as to minimize bias, people in the test-drug group and the placebo group do not know which substance they are receiving; that is, they are "blind." Furthermore, none of the scientists administering the test drug or the placebo knows what the patients are receiving; that is, they also are "blind." Only the project administrator knows who is receiving what. The efficacy of the new drug is determined by its performance compared to the placebo.

The placebo effect occurs in the treatment of many diseases, including ulcers, irritable bowel syndrome, colitis, chronic pain, headache, hay fever, asthma, depression, warts, and high blood pressure. The number of patients responding to placebos for almost any disease or symptom ranges from 30% to 70%; most placebo-controlled drug studies find that about half of all patients respond to placebos. This remarkable finding means that you have a 50–50 chance of being cured simply by believing something will make you better.

Depression is a condition in which the placebo effect can account for as much as 75% of any relief experienced. To determine how the placebo effect could be operating to relieve depression, researchers used positron emission tomography (a PET scan) to visualize the activity of different regions of the brain when depressed individuals

TERMS

placebo effect: healing that results from a person's belief in a treatment that has no medicinal value

psychosomatic illnesses: physical illnesses brought on by negative mental states such as stress or emotional upset

somatic symptom disorder: occurrence of physical symptoms without any bodily disease or injury being present

received antidepressant medication or placebo (Mayberg et al., 2002). The results showed that the pattern of brain activity of patients receiving placebo was almost the same as those receiving antidepressant medications. Apparently, the expectation that their symptoms would improve caused biological changes in the brain that contributed to relief of depression (Kirsch et al., 2008). **Figure 2.4** shows comparisons of the effectiveness of four antidepressant medications and placebos to reduce symptoms of mild to moderate depression. Note that in each instance the placebo is almost as effective as the medication used to treat depression. About 60% of patients respond to the placebo as do those receiving the drug. Since one major characteristic of depression is feeling hopeless and that things cannot improve, these results suggest that believing that one is receiving a medication triggers a sense of hope, which reduces symptoms of depression. Antidepressant drugs and placebos produce similar alterations in brain chemistry, principally, elevations in the neurotransmitters serotonin and norepineprine.

Why, if placebos are so effective in healing, are they not used more by physicians in treating patients? One reason is an ethical dilemma for physicians: A placebo might work for one patient, but not for another. Although the same could be true for a prescribed drug, the physician is protected legally by prescribing a drug that has been clinically tested and approved by the FDA. However, no legal protection exists for a physician prescribing a placebo if the patient decides to sue, claiming that the treatment did not meet accepted medical standards.

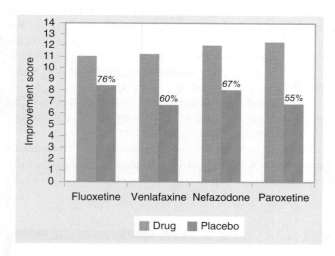

■ **Figure 2.4**

Comparison of Four Antidepressant Medications and Placebo in Improvement of Symptoms of Mild and Moderate Depression
The bars in the graph indicate the degree of improvement in symptoms of depression as determined by the Hamilton Depression Rating Scale (http://www.psy-world.com/hdrs.htm). In each instance the placebo produces considerable improvement.

Data from Kirsch, I., et al. (2008). Initial severity and antidepressant benefits: A meta-analysis of data submitted to the Food and Drug Administration. *PLoS Medicine, 5,* e45. http://www.plosmedicine.org/article/info:doi/10.1371/journal.pmed.0050045

Who knows what might work as a placebo? Perhaps consuming a couple of M&Ms twice a day can cure pain and many other symptoms that people suffer. Often the safest and best path to relief of suffering is to engage the power of the mind.

The Nocebo Effect

A negative, harmful placebo effect is called a **nocebo effect** (from the Latin "I shall harm"), and it is another reason placebo pills are not used in medical practice. Placebos can be dangerous, just as drugs can be dangerous. Patients can become addicted to placebo pills used for pain relief and suffer withdrawal symptoms when they stop using them. Also, like prescription drugs, placebo pills can cause side effects. In one experiment, 40 volunteer asthmatic patients were asked to inhale a placebo spray, which they were told contained an allergen. Twelve of the volunteers had full-blown asthma attacks, and seven had lesser symptoms. The asthma attacks were reversed by inhalation of another placebo spray, which they were told would relieve the symptoms.

Words can produce a placebo effect in the same way as a pill. Because of this fact, you should always seek out health practitioners whom you trust and who use positive, constructive healing suggestions and who encourage you to become involved in self-healing practices. Avoid health practitioners who voice negative and pessimistic recommendations. No one needs to hear negative suggestions such as "You'll probably have to take these pills for the rest of your life," or "I doubt that you'll be able to move around much after an accident like that." In the presence of a physician, many patients become very open to suggestions, both positive and negative, because their minds are intently focused on what the doctor is saying. Such a focused state of mind is similar to that obtained in meditation or hypnosis. It is more helpful to practice being alert and critical when discussing your health concerns or diagnostic test results with a health professional. Of course, this is not always easy to do, especially when the information being conveyed causes distress or fear.

A tragic, but dramatic, example of a nocebo effect involved a patient who died apparently from reading a single word (Hewlett, 1994). This person had a history of chronic lymphocytic leukemia, a form of blood cancer that usually is easily controlled with drugs. The patient had been well for more than 3 years with only intermittent need for medication. However, he had never actually been informed of the original diagnosis of his condition.

One day he was in his physician's office on a routine visit and happened to read the physician's notes, which were lying on the desk. He saw the word *leukemia* in his file. He missed his next scheduled office visit and shortly thereafter showed up in the hospital's emergency room. Within 3 weeks he died in the hospital. No cause of death could be discovered at autopsy, and his leukemia was still

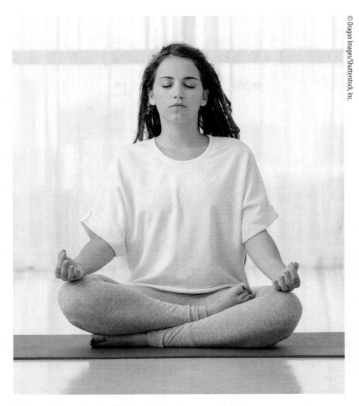

Take a time out to meditate whenever you need to.

in remission. The patient apparently *believed* that he had terminal cancer just from seeing the word *leukemia* in his medical records. The mind *does* heal; the mind *does* kill.

Methods to Promote Mind–Body Harmony and Health

Autogenic Training

Autogenic training uses autosuggestion to establish a balance between the mind and body through changes in the autonomic nervous system. The method has been shown to be effective in relieving anxiety (Miu, Heilman, & Miclea, 2009) and improving the quality of life in people with chronic medical conditions (Sutherland, Andersen, & Morris, 2005).

Autogenic training involves learning to concentrate on one of six basic autogenic phrases for a few minutes each day over a week or more. After weeks or months of practice, one is able to attain a deep sense of relaxation, often within seconds, which can result in healthful physiological changes. The six basic autosuggestions are as follows:

- My arms and legs are heavy.
- My arms and legs are warm.
- My heartbeat is calm and regular.
- My lungs breathe for me.
- My abdomen is warm.
- My forehead is cool.

The exact phrasing of any autogenic suggestion is not critical to its effectiveness. The words carry no particular power. Any suggestion can be rephrased so that it becomes comfortable, believable, and acceptable to the practitioner's mind.

Biofeedback

A classic method for using the mind to alter bodily functions is **biofeedback**. This method employs a recording device to facilitate learned self-control of physiological activities (see the Managing Stress feature "Biofeedback"). The recording device is connected to a region of the body (e.g., forehead, arm), and information about biological activity in that region is "fed back" on a screen or by means of a sound to the person in whose body the activity is taking place. Using this visual or auditory information about the activity, the person can learn to control the activity in a desired way. Biofeedback has been used successfully to treat more than 150 medical conditions, including high blood pressure, back pain, panic attacks, asthma, and headaches (Mayo Clinic, 2016). Biofeedback also can be used to produce changes in the brain's electrical activity (*alpha waves*) to bring about a state of relaxation.

Hypnosis and Healing

Hypnosis (from the Greek *hypnos*, meaning sleep) is a state of concentration and focused attention. The method typically involves attaining a relaxed mental state in which suggestions for imaginative experiences are presented by another person. This is called the hypnotic induction. Hypnotic suggestions can alter perception, sensation, emotion, thought, or behavior and, in this way, the mind can be focused on health issues. **Hypnotherapy** is the use of hypnosis to treat sickness. Hypnosis has been shown to help restore health in many conditions, including reducing pain, facilitating childbirth, decreasing anxieties, managing body weight, and stopping smoking.

The modern use of hypnosis as a medical technique began with the Viennese physician Franz Anton Mesmer,

> **TERMS**
>
> **autogenic training:** the use of autosuggestion to establish a balance between the mind and body through changes in the autonomic nervous system
> **biofeedback:** using an electronic device to "feed back" information about the body to alter a particular physiological function
> **hypnosis:** a state of concentration and focused attention
> **hypnotherapy:** the use of hypnosis to treat sickness
> **nocebo effect:** the opposite of placebo effect; a harmless substance that has harmful, undesirable, and adverse effects on health

Biofeedback

Dan was a first-year graduate student who experienced frequent headaches, for which he sought help from the Student Health Center. Medical tests showed no brain pathology, such as a tumor, or brain infection or injury. Diagnosis: Dan's headaches were related to the stress and anxiety about doing well in graduate school.

Dan's therapy involved meeting with a counselor to discuss ways to manage the stress of graduate school and biofeedback training to deal specifically with his headaches. In biofeedback sessions, three small sensing devices, which monitored the activity of the forehead's frontalis muscle, were attached to Dan's forehead (**Figure 2.5**). The frontalis and certain muscles in the neck involuntarily contract during times of stress, which impedes blood flow to the head, resulting in a headache. Wires from the three sensors were connected to a biofeedback unit, which was placed on a table directly in Dan's view. Whenever Dan's frontalis muscle contracted, the biofeedback unit produced audible clicks. A very tense frontalis produced rapid clicks. A relaxed frontalis produced infrequent, irregular clicks.

Dan was instructed by his biofeedback therapist to try to reduce the number of clicks, a skill that required several training sessions to attain. Paradoxically, not trying to relax his frontalis produced the best results. The therapy proved

successful. Dan seldom got headaches. And when he did, he could relieve them by relaxing the muscles in his forehead.

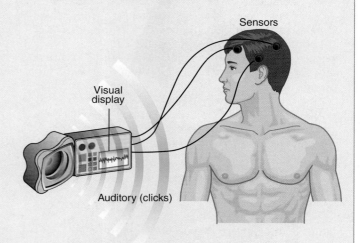

■ Figure 2.5

Biofeedback
The biofeedback device measures muscle tension in the head region. The speaker produces rapid audible clicks when muscles are tense and infrequent and irregular clicks when head muscles are relaxed.

who practiced in the late eighteenth and early nineteenth centuries. History has preserved the term *mesmerism* for the trancelike state that Mesmer produced in his patients (Galdos, 2009).

Mesmer called his technique for healing "animal magnetism" because he had his patients hold onto metal rods that supposedly transmitted healing energy while the patients were in trance. Mesmer was so successful that other physicians in Vienna forced the authorities to order him to stop using his unorthodox methods. In 1778, Mesmer moved to Paris, where he again was successful in attracting patients. Eventually, the French authorities appointed a scientific panel, which included Benjamin Franklin (U.S. ambassador to France at the time), to investigate Mesmer and his methods. The panel concluded that there was no scientific basis to animal magnetism and that Mesmer was a fraud. This conclusion was reached even though the panel did not dispute Mesmer's success in curing many patients. Discredited by physicians and scientists, Mesmer died in obscurity in 1815.

Despite being officially discredited, mesmerism (now called hypnotism) flourished throughout England, Europe, and the United States in the nineteenth century. In 1847, J. W. Robbins, a Massachusetts physician, reported using hypnotherapy to treat eating disorders and to help people stop smoking. Dr. Robbins used aversive suggestions with hypnotized patients and also gave

> We do not see things as they are....We see things as we are.
> *Talmud*

them posthypnotic suggestions. Many of the same procedures are used today in treating these and other disorders.

To be successful therapeutically, hypnosis requires that (1) the participants in the hypnosis encounter are identified as the *hypnotist* and the *client*; (2) suggestions are a key to the procedure; (3) the client (patient) consents to participating in the procedure, especially to receiving and accepting suggestions; and (4) the therapist describes the technique beforehand and how it is supposed to help (Montgomery et al., 2013). Success in hypnosis is greatly influenced by the rapport between client and hypnotherapist so the client can suspend reality and respond to suggestions (Bryant et al., 2012). Effective use of suggestion in healing seems to depend on the degree of mental relaxation involved. For reasons that are not entirely clear, a mind engaged in the conscious thoughts of daily living is not as open to suggestion as one that is internally relaxed by hypnosis, meditation, or other mental relaxation techniques.

Understanding Hypnosis May Help You

Many people have misapprehensions about being hypnotized, and many myths about hypnosis still exist. Perhaps the greatest fear people have is being induced to do something embarrassing, immoral, illegal, or evil when they are hypnotized. Some of the misconceptions and apprehensions about hypnosis are summarized in **Table 2.3**.

Hypnotherapy is potentially a valuable adjunct to medical practice and has a long and successful history. It is not used widely because of time constraints and

Focusing Attention

A wise teacher said that you could read thousands of books about meditation, but none is as good as a demonstration. So, do this: Right now, notice the sensation of the bottoms of your feet touching the insides of the bottoms of your shoes. That sensation is caused by the nerves in the bottoms of your feet signaling your brain that your feet are touching your shoes. That signaling has been going on the entire time you've been reading this page, but you were unlikely to have noticed because your attention was focused on what you were reading—or perhaps on other thoughts—until you were asked to change the focus of your attention to the bottoms of your feet. This shows that you can choose to focus your attention (also called your *conscious awareness*) on what you want to: your feet, signals of discomfort from your body, worries, your to-do list, or memories of a nice time you had with someone special. Meditation is being aware of what your mind is doing on a moment-to-moment basis and shifting the focus of your awareness if you wish to, for example, to your breathing, a repeating sound or prayer, or an image. Instead of your mind being pushed and pulled this way and that by the busyness of your life, meditation allows you to notice that your mind is overly busy—perhaps distressingly so—and to shift your mental process to something that facilitates feeling stable, in control, flexible, and adaptive.

Table 2.3

Myths About What Happens During Hypnosis

Myth: While under hypnosis you lose control of your mind and the hypnotist can make you do anything that he or she wants.

Fact: Despite what is portrayed in movies, a hypnotist cannot control your mind or make you do something against your will or beliefs. A hypnotized person can decide to become "unhypnotized" at any time. Ultimately, all hypnosis is self-hypnosis. The stage hypnotist selects people from the audience who *want* to be hypnotized and be part of the act. People do funny things on the stage because they agree in their minds that it is OK to do them. Similarly, a person follows a therapist's suggestions because of trust and a desire to be helped. No one can control your mind if you do not agree to cooperate voluntarily.

Myth: Hypnosis is like falling asleep. You become unconscious and are unaware of what is happening around you. When you wake up you do not remember what was going on around you while you were hypnotized.

Fact: In hypnosis you do not lose consciousness, and most hypnotized subjects report that they feel very aware. Hypnosis is like focused attention in which you are aware of specific thoughts to the exclusion of others. Just as with deep meditation, you are always in touch with reality and choose to remain in the meditative state or "wake up."

Myth: Hypnotists have special psychic or occult powers, which explains why they can control other people's minds.

Fact: Hypnotists have trained their powers of observation and are skillful at giving suggestions. Those who claim to have special powers should be avoided because they harbor hidden motives and should not be trusted. Always remember that all hypnosis is self-hypnosis.

Myth: Only people with "weak minds" or of low intelligence can be hypnotized.

Fact: Everyone can be hypnotized, although people vary in that ability as they do in all abilities. People with above average intelligence usually enter a state of hypnosis more easily than others. Consider what happens in a movie theater. People laugh, cry, or are terrified by what is happening on the screen. But the images that affect them so powerfully are, in reality, light on the screen. Most moviegoers are in a state of hypnosis and, by adopting the role of "moviegoer," have agreed to allow their emotions to be manipulated by the images. Nevertheless, everyone is in control of their minds. Witness the sudden "unhypnotizing" if someone yells "fire" or if the lights are turned on abruptly. Again, it is worth emphasizing that all hypnosis is self-hypnosis.

Myth: Hypnosis is not useful or effective in improving health or harmful behaviors.

Fact: Hypnosis, or hypnotherapy as it is called when used by trained health professionals, may be very useful in treating a wide range of symptoms. In 1957, the American Medical Association approved hypnotherapy as a valid therapeutic technique. Many physicians and clinical psychologists use hypnotherapy to treat a wide range of physical, emotional, and behavioral problems such as pain, panic attacks, smoking, alcoholism, and posttraumatic stress disorder.

the almost universal belief that the right pill will cure everything. Physicians have to take time to develop a rapport with patients and be willing to take as much time as necessary to answer all questions and make sure the patient is comfortable with being hypnotized. Modern medical practice does not allow for this in an age of managed care and HMOs. Time is money in modern medical practice.

Meditation

Meditation is a long-standing religious and spiritual practice of focused awareness, trance induction, and relaxation that is increasingly used to promote health and healing. Contrary to what some people think, meditation is not a cult, religion, or giving up control over one's mind. It isn't being "zoned out" without thoughts or used to escape reality. Instead, meditation is focusing on, paying attention to, and noticing what your mind

TERMS

Meditation: focusing awareness on a self-produced inner sound ("mantra") or an external sound, or image, or one's breathing to lessen attentiveness to external stimuli

is doing right in this moment without judgment. If you examine what is going on in your mind at any given moment, you will probably find it flitting from one thought to another, called "chatter": "Did I remember to turn off the lights before I left the house?" "My feet are killing me; I shouldn't have worn these shoes." "I wonder what will be on the math test?" "Is it ok to let the kids go to that sleepover this weekend?" Our minds are generally constantly active and often involved in worrying or thinking about emotional upsets, financial concerns, or the tasks and pressures of daily activities.

Quieting the mind is healthy, and meditation is a way to accomplish that. Focused awareness can be achieved in a number of ways, and there are many different kinds of meditation. *Zen meditation* (zazen) involves sitting still with legs crossed while trying to empty the mind of its chatter. *Transcendental meditation* teaches practitioners to focus on a particular phrase (called a **mantra**) that is repeated internally; focusing the mind's attention on a single phrase excludes other random thoughts. *Insight* or *mindfulness meditation* (Vipassana) teaches meditators simply to observe the flow of thoughts that pass through the mind without focusing on any particular one. Buddhists, especially Tibetan Buddhists, often meditate by focusing their attention on a religious image (called a **mandala**). Prayer is a form of meditation in that it focuses awareness on God. Meditation is something that nearly everyone has experienced even if they have not called it meditation.

> Meditation is not what you think.
> *Krishnamurti*

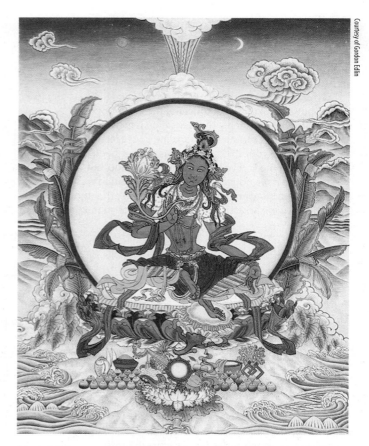

A mandala is a complex visual image used to focus attention and facilitate meditation. ("Green Tara," an original painting by Maile Yawata.)

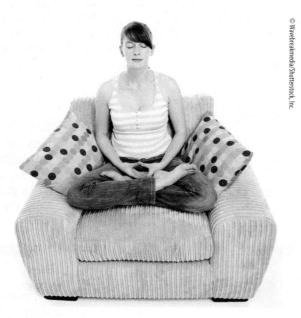

Meditation can be done anywhere, any time.

Make Up Your Own Mantra for Changing Behaviors

Use the power of a mantra to change some aspect of performance or behavior. Choose some behavior or activity that you would like to change or improve. Then create your own mantra. It should not be something complicated, but a small thing that you feel you can achieve. It should be as specific as possible. For example:

Sports: I feel my body getting stronger.
           I feel my body moving more swiftly
           through the water.
           I become less tired each time
           around the track.

Behaviors: I will stop eating when I feel full.
           I will not speak until the anger passes.
           My mind will stay alert during
           classes and exams.

Be creative in designing your own mantra and spend time each day reciting it internally while in a quiet state. You can be a skeptic and the mantra will still work.

Relaxation with Music

Many people know and research has shown (Chanda & Levitin, 2013) that listening to or playing music can be relaxing. Music can focus the mind just as meditation, hypnosis, and prayer do. Thus, listening to or playing music can reduce stress. In medical settings, music can help patients lessen anxiety and stress. One study found that patients undergoing surgery were just as likely to be calmed by music as by sedative drugs (Bradt et al., 2013). Music can help reduce the chronic pain that accompanies rheumatoid arthritis, herniated discs, or fibromyalgia. Music can help those who have experienced stroke, Alzheimer's, and other neurological diseases.

The kind of music that people find helpful varies according to individuals' preferences. In general, soft music is preferred to loud; gentle rhythms and moderate beats that approximate the heart rate (65 to 75 beats per minute) are preferred to vigorous or complex rhythms and fast beats. The "background music" found in doctors' and dentists' offices is known to reduce heart and breathing rates and reduce anxiety.

To use music as a therapy for insomnia, pain, stress, anxiety, or other problem, use the following guidelines:

- Choose music that you enjoy and find relaxing. Many types of classical music, soft jazz, Celtic and Native American music, and chants are suitable. Most people prefer music with flowing rhythms.
- Pick a time and place where you will not be disturbed and can let go of daily concerns. Plan to spend at least an hour in a relaxed state.
- You can listen at low volume or may feel more comfortable using ear-cupping headphones that reduce outside noise and distractions.
- Consider consulting a music therapist for additional advice and help.

Meditation does not have to be done in a religious setting, nor is it complicated.

- Choose a quiet place in your home or outside.
- Find a comfortable sitting position with your back straight. (Lying down is not recommended because it is strongly associated with sleep.)
- Be sure that you have at least 10 to 30 minutes during which you will not be disturbed.
- Busy people often find that meditating before bedtime works best (privacy, quiet).

A good way to begin meditation is to focus your attention on breathing. Begin by becoming aware of the way you are breathing. Is it slow and deep? Is it quick and shallow? Is it through one nostril or both?

As you focus your awareness on your breathing, your mind is highly likely to wander to various thoughts that stream by. When you notice your mind wandering, simply say to yourself, "My mind is wandering," and refocus your awareness on your breathing. Perhaps count your breaths from 1 to 10 to help you focus (counting is similar to a mantra). After some time, it is highly likely that your mind will wander again. When you notice this, do not become frustrated or angry with yourself ("This isn't working!"; "I'm a bad meditator"). The mind's job is to think, and wandering to thoughts in meditation is demonstration of that. So, when your mind wanders to thought, notice and refocus your awareness on your breathing. Meditation is often repeating cycles of focus and wandering (loss of focus). With some practice (Remember: You are good at what you practice), you will become more skilled at focusing on breathing and the calm state of being that it brings, and will be able to let your thoughts stream in the background of your mind without paying much attention to them.

Practicing meditation almost every day can help you manage burnout and stress, increase your sense of well-being, lessen risks of a variety of illnesses and infections, deal with pain, increase your sense of harmony with your social and physical surroundings, get a good night's sleep, improve performance on tasks, and become aware of how your mental processes affect your life. College students take note! A mere 4 days of meditation training for 20 minutes a day can improve cognition and working memory (Zeidan et al., 2010, Chiesa et al., 2011).

Meditation has many documented health benefits—lowered blood pressure, decreased heart rates, less stress, increased blood flow, reduced pain, and relief of many chronic conditions such as asthma, arthritis, and irritable bowel syndrome.

The faster the world becomes, the more we need to slow down.

The Relaxation Response

The **relaxation response** is an automatic physiological response that is the opposite of autonomic nervous system activation (Benson & Klipper, 2000). The relaxation

TERMS

mandala: an artistic, religious design used as an object of meditation

mantra: a sound or phrase that is repeated in the mind to help produce a meditative state

relaxation response: the physiological changes in the body that result from mental relaxation techiques

Positive Thinking Has the Power to Improve Health

- Become more aware of the power your mind has to improve health, hasten healing, and help you perform better in school and in other activities. Belief in yourself, in prayer, or in a particular treatment can facilitate healing and help prevent sickness.
- Use mental images that feel right to you to reduce exam anxiety and to improve performance in sports or other activities. Avoid negative mental images and thoughts such as "I feel lousy," or "I'm too tired to run," or "I just know I can't do that." Use your mind to create positive images and thoughts. You can reverse what seems to be a "bad" day by suggesting to yourself that things are going to change and improve.
- Practice a daily mental relaxation technique in a place that is comfortable and quiet. Use the time to "talk" to your body to promote healing or to change behaviors. Visualize scenes from the past or the future that you know are healthy and constructive. As you become more adept at using your mind, you will find new ways to use mental relaxation in all aspects of your life. (Notice how we inserted a positive suggestion.)

response decreases oxygen consumption, respiratory rate, heart rate, blood pressure, and muscle tension. A variety of mind–body methods can produce the relaxation response, such as mantra meditation, progressive muscle relaxation, and guided imagery. For example, at Harvard Medical School, patients are taught to sit quietly and silently repeat the word "one." Methods that elicit the relaxation response share these features:

- A quiet environment
- A focusing of the mind's attention, such as silently repeating a word or phrase, or focusing one's breathing
- A passive, accepting mental state
- A comfortable physical position

Practicing the relaxation response regularly for 10 to 15 minutes per day increases feelings of well-being and decreases depression, anxiety, and hostility, which is correlated with improved cardiovascular and immune health (Chang et al., 2010).

Suggestion

Any time the mind becomes focused and relaxed, it also becomes more open to suggestion. This can be very beneficial or it can create problems, depending on the kind of suggestions being received by the mind. Suggestions given as warnings, especially to children, who are particularly vulnerable to suggestion, can affect behaviors and cause health problems throughout life. For example, here are some common admonitions given to children that can cause health problems because young children *believe* what they are told.

- Put on your boots when you go out in the snow or you will catch cold.
- If you keep eating cookies, you'll get fat.
- If you don't try harder, you'll be a failure in life.
- If you climb those trees, you'll fall and get hurt.
- If you go out at night, the ghosts will get you.

Each of these suggestions predicts a negative outcome. To a child's mind, which is usually in a trancelike, suggestible state, these negative suggestions become fixed in the unconscious mind and may have a harmful effect even many years later.

The mind can be made more open to suggestion by many things we are exposed to in daily life. For example, movies and television focus attention with both images and sound. As a consequence, they can induce a trance-like state and cause us to cry, laugh, and become angry or upset; they can actually manipulate our emotions through light and sound. No one dies on a movie screen, but we often react as if they did. The violence and horror people watch in movies and on TV often do affect both physical and emotional states. As a result of watching some frightening scene, people may actually become sick days, weeks, or years later when something reminds the subconscious mind of the scene and brings back the fear.

Advertisers know how to take advantage of viewers' suggestible, hypnotic states of mind. Television programs usually are interrupted at an emotional peak in the story by advertising a product while viewers are still in a suggestible state of mind. Many people believe they are not influenced by advertising, but marketing studies indicate otherwise. Most advertisers try to persuade people to buy products they usually do not need. It is important to become more aware of how suggestible you are and to protect yourself from both obvious and subtle suggestions that can damage your health and peace of mind.

A very effective way to use suggestion to promote wellness and change undesirable behaviors is through the use of **image visualization**. Many mind–body healing techniques employ some form of image visualization. For example, frightening scenes from the past, especially from early childhood, can be reexperienced while a person is in a state of mental relaxation brought on by hypnosis or some other technique. As the scenes and emotional upsets are visualized in the mind, they can be reinterpreted and reprogrammed to change their negative effects on health and behaviors. Mental imagery can also be used to reduce pain; hasten healing; improve performance in sports; change smoking, drinking, or eating behaviors; and help control compulsive urges to gamble. At one time or another in our lives, we all daydream or run an "internal movie," fantasizing our hopes and fears. During such fantasies we visualize experiences and create feelings. Image visualization can change body temperature, blood flow, heartbeat,

Image Visualization Reduces Stress

Image visualization is telling yourself a story and "seeing" the images in your mind's eye. An attorney in Los Angeles uses image visualization once in a while during the first few minutes of her lunch break. She closes the door to her office, takes off her shoes, and sits on the floor with her back against a wall. She closes her eyes and takes a few deep breaths. Then she imagines…

…that she is standing at the edge of a meadow that is filled with golden wildflowers. The sun is shining and the air is a very pleasant temperature. On the far side of the meadow is a hill. She imagines herself slowly walking across the meadow toward the hill on a path that has been worn down by previous walks through the flowers. When she reaches the hill, she begins to walk on a gently winding path toward the top. As she walks, she hears the sounds of birds and a nearby stream. Along the side of the path she sees bushes, small trees, a few flowers, and a few stones. Finally, she reaches the top of the hill, where there is a lovely stand of tall trees. There's a clearing in the trees, and on one side of the clearing there's a fallen log. She sits on the log and enjoys the warm sun filtering through the branches of the tall trees. She closes her eyes and rests. After a few minutes, it's time to return, so she opens her eyes, rises, and walks across the clearing to a very large, smooth, white boulder. She looks on the top of the boulder and there's a private message written just for her. She reads the message and then begins to walk down the path to the meadow, still hearing the sounds of the birds and the stream, and still feeling the warm sun. Eventually she reaches the meadow, retraces her path through the golden flowers, and then…

…she opens her eyes and embarks on the rest of her work day.

breathing rate, production of hormones, and other body processes regulated by the brain.

Most psychologists who work with athletes to improve physical performance use image visualization. The so-called inner games of tennis, golf, skiing, and skating are based on image visualization. Baseball players in a batting slump use relaxation and visualization to "see" themselves getting hits. Basketball players use the technique to "see" their free throws going cleanly through the hoop.

Image visualization also can improve sexual responses and enjoyment. Sexual arousal begins in the mind, and negative thoughts or fears can stifle the sexual responses. The sex organs are particularly sensitive to images generated in the mind. Most sex therapists use relaxation techniques and image visualization to help clients improve their sexual experiences. Tension related to sexual performance is usually the main reason for not experiencing the desired sexual sensations. In all areas of your life, begin to use your mental powers more to enhance health and improve performance in daily tasks.

Guided imagery is another application of suggestion to promote health and well-being and to relieve stress. Unlike image visualization, in which the image is created by oneself, in guided imagery, another's verbal suggestions help guide you to create a particular physical response such as reducing stress, lowering blood pressure, or reducing pain. Often, a guided imagery experience begins with the guide suggesting that you take a few moments to settle from the day's usual "busyness" by sitting or lying comfortably, closing your eyes, and taking some deep breaths. Then the guide may suggest images of you being in a peaceful locale, such as beside a mountain stream or at an isolated beach. The guide will describe in great detail the scene and remind you how peaceful and serene you feel. In the mountains you may be guided to see flowers in a meadow or birds flying overhead and to be soothed by the imagined sound of water flowing in a stream. You might be guided to imagine the water carrying away your worries and tension. At the beach you may be guided to sense the warm sun on your skin and hear the sound of waves coming ashore. As the water retreats to the sea it carries away some of your worry, tension, or pain. After a few minutes, your guide will suggest that it is time to leave your serene place and you are guided back to your normal environment. As you return, your guide reminds you how relaxed and good you feel and encourages you to carry that feeling with you as you move through the rest of your day.

Virtual Reality Therapies

It has been known for many centuries that *distraction* is a very effective treatment for pain. That is why meditation, hypnotherapy, prayer, and other methods that focus the mind's attention on something other than pain or other symptoms are so effective. Many Buddhist monks and devout individuals of many faiths learn to focus their attention so completely on a mantra, mandala, breathing, or exalted inner state that they are, quite literally, "out of their bodies." Modern medical researchers are using this aspect of mind to create **virtual reality therapy (VRT)** to treat burns, pain, and phobias (e.g., fear of flying, insects,

TERMS

guided imagery: using verbal suggestions to create one's own mental images that produce relaxation and feelings of harmony, and reduce stress

image visualization: use of mental images to promote healing and change behaviors

virtual reality therapy (VRT): use of computer programs to create virtual worlds that engage the mind in order to overcome pain and fear and to treat symptoms of posttraumatic stress disorder

or heights). Virtual reality therapy involves focusing one's attention on a computer-generated imaginary world. A medical application of VRT exposes burn patients to virtual realities of glaciers, ice, snow, snowmen, and other features of a cold, cold world to distract them from their pain. Another application of VRT is to help stroke patients to improve their gait and posture (Park et al., 2013). While in the fearful virtual world patients are, at the same time, safe in their therapist's office and know that they can remove the headset at any time. Because part of their mind knows they are safe, patients can confront their fears in the virtual world and learn to overcome them.

A very important use of VRT is in the treatment of posttraumatic stress disorder (PTSD), which was experienced by many survivors of the 9/11 attack in New York and by soldiers who served in Iraq (Morina et al., 2015). Examples of environments simulated are virtual Iraq, virtual airplane, virtual nicotine, and virtual 9/11. Patients using VRT can manipulate the virtual environments to lessen their fears and stress. Some manage to reduce their overall anxiety and arousal response so that they become relatively free of PTSD.

The software for virtual reality therapies is costly to develop, and so is the equipment to deliver the therapeutic treatments. Nevertheless, virtual reality therapy has enormous potential to help people overcome a variety of fears and symptoms of fear.

Taking Time Out to Quiet the Mind

Most of us live pretty hectic lives that are full of time pressures and mental stress. Most young people either go to school, work at a job, or do both. In addition to school and work, students engage in extracurricular activities, sports, concerts, smartphone conversations, computer chat rooms, video games, movies, television—the list goes on and on. To do all these things requires a healthy mind and body. Usually, health is something young people take for granted until it disappears. But staying healthy, even when you are young, means finding time to be quiet, to silence stressful thoughts, and to alleviate tensions in the body.

There are many ways to quiet down, and some suggestions and techniques have been presented in this chapter. But the best ones are the ones that you discover for yourself. Find a quiet spot in a park or in your yard where you can sit and reflect on the good things in your life. Forget for a time the problems of the world and what you need to accomplish in life. Just notice things around you, especially the small things. Watching an ant carry a bit of food twice its size is a good thing to do. Looking at the pattern of stars in the night sky is a good thing to do. Experiencing the freshness of new snow and the taste of rain is a good thing to do. Just be quiet as often as you can. It's good for your mental and physical health.

Critical Thinking About Health

1. Identify one time in your life when you have been seriously ill (not counting colds or minor injuries). Describe the nature of the illness and the time it took to become well again. Discuss all of the factors that you think may have contributed to your becoming sick, including stress, emotional problems, poor nutrition, and so forth. Then discuss all of the factors that you believe contributed to your becoming well again, including medical care, prayer, alternative medicines, and other factors. What were the most important factors that led to your becoming sick? What were the most important ones in the healing process?

2. Find a selection of medical journals in the library and look at the drug company advertisements. Try to locate ones that show a comparison of the drug's effectiveness with a placebo. Determine how effective the placebo was from the data given (usually shown in a graph). Then compare the effectiveness of the drug with the placebo. If the placebo was effective, explain why you think it was so effective in this instance. Give your views on whether doctors should prescribe a placebo pill for some conditions before prescribing an active drug.

3. What is the role of religion/spirituality in health? To what degree should religion/spirituality be part of the clinical encounter between patient and physician?

4. Describe any experiences you have had with meditation, hypnosis, yoga, *qigong*, image visualization, or any other form of mental focusing and relaxation. Describe how you became involved with this activity and for what purpose you used it. Did it help you solve a particular health or emotional problem? Would you recommend this technique to others?

Chapter Summary and Highlights

Chapter Summary

Our bodies and brains are intimately interconnected. The brain controls thousands of chemical reactions in the body moment by moment; conversely, the state of the body directly affects thoughts, feelings, and emotions. Optimal health depends on maintaining mind–body harmony so that both work together to keep you feeling well, energetic, strong, and aware of yourself and others. The brain automatically regulates essential functions of the body such as breathing, digestion, blood pressure and flow, and reaction to the environment such as stopping you from walking in front of a moving car or pulling your hand away from a flame. Most brain activities occur without conscious control. But the mind can be trained through various mental and physical techniques to be more effective in healing illnesses and injuries. On the other hand, if your mind is disturbed, anxious, or depressed, it can cause bodily organs to malfunction, thus leading to illness. A dramatic example of the mind's power to affect health is the placebo effect. If a person believes in the power of a pill to cure or prevent disease, taking such a placebo pill will often work as well as a prescribed drug. Belief can heal because the mind has the power to change body chemistry.

Just as the body can be trained to do certain things, the mind also can be trained to calm anxieties and to facilitate healing. Techniques such as meditation, hypnosis, image visualization, and many others increase awareness of thoughts, reduce stress and emotional upset, and even alter body chemistry to promote healing and health. Learning and practicing regularly meditation or another of several mental relaxation techniques can provide life-long tools for improving health and coping with upsetting situations that one encounters in life.

Highlights

- The human mind can cause changes in body chemistry through thoughts and feelings, which may have a positive or negative effect on your health.
- Optimal health is achieved when the mind and body communicate harmoniously.
- Disease can be regarded as disruption of homeostasis or disruption of the harmonious interaction of mind and body.
- The mind and organs of the body communicate continuously via the autonomic nervous system, which maintains vital body functions such as heart rate, level of blood sugar, and temperature.
- Psychosomatic illnesses are physical symptoms caused by stress, anxiety, and emotional upsets.
- Somatic symptom disorders are caused by psychosocial problems.
- The placebo effect often is almost as powerful as drugs in treating symptoms of illness.
- Hypnosis and meditation can play a positive role in healing illnesses.
- Belief, faith, and suggestion all have the power to heal because the mind can change disturbed body functions and reestablish homeostasis.
- A key to maintaining or improving health and wellness is to learn and practice a mental relaxation technique.
- Image visualization can be used to reduce anxiety and stress, modify behaviors, and enhance performance.
- Virtual reality therapies use computer software to treat phobias and severe pain.

For Your Health

Become more adept at using your mind to enhance your health by learning to meditate (Exercise 2.1 in the Workbook). Meditation can help you manage stress, quiet your mind, increase your sense of well-being, enhance harmony with your social and physical surroundings, get a good night's sleep, improve performance on tasks, and become aware of how your mental processes affect your life.

References

Antoni, M. A. (2012). Stress management, PNI, and disease. In S. E. Segerstrom (Ed.), *The Oxford Handbook of Psychoneuroimmunology* (pp. 385–420). Oxford, UK: Oxford University Press.

Bennett, M. P., & Lengacher, C. (2009). Humor and laughter may influence health IV. Humor and immune function. *Evidenced-Based Complementary and Alternative Medicine*, 40, 159–164.

Benson, H., & Klipper, M. (2000). *The relaxation response.* New York: HarperCollins.

Bradt, J., Dileo, C., &, Shim, M. (2013). Music interventions for preoperative anxiety. *Cochrane Database of Systematic Reviews*, Jun 6;6:CD006908. doi: 10.1002/14651858. CD006908.pub2.

Bryant, R. A., et al. (2012). Oxytocin as a moderator of hypnotizability. *Psychoneuroendocrinology*, 37, 162–166.

Chanda, M. L., & Levitin, D. J. (2013). The neurochemistry of music. *Trends in Cognitive Science*, 17, 197–193.

Chang, B. H., et al. (2010). Relaxation response and spirituality: Pathways to improve psychosocial outcomes in cardiac rehabilitation. *Journal of Psychosomatic Research*, 69, 93–100.

Chida, Y., et al. (2009). Religiosity/spirituality and mortality. *Psychotherapy and Psychosomatics*, 78, 81–90.

Chiesa, A., et al. (2011). Does mindfulness training improve cognitive abilities? A review of neuropsychological findings. *Clinical Psychology Review*, 31, 449–464.

Cousins, N. (1979). *Anatomy of an illness.* New York: W. W. Norton.

Dockray, S., & Steptoe, A. (2010). Positive affect and psychobiological processes. *Neuroscience and Biobehavioral Reviews*, 35, 69–75.

Galdos, S. (2009, October 10). The mesmerized mind. *Science News*, 26–29.

Hewlett, C. (1994). Killed by a word. *Lancet*, 344, 695.

Khatchadourian, R. (2010, August 30). The laughing guru. *The New Yorker*, 56–64.

Kirsch, I., et al. (2008). Initial severity and antidepressant benefits: A meta-analysis of data submitted to the Food and Drug Administration. *PLoS Medicine*, 5, e45. Retrieved from http://www.plosmedicine.org/article/info:doi/10.1371/journal.pmed.0050045

Mayberg, H. S., et al. (2002). The functional neuroanatomy of the placebo effect. *American Journal of Psychiatry*, 5, 728–735.

Mayo Clinic. (2016). Biofeedback: Retrieved from https://www.mayoclinic.org/tests-procedures/biofeedback/home/ove-2016972

Medoff, Z. M., & Colloca, L. (2015). Placebo analgesia: Understanding the mechanisms. *Pain Management*, 5, 89–96.

Miu, A. C., Heilman, R. M., & Miclea, M. (2009). Reduced heart rate variability and vagal tone in anxiety: Trait versus state, and the effects of autogenic training. *Autonomic Neuroscience*, 145, 99–103.

Montgomery, G. H., et al. (2013). Hypnosis for cancer care: Over 200 years young. CA *Cancer Journal for Clinicians*, 63, 31–44.

Morina, N., et al. (2015). Can virtual reality exposure therapy gains be generalized to real-life? A meta-analysis of studies applying behavioral assessments. *Behavioral Research and Therapy*, 74, 18–24.

Park, Y. H., et al. (2013). Clinical usefulness of the virtual reality–based postural control training on the gait ability in patients with stroke. *Journal of Exercise and Rehabilitation*, 9, 489–494.

Pressman, S. D., & Black, L. L. (2012). Positive emotions and immunity. In S. E. Segerstrom (Ed.), *The Oxford Handbook of Psychoneuroimmunology* (pp. 92–104). Oxford, UK: Oxford University Press.

Roaldsen, B. L., et al. (2015). Cancer survivors' experiences of humour while navigating through challenging landscapes—a socio-narrative approach. *Scandinavian Journal of Caring Science*, 29, 724–733.

Roberts, L., et al. (2009). Intercessory prayer for the alleviation of ill health. Cochrane Summaries. Retrieved from http://summaries.cochrane.org/CD000368/intercessory-prayer-for-the-alleviation-of-ill-health

Sulmasy, D. P. (2009). Spirituality, religion, and clinical care. *Chest*, 135, 1634–1642.

Sutherland, G., Andersen, M. B., & Morris, T. (2005). Relaxation and health-related quality of life in multiple sclerosis: The example of autogenic training. *Journal of Behavioral Medicine*, 28, 249–256.

Wachholtz, A., & Sambamoorthi, U. (2011). National trends in prayer use as a coping mechanism for health concerns: Changes from 2002 to 2007. *Psychology of Religion and Spirituality*, 3, 67–77.

Wager, T. D., et al. (2004). Placebo-induced changes in fMRI in the anticipation and experience of pain. *Science*, 303, 1162–1167.

Zeidan, F., et al. (2010). Mindfulness meditation improves cognition: Evidence of brief mental training. *Consciousness and Cognition*, 2, 597–605.

Suggested Readings

Benson, H. (2011). *Harvard Medical School stress management: Approaches for preventing and reducing stress.* Cambridge, MA: Harvard Medical School. The founder and former director of Harvard's Cardiac Wellness Programs and Institute for Mind Body Medicine teaches how to identify stress warning signs and to better manage stressful situations using a variety of stress-relief techniques.

Chiesa, A., et al. (2011). Does mindfulness training improve cognitive abilities? A systematic review of neuropsychological findings. *Clinical Psychology Review, 31,* 449–464. Discusses recent research showing that mindfulness meditation can enhance cognitive abilities.

Cohen, K. S. (1997). *The way of qigong.* New York: Ballantine. The definitive guide to *qigong*—what it is, how it works, and what it can do for you.

Dalai Lama. (2005). *The universe in a single atom: The convergence of science and spirituality.* New York: Morgan Road Books. The spiritual head of one of the world's oldest religions, Buddhism, explains why he does not see any conflict between spirituality and science.

Farb, N. A., et al. (2012). The mindful brain and emotion regulation in mood disorders. *Canadian Journal of Psychiatry, 57,* 70–77. Shows that mindfulness can help people with mood disorders such as anxiety and depression by reducing automatic negative self-evaluation, increasing tolerance for negative affect and pain, and engendering self-compassion and empathy.

Kabat-Zinn, J. (2011). *Mindfulness for beginners: Reclaiming the present moment—and your life.* Louisville, CO: Sounds True. Teaches how to transform your relationship to the way you think, feel, love, work, and play and thereby awaken to and embody more completely who you really are. Jon Kabat-Zinn, PhD, is executive director at the Center for Mindfulness in Medicine, Health Care and Society at the University of Massachusetts Medical Center and is the founder and former director of the UMMC Stress Reduction Clinic.

Kornfield, J. (2008). *Meditation for beginners.* Louisville, CO: Sounds True. Presents a complete introduction to "Insight" meditation with step-by-step instruction in breathing, posture, attention, working with difficult emotions, and physical discomfort.

Murray, D., & Stoessl, A. J. (2013). Mechanisms and therapeutic implications of the placebo effect in neurological and psychiatric conditions. *Pharmacology and Therapeutics, 140,* 306–318. Reviews the research on the effectiveness of placebos and their physiological mechanisms of action.

Nash, M. R. (2001, June). The truth and hype of hypnosis. *Scientific American,* 37–54. A good introduction to our scientific understanding of hypnosis.

Sagerstrom, S. C. (2012). *The Oxford handbook of psychoneuroimmunology.* Oxford, UK: Oxford University Press. Discusses the latest research in all aspects of the topic.

Scott, R. A. (2010). *Miracle cures: Saints, pilgrims, and the healing powers of belief.* Berkeley: University of California Press. An academic sociologist examines the evidence for miracle cures over the centuries.

Smith, B. L (2011). Hypnosis today. *American Psychological Association Monitor, 42,* 50. An excellent discussion of the current state of hypnotherapy.

Thompson, G. (2005). *The placebo effect and health: Combining science and compassionate care.* Amherst, NY: Prometheus Books. The author provides a comprehensive examination of the placebo effect.

Recommended Websites

Audio Relaxation CDs and MP3 Downloads
Dr. Emmett E. Miller presents articles on mental well-being and sells CDs and MP3 programs on image visualization, self-hypnosis, and many aspects of wellness and healing.

National Center for Complementary and Integrative Health (NIH) on Meditation: What You Need to Know
Descriptions of several kinds of meditation practices.

Study Help
The University of Toronto's suggestions for mastering academic skills and reducing stress from classes and studying.

University of Maryland Medical Center
http://umm.edu/health/medical/altmed/treatment/hypnotherapy. A very thorough discussion of the method of hypnotherapy.

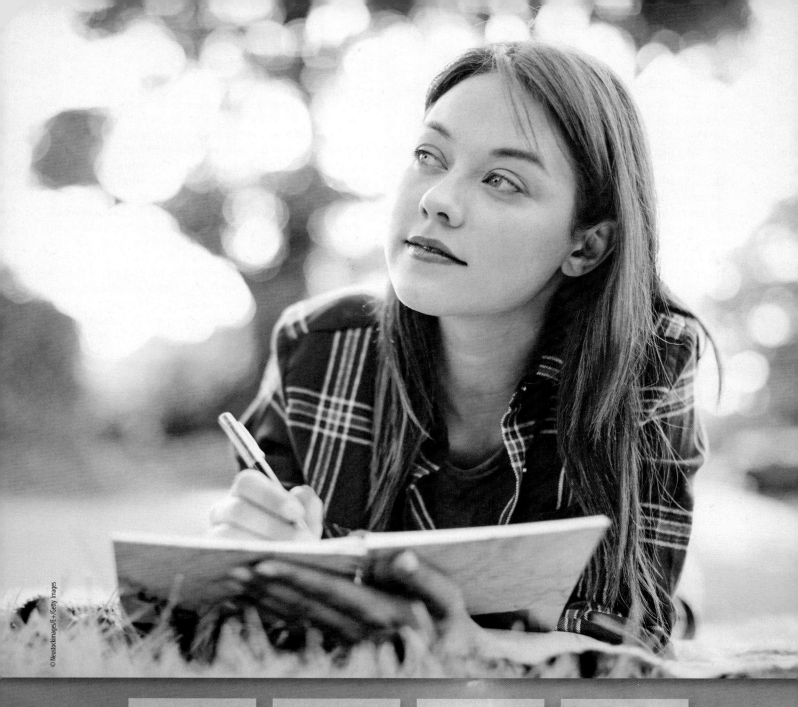

Health Tips

Warning Signs of Stress

Worry, Worry, Worry: How to Stop Stressful Thoughts

Visualization Reduces Exam Anxiety

Global Wellness

Overwork Causes Death in Japan

Managing Stress

Two Monks and the River

Wellness Guide

Assessing Life Changes

The Powerful General and the Monk

CHAPTER 3

Managing Stress: Restoring Mind–Body Harmony

Learning Objectives

1. Define the terms *stress*, *stressor*, *eustress*, and *distress*.

2. Describe the environmental, mental, and emotional components of stress.

3. Describe the physiological components of stress.

4. Describe four ways that stress causes illness.

5. Define problem-focused and emotion-focused coping.

6. Explain how college students can manage overload and test anxiety and practice time management.

Health Instructor (to class): What stresses you?
Student 1: Not enough money.
Student 2: My relationship. It's like a five-unit class.
Student 3: Econ pop quizzes.
Student 4: No, all tests.
Student 5: All of that!

College students are very familiar with stress and its associated feelings of being overwhelmed and by anxiety, frustration, anger, and depression. Along with these, stress can engender sleeplessness, fatigue, gastrointestinal upset, headache, muscular tension, increased susceptibility to infections, and invitations to engage in unhealthy behaviors (e.g., smoking, drinking).

> She would rather light a thousand candles than curse the darkness.
>
> *Adlai Stevenson (Eulogy for Eleanor Roosevelt)*

Stress is a disruption in one's psychobiological balance and sense of harmony within oneself and/or with the social and physical environments. The experience of stress is unpleasant, so when we become stressed, we try to regain psychological and physical balance. If we are successful, not only do we feel better but we also gain confidence in our ability to handle stress in the future. If we are not successful, however, and stress is prolonged or severe, we may feel helpless and become fatigued, worn out, and sick (**Table 3.1**).

In this chapter, we discuss stress and suggest ways to reduce it.

How Stress Occurs

Stress results from the interplay of environmental situations and life events and the mental (cognitive), emotional, and physical reactions to those occurrences (**Figure 3.1**).

Stress experts define stress as "a relationship between the person and the environment that is appraised by the person as taxing or exceeding his or her resources and endangering his or her well-being" (Folkman, 1984). In other words, stress comes from thinking, "This situation puts my well-being at risk and I'm not sure I have the personal, social, economic, or physical resources to meet this challenge and come out OK."

Table 3.1

Disorders That Can Be Caused or Aggravated by Stress

Gastrointestinal disorders	*Musculoskeletal disorders*
Constipation	Rheumatoid arthritis
Diarrhea	Low back pain
Duodenal ulcer	Migraine headache
Ulcerative colitis	Muscle tension
Respiratory disorders	*Metabolic disorders*
Asthma	Hyperthyroidism
Hay fever	Hypothyroidism
Tuberculosis	Diabetes
Colds	Overweight
Flu	Metabolic syndrome
Skin disorders	*Cardiovascular disorders*
Eczema	Coronary artery disease
Pruritus	Essential hypertension
Urticaria	Congestive heart failure
Psoriasis	*Menstrual irregularities*
Eating disorders	*Cancer*
Depression	*Accident proneness*

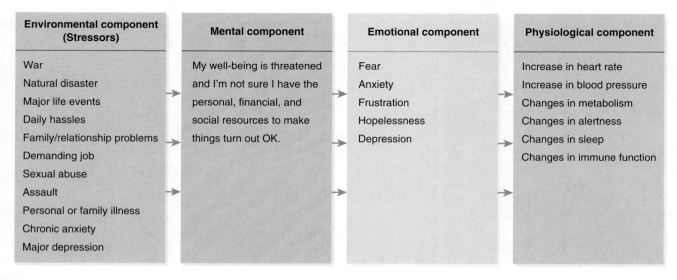

■ **Figure 3.1**

The Components of Stress
Stress results from the interplay of potentially stressful environmental situations and life events and the mental (cognitive), emotional, and physiological reactions to those occurrences.

The Environmental Component of Stress

The environmental component of stress consists of situations and events that bring about stress. **Stressors** can be the day-to-day hassles and complexities that block the efficient and timely accomplishment of daily life tasks, family problems, unpleasant interactions with other people, job/school problems, major external events (war, flood, famine), and major life changes and events (see the Wellness Guide feature "Assessing Life Changes") that become obstacles to achieving desired life goals. Positive experiences, such as starting a new love relationship or graduating from college, although positive, can also be taxing. In general, stressful situations can be classified into these types:

> **Harm-and-loss situations**, which include death of a loved one, theft or damage to one's property, physical injury or loss of a body part, physical assault, or loss of self-esteem.
>
> **Threat situations**, which are perceived as likely to produce harm or loss whether any harm or loss actually occurs. The experience is one of continually watching for and warding off potential dangers.
>
> **Challenge situations**, which are perceived as opportunities for growth, mastery, and gain. The stress that comes from challenging situations is called **eustress** (positive stress), as opposed to **distress** (negative stress) that accompanies harm, loss, and threat.

The Mental Component of Stress

The mental component of stress consists of (1) the appraisal of a situation as absolutely or potentially damaging to one's physical or psychological well-being or a threat to one's survival, and (2) believing that one's personal resources are insufficient to ward off or overcome the threat to one's well-being. The situation can be real, such as breaking up in a relationship, or imagined, such as the possibility of a pop quiz that may or may not happen.

The degree to which a situation is appraised as stressful depends on an individual's psychological makeup. Everyone interprets the world and events differently. Thus, a situation that is upsetting and stressful to one person may not even bother another.

The Emotional Component of Stress

The emotional component of stress consists of unpleasant emotions that arise from one's appraisal of a situation as harmful or threatening and that one's resources for protection are limited or uncertain. These emotions are anxiety, fear, frustration, anger, and depression.

Factors Affecting the Experience of Stress

Several factors influence the degree of stress a person experiences. Among them are predictability, personal control, belief in the outcome, and social support.

Predictability Knowing when a stressful situation will occur produces less stress than not knowing. This is

Warning Signs of Stress

Although stress is pervasive in the life of a college student, it is not always easy to recognize when stress has become a threat to physical or mental health. If you experience any of these signs of stress, it's time to make some changes in your life, and perhaps seek professional help to reduce the stress.

- Trouble falling asleep
- Difficulty staying asleep
- Waking up tired and not well rested
- Changes in eating patterns
- Craving sweet/fatty/salty ("comfort") foods
- More headaches than usual
- Short temper or irritability
- Recurring colds and minor illnesses
- Muscle ache and/or tightness
- Trouble concentrating, remembering, or staying organized
- Depression

because knowing when a stressful event will occur (like taking an exam) allows a person to relax in the interim and prepare to face the challenge, whereas not knowing puts a person on constant alert (like having to face pop quizzes). For example, people whose employment status is secure have less stress than people who must worry constantly about losing their jobs (Scott-Marshall, 2011). During World War II, London was bombed every night, but the London suburbs were not. Londoners had fewer ulcers than suburbanites, presumably because they knew when bombings would occur.

Personal Control Individuals who believe they can influence the course of their lives are likely to experience less stress than are individuals who believe that their fate is determined by factors outside of their control. The crucial factor is belief in one's ability to control situations

TERMS

challenge situations: positive events that may involve major life transitions and may cause stress

distress: stress resulting from unpleasant stressors

eustress: stress resulting from pleasant stressors

harm-and-loss situations: stressful events that include death, loss of property, injury, and illness

stress: the sum of physical and emotional reactions to any stimulus that disturbs the harmony of body and mind

stressor: any physical or psychological situation that produces stress

threat situations: events that cause stress because of a perception that harm or loss may occur and not whether control is actually possible. For example, people who have jobs that involve a lot of pressure to perform but that allow them little opportunity for deciding how the tasks are to be accomplished have more stress than workers who have more control over decisions (Backé et al., 2012).

Belief in the Outcome People who believe that things are likely to improve (optimists) experience less stress than do people who believe that things will get worse (pessimists).

Social Support Having someone to talk to and believing that the person can help manage a stressor by providing physical, emotional, or intellectual help lessens stress (Taylor, 2011). For example, prostate cancer patients experience less stress if they have social support (Lafaye et al., 2014). Also, patients who talk to their surgeons about their fears of an impending surgery have a smaller stress response than patients who go through such procedures feeling uninformed and unsupported do.

The Physiological Component of Stress

The physiological component of stress consists of automatic physiological responses to real or imagined situations that are considered damaging or threatening.

Heart
Increases in heart rate and force of contractions

Blood
Constriction in abdominal viscera and dilation in skeletal muscles

Eye
Contraction of radial muscle of iris and relaxation of ciliary muscle

Intestines
Decreased motility and relaxation of sphincters

Skin
Contraction of pilomotor muscles and contraction of sweat glands

Spleen
Contraction

Brain
Activation of reticular formation

© AbleStock

■ **Figure 3.2**

The Flight-Fight–Freeze Response
All humans display this response when confronted with challenges they interpret as frightening or threatening.

One physiological response to stress is called the **flight-fight–freeze response** (**Figure 3.2**). Its purpose is to enable an individual to deal with a perceived or actual threat by running away or avoiding it (flight), confronting it (fight), or becoming nonvolitionally immobile

The Powerful General and the Monk

The powerful general and his army arrived at the border of a neighboring country. Scouts were sent into the countryside to reconnoiter. After a time a scout returned. Throwing himself off his horse, he knelt at the powerful general's feet and bowed his head.

"What is your report?" barked the powerful general.

"Master," replied the scout. "Hearing that your magnificent and powerful armies have landed, all for miles around have fled."

The powerful general stood proudly and smiled. The scout looked up ever so meekly and continued, "Except the monk."

"What?!?"

"Yes, sire, except the monk. He has not fled."

"Where is this foolish monk?" bellowed the powerful general.

The scout looked up. "In the village, sire, not 15 minutes ride from here. He is in his hut at the top of the hill."

The powerful general, by now enraged, strapped on his sword and armor, mounted his massive white horse, and galloped south along the coast road. At the village he sped up the hill and quickly dismounted in front of the monk's hut. Drawing his sword from its scabbard, the powerful general burst into the hut. There, a small man in clean but tattered robes, with a shaved head, was sitting on a cushion, meditating.

The powerful general placed the tip of his sword at the monk's throat, and in his deepest, most commanding voice said, "You dare not flee before my powerful armies? Do you realize I could run you through with my sword without blinking an eye?"

The monk opened his eyes, looked at the general, and said, "Do you realize that I could let you run me through with your sword without blinking an eye?"

The powerful general thought for a moment. Then he put the sword back in its scabbard, bowed to the monk, and rode away.

and silent (freeze, or "playing dead"). The flight-fight response is coordinated by the sympathetic division of the autonomic nervous system; the freeze response, by the parasympathetic division. The flight-fight response involves the release of adrenaline (also called *epinephrine*) from the adrenal glands (located in the thorax above the kidneys). This elevates the heart rate and blood pressure (to provide more blood to muscles), constricts the blood vessels of the skin (to limit bleeding if wounded), dilates the pupil of the eye (to let in more light, thereby improving vision), increases activity in the reticular formation of the brain (to increase the alert, aroused state), liberates glucose and free fatty acids from body storage sites (to make energy available to the muscles, brain, and other tissues and organs), and activates certain immune cells to prepare to defend the body if wounded. The freeze response includes loss of tone of skeletal muscles (to create disinterest in a predator or to maintain blood flow to the brain if wounded), a drop in blood pressure (to reduce blood loss from wounds), and tightening of the larynx (to inhibit vocalization).

A second physiological response to stress is activation of the **hypothalamo-pituitary-adrenal (HPA) axis** (**Figure 3.3**). The thought that one is in a stressful situation causes the hypothalamus of the brain to release a hormone called *corticotrophin releasing factor* (CRF). This hormone stimulates the pituitary gland (located at the base of the brain) to release a hormone called adrenocorticotropic hormone (ACTH) into the bloodstream. ACTH circulates in the blood and stimulates the pair of adrenal glands to release into the blood yet another hormone called *cortisol*. In the immediate (acute) response to stress, this hormone circulates in the blood, causing tissues to respond to the stressor, generally by providing energy for confrontation (fight) or avoidance (flight), for fighting infection, and for healing wounds. However, in the extended (chronic) response to stress, this hormone alters metabolism, contributing to overweight and type 2 diabetes; suppresses the immune system, thereby increasing susceptibility to infections and cancer; weakens bones; impairs memory; and worsens depression.

The flight-fight–freeze response and activation of the HPA axis are designed for short-term (minutes to

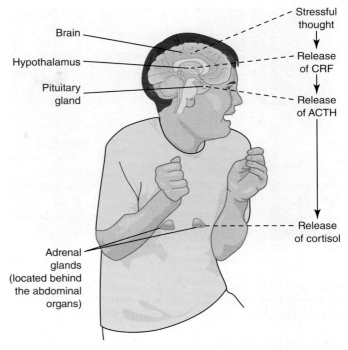

■ Figure 3.3

The Hypothalamo-Pituitary-Adrenal Axis

Stressful thoughts trigger the release of a hormone called *corticotrophin releasing factor* (CRF) from the hypothalamus of the brain. CRF flows in the bloodstream to the pituitary gland, where it stimulates the release of the hormone ACTH. ACTH circulates in the bloodstream to the adrenal glands, where it stimulates the release of cortisol and other stress hormones. In acute stress, cortisol helps prepare the body for fight, flight, wound healing, and infection. In chronic stress, cortisol unbalances metabolism and suppresses the immune system.

TERMS

flight-fight–freeze response: a defensive reaction that prepares the organism for conflict or escape by triggering hormonal, cardiovascular, metabolic, and other changes

hypothalamo-pituitary-adrenal (HPA) axis: a coordinated physiological response to stress involving the hypothalamus of the brain and the pituitary and adrenal glands

---

Overwork Causes Death in Japan

Stress not only can increase a person's susceptibility to infections and sickness but also can cause death, as recognized in Japan. Many people in Japan work long hours and sometimes are asked to take on more work than they can handle. The stress from overwork can raise blood pressure, lower immune system functioning, and cause changes in some people's bodies that result in sudden death. In Japan, sudden death from overwork is called *karoshi*. The major causes of *karoshi* deaths are heart attack and stroke.

In 1987, the Japanese Labor Ministry officially recognized *karoshi* (overwork) as a cause of death. The ministry estimates that about 100 people die each year from overwork and about 60 more are suicide victims. However, the actual number of deaths from overwork is thought to be about 10,000 annually. In 2011, a jury awarded the parents of a Japanese car factory worker $700,000 in damages after a court ruled their son committed suicide because he was overworked.

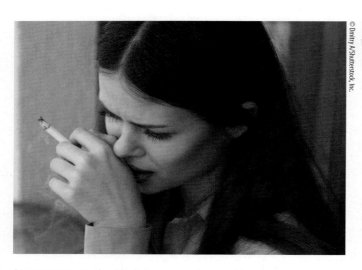

Stress can cause unhealthy behaviors, such as smoking.

Worry, Worry, Worry: How to Stop Stressful Thoughts

If you have the same worrisome thought over and over, try this:

1. Stop the thought when you realize you are having it. Say to yourself, "There's that worry again. Stop!"
2. Replace the thought with a more positive thought.

Here's an example: A student realizes that when he looks at his watch to see how much time remains on a test, he immediately has the thought "There's not enough time." This thought comes over and over again, stressing him and disrupting his focus. He learns thought-stopping. The next time this occurs, he stops. He puts down his pencil, closes his eyes, takes a deep breath, and says to himself, "There's that thought again. I can do this test if I focus." A few seconds later the thought is gone, his mind is clear, and he returns to the exam.

hours) management of a stressful situation. If the individual can think differently or do something to change the perception that the situation is overwhelmingly threatening, stress activation of the nervous system and the secretion of stress hormones stop and the person's mind and body return to balance. This can be accomplished by attempting to change the stressful situation, changing one's interpretation of it, or thinking that the situation is manageable rather than overwhelming. If nothing changes, however, and the stress response continues, then a person can feel anxious, depressed, irritable, fatigued, and burned out, and the risks of becoming both mentally and physically ill increase.

How Stress Contributes to Illness

Stress contributes to illness by (1) causing the mind and body to become exhausted, worn down, and damaged; (2) weakening immunity; and (3) motivating unhealthy behaviors in an attempt to deal with stress (**Figure 3.4**). Some people who have been exposed to a life-threatening, traumatic experience, such as a car crash or combat, can develop posttraumatic stress disorder (PTSD), unpleasant and often debilitating symptoms that persist for months and years after the traumatic experience (discussed later in this chapter).

> Heavy thoughts bring on physical maladies; when the soul is oppressed so is the body.
>
> *Martin Luther*

The General Adaptation Syndrome

Continual physiological response to stressors can bring about a three-stage biological response called the **general adaptation syndrome (GAS)** (**Figure 3.5**).

1. *Stage of alarm:* A person's ability to withstand or resist any type of stressor is lowered by the need to deal with the stressor, whether it is a burn, a broken arm, the loss of a loved one, the fear of failing a class, or the loss of a job.
2. *Stage of resistance:* The body adapts to the continued presence of the stressor by producing more epinephrine, raising blood pressure, increasing alertness, suppressing the immune system, and tensing muscles. If interaction with the stressor is prolonged, the ability to resist becomes depleted.
3. *Stage of exhaustion:* When the ability to resist is depleted, the person becomes ill. Because many months or even years of wear and tear may be required before the body's resistance is exhausted, illness may not appear until long after the initial interaction with the stressor.

Stress Weakens Immunity

A variety of studies have shown that stress can impair the functions of the immune system (Dhabhar, 2011). For example, students who experience considerable stress prior to taking exams show reduced blood levels of immune system cells (e.g., natural killer cells, T cells), thus making exam stress a risk factor for colds and flu. Stress also slows the body's ability to mount an immune response to a vaccine. Furthermore, stress impairs immune functioning in people who have lost their jobs, recently experienced the death of a loved one, or are unhappily married, never married, or recently divorced.

Stress-related impairment of the immune system is mediated by stress hormones, particularly cortisol, which bind to immune system cells and alter their functions. Stress activation of sympathetic nervous system fibers that connect to immune system tissues also alters immune functioning.

> The man who fears suffering is already suffering from what he fears.
>
> *Montaigne*

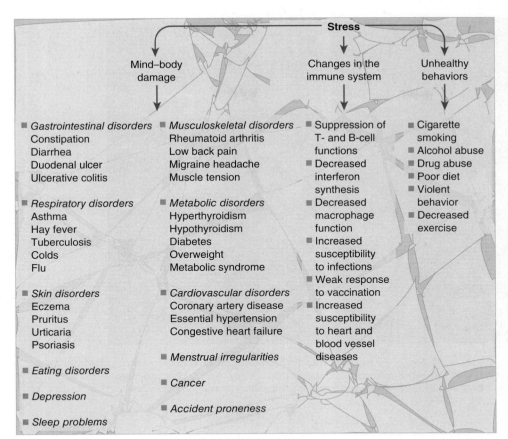

■ Figure 3.4

The Stress–Illness Relationship
Stress contributes to illness by causing the mind and body to become exhausted, worn down, and damaged; by weakening immunity; and by fostering unhealthy behaviors.

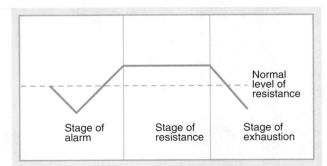

■ Figure 3.5

The General Adaptation Syndrome
In the stage of alarm, the body's normal resistance to stress is lowered from the first interactions with the stressor. In the stage of resistance, the body adapts to the continued presence of the stressor and resistance increases. In the stage of exhaustion, the body loses its ability to resist the stressor any longer and becomes exhausted.

Unhealthy Behaviors

Stress can contribute to ill health by fostering unhealthy behaviors. To manage stressful feelings, some people smoke cigarettes, overeat, undereat, overwork, or drink alcohol and use other drugs. Among U.S. college students, for example, overconsumption of alcohol is often employed to reduce stressful feelings (Conn et al., 2017). Furthermore, people with high levels of stress may not engage in health-promoting activities, such as exercising regularly, eating properly, or getting enough sleep.

Posttraumatic Stress Disorder

Some forms of stress are so severe that they produce a serious, long-lasting condition called **posttraumatic stress disorder (PTSD)**. This condition can result from witnessing or being confronted with events that involve death or serious injury or a threat to the physical or psychological integrity of oneself or others. In such traumatic situations, the person experiences intense fear, helplessness, or horror. The most common source of PTSD in American men is combat in war; in American women, rape and sexual molestation. Other sources of PTSD are living through a natural disaster, experiencing a severe car or plane crash, physical assault, repeated psychological abuse, or a life-threatening illness. Adults who as children experienced traumatic stress have been shown to be at high risk for cardiovascular disease, cancers, asthma, and depression as a result of damage to brain structure from cortisol

TERMS

general adaptation syndrome (GAS): a three-phase biological response to stress

posttraumatic stress disorder (PTSD): physical and mental illnesses resulting from severe trauma

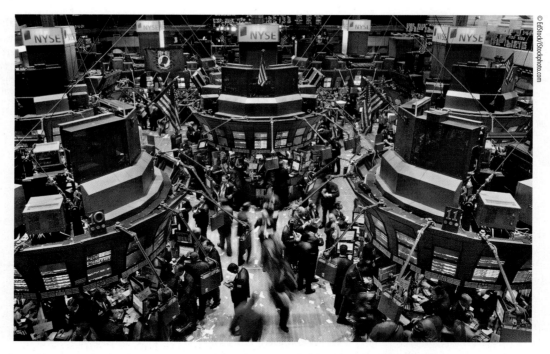

Several heart attacks occur every year on the floor of the New York Stock Exchange, making it one of the highest-density heart attack zones in the United States. The exchange has installed a defibrillator near the bank of phones used to place orders for stock trading, and it has trained workers to use the defibrillator and perform CPR when a heart attack occurs.

and neuroinflammation (Johnson et al., 2013). About 4% of the U.S. population is estimated to have PTSD.

Some of the diagnostic criteria for PTSD include (1) flashbacks to the traumatizing event(s) or recurrent unbidden thoughts and dreams of the experience; (2) persistent avoidance of cues that symbolize the traumatizing event(s); (3) difficulty sleeping, outbursts of anger, and being hyperalert and easily startled; and (4) having little interest in daily activities, feeling cut off from others, and a sense of having a limited future.

Although not known by its current medical name, the symptoms of PTSD were long recognized as an outcome of exposure to combat in war. The Vietnam War ushered in the current concept of PTSD because a large number of returning soldiers had clinically significant symptoms of PTSD. About 20% of military personnel returning from the Iraq and Afghanistan wars have a diagnosis of PTSD.

How the traumatic stress of combat, natural disasters, and physical and sexual assault produces the symptoms of PTSD is not fully understood. Because not everyone exposed to a traumatic situation develops PTSD, researchers suspect that some people are more susceptible, perhaps because of some aspect of temperament, prior stressful experiences, or a history of anxiety or depression. Treatment of PTSD includes psychological therapy and one of a variety of drugs that stabilize mood. Analysis of research findings suggests that children of parents with PTSD are at risk for a variety of psychological and physical problems later in life, most likely due to the effects of parental behavior and intergenerational transmission of increased biological vulnerability to stress hormones (Leen-Feldner et al., 2013).

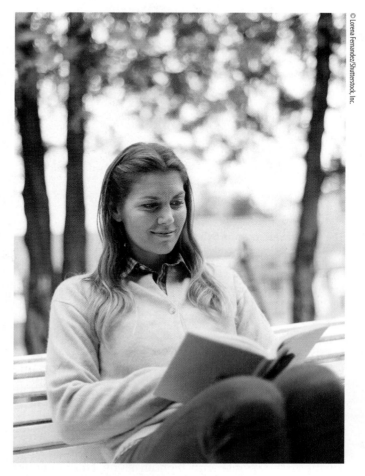

Taking time to relax helps eliminate stress.

Managing Stress

The best ways to manage stress are to replace stressful ways of living with beliefs, attitudes, and behaviors that promote peace, joy, and mind–body harmony. That does not mean you must become reclusive or try to eliminate all sources of conflict and tension in your life. People need challenges to be creative and grow psychologically and spiritually. It may mean, however, changing some self-harming ways of thinking and behaving.

> If you don't learn to laugh at trouble, you won't have anything to laugh at when you are old.
>
> *Will Rogers*

Living healthfully is fundamental to limiting stress. By eating properly; stretching and exercising regularly; getting sufficient sleep; not smoking cigarettes; limiting caffeine, alcohol, and other drugs; and taking "quiet time" to be contemplative, creative, and joyful, you establish a strength of mind–body–spirit that can help buffer the twists, turns, and pulls of stress. When very busy, it's tempting to put off taking care of oneself ("There isn't time; I'll do it later."), so if you must, schedule time for healthful living as you do a class or other regular activity.

Besides living healthfully, managing stress also involves **coping**, which refers to efforts to manage a stressful situation regardless of whether those efforts are successful. In general, there are three types of coping processes (Folkman et al., 1986).

Problem-Focused Coping The stressful situation is appraised as changeable and a plan for improving things is devised and attempted. The key feature of **problem-focused coping** is the belief that one can change things for the better (optimism). Even if it turns out that change is not possible, believing it to be so lessens stress. Believing that one cannot change a *changeable* situation for the better (pessimism) creates a sense of helplessness and hopelessness, which can lead to giving up and depression.

Some ways to practice problem-focused coping include the following:

- Limit or eliminate interaction with the stressor. Be assertive with an annoying roommate, say "no" to unreasonable requests, use earplugs to block out noise, change jobs, change your major.
- Alter your perception of a stressful situation (called *cognitive reappraisal*). By perceiving a situation as less challenging, you lessen the chance of feeling overwhelmed. Ask yourself: "Am I seeing this situation realistically? And even if I am, is it really that threatening?"
- Set attainable goals. Winning may be an athlete's highest goal, but worrying about losing can make one sick. The solution is not to give up sports but to change priorities, perhaps by emphasizing the joy of participation rather than the outcome of competition.
- Focus on your personal strengths, values, and positive qualities. Have confidence in your ability to lessen stress. Give yourself credit for things you have done to lessen stress rather than believing that it was blind luck. This enhances the belief and confidence that you can master many situations that you encounter. Remember that stress is a function of one's belief about managing a challenging situation.
- Seek social support. Talk to friends, family members, counselors, teachers—anyone who you believe can understand, lend a sympathetic ear, and offer sound feedback and advice if you request it. Remember: A problem shared is a problem halved.
- Reduce physical tension. Take a walk, ride a bike, jog, or do yoga, progressive muscle relaxation, or t'ai chi—any physical activity that can release muscle tension and focus your mind on something other than your problems.
- Keep your sense of humor. Laughter and joy are beneficial to the spirit and immune system (Hasan & Hasan, 2009).
- Engage in sensory experiences, such as art, music, or a walk in a garden, through the woods, or along the beach or lake shore (Westlund, 2015).

Emotion-Focused Coping The stressful situation is appraised as not immediately changeable and one decides to accept and work with the reality of the situation, perhaps by waiting for an opportunity to take action or by looking for the good in the bad ("a learning experience"). To facilitate acceptance, one might seek solace and comfort in religion, social contact, being with Nature, or perhaps becoming more involved in helping others.

Some ways to practice **emotion-focused coping** include the following:

- Ease your mind. Employ any of a variety of methods that can stop the physiological stress response and produce instead the "relaxation response." These include meditation, image visualization, guided imagery, journal writing, and prayer. Making one of these methods work for you requires practice and persistence. After learning about the methods, choose one to experiment with almost daily over the course of a week. When you find one or two that you like, make doing them a regular part of your life.
- Let go. Even if only for a few minutes, stop carrying problems in your mind. Give yourself a break from

TERMS

coping: efforts to manage a stressful situation regardless of whether those efforts are successful

emotion-focused coping: appraising and accepting a stressful situation as not immediately changeable and adopting an attitude that lessens anxiety and brings comfort

problem-focused coping: appraising a stressful situation as changeable and making and attempting a plan for changing something to improve things

stress by "leaving it at the river" (see the Managing Stress feature: "Two Monks and the River").

Denial/Distancing/Giving Up The stressful situation is appraised as not amenable to change, and rather than accepting that reality, one chooses not to think about it (denial), to undertake escapist activities (oversleeping, overeating, using drugs and alcohol, or increased TV watching, Web surfing, and videogame playing), or to become fatalistic and helpless (give up).

In general, problem-focused coping is best for dealing with practical problems and situations that can be resisted or overcome with one's personal efforts. Emotion-focused coping is best for dealing with situations not amenable to change but which must be faced, such as the death of a loved one, illness, or coping with a natural disaster. Denial and avoidance tend to be ineffective coping strategies.

College Student Stress

Being in college can be both rewarding and intense. In college you get the opportunity to learn a variety of interesting things, meet new people, prepare yourself for a rewarding job/career, become an honorable person and good citizen, and identify your values, abilities, and preferences. On the other hand, college life has the potential to be stressful (Table 3.2). Students are challenged daily to perform academic tasks, some of which are new (that's why it's called learning) and thus raise doubts about oneself and one's abilities. The college experience is rife with change and unfamiliarity: new classes, new teachers, new people, new living situations. Because college is not home and the people are not family, there may be little support. And, to top it off, rather than getting paid for all their hard work, students do the paying. Furthermore, when younger college students are first on their own, they may not always make the wisest, safest, and healthiest choices.

A healthy lifestyle—eating properly, exercising regularly, getting sufficient restful sleep, having daily quiet time and regular creative relaxation (reading, socializing, art, music)—is fundamental to dealing with college stress. Unfortunately, with so many demands and time pressures, it is tempting to put off choices for living healthfully.

Overload

If they were to occur sequentially, individual stressors in college, such as taking a test, going through a rough time with a romantic partner, or moving to a new residence, although unpleasant, would be generally manageable.

Table 3.2

Examples of College Student Stressors

Academic	***Social***
Competition	Loneliness
Schoolwork (difficult, low motivation)	Obligations, annoyances (family/friends/girl-/boyfriend)
Exams and grades	Not dating
Poor resources (library, computers)	Roommate(s)/housemate(s) problems
Oral presentations/public speaking	Concerns about STDs and/or unintended pregnancy
Professors/coaches (unfair, demanding, unavailable)	***Self***
Choosing and registering for classes	Behavior (habits, temper)
Choosing a major/career	Appearance (unattractive features, grooming)
Time	Ill health/physical symptoms
Deadlines	Forgetting, misplacing, or losing things
Procrastination	Weight/dietary management
Waiting for appointments and in lines	Substance abuse
No time to exercise	Self-confidence/self-esteem
Late for appointments or class	Boredom
Environment	***Money***
Others' behavior (rude, inconsiderate, sexist/racist)	Not enough
Injustice: seeing examples or being a victim of	Bills/overspending
Crowds/large social groups	Job: searching for or interviews
Fears of violence/terrorism	Job/work issues (demanding, annoying)
Weather (snow, heat/humidity, storms)	***Tasks of daily living***
Noise	Tedious chores (shopping, cleaning)
Lack of privacy	Traffic and parking problems
	Car problems (breaking down, repairs)
	Housing (finding/getting or moving)
	Food (unappealing or unhealthful meals)

However, in college, many challenges and changes occur virtually simultaneously. For example, at the end of a semester, a student could face having to write two final papers, take five finals, deal with a bad cold, and move to a new apartment. And the next semester, there would likely be a new set of challenges (an ill parent, a course that makes no sense) along with some of the usual ones (final papers and exams and problematic social relationships).

Being confronted with too many challenges and changes can lead to overload—the feeling that there are too many demands on your time and energy. Your life consists of zipping from here to there to attend to all of your tasks, but what you really want is a week off to hang with your friends and "veg." And if overload grows to feeling overwhelmed, a student might drop a class or two, drop out of school, get depressed, or use alcohol or drugs.

At the heart of overload is the sense of lacking personal control. Individuals who believe they can influence the course of their lives (internal locus of control) are likely to experience less stress than individuals who believe that their fate is determined by factors outside of their control (external locus of control) (Au, 2015). Thus, although it is tempting to focus on things outside of yourself to explain feelings of overload and being overwhelmed, it is more productive to look at yourself. Which is good, because you have more control over yourself than you do over things in your environment.

Here are some antidotes to overload:

1. *Plan ahead.* Knowing when a stressful situation will occur produces less stress than not knowing does. For example, most of the time, you will know at the beginning of a semester when major assignments are due. Plan for them.

2. *Keep a to-do list.* At the beginning of each day, or the night before, write down and prioritize all the things you have to do.

3. *Clarify intentions.* Before you begin each day, take a few moments to be quiet and still and clarify your intentions. Ask yourself, "What do I want/need to make happen today?" "What do I need to do to keep my mind, body, and spirit healthy and well?" Don't think only of accomplishing tasks but also the effects your behaviors will have on yourself and others.

4. *Prioritize tasks.* First things first. Classify tasks according to their urgency and importance (**Figure 3.6**), and do them in this order: (1) urgent and important; (2) not urgent but important; (3) urgent but not important; and (4) not urgent or important. Distinguishing the urgent/important tasks from the urgent/not important ones is often difficult because urgency is a state of mind and makes everything seem important. Before prioritizing items on your to-do list, take a few minutes to become mentally and physically quiet. This will allow you to place truly urgent and important items at the top of your to-do list.

5. *Don't sweat the small stuff.* Eliminate unimportant tasks from your list. Don't do, think about, or worry about anything that doesn't match your most important values and long-term goals. "Keep your eyes on the prize."

Two Monks and the River

Two monks set out on their last day's journey to their monastery. At midmorning they came upon a shallow river, and on the bank there stood a beautiful young maiden.

"May I help you cross?" asked the first monk.

"Why, yes, that would be most kind of you," replied the maiden.

So the first monk hoisted the maiden on his back and carried her across the river. They bowed and went their separate ways.

After an hour or two of walking, the second monk said to the first monk, "I can't believe you did that! I just can't believe it! We take vows of chastity, and you touched a woman. You even asked her! What are we going to tell the abbot when we get home? He's going to ask how our journey was, and we can't lie. What are we going to say?"

Another couple of hours passed and the second monk erupted again. "How could you do that? She didn't even ask. You offered! The abbot's going to be incredibly angry."

By late afternoon the two were nearing their home, and the second monk, now filled with anxiety, said, "I can't believe you did that! You touched a woman. You even carried her on your back. What are we going to tell the abbot?"

The first monk stopped, looked at the second monk and said, "Listen, it's true that I carried that maiden across the river. But I left her at the river bank hours ago. You've been carrying her all day."

TERMS

overload: the feeling that there are too many demands on one's time and energy from being confronted with too many challenges

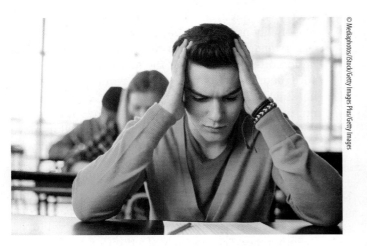

Academic pressures and test taking can produce anxiety and stress.

© Mediaphotos/iStock/Getty Images Plus/Getty Images

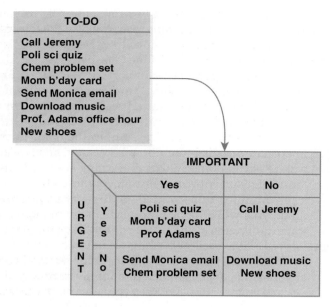

Figure 3.6

Prioritizing Tasks

Classify tasks from your to-do list according to their urgency and importance and do them in this order: (1) urgent and important; (2) not urgent and important; (3) urgent but not important; and (4) not urgent or important. Move tasks labeled "urgent and not important" to other categories because urgency is a state of mind and makes things seem important even if they are not.

6. *Schedule downtime.* Even if it's only a few moments a day, take time for activities that you find meaningful and fun, or just chill.

7. *Sleep.* Not sleeping enough reduces performance and efficiency on tasks by as much as 50%, which makes tasks take longer and contributes to the sense of overload.

8. *Don't "Just do it."* "Just do it" is a slogan for selling sports shoes, not living a life. Students often erroneously believe that the solution to overload is to put in more effort ("just do it"). Because they already are maxed out, putting in more effort cannot succeed, although a list of undone tasks can contribute to a loss of confidence and self-esteem.

Time Management

A major cause of college student stress is the sense that there's too much to do and not enough time to do it. Because you can't make more time, the way to ease this pressure is to make the best use of the time you have. Here are some tips for time management:

- *Perform a time audit.* For at least three representative days in your week (a whole week is better), write down everything you do during each of the 24 hours. Make a chart (**Table 3.3**). Identify windows of time that could be put to better use and alter your activities accordingly.

Table 3.3

Time Diary

Time	Activity
6:00 A.M.	Wake up
6:15 A.M.	Shower/dress/eat
7:00 A.M.	Go to school
8:00 A.M.	Chem lecture
9:30 A.M.	Hang out in library/snack
10:30 A.M.	Psych lecture
12:00 P.M.	Work
5:00 P.M.	Go home

Directions: Record your activities for three representative days. Enter data two to three times a day. For example, at noon, record your activities since awakening; at 5:00 P.M., record your activities since noon; at bedtime, record your activities since 5:00 P.M. Calculate the average daily hours awake, asleep, at school, studying/schoolwork, at work, with family, with friends, with self, commuting, other.

- *Be energy efficient.* Schedule important activities for the times of the day when you are most alert and attentive. For example, if you're a morning person, take morning classes and study in between them. Schedule exercise and socializing for the afternoon. Night people might do the opposite.

- *Resist multitasking.* Try to do only one thing at a time. Multitasking appears to be time efficient, but it also creates a sense of urgency, which produces anxiety and stimulates the secretion of stress hormones, thus contributing to stress and decreased performance.

- *Control interruptions.* Discourage drop-in visiting; don't answer texts, the phone, or instant messages (if it's important, the person will try again); stay away from TV, computer games, and the Internet.

- *Tame any tendencies toward perfectionism.* Don't waste time trying to make everything perfect. Every task has a point of diminishing returns—when the time and energy you put in is out of proportion to what you can reasonably hope to get back.

- *Understand any tendencies to procrastinate.* Procrastination often grows out of the fear of failure or exposure (people seeing you or your work and judging it harshly). When you hear your litany of excuses for not working at a task, ask yourself what you fear. Be your own best friend and encourage yourself to move ahead. Rather than focus on the end product of your efforts, do *one thing* that will move you ahead. If you have not begun to study for an upcoming exam, don't think about the exam. Instead, promise yourself that you will take your textbook out of your backpack today. That's all. Tomorrow, promise yourself you will open it. Remember: "The journey of a thousand miles starts with a single step."

Test Anxiety

It is a rare college student who does not get nervous when taking tests. People in American society equate educational success, academic degrees, and professional licenses with the attainment of important life goals, particularly financial ones. As a consequence, competition among students at all levels is intense. Students believe that grades and exam scores will determine how successful their lives will be in terms of jobs, careers, and money.

Many students experience health problems because of academic pressures and anxiety about exams. They may suffer from headaches, stomach and bowel problems, disordered eating, recurrent infections, and other symptoms of stress. Students whose exam anxiety affects their health need to make personal adjustments to reduce the anxiety while they pursue their goals.

Test anxiety is a sense of unease and apprehension—frequently accompanied by physiological symptoms such as upset stomach, restlessness, sleep problems, irritability, and "nervous" eating—that precedes the taking of an exam. Besides creating physical illness, test anxiety can make it difficult to concentrate, which increases the likelihood of forgetting (blocking) and making "careless" errors.

Test anxiety is a form of performance anxiety, which can occur in any activity in which someone cares about the outcome of her or his performance. (If the person didn't care about the outcome, then he or she would not be nervous about it.) Students, athletes, musicians, actors, and people who interview for jobs are all familiar with performance anxiety.

Being somewhat nervous about how well you are going to do leads to performing well. Unfortunately, being too nervous reduces performance on the task (**Figure 3.7**). With regard to tests, being a little nervous can motivate you to study prior to the test and to focus your attention while taking the test. Being too nervous prior to the test can lead to procrastination and during the test can distract you from the test.

Whenever you are performing a task (and you care about the outcome), your goal is to be just nervous enough to be at peak performance but not so nervous that you panic. The only way to know where this peak is for you is by experience. This is why, after having taken dozens of tests, students become expert test-takers. And this is why during the first couple of years of college, many students are petrified of tests.

Test anxiety is caused by a test-taker's internal mental messages, or self-talk, which focus on imaginary "terrible" outcomes of doing poorly on the exam. Some examples include the following:

- *Exaggerating the importance of the test:* "If I do poorly on this test, I'll do poorly in the class. If I do poorly in the class, I won't get into law school. If I don't get into law school, I'll be a failure and die of shame."
- *Fear of autonomy and exposure:* "If I do well, everyone will notice me and I will be embarrassed."
- *Fear of abandonment:* "If I do poorly, my friends and family will dislike me."
- *Confusing one's performance on an exam with one's self-worth:* "If I do poorly on the exam, it will prove that I'm a loser."

Solutions to Text Anxiety Acknowledge that you get nervous before tests and try to become aware of the roots of your test anxiety. Keep a journal of pretest feelings and symptoms. Be attentive for the images and negative messages in your internal self-talk. If you tell yourself, "You're not smart enough to do well," perhaps respond by saying to yourself, "That's your opinion. Mine is that I know I can do this." Remember: If you don't prepare adequately for the exam by studying, and you care about your performance, then it's realistic to feel anxious about the possibility of doing poorly.

Here are some other suggestions for managing test anxiety:

- Realistically appraise the importance of an exam. Remind yourself that a test is only a test and not a measure of your self-worth.
- Remind yourself that focusing on the grade will distract you from learning the material.
- As part of test preparation, give yourself periods of quiet time in which to relax and visualize yourself taking the test (see the Health Tips feature "Visualization Reduces Exam Anxiety"). In your image, see yourself taking the exam confidently and masterfully. See yourself coming across a difficult question and taking that experience in stride and moving on to another question that you can respond to with confidence.
- Focus your awareness on the test by getting your test-taking materials together before test time. Sharpen your pencils and get your Scantron or blue book and

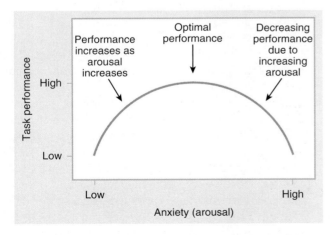

■ Figure 3.7

Performance Is Affected by Anxiety/Arousal
Performance on a task is affected by how anxious a person is about how well she or he is going to do. Being somewhat anxious leads to better performance until an optimum level of performance is reached. Being too anxious distracts the mind and reduces performance.

Visualization Reduces Exam Anxiety

The following exercise can reduce the stress and anxiety of taking exams. It can result in improved scores and a reduction in symptoms produced by stress.

1. Find a comfortable place in your house or room and a time when you will not be disturbed by other people. Sit in a comfortable chair or lie down on a couch or floor. The main thing is to get physically comfortable. If music helps you relax, play some of your favorite music softly.

2. Close your eyes and ask your mind to recall a place and time where you felt contented. It might be a vacation time, being with someone, or being alone in a beautiful environment. Use your imagination and memory to reconstruct the scene where you felt happy and healthy. Notice that you had no concerns there at that time. Let yourself become involved with the scene. The process is similar to having a daydream or a fantasy. While your mind is focused on pleasurable memories, your body automatically relaxes.

3. When you feel quite relaxed, refocus your mind on the upcoming exam. See yourself taking the exam while feeling relaxed and confident. Because your mind and body are relaxed and comfortable, your mind automatically associates the same feelings with the image of taking the exam. Visualize the exam room, the other students, yourself answering the questions; let your mind focus on as many details as possible.

4. Now project your mind into the future to the actual day and place of the exam. Notice how relaxed you feel as you take the exam; the anxiety you used to experience seems to have vanished. Continue with the visualization until you see yourself turning in the exam and feeling confident and pleased with your performance.

5. Do this exercise for several days prior to any exam that causes anxiety. You will be surprised at the absence of nervousness and stress on exam day. You will be even more pleased at the improvement in your grades.

write your name on it. Arrive at the exam 5 to 10 minutes early and let yourself relax.

- Don't get into a frenzy before the test. Don't cram. That only increases anxiety.
- Get a good night's sleep. Eat a balanced meal (protein and complex carbohydrate; not sugary/fatty snacks) one or two hours before the exam.
- Once in the test situation, stop worrying. Try to flow. If you block, put down your pencil, put your feet flat on the floor, close your eyes, and focus your awareness on your breathing. After 20 to 30 seconds, when you're ready, go back to the exam.
- Realize that test-taking is a skill only partially related to how much one knows and understands. Like any skill, one improves with practice.

What You Can Do About Stress

In the fast-paced, competitive world we live in, it's almost impossible not to experience stress and its many physiological and psychological manifestations. When stressed, we generally identify its causes as the hassles, obstacles, time pressures, unpleasantness in generally pleasant relationships, interactions with unpleasant others, and other situations that disrupt our feelings of inner harmony. What we often fail to recognize, however, is that we often contribute to our stress by how we think about and respond to what we experience. It is not always possible to avoid or escape stressful situations. Neither is it generally possible to change others so that they behave in ways we desire. In the face of stress, a wise course is to become mindful of how your thoughts contribute to feeling stressed. Becoming increasingly aware of how your mind works can help you decrease the time your mind swirls around in the throes of stress.

Critical Thinking About Health

1. Three groups of people were vaccinated against a test substance (one that could not make anyone sick). Group 1 consisted of students during final exams; group 2, people complaining of loneliness; group 3, people whose spouse had cancer. Each group was further subdivided into two subgroups. One subgroup in each major group was given 6 weeks of weekly support group meetings plus education about reducing the stress of their circumstance. The other subgroup in each major group was given no support or education. The accompanying figure shows the results of the strength of the immune response to the test vaccine.

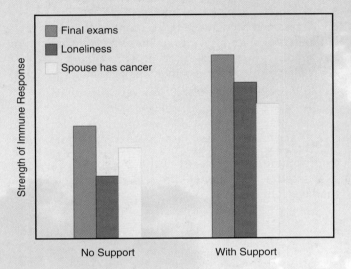

   a. Explain the results of the experiment.
   b. Suggest a hypothesis to explain the results of the experiment.
   c. What do the results suggest about how you can better deal with stress in your life?

2. Johann Wolfgang von Goethe (1749–1832), the German author of *Faust* and other literary works, once wrote: "Things which matter most must never be at the mercy of things which matter least."

   a. What is your interpretation of Goethe's idea?
   b. How does letting things which matter most be at the mercy of things which matter least contribute to stress?
   c. How susceptible are you to stress from letting things which matter most be at the mercy of things which matter least? What could you change to reduce that stress?

3. Offer an explanation for the following: In the 1980s, researchers studied the health of adults living in two communities that were separated by a river. North River was a prosperous suburb, and South River was an industrial region in which the major employer, an auto plant, had shut down. The research showed that after the auto plant closed, children living in South River had many more doctor visits for infections and allergies than did children in North River. Also, adults in South River had more motor vehicle accidents and colds and flu during winter months than adults in North River did.

4. On the Recent Life Changes Questionnaire, the death of a child, spouse, sibling, or parent carries the highest LCU values.

   a. Offer a hypothesis to explain that result. In your hypothesis, take into account the nature of those kinds of relationships and what is lost when someone dies.
   b. Given that the loss of a loved one is associated with the highest LCU values, how should someone who experiences that kind of loss navigate life so as to reduce his or her stress and the risk of becoming ill?
   c. What is the best way to cope with the loss of a loved one?

5. Do you experience test anxiety to such a degree that you become physically or emotionally upset before or after taking an exam? If so, describe your symptoms and feelings. If you're anxious about an exam coming up in the next few weeks, try the exercise described in the Managing Stress box entitled "Visualization Reduces Exam Anxiety" for at least a week before taking the exam. After the exam, describe your experience in detail and indicate whether you performed better than you expected on the exam.

Chapter Summary and Highlights

Chapter Summary

Stress is an integral part of everyone's life. Stress occurs when something new is encountered, when you cannot perform a required task correctly, when you fail a test at school, or when a project does not turn out the way you want it to. Stress occurs when you are criticized, bullied, laughed at, or physically abused. On the one hand, stress plays an essential role in helping us learn, grow, and become more capable and confident. Stress is necessary for persons to learn how to handle difficult situations that are encountered throughout life. On the other hand, prolonged or excessive stress is physically and mentally destructive. Stress may lead to high blood pressure, to digestive problems, to overeating and obesity, to sexual difficulties, and, in fact, stress probably contributes in some measure to most mental and physical illnesses.

In the absence of disrupting influences or excessive stress, the thousands of chemical reactions needed to maintain a healthy brain and body are automatically regulated by a process called *homeostasis*. The brain sends signals via the nervous and hormone systems to all the organs of the body to keep them functioning at precise, healthy levels. It is only when homeostasis goes awry as a result of stress or other disruptive factors that symptoms and sickness may occur. Maintaining mind–body harmony is another vital key to well-being. Things that affect mind–body harmony include relations with friends and family as well as being conscious of the environment you live in. Do you spend time gardening or hiking or just walking somewhere quiet and peaceful? These simple activities reduce stress, foster mind–body harmony, and help keep you healthy.

Highlights

- Stress is the disruption of mind–body harmony brought about by trauma, threats to life, or obstacles to carrying out daily tasks, accomplishing life goals, or achieving desired changes in life.
- Stressors are situations and circumstances that cause stress.
- The mental component of stress consists of the interpretation of a situation as threatening and the appraisal that one's personal resources are insufficient to meet the demands of dealing with the stressful situation.
- The physiological components of stress are the flight-fright-or-freeze response and activation of the hypothalamo-pituitary-adrenal axis, with consequent secretion of stress hormones, especially cortisol.
- Stress contributes to illness by wearing down the mind and body (general adaptation syndrome), impairing immunity, and fostering unhealthy behaviors.
- Posttraumatic stress disorder is a serious medical condition resulting from exposure to traumatic events and near-death experiences.
- Stress can be reduced by disengaging from stressors and/or by altering perceptions and goals, thereby reducing the potential for stress-related illness.
- Stress can be reduced by techniques that produce a peaceful state of being, such as image visualization, meditation, exercise, yoga, and just taking it easy.
- College student stress includes overload, time pressures, and test anxiety.

For Your Health

To manage stress it is helpful to know what stresses you and how much stress something causes. Find out more about your stress by filling in the "My Stressors" Questionnaire (Exercise 3.1 in the Workbook). The other exercises for this chapter can help you understand and manage your stress.

References

Au, E. W. (2015). Locus of control, self-efficacy, and the mediating effect of outcome control: Predicting course-level and global outcomes in an academic context. *Anxiety, Stress, and Coping, 28,* 425–444.

Backé, E. M., et al. (2012). The role of psychosocial stress at work for the development of cardiovascular diseases: A systematic review. *International Archive of Occupational and Environmental Health, 85,* 67–79.

Conn, B. M., et al. (2017). Acculturative stress as a moderator of the effect of drinking motives on alcohol use and problems among young adults. *Addictive Behaviors, 75,* 85–94.

Dhabhar, F. S., & McEwan, B. S. (2007). Bi-directional effects of stress on immune function. In Robert Ader (Ed.), *Psychoneuroimmunology* (4th ed.). Boston: Elsevier Academic Press.

Folkman, S. J. (1984). Personal control and stress and coping processes: A theoretical analysis. *Journal of Personality and Social Psychology, 46,* 839–852.

Folkman, S., et al. (1986). Dynamics of a stressful encounter: Cognitive appraisal, coping, and encounter outcomes. *Journal of Personality and Social Psychology, 50,* 992–1003.

Hasan, H., & Hasan, T. F. (2009). Laugh yourself into a healthier person: A cross-cultural analysis of the effects of varying levels of laughter on health. *International Journal of Medical Science, 28,* 200–211.

Johnson, S. B., et al. (2013). The science of early life toxic stress for pediatric practice and advocacy. *Pediatrics, 131,* 319–327.

Lafaye, A., et al. (2014, July). Dyadic effects of coping strategies on emotional state and quality of life in prostate cancer patients and their spouses. *Psychooncology, 23*(7), 797–803. Epub ahead of print, 3 February.

Leen-Feldner, E. W., et al. (2013). Offspring psychological and biological correlates of parental posttraumatic stress: Review of the literature and research agenda. *Clinical Psychology Reviews, 33,* 1106–1133.

Miller, M. A., & Rahe, R. H. (1997). Life changes scaling for the 1990s. *Journal of Psychosomatic Research, 43,* 279–292.

Scott-Marshall, H. (2011). The health consequences of precarious employment experiences. *Work, 38,* 369–382.

Taylor, S. E. (2011). Affiliation and stress. In S. Folkman (Ed.), *The Oxford handbook of stress, health, and coping* (pp. 86–100). Oxford, UK: Oxford University Press.

Westlund, S. (2015). 'Becoming human again': Exploring connections between nature and recovery from stress and post-traumatic distress. *Work, 50,* 161–174.

Suggested Readings

Ader, R. (Ed.). (2007). *Psychoneuroimmunology* (4th ed.). Boston: Elsevier Academic Press. A complete and thorough discussion of all aspects of psychoneuroimmunology.

Baum, A., et al. (2011). The molecular biology of stress. In R. J. Contrada & A. Baum (Eds.), *The handbook of stress science: Biology, psychology, and health* (pp. 87–99). New York: Springer. Describes changes in the basic biology of cells brought about by stress.

Contrada, R. J., & Baum, A. (2011). *The handbook of stress science: Biology, psychology, and health.* New York: Springer. Presents a detailed overview of key topics in stress, including how stress influences physical health, such as its effects on the nervous, endocrine, cardiovascular, and immune systems.

Davis, M. (2008). *The relaxation and stress reduction workbook.* Oakland, CA: New Harbinger. Offers many self-assessment tools and calming techniques to help overcome anxiety and promote physical and emotional well-being.

Folkman, S. (2011). *The Oxford handbook of stress, health, and coping.* Oxford, UK: Oxford University Press. Thorough and most up-to-date information that science has to offer on stress, health, and coping.

Goyal, M., et al. (2014, January). *Meditation programs for psychological stress and well-being.* Rockville, MD: Agency for Healthcare Research and Quality. Report No.: 13(14)-EHC116-EF. Retrieved from http://www.ncbi.nlm.nih.gov/books/NBK180102/

Kabat-Zinn, J. (1990). *Full catastrophe living: Using the wisdom of your body and mind to face stress, pain, and illness.* New York: Delta. In this venerable book, the founder of the Stress Reduction Clinic at the University of Massachusetts Medical Center presents a sound introduction for anyone who has considered meditating but was afraid it would be too difficult or would include religious practices they found foreign.

McEwan, B. S. (2013). The brain on stress: Toward an integrative approach to brain, body, and behavior. *Perspectives on Psychological Science, 8,* 673–675. A renowned stress scientist explains how stress experiences are embedded in the biology of the brain to determine whether events in the social and physical environments will lead to successful adaptation or impaired mental and physical health.

Seaward, B. L. (2013). *Managing stress.* Burlington, MA: Jones & Bartlett Learning. Provides a comprehensive approach to stress management, honoring the integration, balance, and harmony of mind, body, spirit, and emotions.

Segerstrom, S. (2012). *The Oxford handbook of psychoneuroimmunology.* Oxford, UK: Oxford University Press. Perspectives on the state-of-the-art applications of psychological theory to psychoneuroimmunology from experts in the field.

Sherin, J. E., & Nemeroff, C. B. (2011). Post-traumatic stress disorder: The neurobiological impact of psychological trauma. *Dialogues in Clinical Neuroscience, 13,* 263–278.

Recommended Websites

Anchoring

An online tutorial on how to quiet your mind, by Eric Golanty, PhD, coauthor of *Health and Wellness* and professor of health at Las Positas College.

College Student Stress

The University of Chicago's list of online resources.

Mind/Body Health Stress

Explains stress and offers methods for lessening it; from the American Psychological Association.

Stress Resources

U.S. National Library of Medicine.

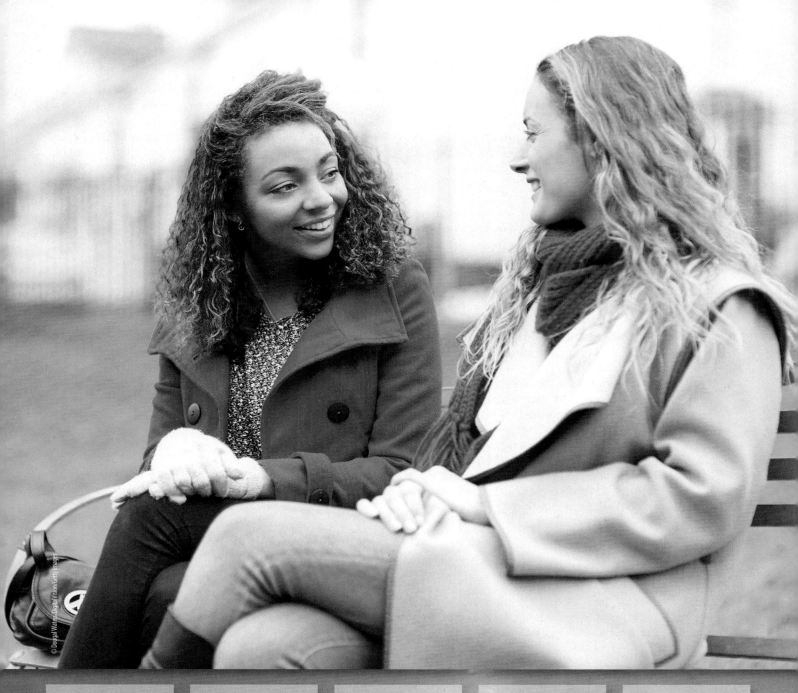

Health Tips

Tips for Meeting Basic Human Needs

Some Tips for Dealing with Anger and Conflict

Wiped Out?

Dollars & Health Sense

Drugs for Coping with Everyday Life

Global Wellness

Depression Is Worldwide

Managing Stress

Do it the "Write" Way

If a Friend Is Considering Suicide

Wellness Guide

Self-Compassion for Academic Success and Lifelong Well-Being

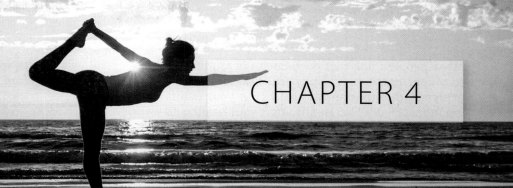

Mental Health

Learning Objectives

1. List the three components of mental health.

2. Define *mental illness*.

3. Describe the role of meeting basic human needs and mental health.

4. Describe the relationship among thoughts, emotions, and mental health.

5. List and describe strategies for coping with emotional distress.

6. Define defense mechanisms.

7. List and describe four common anxiety disorders.

8. List five signs of depression.

9. Discuss the importance of sleep for well-being.

10. List and describe seven facets of sleep hygiene.

Many people think that good health is primarily related to proper nutrition and physical fitness. Nutrition and exercise are important to health, but your mental and emotional health also greatly affect your health and well-being. When your thoughts, feelings, and behaviors are in harmony within yourself and you live harmoniously within your social and physical environments, you are more likely to feel good and be in good health than if you are chronically angry, frightened, tense, depressed, and at odds with your surroundings.

> Forgiveness benefits the forgiver much more than the forgiven.
>
> *Vusi Mahlassela, South African musician*

The term *mental* refers to the totality of brain functions that produce thoughts, feelings, and intentional behaviors. **Mental health** is "a state of well-being in which every individual realizes his or her own potential, can cope with the normal stresses of life, can work productively and fruitfully, and is able to make a contribution to her or his community" (World Health Organization, 2014). Just as with physical health, the World Health Organization considers mental health to reflect the totality of a person's life and not solely the absence of a specific mental illness.

Mental and emotional health and well-being has three components (Centers for Disease Control and Prevention, 2017):

1. *Psychological well-being*, including self-acceptance, openness to new experiences, optimism, hopefulness, purpose in life, spirituality, self-direction, positive relationships, and personal self-worth
2. *Emotional well-being*, including joy, happiness, cheerfulness, contentment, and satisfaction with one's life
3. *Social well-being*, including believing that people are basically good, feeling socially accepted, belonging and being involved in a community, and believing that society can get better for all

Mental illness refers to alterations in thinking, emotions, and/or intentional behaviors that produce psychological distress, medical illness, and/or impaired functioning. Mental illness can result from aberrant learning experiences; childhood abuse, abandonment, neglect, and rejection; or exposure to traumatic experiences, such as being harmed, threatened, or exposed to war or a natural disaster. Because mental functions are carried out by the brain, mental illness can be associated with disease (such as syphilis), infection, drug/toxin-induced alterations in brain biology, biological changes in the brain (such as Alzheimer's disease), and abnormal hereditary conditions.

According to the U.S. National Institute of Mental Health (2016), approximately 18% of American adults are diagnosed with a (non-drug-related) mental illness each year; the annual prevalence of mental illness among children aged 8 to 15 years is 13%. Mental illness affects approximately 500,000,000 adults worldwide (Whiteford, 2015).

Basic Needs and Mental Health

Much of a person's behavior is motivated by attempts to meet her or his basic human needs. When individuals succeed in meeting their basic needs, they experience pleasant emotions, such as joy, pleasure, satisfaction, and contentment. When they do not, however, they experience unpleasant emotions, such as frustration, anger, sadness, grief, and shame. The purpose of unpleasant emotions is to motivate behaviors that are expected to meet one or more basic needs. For example, anger motivates resisting a threat to oneself or someone or something one cares about; shame and guilt motivate atoning for a social misdeed.

Although basic needs are intrinsic to humans, the ways in which people satisfy them are not. Everyone may need to eat, but not everyone obtains food in the same way. Neither does everyone choose to eat the same kind of food. Similarly, people engage in a variety of activities, occupations, relationships, and recreational pursuits to meet their needs.

Infants have a limited need-fulfilling repertoire. A child can cry when hungry or distressed and can smile or coo to invite touch and play. Beginning in childhood, individuals learn to understand the nature of their needs and develop strategies for interacting with the environment to meet them.

Scientists postulate that there are three categories of basic human needs (Gilbert, 2015) (**Figure 4.1**):

1. Detecting threats to survival and generating strategies for defense and safety
2. Seeking and acquiring mental, emotional, and spiritual stimulation, self-esteem, and sexual and reproductive experiences
3. Seeking contentment, pleasant interpersonal bonding, kindness, safety, and soothing when upset

Mental and emotional health are functions of how successfully a person meets her or his basic needs and deals with circumstances in which these needs are not met. Thoughts, beliefs, and attitudes that help us appropriately interpret and respond to internal needs, as well as environmental challenges, are involved. Mental health is built on emotional experiences that accurately help us interpret the environment and our interactions with it. Mental health also requires a biologically healthy brain and nervous system, not one that is undernourished, diseased, or disequilibrated with drugs or alcohol.

A foundation of mental health is perceiving and interpreting the world realistically. The more your mental processes are in sync with the ways in which your social and physical environments work, the more

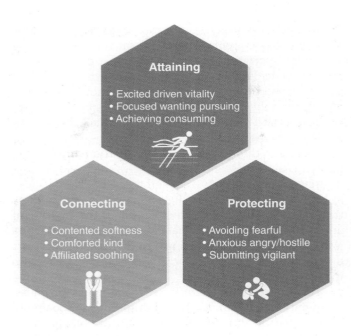

■ **Figure 4.1**

Categories of Basic Human Needs
Modified from: Gilbert, P. (2015). Affiliative and prosocial motives and emotions in mental health. Dialogues in *Clinical Neuroscience, 17,* 381–389.

likely you will devise strategies that can get your basic needs met.

To be mentally healthy, we do not have to be like everyone else. Being true to ourselves leads to greater satisfaction in life than social conformity does. Also, being mentally healthy does not mean that we never feel angry, anxious, lonely, depressed, confused, or overwhelmed. These are normal human emotions. Furthermore, being mentally healthy does not mean that we never need support, advice, or other kinds of help. In fact, inner strength is being able to recognize our limits and to seek and accept help so we can restore harmony when our mental and emotional resources are taxed.

Thoughts, Emotions, and Mental Health

How we see the world is determined by the mental process called **cognition** (from the Latin *cognito,* meaning "I know"). Cognition includes the following mental processes:

- *Perception:* interpreting data gathered by the senses (sight, smell, hearing, taste, touch, movement)
- *Learning:* integrating new perceptions with previous ones and storing them in memory as values, beliefs, attitudes, and action patterns
- *Reasoning:* does this make sense?
- *Problem solving:* formulating plans of action

Cognitions include beliefs, attitudes, and values. *Beliefs* are thoughts and ideas that are assumed to be true. Beliefs can be taken on faith or they can originate from having been tested against reality. Beliefs help us make sense of our experiences and guide behaviors that are intended to satisfy our wants and needs; avoid suffering, pain, and death; and produce harmonious interactions with the social and physical environments. In general, you have beliefs about (1) yourself as a unique physical and psychological entity, (2) how the social and physical/biological environments work, and (3) the consequences of particular *interactions* with the social and physical environments. *Attitudes* are beliefs that are associated with a positive or negative judgment or evaluation of an idea, person, object, or group. *Values* are a category of beliefs pertaining to concepts of right and wrong; good and bad; moral and immoral. Values represent what are considered to be basic, universal truths derived from "natural law," "the universe," or a deity. Furthermore, values are believed to endure over time and transcend specific situations and an individual's unique attitudes.

Beliefs are often associated with emotions (**Figure 4.2**). **Emotions** are patterns of brain activity that can arise spontaneously or in response to what you experience, have experienced, or believe you may experience. Emotions generate a sense of pleasantness or unpleasantness, which helps you evaluate as positive or negative an anticipated or actual experience and the outcome of a planned or an actual behavior. The subjective experiencing of an emotion is a *feeling.*

Besides providing an evaluation of an experience, emotions provide the energy or motivation for behavior. In general, pleasant emotions (e.g., joy, interest, contentment, and love) motivate the pursuit of novel, creative, enjoyable activities, whereas unpleasant emotions (e.g., anger, fear, anxiety, disgust, guilt) can help one evaluate the outcome of a behavior and/or motivate avoidance or aversion to perceived threats to one's sense of well-being, physical safety, or survival.

TERMS

cognition: the act or process of knowing

emotions: patterns of brain activity that can arise spontaneously or in response to what is experienced, has been experienced, or believed to be experienced.

mental health: a sense of optimism, vitality, and well-being, and intentional behaviors that lead to productive activities, fulfilling relationships with others, and the ability to adapt to change and to cope with adversity

mental illness: alterations in thinking, emotions, and/or intentional behaviors that produce psychological distress and/or impaired functioning

Tips for Meeting Basic Human Needs

Meeting life situations with equanimity and compassion

Being open to new ideas and experiences

Being grateful for the good things in your life

Setting attainable, realistic goals for yourself

Perseverance and patience

Not being incapacitated by survival emotions of anger, fear, disgust, shame, and guilt

Being kind to and tolerant of oneself in times of adversity, defeat, and failure

Getting satisfaction from simple, everyday pleasures

Giving love and accepting others the way they are

Engaging in satisfying personal relationships

Respecting and appreciating diversity of body, mind, and spirit among people

Not trying to control others' thoughts, emotions, and behaviors

Accepting your responsibilities and taking action when problems arise

In some scientific classifications, pleasant emotions are referred to as *positive* and unpleasant emotions as *negative*. It is important to recognize that these classifications refer to the feeling tone and not that the emotions themselves are good or bad. Even unpleasant emotions are beneficial when they signal that someone or something may be harmful and therefore avoided or subdued. In this way, unpleasant emotions are self-protective.

Consider this example of the relationship among thoughts, emotions, and behavior. Jill is supposed to meet Andrew so they can go to a concert together. Andrew looks at his watch and sees that Jill is 30 minutes late. Andrew thinks, "Jill's being rude," which produces the emotion of anger. Notice that Andrew has no idea why Jill is late; he is assuming that Jill is rejecting him. By the time Jill shows up 10 minutes later, Andrew is boiling mad and refuses to talk to her.

Had Andrew thought differently about Jill's tardiness, he might have felt and behaved differently. Choosing to see a situation from a different point of view is called **cognitive reframing**. For example, using cognitive reframing, Andrew could have realized that his reaction to his fantasy about Jill's motive comes from *his* mind and not necessarily the real world. Having realized this, he could

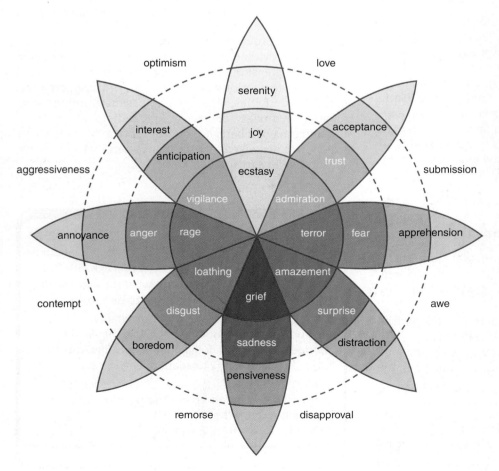

■ **Figure 4.2**

Basic Human Emotions

This image of the "emotion wheel" illustrates psychologist Robert Plutchik's (1991) classification of human emotions into eight basic types, or primary emotions: anger, fear, sadness, disgust, surprise, anticipation, trust, and joy. Each basic emotion is represented by an arm on the emotion wheel. The three parts of each arm represent a basic emotion's intensity, for example, joy intensifies to ecstasy. Plutchik proposed that the basic emotions are biologically based, having evolved to help human survival.

change his thought to something like, "I hope Jill isn't late because something bad happened to her," and his emotion upon seeing her might have been joy and relief that she was OK. He might even have hugged her.

Cognitive behavioral therapy (CBT) is a method for helping people in psychological distress by encouraging them to examine and change the thoughts that contribute to that distress. The method is based on the premise that erroneous beliefs about oneself and the world produce distressing emotions and maladaptive behaviors. Both the distressing emotions and maladaptive behaviors produce symptoms, which clinicians diagnose as mental illness. For example, someone with a healthy body weight may erroneously believe that he or she is grossly overweight. This thought might lead to the development of an unhealthy eating disorder.

Often maladaptive beliefs are "automatic"; that is, they arise in particular situations independent of reason or logic and occasionally they are unconscious. Therapeutic strategies involve the patient and therapist working together to identify and challenge the validity of maladaptive beliefs and to replace them with more realistic ones. This leads to relief of emotional distress and reduction in problematic behaviors that arise from it. CBT is efficacious in treating anxiety disorders, sleep problems, somatic symptom disorders, bulimia, anger control problems, general stress, and depression. It is not uncommon for mindfulness training or self-compassion training to be integrated with CBT to enhance therapeutic efficacy. Delivery of CBT over the Internet or via mobile device can be successful in certain situations (Sijbrandij, 2016; Vigerland, 2016).

Positive Thoughts and Emotions Contribute to Health

Much research shows that negative thoughts, stress, and unpleasant emotions, such as fear, anxiety, anger/hostility, and depression, can damage health. This occurs because those emotions are self-protective responses to perceived threats. Although intended for protection, if chronic and maladaptive they may instead increase the risk of illness by focusing attention on real (as in a war zone) or imagined (anticipating a pop quiz) threat. This can activate biological stress responses and immune inflammatory responses, which can damage internal organs.

On the other hand, it is also likely that positive thoughts and emotions, such as joy, interest, contentment, and love, can promote health (D'raven et al., 2014). For example, researchers analyzing early-in-life personal writings of 180 elderly American nuns found that those whose writings had the highest degree of positive emotional content lived the longest (**Figure 4.3**) (Danner, Snowdon, & Friesen, 2001). Several studies have shown that positive emotions such as optimism and contentment lessened

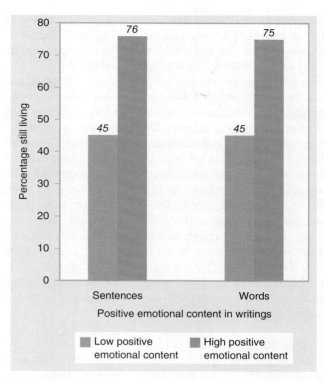

■ **Figure 4.3**

Percentage Surviving at Age 80 of Nuns with Low or High Degree of Emotional Content in Writings in Early Life
Adapted from Danner, D.D., Snowdon, D.A., & Friesen, W.V. (2001). Positive emotions in early life and longevity: Findings from the nun study. *Journal of Personality and Social Psychology, 80*, 804–813.

the risk of cardiovascular disease (Sin, 2016). Higher degrees of hope and curiosity have been found to be associated with a decreased likelihood of having or developing hypertension, diabetes, and respiratory tract infections (Tugade, 2011). Positive thoughts and emotions, such as gratitude, forgiveness, and compassion, can influence health and illness by fostering healthy behaviors and helping to avoid unhealthy ones.

Compassion

Undesired experiences that cause pain and suffering are a part of life. Among these are personal harm and injury, tragedy, trauma, loss, and betrayal. Compassion is

TERMS

cognitive behavioral therapy (CBT): treatment of psychological distress by examining and changing thoughts that underlie it

cognitive reframing: choosing to see a situation from a different point of view

a response to suffering in which one experiences empathy for another's or one's own suffering and commits to relieving that suffering. Other words for compassion are *caring* and *helpfulness.* The Latin root of the English word compassion is *compati,* meaning "to suffer with." Compassion increases positive feelings such as liking and contentment and decreases threat-activated emotions such as anger, fear, and disgust. Many studies have shown that both giving and receiving compassion is beneficial to health. This is because the positive emotions that result from compassion reduce inflammation and other physiological responses increase in response to stress and the perceived threat. Self-compassion is having a positive and caring attitude toward oneself, which can be strengthened through various practices (see the Wellness Guide "Self-Compassion for Academic Success and Lifelong Well-Being"). As a result of this caring attitude, self-compassion contributes to both mental and physical health by motivating self-care attitudes and behaviors (Dunne et al., 2016).

Gratitude

Gratitude is a feeling of thankfulness or appreciation associated with the realization that you've been helped, supported, or affirmed by something outside yourself. The first-century Roman philosopher Cicero referred to gratitude as the mother of all virtues, and the Roman philosopher Seneca believed gratitude to be a fundamental motivational drive, critical for building interpersonal relationships. Most people don't think about gratitude very much because the human brain is biologically constructed to be on the alert for danger, so we tend to focus on stress and life's difficulties. Gratitude is about feeling appreciative and even in awe at the good fortune we've experienced. Gratitude can enhance health and well-being by lessening

disease-related inflammation (Redwine et al., 2016), lowering blood pressure, and fostering self-care (e.g., exercising, good sleep habits). Gratitude is associated with vitality, joy, pleasure, optimism, and happiness, all psychological traits that reduce the biological stress response that includes tissue-damaging inflammation. Gratitude also fosters healthy social relationships by motivating generosity, compassion, and forgiveness. It also reduces social anxiety and loneliness (Caputo, 2015). One way to enhance the capacity for gratitude is to set aside a few minutes each day or a few days a week to list three things for which you are grateful or to write in a journal a few sentences about those things for which you are grateful. You can do the list or the writing as the last thing you do before going to bed. Doing it this way often gets you thinking in the morning about what you'll write about later that day.

Forgiveness

If you've been hurt or harmed by someone, it's natural to be bitter and perhaps hold a grudge. Bitterness and grudges are forms of anger intended to defend yourself from future hurt. Unfortunately, bitterness and grudges can be heavy psychological burdens capable of triggering biological stress reactions, which in the long run can be unhealthy. One antidote to carrying a grudge is forgiveness. This does not mean forgetting what happened and excusing inappropriate, hurtful behavior. Forgiveness is not about the other person; it's about you. The expressions "turn the other cheek" or "forgive your transgressors" mean letting go of the hurt and anger (as much as you are able to) so you do not hurt yourself with your own psychology. In other words, the reason to forgive is to give yourself peace of mind. Studies show that forgiveness can lead to healthier relationships; greater spiritual and psychological well-being; less anxiety, stress, and hostility;

Self-Compassion for Academic Success and Lifelong Well-Being

The college student experience can be one of the most rewarding in life, and also one of the most challenging. One way to assist in getting the most out of college and preparing oneself for the inevitable up and downs of life is the practice of self-compassion.

Self-compassion is a psychological term that refers to the process of liking and caring for oneself and offering support and kindness to oneself in times of failure, setback, and distress. Some people are self-compassion "naturals." They take care of themselves the way they would a loved family member or a close friend. They do their best to live healthfully and forgive themselves and others when goof-ups occur. Other people may be pretty good at being caring and supportive with others but with themselves they are less so, for example, not practicing healthy behaviors that they know are good for them or not following through on school assignments; when mistakes and

setbacks occur, they can be intolerantly self-critical ("activating the inner critic"). Studies show that self-compassion is related to a higher sense of well-being and less risk of being stymied by anxiety, depression, stress, and fear of failure (Gunnell et al., 2017). Self-compassion training has been successful at enhancing psychological resilience among students (Smeets et al., 2014) and collegiate athletes (Mosewich et al., 2013).

Psychologists have identified three components to self-compassion:

1. Self-kindness rather than harsh self-criticism.
2. Acceptance of the truth that all humans make mistakes; no one is perfect.
3. Being emotionally balanced by not misattributing setbacks to one's flaws.

You can determine your own level of self-compassion using Professor Kristin Neff's Self-Compassion Scale (self-compassion.org/test-how-self-compassionate-you-are). If you decide to improve your self-compassion skills, you can follow Professor Neff's online tutorials (self-compassion.org).

Do it the "Write" Way

When we're stressed and troubled, quite often we get so caught up in our emotions that we lose perspective on what's going on. We only know that we're distressed. This is where writing down thoughts and feelings can help.

Research has shown that writing about one's traumatic experiences can lessen stress, improve immune functioning, and foster health and well-being. Apparently, writing about psychologically painful experiences releases the stress and anxiety associated with trying to keep painful unpleasant feelings out of conscious awareness. Writing about trauma helps one sort, understand, and put the experience into the past.

You don't have to experience a trauma to benefit from writing out your thoughts and feelings. Doing so can help you clarify why you feel a certain way and how your thoughts, perceptions, and reactions to situations are affecting your life. Writing forces you to look at your life honestly. Also, writing lets you express yourself privately without concern about someone else's reaction.

"Write for health" by making regular entries in a journal, which is similar to a diary except you express thoughts and feelings instead of record daily events.
- Use a special notebook for your journal.
- Write in a quiet place.
- Keep your journal private so you can be honest with yourself.
- Write continuously. Don't worry about grammar or spelling.
- Be expressive. Don't worry about making sense.

lower blood pressure; fewer symptoms of depression; a stronger immune system; improved heart health; and higher self-esteem (Mayo Clinic, 2016). A study with college students showed that meditation practice can support forgiveness (Oman et al., 2008). A self-test for forgiveness is the Heartland Forgiveness Scale (www.heartlandforgiveness.com).

Developing Coping Strategies

Coping strategies are ways to deal with the emotional distress that comes from not having your needs met. In general, there are three coping strategies: You can alter (1) the interaction with the cause of the distress, (2) thoughts and beliefs regarding the significance of the need that is not being met, or (3) the distressing feeling, without changing the situation or how you think about it.

To reduce emotional distress by changing your interaction with the situation, you could do any of the following:
- Attack the situation head-on ("I'm nervous about meeting new people, but I'll go to the party anyway").
- Avoid the situation ("I'm nervous they won't like me. I'll go some other time").
- Adapt to the situation ("Even though I get nervous in social situations, that's OK. So what?").

To change your thoughts and beliefs about the significance of the unmet need, you could:
- Judge your situation to be less distressing than someone else's ("At least I'm meeting people. Poor John works so much he doesn't get to meet anyone").
- See your distress as necessary or temporary ("This is the way it is," or "Eventually I'll find somebody and I won't have to go through this anymore").
- Focus on positive aspects of a situation and minimize the negative ("If I go, I'll probably have a great time").
- Devalue the goal and believe you will do fine no matter the outcome ("If he says no, it won't be the end of the world").

Reducing emotional distress by changing or reducing the intensity of the feeling itself could involve releasing emotional energy through an alternative activity:
- Exercise helps with frustration and anger.
- Meditation helps with sadness and anger.
- Talking to a receptive and empathic person can help with grief, shame, and anxiety.

Changing feelings with alcohol or drugs usually makes things worse.

Defense Mechanisms

Defense mechanisms are mental processes people use to distort the perception and awareness of reality to avoid unpleasant thoughts, memories, emotions, and situations (Table 4.1). A common defense mechanism is denial, which is not believing a truth. An example of denial is a smoker not believing she is at risk for lung cancer even though she knows that smoking causes cancer. This person denies reality to prevent awareness of the truth, possibly to avoid the fear of death.

Defense mechanisms protect us from thoughts and beliefs that we find threatening; we distort reality to feel safe. Strategies for meeting needs that are based on a faulty foundation generally result in needs not being met. This may lead to disappointment, depression, self-blame, withdrawal or avoidance of involvement in similar situations, and substance abuse.

Distorting reality is not always bad. Sometimes it is necessary because of feeling overwhelmed, trauma, or abuse. In such instances, denial helps a person cope with

TERMS

coping strategies: ways people devise to prevent, avoid, or control the emotional distress of unfulfilled needs

defense mechanisms: mental strategies for avoiding unpleasant thoughts and emotions

Table 4.1

Common Defense Mechanisms

Defense	Description	Example
Denial	Absolute rejection of a truth or of objective reality	A college student who drinks a six-pack of beer a day but believes that he has no problem with alcohol
Repression	Keeping distressing thoughts and feelings unconscious	A rape victim who has no memory of the assault
Projection	Attributing one's own thoughts and feelings to someone else	A student dislikes her roommate but believes the roommate dislikes her
Displacement	Diverting an emotion from the original target or source to another	You are angry with your parents but yell at your best friends
Reaction formation	Believing and experiencing the opposite of how you truly feel	You are friendly with someone you dislike
Rationalization	Creating a plausible but false reason for your behavior	Believing that failing a course was due to the teacher's poor teaching and not your ineffective studying
Identification	Imagining that someone's or some group's attributes are your own	Feeling superior because one's favorite sports team is successful
Isolation and dissociation	Compartmentalizing thoughts and feelings in different parts of awareness	A successful professional negotiator frequently feuds with his neighbors

what would otherwise be a highly stressful psychological situation. Other times, denial can be a way to take a mental vacation. From the perspective of mental health, however, the key is knowing when you are "on a fantasy trip" and when you are not and not letting certain defensive ways of thought become habitual and block pursuit of a healthy and meaningful life. You can do this by learning to observe how your mind works. Such self-knowledge is a goal of meditation, yoga, modern psychotherapies, and other practices that help to focus on awareness and engage one's consciousness.

Facilitating Coping

Even when emotions make us aware that something in our lives is not going well, we do not always know what the problem is, what the best way to deal with it is, or how to overcome fear of change or longstanding inertia. People should not suffer in silence or believe themselves to be flawed or "crazy." Support and advice are available from trusted family members, friends, teachers, clergy, and mental health professionals, such as counselors, psychotherapists, and physicians. Reaching out to such people helps those in distress gain a new perspective on their problems and to see a workable solution.

Psychotherapists are professionals who have undergone considerable training to help people deal with their emotional distress. Whether a person has feelings of inferiority, is troubled by painful dependency in a love relationship, or is immobilized by fear, a psychotherapist can facilitate change that can make a person's life better. The change comes about not only by talking but also by helping the distressed person adopt new behaviors and attitudes. It is one thing to know intellectually the source of a personal problem and even what to do about it, but it may be quite another to face unpleasant emotions and adopt new behaviors ("the map is not the road").

The value of psychotherapy, regardless of the method, is that the distressed person has faith in the professional's ability to facilitate change. This faith produces a situation of trust that enables the distressed person to be honest about himself or herself and to disclose painful and unflattering thoughts, memories, and emotions that would not likely be shared with a friend or relative.

Anger

Anger occurs when we feel attacked, blamed, hurt, or have experienced a loss; when we *imagine* we've been attacked, blamed, hurt, or have experienced a loss; when we imagine we *may* be attacked, blamed, hurt, or experience a loss; or when the pursuit of an important goal is blocked (frustration). Sometimes we get angry because we perceive something as threatening that really isn't. In this case, we make ourselves angry by what we think.

Anger is an excitatory emotion, providing the motivational energy to protect ourselves or things we care about or to overcome obstacles to our goals. We use anger to stop physical or psychological abuse and to protect ourselves from the hurt of loss.

Whereas anger tends to be situational, **hostility** is a personal trait characterized by an ongoing mistrust of others, cynicism, a personal emotional style of anger mixed with disgust and contempt, and a tendency to act out those feelings with overt aggression, snide comments, or criticism. Studies show that hostility is related to an increased risk of heart disease (Suls, 2013).

One constructive way to work with anger is to examine and alter anger-generating thoughts. For example, to deal with frustration you can reassess the merits of the goal you cannot attain or reconsider the strategy you've employed for attaining it. It may feel right to blame someone else for your troubles, but a reevaluation of how you contribute to the situation may be more productive. It is far easier to change yourself than someone else.

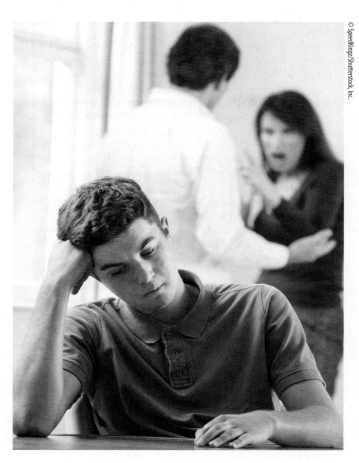

Family arguments disrupt the emotional well-being of parents and children.

Another strategy for dealing with anger is forgiveness. By forgiving, you are not saying that another's transgression is OK or even that you want to have a relationship with that person. When you forgive, you release yourself of the psychological weight and physiological tension of internalized anger. You open the pathway to attaining psychological closure on the incident and the peace of mind that can follow. Furthermore, you contribute to your own health and well-being (Webb, 2013).

The next time you feel angry, take a "time-out" for a few seconds, minutes, or days if necessary. Ask yourself what you've experienced that's led you to be angry. Are you really being harmed or threatened or are you making yourself angry because you've interpreted a situation as such? If you feel frustrated about not being able to accomplish a goal, is your goal realistically attainable? Have you expected too much of yourself? Have you expected too much of someone else? Is your strategy for attaining your goal workable? Is something else better? Did you communicate your goals, needs, plans, and desires to people whose help you wanted or expected?

Social Support Contributes to Health

Social support refers to the resources that one receives from others, particularly people in one's immediate social network with whom one has emotional bonds and/or social ties, such as family, friends, schoolmates, coworkers, fellow church members, and professional helpers within one's community. There are several kinds of social support, including:

- Emotional support, including reassurance, acceptance, love, trust, and intimacy. When you feel cared for, accepted, and understood, you feel less alone, your self-esteem is enhanced, and you feel more confident and optimistic about managing your life. When you offer emotional support, you feel trustworthy and derive the pleasure and satisfaction of helping another.
- Instrumental support, including tangible help and material and financial assistance. Sometimes you need someone to take you to the doctor, bring you a meal, or loan you some money.
- Informational support, including specific information and knowledge of resources in the environment. Lack of information can block decision making, leading to ruminating and worry about your situation instead of acting.
- Appraisal support, including help with decision making. Sometimes you aren't sure what course of action to take, so you ask knowledgeable and trusted others for their opinions and advice.
- Inclusional support, including encouraging feelings of belonging to the community or a group and access to social contacts and group activities. Belonging to groups alleviates loneliness and provides opportunities for fun, recreation, and the giving and receiving of help.

Numerous studies have shown that people with abundant social support live longer and more healthfully (Tay et al., 2013). Social support contributes to health in several ways. First, social support encourages people to live healthfully. When you decide to exercise regularly, eat less junk food, or stop smoking, the encouragement, advice, and support from family and friends can help you stay on track with your plans. Also, when you are stressed or sick, social support can help you take care of yourself, including obtaining help from health professionals and following medical instructions. Second, social support can make you feel good. When others care about you, you feel good about yourself, you are more optimistic about accomplishing your goals, and you are less lonely, anxious, and depressed. All of these factors contribute to

▌TERMS▐

hostility: a personal trait characterized by an ongoing mistrust of others, cynicism, a personal emotional style of anger mixed with disgust and contempt, and a tendency to act out those feelings with overt aggression, snide comments, or criticism

social support: resources that one receives from others, particularly people in one's immediate social network with whom one has emotional bonds and/or social ties

Some Tips for Dealing with Anger and Conflict

Here are some suggestions for dealing with anger constructively.

- *Acknowledge your anger.* Pay attention to anger in yourself when you become aware of it. Then take some time to determine which of your thoughts are causing it. Are you hurt, frustrated, frightened? What happened that made you angry?
- *Own your anger.* Try not to blame someone else for your angry feeling by means of thoughts or statements like "It's all your fault!" or "If it weren't for you," or "If only you'd have …" Don't put it onto someone else unless you're sure it belongs there.
- *Chill.* Even if you are very angry, try not to act immediately on those feelings. Instead, set aside a time to think about them and how best to express them.
- *Resolve the anger.* Try not to let anger build up over time. If you do, you may become resentful, which may cause you to distance yourself emotionally or physically or to displace the anger onto someone else, like a child or a coworker.
- *Don't ambush.* Attacking with anger when it's least expected is unfair and invites resentment or a counterattack, not reconciliation.
- *Be specific.* When you're talking about emotional conflicts, name exactly what's causing the anger and stick to that issue. Don't bring up past hurts. Don't discuss second and third topics until the first one is settled. If other issues arise, write them down so you can discuss them later. Make it a habit to keep pencil and paper handy when issues are discussed. Don't give in to the temptation to bring up secondary issues to retaliate for hurt feelings or as a way to avoid resolving the issue at hand.
- *Don't hit below the belt.* In an argument, don't attack the other person with a statement you know will hurt because you think you're losing the argument.
- *Attack the problem, not the other person.* Don't engage in character assassination with put-downs and accusations. Use "I" statements to communicate resentments. If someone attacks with a put-down, rather than retaliate, you can say, "Ouch, that hurt." This can be a cue to redress the attack and go on with the issue under discussion. If this doesn't happen, the discussion will probably be sidetracked from the main point to the put-down, and a fight about hurt feelings may ensue.
- *Be respectful and respectable.* When working to resolve an issue, try to maintain an attitude of respect. Try to understand the other's point of view. Ask the other person to respect you and your feelings, even though you disagree.
- *Take some time.* Sometimes you can sense that an anger-causing issue isn't getting resolved. It's all right to acknowledge that and to take a few hours or days to reconsider things, and then discuss the issue again. Sometimes emotions are too intense and it's not possible to think clearly. Sometimes you just need time to reflect and figure things out.
- *Physical affection is acceptable.* Sex or any other affectionate behavior before an issue is resolved is acceptable, as long as it's not taken as a sign that the issue is resolved. Affectionate behavior shows that arguing about something can be accommodated within a caring relationship.
- *Both sides win.* After an issue has been discussed and the partners seem agreed on the outcome, if one or both feels a grudge, then the argument has produced a winner and a loser, and the relationship has been harmed. Holding a grudge is a sign that the issue is not resolved. Try again.

better health. Third, social support diminishes the body's stress responses and strengthens the immune system, thus lessening your risk of illness.

In many ways, social support is reciprocal. People get as they give. Thus, you become a worthy recipient of social support when you are a willing giver of it. There are

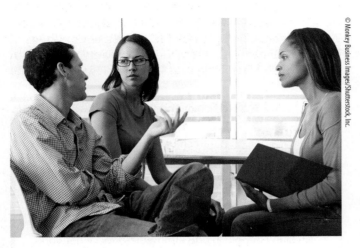

Talking with a counselor can help solve emotional problems.

times in life when you become removed from your established sources of social support, for example, when going away to college or relocating for a job. These are times for making an effort to reestablish a supportive network. One proven strategy for developing a supportive social network is to become involved in activities, groups, and organizations that interest you at campus or within the community. For example, join an exercise class or a hobby group; volunteer at a hospital, museum, church, or community center; or get involved in a cause that you believe in. Groups generally want new members, and you will be meeting and doing things with people with interests similar to yours. Some of the most rewarding activity is that which helps others.

People differ in their willingness to seek and accept social support. Some prefer to meet challenges on their own, seeking help only when absolutely necessary, whereas others are more inclined to offer and accept the support of others. In either case, believing that support is available if needed, called **perceived social support**, contributes to feeling valued and able to meet life's stresses without becoming overwhelmed, whether or not support actually exists.

Fears, Phobias, and Anxiety

Everybody experiences fear at some time or another. Fear is a powerful emotion that arises in situations that are interpreted as dangerous. The purpose of fear is to alert you to take protective action—usually to fight, flee, or seek assistance. For example, if you were hiking in the woods and encountered a snake, you would naturally interpret this situation as dangerous, which would produce the emotion of fear, which, in turn, would motivate some self-preserving behavior—probably an attempt to escape. If, however, you recognize that the snake is harmless, interpreting the situation as dangerous and thus triggering the emotion of fear would be erroneous. Notice how important the cognitive act of interpretation is in experiencing fear.

A *phobia* involves an intense, irrational fear. The word *phobia* comes from the Greek *phobos*, meaning "to take flight." Thus, a phobia causes us to avoid the object or situation that we fear—to flee from it both metaphorically and actually. The phobia can be a fear of anything: spiders, worms, snakes, bees, roses, a color, flying, boats, darkness—the list of phobias is very long. Some common phobias are *acrophobia* (fear of heights), *mysophobia* (fear of dirt and germs), *ophediophobia* (fear of snakes), and *zoophobia* (fear of animals). A particularly disabling phobia is *agoraphobia,* which is a fear of open spaces. People with agoraphobia are often so fear-stricken that they are unable to leave their homes to even run an errand or go shopping.

A person with a phobia almost always knows that the fear is irrational and illogical, yet is unable to control the feelings of anxiety even when thinking about the feared object or situation. Phobias often are triggered in childhood by a frightening event that may or may not be consciously remembered. For example, being stung by a bee while sniffing a rose in the garden at age 4 may result years later in fear produced by the smell of roses or an exaggerrated fear of bees.

Specific phobias, including agoraphobia, can be treated by a variety of image visualization techniques, with hypnotherapy to uncover the unconscious sensitizing event or events, and by systematic desensitization therapy. Because a phobia exists only in the mind, the mind is where the healing must take place. Imagination is a powerful tool. By imagining the thing that is feared while safe and relaxed at home or in the therapist's office, the mind gradually learns to be comfortable with the object or situation that evokes fear. For example, a person with agoraphobia might begin at home by lying down and visualizing opening the door and looking out. After several days of open-door visualization, he or she might further imagine walking down the stairs, and so on, until he or she can visualize going to the corner while feeling safe and comfortable. After imagining the trip outside, the next step is to actually open the door and step outside. The key to systematic desensitization is to monitor the anxiety and only take the step that feels safe. A trusted counselor or friend is essential in this process.

If fear is the response to a situation interpreted as threatening, **anxiety** is the response to an *imaginary situation*—usually something in the future that has not yet happened—that is interpreted as threatening. The purpose of anxiety is to warn you of *potentially* threatening situations, and it can take many forms. For example, anxiety about encountering a snake while on a hike, while heightening your awareness of this potential danger, could make the hike very unpleasant or prevent the hike from taking place at all, even if there were no snakes to encounter.

Anxiety is a normal part of life. It helps us anticipate and prepare for life's challenges. Some degree of anxiety can increase performance on a task, because it can help focus attention and motivate preparation. However, some people experience anxiety to a degree that impairs normal, daily functioning and health. This kind of anxiety tends to be more physiologically and psychologically intense than common anxiety is, and it can seem out of proportion, or even unrelated, to a specific situation. More than 19 million adult Americans experience one or another of the major types of anxiety disorders (Table 4.2). Each year, about 20% of North American college students are diagnosed or treated by a professional for anxiety (American College Health Association, 2017).

Social anxiety disorder is characterized by an ongoing, pervasive fear of being observed and evaluated by others in almost all social situations most of the time. Individuals diagnosed with social phobia are constantly apprehensive that they will do or say something to embarrass or humiliate themselves. They compensate for these feelings by avoiding most social situations or interactions with others or, if unavoidable, enduring them with great anxiety and stress. Affected persons typically have few friends, drop out of school, have difficulty in work environments or in holding jobs, drink alcohol or use drugs to dull the anxiety, and often develop other psychological problems.

Social anxiety disorder affects about 6% of Americans. It should be emphasized that a diagnosis of social anxiety disorder entails more than just being shy or nervous in personal interactions at work or in social settings. It usually involves isolating oneself from even simple kinds of interactions: being unable to talk to authority figures such as a teacher or boss, avoiding informal interactions with

> **TERMS**
>
> anxiety: the fear of an imaginary threat
> perceived social support: believing that support from one's social network is available if needed
> phobia: a powerful and irrational fear of something
> social anxiety disorder: fear of being observed and evaluated by others in social situations

Table 4.2

Kinds of Anxiety Disorders

Condition	Description
Social anxiety disorder (social phobia)	Persistent, intense, and chronic fear of being watched and judged by others and being embarrassed or humiliated by one's own actions, an overwhelming and excessive self-consciousness in everyday social situations such as speaking in formal or informal situations, eating or drinking in front of others, or, in its most severe form, being around other people for any reason. Fear may be so severe that it interferes with work, school, and other ordinary activities. Accompanying physical symptoms include blushing, profuse sweating, trembling, nausea, and difficulty talking.
Panic disorder	Unexpected and repeated episodes of intense fear accompanied by physical symptoms that may include chest pain, nausea, heart palpitations or pounding, shortness of breath, abdominal distress, and feeling sweaty, weak, faint, dizzy, flushed, or chilled. Feelings of terror may strike suddenly and repeatedly with no warning. The hands may tingle or feel numb. There may be smothering sensations, a sense of unreality, or fear of impending doom or loss of control.
Generalized anxiety disorder	Chronic anxiety and exaggerated worry and tension, even when there is little or nothing to provoke it. Anxiety is often accompanied by fatigue, headaches, muscle tension, muscle aches, difficulty swallowing, trembling, twitching, irritability, sweating, and hot flashes.
Obsessive-compulsive disorder (OCD)	Recurrent, unwanted thoughts (obsessions) and/or repetitive behaviors (compulsions) such as handwashing, counting, checking, or cleaning, often performed with the hope of preventing obsessive thoughts or making them go away. Performing these rituals provides only temporary relief, and not performing them markedly increases anxiety.
Posttraumatic stress disorder (PTSD)	Persistent, frightening thoughts and memories of a prior traumatic experience in which grave physical harm occurred or was threatened and feeling emotionally numb, especially with people to whom one was once close. People with PTSD may experience sleep problems, feel detached or numb, or be easily startled.

coworkers, not accepting social invitations, and being unable to talk even in small groups. However, drug company advertisements would have you believe that almost any form of shyness means you suffer from social anxiety disorder and need to take their drug. It might be wise to ignore such advertisements.

Panic disorder is a condition that involves sudden, terrifying *panic attacks* that generally occur without warning. Panic attacks tend to affect otherwise healthy young adults; they are characterized by the sudden appearance of intense fear, pounding heart, shortness of breath, paralyzing terror, sweating, and fear of dying or losing control. Because of these symptoms, panic disorder was formerly known as irritable heart or hyperventilation syndrome. Because the antecedents of a panic attack are often not identifiable, it is very unlike a phobia (fear of specific things such as snakes or air travel) or other kinds of anxiety disorders.

Panic disorder affects about 7% of healthy adult Americans and seriously disrupts their quality of life. Persons with panic disorder often wind up in hospital emergency rooms suffering from dizziness, bowel distress, and symptoms of a heart attack. In the case of a panic disorder, all medical diagnostic tests are negative for disease, but the symptoms reoccur. Although the cause of panic disorder is still unknown, research suggests that a disturbance of neurotransmitters in the brain is responsible, which may be the reason that some people with panic disorder are helped by medications.

Because of the unexpected suddenness and intensity of panic attacks, people with panic disorder often are helped simply by learning that they have an illness and are not crazy. This knowledge opens the way to adopting other helpful measures, including identifying thoughts and situations that might trigger a panic attack (e.g., an upcoming exam, family problems, or noticing a strong heartbeat or shallow breathing, which could suggest the onset of a panic attack).

Generalized anxiety disorder is characterized by persistent and excessive worry and feelings of anxiety. The condition is distinct from phobia, panic disorder, or social anxiety disorder (see Table 4.2), with its own set of diagnostic criteria:

- Excessive worry and anxiety over work or school performance that has continued for at least 6 months.
- Unable to control or cope with the anxiety and feels that it interferes with performance at work or other aspects of daily life.
- The anxiety must be accompanied by at least three of the following: restlessness or being on edge, fatigue, difficulty concentrating, irritability, muscle tension, and problems sleeping.
- The anxiety is not caused by the effects of any drug (legal or illegal) and is not caused by a physiological condition (e.g., hyperthyroidism).

Where does normal worry end and excessive anxiety begin? There does not seem to be any clear or easy answer to this question. For example, many people have ongoing worries (generalized anxiety) about being able to pay their bills, keep their jobs, or get good grades in school. Anxious people may have trouble sleeping or be on edge most of the time. Is one person mentally ill and another mentally well depending on how anxious they are about their money, job, or school problems? This is the dilemma for psychotherapists who treat people with ongoing worries.

Drugs for Coping with Everyday Life

A TV advertisement for a prescription drug shows a woman in her kitchen with dirty dishes in the sink, toys on the floor, and food on the counters waiting to be prepared. Viewers hear the woman's inner voice anxiously complaining about all the things she has to do and how hard it is to cope. No doubt about it, she's stressed. The ad tells viewers that overreactions to life's challenges could be a sign of an anxiety disorder and to see a doctor about getting medication. The ad closes with a shot of the same woman in the same kitchen, now clean and neat. Instead of complaining, her inner voice is singing. All thanks to the drug being advertised.

The makers of this ad are using the strategy of defining normal aspects of living as illnesses to increase sales of a prescription medication. This strategy has also been applied to shyness and sleeplessness (Moloney et al., 2011). In each case, the drugs being advertised were initially approved for treatment of a recognized illness. However, the marketing of the drug focuses on symptoms that are part and parcel of everyday life and for which drugs are inappropriate because they do not resolve the issues causing the problem, and their side effects, and in some cases addiction potential, pose health risks.

Here is another example of "medicalizing" a common experience to sell a drug intended for something else. The prescription drug modafinil (Provigil) was approved by the FDA for treatment of narcolepsy, a serious medical condition characterized by sudden and unintentional falling asleep during wakeful activity, and to ameliorate a specific kind of sleep disturbance in some shift workers. However, until the FDA told its manufacturer to stop, advertising for modafinil claimed that the drug was suitable for fatigue, tiredness, sleepiness, decreased activity, or lack of energy—symptoms characteristic of a large percentage of American college students and many people with legitimate psychological disorders such as depression. People who are drowsy while awake because they cheat on sleep do not have a disease; they are experiencing the predictable consequences of a choice. Rather than taking a drug and risking side effects and possible permanent alterations in brain biology, drowsy people would feel better if they turned off their TVs and computers and got more sleep.

Always remember: Pharmaceutical companies are massive corporations with the goal of making money. Your health is their concern only insofar as it enhances profits. You are the one responsible for your health. Until manipulation is no longer a part of drug company advertising, you are better off ignoring it.

Obsessive-Compulsive Disorder

Obsessive-compulsive disorder (OCD) is characterized by persistent, unwelcome thoughts or images *(obsessions)* that often are accompanied by an uncontrollable, urgent need to engage in certain behaviors *(compulsions)*. Rituals such as handwashing, counting, checking, or cleaning are often performed in hope of preventing obsessive thoughts or making them go away. Performing these rituals, however, provides only temporary relief, and not performing them markedly increases anxiety. OCD affects about 2% of the U.S. population. The condition typically begins during adolescence or late childhood. It is sometimes accompanied by depression, eating disorders, substance abuse, attention deficit hyperactivity disorder, or other anxiety disorders. Symptoms of OCD can also coexist and may even be part of a spectrum of neurological disorders, such as Tourette's syndrome. OCD likely has a neurobiological basis and is not caused by family problems or by attitudes learned in childhood, such as an inordinate emphasis on cleanliness or a belief that certain thoughts are dangerous or unacceptable. Treatments for OCD involve medications and cognitive behavioral therapy (CBT).

Depression

In the course of their lifetime, about 17% of Americans experience an episode of **major depression**, characterized by feelings of helplessness, hopelessness, reduced interest in previously enjoyable activities, and a variety of other symptoms (**Table 4.3**). If asked how they feel, depressed people usually say something like, "Life's a drag" or "What's the use of doing anything?" One hallmark of depression is a helpless/hopeless attitude.

The American College Health Association (2017) reports that nearly half of college students feel sufficiently depressed at some point during the school year that they have trouble functioning; about 17% are depressed enough to require treatment. College students with depression experience most of the same symptoms other American adults do, including some specific to students:

- Withdrawal from formerly pleasurable social activities
- A drop in grades
- Inability to concentrate on schoolwork; reading material becomes overwhelming

TERMS

generalized anxiety disorder: persistent and often nonspecific worry and anxiety

major depression: a mental state characterized by feelings of helplessness, hopelessness, and self-recrimination

obsessive-compulsive disorder (OCD): persistent, unwelcome thoughts or images and the urgent, uncontrollable need to engage in certain rituals

panic disorder: severe anxiety accompanied by physical symptoms

Table 4.3

Common Symptoms of Depression

Psychological symptoms	Behavioral symptoms	Physical symptoms
Depressed mood	Crying spells	Fatigue
Irritability	Interpersonal confrontation	Reduced or too much sleep
Anxiety/nervousness	Anger attacks/outbursts	Decreased or increased appetite
Reduced concentration	Avoidance of anxiety-provoking situations	Weight loss/gain
Lack of interest/motivation	Social withdrawal	Aches and pains
Inability to enjoy things	Workaholism	Muscle tension
Reduced interest in sex	Tobacco/alcohol/drug use or abuse	Heart palpitations
Hypersensitivity to criticism/rejection	Self-sacrifice/victimization	Burning or tingling sensations
Indecisiveness	Suicide attempts/gestures	
Pessimism/hopelessness		
Feelings of helplessness		
Preoccupation with oneself		
Thoughts of death or suicide		

- Sleep disturbances (sleeping much more or less soundly than usual) not related to studying or cramming for tests
- Consuming more alcohol than usual

Often, a depressed student does not recognize that something is amiss. Instead, a parent, friend, roommate, or residence hall advisor may notice depressive symptoms and encourage the student to seek help.

Depression can occur as a normal response to the loss of something that a person values or is attached to, such as a loved one, a job, good health, or self-esteem (e.g., when a person does not succeed at a task she or he deems important). When individuals experience a loss, it is normal to feel sad and depressed and to grieve the loss. Sadness and grief are the human spirit's way to heal the hurt of loss and open the way for new attachments. When normal depression is associated with a loss, the depressed individual may be simultaneously aware that the experience is transitory and, along with grief, feel that

there is hope for the future. This kind of depression tends to lift after the grieving ends.

In contrast to the normal depression that may accompany loss, some people experience a long-lasting depressive state or periodic episodes of deep depression that are not self-limiting and may hinder and even jeopardize a person's life. These depressions may be a response to stress, severe psychological trauma, injury, disease, biological malfunctions of some part of the brain, or a combination of factors. In some persons, major episodes of depression are accompanied by periods of excited euphoria (*mania*), resulting in a condition referred to as **bipolar disorder**.

Some individuals are susceptible to depression during the winter months because a lack of sunlight disturbs the production of neurotransmitters in the brain that affect mood. This **seasonal affective disorder (SAD)** is sometimes remedied by increased exposure to stronger-than-normal indoor lighting that mimics sunlight or relocation to southern latitudes where there is more wintertime light.

Depression can also accompany the experience of being very sick or injured. In such cases, depression results from a combination of factors, such as grieving the loss of health; coping with the stress of being sick; lack of exercise and normal routine; disruption of regular social activities; or alterations in physiology that may change brain chemistry. Medications may also make one susceptible to depression. Some people experience a mild form of depression called **dysthymia**. Like major depression, dysthymia is associated with disturbances in sleep, appetite, and the ability to concentrate.

One of the characteristics of severe depression is a considerable degree of negative thinking, characterized by severe self-criticism; negative views about the self, the world, and the future; and a variety of logic errors

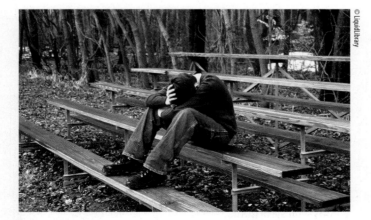

© Liquidlibrary

Many things may make us feel depressed temporarily.

Depression Is Worldwide

> Missing my dear mother, as a son,
> my liver and intestines are painfully broken!
> Crying for my old mother, as a son,
> my tears pour into my chest!
> Thinking about my old mother, as a son,
> to swallow food and tea is difficult!
> Searching for my old mother, as a son,
> I cannot sleep day and night!
>
> Si-Lang, *Searching for Mother*
> Tenth-Century Beijing Opera

Melancholy and depression know no geographic boundaries, as this thousand-year-old Chinese aria describing the physical aspects of depression shows. Depression has been documented in virtually all cultures, although its prevalence varies. Depression in Asia, for example, is less prevalent than in North America and Europe (**Table 4.4**). Rates of depression in the United States even vary by cultural group: The lifetime prevalence of depression among people of African and Hispanic ancestry is about 12%; among people of European ancestry, it's 17%.

Besides prevalence rates, depression manifests differently among cultures. Several Native American cultures tend to experience depression as social loneliness. A typical Caucasian North American or European is likely to experience depression in terms of psychological symptoms, such as melancholy, moodiness, and lack of interest in pleasure. However, in Asian cultures, depression tends to be experienced as physical complaints (as in the Chinese aria above), such as fatigue, loss of appetite, and sleep problems.

Help-seeking behavior for depression also varies among cultures. Latin American men and mainland Chinese tend not to seek help for depression, fearing that doing so will stigmatize them as weak. In Japan and Hong Kong, where depression tends to be experienced as a physical ailment, people tend to consult with a doctor for relief of physical symptoms. Latin American women and European Americans are more likely to consult mental health practitioners.

Table 4.4

Prevalence of Depression in Selected Countries of the World

Region	Burden of depressive illness
Eastern Europe	1,350
North Africa–Middle East	1,300
Latin America–Tropical	1,200
Western Europe	1,100
North America—High Income	1,000
Latin America–Southern	1,000
Asia–East	900
Central Europe	900
Australia	750
East Asia	770
Sub-Saharan Africa–West	700
Asia Pacific—High Income	600

Note: Burden of depressive illness is the number of affected individuals multiplied by the severity of illness.

Data from Ferrari, A. J. et al. (Nov 5, 2013). Burden of depressive disorders by country, sex, age, and year: Findings from the Global Burden of Disease Study 2010. *PlosMedicine* (http://www.plosmedicine.org/article /info%3Adoi %2F10.1371%2Fjournal.pmed.1001547)

---

in assessing the self and the world. Some of these logic errors include the following:

- *All-or-none thinking:* seeing things as polar extremes (e.g., all good and all bad)
- *Overgeneralizing:* interpreting one setback as evidence that *every* similar situation will *forever* turn out badly
- *Negative filtering:* focusing only on the negative while filtering out the positive
- *Disqualifying the positive:* transforming positive occurrences into negative experiences

Becoming aware of negative thoughts (often called *negative self-talk*) opens the way to adopting positive self-images and more realistic appraisals of the world. These, in turn, help to lessen the depressive state. Cognitive behavioral therapy is a very successful method for helping depressed people change their negative thought patterns.

Another characteristic of depression is that it can intensify itself, thus creating a depressive cycle. The depressed person's negative thoughts, social withdrawal, and loss of interest in pleasurable experiences serve to reinforce feelings of worthlessness, helplessness, gloom, and doom. Recovery from depression requires both interrupting the depressive cycle and correcting the life situation that brought on the depression. Recreational activity can divert attention from negative thinking and weaken the depression cycle.

One way to deal with depression is to get life moving again. This is accomplished by establishing and achieving simple, attainable goals that can be done in a brief period of time. The goals should involve movement that

TERMS

bipolar disorder: episodes of depression followed by episodes of mania

dysthymia: a long-lasting, mild form of depression

seasonal affective disorder (SAD): depressive symptoms that appear in autumn or winter and remit spontaneously in spring

If a Friend Is Considering Suicide

Occasionally a person expresses thoughts of suicide to a friend or relative. This can be extremely distressing to the listener, who may react with disbelief, panic, or avoidance. In attempting to deal with his or her own uncomfortable feelings, a listener might say things like, "Cheer up, you've got a lot to live for," or "You're better off than I am," or "You can't be serious!" These and similar statements have the effect of denying the distressed person's feelings. Psychologists recommend instead that listeners speak directly to suicidal thoughts ("Tell me more about why you want to kill yourself"), offer the distressed person nonjudgmental empathy and concern, and firmly but patiently direct the distressed person to professional help immediately.

Often suicidal individuals offer excuses for not seeing a professional and may even try to blackmail a friend into silence with threats ("I'll kill myself if you tell anyone"). The friend must hold firm and, if necessary, make an appointment with a counselor or psychiatrist at the student health center or hospital emergency room and deliver the distressed person there, or telephone a suicide prevention hotline.

restores fundamental breathing and other mind–body rhythms, which may alter the chemistry of the brain to facilitate pleasant (instead of unpleasant) moods. Many a depressed person has found relief in taking up a regular exercise program.

Also, depressed individuals should interact with people who offer support. Remaining in seclusion only reinforces feelings of loss and worthlessness. A depressed person should not engage in long conversations with friends and family about how lousy life is.

Several types of medication are available to treat depression (Gartlehner et al., 2016). The most widely prescribed medications are *selective serotonin reuptake inhibitors* (SSRIs). Other medications include tricyclic antidepressants and monoamine oxidase inhibitors. In many cases, successful treatment of mild depression with SSRIs is likely due to a placebo effect rather than a pharmacological effect of the drug (Fournier et al., 2010). One possible reason for this is that a major characteristic of depression is a helpless/hopeless attitude, which can be altered to a more positive, optimistic outlook with the expectation of relief offered by medication. Because all drugs have side effects, and SSRIs in particular have been linked to an increased risk of suicide, particularly among young people, the risk of harm when taking these drugs must always be considered. In moderate to severe depression, SSRIs seem to be more helpful than placebo. That many medications for mild depression are no more effective than placebo shows that recovery from mild depression is more psychological than biological; belief that relief is at hand is a powerful healer of depression.

Because depression involves inactivity, withdrawal, hopelessness, and self-defeating thoughts and behaviors, it is often difficult for individuals to activate themselves on a program of self-healing. At such times, the encouragement of a caring friend or family member and the guidance of a therapist, counselor, or other helper can be invaluable. Others can help a depressed person confront the causes of the depression and become aware of and try to minimize negative self-talk—negative views about the self, the world, and the future; self-critical inner dialogue; and logic errors in the assessment of self and events.

Suicide

One of the most worrisome aspects of depression is the risk of suicide. Besides depression, the risk of suicide is associated with panic disorder, social phobia, PTSD, bipolar disorder, and adult attention deficit hyperactivity disorder. In the United States, suicide ranks among the 10 most frequent causes of death, accounting for approximately 42,000 deaths per year. The number of reported suicides is thought to represent only 10% to 20% of suicide attempts. Among the 10 leading causes of death, the mortality rates of all but suicide have decreased in the past 20 years. People over age 50 make up the largest age group of suicides. Among young people (15 to 24 years old), suicide ranks third behind accidents and homicide as a cause of death.

Suicide is the second leading cause of death among college students, although the suicide rate among college students is about half that of their non-college-age peers (7.5 per 100,000 vs. 15 per 100,000). About 11% of college students admit to having seriously thought about or attempted suicide within the prior 12 months (American College Health Association, 2017). Very often, attempts occur on the same day or shortly after an acute life crisis. To help avert student suicides, many colleges have developed and are making students aware of helping services. Two risk factors for suicide to which college students are particularly susceptible are social isolation and feeling ineffective. Until they can build an on-campus supportive social network, students away from home may feel lonely, insecure, and unworthy of others' attention, all of which can lead to feeling depressed. Furthermore, without a social network, they may be less able to find support when they are anxious and depressed. Feeling ineffective at school because of grade competition and a constant sense of not being able to keep up with coursework can result in feeling helpless, guilty, and ashamed.

Suicide is not a disease, nor is it a disorder that can be inherited. Suicides are not caused by the weather or a full moon. Generally, people consider suicide because they feel overwhelmed and painfully distressed by life, helpless to improve matters, and hopeless that life can improve. Sometimes people attempt suicide not because they really want to die but because they want to express anger at others or signal others for help. In such instances, suicide attempts are characterized by limited self-destructive acts, such as taking less than a lethal dose of sleeping pills or arranging that the attempt be discovered in time for the person to be saved.

At the time a person contemplates suicide, life seems absolutely hopeless. But few life problems are beyond solution. Life crises improve and distressing emotions pass. Time does heal many hurts. And the experience gained by working through a distressing time of life can bring confidence, insight, and understanding. Acquiring experience and understanding, a person is better able to cope with life's problems and is better able to help others deal with their challenges.

If you're thinking about suicide, are worried about a friend or loved one, or would like emotional support, the National Suicide Prevention Lifeline (1-800-273-8255; https://suicidepreventionlifeline.org) is a national network of local crisis centers that provide free and confidential emotional support to people in suicidal crisis or emotional distress 24 hours a day, 7 days a week. The Lifeline is free, confidential, and available in Spanish and for the hearing impaired.

Adult Attention Deficit Hyperactivity Disorder (ADHD)

Adult attention deficit hyperactivity disorder (ADHD) is characterized by difficulty focusing on activities, organizing and finishing tasks, managing one's time, following instructions and/or being overly restless, "on the go," and perceived as not thinking before acting or speaking. About 4% of adults are believed to have ADHD. Nearly 9% of American college students have ADHD (American College Health Association, 2017). Untreated ADHD in adults is associated with impaired physical and mental health, lower socioeconomic status, lower rates of professional employment, more frequent job changes, more work difficulties, and more spousal separations and divorce. Also, adults with ADHD have more automobile collisions, speeding violations, and driver's license suspensions. Moreover, adults with ADHD are likely to be distressed by the persistent discomfort of their symptoms and the personal and social problems that arise from them.

In many adults, ADHD persists from childhood, when they experienced difficulties in educational performance, discipline problems, and being labeled as intentional underachievers and lacking in intelligence. This blaming and lack of understanding and empathy often damaged self-esteem, creating another problem that contributed to difficulties in performance in adulthood.

ADHD is not intentional but most likely a consequence of biological conditions in the brain. Compared with other adults, those with ADHD show differences in brain dopamine and noradrenaline neurotransmitter

---

Table 4.5

Success Strategies for Students with ADHD

Keep a day-planner and a to-do list

Use a backpack as an organizer. Put pens and pencils in outside pockets, notebook in another pocket, and homework in another. Keep books inside.

Keep an assignment notebook. Daily, list all assignments, quizzes, and exams, and check them off when completed.

Create a two-pocket homework folder. Label one pocket "Work to Be Done" and put all assignment sheets therein. Label the other pocket "Work Completed" and put all finished assignments therein. Check the folder every day.

Help yourself pay attention in class. Sit close to the instructor to lessen distractions. Use a voice recorder for lectures and studying.

Let others help you. If friends and instructors know about your ADHD, they are more likely to help you stay organized and on top of your tasks.

---

systems and anatomical/functional differences in the frontal regions of the brain, which are responsible for attention and working memory (Rubia et al., 2014).

College students with undiagnosed ADHD generally struggle to complete school assignments, manage their time, get good grades, and even complete their degrees. With medications, coaching, counseling, and living healthfully, however, students with ADHD can learn to stay organized and manage the tasks of college (Table 4.5). Some adults with ADHD find ways to direct their bountiful energy, curiosity, and desire for novelty to achieve success in careers as physicians, journalists, attorneys, salespeople, and in the arts.

Autism Spectrum Disorders

Autism spectrum disorders (ASD), also called *pervasive developmental disorders*, are a group of conditions characterized by varying degrees of impairment in communication skills and social interactions and restricted, repetitive, and stereotyped patterns of behavior. People with an ASD can seem to be absorbed in themselves and separate from interaction with others. The word *autism* is derived from the Greek *autos*, meaning "self," and *ismos*, meaning "state of being."

TERMS

adult attention deficit hyperactivity disorder (ADHD): difficulty focusing on activities, organizing and finishing tasks, managing one's time, following instructions and/or being overly restless, "on the go," and perceived as not thinking before acting or speaking

austism spectrum disorders (ASD): a group of conditions characterized by degrees of impairment in interpersonal interaction

Approximately 1 in 75 children throughout the world is diagnosed with an ASD—a prevalence exceeding that of diabetes, spina bifida, or Down syndrome. In most cases, problems in communication and social skills become noticeable early on as the child lags behind age peers. Parents may report normal development that suddenly changes as the child starts to reject people, act strangely, and lose previously acquired language and social skills.

There is no single best treatment for all children with an ASD. Parents and health practitioners must approach helping affected children with an openness to experimenting with a variety of treatment options. Perhaps most successful so far are programs that involve well-planned, structured teaching of specific skills, although success is variable. Common treatment modalities include the following:

- Behavior and communication approaches, which encourage positive behaviors and discourage negative behaviors in order to improve a variety of skills. The child's progress is tracked and measured.
- Dietary approaches, which include removing certain types of foods from a child's diet and using vitamin or mineral supplements.
- Medication, which includes drugs to manage high energy levels, inability to focus, depression, or seizures, and tendencies for severe tantrums, aggression, and self-injury.
- Complementary and alternative medicine, which includes special diets, chelation (a treatment to remove heavy metals like lead from the body), biologicals (e.g., secretin), or body-based systems (like deep pressure massage).

The nonspecific approach to treating ASD reflects both the wide variety of manifestations of the condition and a likely multiplicity of causes. For most of the twentieth century, the cause of autism was thought to be improper parenting leading to impaired social development. Research eventually disproved that hypothesis, opening the way to consideration of biological factors. For example, a popular hypothesis—not supported by research—is that mercury used as a preservative in vaccines impairs brain development in some susceptible children. And although ASD is not related to the inheritance of a single gene, the condition is associated with a variety of genetic abnormalities that seem to occur after conception, perhaps due to the toxic effects of environmental pollutants on the developing brain. For example, abnormal immune function may increase the risk of ASD.

Sleep and Dreams

Mental health depends on sleep and dreaming. All living things exhibit cycles of rest and activity, which in humans are represented by the daily sleep–wake cycle. Everyone has a sleep–wake cycle that corresponds to his or her optimal degree of physical, mental, and spiritual well-being. The optimum sleep for most adults is 7 to 8 hours per night, with some needing less sleep and others more. The duration of sleep is less significant than whether an individual awakens feeling refreshed, vital, and able to function optimally. Nearly 80% of American college students report not getting enough sleep on most days of the week to feel rested the next morning (American College Health Association, 2017).

Adequate sleep enhances attentiveness, concentration, mood, and motivation. Inadequate sleep, on the other hand, impairs concentration, memory, and the ability to be productive, good-humored, satisfied with life, and even to laugh at a joke! Lack of sleep can gravely impair judgment: Sleeplessness is second only to drunkenness as a cause of automobile accidents. Inadequate sleep is linked to all-cause and cardiovascular mortality, susceptibility to stress, excess body weight, and perturbed immune functioning.

Sleep is a basic biological function. There are two basic types of sleep: rapid eye movement (REM) sleep and non-REM sleep (consisting of three stages: called 1, 2, and 3). Each stage has a specific brain wave pattern and activity. You cycle through all stages of REM and non-REM sleep several times during a typical night, with increasingly longer, deeper REM periods occurring toward the end of the sleep cycle. In REM sleep your eyes move rapidly from side to side behind closed eyelids, brain wave activity becomes closer to that seen in wakefulness, breathing becomes faster and irregular, and heart rate and blood pressure increase to near waking levels. Most dreaming occurs during REM sleep, although some can also occur in non-REM sleep. When dreaming, your arm and leg muscles become temporarily paralyzed, which prevents you from acting out your dreams. As you age, you sleep less of your time in REM sleep. Memory consolidation most likely requires both non-REM and REM sleep. Sleep centers in the brain control sleep behavior, much as appetite centers in the brain control eating behavior. When you don't get adequate sleep, your brain creates an urge to sleep, which can be irresistible if you are sufficiently sleep-deprived. Human sleep is composed of five stages, through which one cycles every 90 to 120 minutes during a sleep episode (**Figure 4.4**).

Good sleep requires diminished physiological and psychological arousal caused by heightened sympathetic nervous system activity (e.g., caused by caffeine, a prebedtime cigarette, or anger, worry, and stress). Exposure to bright light, such as from a computer screen, can delay falling to sleep. Reading bedtime stories to children is a time-honored way to diminish their sympathetic nervous system arousal and provide a transition to sleep. Methods common to adults include reading before bedtime, prayer or meditation, taking a warm bath, and having a light snack. Drinking alcohol, while possibly contributing to drowsiness, actually impairs falling asleep and getting restful sleep.

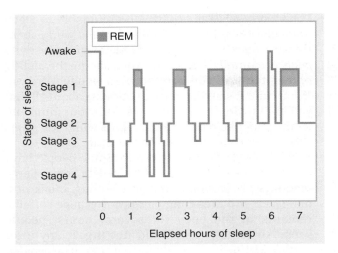

■ **Figure 4.4**

The Human Sleep Cycle
The graph shows changes in brain activity during sleep as measured by an EEG (electroencephalogram).

Modified from U.S. Coast Guard. (2003, January). *Crew Endurance Management Practices: A Guide for Maritime Operations.*

Sleep researchers believe that a majority of Americans are sleeping 60 to 90 minutes a night less than the 7 or 8 hours that would leave them refreshed and energetic during the day (**Figure 4.5**). Individuals "cheat on their sleep" to create time for other things in their busy schedules. Sleep is considered expendable, and not sleeping is considered a sign of ambition and drive.

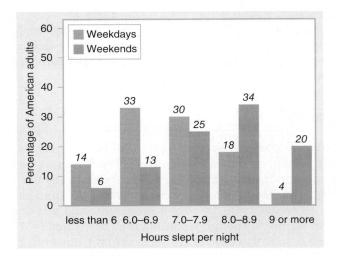

■ **Figure 4.5**

Number of Hours Slept per Night on Weekdays and Weekends by American Adults
Notice that many people are getting less than the recommended 7 to 8 hours a night on weekdays and are making up for it by sleeping more on weekends.

Data from National Sleep Foundation. (2012). Sleep in America 2012 Bedroom poll. Retrieved from http://www.sleepfoundation.org

Furthermore, around-the-clock TV, radio entertainment, and the Internet can distract people from sleeping. Before the advent of the electric light bulb in the late 1800s, people tended to sleep about 9 hours a night. When it got dark, people slept. Because sleep is so strongly linked to one's total state of well-being, focusing on healthy sleep habits can produce greater mind–body harmony.

College Students and Sleep

Deprive, deprive, deprive, deprive, crash. This is a very common sleep pattern among college students. During the week, students deprive themselves of sleep to complete their academic tasks, work, interact with electronic media, and socialize, and on the weekend they pay back their "sleep debt" with one or two extended episodes of sleep. Because this pattern is prevalent, it may seem normal, but it has drawbacks. For example, shortened sleep time, erratic sleep/wake schedules, and poor sleep quality are associated with lower academic performance, thus creating the irony that the motivation to sleep less to produce more is counterproductive (Gruber et al., 2010). Sleeping only 4 to 6 hours a night can reduce the ability to pay attention, react to a stimulus, think quickly, not make mistakes, and multitask.

Many college students experience times of disturbed or nonrestful sleep. They go to bed, but instead of falling asleep, they lie awake thinking about their to-do list, personal problems, an upcoming exam or speech, and just about anything else that enters their minds. Or they fall asleep, but after a few hours they awaken—ruminating—and cannot readily go back to sleep. Having not gotten a good night's sleep (or two or three), when awake they are irritable, depressed, tired, have low motivation (even for things they like), and have diminished concentration.

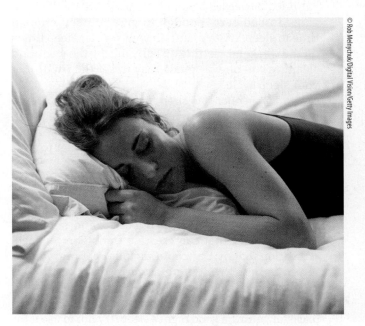

Sufficient sleep and dreams are essential to mental health.

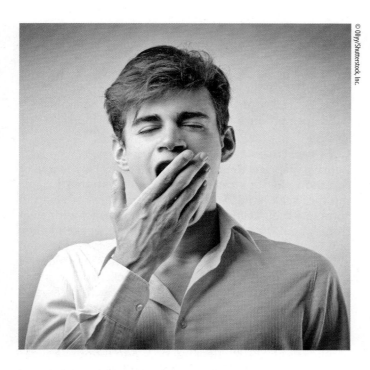

© Ollyy/Shutterstock, Inc.

Frequently, when academic pressures relent and stress subsides, normal, restorative sleep returns. It is possible, however, that the factors producing disturbed sleep become habitual, causing chronic insomnia (see the following section).

Getting a Good Night's Sleep

Here are some suggestions for getting a good night's sleep.

- *Establish a regular sleep time.* Give your own natural sleep cycle a chance to be in synchrony with the day–night cycle by going to bed at the same time each night (within an hour more or less) and arising *without being awakened by an alarm clock.* This will mean going to bed early enough to give yourself enough time to sleep. Try to maintain your regular sleep times on the weekend. Getting up early during the week and sleeping late on weekends may upset the rhythm of your sleep cycle.
- *Create a proper (for you) sleep environment.* Sleep occurs best when the sleeping environment is dark, quiet, free of distractions, and not too warm. If you use radio or TV to help you fall asleep, use an autotimer to shut off the noise after falling asleep.
- *Wind down before going to bed.* About 30 to 60 minutes before bedtime, stop any activities that cause mental or physical arousal, such as work or exercise, talking or texting, and playing video games, and take up a "quiet" activity that can create a transition to sleep. Transitional activities could include reading, watching "mindless" TV, taking a warm bath or shower, meditation, or making love.
- *Make the bedroom for sleeping only.* Make the bedroom your place for getting a good night's sleep. Try not to use it for work or for discussing problems with your partner.

- *Don't worry while in bed.* If you are unable to sleep after about 30 minutes in bed because of worry about things in your life, get up and do some limited activity such as reading a magazine article, doing the dishes, or meditating. Go back to bed when you feel drowsy. If you cannot sleep because of thinking about all that you have to do, write down what's on your mind and let the paper hold onto the thoughts while you sleep. You can retrieve them in the morning.
- *Avoid alcohol, caffeine, and tobacco.* Some people have a glass of beer or wine before bed to relax. Large amounts of alcohol, although sedating, block normal sleep and dreaming patterns. Because caffeine remains in the body for several hours, people sensitive to caffeine should not ingest any after noon. Nicotine is a stimulant, so it should be avoided before bedtime.
- *Exercise regularly.* Exercising 20 to 30 minutes three or four times a week enhances the ability to sleep. You should not exercise vigorously within 3 hours of bedtime, however, because of the possibility of becoming too aroused to sleep.

Sleep Problems

Because of life's never-ending array of challenges, just about everyone has trouble sleeping once in a while. Experiences that commonly disrupt sleeping patterns include being sick, jet-lagged, nervous about an upcoming exam, or excited about something new; having consumed too much food, alcohol, or caffeine; or losing a loved one. Fortunately, most people tend to adjust to these situations, and their sleep rhythms return to normal (for them). A large percentage of Americans, however, have problems with sleeping that last several weeks to years. The most common sleep problems are not sleeping enough (insomnia), sleeping during the day (excessive daytime sleepiness), and unusual activities associated with sleep (parasomnias).

Insomnia

The majority of people with long-term sleep problems have **insomnia**. They have trouble falling asleep or staying asleep, or they awaken after a few hours of sleep and cannot go back to sleep. The daytime results of insomnia are fatigue, the desire to nap, impaired ability to concentrate, impaired judgment, and a lack of zest for life. Although insomnia may be related to disease or injury in the brain's sleep centers, most often it is the result of a physical illness, chronic pain, stress, depression, anxiety, obsessive-compulsive ruminations, panic attacks, posttraumatic stress disorder, or drug or alcohol abuse.

Sometimes, as a result of insomnia, individuals have a difficult time staying awake during the day. They may feel sleepy most of the time, may nod off easily during a routine activity, or may nap at the slightest opportunity.

Because they get insufficient sleep at night, about 20% of college students can fall asleep almost instantaneously if permitted to lie down in a darkened room. An extreme tendency to fall asleep during the day is called **narcolepsy**.

Insomnia is related to a variety of physical health problems, including more sick days, high blood pressure, type 2 diabetes, chronic respiratory disease, arthritis, pain, and headache. Insomnia increases the risks of depression, anxiety, and substance abuse. Because lack of sleep is a form of stress, and thus promotes the production of stress hormones, it tends to perpetuate itself. Furthermore, stress hormones may be responsible for the relationship of insomnia and being overweight, especially in children (Magee & Hale, 2012).

People with insomnia may try to improve their situation by going to bed early, staying in bed longer even though not sleeping, or trying to nap. Some try alcohol and sleep medications. In general, these strategies fail because they disrupt the biology of sleep and do not address the root causes of insomnia: negative expectations about one's ability to get to sleep and the consequent physiological arousal created by those thoughts. In other words, worrying about not sleeping is psychophysiologically stimulating, and thus it defeats getting to sleep. To overcome insomnia, one must follow the suggestions for adequate sleep hygiene, practice some form of relaxation (e.g., meditation, progressive muscle relaxation), and become aware of and change one's worry about getting to sleep. For example, instead of worry, one acknowledges that one worries ("There's that worry, again") and then reminds oneself that the worry is both unnecessary ("It's not true that I will fail at getting to sleep again") and counterproductive ("These thoughts aren't helping me"). Changing one's thoughts about sleep and learning proper sleep hygiene are more effective for insomnia than medications are (Mitchell et al., 2012). Moreover, many prescription sleep drugs (hypnotics, antidepressants, barbiturates) can be dangerous (MayoClinic.com, 2017).

Parasomnias

Parasomnias occur in many forms and have the potential to interrupt restful sleep. Common parasomnias include the following:

- *Nightmares*, dreams that arouse feelings of fear, terror, anxiety, or panic.
- *Somnambulism*, also known as sleepwalking. This is a condition occurring primarily in children and often associated with anxiety, fatigue, or stress. The person performs motor activity, usually leaving bed and walking around, while sleeping and has no memory of it on awakening. Other vigorous behaviors, such as punching, kicking, and night terrors (episodes that begin with a loud cry followed by rapid heart rate, sweating, and feelings of panic), will also interrupt sleep.

Wiped Out?

Fatigue is feeling tired, lacking energy, or acting weary. If you run a marathon, you are likely to be very tired afterward, but you will recover your strength and bounce back after you rest. If you are sick, you may feel lethargic and tired until you get better. However, if you are like many college students and day after day you don't get sufficient sleep or you live under constant stress, you are likely to feel unrelentingly worn out and bone tired. To feel spunky again, you need to establish good sleep patterns; take a little time each day to relax; eat properly; say "no" to invitations to overextend yourself; stay away from tobacco, alcohol, and other drugs; stop talking on the phone, texting, or videogaming 60 minutes before bedtime; and turn off your cell phone while you are asleep.

- *Sleep apnea*, in which breathing stops or gets very shallow for about 10 to 20 seconds and then resumes with a snort or choking sound. These pauses can occur 20 to 30 times or more an hour.
- *Restless legs syndrome* (RLS), characterized by a powerful urge to move the legs, often described as a creeping, crawling, tingling, or burning sensation. The urge to move and unpleasant feelings occur when resting and inactive, thus making it hard to fall asleep and stay asleep.

Because the majority of sleep problems represent some form of disharmony within ourselves or with our surroundings, restoring harmony is a way to return to our natural rest–activity cycle. This can be accomplished by employing mind–body health practices such as meditation, exercise, and proper nutrition. For extreme sleep disorders, professional help should be sought.

Understanding Your Dreams

We all dream while we sleep. Even animals dream. Although some people deny they dream, this is because they do not recall their dreams when awake. On the other hand, some people have vivid recall of the several dreams they have each night (a skill that can be learned).

Dreams tend to occur in the stage of sleep called **rapid eye movement (REM) sleep** (see Figure 4.4). REM

TERMS

insomnia: prolonged inability to obtain adequate sleep

narcolepsy: extreme tendency to fall asleep during the day

parasomnias: activities that interrupt restful sleep

rapid eye movement (REM) sleep: stage of sleep in which dreams occur

sleep encompasses about 25% of sleep time, and it dominates sleep time in the last half of the night.

No one knows why we dream. Some researchers have suggested that REM sleep states are necessary for brain growth, daily information processing, and cellular rejuvenation. Others believe that dreams are the brain's way of processing and eliminating information and memories that are no longer useful. Whatever the reasons, dreams are necessary for health. Experimental subjects who were deprived of the chance to dream (they were awakened by experimenters during REM sleep) developed bizarre behaviors and psychotic symptoms. The individuals returned to normal after at least one night of catching up on the missed REM time.

For thousands of years dreams have been used in many cultures to restore mental and physical health. The temples of Asclepius were used by ancient Greeks for more than a thousand years as places where people went to have healing dreams and to have them interpreted by the priests and priestesses.

Indications that dreams can be healthy come from studies of the Senoi, a Malaysian tribe known as the "dream people." The Senoi live in a nonaggressive, noncombative, communal society. The tribe's members have a remarkable degree of mental and emotional health, which is attributed by some to the daily ritual of discussing and interpreting their dreams. Both children and adults gather each morning to recount their dreams to one another, singly and in groups. According to Senoi custom, the events, anxieties, and people in a dream are real and must be acknowledged and dealt with. Such behavior is similar to our custom of looking for meaning in dreams, especially as a component of psychotherapy.

Critical Thinking About Health

1. Dr. Razmataz's book, *30 Days to Exceptional Mental Health,* had been on the best-seller charts for 10 weeks, but after his appearance on TV's *Inside This Week,* sales went through the roof. Entertainers, business executives, professional athletes, and political leaders extolled the value of his program to lessen needless worry, improve sleep, and enhance mood, self-esteem, memory, and mental acuity.

   Dr. Razmataz based his program on 10 years of research he conducted as director of the Ersatz Mental Health Clinic. In his book and his media appearances, Dr. Razmataz explained that the type and severity of a particular mental illness were caused by either the over- or underactivity of the genes that controlled the production of the six basic neurotransmitter chemicals in the brain. The key to his method was determining a patient's genetic profile and matching it to one of six specific organic food diets.

   a. What factors are mentioned in the description above that might suggest to someone that Dr. Razmataz's method is credible and efficacious?

   b. Which of these factors do you find influence you when you are making a health decision?

   c. What additional information, if any, would you want before trying Dr. Razmataz's method yourself or recommending it to someone else? How would you find such information?

2. List five characteristics of a mentally healthy person. If you were a parent, how would you ensure that your child(ren) grow(s) up to manifest the five characteristics on your list? Also discuss how individuals can contribute to the mental health of people in their community.

3. John hasn't liked being Margie's supervisor since her first day of work. She just doesn't get it. And because she's the boss's niece, there is little he can do. In the past 6 months, whenever Margie is on John's shift-team, he finds himself so distressed that he doesn't want to go to work.

   a. The chapter describes several ways to cope with emotional distress, including (1) changing the situation that is causing the distress, (2) altering the significance one places on the distressing situation, and (3) lessening the distressing emotions. Discuss how John could employ each of these coping strategies to lessen his emotional distress. Also, describe the consequences for John of implementing each coping strategy.

   b. When you experience emotional distress, which of the three coping strategies do you employ most often? Do you notice situations in which one coping strategy works better than others?

4. Many people equate mental and emotional well-being with happiness. If they feel happy, they identify themselves as emotionally well. In your opinion, what is the relationship of emotional well-being and happiness? How do unpleasant emotions, such as sadness, grief, shame, guilt, and anger affect one's sense of emotional well-being? Would you argue that the path to mental and emotional well-being is the pursuit of happiness? If not, in your view, what constitutes the path to mental and emotional well-being?

Chapter Summary and Highlights

Chapter Summary

Mental health and mental illness are more difficult to recognize and define as compared to physical health and physical illness. Symptoms of physical illness are usually specific and clearly measurable or observable—elevated temperature, coughing, nausea, or diarrhea. Symptoms of mental illness are often less well defined or consistent. We all feel "down-in-the-dumps" sometimes, but that is very different from clinical depression, which is a form of mental illness. Normal emotions run the gamut from joy, happiness, pleasure, and contentment to sadness, anger, hostility, and despair. All of us experience mood swings all of the time, and these are normal emotional reactions to things we are experiencing. However, the extremes in mood swings experienced by a person with a manic-depressive disorder are uncontrolled and disabling unless treated. Trained counselors and mental health professionals can help you recognize and cope with emotions that upset and disturb your mental equilibrium. Mental wellness is characterized by feelings of happiness, optimism, vitality, and appreciation of life.

Strong social support from family, friends, teachers, and spiritual figures fosters mental health. Living in a family unit with parents and siblings who care for and express love for one another also helps prevent serious negative mood swings. Sometimes a few good jokes can wipe out despondency and despair. So you did not get the meet-up that you desired so intensely. So what? You will have many more dates and dances in your life. Negative emotions can be controlled if you make the effort. For example, anger is an emotion that everyone experiences. You often hear the expression "She/he made me so angry!" In fact, if you think about it for a moment, you will see that everyone who is angry has made themselves angry. Something has happened or been said that you decided to react to with anger. You could just as easily have smiled and walked away. Mental health begins with taking control of your emotions and deciding which ones allow you to live in harmony with yourself and with those around you.

Highlights

- Mental health is when your mental functions produce a sense of optimism, vitality, and well-being and when your intentional behaviors lead to productive activities (including healthy behaviors), fulfilling relationships with others, and the ability to adapt to change and to cope with adversity.
- Mental illness refers to alterations in thinking, emotions, and/or intentional behaviors that produce psychological distress and/or impaired functioning.
- Mental and emotional health depend on how well individuals meet their maintenance and growth needs and cope with situations in which their needs are not met.
- People understand their needs by interpreting what they sense from the environment and in their bodies. As they mature, people develop ideas about and learn strategies to meet their emotional needs.
- Emotions tell us whether we are satisfied by, and the level of satisfaction from, our experiences, plans, and outcomes of behavior.
- Emotional distress occurs when needs are not met. People cope with emotional distress by changing their modes of interaction with the environment, changing the importance of their unmet needs, or changing the distressing feelings.
- Positive thoughts and emotions, including beliefs in one's worth (self-esteem) and abilities (self-efficacy and agency), motivate people to engage in healthy behaviors and to avoid unhealthy ones.
- Optimism is associated with perceiving negative events as specific, temporary obstacles to be overcome, whereas pessimism is associated with explaining negative events as self-caused, stable, and global.
- Counselors, therapists, and others can help clarify the source of emotional distress and find healthy ways to cope with it.
- Social support enables individuals to receive resources to help during difficult times.
- Phobias are exaggerated and often unrealistic fears.
- Anxiety disorders include social anxiety disorder, panic disorder, generalized anxiety disorder, and obsessive-compulsive disorder.
- Depression is often characterized by feelings of dejection, guilt, hopelessness, self-recrimination, loss of appetite, insomnia, loss of interest in sexual activity, withdrawal from friends, inability to concentrate, lowered self-esteem, and a focus on the negative.
- Suicide is the third leading cause of death among persons aged 15 to 24 years, of all races and both genders.
- Many of the signs of depression occur in someone suicidal. Many suicidal people talk about suicide when life appears hopeless.
- Adult attention deficit hyperactivity disorder is the result of conditions in the brain.
- Unresolved anger and hostility are risk factors for heart disease.
- Sleep and dreams are fundamental to human health. Sleep has five stages. REM sleep, during which dreams occur, happens during the cycle of sleep from deep to lighter stages.
- Many people use their dreams to help them understand and deal with distressing situations and confusing emotions.

For Your Health

The mind is a major contributor to one's health. Keeping a journal (Exercise 4.1 in the Workbook) is a good way to become more aware of your thoughts and feelings and how they affect your life. The other exercises for this chapter can help you understand yourself also.

References

American College Health Association. (2017). *American College Health Association National College Health Assessment II: Undergraduate students: Reference group executive summary, spring 2017.* Hanover, MD: Author. Retrieved from http://www.acha-ncha.org/docs/ACHA-NCHA-II_UNDERGRAD_ReferenceGroup_Executive Summary_Spring2013.pdf

Caputo, A. (2015). The relationship between gratitude and loneliness: The potential benefits of gratitude for promoting social bonds. *Europe's Journal of Psychology, 11,* 323–334.

Centers for Disease Control and Prevention. (2017). Mental health basics. Retrieved from https://www.cdc.gov/mentalhealth/basics.htm

Danner, D. D., Snowdon, D. A., & Friesen, W. V. (2001). Positive emotions in early life and longevity: Findings from the nun study. *Journal of Personality and Social Psychology, 80,* 804–813.

Dunne, S., et al. (2016, April 26). Self-compassion, physical health, and the mediating role of health-promoting behaviors. *Journal of Health Psychology.* doi: 10.1177/1359105316643377

D'raven, L. T., et al. (2014). Happiness intervention decreases pain and depression, boosts happiness among primary care patients. *Primary Health Care Research and Development, 15,* 1–13.

Fournier, J. S., et al. (2010). Antidepressant drug effects and depression severity. *Journal of the American Medical Association, 303,* 47–53.

Gartlehner, G., et al. (2016). Comparative benefits and harms of antidepressant, psychological, complementary, and exercise treatments for major depression: An evidence report for a clinical practice guideline from the American College of Physicians. *Annals of Internal Medicine, 164,* 331–341.

Gilbert, P. (2015). Affiliative and prosocial motives and emotions in mental health. *Dialogues in Clinical Neuroscience, 17,* 381–389.

Gruber, R., et al. (2010). Sleep and academic success: Mechanisms, empirical evidence, and interventional strategies. *Adolescent Medicine State of the Art Reviews, 21,* 522–541.

Gunnell, K. E., et al. (2017). Don't be so hard on yourself! Changes in self-compassion during the first year of university are associated with changes in well-being. *Personality and Individual Differences, 107,* 43–48.

Magee, L., & Hale, L. (2012). Longitudinal associations between sleep duration and subsequent weight gain: A systematic review. *Sleep Medicine Review, 16,* 231–241.

Mayo Clinic. (2016). Forgiveness: Letting go of grudges and bitterness. Retrieved from https://www.mayoclinic.org/healthy-lifestyle/adult-health/in-depth/forgiveness/art-20047692

MayoClinic.com. (2017). Prescription sleeping pills: What's right for you? Retrieved from http://www.mayoclinic.org/diseases-conditions/insomnia/in-depth/sleeping-pills/art-20043959

Mitchell, M. D., et al. (2012). Comparative effectiveness of cognitive behavioral therapy for insomnia: A systematic review. *BMC Family Practice, 13,* 40.

Moloney, M. E., et al. (2011). The medicalization of sleeplessness: A public health concern. *American Journal of Public Health, 101,* 1429–1435.

Mosewich, A. D., et al. (2013). Applying self-compassion in sport: An intervention with women athletes. *Journal of Sport and Exercise Psychology, 35,* 514–524.

Oman, D., et al. (2008). Meditation lowers stress and supports forgiveness among college students. *Journal of American College Health, 56,* 569–578.

Plutchik, R. (1991, July/August). The nature of emotions. *American Scientist.* Retrieved from https://americanscientist.org/articles/01articles/Plutchik.html

Redwine, L. S., et al. (2016). Pilot randomized study of a gratitude journaling intervention on heart rate variability and inflammatory biomarkers in patients with Stage B heart failure. *Psychosomatic Medicine, 78,* 667–676.

Rubia, K., et al. (2014). Brain abnormalities in attention-deficit hyperactivity disorder: A review. *Reviews in Neurology, 58,* Supplement 1, S3–S16.

Sijbrandij, M., et al. (2016). Effectiveness of Internet-delivered cognitive behavioral therapy for post-traumatic stress disorder: A systematic review and meta-analysis. *Depression and Anxiety, 33,* 783–791.

Sin, N. L. (2016). The protective role of positive well-being in cardiovascular disease: Review of current evidence, mechanisms, and clinical implications. *Current Cardiology Reports, 18,* 106–112.

Smeets, E., et al. (2014). Meeting suffering with kindness: Effects of a brief-self-compassion intervention for female college students. *Journal of Clinical Psychology, 70,* 794–807.

Suls, J. (2013). Anger and the heart: Perspectives on cardiac risk, mechanisms and interventions. *Progress in Cardiovascular Disease, 55,* 538–547.

Tay, L., et al. (2013). Social relations, health behaviors, and health outcomes: A survey and synthesis. *Applied Psychology. Health and Well-Being, 5,* 28–78.

Tugade, M. M. (2011). Affiliation and stress. In S. Folkman (Ed.), The Oxford handbook of stress, health, and coping (pp. 186–199). Oxford, UK: Oxford University Press.

U.S. National Institute of Mental Health. (2017). Statistics. Retrieved from https://www.nimh.nih.gov/health/statistics/index.shtml

Vigerland, S. (2016). Internet-delivered cognitive behavior therapy for children and adolescents: A systematic review and meta-analysis. *Clinical Psychology Reviews, 50,* 1–10.

Webb, J. R. (2013). Forgiveness and health: Assessing the mediating effect of health behavior, social support, and interpersonal functioning. *Journal of Psychology, 147,* 391–414.

Whiteford, H. S. (2015). The global burden of mental, neurological and substance use disorders: An analysis from the Global Burden of Disease Study 2010. *PLoS One, 10*(2):e0116820. Retrieved from https://www.ncbi.nlm.nih.gov/pmc/articles/PMC4320057/

World Health Organization. (2014). Mental health: A state of well-being. Retrieved from www.who.int/features/factfiles/mental_health/en/

Suggested Readings

Acocella, J. (2000, May 8). The empty couch—what is lost when psychiatry turns to drugs. *The New Yorker,* 82–118. A thoughtful article addressing the serious problems stemming from excessive use of therapeutic drugs in the treatment of mental disorders.

Belkmayer, R. H., & Agram, G. (2008). Major depressive disorder. *New England Journal of Medicine, 358,* 55–68. Discusses the roles of genetics, neurotransmitter biology, and stress biology on the development of severe clinical depression.

Bourne, E. J. (2015). *The anxiety and phobia workbook.* Oakland, CA: New Harbinger. Presents step-by-step guidelines, questionnaires, and exercises to help sufferers learn skills and make lifestyle changes to help them get relief from the most distressing symptoms.

Cartwright, R. D. (2012). *The twenty-four hour mind: The role of sleep and dreaming in our emotional lives.* New York: Oxford University Press. An internationally renowned sleep scientist discusses decades of research in the scientific study of sleep and sleep disorders and how the human mind works during sleep.

Chrita, A. L., et al. (2015). Current understanding of the neurobiology of major depressive disorder. *Romanian Journal of Morphology and Embryology, 56(2 Suppl.),* 651–658. Retrieved from www.rjme.ro/RJME/resources/files/561215651658.pdf

Goleman, D. (2003). *Healing emotions: Conversations with the Dalai Lama on mindfulness, emotions, and health.* Boston: Shambhala. The world's leading Western physicians, psychologists, and meditation teachers discuss with the Dalai Lama contemporary research on the interrelationship between emotional states and physical well-being in the context of ancient Buddhist thinking.

Koerner, B. I. (2002, July/August). Disorders made to order. *Mother Jones, 75.* Retrieved from http://www.motherjones.com/news/feature/2002/07/disorders.html. Explains the marketing strategy of pharmamaceutical companies to define symptoms of everyday life as a new mental illness and then sell pills to cure it.

Mayo Clinic. (2017). Letting go of grudges and bitterness. Retrieved from https://mayoclinic.org/healthy-life-style/adult-health/in-depth/forgiveness/art-20047692. Shows how to embrace forgiveness and move forward rather than holding on to anger and resentment.

PBS NewsHour. (2011, April 20). *Autism's causes: How close are we to solving the puzzle?* Retrieved from http://www.pbs.org/newshour/bb/health/jan-june11/autism3causes_04-20.html. A TV news report summarizing progress in elucidating the causes of autism.

Ramar, K., & Olson, E. J. (2013). Management of common sleep disorders. *American Family Physician, 88,* 231–237. A thorough discussion of current treatment strategies for managing sleep disorders.

Surman, C., et al. (2014). Fast minds: How to thrive if you have ADHD (or think you might). Berkeley, CA: Berkeley Trade. Helps people with ADHD or some of its characteristics develop personalized strategies to manage their lives.

U.S. National Institute of Mental Health. (2012). Depression and college students. Retrieved from http://www.nimh.nih.gov/health/publications/depression-and-college-students/index.shtml

U.S. National Institute of Mental Health. (2017). Suicide. A guide to information about suicide in the United States. Retrieved from https://www.nimh.nih.gov/health/statistics/suicide/index.html

Recommended Websites and Phone Numbers

American Sleep Association
Information and resources on all aspects of sleep and sleep problems.

Depression Screening Tests
From Mental Health America.

MedlinePlus on Mental Health and Behavior Topics
The National Library of Medicine's web page of resources on a variety of mental health topics.

Mental Health America
Help Line: 800-950-6264
The nation's largest organization offering help to patients and families.

Mind/Body Health: Interactive
Explains how mental health affects the physical health with interactive animations and additional resources. Presented by the American Psychological Association.

National Mental Health Consumers' Self-Help Clearinghouse
800-553-4539
Provides support for persons in search of self-help and advocacy resources.

National Sleep Foundation
Information and resources on all aspects of sleep and sleep problems.

National Suicide Prevention Lifeline
800-273-8255
This confidential hotline is staffed 24/7 by trained counselors.

PART TWO

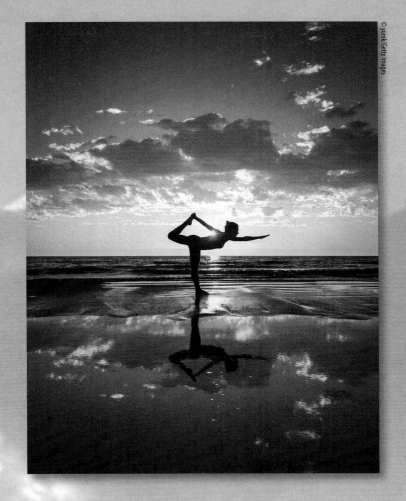

© yuruk/Getty Images

Eating and Exercising Toward a Healthy Lifestyle

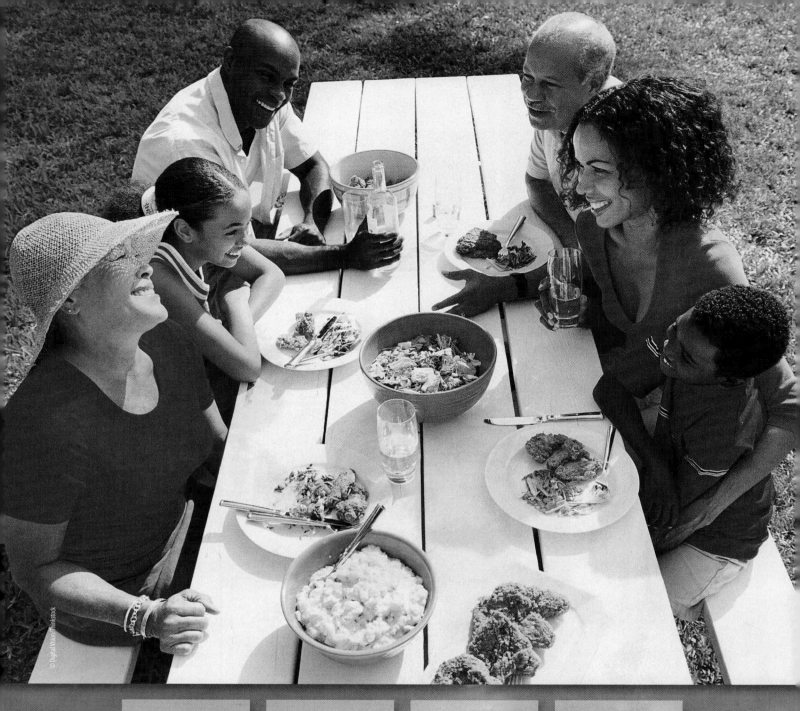

Health Tips

Healthier Eating: One Step at a Time

Power Up! Do Breakfast

Estimating Your Daily Calorie Needs

Dollars & Health Sense

Ways to Reduce Food Waste

Global Wellness

There's Good News and There's Bad News

The Mediterranean Diet

Wellness Guide

Taking Care of Your Teeth and Gums

Rules for Organic Labeling

Guidelines for Food Safety

Tips for Eating Healthy When Eating Out

CHAPTER 5

Choosing a Healthy Diet

Learning Objectives

1. List several factors that influence dietary choices.

2. Define *nutrient-dense food* and *calorie-dense food*.

3. Describe the dietary guidelines proposed by the U.S. government and health organizations.

4. Describe the ingredients and nutrition facts labels on manufactured foods.

5. Describe the three functions of food.

6. List the three functions of biological energy.

7. List the seven components of food, and identify common foods that contain each component.

8. Describe the kinds of vegetarian diets and several reasons for vegetarianism.

Everyone knows it's important for health to eat right. But how do you do that? Given that the average American supermarket carries 39,500 items, the obvious key to eating healthfully is to choose wisely. To do that you need to know what constitutes a healthy diet and the social and economic forces that influence your food choices; for example, family, ethnic, and cultural eating patterns; social factors (eating what friends eat); food fads; and time pressures that limit thoughtful food shopping and meal preparation and make fast food and snacks attractive. Stress also influences food choices by encouraging consumption of foods high in fat and sugar to soothe jangled nerves and emotions (i.e., "comfort foods") (Roberts et al., 2014). Other factors that affect food choices are the cost and availability of healthy foods and the billions of dollars a year spent on the marketing and advertising of food products.

Healthful living requires consumption of foods—preferably in their natural state—that are **nutrient dense**, which means that they provide high levels of nutrients, like vitamins and minerals, per calorie of energy compared to other foods. For example, even though they offer approximately the same amount of energy (about 100 calories), an apple is more nutrient dense than a serving of 10 potato chips because it provides more fiber, vitamin C, and several other vitamins than the chips do, with no added fat and salt. According to the U.S. Department of Agriculture (2015), "all vegetables, fruits, whole grains, seafood, eggs, beans and peas, unsalted nuts and seeds, fat-free and low-fat dairy products, and lean meats and poultry—when prepared with little or no added solid fats, sugars, refined starches, and sodium—are nutrient-dense foods."

Unfortunately, the U.S. food supply contains an abundance of inexpensive foods that are **calorie dense** instead of nutrient dense. Calorie-dense foods offer considerable energy in the form of (usually added) sugar and saturated fat but lack reasonable quantities of nutrients. Calorie-dense foods include many pastries, candies, and most fast foods and **processed foods**, which are industrial products derived from natural foods to which salt, sugar, oils and fats, and other chemicals, such as flavorings, colorings, sweeteners, and thickeners, are added to alter taste, color, palatability, and resistance to spoilage and to disguise any undesirable qualities arising from the manufacturing process (Martinez Stelle et al., 2015). Overconsumption of calorie-dense foods creates the paradox in that many people are simultaneously overfed and undernourished, and it also increases the risk for overweight, heart disease, high blood pressure, diabetes, kidney disease, and some cancers (Murray et al., 2016). About 67% of the North American food supply is manufactured food. The remaining 33% is in its natural state.

Dietary Guidelines for Eating Right

Many people realize that their eating pattern is not as healthy as it could be (**Figure 5.1**), and most would probably want to make healthier food choices. But the plethora of claims and counterclaims about what consumers should eat are as likely to confuse as enlighten.

Nutrition scientists and doctors try to educate the public about healthy eating, but often their explanations are too technical for most people to comprehend readily (Buckton et al., 2015). Moreover, the quest for authoritative nutritional guidance can be thwarted by the efforts of self-professed experts and commercial interests whose goals are profits rather than health education.

Scientists have identified the kinds, amounts, and proportions of foods that make up a healthy diet (**Table 5.1**). Also, modern food production and distribution systems can potentially provide human populations with a variety of good tasting nutritious food. To help consumers develop strategies for eating healthfully, the World Health Organization, the U.S.

> The destiny of a nation depends on the manner in which it feeds itself.
>
> *Jean Anthelme Brillat-Savarin (1755–1826)*

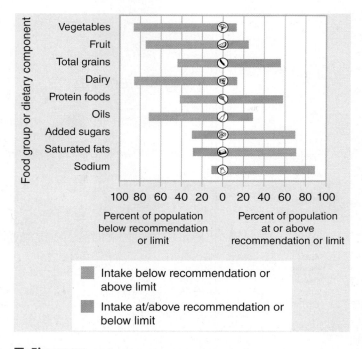

■ **Figure 5.1**

Dietary Intakes Compared to Recommendations. Percent of the U.S. Population Ages 1 Year and Older Who Are Below, At, or Above Each Dietary Goal or Limit

The "0" line is the goal intake. Orange sections of a bar indicate consumption below goal intake; blue sections indicate consumption above goal intake.

U.S. Department of Agriculture, Dietary Guidelines for Americans, 2015–2020.

TERMS

calorie dense: food items that contain considerable calories but are of little nutritional value

nutrient dense: food items that are high in nutrition in proportion to their calorie content

processed foods: industrial products derived from natural foods to which salt, sugar, oils and fats, and other chemicals are added to modify taste and consistency

Table 5.1

Healthy Eating Pattern: Recommended Intake Amounts in U.S.

Calorie Level of Pattern[a]	1,600	2,000	2,400
Food Group[b]			
Vegetables	**2 c-eq**	**2½ c-eq**	**3 c-eq**
Dark-green vegetables (c-eq/wk)	1½	1½	2
Red and orange vegetables (c-eq/wk)	4	5½	6
Legumes (beans and peas) (c-eq/wk)	1	1½	2
Starchy vegetables (c-eq/wk)	4	5	6
Other vegetables (c-eq/wk)	3½	4	5
Fruits	**1½ c-eq**	**2 c-eq**	**2 c-eq**
Grains	**5 oz-eq**	**6 oz-eq**	**8 oz-eq**
Whole grains[d] (oz-eq/day)	3	3	4
Refined grains (oz-eq/day)	2	3	4
Dairy	**3 c-eq**	**3 c-eq**	**3 c-eq**
Protein Foods	**5 oz-eq**	**5½ oz-eq**	**6½ oz-eq**
Seafood (oz-eq/wk)	8	8	10
Meats, poultry, eggs (oz-eq/wk)	23	26	31
Nuts, seeds, soy products (oz-eq/wk)	4	5	5
Oils	**22 g**	**27 g**	**31 g**
Limit on Calories for Other Uses (% of calories)[e,f]	130 (8%)	270 (14%)	350 (15%)

[a] Patterns from 1,600 to 3,200 calories are designed to meet the nutritional needs of children 9 years and older and adults. If a child 4 to 8 years of age needs more calories and, therefore, is following a pattern at 1,600 calories or more, his/her recommended amount from the dairy group should be 2.5 cups per day. Children 9 years and older and adults should not use the 1,000-, 1,200-, or 1,400-calorie patterns.

[b] Foods in each group and subgroup are:

Vegetables
- Dark-green vegetables: All fresh, frozen, and canned dark-green leafy vegetables and broccoli, cooked or raw: for example, broccoli; spinach; romaine; kale; collard, turnip, and mustard greens.
- Red and orange vegetables: All fresh, frozen, and canned red and orange vegetables or juice, cooked or raw: for example, tomatoes, tomato juice, red peppers, carrots, sweet potatoes, winter squash, and pumpkin.
- Legumes (beans and peas): All cooked from dry or canned beans and peas: for example, kidney beans, white beans, black beans, lentils, chickpeas, pinto beans, split peas, and edamame (green soybeans). Does not include green beans or green peas.
- Starchy vegetables: All fresh, frozen, and canned starchy vegetables: for example, white potatoes, corn, green peas, green lima beans, plantains, and cassava.
- Other vegetables: All other fresh, frozen, and canned vegetables, cooked or raw: for example, iceberg lettuce, green beans, onions, cucumbers, cabbage, celery, zucchini, mushrooms, and green peppers.

Fruits
- All fresh, frozen, canned, and dried fruits and fruit juices: for example, oranges and orange juice, apples and apple juice, bananas, grapes, melons, berries, and raisins.

Grains
- Whole grains: All whole-grain products and whole grains used as ingredients: for example, whole-wheat bread, whole-grain cereals and crackers, oatmeal, quinoa, popcorn, and brown rice.
- Refined grains: All refined-grain products and refined grains used as ingredients: for example, white breads, refined grain cereals and crackers, pasta, and white rice. Refined grain choices should be enriched.

Dairy
- All milk, including lactose-free and lactose-reduced products and fortified soy beverages (soymilk), yogurt, frozen yogurt, dairy desserts, and cheeses. Most choices should be fat-free or low-fat. Cream, sour cream, and cream cheese are not included due to their low calcium content.

Protein Foods
- All seafood, meats, poultry, eggs, soy products, nuts, and seeds. Meats and poultry should be lean or low-fat and nuts should be unsalted. Legumes (beans and peas) can be considered part of this group as well as the vegetable group, but should be counted in one group only.

[c] Food group amounts shown in cup-I or ounce-equivalents (oz-eq). Oils are shown in grams (g). Quantity equivalents for each food group are:
- Vegetables and fruits, 1 cup-equivalent is: 1 cup raw or cooked vegetable or fruit, 1 cup vegetable or fruit juice, 2 cups leafy salad greens, ½ cup dried fruit or vegetable.
- Grains, 1 ounce-equivalent is: ½ cup cooked rice, pasta, or cereal; 1 ounce dry pasta or rice; 1 medium (1 ounce) slice bread; 1 ounce of ready-to-eat cereal (about 1 cup of flaked cereal).
- Dairy, 1 cup-equivalent is: 1 cup milk, yogurt, or fortified soymilk; 1½ ounces natural cheese such as cheddar cheese or 2 ounces of processed cheese. Protein foods, 1 ounce-equivalent is: 1 ounce lean meat, poultry, or seafood; 1 egg; ¼ cup cooked beans or tofu; 1 Tbsp peanut butter; ½ ounce nuts or seeds.

[d] Amounts of whole grains in the patterns for children are less than the minimum of 3 oz-eq in all patterns recommended for adults.

[e] All foods are assumed to be in nutrient-dense forms, lean or low-fat, and prepared without added fats, sugars, refined starches, or salt. If all food choices to meet food group recommendations are in nutrient-dense forms, a small number of calories remain within the overall calorie limit of the pattern (i.e., limit on calories for other uses). The number of these calories depends on the overall calorie limit in the pattern and the amounts of food from each food group required to meet nutritional goals. Nutritional goals are higher for the 1,200- to 1,600-calorie patterns than for the 1,000-calorie pattern, so the limit on calories for other uses is lower in the 1,200- to 1,600-calorie patterns. Calories up to the specified limit can be used for added sugars, added refined starches, solid fats, alcohol, or to eat more than the recommended amount of food in a food group. The overall eating pattern also should not exceed the limits of less than 10 percent of calories from added sugars and less than 10 percent of calories from saturated fats. At most calorie levels, amounts that can be accommodated are less than these limits. For adults of legal drinking age who choose to drink alcohol, a limit of up to 1 drink per day for women and up to 2 drinks per day for men within limits on calories for other uses applies; and calories from protein, carbohydrate, and total fats should be within the Acceptable Macronutrient Distribution Ranges (AMDRs).

[f] Values are rounded.

Reproduced from U.S. Department of Agriculture, *Dietary Guidelines for Americans, 2015–2020*. Retrieved from health.gov/dietaryguidelines/2015/guidelines/appendix-3/

and Canadian governments, and health organizations, such as the American Heart Association and the American Cancer Society, put forth specific guidelines for healthful nutrition. These guidelines are based on the latest scientific evidence for good nutrition, created by examining the biological effects of specific dietary components and by comparing eating patterns and disease frequencies in different populations. For example, compared to the common American diet, also called the standard Western diet, which is based on meats, refined-flour products, and industrial products such as fast food and packaged fatty or sugary snacks and sweets, the traditional Asian and Mediterranean diets, which are based on whole unprocessed grains (rice, whole-wheat flour), beans, fresh vegetables and fruits, and fish, are associated with less heart disease and several kinds of cancer because they maintain healthy body weight, lessen inflammation and insulin resistance,and improve blood vessel functioning (see the Global Wellness box, "The Mediterranean Diet," on p. 96).

Every 5 years, the U.S. Department of Agriculture (USDA) issues dietary guidelines for the American people (U.S. Department of Agriculture, 2015) designed to promote wellness and prevent illnesses that result from poor nutrition, including:

- Heart disease, cancer of various organs, type 2 diabetes, and overweight from diets high in sugar and fat
- Cancer of the colon from consumption of too much processed and cooked red meat
- Diseases of the gastrointestinal tract from not consuming sufficient fiber
- High blood pressure from consuming too much salt
- Tooth decay and overweight from consuming too much sugar, added to almost every packaged food product (Popkin & Hawkes, 2016)

The guidelines also stress the importance of physical activity in maintaining a healthy body weight.

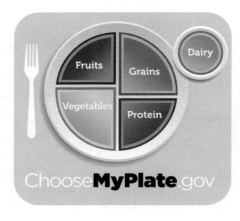

■ **Figure 5.2**

MyPlate

MyPlate can help you eat balanced meals.

Courtesy of U.S. Department of Agriculture.

To help consumers remember the most important dietary recommendations, the USDA has developed **MyPlate** (**Figure 5.2**), a graphic consisting of a plate divided into four sections for fruits, vegetables, protein, and grains with a dairy cup beside it. MyPlate is intended to encourage consumers to follow these guidelines:

- Enjoy food, but avoid oversized portions.
- Make nearly half your plate fruits and vegetables of all colors. (Potatoes and french fries don't count.)
- Make at least half your grains whole grains.
- Consume one to two servings per day of fat-free or low-fat (1%) milk.
- Drink water instead of sugary drinks.
- Choose packaged and frozen food items that contain less salt/sodium (check the product label).
- For protein, choose fish, poultry, beans, and nuts; limit red meat, bacon, cold cuts, and other processed meat.

The USDA also has produced the DASH Diet (Dietary Approaches to Stop Hypertension) for people with high blood pressure (**Figure 5.3**).

There's Good News and There's Bad News

The good news is that in recent years the diet of much of the world's human population has gotten healthier (Imamura et al., 2015). The bad news is that during that same time period the diet of much of the world's population has gotten less healthy. How could that be?

The answer is that, on the whole, the people of the world are consuming more healthy foods *and* more unhealthy foods. Researchers compared the dietary patterns of adults in 187 countries in the years 1990 and 2010, considering 10 healthy and 7 unhealthy dietary constituents. In high-income countries, consumption of healthy dietary constituents increased and that of unhealthy items declined a bit. In low-income countries, however, consumption of healthier dietary constituents decreased and that of unhealthy dietary items increased. Also, even though consumption of unhealthy dietary items decreased among residents of high-income countries, their

diets still had greater amounts of unhealthy items than those in low-income countries did. A diet high in unhealthy constituents is the major risk factor for heart and blood vessel disease, the two most common causes of death in the world (World Health Organization, 2015).

Healthy Dietary Constituents	Unhealthy Dietary Constituents
Fruits	High sodium
Vegetables	High trans fats
Beans and legumes	Processed meats
Whole grains	Red meat
Nuts and seeds	Sugar-sweetened beverages
Milk	Saturated fat
Fiber	Cholesterol
Calcium	
Omega-3 fatty acids	
Polyunsaturated fatty acids	
Fish	

The DASH eating plan shown below is based on 2,000 calories a day. The number of daily servings in a food group may vary from those listed, depending on your caloric needs. Use this chart to help you plan your menus or take it with you when you go to the store.

Food Group	Daily Servings (except as noted)	Serving Sizes	Examples and Notes	Significance of Each Food Group to the DASH Eating Plan
Grains and grain products	6–8	1 slice bread 1 oz dry cereal* 1/2 cup cooked rice, pasta, or cereal	Whole-wheat bread, English muffin, pita bread, bagel, cereals, grits, oatmeal, crackers, unsalted pretzels, and popcorn	Major sources of energy and fiber
Vegetables	4–5	1 cup raw leafy vegetable 1/2 cup cooked vegetable 6 oz vegetable juice	Tomatoes, potatoes, carrots, green peas, squash, broccoli, turnip greens, collards, kale, spinach, artichokes, green beans, lima beans, sweet potatoes	Rich sources of potassium, magnesium, and fiber
Fruits	4–5	4 oz fruit juice 1 medium fruit 1/4 cup dried fruit 1/2 cup fresh, frozen, or canned fruit	Apricots, bananas, dates, grapes, oranges, orange juice, grapefruit, grapefruit juice, mangoes, melons, peaches, pineapples, prunes, raisins, strawberries, tangerines	Important sources of potassium, magnesium, and fiber
Low-fat or fat-free dairy foods	2–3	8 oz milk 1 cup yogurt 1 1/2 oz cheese	Fat-free (skim) or low-fat (1%) milk, fat-free or low-fat buttermilk, fat-free or low-fat regular or frozen yogurt, low-fat and fat-free cheese	Major sources of calcium and protein
Lean meats, poultry, and fish	6 or less	3 oz cooked meats, poultry, or fish	Select only lean; trim away visible fats; broil, roast, or boil instead of frying; remove skin from poultry	Rich sources of protein and magnesium
Nuts, seeds, and dry beans	4–5 per week	1/3 cup or 1 1/2 oz nuts 2 Tbsp or 1/2 oz seeds 1/2 cup cooked dry beans, peas	Almonds, filberts, mixed nuts, peanuts, walnuts, sunflower seeds, kidney beans, lentils	Rich sources of energy, magnesium, potassium, protein, and fiber
Fats and oils†	2–3	1 tsp soft margarine 1 Tbsp low-fat mayonnaise 2 Tbsp light salad dressing 1 tsp vegetable oil	Soft margarine, low-fat mayonnaise, light salad dressing, vegetable oil (such as olive, corn, canola, or safflower)	DASH has 27% of calories as fat, including fat in or added to foods
Sweets	5 per week	1 Tbsp sugar 1 Tbsp jelly or jam 1/2 oz jelly beans 8 oz lemonade	Maple syrup, sugar, jelly, jam, fruit-flavored gelatin, jelly beans, hard candy, fruit punch, sorbet, ices	Sweets should be low in fat
Maximum sodium limit	2,300 mg per day			

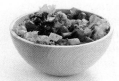

© Hemera/Thinkstock

■ **Figure 5.3**
The DASH Eating Plan

*Equals 1/2–1 1/4 cups, depending on cereal type. Check the product's Nutrition Facts label.
†Fat content changes serving counts for fats and oils: for example, 1 Tbsp of regular salad dressing equals 1 serving.
Reproduced from U.S. Department of Health and Human Services, National Institutes of Health, National Heart, Lung, and Blood Instutite (2015). What is the DASH Eating Plan? Available at http://www.nhlbi.nih.gov/health/health-topics/topics/dash/.

Food Labels: Know What You're Putting into Your Body

Few people in developed countries grow their own food or obtain it directly from growers and preparers. Instead, they get much of their food prepackaged with added sugar, salt,

TERMS

MyPlate: a graphic to remind people of the composition of a healthy diet

artificial flavorings, and preservatives or prepared in restaurants with ingredients of which the quality, amounts, purity, and sources are unknown to them. Thus, it can be very difficult for consumers to judge the nutritional value and sometimes safety of food products they consume.

To help consumers assess the quality and safety of food products, the U.S. and many other governments require food manufactures to provide certain information about a product on its packaging label. In the United States, the information consists of the name and address of the manufacturer, packer, or distributor; the ingredients label; the Nutrition Facts label; and any required allergy labeling. The package can also state if the product is gluten free and include any health claims supported by scientific research.

The **ingredients label** (**Figure 5.4**) lists the chemical composition of the food, that is, all the substances that the manufacturer uses, including other foods (e.g., grains, eggs), natural and artificial sweeteners, natural and artificial fats, water, natural and artificial thickeners, natural and artificial flavorings, food colorings, and preservatives. The ingredients label lists substances in descending order by weight; the substance in the greatest amount is listed first and that in the least amount is listed last.

The ingredients label does not specify how much—either by weight or percentage—of an ingredient is in a food product, only its amount relative to the other ingredients. Also, by listing each individual substance,

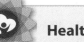

Healthier Eating: One Step at a Time

If you want to improve your diet, make one healthful change at a time. Here are some suggestions:

- Eat a breakfast consisting of at least a whole-grain product and a fruit.
- Substitute one daily serving of real fruit juice or tea (not colored sugar water or an energy drink) for a soda.
- Substitute one daily serving of a fruit or nuts for a candy bar or a handful (or two) of chips.
- Substitute a lean meat sandwich with tomato on whole-wheat bread for a fast-food hamburger, fried fish entree, taco, pizza, or burrito.

Ingredients: Wheat flour, sugar, rolled oats, corn sweetener, molasses, partially hydrogenated safflower oil, salt, pantothenic acid, reduced iron, yellow no. 6, yellow no. 5, pyridoxine, ascorbic acid (vitamin C), BHT, riboflavin, folic acid.

■ **Figure 5.4**

The Ingredients Label
The U.S. government requires that food manufacturers list the substances within their products by weight from greatest to least.

The Mediterranean Diet

A key to healthy eating

The Mediterranean diet is associated with longer life and reduced risk of heart disease and cancer. It's a diet based on whole grains, fresh fruits and vegetables, minimal animal and trans fat, and little red meat.

What is a Mediterranean diet?
- Meals based on whole-grain foods: breads, pasta, couscous, polenta, bulgur
- Abundant fresh vegetables and fruits
- Generous amounts of beans, nuts, and seeds
- Olive oil as the principal source of fat
- Use of garlic, onions, and herbs as condiments
- Moderate use of fish
- Moderate use of dairy
- Minimal use of red meat
- Low-to-moderate intake of alcohol

What makes the Mediterranean diet healthy?
- Low in saturated fat and cholesterol
- Energy supplied by unsaturated fat (in olive oil and nuts)
- No trans fats (artificial fats in packaged pastries and margarine)
- High in fiber
- High in antioxidants
- Low in refined sugar and flour
- High in plant-based vitamins and micronutrients

Researchers in France have determined that the Mediterranean diet lowers the risk of heart disease and many types of cancer. Even though a large percentage of calories is derived from fat, mono- and polyunsaturated fats predominate, the kind that raise HDL (so-called good cholesterol). Almost absent are animal fats (saturated fats and cholesterol) and manufactured trans fats, which raise LDL (so-called bad cholesterol). The Mediterranean diet's high levels of antioxidants and other micronutrients reduce the risk of cardiovascular disease and cancer.

The typical American dinner, with a slab of meat in the center and one or two "sides," consisting of an overcooked vegetable and a butter-drenched potato, is a far cry from a typical Mediterranean dinner: pasta made of unrefined flour topped with a variety of minimally cooked vegetables (tomatoes, onions, peppers), some beans (peas, fava beans), and a sprinkle of hard cheese (Parmesan or Romano). For dessert, the Mediterranean diet calls for almonds and fresh fruit instead of cake, cookies, or ice cream.

It's too much to ask Americans to replace generations of dietary habits overnight. However, there are ways to incorporate some of the healthier aspects of the Mediterranean diet without radically changing customary eating patterns:
- Cut back on fast food, which is generally 50% saturated fat and cholesterol.
- Replace cake/ice cream desserts with fruit salad and nuts.
- Replace meat-centered meals with grain- and bean-centered ones.
- Replace doughnuts and sugar-laden snacks with fruit and mixed nuts.

Bon appetit!

the ingredients label may not indicate the true relative amount of sugar or fat in a product. For example, a snack product's ingredients label could list separately sucrose, fructose, high-fructose corn syrup, and corn sweetener, all of which are sugars. As noted earlier, the ingredients label must also contain food allergy information. About 160 foods are known to cause food allergies in sensitive individuals, although 8 foods account for 90% of all food allergies. They are milk, egg, fish, crustacean shellfish, tree nuts, wheat, peanuts, and soybeans. If one or more of these foods is an ingredient in a food product or the product contains a protein derived from one or more

of them, either the ingredients label must identify that ingredient in parentheses following the common or usual name of the major food allergen in the list of ingredients or below the ingredients list with the word "Contains" followed by the name of the food source from which the major food allergen is derived (e.g., "Contains Wheat, Milk, Egg, and Soy"). The allergy notification is to appear immediately after or adjacent to the list of ingredients, in a type size that is no smaller than the type size used for the list of ingredients. Allergens other than the major food allergens are not subject to labeling requirements.

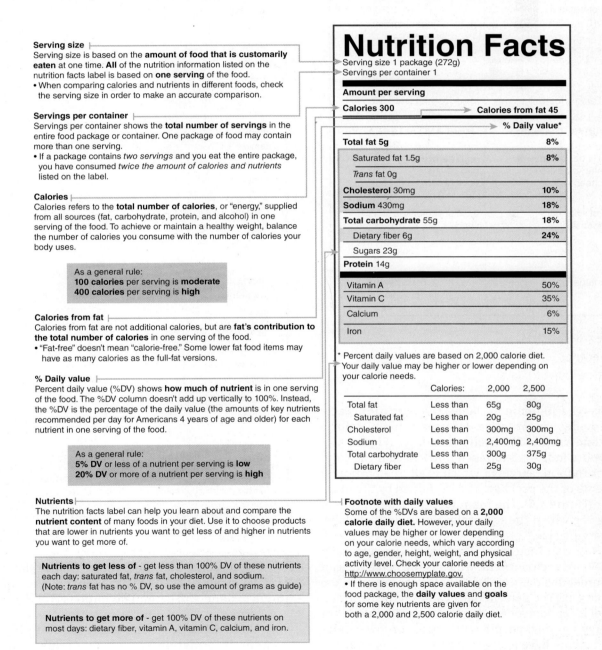

■ Figure 5.5

The Nutrition Facts Label

More from the Food and Drug Administration: http://www.fda.gov/food/ingredientspackaginglabeling/labelingnutrition/ucm274593.htm

Reproduced from U.S. Food and Drug Administration (2017). How to Understand and Use the Nutrition Facts Label.

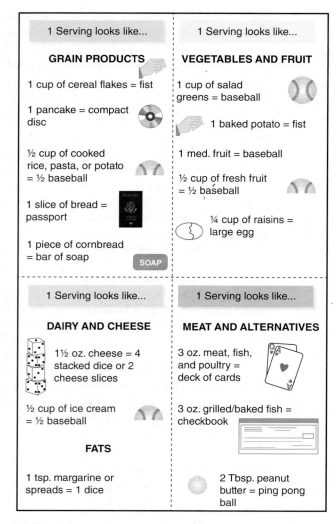

■ **Figure 5.6**

What's a Serving?

Table 5.2

Daily Values (DVs) for Adults and Children Over Four Years of Age Based on a Caloric Intake of 2,000 Calories

Food Component	DV
Total Fat	65 grams (g)
Saturated Fat	20 g
Cholesterol	300 milligrams (mg)
Sodium	2,400 mg
Potassium	3,500 mg
Total Carbohydrate	300 g
Dietary Fiber	25 g
Protein	50 g
Vitamin A	5,000 International Units (IU)
Vitamin C	60 mg
Calcium	1,000 mg
Iron	18 mg
Vitamin D	400 IU
Vitamin E	30 IU
Vitamin K	80 micrograms µg
Thiamin	1.5 mg
Riboflavin	1.7 mg
Niacin	20 mg
Vitamin B6	2 mg
Folate	400 µg
Vitamin B12	6 µg
Biotin	300 µg
Pantothenic acid	10 mg
Phosphorus	1,000 mg
Iodine	150 µg
Magnesium	400 mg
Zinc	15 mg
Selenium	70 µg
Copper	2 mg
Manganese	2 mg
Chromium	120 µg
Molybdenum	75 µg
Chloride	3,400 mg

Reproduced from U.S. Food and Drug Administration (http://www.fda.gov/Food/GuidanceRegulation/GuidanceDocumentsRegulatory Information/LabelingNutrition/ucm064928.htm) U.S. National Institutes of Health, 2017) Nutrient Recommendations: Dietary Reference Intakes. https://ods.od.nih.gov/Health_information/Dietary_Reference_intakes.aspx

Unlike the ingredients label, the **Nutrition Facts label** provides *quantitative* information on calorie content and certain nutrients in a food (**Figure 5.5**). The amounts indicated for each nutrient and the calorie count are for a "serving," which is all or a portion of the contents of the package, as determined by the manufacturer (**Figure 5.6**). The manufacturer's definition of a serving is given at the top of the Nutrition Facts label as the "serving size."

The Nutrition Facts label also lists the **percent daily value (PDV)** for each nutrient, which is the percentage of the recommended daily amount that is contained in the food (**Table 5.2**). (The percent daily value on the Nutrition Facts label is for someone who requires 2,000 calories of food energy per day; people with higher or lower calorie requirements have a larger or smaller PDV.) Near the bottom of the Nutrition Facts label is the recommended daily amount of nutrients, listed by weight (in grams) for 2,000-calorie-per-day diets.

To help consumers determine health-related claims on food labels, the U.S. government requires manufacturers to adhere to certain definitions (**Table 5.3**).

Restaurants and similar retail food establishments with 20 or more locations are required to list calorie content information for standard menu items on restaurant menus and menu boards, including drive-through menu boards. Other nutrient information—total calories, fat, saturated fat, cholesterol, sodium,

Table 5.3

What Words on Product Labels Mean

Calorie free	Fewer than 5 calories per serving
Low calorie	No more than 40 calories for a given reference amount (except sugar substitutes)
Light (lite)	⅓ less calories or no more than ½ the fat of the higher-calorie, higher-fat version; or no more than ½ the sodium of the higher-sodium version
Fat free	Less than 0.5 g of fat per serving
Low fat	3 g or less of total fat for a given reference amount
Reduced or less fat	At least 25% less fat per serving than the higher-fat version
Lean	Less than 10 g of fat, 4 g of saturated fat, and 95 mg of cholesterol per serving
Extra lean	Less than 5 g of fat, 2 g of saturated fat, and 95 mg of cholesterol per serving
Low in saturated fat	1 g saturated fat (or less) per serving and not more than 15% of calories from saturated fatty acids
Saturated fat free	Less than 0.5 g saturated fat for a given reference amount, and no more than 0.5 g of trans fatty acids
Cholesterol free	Less than 2 mg of cholesterol and 2 g (or less) of saturated fat per serving
Low cholesterol	20 mg of cholesterol (or less) and 2 g of saturated fat (or less) per serving
Reduced cholesterol	At least 25% less cholesterol than the higher-cholesterol version, and 2 g (or less) of saturated fat per serving
Sodium free (no sodium)	Less than 5 mg of sodium per serving, and no sodium chloride (NaCl) in ingredients
Very low sodium	35 mg of sodium (or less) per serving
Low sodium	140 mg of sodium (or less) per serving
Light in sodium or lightly salted	At least 50% less sodium than the regular product
No salt added or unsalted	No salt added during processing
Reduced or less sodium	At least 25% less sodium per serving than the higher-sodium version
Sugar free	Less than 0.5 g of sugar per serving
High fiber	5 g of fiber (or more) per serving
Good source of fiber	2.5 to 4.9 g of fiber per serving
Gluten free	Not derived from wheat, rye, barley, or crossbreeds of these grains and does not contain more than 20 parts per million of gluten from added ingredients

total carbohydrates, sugars, fiber, and total protein—hasto be made available in writing upon request. Vending machine operators who own or operate 20 or more vending machines must disclose calorie content for certain items.

While not required to be on a product label, most packaged foods carry a **date label**, distinguished by the words "Sell by," "Use by," "Best by," or "Best Used by." Most consumers interpret a date label as "use it by that time or expose yourself and your family to a health risk." This interpretation is incorrect. Date labels are not expiration dates for health reasons, except for infant formula; there are no U.S. standards for date markings on food product labels. Generally, they refer to the manufacturer's or a store's assessment of when the product is at peak quality. In a few states and in some countries, date labels have a specific meaning by law, but rarely do they indicate a health risk.

Besides date labels, packaged and canned foods can carry strings of numbers and letters and very specific dates. These are codes that refer to when the product was manufactured. They enable manufacturers and retailers to rotate their stock as well as locate their products in the event of a recall.

Because people misinterpret the dates on products to mean "no longer safe," they tend not to buy them even if they are still safe to consume after the sell by date. Manufacturers and retailers remove the products, thus contributing to the wasting of 15% to 20% of the country's food supply. The average American family of four wastes more than $1,500 worth of food per year (see the Dollars & Health Sense box, "Ways to Reduce Food Waste"). In 2017, the major food manufacturers announced that they will follow U.S. Department of Agriculture guidelines to apply only one date label, "Best if Used By/Before," to indicate when a product will be of best flavor or quality. It is not a purchase or safety date.

The Three Functions of Food

Food has three functions:
1. To provide the chemical constituents of the body
2. To provide the energy for life
3. To be pleasurable, including satisfying hunger; being appealing in its smell, taste, sight, and texture; and being associated with enjoyable social activities

TERMS

date label: a manufacturer's or a store's assessment of when a food product is at peak quality; not related to when the product poses a potential health risk

ingredients label: label on a manufactured food that lists the ingredients in descending order by weight

Nutrition Facts label: label on a manufactured food that lists the quantity of certain nutrients in the food and the percent daily value for those nutrients

percent daily value (PDV): percentage of the recommended daily amount of a particular nutrient found in a food

Providing Chemical Constituents

Your body is made up of billions of atoms and molecules arranged in particular combinations and proportions. Most of the atoms and molecules that now make up your body were not part of you even a few weeks ago because living things continually exchange their chemical constituents with the environment. The food you consume provides your body with replacement chemicals, which are utilized to manufacture the biological substances that make you *you*. Your body can manufacture most of the chemicals it needs, but it cannot manufacture 40 of them. These are called the **essential nutrients** (**Table 5.4**). Failure to obtain adequate amounts of any essential nutrient can result in weakness, ill-health, or a deficiency disease such as goiter from lack of iodine. Inadequate intake of vitamin A is the most common cause of blindness in children worldwide (World Health Organization, 2016).

Researchers have determined the daily amount of the essential and other nutrients consistent with good health. Many countries and the World Health Organization have produced dietary recommendations based on this research. In the United States, these recommendations, called **Dietary Reference Intakes**, or **DRIs**, are issued by the Food and Nutrition Board of the National Academy of Science's Institute of Medicine (U.S. Department of Agriculture, 2017). DRIs are issued for men and women in reasonably good health, pregnant

Table 5.4

The Essential Nutrients*

Amino acids	Fats	Water	Vitamins	Minerals
Isoleucine	Linoleic acid		Ascorbic acid (vitamin C)	Calcium
Leucine	Linolenic acid		Biotin	Chlorine
Lysine			Cobalamin (vitamin B$_{12}$)	Chromium
Methionine			Folic acid	Cobalt
Phenylalanine			Niacin (vitamin B$_3$)	Copper
Threonine			Pantothenic acid	Iodine
Tryptophan			Pyridoxine (vitamin B$_6$)	Iron
Valine			Riboflavin (vitamin B$_2$)	Magnesium
Arginine[†]			Thiamine (vitamin B$_1$)	Manganese
Histidine[†]			Vitamin A	Molybdenum
			Vitamin D	Phosphorus
			Vitamin E	Potassium
			Vitamin K	Selenium
				Sodium
				Sulfur
				Zinc

*Must be obtained from food.
[†]Not essential for adults; needed for growth in children.

Ways to Reduce Food Waste

Plan

Make a weekly menu. Prepare a shopping list noting how many meals you'll make with each item and buy no more than what you expect to use. Keep a list of meals and their ingredients that you enjoy. Avoid buying foods you already have. Buying in bulk is thrifty only if you use the food before it spoils.

Store

Store fruits and vegetables for maximum freshness. Freeze, preserve, or can surplus fruits and vegetables. To slow ripening, store bananas, apples, and tomatoes by themselves, and store fruits and vegetables in different bins. Wash berries prior to eating to prevent mold.

Prep

Wash, dry, chop, dice, slice, and place fresh food items in clear storage containers soon after shopping for use later in the week. Prep and freeze meals ahead of time. Freeze bread, sliced fruit, or meat you know won't eat soon.

Save Money

Cook or eat what you already have at home before buying more (soups, casseroles, stir fries, sauces, baked goods, pancakes, or smoothies). Use the edible parts of food that you normally do not eat (stale bread for croutons, sautéed beet tops, vegetable scraps for stock). Have "eat the leftovers" night each week. At restaurants, order only what you can finish; be aware of side dishes included with entrees; take home the leftovers for your next meal.

Divert from Landfills

Donate to food banks nutritious, safe, and untouched food. Compost food scraps rather than throw them away.

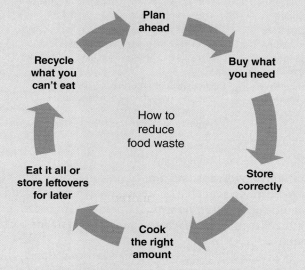

Data from U.S. Environmental Protection Agency. (2017). Reducing food waste at home. Retrieved from https://www.epa.gov/recycle/reducing-wasted-food-home.

Table 5.5

Examples of Daily Reference Intakes (DRIs)

Nutrient	Recommended Daily Intake 21-year-old female*	21-year-old male**
Carbohydrate	277–400 g	319–461 g
Total fiber	25 g	38 g
Protein	47 g	60 g
Linoleic acid	Low with adequate diet	17 g
Saturated fatty acids	As low as possible while consuming a nutritionally adequate diet	
Dietary cholesterol	As low as possible while consuming a nutritionally adequate diet	
Total water***	2.7 L (about 11 cups)	3.7 L (about 16 cups)
Vitamin A	700 mcg	900 mcg
Vitamin C	75 mg	90 mg
Vitamin D	15 mcg	15 mcg
Vitamin B_6	1 mg	1 mg
Vitamin E	15 mg	15 mg
Vitamin K	90 mcg	120 mcg
Vitamin B_{12}	2 mcg	2 mcg
Thiamin	1 mg	1 mg
Riboflavin	1 mg	1 mg
Folate	400 mcg	400 mcg
Niacin	14 mg	16 mg
Choline	425 mg	550 mg
Pantothenic acid	5 mg	5 mg
Biotin	30 mcg	30 mcg
Calcium	1,000 mg	1,000 mg
Chloride	2.3 g	2.3 g
Chromium	25 mcg	35 mcg
Copper	900 mcg	900 mcg
Fluoride	3 mg	4 mg
Iodine	150 mcg	150 mcg
Iron	18 mg	8 mg
Magnesium	310 mg	400 mg
Manganese	1.8 mg	1.8 mg
Molybdenum	45 mcg	45 mcg
Phosphorus	700 mg	700 mg
Potassium	4.7 g	4.7 g
Selenium	55 mcg	55 mcg
Sodium	1.5 g	1.5 g
Zinc	11 mg	8 mg

g = gram; mcg = microgram; mg = milligram

* Female: height = 5 feet 5 inches, weight = 140 pounds, Body Mass Index = 23.4, Estimated Energy Requirement = 2,204 Cal/da

** Male: height = 5 feet 9 inches, weight = 165 pounds, Body Mass Index = 24.5, Estimated Energy Requirement = 2,835 Cal/da

*** Total water = water from food, beverages, and drinking water

Nutrients not included in the table: carotenoids, arsenic, boron, nickel, silicon, sulfate, vanadium

Reproduced from U.S. Department of Agriculture, National Agricultural Library, Interactive DRI for Health Professionals. Retrieved from: www.nal.usda.gov/fnic/interactiveDRI/index.php

and lactating women, and children (**Table 5.5**). The DRIs are derived from the following:

- Recommended Dietary Allowance (RDA): The average daily level of intake established by research that is sufficient to meet the nutrient requirements for 97% to 98% of healthy individuals.
- Adequate Intake (AI): The intake level of a nutrient estimated to ensure nutritional adequacy when scientific evidence is insufficient to state an RDA.

TERMS

Dietary Reference Intakes (DRIs): recommended nutrient intakes intended to prevent chronic diseases

essential nutrients: chemical substances obtained from food and needed by the body for growth, maintenance, or repair of tissues; not made by the body; must be obtained from food

Power Up! Do Breakfast

Even if you get by on only a few hours of sleep, when you wake up it has still been 5, 10, or even more hours since you last ate. Your biological gas tank is nearly empty. If you're like many other students, as soon as you get out of bed you get ready to face the day and dash out the door without eating breakfast.

Yes, you could get a wake-up jolt from stopping en route for a pastry and a sweetened, caffeinated coffee drink. This is not the best option. In a couple of hours you'll be hungry because all that sugar got metabolized and you'll be drowsy from low blood sugar and the caffeine wearing off.

Better to start the day by powering up your body and mind with a few hundred calories of nutritious food so you can function maximally right out of the gate. It doesn't have to be a big, sit-down breakfast of OJ and bacon and eggs or pancakes and sausage, although that'll work. You can do fine with investing 10 minutes to gobble down a whole-grain food (oatmeal, whole wheat toast, or bagel), a piece of fruit or 100% juice (none of the sugary stuff), and some protein (milk or yogurt). If you can't find 10 minutes, pack up some healthy items the night before and grab-and-go as you head out the door. That way you'll get the slow-release energy provided by the complex carbs in the whole-wheat foods and be better able to function physically, mentally, and emotionally to the max from the vitamins, minerals, and amino acids from the fruit and protein.

- Tolerable Upper Intake Level (UL): The daily amount of a nutrient above which the risk of adverse health effects occurs.
- Estimated Average Requirement (EAR): An amount of a nutrient that is estimated to meet the requirement of 50% of the healthy individuals in a group.

For almost all nutrients, the DRI is the basis for Daily Value (DV) on a commercial food's Nutrition Facts label.

Many Americans overconsume DRI amounts of sodium (salt) and saturated fat and underconsume DRI amounts of calcium, magnesium, vitamin A, vitamin C, vitamin D, vitamin E, folate, potassium, and fiber (U.S. Department of Agriculture, 2015). In addition, many pregnant women do not consumer sufficient iron. You can determine your personal DRI at the USDA website (https://www.nal.usda.gov/fnic/interactiveDRI/). You can see how your usual diet conforms to DRI recommendations by keeping a food diary (see Workbook Chapter 5) and analyzing it with USDA's FoodTracker (https://www.supertracker.usda.gov/foodtracker.aspx).

Energy for Life

Food also provides energy to the body. The ultimate source of energy for complex organisms is sunlight, which is captured by green plants and converted to chemical energy that is stored as plant material. When humans eat plant matter or tissue from plant-eating animals, they obtain this stored chemical energy. Biological energy is used most efficiently when liberated in the presence of oxygen, which is one reason you breathe. In the process, the food material is converted to carbon dioxide, water, and other waste products and eliminated from the body in expired air, urine, feces, and sweat.

Energy transformations in living things are discussed in terms of calories. A **calorie** is the amount of heat energy required to raise 1 gram of water from 14.5°C to 15.5°C. A **nutritional calorie**, which is what weight watchers watch, is 1,000 calories, or a **kilocalorie**. Discussions of human nutrition and physical fitness frequently use the word *calorie* when actually referring to a kilocalorie. This text follows the same convention.

Nutrients can be grouped into six categories: carbohydrates, fats, proteins, vitamins, minerals, and water. Of these groups, fats and carbohydrates are the major forms of food energy. Fats provide 9 calories of energy per gram of fat, and carbohydrates provide 4 calories of energy per gram of carbohydrate. Although protein is capable of supplying 4 calories of energy per gram, its primary functions are to provide the body's architecture and to carry out maintenance functions. Virtually every cell in the body is capable of the series of chemical transformations necessary to extract chemical energy from these nutrient molecules. The biological process of deriving energy and obtaining material for the manufacture of cellular molecules is called **metabolism**.

Alcohol supplies about 7 calories per gram. This means a standard mixed drink, a beer, or a glass of wine has about 120 to 150 calories. Consuming two to three drinks every day without a compensatory reduction in food calories or an increase in exercise can lead to an increase in body weight. Yes, a beer belly can actually be a beer belly.

Estimating Your Daily Calorie Needs

Step 1: What is your height?
I am _____ feet _____ inches tall.

Step 2: How many body mass units do you have? Calculate them this way:
Women: Allow 100 body mass units for first 5 feet of height + 5 body mass units for each additional inch.
Men: Allow 106 body mass units for first 5 feet of height and 6 body mass units for each additional inch.
My total body mass units = _____

Step 3: What is your activity factor?
Sedentary = 13
Active = 15
Very active = 17

Step 4: What is your estimated daily calorie need?
Multiply your body mass units by your activity factor = _____

Energy is needed to support three major processes, (1) **basal** (or resting) **metabolism**, which is the energy required to keep the body alive; (2) physical activity, the things you do when you're not completely at rest; and (3) growth and repair. The energy to support basal metabolism keeps cells functioning, maintains the body temperature within its normal limits, and keeps the heart, lungs, kidneys, and other internal organs functioning. The daily amount of energy required to support basal metabolism is called the **basal metabolic rate (BMR)**, or resting metabolic rate (RMR). The BMR for adult women is about 1,100 calories per day, and for adult men it is 1,300 calories per day.

In addition to the energy you need for basal metabolism, you use energy in physical activity: walking, running, working, and so on. The amount of energy expended for these activities depends on how strenuous the activity is, how long it is engaged in, the body's size, and the environmental temperature. It takes more energy to be active in hot weather than in moderate temperatures, and it takes more energy to maintain body temperature when the weather is cold.

Energy is also needed whenever the body produces more cells than are needed to replace ones that periodically die. Thus, all young people need additional energy for growth. Energy is also needed to produce new cells to repair wounds and injuries.

Energy requirements for individuals vary depending on body size and composition, physical activity, growth needs during adolescence and young adulthood, pregnancy or breastfeeding status, and injury or illness. The DRI for adult American men is about 2,800 calories per day; for nonpregnant, nonlactating adult American women, it is about 2,300. Nutritionists recommend that carbohydrates from whole grains, vegetables, and fruits be the principal source of energy, supplying about 50% of total calories consumed. Fats should make up no more than 30% of total calories consumed. Protein is generally not recommended as a source of energy but only as a source of building blocks for the body's tissues and organs.

People who are interested in weight management need to keep in mind that a large percentage of daily energy is required just to stay alive. That's why cutting back on food (energy) is a limited and generally unsuccessful strategy for weight management. All successful weight management focuses on the physical activity portion of energy use. That's something you can increase that will consume energy without affecting basic life functions.

Pleasures of Eating

Everyone has experienced the feeling of hunger and its appeasement by eating something. But hunger is not the only reason for eating. Most of the time we eat because it is "time to eat," because we have been presented with food, because it feels good to be eating something—especially something fatty or sweet—or because eating is an enjoyable social ritual. The ready availability of food is unique to modern societies; a hundred years ago there were no supermarkets, fast-food restaurants, or convenience stores on every block. Thus, we can consume food for a variety of reasons. Also, advertising encourages us to eat more, and often products that aren't particularly healthy.

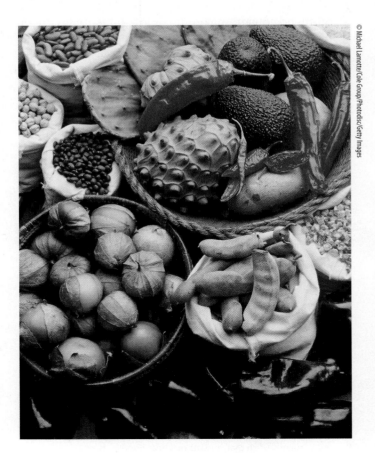

Natural, unprocessed foods provide the best nutrition.

© Michael Lamotte/Cole Group/Photodisc/Getty Images

TERMS

basal metabolic rate (BMR): the amount of energy needed to keep the body functioning while at rest

basal metabolism: the minimum amount of energy needed to keep the body alive

calorie: the amount of energy required to raise 1 g of water from 14.5°C to 15.5°C

kilocalorie: unit of energy; the amount of heat needed to raise 1 kilogram of water 1°C, equivalent to 1,000 calories

metabolism: the process of obtaining energy and matter from the chemical breakdown of molecules obtained from food or from the body

nutritional calorie: unit of energy; often used interchangeably with the term *kilocalorie*

The Seven Components of Food

Food is composed of seven kinds of chemical substances: proteins, carbohydrates, lipids (fats), vitamins, minerals, phytochemicals, and water. Dietary proteins, most types of carbohydrates, and most lipids cannot be used by the body until they are broken down in the digestive system into smaller chemical units (**Figure 5.7**). In fact, only vitamins, minerals, a few kinds of carbohydrates, phytochemicals, and water are absorbed into the body as is.

Proteins

About 20% of your body mass is **protein**. Much of the body's structural components and many of its vital functions are carried out by proteins.

Proteins are made up of chemical units called **amino acids**, which come in 20 different forms. Amino acids are classified as **essential** and **nonessential**. Adults require eight essential amino acids; those eight and two others are required by infants. Animal sources of protein include milk and milk products, meat, fish, poultry, and eggs. Plant sources include breads and cereal products, legumes, nuts, and seeds. The body can transform essential amino acids to nonessential ones as needed.

Amino acids are not stored in the body in any appreciable amounts; therefore, proper nutrition requires eating enough high-quality protein just about every day to meet the body's needs for essential amino acids. The recommended consumption of protein for adult women is 46 grams per day and adult men about 55 grams.

A hamburger patty has about 20 grams of protein. The average North American adult consumes about twice the recommended amount; the unneeded protein is broken down by the body and excreted in urine or stored as fat.

Because the amino acid composition of most animal protein is similar, people tend to acquire adequate amounts and proportions of the essential amino acids from animal tissue, such as fish, meat, eggs, and dairy products. Most vegetable proteins, however, are deficient in one or more of the essential amino acids, so individuals who eat little or no meat or dairy products must eat foods in which an amino acid deficiency in one food is compensated for by an amino acid surplus in another. For example, wheat, rice, and oats contain very little of the essential amino acid lysine but have large amounts of the essential amino acids methionine and tryptophan. Soybeans and other legumes are relatively high in lysine but are low in methionine and tryptophan. Meals consisting of both grains and legumes (e.g., rice and beans, corn and beans, wheat and soybeans) can supply adequate amounts of these essential amino acids. **Protein complementarity** is the practice of combining sources of protein such that amino acid deficiencies in one source are counterbalanced, or *complemented*, by abundances in another source.

Meat, dairy products, and eggs provide the essential amino acids, but they can be high in saturated fat, and thus contribute to heart disease, cancer, and other fat-related health problems. For this reason, nutritionists recommend consuming nonfat or low-fat dairy products, using butter as a spread and not as an ingredient for cooking, and being mindful of the amount of ice cream eaten. Nutritionists also favor trimming fat from meat before cooking, selecting meat with a low fat content, and eating poultry (with skin removed because it contains fat) and fish, which have proportionately less fat than red meats. They also recommend using meat sparingly by adding it

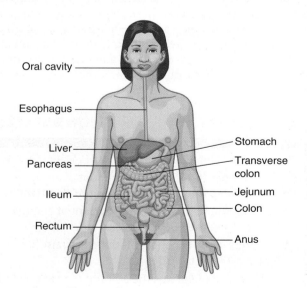

■ Figure 5.7

Human Digestive System
Teeth and glandular secretions in the mouth help break up food, which the esophagus transports to the stomach. The stomach breaks down some of the food molecules and passes the food to the rest of the digestive tube: the duodenum, jejunum, ileum, colon, and rectum. The pancreas secretes enzymes and fluid into the duodenum to help the digestive process. The liver controls the release of absorbed nutrients into the body. Undigested material is eliminated from the body at the anus.

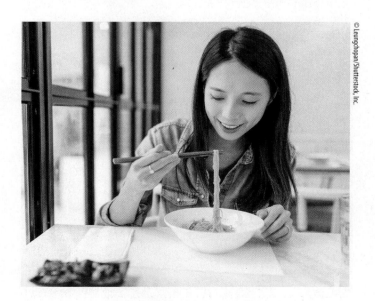

© Leungchopan/Shutterstock, Inc.

Ramen, a Japanese dish that consists of wheat noodles, is a healthy alternative to eating fatty fast food.

to grain- or bean-based dishes, rather than making it the center of the meal.

A small but measurable association has been found between the regular consumption of red meat and processed meats and the risk of developing colorectal cancer (Alexander, 2015), the third most commonly diagnosed cancer and the fourth-leading cause of cancer death in the world. Consuming fish or chicken do not increase the risk of death from colon cancer. Red meat includes beef, veal, pork, lamb, mutton, horse, and goat. *Processed meat* refers to meat that has been transformed through salting, curing, fermentation, smoking, or other methods to enhance flavor or improve preservation. Most processed meats contain pork or beef; some may contain other red meats, poultry, offal, or meat by-products, such as blood. Examples of processed meat include hot dogs (frankfurters), ham, sausages, corned beef, and biltong or beef jerky, as well as canned meat and meat-based preparations and sauces.

Scientists do not know the reason(s) for the observed association of meat and processed meat consumption and cancer but offer the following plausible explanations: (1) cooking (especially charring) meat can produce cancer-causing agents called heterocyclic amines (HCAs), which harm the colon; (2) when red and processed meats are at the center of the diet, they replace vegetables and legumes (beans), so the variety of healthful nutrients found in plants is not consumed; (3) bacteria in the colon convert substances necessary for the digestion of fats (bile acids) into cancer-causing agents; (4) nitrates and nitrate chemicals (*N-nitroso compounds*, or *NOCs*) used as preservatives in processed meats can damage DNA in colon cells, resulting in an increased risk of cancer (O'Keefe et al., 2016). Besides increasing the risk of colorectal cancer, meat consumption poses other risks to health. For example, meat is the vector for spongiform encephalopathy (mad cow disease) and other foodborne illnesses. High-intensity meat production also is detrimental to the environment. The production of 1 pound of meat requires 15,000 to 20,000 gallons of water. Cattle are fed corn and soy, the excess production of which degrades the land and introduces pesticides into the food supply. The methane produced by cattle digestive processes contributes significantly to global warming.

> Vegetables aren't my meat and potatoes.
>
> *Yogi Berra*

Athletes are often encouraged to consume more than the DRI of protein to increase endurance, body strength, and repair of injury, with emphasis on benefits from consuming protein around the time of muscular exertion. For athletes, the American Society of Sports Medicine and the Academy of Nutrition and Dietetics of Canada (2016) recommend intakes of 1.2 to 2.0 grams of high-quality protein per kilogram of body weight consumed on days of strenuous training and activity and on the day after. That protein can come from lean meat, fish, poultry, eggs, vegetables, grains, beans, and dairy. It is not necessary to consume protein powders or high-protein liquids. Regular food will do.

Carbohydrates

Carbohydrates are a major source of food energy and also are used to manufacture some cell components, such as the hereditary material *deoxyribonucleic acid (DNA)*. Because the body can manufacture them from other substances, carbohydrates are not considered essential nutrients. However, not eating enough carbohydrates, recommended by some ill-conceived reducing diets, can force the body to break down muscle tissue to supply energy necessary for life functions.

Most animals have a "sweet tooth" to motivate consumption of energy-rich foods, and humans are no exception. That's why food manufacturers often add sugars and other sweeteners (such as high-fructose corn syrup (HFCS)) to their products. Indeed, about 70% of packaged food products in the United States and Canada contain added sugar (Popkin & Hawkes, 2016). Because added sugar provides calories but no essential nutrients, sugar is usually described as contributing "empty calories" to the diet. Excess calories from added sugar are converted to body fat, which may contribute to overweight, obesity, heart disease, diabetes, and dental caries.

The average American adult consumes about 80 grams of added sugar per day. The American Heart Association recommends that adult men consume no more than 38 grams of added sugar per day and adult women and teens no more than 25 grams. A 12-ounce soda contains 46 grams of added sugar; a 16-ounce bottle of sweet tea contains 50 grams. A serving of bottled spaghetti sauce contains 12 grams.

TERMS

amino acids: compounds containing nitrogen that are the building blocks of protein

carbohydrates: biological substances composed of one or more sugar molecules

essential amino acids: amino acids that cannot be synthesized by the body and must be provided by food

nonessential amino acids: eleven amino acids synthesized by humans and are not required in the diet

protein: biological molecules composed of chains of amino acids

protein complementarity: combining sources of dietary protein such that amino acid deficiencies in one are counterbalanced by abundances in another

Taking Care of Your Teeth and Gums

Taking care of your teeth and gums means adopting practices for oral health that prevent tooth decay (dental caries) and gum disease (gingivitis and periodontitis). Tooth decay and gum disease are caused by the action of a variety of bacteria that live in the mouth, which produce acids by breaking down the sugars in food. The acids attack the enamel of teeth, causing tooth decay. Other bacteria are involved in the conversion of sugars and some of the material in saliva into a gelatinous substance called *plaque*, which sticks to teeth and gums and fosters more bacterial growth and decay.

Tooth and gum disease could be prevented if (1) the bacteria responsible could be removed from the mouth, (2) the sugars and other substances bacteria use to produce acids and plaque were removed from the mouth, or (3) teeth were protected from the bacterial products.

It is not yet possible to keep all tooth and gum disease–causing bacteria from the mouth or to render them harmless. So, keeping the mouth free of sugar and plaque is the best way to prevent tooth and gum problems. You can accomplish this by doing the following:

- Not eating sugar and sugar-containing foods between meals
- Consuming sweets in liquid rather than solid form when possible
- Avoiding sticky or slowly dissolving sweets
- Brushing teeth after each meal
- Rinsing the mouth with warm water when unable to brush after a snack or meal
- Obtaining fluoride (to increase resistance to tooth decay) from toothpastes, mouthwashes, and drinking water
- Getting periodic dental checkups

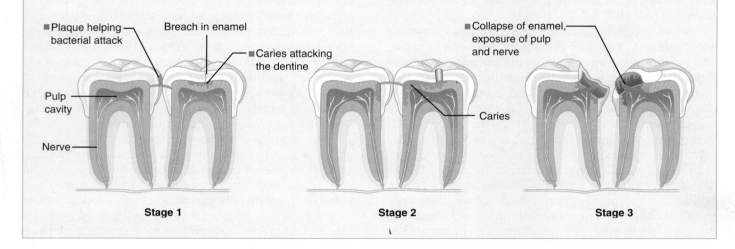

■Plaque helping bacterial attack

Breach in enamel

■Caries attacking the dentine

Pulp cavity

Nerve

Stage 1

■Collapse of enamel, exposure of pulp and nerve

Caries

Stage 2

Stage 3

The Nutrition Facts panel on a manufacured food product lists as "sugar" both the sugar that occurs naturally in the food and the sugar added by the manufacturer. Thus, consumers must do more work to determine the kinds and amounts of added sugar. A product's ingredients label lists all the forms of added sugar but not how much of each (**Figure 5.8**). The amount of added sugar requires consulting web sites that list such values.

Simple Sugars

There are two principal types of carbohydrates: **simple sugars**, found predominantly in fruit, and **complex carbohydrates**, found in grains, fruit, and the stems, leaves, and roots of vegetables.

Glucose is the most common simple sugar; it is found in all plants and animals. Glucose circulates in the bloodstream and is commonly referred to as "blood sugar." Another simple sugar is fructose, which is found in fruits and honey. **Fructose** is one of the sweetest sugars, which means you can eat less fructose than other simple sugars and taste an equivalent amount of sweetness.

Sucrose, which is common table sugar (the "refined" sugar added to many packaged foods), is a combination of glucose and fructose. Sucrose is digested by breaking apart the glucose and fructose portions. Because fructose is sweeter than sucrose, you can reduce the amount of sugar in your diet without cutting out sweet tastes by replacing pastries with fresh fruit and table sugar with honey. Besides more sweet taste, you will be gaining other nutrients in the fruit and honey that are not present in refined sucrose.

Lactose, a sugar found principally in milk and milk products, is made of the simple sugars glucose and galactose joined together. To free the glucose and galactose parts to provide energy for growth and development, lactose is broken apart in the digestive systems of nearly all babies by a protein called **lactase**. Following the genetic blueprint of early humans who did not domesticate cattle for milk production, in many peoples of the modern world the gene(s) responsible for making lactase in early life are permanently switched off in older children and adults (University of California, Berkeley, 2007). When these

Agave nectar	Date sugar	Molasses
	Dehydrated cane juice	Muscovado
Barbados sugar	Demerara sugar	
Barley malt	Dextrin	Palm sugar
Barley malt syrup	Dextrose	Panocha
Beet sugar		Powdered sugar
Brown sugar	Fructose	
Buttered syrup	Fruit juice concentrate	Raw sugar
		Refiner's syrup
Cane juice	Glucose	Rice syrup
Cane juice crystals		
Cane sugar	HFCS (high-fructose corn syrup)	Saccharose
Caramel	Honey	Sorghum syrup
Carob syrup		Sucrose
Caster sugar	Icing sugar	Sugar (granulated)
Coconut palm sugar	Invert sugar	Sweet sorghum
Coconut sugar		Syrup
Confectioner's sugar	Malt sugar	
Corn sweetener	Maltodextrin	Treacle
Corn syrup	Maltol	Turbinado sugar
Corn syrup solids	Maltose	
	Mannose	Yellow sugar
	Maple syrup	

■ **Figure 5.8**
Names for Sugars Added to Commercial Foods

individuals consume milk, cream, ice cream, or other milk products, they experience gastrointestinal upset, diarrhea, and, occasionally, severe illness. These individuals can supplement their diets with products containing lactase (e.g., Lactaid) or by eating yogurt, cheese, and other dairy products in which the lactose has been broken down by the fermentation process. Because dairy products are a major source of calcium in the North American diet, people who avoid dairy products should consume calcium-rich vegetables (e.g., broccoli and peas), calcium-fortified foods, and possibly take calcium supplements.

Complex Carbohydrates

Complex carbohydrates come primarily from grains (wheat, rice, corn, oats, barley); legumes (peas, beans); the leaves, stems, and roots of plants; and some animal tissue. There are two main classes of complex carbohydrates: **starch**, which is digestible, and **fiber**, which is not digestible.

Starch consists of many glucose molecules linked together. It is a way organisms store glucose efficiently until it is needed. In plants, starch is usually contained in granules within seeds, pods, or roots. Wheat flour, for example, is made by crushing wheat grain, which separates the outer husk (the bran) from the middle, starch-containing portion (the endosperm) and the inner germ. The white flour commonly used in baking is "70% extraction," which means that 70% of the original grain remains after crushing. In the milling of 70% extraction flour, many nutrients in the wheat grain are lost, so flour manufacturers add back several vitamins and minerals to produce "enriched flour." A "whole-grain flour," on the other hand, is 90% to 95% extraction and does not have to be enriched. Bread made with whole-wheat flour is brown, but not all brown bread is whole-wheat bread because some manufacturers add molasses or honey to white-flour dough to

give it a brown color. **Gluten** is a mixture of proteins that occur naturally in wheat, rye, barley, and crossbreeds of these grains. Several million people in North America and many more in the world can become ill when they consume gluten either because of a genetic predisposition to a condition called *celiac disease* or some other gluten-related condition that damages the lining of the small

TERMS

complex carbohydrates: a class of carbohydrates called polysaccharides; foods composed of starch and cellulose

fiber: a group of compounds that make up the framework of plants; fiber cannot be digested

fructose: a simple sugar found in fruits and honey

glucose: the principal source of energy in all cells; also called dextrose

gluten: a mixture of proteins that occur naturally in wheat, rye, barley and crossbreeds of these grains, which can damage the small intestine

lactase: enzyme secreted by glands in the small intestine that converts lactose (milk sugar) into simple sugars

lactose: a sugar formed by glucose and galactose chemically bonded together; found primarily in milk

simple sugars: a class of carbohydrates called monosaccharides; all carbohydrates must be reduced to simple sugars to be digested

starch: complex chain of glucose molecules

sucrose: common refined table sugar; a molecule of glucose and a molecule of fructose chemically bonded together

intestine. Without a healthy intestinal lining, the body cannot absorb needed nutrients, possibly resulting in anemia (a lower than normal number of red blood cells), growth retardation, infertility, miscarriages, short stature, osteoporosis (a disease in which bones become fragile and more likely to break), diabetes, autoimmune thyroid disease, and intestinal cancers. To aid consumers who are at risk for gluten-related illness, the words "gluten-free" on a food label or restaurant menu mean it has less than 20 parts per million of gluten. Keep in mind that "gluten free" does not necessarily mean healthier for people who are not sensitive to gluten. A gluten-free food product can still have a paucity of nutrients.

Starch is also found in potatoes, which have an undeserved reputation for being fattening. Potatoes are no more fattening than any other starchy food unless they are cooked in large amounts of fat or oil, which is used in making french fries and potato chips. One large potato has about 100 calories, less than a medium-sized soft drink. French fries made from a medium potato, however, contain over 300 calories.

Animals and humans produce a starch in muscle and liver tissue called **glycogen**. When energy is needed, the glycogen breaks down and its constituent glucose molecules are liberated. Athletes sometimes eat large quantities of carbohydrates the day before competition to build up their supply of glycogen, a practice known as *carbohydrate loading*.

Fiber is the second main class of complex carbohydrates. There are two kinds of fiber: **insoluble fiber**, which cannot dissolve in water, and **soluble fiber**, which can. Insoluble fiber is made up of **cellulose** and **hemicellulose**, substances that offer rigidity to plant material (wood; stems; the outer coverings of nuts, seeds, grains; the peels and skins of fruits and vegetables). Soluble fiber is composed of pectins, gums, and mucilages. The differences in insoluble and soluble fiber are not significant for health. Nutritionists recommend that individuals consume 20 to 35 grams of fiber daily, regardless of its type (**Table 5.6**).

Fiber adds bulk to the feces, thereby preventing constipation and related disorders, such as hemorrhoids and hiatal hernia, which can result from prolonged increase in intra-abdominal pressure while defecating. Fiber also facilitates the transport of waste material through the digestive tract, lessening the risk of appendicitis, diverticular disease (out-pocketings in the wall of the lower intestine), and cancer of the colon and rectum. High-fiber diets may also help to lessen the risk of heart disease and some cancers.

Because they contain complex carbohydrates, fiber, vitamins, and other nutrients, whole-grain foods are superior to manufactured and restaurant foods composed of refined grains (**Table 5.7**). Moreover, consumption of foods made of refined flour, which are nutritionally inferior, means that healthy whole-grain foods will not be consumed.

Table 5.6

Fiber Content of Various Foods

Food	Amount	Fiber (g)
Whole-wheat bread	1 slice	1.6
Rye bread	1 slice	1.0
White bread	1 slice	0.6
Brown rice (cooked)	½ cup	2.4
White rice (cooked)	½ cup	0.1
Spaghetti (cooked)	½ cup	0.8
Kidney beans (cooked)	½ cup	5.8
Lima beans (cooked)	½ cup	4.9
Potato (baked)	Medium	3.8
Corn	½ cup	3.9
Spinach	½ cup	2.0
Lettuce	½ cup	0.3
Strawberries	¾ cup	2.0
Banana	Medium	2.0
Apple (with skin)	Medium	2.6
Orange	Small	1.2

Extensive data for fiber in foods:

Dietary Fiber Chart: http://www.wehealny.org/healthinfo/dietaryfiber/fibercontentchart.html

Fiber Content Calculator: http://www.globalrph.com/fiber_content.htm

USDA Nutritional Data Lab: http://www.nal.usda.gov/fnic/foodcomp/search/

Some foods contain fortified or functional fiber (sometimes referred to as "fake fiber"), which is not actual plant fiber but chemicals extracted from plants or manufactured in factories. Manufacturers add these substances to their food products in order to augment sales by making "high-fiber" claims. Generally, functional fiber is found in highly processed foods such as white bread, yogurt, ice cream, sugary cereals, energy bars, and even juices and waters. Even though it has little nutritive value, functional fiber can be counted in the total fiber listed on the Nutrition Facts label and listed on the product's ingredients label as inulin, pectin, polydextrose, methylcellulose, and/or maltodextrin. Examples of natural fiber listed on the ingredients label are wheat bran, corn bran, and oats.

Lipids (Fats)

Lipids are a diverse group of substances that have the common chemical property of not readily mixing or dissolving in water. Some of these substances include **cholesterol** and **lecithin**, which are essential constituents of cell membranes; the steroid hormones produced by the reproductive organs and adrenal glands; vitamins A, D, E, and K; and bile acids, which aid the digestion of fats. Despite the current anti-fat trend, lipids are an essential part of the diet. They supply calories, provide flavor and texture to food, and during digestion provide feelings of satiety and well-being. One kind of fat, **linoleic acid**, found in vegetable oils such as safflower, sunflower, and corn, is

Table 5.7

Whole-Grain and Refined-Grain Foods

Whole-grain foods	Refined-grain foods
Brown rice	Cornbread*
Buckwheat	Corn tortillas*
Bulgur (cracked wheat)	Couscous*
Oatmeal	Crackers*
Popcorn	Flour tortillas
	Grits
Ready-to-eat breakfast cereals	
Whole-wheat cereal flakes	*Pasta**
Muesli	Noodles*
Whole-grain barley	Spaghetti
Whole-grain cornmeal	Macaroni
Whole rye	Pitas*
Whole-wheat bread	Pretzels
Whole-wheat crackers	
Whole-wheat pasta	*Ready-to-eat breakfast cereals*
Whole-wheat sandwich	Corn flakes
buns and rolls	White bread
Whole-wheat tortillas	White sandwich buns and rolls
Wild rice	White rice
Less common whole grains	
Amaranth	
Millet	
Quinoa	
Sorghum	
Triticale	

Note: Whole-grain foods contain the entire grain kernel: bran, germ, and endosperm. Refined-grain foods are foods in which the bran and germ are removed to produce a finer texture and longer shelf life; the refining process removes fiber, iron, and many B vitamins. Most refined grains are enriched; certain B vitamins (thiamin, riboflavin, niacin, folic acid) and iron are added back after processing. Fiber is not added back. Some food products are made from mixtures of whole grains and refined grains. Some grain products contain significant amounts of bran. Bran provides fiber, which is important for health. However, products with added bran or bran alone (e.g., oat bran) are not necessarily whole-grain products.

*Most of these products are made from refined grains. Some are made from whole grains. Check the ingredients list for the words "whole grain" or "whole wheat" to decide if they are made from a whole grain. Some foods are made from a mixture of whole and refined grains.

Modified from U.S. Department of Agriculture. (2017). What foods are in the grains group? Retrieved from http://www.choosemyplate.gov/grains

A saturated fatty acid carries all the hydrogen atoms it can. A monounsaturated fatty acid (MUFA) carries one less than all the hydrogen atoms it possibly could. A polyunsaturated fatty acid lacks two or more hydrogen atoms. A dietary fat is classified as saturated, monounsaturated, or polyunsaturated depending on the type of fatty acids it contains in greatest quantity.

Saturated fats are found in whole milk and products made from whole milk; egg yolks; meat; meat fat; coconut and palm oils; chocolate; regular margarine; and hydrogenated vegetable shortenings. Sources of monounsaturated fats include olive oil and some nuts. Polyunsaturated fats are found in safflower, cottonseed, corn, soybean, and sesame seed oils, and fatty fish (**Figure 5.9**).

Diets high in saturated fat increase the risk of heart disease, some cancers, and overweight. Dietary guidelines recommend that adults saturated fat intake be 10% or less of total calories. Conversely, polyunsaturated fats tend to lessen the risk of heart and blood vessel disease, which is why nutritionists recommend consuming vegetable oils, nuts, and fish.

TERMS

cellulose: a carbohydrate forming the skeleton of most plant structures and plant cells; the most abundant polysaccharide in nature and the source of dietary fiber

cholesterol: a fatlike compound occurring in bile, blood, brain, nerve tissue, liver, and other parts of the body

fatty acids: naturally occurring in fats, either saturated or unsaturated (monounsaturated or polyunsaturated)

glycogen: the form in which carbohydrate is stored in humans and animals

hemicellulose: substances found in plant cell walls that are composed of various sugars chemically linked together

insoluble fiber: cannot be dissolved in water

lecithin: an essential component of cell membranes

linoleic acid: an essential fat that must be obtained from food

lipids: fats such as cholesterol and triglycerides

monounsaturated fatty acid: carries one less than all the hydrogen atoms it possibly could

polyunsaturated fatty acid: carries at least two fewer hydrogen atoms than it would if saturated

saturated fat: generally solid at room temperature; comes from animal sources

soluble fiber: can be dissolved in water

triglyceride: dietary fat composed of fatty acids

essential, and must be obtained in food. Deficiencies in this substance can produce skin lesions.

Much of the fat consumed in the diet is **triglyceride**, which is composed of **fatty acids**. These substances are further classified as **saturated**, **monounsaturated**, or **polyunsaturated**, depending on their chemistry. Saturation refers to the number of hydrogen atoms (and therefore the amount of energy) contained in a fatty acid.

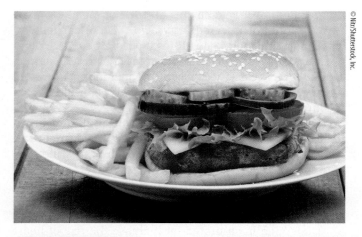

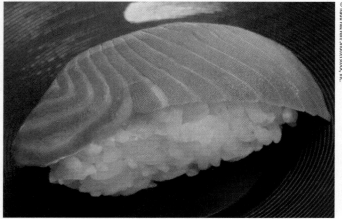

■ **Figure 5.9**

Unhealthy and Healthy Fats

Trans and saturated fats in fast and packaged food are less healthy than polyunsaturated fats found in fish, nuts, and vegetable oils.

Food manufacturers and restaurants sometimes use chemicals derived from vegetable oils called **trans fatty acids**, trans fats or, *partially hydrogenated vegetable oils* (PHVO). Because trans fats are unhealthy, many food product manufacturers and restaurants no longer use them. Certain trans fats are components of natural foods, and because some manufacturers use them in small quantities, the total amount of trans fat is listed on a product's Nutrition Facts label. Many countries have legally banned PHVO from their food supply. The U.S. Food and Drug Administration has banned all use of PHVO in the American food supply.

Fat substitutes ("Simplesse") are chemicals added primarily to packaged pastries, snack foods, sour cream, yogurt, and salad dressings to provide the taste and texture of fat without contributing calories. The purported benefit of fat substitutes that they contribute to weight management—apparently is overstated because consumers tend to compensate for the lack of energy derived from fat by ingesting greater amounts of carbohydrates.

Vitamins

Vitamins are substances that facilitate a variety of biological processes. Vitamins do not provide building blocks for the manufacture of the body's tissues nor do they provide calories to fuel the body's functions. Instead, like working on an assembly line, they carry out the same tasks over and over again until they "wear out" and need to be replaced. This is why the body requires much smaller amounts of vitamins than it does proteins, carbohydrates, and fats. The body requires 13 essential vitamins; they must be obtained from food (**Table 5.8**). Vitamins are classified as **water-soluble** or **fat-soluble**, depending on their chemistry.

Vitamins A (and its dietary precursor, beta-carotene), C, and E are classed as **antioxidants** because they have the capacity to neutralize the effects of chemicals called *free radicals,* which can damage biological structures via chemical oxidation. Antioxidant vitamins are found in a variety of fruits and vegetables (not beans) and can be obtained in vitamin supplements. People who consume foods containing large amounts of antioxidant vitamins have less risk of cancer, heart disease, and cataracts than people who consume small amounts. However, in laboratory studies, antioxidant vitamins C, E, and beta-carotene have not been shown to prevent cancer or cataracts and in large doses may be harmful. This illustrates (once again) that healthy nutrition is a matter of consuming whole, fresh foods rather than large amounts of individual nutrients.

Folic acid (also called *folate* or *folacin*), a vitamin found in dark-green leafy vegetables, beans, and fruits, helps prevent spina bifida and other neural tube defects in newborn babies. The diets of most American women and elderly persons of both sexes are deficient in folic acid (on average, 200 micrograms per day are consumed; 400 micrograms are recommended), so the federal government requires that manufacturers of cereal-based foods (e.g., breads, breakfast cereals, pastas) fortify their products with it. There is debate whether the amount of folic acid in fortified foods is too low, so pregnant women are advised to ask their prenatal healthcare providers about taking folic acid supplements.

Some people are deficient in vitamin D, which is made in the skin in response to the action of sunlight. People who live in northern or southern latitudes, who have dark skin, or who remain indoors for most of the day are most at risk for low levels of vitamin D. Vitamin D helps the body absorb and retain calcium and phosphorus, thus fostering strong bones and teeth. Vitamin D also helps maintain muscle strength, especially in the elderly. It enables the body to fight infections and some cancers, and may lessen the risk of heart disease. Adequate levels of vitamin D can be obtained in light-skinned individuals through 15 minutes' exposure to midday sun; dark-skinned individuals may require more sun exposure. Most foods are naturally low in vitamin D, but adequate amounts can be obtained from food fortified with vitamin D or from vitamin D supplements.

Table 5.8

Water-Soluble and Fat-Soluble Vitamins

Water-soluble vitamin	Why needed?	Primary sources	Deficiency results in
Ascorbic acid (vitamin C)	Tooth and bone formation; production of connective tissue; promotion of wound healing; may enhance immunity	Citrus fruits, tomatoes, peppers, cabbage, potatoes, melons	Scurvy (degeneration of bones, teeth, and gums)
Biotin	Involved in fat and amino acid synthesis and breakdown	Yeast, liver, milk, most vegetables, bananas, grapefruit	Skin problems; fatigue; muscle pains; nausea
Cobalamin (vitamin B_{12})	Involved in single carbon atom transfers; essential for DNA synthesis	Muscle meats, eggs, milk, and dairy products (not in vegetables)	Pernicious anemia; nervous system malfunctions
Folacin (folic acid)	Essential for synthesis of DNA and other molecules	Green leafy vegetables, organ meats, whole-wheat products	Anemia; diarrhea and other gastrointestinal problems
Niacin	Involved in energy production and synthesis of cell molecules	Grains, meats, legumes	Pellagra (skin, gastrointestinal, and mental disorders)
Pantothenic acid	Involved in energy production and synthesis and breakdown of many biological molecules	Yeast, meats and fish, nearly all vegetables and fruits	Vomiting; abdominal cramps; malaise; insomnia
Pyridoxine (vitamin B_6)	Essential for synthesis and breakdown of amino acids and manufacture of unsaturated fats from saturated fats	Meats, whole grains, most vegetables	Weakness; irritability; trouble sleeping and walking; skin problems
Riboflavin (vitamin B_2)	Involved in energy production; important for health of the eyes	Milk and dairy foods, meats, eggs, vegetables, grains	Eye and skin problems
Thiamin (vitamin B_1)	Essential for breakdown of food molecules and production of energy	Meats, legumes, grains, some vegetables	Beri-beri (nerve damage, weakness, heart failure)
Fat-soluble vitamin	**Why needed?**	**Primary sources**	**Deficiency or excess results in**
Vitamin A (retinol)	Essential for maintenance of eyes and skin; influences bone and tooth formation	Liver, kidney, yellow and green leafy vegetables, apricots	Deficiency: night blindness; eye damage; skin dryness. Excess: loss of appetite; skin problems; swelling of ankles and feet
Vitamin D (calciferol)	Regulates calcium metabolism; important for growth of bones and teeth	Cod liver oil, dairy products, eggs	Deficiency: rickets (bone deformities) in children; bone destruction in adults. Excess: thirst; nausea; weight loss; kidney damage
Vitamin E (tocopherol)	Prevents damage to cells from oxidation; prevents red blood cell destruction	Wheat germ, vegetable oils, vegetables, egg yolk, nuts	Deficiency: anemia, possibly nerve cell destruction
Vitamin K (phylloquinone)	Helps with blood clotting	Liver, vegetable oils, green leafy vegetables, tomatoes	Deficiency: severe bleeding

Minerals

Many body functions require one or more inorganic elements called **minerals** (Table 5.9). Sodium, potassium, and chlorine, for example, are essential for maintaining cell membranes, conducting nerve impulses, and contracting muscles. Magnesium, copper, and cobalt facilitate certain biochemical reactions; iron is essential for the oxygen-carrying function of hemoglobin; iodine is needed to produce thyroid hormone; and calcium and phosphorus make up bones and teeth. Selenium may reduce the risk of cancer, perhaps because of its activity as an antioxidant.

Minerals are found in most foods, especially fresh vegetables. Women and young people are susceptible to iron deficiency, so they must eat iron-rich foods, such as eggs, lean meats, brans, whole grains, and green leafy vegetables. Most women and elderly people ingest too little calcium, which is found in dairy products and some green leafy vegetables such as broccoli and turnip greens

TERMS

antioxidants: substances that in small amounts inhibit the oxidation of other compounds

fat-soluble vitamins: soluble in fat; there are four fat-soluble vitamins

fat substitutes: chemicals added to packaged foods to provide the taste and texture of fat but few or no calories

minerals: inorganic elements found in the body both in combination with organic compounds and alone

trans fatty acid: also trans fat, an artificial fat manufactured by chemically modifying monounsaturated and polyunsaturated fatty acids

vitamins: essential organic substances needed daily in small amounts to perform specific functions in the body

water-soluble vitamins: soluble in water; there are nine water-soluble vitamins

Table 5.9

Essential Minerals

Mineral	Why needed?	Primary sources	Deficiency results in
Calcium	Bone and tooth formation; blood clotting; nerve transmission	Milk, cheese, dark-green vegetables, dried legumes	Stunted growth; rickets, osteoporosis; convulsions
Chlorine	Formation of gastric juice; acid–base balance	Common salt	Muscle cramps; mental apathy; reduced appetite
Chromium	Glucose and energy metabolism	Fats, vegetable oils, meats	Impaired ability to metabolize glucose
Cobalt	Constituent of vitamin B_{12}	Organ and muscle meats	Not reported in humans
Copper	Constituent of enzymes of iron metabolism	Meats, drinking water	Anemia (rare)
Iodine	Constituent of thyroid hormones	Marine fish and shellfish, dairy products, many vegetables	Goiter (enlarged thyroid)
Iron	Constituent of hemoglobin and enzymes of energy metabolism	Eggs, lean meats, legumes, whole grains, green leafy vegetables	Iron-deficiency anemia (weakness, reduced resistance to infection)
Magnesium	Activates enzymes; involved in protein synthesis	Whole grains, green leafy vegetables	Growth failure; behavioral disturbances; weakness, spasms
Manganese	Constituent of enzymes involved in fat synthesis	Widely distributed in foods	In animals: disturbances of nervous system, reproductive abnormalities
Molybdenum	Constituent of some enzymes	Legumes, cereals, organ meats	Not reported in humans
Phosphorus	Bone and tooth formation; acid–base balance	Milk, cheese, meat, poultry, grains	Weakness; demineralization of bone
Potassium	Acid–base balance; body water balance; nerve function	Meats, milk, many fruits	Muscular weakness; paralysis
Selenium	Functions in close association with vitamin E	Seafood, meat, grains	Anemia (rare)
Sodium	Acid–base balance; body water balance; nerve function	Common salt	Muscle cramps; mental apathy; reduced appetite
Sulfur	Constituent of active tissue compounds, cartilage, and tendon	Sulfur amino acids (methionine and cysteine) in dietary proteins	Related to intake and deficiency of sulfur amino acids
Zinc	Constituent of enzymes involved in digestion	Widely distributed in foods	Growth failure

(Table 5.10). Because sodas tend to replace milk—and therefore calcium—in the diet, nutritionists recommend that soda consumption be limited (if not eliminated) in the diets of children and adolescents to strengthen bones in both early and later life.

Salt

Adults need about 3 grams of dietary salt per day (about a teaspoon) or they will become sick and possibly die. Salt is so important to life that you crave it when you don't have enough in your body. When crystalline salt dissolves in water, it breaks into a unit of the chemical sodium and a unit of the chemical chloride. Salt is about 40% sodium. Every cell in the body needs sodium in order to function properly.

If salt is so important, then why do we hear that it is unhealthy to consume too much of it? The reason is that too much sodium can contribute to high blood pressure, a major risk factor for heart disease, stroke, and kidney failure.

The recommended upper limit of salt consumption per day for non–African American adults younger than 40 years of age is 5.8 grams (about 2,300 mg of sodium); for all African Americans and adults older than age 40, it's 3.8 grams (1,500 mg of sodium). The average U.S. adult

Table 5.10

Calcium in Various Foods

The recommended daily value for adults is 1,000 mg.

Food	Serving size	Milligrams (mg) calcium
Tofu, calcium processed	⅓ cup	581
Yogurt, plain	8 oz container	411
Milk, skim and low-fat	1 cup	301
Sesame seeds, whole roasted	1 oz	297
Cheese, Swiss	1 oz	288
Cheese, cheddar	1 oz	216
Cheese, mozzarella	1 oz	194
Soybeans, cooked	½ cup	131
Turnip greens, cooked	½ cup	116
Blackeyed peas, cooked	½ cup	115
All-bran cereal	½ cup	106
Collard greens	½ cup	101
Sardines, canned	1 oz	105
Salmon, canned (with bones)	1 oz	59
Sodas	12 oz	0

consumes close to 8 grams of salt per day. It's estimated that reducing salt intake by an average of 3 grams per day would save several hundred thousand U.S. lives and over $10 billion in healthcare costs each year.

About 75% of the salt in the U.S. diet comes from manufactured, processed, and fast foods. A typical fast-food meal contains about 1,000 mg of sodium; some, twice that much. To enhance taste, salt is added to many packaged foods including ketchup, mustard, salsa, and packaged and frozen meat, fish, and poultry. Health experts recommend a 50% reduction in the amount of sodium in processed, fast-food, and restaurant meals and improved food labeling to help consumers know the amount of sodium contained in food products and when a food is high in sodium. To reach international target goals of reducing salt in the diet by at least 25% by 2025, more than 75 countries have instituted salt-reduction strategies. These include engaging with industry to lessen salt added to products, establishing targets for sodium content of foods, educating consumers about healthy salt consumption, mandating front-of-package sodium labeling, taxing high-salt foods, and providing healthy salt content in foods served in public institutions (Trieu et al., 2015). The UK instituted salt-reduction policies in 2003, which is credited with a considerable reduction within 10 years of average blood pressure and the number of deaths from heart disease and stroke (He et al., 2014).

Phytochemicals

Many vegetables and fruits contain chemical substances, referred to as **phytochemicals**, that are not nutrients per se but that positively affect human physiology (Table 5.11). Phytochemicals may help the body destroy and eliminate toxins acquired from the environment or tissue-damaging by-products of metabolism, such as oxygen free radicals. For example, cruciferous vegetables (e.g., broccoli, kale, cauliflower, brussels sprouts, cabbage, mustard greens) are rich in the cancer-preventing phytochemicals *sulforaphane* and *isothiocyanates*. Tomatoes and tomato products (ketchup, tomato sauce), pink grapefruit, papaya, peaches, and watermelon contain a phytochemical called *lycopene,* which protects against oxidative damage and reduces the risk of cancer and heart disease. *Lutein,* found in dark leafy and brightly colored vegetables, reduces the risk of heart disease and the eye disease of age-related macular degeneration. Green and black tea, onions, apples, and grapes contain a family of phytochemicals called *flavonoids,* which also protect against cancer and heart disease. Dates, figs, and other dried fruits contain *polyphenols,* which are powerful antioxidants.

Water

Water is the principal constituent of blood and is the major component of all cells. Water provides the medium in which all biological chemical activities take place.

Body water is maintained at a relatively constant level by the nervous, hormone, and urinary systems.

Table 5.11

Phytochemicals in Fruits and Vegetables and Their Possible Benefits

Food	Phytochemicals	Possible benefits
Blueberries, strawberries, raspberries, blackberries, currants, etc.	Anthocyanidins, ellagic acid	Antioxidants Cancer prevention
Chili peppers	Capsaicin	Possible antioxidant Topical pain relief
Citrus fruits Oranges, grapefruit, lemon, limes, etc.	Flavanones (tangeretic, nobiletin, hesperitin) Carotenoids	Antioxidants
Cruciferous vegetables Broccoli, kale, cauliflower, brussels sprouts, cabbage, mustard greens	Indoles Isothiocyanates Sulforaphane Carotenoids	Antioxidants Anticancer properties
Garlic family Garlic, onions, shallots, leeks, chives, scallions	Allylic sulfides Flavonoids (quercetin)	Anticancer properties
Soy	Daidzein, equol, genestein, enterolactone, and other plant estrogens	Reduce risk of breast, prostate cancer; reduce risk of heart disease

If body water volume is low, a person experiences thirst, which motivates drinking. A low volume of body water activates hormonal mechanisms that reduce the production of urine. Excess body water volume activates certain hormonal mechanisms that increase the output of urine. Increasing urine output is the function of diuretics, drugs often given to reduce blood pressure, fluid volume after a heart attack, or feelings of bloatedness. The popular maxim that you should drink eight glasses of water a day is partially correct. The average adult loses about that much body water through sweat, moisture in expired air, urine, and feces. This loss is partly offset by drinking water and obtaining water in other fluids and foods.

Body water should be replaced by consuming pure water, milk, tea, or real juice. So-called enhanced waters are not pure. They contain a few grams of sugar, a small amount of vitamins, and often caffeine. Soda also is a poor substitute for water, as it may affect calcium metabolism and bone mass. Also, consuming soda replaces milk, giving the body less calcium with which to strengthen bones.

TERMS

phytochemicals: non-nutrient health-promoting chemicals produced by plants

Liquids containing caffeine (coffee, tea, sodas) and alcohol are diuretics, which means that some of the fluid ingested is lost in additional urine output.

Many people drink bottled water in the belief that it is more healthful than tap water. Not all bottled water comes from "natural" sources as the name of the product may suggest. The source of some bottled water products is a municipal water tap. One should look on the product label to ascertain the source of the water inside.

Dietary Supplements

More than 60,000 products are available in the United States as **dietary supplements**. By definition, dietary supplements are food derivatives ingested to provide one or more of the 40 essential nutrients, such as a particular vitamin, mineral, or amino acid. Besides food supplements, dietary supplements include a variety of plant or animal extracts, enzymes, amino acids, herbs, hormones, and nucleic acids (DNA and RNA), the use of which is intended to alter one or more of the body's biological systems to produce a specific physiological or psychological effect **Table 5.12**. For example, someone might take capsules containing omega-3 fatty acids (fish oil) to try to prevent a heart attack (or *another* heart attack) or stroke by lowering serum lipids. Or someone may drink herbal tea to feel energized. Unlike drugs, dietary supplements are not permitted by the FDA to be marketed for the purpose of treating, diagnosing, preventing, or curing diseases. That means supplements should not make disease claims, such as "lowers high cholesterol" or "treats heart disease."

When a dietary supplement is used to augment the nutritional quality of the diet, it is considered a food. When a dietary supplement is used to bring about a particular biological change, it is considered a drug and referred to as a **nutraceutical**. About 100 million Americans spend a total of $32 billion each year on dietary supplements.

A varied diet that conforms to the recommendations of MyPlate (Figure 5.2) is likely to provide most people with sufficient essential nutrients for good health. For these people, a nutritional dietary supplement is probably unnecessary, although some may want to take one as a form of "dietary insurance" (Harvard School of Public Health, 2017). People who suspect that their diets are nutritionally inadequate may benefit from taking a daily multivitamin and mineral supplement. For example:

- People who skip meals and eat a lot of processed and fast food
- People who consume an unusual or low-calorie diet for weight loss
- People who consume nutritionally inadequate diets for reasons of economic hardship
- Athletes who are concerned about body size
- People who consume large amounts of coffee and/or alcohol

Others who may benefit from dietary supplements include strict vegetarians, who may need vitamin B_{12} because that vitamin comes primarily from animal tissue; people who are lactose intolerant (have difficulty digesting dairy products); and women of childbearing age who tend to consume insufficient amounts of folic acid and iron. When supplementing the diet with vitamins and minerals, remember that more is not necessarily better. In high doses, vitamins A, D, K, B_3 (niacin), and B_6 (pyridoxine) may be toxic.

Supplements containing enzymes, other proteins, and nucleic acids are not absorbed intact from the digestive tract; instead, they are broken down into smaller subunits. When a supplement is intended for use in the digestive tract, such as lactase, this is of little concern because the substance acts prior to being digested. However, an enzyme or nucleic acid will not be absorbed intact into the body, so using them is a waste of money.

Whether a substance is natural or synthetic makes no difference chemically as long as the manufacturer has taken care to be sure that the product is pure. Many individuals have been made ill and some have died from consuming an impure or adulterated supplement. Moreover, just because a product is labeled "natural" or "comes from plants" does not mean it is safe or effective. A "natural" or "plant" product can have a large number of impurities and may be toxic.

Unlike prescription and over-the-counter medicines, dietary supplements do not have to be tested before going on the market, so consumers have no assurance of a supplement's contents, that it has no impurities, that it is not harmful, or that it actually does anything beneficial. Some supplements have been found to be contaminated with toxic plant material, heavy metals, bacteria, or prescription medications and illegal drugs (Sax, 2015). Contaminants are never listed on the product label.

Supplement manufacturers are supposed to promise that their products are safe and that ingredients are accurately listed on the product label. However, there is no oversight of supplements as there is for prescription drugs.

Table 5.12

Some Dietary Supplements That Have Been Scientifically Tested and Found to Be Effective

Supplement	Use
Glucosamine	Reduce symptoms of arthritis
Echinacea	Enhance immune functioning
Garlic	Reduce risk of heart disease
Gingko biloba	Slow the progression of some forms of dementia
Omega-3 fatty acids	Prevent heart disease and stroke
S-adenosyl methionine (SAM-e)	Relieve mild to moderate depression
St. John's wort	Relieve mild to moderate depression
Saw palmetto	Treat prostate disease

Find a comprehensive list at http://www.nlm.nih.gov/medlineplus/druginfo/herb_All.html

Rules for Organic Labeling

The U.S. Department of Agriculture (USDA) sets standards for foods labeled "organic." Foods labeled "100% organic" and "organic" cannot be produced using sewage sludge, ionizing radiation, artificial growth hormones, genetically modified crops, and most synthetic fertilizers and pesticides. The labeling requirements apply to both fresh products and processed foods. Foods that are sold, labeled, or represented as organic have to be produced and processed in accordance with the USDA standards, and they may carry the "USDA Organic" seal.

The labeling requirements are based on the percentage of organic ingredients in a product. Foods and food products labeled "100% organic" must contain (excluding water and salt) only organically produced ingredients. Products labeled "organic" must consist of at least 95% organically produced ingredients. Any remaining ingredients must consist of nonagricultural substances approved on the national list of products that are not commercially available in organic form.

Processed products that contain at least 70% organic ingredients can use the phrase "made with organic ingredients" and list up to three of the organic ingredients or food groups on the product label. For example, soup made with at least 70% organic ingredients and only organic vegetables may be labeled either "soup made with organic peas, potatoes, and carrots" or "soup made with organic vegetables." Processed products that contain less than 70% organic ingredients cannot use the term "organic" anywhere on the principal display panel. However, they may identify the specific ingredients that are organically produced under ingredients on the information panel.

Data from USDA National Organic Program. Retrieved from http//www.ams.usda.gov/nop/

Although the FDA requires supplement manufacturers to report supplement-related adverse events, they rarely do. In the United States, only a few hundred of the estimated 50,000 annual supplement-related adverse events are reported. The FDA warns consumers of problems with supplements on this web page: www.fda.gov/For_Consumers/ConsumerUpdates/default.htm. A private organization called the United States Pharmacopeial Convention (USP) verifies the equality, purity, identity, and strength of dietary supplements on this web page: http://www.usp.org/usp-verification-services/.

Food Additives

Almost all manufactured foods contain chemicals that are added during production to alter taste (sweeteners and salt), texture (thickeners), color (petroleum- or plant-derived dyes and colorings), stability (preservatives), and nutrient composition (nutraceuticals and functional foods) (**Table 5.13**). The U.S. Food and Drug Administration Center for Food Safety and Applied Nutrition (CFSAN) lists approximately 4,000 substances added directly to food (www.fda.gov/food/ingredientspackaginglabeling/foodadditivesingredients/ucm115326.htm).

Some additives promote health. For example, vitamins and minerals are added to highly processed white flour to replace nutrients lost in its production. Many so-called functional foods (see the Functional Foods section in this chapter) contain added substances that claim (often without supporting scientific evidence) to enhance health.

Many food additives are nutritionally unnecessary, and some may adversely affect health. For example, sugar and salt are added to many foods to intensify taste and thereby increase sales. Unfortunately, overconsumption of sugar and salt can have severe health consequences. The U.S. Food and Drug Administration, the European Food Safety Authority, and many international agencies monitor the safety of chemicals added to food. Some chemical additives, such as food colorings, must be tested for safety by the manufacturer prior to being approved for use in foods. On the other hand, many kinds of food additives are not tested rigorously for safety before entering the food supply; safety issues arise only after an additive has been in use and a deleterious effect on consumers' health is suspected. At that point the suspect chemical can undergo rigorous testing, and if found harmful, food safety agencies can order that it be not approved from food products. Food safety regulations refer to untested additives that have been in use for a long time and that are not suspected of causing harm as *generally regarded as safe* (GRAS). A suspected or potentially harmful chemical additive can be considered generally safe if it is present in foods in very low amounts, referred to as *acceptable daily intake levels* (ADI).

Manufacturers are required to list all the additives in the order of their relative proportions on the ingredients label. Do not assume that the words "natural," "organic," or "health food" mean that foods are free from additives or extra sugar and salt. The only way to be certain of the contents of a food is to know how it was produced.

Preservatives

About 20% of the world's food supply is lost to spoilage each year. Common preservatives include BHA

TERMS

dietary supplements: products that provide one or more of the 40 essential nutrients or nonessential vitamins, minerals, enzymes, amino acids, herbs, hormones, and nucleic acids

nutraceutical: a dietary supplement intended to prevent or treat an illness or disease

Table 5.13

Some Types of Food Additives

Type of Additive	Function	Common Sources	Common Label Names
Preservatives	Prevent or slow spoilage, changes in color, texture, flavor	Jellies, baked goods, cured meats, snacks, cereals, sauces	Ascorbic acid, citric acid, sodium benzoate, calcium propionate, sodium nitrite, calcium sorbate, BHA, BHT
Sweeteners	Add sweet taste	Many processed foods, candy, baked goods, beverages	Sucrose, high fructose corn syrup, corn syrup, aspartame, acesulfame, fructose
Colorings	Offset color loss due to light, air, temperature, moisture and storage; provide, correct and enhance natural color	Candies, snack foods, pie fillings, cheese, puddings, soft drinks, jams/jellies	FD&C Blue Nos. 1 and 2, FD&C Green No. 3, FD&C Red Nos. 3 and 40, FD&C Yellow Nos. 5 and 6, Orange B, Citrus Red No. 2, annatto extract, beta-carotene, grape skin extract, cochineal extract or carmine, paprika oleoresin, caramel color, fruit and vegetable juices, saffron
Flavorings	Spices, natural and artificial flavors	Ice cream, pudding, cake mixes, salad dressing, soft drinks, candy, BBQ sauce	Natural flavoring, artificial flavor, and spices
Flavor Enhancers	Enhance flavors already present without providing a separate flavor	Many processed foods	Monosodium glutamate (MSG), salt, autolyzed yeast extract
Fat Replacements	Provide expected texture and a creamy "mouth-feel"	Baked goods, dressings, frozen desserts, candy, cake mixes, dairy products	Cellulose gel, guar gum carrageenan, food starch, polydextrose, whey protein
Emulsifiers	Prevent separation, reduce stickiness, smooth mixing of ingredients	Salad dressings, peanut butter, chocolate, frozen desserts	Soy lecithin, mono- and diglycerides, egg yolks, sorbitan monostearate
Stabilizers, Thickeners	Produce uniform texture, improve "mouth-feel"	Frozen desserts, sauces, dairy products, cakes, jams, pudding, dressings	Gelatin, pectin, guar gum, carrageenan, xanthan gum, whey

Data from U.S. Food and Drug Administration (2017). Overview of Food Ingredients, Additives & Colors. www.fda.gov/Food/IngredientsPackagingLabeling/FoodAdditivesIngredients/ucm094211.htm#types

(butylated hydroxyanisole), BHT (butylated hydroxytoluene), and sodium nitrite. Each of these substances can be toxic and damaging to humans if consumed in excess; however, in amounts commonly present in food, they are presumed safe.

Sulfites in the form of sulfur dioxide, sodium sulfite, sodium or potassium bisulfite, and sodium or potassium metabisulfite are added to many foods to kill bacteria and to slow the food's chemical breakdown. Sulfites are commonly added to wine and to dehydrated soups, vegetables, and dried fruit (apples, apricots, raisins, pears, and peaches). To keep vegetables looking fresh, they are also used in restaurant salad bars. Some individuals, particularly those with asthma, may be extremely sensitive to sulfites and may experience nausea, diarrhea, respiratory distress, and skin eruptions. Such problems have led to banning the use of sulfites in restaurants.

Dyes and Colorings

Dyes and colorings are added to foods to provide uniform color, to enhance a food's visual appeal, and to offset color loss due to exposure to light, air, temperature extremes, moisture, and storage conditions. Without color additives, colas wouldn't be brown and mint ice cream wouldn't be green.

The FDA is responsible for ensuring that foods containing dyes and colorings are safe to consume, contain only approved ingredients, and are accurately labeled.

Some colorings are derived from petroleum and coal (FD&C Blue Nos. 1 and 2, FD&C Green No. 3, FD&C Red Nos. 3 and 40, FD&C Yellow Nos. 5 and 6, Orange B, Citrus Red No. 2); others are derived from vegetables, minerals, or animals, such as caramel color, which is derived from sugar. Some petroleum-based dyes have been linked to hyperactivity and behavior problems in children (Center for Science in the Public Interest, 2016).

Artificial Sweeteners

Artificial sweeteners are chemicals capable of producing the sensation of sweetness far more effectively—from 200 to 10,000 times more, depending on the chemical—than sucrose, fructose, glucose, and other natural sugars. Six chemicals are approved for use as artificial sweeteners in North America: aspartame, saccharin, acesulfame-K, neotame, advantame, and sucralose; the chemical stevia is a low-calorie sweetener.

> **TERMS**
>
> sulfites: used as preservatives for salad, fresh fruits and vegetables, wine, beer, and dried fruit; in susceptible individuals, especially those with asthma, they can cause a severe reaction

Guidelines for Food Safety

When Purchasing Food

1. Purchase meat and poultry products after all other groceries have been selected and keep packages of raw meat and poultry separate from other foods, particularly foods that will be eaten without further cooking. Consider using plastic bags to enclose individual packages of raw meat and poultry.
2. Make sure meat and poultry products—whether raw, prepackaged, or cooked from the deli—are refrigerated when purchased.
3. USDA strongly advises against purchasing fresh, prestuffed whole birds.
4. Canned goods should be free of dents, cracks, or bulging lids.
5. Take food straight home to the refrigerator. If travel time will exceed one hour, pack perishable foods in a cooler with ice and keep groceries and cooler in the passenger area of the car during warm weather.

When Storing Food at Home

1. Verify the temperature of your refrigerator and freezer with an appliance thermometer—refrigerators should run at 40°F (4°C) or below; freezers at 0°F (−18°C). Most foodborne bacteria grow slowly at 40°F, which is a safe refrigerator temperature. Freezer temperatures of 0°F (−18°C) or below stop bacterial growth (U.S. Food and Drug Administration, 2015).
2. At home, refrigerate or freeze meat and poultry immediately.
3. To prevent raw juices from dripping on other foods in the refrigerator, use plastic bags or place meat and poultry on a plate.
4. Wash hands with soap and water for 20 seconds before and after handling any raw meat, poultry, or seafood products.
5. Store canned goods in a cool, clean, dry place. Avoid extreme heat or cold, which can be harmful to canned goods.
6. Never store any foods directly under a sink and always keep foods off the floor and separate from cleaning supplies.

When Getting Food Ready to Prepare

1. The importance of hand washing cannot be overemphasized. This simple practice is the most economical, yet often forgotten, way to prevent contamination or cross-contamination.
2. Wash hands (gloved or not) with soap and water for 20 seconds: (a) before beginning preparation; (b) after handling raw meat, poultry, seafood, or eggs; (c) after touching animals; (d) after using the bathroom; (e) after changing diapers; and (f) after blowing the nose.
3. Don't let juices from raw meat, poultry, or seafood come in contact with cooked foods or foods that will be eaten raw, such as fruits or salad ingredients.
4. Wash hands, counters, equipment, utensils, and cutting boards with soap and water immediately after use. Counters, equipment, utensils, and cutting boards can be sanitized with a chlorine solution of 1 teaspoon liquid household bleach per quart of water. Let the solution stand on the board after washing, or follow the instructions on sanitizing products.
5. Thaw meat in the refrigerator, never on the counter. It is also safe to thaw in cold water in an airtight plastic wrapper or bag, changing the water every 30 minutes until meat is thawed; or thaw in the microwave and cook the product immediately.
6. Marinate foods in the refrigerator, never on the counter.
7. The USDA recommends that if you choose to stuff whole poultry, you must use a meat thermometer to check the internal temperature of the stuffing. The internal temperature in the center of the stuffing should reach 165°F (74°C) before removing it from the oven. If you don't have a meat thermometer, cook the stuffing outside the bird. Also, don't put hot stuffing into a frozen bird. By the time it thaws, it will be contaminated inside.

When Cooking

1. Always cook thoroughly. If harmful bacteria are present, only thorough cooking will destroy them; freezing or rinsing the foods in cold water is not sufficient to destroy bacteria.
2. Use a meat thermometer to determine if your meat, poultry, or casserole has reached a safe internal temperature (145°F (63°C) for roasts and steaks, 180°F (82°C) for whole poultry, 160°F (71°C) for ground meat, and 165°F (74°C) for leftovers). Check the product in several spots to ensure that a safe temperature has been reached and that harmful bacteria, such as *Salmonella* and certain strains of *E. coli,* have been destroyed.
3. Avoid interrupted cooking. Never refrigerate partially cooked food to later finish cooking on the grill or in the oven. Meat and poultry products must be cooked thoroughly the first time, and then they may be refrigerated and safely reheated.
4. When microwaving foods, carefully follow the manufacturer's instructions. Use microwave-safe containers, cover, rotate, and allow for the standing time, which contributes to thorough cooking.

When Serving

1. Wash hands with soap and water before serving or eating food.
2. Serve cooked products on clean plates with clean utensils and clean hands. Never put cooked foods on a dish that has held raw products unless the dish is first washed with soap and hot water.
3. Hold hot foods above 140°F (60°C) and cold foods below 40°F (4°C).
4. Never leave foods, raw or cooked, at room temperature longer than two hours. On a hot day with temperatures at 90°F or warmer, this time decreases to one hour.

When Handling Leftovers

1. Wash hands before and after handling leftovers. Use clean utensils and surfaces.
2. Divide leftovers into small units and store in shallow containers for quick cooling. Refrigerate within two hours of cooking.
3. Discard anything left out too long.
4. Never taste a food to determine if it is safe.
5. When reheating leftovers, reheat thoroughly to a temperature of 165°F (74°C), or until hot and steamy. Bring soups, sauces, and gravies to a rolling boil.
6. If in doubt, throw it out.

Data from Food Safety and Inspection Service, U.S. Department of Agriculture (2008). Kitchen Companion: Your Safe Food Handbook. Retrieved from http://www.fsis.usda.gov/Fact_Sheets/Kitchen_Companion/

Tips for Eating Healthy When Eating Out

Full-service and fast-food restaurants, convenience stores, and grocery stores offer a variety of meal options. Typically, these meals are higher in calories, saturated fat, sodium, and added sugars than the food you prepare at home. Think about ways to make healthier choices when eating food away from home.

- **Consider your drink**

  Choose water, unsweetened tea, and other drinks without added sugars to complement your meal. If you drink alcohol, choose drinks lower in added sugars and be aware of the alcohol content of your beverage. Keep in mind that many coffee drinks may be high in saturated fat and added sugar.

- **Savor a salad**

  Start your meal with a salad packed with vegetables to help you feel satisfied sooner. Ask for dressing on the side and use a small amount of it.

- **Share a dish**

  Share a dish with a friend or family member. Or, ask the server to pack up half of your entree before it comes to the table to control the amount you eat.

- **Customize your meal**

  Order a side dish or an appetizer-sized portion instead of a regular entree. They're usually served on smaller plates and in smaller amounts.

- **Pack your snack**

  Pack fruit, sliced vegetables, low-fat string cheese, or unsalted nuts to eat during road trips or long commutes. No need to stop for other food when these snacks are ready-to-eat.

- **Fill your plate with vegetables and fruit**

  Stir-fries, kabobs, or vegetarian menu items usually have more vegetables. Select fruits as a side dish or dessert.

- **Compare the calories, fat, and sodium**

  Many menus now include nutrition information. Look for items that are lower in calories, saturated fat, and sodium. Check with your server if you don't see them on the menu. For more information, check www.FDA.gov.

- **Pass on the buffet**

  Have an item from the menu and avoid the "all-you-can-eat" buffet. Steamed, grilled, or broiled dishes have fewer calories than foods that are fried in oil or cooked in butter.

- **Get your whole grains**

  Request 100% whole-wheat breads, rolls, and pasta when choosing sandwiches, burgers, or main dishes.

- **Quit the "clean your plate club"**

  You don't have to eat everything on your plate. Take leftovers home and refrigerate within 2 hours. Leftovers in the refrigerator are safe to eat for about 3 to 4 days.

Reproduced from U.S. Department of Agriculture. Tips for Eating Healthy When Eating Out. Retrieved from http://www.choosemyplate.gov/healthy-eating-tips/tips-for-eating-out.html

---

Although touted as aids to weight control, diabetes management, and moderating tooth decay, artificial sweeteners have yet to be shown to promote health in any way. Thinking that artificial sweeteners are healthy, people may choose artificially sweetened junk foods in place of natural foods. Some may think that since they consume artificial sweeteners they can have more pastries or other sweets or fatty foods such as french fries. Furthermore, artificial sweeteners may alter physiological mechanisms that lead to increases in abdominal fat deposition and weight, overweight, and obesity and the risk of high blood pressure, metabolic syndrome, diabetes, depression, kidney dysfunction, heart attack, stroke, and even cardiovascular and total mortality. Much remains to be studied about the safety of artificial sweeteners (Fowler, 2016).

Functional Foods

When vitamins, minerals, herbs, or other substances are added to foods to allow the manufacturer to make health claims, the food is called a **functional food**. Americans have been eating functional foods since 1924, when iodine was added to salt to prevent goiter, a disease of the thyroid gland caused by iodine deficiency. For many years after that, some foods (such as enriched flour) were fortified with extra vitamins and minerals but without the manufacturer making health claims. That changed in 1993, when the FDA ruled that milk and yogurt, which contain high amounts of calcium, could carry labels claiming that the products helped prevent osteoporosis. Non-dairy food manufacturers quickly began adding calcium to their products—orange juice, waffles, potato chips—so they, too, could make health claims.

Since then, food manufactures have found that adding substances to foods in order to make health claims is good business, even if the added substances have not been shown scientifically to be helpful. Thus, we now have sodas with ginseng (for relaxation), cereals with psyllium husk (to protect against heart disease or cancer), margarine with plant-derived sterols (to lower cholesterol), ice cream with echinacea (to help the immune system), and soups with St. John's wort (to combat depression).

Neither the health claims nor the purity and amount of additives in functional foods are tested or regulated by the Food and Drug Administration (FDA). Herbs added to foods may be dangerous because amounts are not well controlled and, in some instances (e.g., St. John's wort), the herb can interfere with the action of certain medications. Some people may mistakenly believe that more is better and risk overdose with a vitamin, mineral, or plant product by ingesting both dietary supplements and a functional food. Moreover, functional foods often cost more, sometimes a lot more, than equivalent foods without added chemicals do.

Food Safety

Hundreds of yearly outbreaks of food poisoning in the United States from bacterial and viral contamination of commercial beef, poultry, fruit, and vegetables have raised concerns about the safety of the food supply. In the United States, there are 48 million cases of foodborne illness annually, resulting in 128,000 hospitalizations and 3,000 deaths. Six pathogens—*Salmonella*, *Clostridium perfringens*, *Campylobacter*, norovirus, *Staphylococcus aureus*, and *Toxoplasma*—account for most of the infections and approximately 1,600 deaths each year (Table 5.14).

> **TERMS**
>
> **functional food:** a food to which additional vitamins, minerals, herbs, or other substances are added to allow the manufacturer to make health claims

Table 5.14

Pathogens That Cause Foodborne Illness

Pathogen	Found	Transmission	Symptoms
Campylobacter jejuni	Intestinal tracts of animals and birds, raw milk, untreated water, and sewage sludge.	Contaminated water, raw milk, and raw or undercooked meat, poultry, or shellfish.	Fever, headache, and muscle pain followed by diarrhea (sometimes bloody), abdominal pain, and nausea. Symptoms appear 2 to 5 days after eating; may last 7 to 10 days.
Clostridium botulinum	Widely distributed in nature; in soil, water, on plants, and in intestinal tracts of animals and fish. Grows only in little or no oxygen.	Bacteria produce a toxin that causes illness. Improperly canned foods, garlic in oil, vacuum-packed and tightly wrapped food.	Toxin affects the nervous system. Symptoms usually appear 18 to 36 hours after eating but can sometimes appear as few as 4 hours or as many as 8 days after eating; double vision, droopy eyelids, trouble speaking and swallowing, and difficulty breathing. Fatal in 3 to 10 days if not treated.
Clostridium perfringens	Soil, dust, sewage, and intestinal tracts of animals and humans. Grows only in little or no oxygen.	Called "the cafeteria germ" because many outbreaks result from food left for long periods in steam tables or at room temperature. Bacteria destroyed by cooking, but some toxin-producing spores may survive.	Diarrhea and gas pains may appear 8 to 24 hours after eating; usually last about 1 day, but less severe symptoms may persist for 1 to 2 weeks.
Escherichia coli O157:H7	Intestinal tracts of some mammals, raw milk, unchlorinated water; one of several strains of *E. coli* that can cause human illness.	Contaminated water, raw milk, raw or rare ground beef, unpasteurized apple juice or cider, uncooked fruits and vegetables; person to person.	Diarrhea or bloody diarrhea, abdominal cramps, nausea, and malaise; can begin 2 to 5 days after food is eaten, lasting about 8 days. Some, especially the very young, have developed hemolytic-uremic syndrome (HUS), which causes acute kidney failure. A similar illness, thrombotic thrombocytopenic purpura (TTP), may occur in adults.
Listeria monocytogenes	Intestinal tracts of humans and animals, milk, soil, leafy vegetables; can grow slowly at refrigerator temperatures.	Ready-to-eat foods such as hot dogs, luncheon meats, cold cuts, fermented or dry sausage, and other deli-style meat and poultry, soft cheeses, and unpasteurized milk.	Fever, chills, headache, backache, sometimes upset stomach, abdominal pain and diarrhea; may take up to 3 weeks to become ill; may later develop more serious illness in at-risk patients (pregnant women and newborns, older adults, and people with weakened immune systems).
Norovirus	Human intestinal tract.	Person to person.	Nausea, vomiting, diarrhea, resolving in 1 to 2 days.
Salmonella (more than 2,300 types)	Intestinal tracts and feces of animals; *Salmonella enteritidis* in eggs.	Raw or undercooked eggs, poultry, and meat; raw milk and dairy products; seafood; and food handlers.	Stomach pain, diarrhea, nausea, chills, fever, and headache usually appear 8 to 72 hours after eating; may last 1 to 2 days.
Shigella (more than 30 types)	Human intestinal tract; rarely found in other animals.	Person to person by fecal–oral route; fecal contamination of food and water. Most outbreaks result from food, especially salads, prepared and handled by workers using poor personal hygiene.	Disease referred to as *shigellosis* or bacillary dysentery. Diarrhea containing blood and mucus, fever, abdominal cramps, chills, and vomiting; 12 to 50 hours from ingestion of bacteria; can last a few days to 2 weeks.
Staphylococcus aureus	On humans (skin, infected cuts, pimples, noses, and throats).	Person to person from improper food handling. Multiply rapidly at room temperature to produce a toxin that causes illness.	Severe nausea, abdominal cramps, vomiting, and diarrhea occur 1 to 6 hours after eating; recovery within 2 to 3 days—longer if severe dehydration occurs.

Data from U.S. Department of Agriculture. (2013). Foodborne illness: What consumers need to know. https://www.fsis.usda.gov/wps/portal/fsis/topics/food-safety-education/get-answers/food-safety-fact-sheets/foodborne-illness-and-disease/foodborne-illness-what-consumers-need-to-know/ct_index

Symptoms of bacterial food poisoning are headache, nausea, fever, abdominal cramps, and diarrhea.

The foods most likely to be contaminated with infectious microorganisms are raw meat and poultry, raw eggs, unpasteurized milk, and raw shellfish. Foods that mingle the products of many individual animals, such as bulk raw milk, pooled raw eggs, or ground beef, are particularly hazardous because a pathogen present in an individual animal can contaminate the entire mix. For example, a single hamburger may contain meat from hundreds of animals. A single restaurant omelet may contain eggs from hundreds of chickens. A glass of raw milk may contain milk from hundreds of cows.

Besides animal products, uncooked fruits and vegetables also carry pathogenic microorganisms from improper handling and processing, for example, using contaminated water to wash fresh produce after it is harvested. Another source of contamination is fresh manure used to fertilize food crops. Unpasteurized fruit juice can also be contaminated if there are pathogens in or on the fruit that is used to make it.

In 2011, Congress passed the Food Safety Modernization Act (FSMA), which gave the FDA authority to put greater emphasis on preventing, rather than responding to, outbreaks of foodborne illness. The law requires food companies to develop and implement food safety plans and permits the FDA to require recalls when food safety problems occur and to develop systems to ensure that imported foods are as safe for consumers as foods produced in the United States. It also is recognized that the FDA and U.S. Department of Agriculture do not have the staff to oversee nearly 60,000 food manufacturers and processors and billions of tons of imported food. That's why it's imperative for consumers to follow food safety guidelines when they purchase, store, and prepare food (see the Wellness Guide: Guidelines for Food Safety).

One method of protecting food involves exposing it to **gamma irradiation** to destroy fungi, bacteria, and

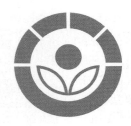

■ **Figure 5.10**

The Radura Symbol
The radura symbol is used internationally to indicate that a food has been treated with irradiation.

other microorganisms. The U.S. government allows irradiation for sterilizing insects, extending shelf life, controlling pathogens and parasites, and inhibiting the sprouting of vegetables. Irradiation also is approved for red meat, poultry, pork, fruits and vegetables, some spices, seeds, herbs and seasonings, eggs, and wheat. At approved doses, irradiation does not eliminate toxins, prions (agents that cause mad cow disease), and many types of viruses. Irradiation does not prevent subsequent contamination of food by food-service workers or consumers, a major source of bacterial and viral contamination.

Keep in mind that irradiation *does not* make food radioactive and therefore consumers are not at risk from radiation. The U.S. government requires a written radiation disclosure statement on the label of irradiated foods; the use of the radura symbol (**Figure 5.10**), however, is optional.

Some opponents of food irradiation argue that the method has not been proven safe in all instances. Their concern is that irradiation may produce cancer-causing or toxic by-products or mutant strains of toxic, radiation-resistant microorganisms. Furthermore, vitamins can be destroyed by irradiation.

Genetically Modified Foods

Genetically modified foods, referred to as *genetically modified organisms* or *GMOs*, are agricultural plants and animals in which one or more genes have been altered using modern biotechnological methods. Other words for genetically modified are *genetic engineering* and *transgenic*.

Prior to the invention of GMOs in the 1990s, most plants and animals in the North American food supply were created by breeders who mated individuals with particular traits to produce offspring with those traits. For example, suppose you want a big, good-tasting tomato. You start by finding a tomato plant in Nature that produces good-tasting tomatoes. Then you find a different tomato plant that produces large tomatoes. You crossbreed the two plants, and plant the offspring

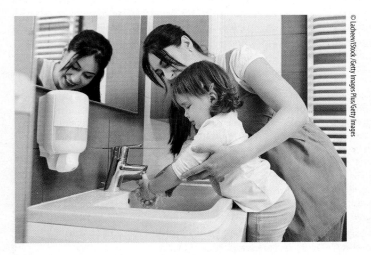

© Lacheev/iStock /Getty Images Plus/Getty Images

Hand washing is essential to safe food preparation.

seeds. After many tries (and possibly many growing seasons), you have the large, good-tasting tomatoes you originally wanted.

Compared to conventional plant and animal breeding, which requires combining genes from organisms of the same species, genetically modified organisms can be engineered with genes from *different* species. For example, genes from a daffodil and a particular bacterium have been inserted into a type of rice so it contains vitamin A, which in Nature it does not. This was done to help prevent childhood blindness in the developing world.

The major genetically modified crops grown commercially are herbicide- and insecticide-resistant soybeans, corn, cotton, and canola. Other crops grown commercially and/or field-tested are sweet potato resistant to a virus that could destroy most of the African harvest, rice with increased iron and vitamins that may alleviate chronic malnutrition in Asian countries, and a variety of plants that are able to survive weather extremes. There are bananas that produce human vaccines against infectious diseases such as hepatitis B, fish that mature more quickly, fruit and nut trees that yield fruit years earlier, plants that produce new plastics with unique properties, and yeast that produce fuel oil.

Technologies for genetically modifying foods offer dramatic promise for meeting some of the greatest challenges for the future. Like all new technologies, they also pose some risks, both known and unknown. With concern about possible health and environmental effects of consuming genetically modified plants and the food products derived from them, the European Union and Japan have banned all GMOs in foods. On the other hand, China, India, Brazil, and many other countries have embraced GMOs and see them as a solution to food shortages and agricultural inefficiency. Some of the problems and concerns about GMOs include the following:

- Planting crops that are resistant to herbicides poses a major threat to the environment and possibly to people. To control weeds, every year growers spray hundreds of millions of pounds of herbicide onto crops. Often other toxic chemicals are added to Roundup (glyphosate) to make it more effective and long lasting. This promotes contamination of soil and water. Roundup contaminates farm workers and others regularly exposed to the herbicide.
- Inserting nonnative genes into plants and animals may increase the risk that the genetically modified organism causes allergic reactions, a valid but, as yet, unobserved danger. People have been eating genetically modified corn and soy for more than a decade. In the United States, no adverse health effects on the American population have been observed.
- Pollen from GMOs can be blown by wind onto nearby fields and can contaminate other crops. Farmers trying to grow organic corn have had their corn contaminated by pollen from nearby genetically modified corn. Small organic farms may find it difficult to avoid contamination of their crops.
- Genetic engineering is regarded as "evil," "dangerous," and "sinful" by some opponents of GMOs. These critics often refer to foods produced from genetically engineered plants as "Frankenfoods."

One way to lessen any health and environmental risks of GMOs is to test them thoroughly before they are used. Since testing and regulation can reduce some risks, but not all, buying foods labeled "organic" helps avoid GMO products. A majority of the U.S. population wants GMO foods to be labeled as such. Fearing that labeling products as genetically modified would drive away many consumers and arguing that most Americans have been consuming genetically modified foods for many years without, as yet identified, ill effects, agribusiness companies resist GMO labeling.

Fast Food

Student: *You're always telling us not to eat fast food. If it's so bad, why is it so cheap, easy to get, and taste so good?*

Health Instructor: *Just because fast food is everywhere, convenient, inexpensive, and concocted by chemists to appeal to the human taste system doesn't mean it's healthy.*

Despite the fact that about 75% of American adults say that fast food is "not too good for you" or "not good at all for you" (Gallup Poll, 2013), each week, approximately 50% of American adults consume fast food at least one time; about 4% consume fast food daily. The reasons for patronizing such establishments are low cost, convenience (they are everywhere—more than 200,000 worldwide), perceived lack of time to shop and prepare meals at home, fast food's taste and texture, and the need to feed children quickly. One-third of American children and adolescents consume fast food every day (Vikraman et al., 2015).

Compared to nonregular fast-food consumers, those who regularly consume fast food ingest between 150 and 200 more calories per day, which can contribute to a gain of several pounds in a year. Moreover, the large amounts of salt, fat, and sugar in fast food set these consumers on a course for high blood pressure, type 2 diabetes, heart disease, and blocked arteries (Bahadoran et al., 2015).

TERMS

gamma irradiation: nonchemical method of food preservation

genetically modified food: agricultural plants and animals into which one or more genes from other organisms have been inserted (also called genetically modified organisms, or GMOs)

Convenience notwithstanding, fast-food items must be chosen carefully because many contain high quantities of saturated fat, cholesterol, and salt; few complex carbohydrates; and low levels of vitamins A and C (Table 5.15). The major fast-food companies have responded to consumers' concerns about nutrition by offering salads, baked potatoes, roast beef, and broiled chicken. Roast beef has less fat than hamburger, and broiled chicken breast has less fat than deep-fried chicken. Be cautious, though. Fish, a low-fat food, if breaded and fried, may be 50% fat. Salads and baked potatoes can be carriers of high-fat toppings.

Since fast food is so popular and prevalent, it is healthful to know the nutrient content of the fast food you consume. You can do that by doing the following (if you do not patronize such establishments, do the following as a service to someone who does and share the information with her or him).

- Choose a fast-food meal that is typical for you and list the meal's components (e.g., burger, fries, and milk shake).
- For each of your meal's components, determine the total calories, grams of protein, total grams of fat, total grams of saturated fat, milligrams of cholesterol, milligrams of salt, and grams of fiber. You can get this information from the establishment's website, in-store brochure, or the following website: http://fastfoodnutrition.org.
- Calculate the dollar cost of the energy content of the meal by dividing the total calories by the total cost. This tells you how much bang (i.e., energy) you are getting for your buck.
- Calculate the percentage of your estimated daily calories contributed by this meal (divide the calories in your meal by your daily calorie need). (Refer to the Health Tips box, "Estimating Your Daily Calorie Needs" on page 102.)

Vegetarian Diets

Vegetarianism has existed as long as humankind has and has been advocated by such famous people as Leonardo da Vinci, Benjamin Franklin George Bernard Shaw, Mahatma Gandhi, Albert Einstein, Steve Jobs, Paul McCartney, and Ellen Degeneres. People choose to be vegetarians for various reasons, including:

1. To avoid killing animals—either killing them oneself or killing by others. Some people who have a strong affection for other animals and feel a certain biological and spiritual kinship with them object to killing them for food.
2. To contribute to the more efficient utilization of world protein supplies. It takes approximately 10 pounds of livestock feed, usually corn or soybeans, to produce 1 pound of meat. Obviously, the 10 pounds of corn or soybeans could feed more people than 1 pound of meat can. With the population of Earth doubling approximately every 30 years, some people feel a moral obligation to avoid overconsuming food resources in the hope that ways will be found to distribute the world food supply more equitably.
3. To live longer and healthier lives. A study of over 34,000 Seventh Day Adventists in California, most of whom were vegetarians, showed that vegetarian dietary patterns were associated with less overweight and obesity, lower prevalence and incidence of diabetes, lower prevalence of high blood pressure, lower all-cause mortality, and in some instances, lower risk of cancer. Other studies have shown that vegetarian Adventists take fewer medications and experience fewer medical procedures. The explanation: Compared to a non-vegetarian diet, a vegetarian diet prevents heart disease and cancer because it has less saturated fat and cholesterol,

Table 5.15

Approximate Composition of Selected Fast-Food Items

Food	Total calories	Total fat (grams)	Calories from fat	Cholesterol (milligrams)	Sodium (milligrams)
Adult-size hamburger (beef)	600	29	260	75	1,040
Adult-size burrito (beef)	410	16	140	30	1,140
French fries (medium/salted)	450	22	200	0	290
Turkey sub sandwich	280	4	30	20	730
Fried chicken breast	360	21	190	110	1,080
Cheese pizza (6″ personal)	590	25	220	50	1,350
Caesar salad (no dressing)	90	5	45	10	180
Caesar salad (with dressing)	390	21	190	50	820
Chocolate shake	690	18	160	40	380
Blended coffee drink with whipped cream	420	9	180	55	270

Data from Fast Food Nutrition. (2014). Retrieved from http://www.fastfoodnutrition.org/. The nutritional content of items from each of the major fast food chains can also be found on each company's website. (Mobile App with fast food facts available.)

and more fiber, antioxidant vitamins, and plant-derived chemicals that are good for health (Orlich et al., 2014).

4. To encourage food and environmental sustainability. A plant-based diet reduces the demand for raised livestock, which is a major stress on ecosystems and on the planet as whole.

There are several kinds of **vegetarian** diets: strict or **veganism**, which excludes all animal products, including milk, cheeses, eggs, and other dairy products; **lacto-vegetarianism**, which excludes meat, poultry, fish, and eggs but includes dairy products; **lacto-ovo-vegetarianism**, which excludes meats, poultry, and seafood but includes eggs and dairy products; and **ovo-vegetarianism**, which excludes meat, poultry, sea food, and dairy but includes eggs. Properly planned vegetarian diets can meet the body's nutritional needs, especially by combining sources of protein to ensure adequate intake of the essential amino acids. Vegans may need vitamin B_{12} (cobalamin) supplements.

How Food Affects the Brain

The brain requires nutrients to function properly. For example, adequate protein in the diet provides nutrients for the manufacture of the neurotransmitters acetylcholine (choline), dopamine, epinephrine, and norepinephrine (from tyrosine), gama-aminobutyric acid (from glutamine), histamine (from histidine), and serotonin (from tryptophan).

> Don't buy much from the center aisles of the supermarket. Avoid packaged food with more than five ingredients and anything with a cartoon on it.
>
> *Marian Nestle*
> *What to Eat*

To some degree, moods, feelings of vitality, and sleep patterns may depend on the amount of neurotransmitter molecules ingested and therefore depend indirectly on meals (Hogenelst et al., 2015). Tyrosine may help to relieve depression and choline may help to modify certain postural and motor disturbances.

Also, some individuals can experience a strong, uncontrollable preference (craving and compulsive consumption) for certain foods or certain kinds of foods, particularly foods high in fat, sugar, and salt. When craving, these individuals show patterns of brain activity similar to those observed in drug addiction (Carter et al., 2016). Apparently, prior exposure to the craved foods activates the brain's reward centers, and conditions the susceptible person to certain patterns of eating behaviors.

The thoughts, moods, and body sensations of some individuals are sensitive to the amount of fat and sugar they ingest. We all know of individuals who use certain foods—chocolate, fatty, and sugary foods ("comfort foods")—to lessen the experience of stress or emotional upset or for consolation when feeling sad, lonely, or fatigued. Some individuals experience anxiety, fatigue, weakness, depressed mood, and an inability to concentrate shortly after consuming a couple of doughnuts or a candy bar. This response, called **reactive hypoglycemia**, is often the result of a sharp drop in blood sugar when insulin is secreted; this drop, in turn, is produced in response to the large load of sugar in the blood. Something akin to reactive hypoglycemia may be at the root of an eating pattern common to many: consumption of a high-sugar food at breakfast, followed two hours later by a reactive blood sugar low, which motivates a midmorning sugar "hit." The cycle is repeated at noon and midafternoon, and at dinner and late in the evening. To break this cycle, it helps to consume complex carbohydrates with protein and some fat, thereby moderating the rate at which simple sugars enter the body.

Because the human brain develops extensively during the late fetal period and the first 3 postnatal years, optimal brain development is dependent on key nutrients derived from the mother, such as glucose and oxygen for cellular energy production; protein for the manufacture of cellular material and amino acids for neurotransmitters; several vitamins; and the minerals iron, zinc, iodine, and copper. Nutrient deficiencies in early development can result in a variety of difficulties in late childhood and adulthood. Among these are impaired memory and cognition, slower neural processing, increased wariness, movement abnormalities, and susceptibility to depression (Georgieff et al., 2015). Maternal starvation during pregnancy is associated with an increased risk in children of schizophrenia, antisocial personality, and affective disorders (McGrath, Brown, & St. Clair, 2011).

By contrast, adequate fetal nutrition can have lifelong beneficial effects. Fetal intake of polyunsaturated fatty acids has beneficial effects on memory function by the time a child reaches school age (Boucher et al., 2011).

▌TERMS▐

lacto-ovo-vegetarian: one who excludes meats, poultry, and fish but includes eggs and dairy products from diet

lacto-vegetarian: one who excludes meat, poultry, fish, and eggs but includes dairy products from diet

ovo-vegetarian: one who excludes meats, poultry, fish, and dairy but eats eggs

reactive hypoglycemia: occurring after the ingestion of carbohydrate, with consequent release of insulin

vegan: one who excludes all animal products from the diet, including milk, cheese, eggs, and other dairy products

vegetarian: one who consumes no meat, poultry, or fish

Critical Thinking About Health

1. Everyone aboard the Zoracian space vehicle XTA-9781 was thrilled when their ship's sensors indicated life forms on a small planet orbiting a medium-sized star in the Milky Way galaxy. To make contact with and explore the planet, a landing party of six underwent molecular rearrangement to take on human form both to survive on Earth and communicate and interact with any Earthlings they encountered.

   "When you reach the surface," explained the mission commander, "you will have about eight of their time segments before you must refuel. Energy packets can be obtained in large, stationary pods the locals call supermarkets."

   The crew of the landing party nodded. It seemed similar enough to refueling on their home planet of Zorax not to cause confusion.

   "Except for one thing," the commander cautioned. "There are thousands of kinds of energy packets, from which you will have to choose the appropriate ones."

   "Appropriate ones?" asked the assistant crew-chief.

   "Yes. None of the fuel packets are efficient. You will have to sort and select."

   The crew shifted nervously.

   "Do not worry," said the commander, handing each member of the crew a copy of the U.S. Department of Agriculture's *Dietary Guidelines for Americans 2015–2020*. "Their leaders have prepared refueling guidelines. Take these and use them when the time comes."

   a. How would you explain to the Zoracian landing party why, with the great abundance of food choices in American supermarkets, the U.S. government advises its citizens how to eat properly?

   b. From the Zoracians' point of view, the American food supply, although abundant with many kinds of foods, is inefficient with regard to refueling. Explain why the American food supply is so diverse yet nutritionally inefficient.

   c. What factors influence your food selection?

2. A crusading nutrition journalist points out that the food label on a soup company's best-selling product indicates that the product has 6 grams of fat. Fearing that consumers will stop buying the product, the company responds, and within weeks the label indicates that the product has 3 grams of fat. The company has changed nothing in the product.

   a. Why does the label show that the product contains half the fat?

   b. What limits, if any, would you advocate be placed on what food manufacturers can put on product labels? Where would you draw the line between free enterprise, *caveat emptor* (buyer beware), and the public good?

   c. How much attention do you pay to what is written on food product labels?

3. Explain how an herbicide (weed-killing chemical) could wind up in the breast milk of a woman living hundreds of miles away from the site of herbicide application. Are you concerned about pesticides and additives in the food supply? Why or why not?

Chapter Summary and Highlights

Chapter Summary

Nearly everyone loves to eat—some more than others. Obtaining and consuming food is a basic need of all living organisms, including human beings. At one time, people hunted for and gathered food from the wild; now food is supplied by a gigantic food industry that would like you to buy and consume everything it manufactures regardless of its nutritional value or contribution to health. Government agencies try to help you eat properly by issuing nutritional guidelines and by requiring food manufacturers to list ingredients and nutritional values on all food products and packages. But judging from the epidemic of overweight and obesity in the United States and other countries, overconsumption of food, especially food of low nutritional value, has become the norm. To be healthy you need to become a smart and careful food shopper, both in supermarkets and in restaurants. Many diets and food choices can be healthy. You can decide to be a strict vegetarian or you can decide to add fish to a vegetarian diet. You can eat some kinds of meat, but not others. The important thing is to eat a balanced diet, which means that you are getting all the essential ingredients that your body needs—proteins, carbohydrates, fats, water, vitamins, essential minerals, and phytochemicals. A balanced diet, regardless of food sources, provides all the chemical ingredients your body needs to grow and function.

Eating healthfully does not mean you must never have a soda, a doughnut, a hamburger, a hot dog, or some kind of "junk" food. Everyone can overeat sometime; most of us overeat on holidays. Health is achieved by eating a modest amount of quality, fresh foods most of the time. Do not feed with food negative emotions, boredom, or unhappiness. Avoid foods grown with lots of chemicals and pesticides. As much as possible, buy fresh organic fruits, vegetables, and meats. Paying more for quality may also help you to eat less. When shopping for food in a supermarket, follow this rule: Shop mostly from the edges of the market, and buy as little as possible from the inside shelves. Produce, dairy, meats, and fresh breads are almost always arranged along the walls of the market. Inside aisles and shelves contain processed foods. Buy as little of the packaged, canned, bottled, and frozen foods as possible. Your body and brain will thank you.

Highlights

- The U.S. government and a variety of health organizations have created dietary guidelines to help people make nutritional choices to prevent heart disease, cancer, and other diseases based on the consumption of whole grains, fruits, and vegetables while limiting the consumption of meats, whole-fat dairy products, salt, and fatty, sugary snacks and sweets.
- MyPlate emphasizes the consumption of polyunsaturated fats, fruits, and vegetables rather than refined-grain products, meats, and sweets.
- The ingredients label on a food product lists the components of the product in descending order by weight.
- The Nutrition Facts label provides information on the amounts of certain nutrients in a food product.
- Food has three functions: to provide chemical constituents of the body, energy, and pleasure.
- Food is composed of seven components: protein, carbohydrate, fat, water, vitamins, minerals, and phytochemicals.
- Dietary supplements are unregulated substances that are used to augment the nutritional adequacy of the diet and as drugs to heal or prevent illness.
- Manufactured foods contain a variety of additives that alter their texture, flavor, color, and stability. Preservatives keep foods from spoiling through the use of sulfites.
- One nonchemical method of food preservation involves exposing food to gamma irradiation to destroy microorganisms.
- Artificial sweeteners are widely used, most commonly in diet soft drinks.
- There are several reasons for being a vegetarian, including increased interest in health, ecology, and world issues; economical issues; and the philosophy of not killing animals. A strict vegetarian, or vegan, diet eliminates all animal products, including milk, cheese, eggs, and other dairy products.

For Your Health

As the saying goes, "You are what you eat." Keep a Food Diary (Exercise 5.1 in the Workbook) to determine your typical dietary intake. The other exercises for Chapter 5 help you learn a variety of things about your diet.

References

Alexander, D. D., et al. (2015). Red meat and colorectal cancer: A quantitative update on the state of the epidemiological science. *Journal of the American College of Nutrition, 34*, 521–543.

American College of Sports Medicine/Academy of Nutrition and Dietetics Canada. (2016). Nutrition and Athletic Performance. *Medicine & Science in Sports & Exercise, 48*, 543–568. Retrieved from http://journals.lww.com/acsm-msse/Fulltext/2016/03000/Nutrition_and_Athletic_Performance.25.aspx

Bahadoran, Z., et al. (2015). Fast food pattern and cardiometabolic disorders: A review of current studies. *Health Promotion Perspectives, 5*, 231–240.

Boucher, O., et al. (2011). Neurophysiologic and neurobehavioral evidence of beneficial effects of prenatal omega-3 fatty acid intake on memory function at school age. *American Journal of Clinical Nutrition, 93*, 1025–1037.

Buckton, C. H., et al. (2015). Language is the source of misunderstandings: impact of terminology on public perceptions of health promotion messages. *BMC Public Health, 15*, 579. doi: 10.1186/s12889-015-1884-1. Retrieved from https://www.ncbi.nlm.nih.gov/pmc/articles/PMC4476206/pdf/12889_2015_Article_1884.pdf

Carter, A., et al. (2016). The neurobiology of "food addiction" and its implications for obesity treatment and policy. *Annual Review of Nutrition, 36*, 105–128.

Center for Science in the Public Interest. (2016). Seeing red: Time for action on food dyes. Retrieved from https://cspinet.org/resource/seeing-red-time-action-food-dyes

Fast Food Nutrition. (2014). Retrieved from http://www.fastfoodnutrition.org/

Fowler, S. P. (2016). Low-calorie sweetener use and energy balance: Results from experimental studies in animals, and large-scale prospective studies in humans. *Physiology and Behavior, 164*, 517–523.

Gallup Poll. (2013). Nutrition and Food. www.gallup.com/poll/6424/nutrition-food.aspx

Georgieff, M. K., et al. (2015). Early life nutrition and neural plasticity. *Developmental Psychology, 27*, 411–423.

Gilsing, A. M., et al. (2015). Vegetarianism, low meat consumption and the risk of colorectal cancer in a population-based cohort study. *Scientific Reports, 5*, 13484. doi: 10.1038/srep13484

Harvard School of Public Health. (2017). Nutrition source: Vitamins. https://www.hsph.harvard.edu /nutritionsource/what-should-you-eat/vitamins/

He, F. J., et al. (2014). Salt reduction in England from 2003 to 2011: Its relationship to blood pressure, stroke and ischemic heart disease mortality. *BMJ Open, 4, e004549.* doi: 10.1136/bmjopen-2013-004549

Hogenelst, K., et al. (2015). The effects of tryptophan on everyday interpersonal encounters and social cognitions in individuals with a family history of depression. *International Journal of Neuropsychopharmacology, 18(8),* pii: pyv012. doi: 10.1093/ijnp/pyv012

Imamura, F., et al. (2015). Dietary quality among men and women in 187 countries in 1990 and 2010: A systematic assessment. *Lancet Global Health, 3,* e132–e142.

Martinez Steele, E., et al. (2015). Ultra-processed foods and added sugars in the US diet: Evidence from a nationally representative cross-sectional study. *British Medical Journal Open, 6,* e009892. doi:10.1136 /bmjopen-2015-009892

McGrath, J., Brown, A., & St. Clair, D. (2011). Prevention and schizophrenia—the role of dietary factors. *Schizophrenia Bulletin, 37,* 272–283.

Murray, C. J. L., et al. (2016). Global burden of stroke and risk factors in 188 countries, during 1990–2013: A systematic analysis for the Global Burden of Disease Study 2013. *Lancet Neurology, 15,* 913–924.

O'Keefe, S. J., et al. (2016). Diet, microorganisms and their metabolites, and colon cancer. *Nature Reviews of Gastroenterology and Hepatology, 13,* 691–706.

Orlich, M. J., et al. (2014). Vegetarian diets in the Adventist Health Study 2: A review of initial published findings. *American Journal of Clinical Nutrition, 100,* 353S–358S.

Popkin, B. M., & Hawkes, C. (2016). Sweetening of the global diet, particularly beverages: Patterns, trends, and policy responses. *Lancet Diabetes & Endocrinology, 4,* 174–186.

Roberts, C. J., et al. (2014). Increases in weight during chronic stress are partially associated with a switch in food choice towards increased carbohydrate and saturated fat intake. *European Eating Disorders Review, 22,* 77–82.

Sax, J. K. (2015). Dietary supplements are not all safe and not all food: How the low cost of dietary supplements preys on the consumer. *American Journal of Law & Medicine, 41,* 374–394.

Trieu, K., et al. (2015). Salt reduction initiatives around the world: A systematic review of progress towards the global target. *PLoS ONE, 10,* e0130247. doi: 10.1371 /journal.pone.0130247

University of California, Berkeley. (2007). Got lactase? Retrieved from http://evolution.berkeley.edu /evolibrary/news/070401_lactose

U.S. Department of Agriculture. (2015). *Dietary Guidelines for Americans 2015–2020.* health.gov /dietaryguidelines/2015/guidelines/

U.S. Department of Agriculture. (2017). What Foods are in the grains group? Retrieved from http://www .choosemyplate.gov/food-groups/grains.html

U.S. Department of Agriculture, National Agricultural Library (2017a). DRI Tables and Application Reports. nal.usda.gov/fnic/dri-tables-and-application-reports

U.S. Department of Agriculture, Food Safety and Inspection Service. (2017b). Kitchen companion. Your safe food handbook. https://www.fsis.usda.gov /wps/portal/fsis/topics/food-safety-education/get -answers/food-safety-fact-sheets/safe-food-han -dling/kitchen-companion-your-safe-food-handbook /ct_index

U.S. Department of Agriculture. (2013a). Foodborne illness: what consumers need to know. https:// www.fsis.usda.gov/wps/portal/fsis/topics/food- safety-education/get-answers/food-safety-fact -sheets/foodborne-illness-and-disease/foodborne -illness-what-consumers-need-to-know/ct_index

U.S. Department of Agriculture. (2015). *Dietary guidelines for Americans 2015–2020* (8th ed). Retrieved from http:// www.health.gov/dietaryguidelines/2015/guidelines

U.S. Department of Health and Human Services, National Institutes of Health, National Heart, Lung, and Blood Institute. (2012). What is the DASH eating plan? Retrieved from http://www.nhlbi.nih.gov/health /health-topics/topics/dash

U.S. Food and Drug Administration. (2015). Are you storing food safely? Retrieved from http://www.fda.gov /ForConsumers/ConsumerUpdates/ucm093704.htm

Vikraman S., et al. (2015). Caloric intake from fast food among children and adolescents in the United States, 2011–2012. NCHS Data Brief, no 213. Hyattsville, MD: National Center for Health Statistics. Retrieved from https://www.cdc.gov/nchs/products/databriefs /db213.htm

World Health Organization. (2015). Micronutrient deficiencies: Vitamin A deficiency. Retrieved from http:// www.who.int/nutrition/topics/vad/en/

Suggested Readings

Alsaffar, A. A. (2016). Sustainable diets: The interaction between food industry-nutrition-health and the environment. *Food Science and Technology, 22,* 102–111. Explores the interactions of the food industry, nutrition, and the environment on achieving a healthy diet, entailing minimal consumption of highly processed and packaged foods and those that have low environmental impacts.

American College of Sports Medicine/Academy of Nutrition and Dietetics Canada. (2016). Nutrition and Athletic Performance. *Medicine & Science in Sports & Exercise, 48,* 543–568. Retrieved from http://journals.lww.com/acsm-msse/Fulltext/2016/03000/Nutrition_and_Athletic_Performance.25.aspx

Brown University Health Promotion. (2014). Being a vegetarian. Retrieved from http://www.brown.edu/Student_Services/Health_Services/Health_Education/nutrition_&_eating_concerns/being_a_vegetarian.php

Ehrenberg, R. (2016, February). GMOs under scrutiny. *Science News.* A thorough discussion of the history, promise, and pitfalls of GMO foods.

Food Product Dating. Retrieved from https://www.fsis.usda.gov/wps/portal/fsis/topics/food-safety-education/get-answers/food-safety-fact-sheets/food-labeling/food-product-dating/food-product-dating. Discusses the legal rules regarding date labels on food products.

Freedman, D. H. (2013, August 20). The truth about genetically modified food. *Scientific American.* Retrieved from http://www.scientificamerican.com/article/the-truth-about-genetically-modified-food/?print=true. Proponents of genetically modified crops say the technology is the only way to feed a warming, increasingly populous world. Critics say we tamper with nature at our peril. Who is right?

Harvard Medical School. (2009, October). Becoming a vegetarian. *Harvard Women's Health Watch.* Avoiding meat is only one part of the picture. A healthy vegetarian diet should be chock-full of foods with known benefits. Read this before embarking on a vegetarian diet.

Kelly Dry Law. (2017). Food and drug law access. Retrieved from www.fooddruglaw.com. Provides news and commentary concerning food and drug law and public policy developments administered by the Food and Drug Administration (FDA), the U.S. Department of Agriculture (USDA), the European Commission, Member States in the European Union (EU), and similar authorities throughout the world affecting companies that manufacture, import, market, distribute, or sell foods, dietary supplements, cosmetics, drugs and/or medical devices.

Mayo Clinic. (2017). Organic foods: Are they safer? More nutritious? Retrieved from www.mayoclinic.org/healthy-lifestyle/nutrition-and-healthy-eating/in-depth/organic-food/art-20043880. All about organic foods.

National Institutes of Health Office of Dietary Supplements. (2017). Dietary supplements: What you need to know. ods.od.nih.gov/HealthInformation/DS_WhatYouNeedToKnow.aspx. Provides consumers with a variety of fact sheets with a current overview of individual vitamins, minerals, and other dietary supplements.

Nestle, M. (2007). *Food politics: How the food industry influences nutrition and health.* Berkeley: University of California Press. A noted professor of nutrition analyzes how the food industry, in its search for profits, contributes to ill health.

Nestle, M. (2010). *Safe food: The politics of food safety, updated and expanded.* Berkeley: University of California Press. Shows the many influences on the system that supposedly guarantees the safety of the U.S. food supply.

Nestle, M. (2013). *What to eat.* Berkeley: University of California Press. A noted professor of nutrition shows how to navigate supermarket aisles healthfully by resisting marketers' attempts to influence the purchase of unhealthy foods and using common sense to make healthy choices.

Robbins, J. (2010). *The food revolution: How your diet can help save your life and our world.* San Francisco: Conari Press. Describes how vegetarianism can improve health, help stop global warming, feed the hungry, prevent cruelty to animals, and avoid genetically modified foods.

Schlosser, E. (2001). *Fast food nation*. New York: Houghton Mifflin. Everything you ever wanted to know (and not know) about fast food: its history, role in the economy, and contribution to the epidemic of obesity.

Song, M., et al. (2015). Nutrients, foods, and colorectal cancer prevention. *Gastroenterology, 148,* 1244–1260. Retrieved from https://www.ncbi.nlm.nih.gov/pmc/articles/PMC4409470/. Good review for students to check out.

Specter, M. (2015, November 2). Freedom from fries: Can fast food be good for you? *The New Yorker.* Retrieved from https://www.newyorker.com/magazine/2015/11/02/freedom-from-fries. Profiles the history and current state of the U.S. quick-meal system.

Tilman, D., et al. (2015, Fall). The future of food, health and the environment of a full Earth. *Daedalus.* doi:10.1162/DAED_e_00349. Considered opinions about human health and living conditions in 2035 when the world's human population is 11 billion people, food and water are scarce, and climate change is in full swing.

U.S. Food and Drug Administration. (2017). Learn about the Nutrition Facts label. Retrieved from www.accessdata.fda.gov/scripts/InteractiveNutritionFactsLabel/#intro. The FDA's online tutorial on how to read the Nutrition Facts label.

Willett, W. C., & Skerrett, P. J. (2005). *Eat, drink and be healthy.* New York: Free Press. Two prominent nutritionists explain healthy eating.

Recommended Websites

American Cancer Society
Discusses the importance of nutrition in cancer prevention.

American Dietetic Association
Provides information and daily tips.

American Heart Association
Provides information on the association's eating plan.

Food Politics
Professor Marion Nestle of the Department of Nutrition at New York University blogs about nutrition, the food industry, and health.

Herbs and Botanical Information
Provides scientific information on more than 130 botanical agents used in health and disease.

Nutritional Analysis Tool (NAT)
Allows analysis of foods for various nutrients.

Nutrition.gov
Provides easy access to all online federal government information on nutrition, including healthy eating, physical activity, and food safety.

Nutrition Source
The Department of Nutrition at the Harvard School of Public Health provides a comprehensive website designed to inform and educate the public, journalists, and nutrition professionals about the latest news and issues concerning diet and health.

Quackwatch
Offers information on safety and health issues of dietary supplements.

U.S. Department of Agriculture. Dietary Supplements: Safety and Health Claims
Tips and resources that we hope will help you be a savvy dietary supplement user.

U.S. Department of Agriculture Food Safety and Inspection Service
Includes consumer advice on foodborne illnesses.

U.S. Department of Agriculture National Organic Program
Provides information on organic food.

U.S. Food and Drug Administration Center for Food Safety and Applied Nutrition
Provides information on food safety, food additives, dietary supplements, and food biotechnology.

U.S. Food and Drug Administration Food Labeling Publications Page
Labeling requirements for prepared foods such as breads, cereals, canned and frozen foods, snacks, desserts, drinks, etc.

Vegetarian Resource Group
Provides nutrition information, recipes, and FAQs.

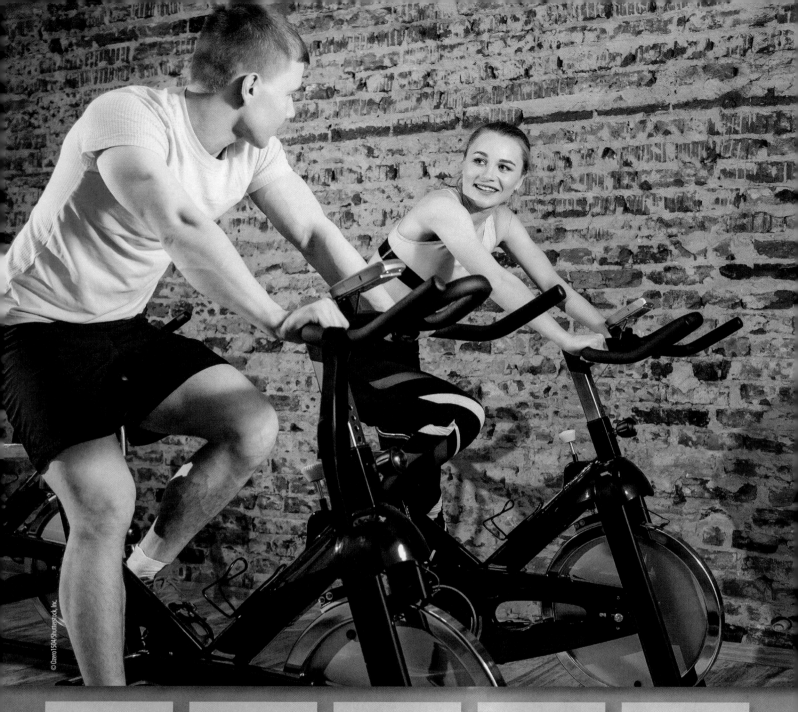

© Ozero1504/Shutterstock, Inc.

Health Tips

Walk the Walk

Mindful Eating

Inform Yourself: Don't Buy Worthless and Sometimes Harmful Weight-Loss Products

Dollars & Health Sense

Junk Food Marketing and Overweight Childhood

Global Wellness

Eating Disorders Are a Worldwide Concern

Managing Stress

Treating the Underlying Emotional Causes of Obesity

Wellness Guide

Uncle Joe's Successful Weight Loss

Overweight has become a monumental health problem in the United States and the world. Approximately 130 million American adults—about 68% of the population—are considered overweight (**Figure 6.1**). One-third of U.S. children between the ages of 6 and 19 are also overweight. An estimated 1.9 billion adults worldwide are overweight (World Health Organization, 2016).

> There is no sincerer love than the love of food.
>
> *George Bernard Shaw*

Many people consider overweight to be primarily a cosmetic issue. Although feeling attractive is important, overweight is a serious health issue. Overweight individuals are predisposed to a variety of illnesses (**Figure 6.2**), including heart disease and type 2 diabetes, which can result in blindness, kidney failure, and nonhealing skin ulcers, and is the leading cause of nontraumatic amputation in the United States. Because of their large body size, overweight individuals tend to have more job-related injuries and an increased risk of becoming disabled from arthritis, gait disturbances, back pain, and general instability. Overweight also predisposes individuals to the *metabolic syndrome,* which is characterized by high body fat primarily located around the abdomen, high blood sugar and triglycerides, high blood pressure, and the inability to respond to insulin. On average, people who are overweight live several years less than healthy-weight age peers. Annually, about 160,000 Americans die prematurely from complications of being overweight. Annual U.S. healthcare costs related to overweight are over $150 billion.

The percentage of Americans who are overweight has been increasing steadily since about 1970 (**Figure 6.3**). The reasons for this increase in overweight include the following:

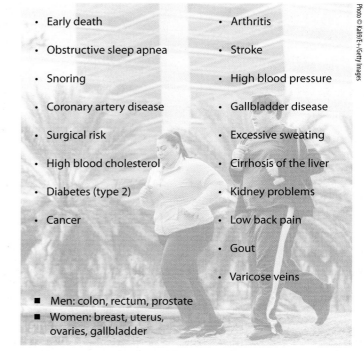

- Early death
- Obstructive sleep apnea
- Snoring
- Coronary artery disease
- Surgical risk
- High blood cholesterol
- Diabetes (type 2)
- Cancer

- Arthritis
- Stroke
- High blood pressure
- Gallbladder disease
- Excessive sweating
- Cirrhosis of the liver
- Kidney problems
- Low back pain
- Gout
- Varicose veins

- ■ Men: colon, rectum, prostate
- ■ Women: breast, uterus, ovaries, gallbladder

■ Figure 6.2

Health Consequences of Overweight
Overweight and obese people have a greater likelihood of developing certain health problems than do people of normal weight.

- An overconsumption of calorie-dense foods in relation to energy expenditure. Between 1971 and 2010, average daily energy intake per American man rose from 2,453 calories to 2,564 calories (111 more per day), and per American woman rose from 1,540 calories to 1,803 calories (263 more per day) without a compensatory increase in calorie use through physical activity (Ford & Dietz, 2013).

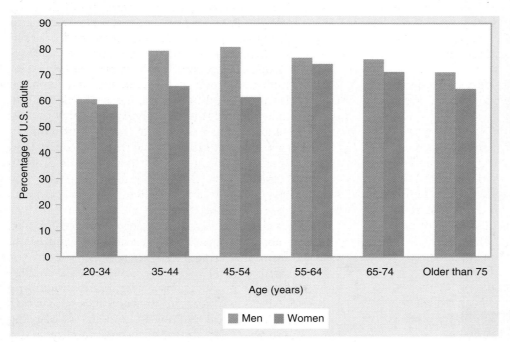

Men   Women

■ Figure 6.1

Prevalence of Overweight in the United States
Overweight is defined as a body mass index (BMI) greater than 25.0.

Data from U.S. Centers for Disease Control and Prevention. (2016). Health, United States, 2015. Retrieved from https://www.cdc.gov/nchs/data/hus/2015/059.pdf

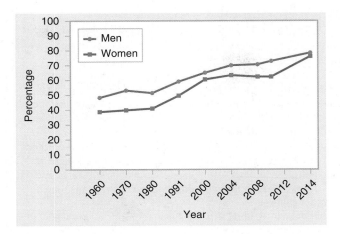

■ Figure 6.3

Overweight in the United States
The percentage of adult Americans who are overweight (BMI > 25), by year.

Data from Ogden, C. D. et al. (2016). Prevalence of overweight, obesity, and extreme obesity among adults aged 20 and over: United States, 1960–1962 through 2013–2014. National Center for Health Statistics, Health E-Stats. Retrieved from https://www.cdc.gov/nchs/data/hestat/obesity_adult_13_14/obesity_adult_13_14.pdf

- An abundance (and relentless marketing) of inexpensive, palatable foods that contribute to weight gain (highly processed foods and snack foods, sodas, and fast food). Fast-food consumption (more than twice per week) is strongly associated with weight gain (Rosenheck, 2008). The prevalence of overweight is proportional to the number of residents per fast-food store and the number of fast-food restaurants in a community (Fleischhacker et al., 2011).
- An increase in portion sizes; for example, in the past 25 years a "regular" soft drink increased in size from 10 to 16 ounces. A supersized soda contains 64 ounces. Also in that time period, the energy content of a typical burger and fries or a serving of Mexican food has increased by 150 calories. Since the 1970s, the size of portions in home and restaurant meals and packaged foods has increased considerably (Benton, 2015).
- A reduction in jobs that require physical labor.
- A decrease in the amount of work and leisure movement activity.
- An increase in suburban living, with an associated reliance on automobile travel rather than walking or bicycling. One study found that each additional hour spent in a car per day was associated with a 6% increase in the likelihood of obesity and each additional kilometer walked per day was associated with a 4.8% reduction in the likelihood of obesity (Frank, Andresen, & Schmid, 2004).
- Reductions in school physical education and after-school physical activities.
- An increase in time spent watching TV, using the computer or mobile device, and playing video games.
- An increase in the pace of life, which creates a demand for prepackaged and fast food.

- An increase in the stress of life, which fosters eating high-fat, high-sugar "comfort foods" resulting in metabolism that can lead to weight gain as part of the metabolic syndrome (Burgess et al., 2014).

Among American college students, about 39% of women and 32% of men consider themselves overweight; 53% are trying to lose weight. (American College Health Association, 2016a, 2016b). Some of these students may have been overweight when they started college, whereas others gained weight after entering college. Some reasons for weight gain in college include the following:

- Being away from home and thus having greater independence in food choices (which may not always be the healthiest)
- Fragmented schedules that promote skipping meals, especially breakfast, and the resultant consumption of high-calorie snacks and fast food when hungry
- Little time invested in physical activity due to academic and paid work responsibilities
- Exposure to factors that promote food consumption, for example, soda and snack vending machines on campus, unlimited access to dorm/dining facility food, and academic and social stress

Judging from the number of books and magazine articles extolling various "surefire" weight-loss methods and of infomercials peddling dietary supplements and exercise gear, it would appear that the U.S. national pastime is weight control. Indeed, about 25% of adult American women and men are on so-called reducing diets (so-called because they generally fail to reduce weight in the long run). Concern about body weight (more typically, body *fatness*) fuels a $64 billion weight-loss industry.

With all the passion for losing weight, it is no wonder that many people view body fat as an enemy. However, the human body has evolved over time in environments of food scarcity; hence, the ability to store fat easily and efficiently is a valuable physiological function that served our ancestors well for thousands of years. Only in recent decades in primarily industrially developed economies and increasingly developed ones, have high-calorie consumable-as-food products become so plentiful and easy to obtain as to cause fat-related health problems. People no longer have to spend most of their time and energy gathering berries and seeds and hoping that a hunting party will return with meat or even plow the back 40 and feed the chickens. Nowadays all they have to do is drive to the supermarket or the fast-food outlet, where for a very low cost they can obtain nearly all of their daily calories (**Table 6.1**).

Body weight issues are not solely about food intake. They are about food intake in relation to a number of other factors, including a sedentary lifestyle and lack of movement activities, heredity, advertising of weight-promoting food products, lack of guidance regarding proper nutrition, confusing information about the effects of food on health and well-being, the custom of using body shape as a measure of social desirability, and a

Junk Food Marketing and Overweight Childhood

Approximately 18% of American children between the ages of 6 and 19 are very overweight, a tripling in prevalence since 1980 (see accompanying figure). Although a variety of social factors have been offered to explain it, marketing of high-calorie, low-nutrient "junk" food to kids is a major contributor to this disturbing trend (Partridge et al., 2016).

About 30% of the calories in an average child's diet come from sweets, salty snacks, fast food, and sodas. Beverage companies spend millions of dollars per year to market their products to youth via TV (American children see between 10 and 20 food-related TV commercials per day). Many, many more marketing dollars are spent on getting products into TV shows as props (e.g., a character consumes a particular brand of soda), product-related toys, games, Websites, special events sponsorship, and the licensing of popular characters to sell products. Studies show that children prefer foods that are associated with a particular character or brand, even if equivalent alternatives are offered (Boyland & Halford, 2013). Numerous firms, on behalf of advertising agencies and food manufacturers, conduct extensive research to elucidate the psychological factors that influence children's food choices and their strategies for obtaining the foods they desire.

In 2006, 18 food and fast-food companies joined together to found the Children's Food and Beverage Advertising Initiative (CFBAI) to decrease the amount of advertising of junk food to children under age 12. However, a 2016 report (Harris et al., 2015) noted the following:

- In 2014, 44% of ads seen by children under age 12 promoted brands that companies pledged not to advertise directly to children, including Nature Valley Snack Bars, Pop-Tarts, and Tostitos. Preschoolers viewed 8% fewer of these ads than did older children.
- Between 2010 and 2014, ads for snack foods viewed by Hispanic children on Spanish-language TV increased from 39% to 89%.
- In 2014, African American teens were exposed to an average 3.1 snack food TV ads per day, compared to 1.5 ads per day for white teens. Doritos, Oreo cookies, and Pop-Tarts showed the largest racial disparities.

Obviously, promises by CFBAI companies offer little comfort to parents and health professionals who want to improve healthy food alternatives to their children.

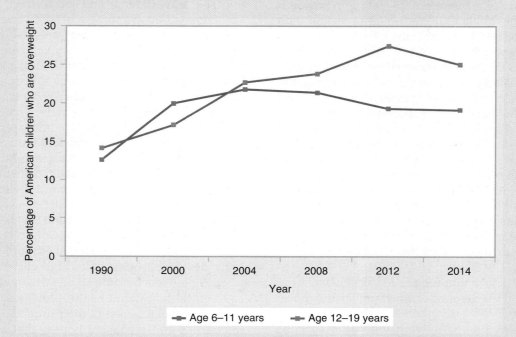

Prevalence of Overweight in U.S. Children, 1990–2014
Overweight is defined as a BMI (body mass index: mass in kilogram/height-squared in meters) at or above the 95th percentile on BMI-for-age growth charts. Data are from the U.S. Centers for Disease Control and Prevention's National Health and Nutrition Examination Survey (NHANES), which is designed to assess the health and nutritional status of adults and children in the United States. The survey is unique in that it combines interviews and physical examinations.

Data from Ogden, C. L., et al. (2016). Trends in obesity prevalence among children and adolescents in the United States, 1988–1994 through 2013–2014. *Journal of the American Medical Association, 315*, 2292–2299.

hectic, stressful lifestyle. In such a complex environment, the overavailability of cheap, fatty, salty, sugary products allows them to be used for a variety of purposes other than to provide calories when hungry.

Exposure to certain industrial chemicals, referred to as *obesogens*, may also affect one's susceptibility to being overweight (overfat) by upsetting the body's fat-storage systems. For example, obesogens can cause the body to

Table 6.1

Percentage of Daily Calories Provided by Typical Fast-Food Meals

	Percentage of daily calories for three different daily calorie levels		
Meal	1,600 calories/day	2,000 calories/day	2,500 calories/day
Quarter Pounder French fries Milkshake	73	58	47
Whopper French fries Diet soft drink	66	54	43
Two slices of pizza Diet soft drink	33	25	20

make more fat cells (Janesick & Blumberg, 2011). These cells not only store fat but also manufacture hormones that increase appetite and decrease energy use. Suspected obesogens include bisphenol A (BPA), bis(2-ethylhexyl) phthalate (DEHP), diethylstilbesterol, mono(2-ethylhexyl) phthalate, perfluorooctanoic acid, tributyltin, and triphenyltin. Most obesogens are chemicals used to manufacture plastics; others are pesticides, wood preservatives, and slime inhibitors in industrial water systems.

In contrast to those who are cautions about overweight, some—almost always men—are concerned about perceived underweight. Although not unhealthy, they imagine themselves to be less attractive and masculine and desire to gain several pounds of muscle. Many men who want to gain weight think that women prefer men who are much more muscular than these men perceive themselves to be. However, women generally prefer men with ordinary body sizes without added muscle. There are biological limits to how muscular one can become. One can try to maximize one's potential for muscularity by engaging in strength training and consuming healthy foods to support that activity. Special diets of "superfoods" and supplements in and of themselves will not produce increased muscularity, advertising claims notwithstanding. And drugs that are purported to bring about weight (muscle) gain are either worthless (chromium, creatine, protein powders) or dangerous (ephedra, anabolic steroids).

What Is Healthy Weight?

In most instances, concerns about being overweight are really concerns about being *overfat*. There is a difference. Some professional male athletes, for example, weigh much more than the recommended weight standards for persons of similar height. Yet as little as 1% of their body weight may be fat. Most of the nonwater body weight of a well-conditioned athlete is muscle and bone. Female body builders, who are the leanest of all female athletes, have

about 8% to 13% of their total body weight as fat. This probably represents the lower limit of fat for a healthy woman.

Body fat is composed of two parts: **essential fat**—fat necessary for normal physiological functioning, such as nerve conduction—and **storage fat**. Essential fat constitutes about 5% to 10% of body weight in men and about 8% to 15% of body weight in women. This sex difference, which is presumably caused by hormones, is due to the biologically based deposition of greater amounts of fat on the hips, thighs, and breasts in females. Storage fat, also called depot fat, constitutes only a small percentage of the total body weight of lean individuals and 5% to 25% of the body weight of the majority of the population. **Obesity** is the medical term for storage fat exceeding about 30% of body weight.

Social standards for the most "desirable" or "ideal" body weight or body composition (fat percentage) vary. For example, in some cultures, women with significant storage fat are considered physically attractive and sexually desirable, and fatness in children is considered a sign of robust health. In North America, attitudes about desirable adult body configuration fluctuate over time and are often keyed to fashion trends. In the 1920s, the ideal female body shape was "tubular," with emphasis on small breasts and slim hips. In the 1950s, the ideals were a large body size characterized by "full-figured" women and "he-men."

Today, the ideal female body shape is "hourglass," with emphasis on ample breasts and hips and a small waist (i.e., *Shape* magazine cover model); the male ideal is slim and muscular with visible, taut ("six-pack") abdominal muscles (*Muscle and Fitness* magazine cover model).

Health-related body weight is gauged by health professionals and scientists with the **body mass index (BMI)**, which is calculated by dividing a person's weight in kilograms by his or her height in meters squared (**Table 6.2**). Studies show that good health is associated with having a BMI between 19 and 25 (**Figure 6.4**). People with BMI greater than 25 have higher risks for type 2 diabetes, gallbladder disease, varicose veins, arthritis, heart disease, stroke, high blood pressure, breathing problems, and accident proneness (because of a large body). People who are extremely overweight often face stigmas, such as job discrimination, and lower social acceptance, and they tend to have lower self-esteem.

TERMS

body mass index (BMI): a measure of body fatness, calculated by dividing body weight (in kilograms) by the square of height (in meters)

essential fat: necessary body fat required for normal physiological functioning

obesity: storage fat exceeding 30% of body weight

storage fat: also called depot fat; energy stored as fat in various parts of the body

Table 6.2

Body Mass Index (BMI) Table

BMI	19	20	21	22	23	24	25	26	27	28	29	30	31	32	33	34	35
Height								Weight (in pounds)									
4′10″ (58″)	91	96	100	105	110	115	119	124	129	134	138	143	148	153	158	162	167
4′11″ (59″)	94	99	104	109	114	119	124	128	133	138	143	148	153	158	163	168	173
5′ (60″)	97	102	107	112	118	123	128	133	138	143	153	158	163	168	174	179
5′1″ (61″)	100	106	111	116	122	127	132	137	143	148	153	158	164	169	174	180	185
5′2″ (62″)	104	109	115	120	126	131	136	142	147	153	158	164	169	175	180	186	191
5′3″ (63″)	107	113	118	124	130	135	141	146	152	158	163	169	175	180	186	191	197
5′4″ (64″)	110	116	122	128	134	140	145	151	157	163	169	174	180	186	192	197	204
5′5″ (65″)	114	120	126	132	138	144	150	156	162	168	174	180	186	192	198	204	210
5′6″ (66″)	118	124	130	136	142	148	155	161	167	173	179	186	192	198	204	210	216
5′7″ (67″)	121	127	134	140	146	153	159	166	172	178	185	191	198	204	211	217	223
5′8″ (68″)	125	131	138	144	151	158	164	171	177	184	190	197	203	210	216	223	230
5′9″ (69″)	128	135	142	149	155	162	169	176	182	189	196	203	209	216	223	230	236
5′10″ (70″)	132	139	146	153	160	167	174	181	188	195	202	209	216	222	229	236	243
5′11″ (71″)	136	143	150	157	165	172	179	186	193	200	208	215	222	229	236	243	250
6′ (72″)	140	147	154	162	169	177	184	191	199	206	213	221	228	235	242	250	258
6′1″ (73″)	144	151	159	166	174	182	189	197	204	212	219	227	235	242	250	257	265
6′2″ (74″)	148	155	163	171	179	186	194	202	210	218	225	233	241	249	256	264	272
6′3″ (75″)	152	160	168	176	184	192	200	208	216	224	232	240	248	256	264	272	279

Directions: Find your height in the left column. Go across the row to find your weight. Go up the column to the top row to find your BMI. Healthy BMI = 18–24.99. Overweight BMI = 25–29.99. Unhealthy BMI ("obese") = 30+.

Reproduced from U.S. Department of Health and Human Services, National Institutes of Health, National Heart, Lung, and Blood Institute. Body Mass Index Table 1. Retrieved from http://www.nhlbi.nih.gov/health/education/lose_wt/BMI/bmi_tbl.htm

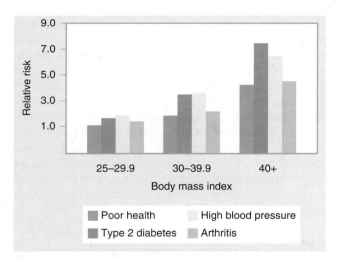

■ Figure 6.4

Relative Health Risks of Various Body Mass Indexes
The risks for poor health, type 2 diabetes, high blood pressure, and arthritis increase as body mass index increases. Relative risk means that the risk for each BMI is standardized to the BMI range of 18.5 to 24.9, which is considered healthy.

Modified from Mokdad, A. H., et al. (2003). Prevalence of obesity, diabetes, and obesity-related health risk factors, 2001. *Journal of the American Medical Association, 289*(1): 76–79.

Another health-related index of body size is the waist-to-hip ratio, which is calculated by dividing the circumference at the waist by the circumference at the hips. For example, someone with a 28-inch waist circumference and 37-inch hip circumference would have a waist-to-hip ratio of 0.75. Health problems are less likely in women whose waist-to-hip ratio is less than 0.8 and in men whose waist-to-hip ratio is less than 0.95. In other words, it is healthier for a body to be pear-shaped than apple-shaped, and it's healthier *not* to have a beer belly (**Figure 6.5**). Doctors sometimes use only the waist circumference as an indicator of health risks associated with being overweight. A waist circumference greater than 40 inches in men and 35 inches in women is associated with greater health risk.

The Regulation of Body Fat

The body has a multifaceted, complex system for acquiring and storing the energy for life. The body acquires its energy from food: 4 calories per gram of protein or carbohydrate, 7 calories per gram of alcohol, and 9 calories per gram of fat. Calories leave the body as energy expended to fuel basal (resting) metabolism, digestion, physical activity, growth, and injury repair and to maintain body temperature. Calories from food that are not used right away are stored either as glycogen, a complex carbohydrate that is found in liver and muscle, or as **triglyceride**, a fat that is found in adipose tissue located on the body in all-too-familiar places. At 9 calories per gram, fat is the most efficient form of energy storage (1 pound of

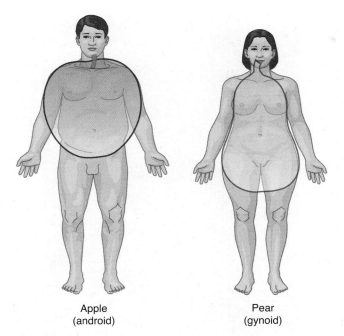

Apple
(android)

Pear
(gynoid)

■ **Figure 6.5**

Apple or Pear?

Apple-shaped people carry much of their body fat above the waist. Pear-shaped people carry their body fat on the hips and thighs. Studies show that it's healthier to be pear-shaped than apple-shaped.

fat will fuel a 40-mile walk), and fat has other biological advantages: it's lightweight, compact, spongy, and a good thermal insulator.

The body's energy-acquisition system has two main components: the homeostatic eating system and the hedonic, or pleasure, eating system. The **homeostatic eating system**, located in the hypothalamus region of the brain, maintains a relatively constant level of body fat. When energy levels fall, either from utilizing food attained in recent meals or by mobilizing energy stored as fat, the body signals that deficit to the brain via certain hormones, which triggers hunger, which motivates eating. When energy (fat) levels are restored, the body signals that situation to the brain, which creates the feeling of fullness (called *satiety*). That causes sensations of hunger to lessen and attention is turned to other matters.

The level of body fat maintained by the homeostatic eating system is determined by heredity and developmental influences and is relatively constant over time; it is sometimes referred to as the *body weight set point* or *fatness set point*. If a person eats more than usual in a short period of time and gains several pounds of weight (fat), for example, while vacationing on a cruise ship, when the person returns to usual life the brain automatically reduces hunger and appetite, the person eats less without thinking about it, and the extra weight is shed until the set point weight is attained. Alternatively, if a person uses more energy than usual in a short period of time and loses several pounds of fat, for example, by being very

sick for 3 weeks, when healthy again the person will eat more without trying to and in a few weeks body weight will return to the set point.

Unlike the homeostatic eating system, which responds to levels of nutrients and energy in the body, the **hedonic eating system**, also called the *pleasure eating system*, responds to food-related thoughts and emotions that are independent of hunger. For example, you can walk into the mall and smell freshly baked chocolate chip cookies and not resist consuming one or more even if you have just eaten and are full. Or you can go to a restaurant with friends or eat dinner with your family at "dinnertime" even if you are not hungry. On the other hand, you could be hungry, but you really dislike the pizza toppings your friends have ordered and you lose your appetite. Or you invite a new love interest to dinner and are too distracted by your emotions to eat.

The hedonic eating system is a network of nerve cells located in various regions of the brain that are involved in reward (feeling good when you get what you desire) and deprivation (feeling bad and/or craving when you don't) (Yu et al., 2015). Rather than being governed by built-in biological mechanisms for maintaining levels of energy and nutrients, hedonic eating is motivated by the psychological desire to experience a certain kind of pleasure, most often associated with consuming so called **palatable foods**, which create the sensations of salty, fatty, and sweet.

Hedonic eating is the body's way of "saving for a rainy day." Even if you're getting enough food to keep you healthy and aren't often hungry, hedonic eating takes advantage of opportunities to fatten up in case you encounter a lengthy time of food scarcity. However, when food is abundant and easy to attain (as in most economically developed and developing countries), hedonic eating is responsible for many, many people being overweight (overfat) and susceptible to the diseases that result from it, social stigma for being perceived as lazy and gluttonous, and self-doubt. Also, because hedonic eating is not governed by the level of energy in the body, it can be put to other uses, for example, to avoid thinking about one's problems or to feel socially accepted by friends and family by happily

TERMS

hedonic eating system: motivation to eat by the desire to experience a psychological reward, or pleasure from consuming food

homeostatic eating system: integrated neurological and hormonal control of eating behavior based on the body's need for energy (calories)

palatable foods: those which create the sensations of salty, fatty, and sweet

triglyceride: a storage form of fat

consuming the same kinds of foods they do (Boggiano et al., 2015). Nicknames for psychological and social motivations for hedonic eating include "emotional eating," "stress-induced eating," "food addiction," "eating comfort foods," "medicating with food," and "grazing." As long as you are generally healthy, your homeostatic eating system is working properly, *and you pay attention to it* when it signals fullness, you are unlikely to develop a weight (fat) problem because your homeostatic eating system will ensure that your calorie intake will pretty much equal your calorie output; this is called being in a state of **energy balance**. However, you only have to exceed energy balance a little bit to develop a weight problem over time. Consider this example:

> Marci is a 26-year-old woman of normal weight with a BMI of 23 who recently changed jobs. Previously the office manager in a small real estate company, she now works as an executive assistant in a much larger firm. Two consequences of this change are (1) Marci now spends more time sitting at her desk typing and answering the phone than in her former job, where she moved around to do virtually every office task; and (2) she now goes to lunch with office mates. The combination of less movement and restaurant lunches has increased Marci's daily calorie intake over expenditure an average of 10%.

What's 10%? For Marci, that's about 160 calories per working day, or 3,200 calories a month. Because a pound of body fat has 3,500 calories, that's enough for Marci to gain about 10 pounds per year. You can see what a few years at this job might do to Marci's waistline. When the office crew goes to lunch, often their intention is to socialize and get away from the stress of the office; they don't intend to consume lots of food. However, the desire to be social, the smell of food, and generous portions make it easy to ignore satiety signals from the homeostatic eating signals from the brain and to overeat.

> The trouble with Italian cooking is that after five or six days you're hungry again.
>
> *Henry Miller, author*

Of course, Marci could prevent gaining those 10 pounds a year by being more mindful of her lunchtime eating behaviors and walking a few more minutes each day. By consuming one less cookie or half of a 12-ounce soda, she would consume 80 fewer food calories per day. Also, if she parked her car a 10-minute walk from her workplace, she would utilize 80 calories more than usual. Eating 80 calories less and walking off 80 calories more would stop the accumulation of 160 calories of fat per day and those 10 extra pounds each year. If she doesn't eat less and exercise more, however, her body is likely to store those excess calories as fat. Over time, her body will probably adjust to the higher weight as its "new normal" fatness set point, and in a couple of years she is likely to find herself with a BMI near 27 and in need of a new wardrobe. If that happens and she

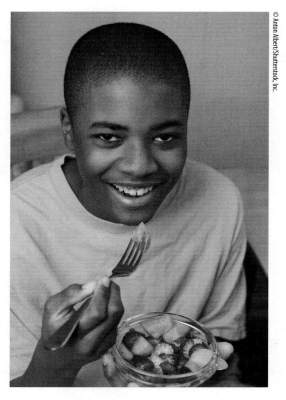

If you have to snack, choose healthy foods such as fruits and vegetables.

decides to lose that extra fat, she's likely to find that to be a serious challenge.

That's because the body doesn't like to let go of fat it has accumulated, or as scientists say, the body defends against fat loss. Remember, over many thousands of years of evolution, the body has developed the capacity to store fat easily, in case you ever have periods of little or no food as your ancient ancestors did. Of course, that almost never happens to people who live in economically advantaged societies, but those built-in, efficient fat-storage mechanisms are still present. So, once fat is deposited in adipose tissue, the body holds on to it. The main ways the body defends against fat loss are to increase the efficiency with which the body uses energy, decreasing the resting metabolic rate and increasing the efficiency with which the muscles do work. Also, even if a person is successful at losing weight, the body responds to the weight loss as if the person's life is in danger from semi-starvation and will increase hunger and appetite to recover that lost weight.

Generally, sensible and consistent weight-loss efforts produce a 5% to 10% reduction in body weight (fat) over the first 6 months of trying, with no further weight loss after that. This is the reason that people are encouraged not to gain weight in the first place. Fortunately, even a 3% reduction in body weight (fat) can significantly improve health status even though reduction in body size is not significant.

Calorie-Restriction Diets Rarely Work

To a nutritionist, the word *diet* means what an individual usually eats and drinks. To almost everyone else, the word *diet* means restricting calories or eating unusual foods to lose weight, as in "I'm on a diet."

It's logical to think that consuming less food than usual will produce weight loss because overeating is generally identified as the reason for weight gain. Although logical, consuming fewer calories than usual works only in medically supervised weight-loss programs or when people are in a continuous state of near starvation, for example, in environments where food is chronically scarce. When living in an environment in which food is plentiful, however, people are unable *not* to eat what they want for very long because semistarvation turns on biological and psychological mechanisms designed to conserve both body fat and energy expenditure, and being hungry and craving your favorite foods is no fun. Whereas calorie-restriction diets initially tend to be moderately successful, resulting in a loss of a few pounds in the first few weeks, within a few months after the diet begins, the body resists further weight loss even if the calorie-restriction diet is maintained (**Figure 6.6**).

Besides the fact that the body defends against weight (fat) loss, calorie-restriction diets fail for the following reasons:

- Dieters focus on food and not on increasing physical activity. Increasing energy expenditure, rather than decreasing energy intake, is the key to successful weight loss and long-term healthy weight management.

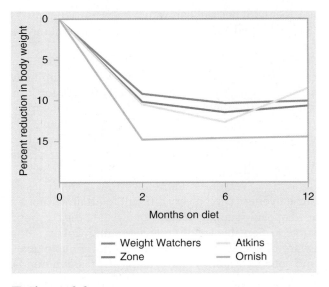

■ **Figure 6.6**

Weight Loss from Adherence to Several Popular Diet Programs
The Ornish diet is vegetarian.

Modified from Dansinger, M. I., et al. (2005). Comparison of the Atkins, Ornish, Weight Watchers, and Zone diets for weight loss and heart disease risk reduction. *Journal of the American Medical Association, 293*, 43–53.

- Because continued adherence to a calorie-restricting plan does not produce commensurate reduction in weight loss, dieters become disillusioned and discouraged and stop following the plan (**Figure 6.7**). Moreover, any weight lost while on the diet tends to be regained. Among those who lose weight by restricting calories, about 50% regain the lost weight within 1 year after stopping the diet, and nearly all regain the lost weight within 4 years.
- Dieters become bored eating the same required foods. This is especially true of diets recommending principally one kind of food (e.g., liquid diet programs, grapefruit, steak, papaya, cottage cheese).
- Dieters become frustrated not being able to eat the kinds and quantities of foods they prefer.
- Dieters are constantly hungry. They become obsessed with food. They even dream about food.
- Prepackaged, special diet foods can be expensive.

Popular Weight-Loss Programs

Popular weight-loss programs generally are of the following types:

- *Low-calorie:* These reduce portion size to limit calories consumed. Examples are Weight Watchers, Nutrisystem, Jenny Craig, Optifast, Medifast, and eDiets. The benefit of these programs is that they are balanced

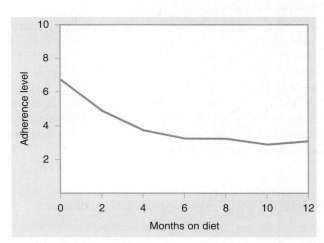

■ **Figure 6.7**

Adherence to Popular Weight-Management Diets
Dieters' self-reports show a gradual decline in adherence to a weight-management diet over 12 months. This pattern is similar for the Atkins, Zone, Weight Watchers, and Ornish diets.

Modified from Dansinger, M. I., et al. (2005). Comparison of the Atkins, Ornish, Weight Watchers, and Zone diets for weight loss and heart disease risk reduction. *Journal of the American Medical Association, 293*, 43–53.

TERMS

energy balance: when energy consumed as food equals the energy expended in living

nutritionally. The drawbacks are that they produce at best a modest loss of weight (5% to 10% of prediet weight) and the reduction in calories makes people hungry and thus leads to discontinuation of the program.

- *Low-carbohydrate:* These reduce intake of breads, rice, pasta, potatoes, sweets, snack foods, and, depending on the plan, vegetables and fruits. To make up for the exclusion of carbohydrate, the programs recommend foods high in protein and fat. Examples are the Atkins and South Beach programs. The benefit of this kind of eating plan is that it reduces the consumption of refined complex carbohydrates, simple sugars, and high-fructose corn syrup found in packaged, fast, and junk foods. Also, protein and fat tend to reduce appetite more effectively than *refined* carbohydrate does. The disadvantage of a low-carb diet is the consumption of high amounts of fat and cholesterol, which are risk factors for heart and blood vessel disease.
- *Low fat:* These diets recommend high complex carbohydrate and little fat. An example is the Ornish diet. A major benefit is that the diet is "heart healthy." A drawback is that in our present food environment, calories from unhealthy refined carbohydrate products are plentiful and heavily marketed, whereas complex carbohydrates from whole grains, fruits, vegetables, and beans are perceived as more expensive than junk and fast food, more difficult to obtain, and less palatable.

When diet programs work, it is generally because they reduce the number of calories consumed and not because of the types and proportions of food consumed. For example, just about any diet plan that delivers approximately 1,450 calories per day represents about a 300- to 700-calorie per day difference between calories ingested and calories expended. This difference can produce a loss of about 1 to 1.5 pounds a week until the body's weight-loss-resistance mechanisms kick in.

Sensible Weight Management

If calorie-restricting diets by themselves do not produce lasting weight loss, what does? Results from studies in the National Weight Control Registry show that American adults who lost weight and *kept it off for several years* did so by engaging in an hour of moderate physical activity daily; consuming five small high-carbohydrate, low-fat meals or snacks; regularly monitoring their weight and exercise activities; and virtually never eating fast food (National Weight Control Registry, 2017). Many studies have shown that significant safe weight loss is associated with limiting calorie intake to 1,200 calories per day for women and 1,500 calories per day for men, limiting fat consumption to less than 30% of calories, consuming recommended amounts of dietary fiber, engaging in physical activity at least 150 minutes per week, and getting involved in counseling and/or group support (Ramage et al., 2014).

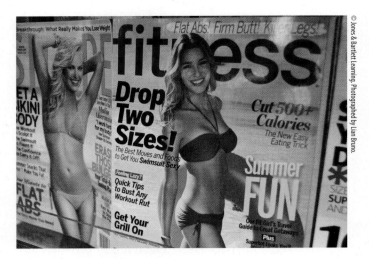

Although most people want to feel good about their bodies, advertisements often portray unrealistic images that can lead to unhealthy diets and eating habits.

Maintaining weight loss is associated with continued application of weight-loss knowledge and skills, continued weight vigilance, and long-term lifestyle changes, especially calorie control, regular physical activity, and professional guidance.

Rather than adopting unusual weight-loss regimens in the search for the "ideal" body size, sensible and successful weight-losers live healthfully and let their bodies find the weight that is right for them, which involves the following:

- *Forget slim, go for health.* Images in media and advertising suggest that a healthy body is slim and muscular. However, a variety of body sizes, shapes, and fat compositions are healthy. For example, someone who is 5 feet 4 inches tall can weigh between 110 pounds (BMI = 19) and 148 pounds (BMI = 25) and still have a healthy body weight.
- *Set realistic goals.* A major obstacle to weight loss is setting a goal of attaining a youthful, former, slim body size—and quickly. Because the body resists fat loss, with patient adherence to a sensible plan, most people can expect to lose about 5% to 10% of their body weight, which, although probably not sufficient to return them to slimness, nevertheless will lessen risks for heart and other serious diseases, and result in feeling better. Everyone must realize that stereotypes of attractiveness can be very difficult to attain without a predisposing genetic makeup or a visit to the cosmetic surgeon. Sensible weight management involves being aware of social pressures toward unattainable goals and not succumbing to advertising and fashion trends.
- *Eat only when hungry and don't overeat.* Use a food diary (see workbook Chapter 5) and pay attention to hunger and satiety signals from your body. Be aware of habits and customs that influence your eating behavior: Do you eat at predetermined times of day (mealtime, between classes, on the way to work) regardless of your state of hunger? Do you eat *everything* on your

Walk the Walk

Count the number of steps you take each day using a pedometer, accelerometer, fitness monitor, or smartphone app. Shoot for 10,000 steps per day (about 5 miles)—15,000 steps is even better.

Table 6.3

Nongym Ways to Increase Physical Activity

Take stairs whenever possible.

Count steps with a pedometer; aim for 10,000 steps a day (15,000 is better).

When feasible, park your car so that you walk 10 minutes to and from your final destination.

Get off of public transportation and walk 10 minutes to your destination.

Walk 20–30 minutes on lunch break.

Exercise/walk with friends or in a group.

Stretch for 5 minutes while on a break at work or before bed.

Strengthen muscles (isometrics, push-ups) 2–3 times a week.

---

plate? Do you work or study while eating and vice versa? Be aware of satiety signals from your body. Can you say to yourself, "That's enough for now"?

- *Eat healthy foods.* Base your diet on whole-grain foods, beans, nuts, and fresh fruits and vegetables. This will add nutrients to your diet and limit the consumption of calorie-laden, nutritionally inferior fast and junk food.
- *Exercise.* Move your body around for at least 30 minutes per day, four to five times a week. Sixty minutes is better. You don't have to work out in a gym or engage in any activity in which you breathe hard and sweat (**Table 6.3**). Take a walk. Use a standing desk. The goal is simply to expend energy by moving your body. Even nonexercise movements such as standing, toe-tapping, walking from room to room, talking, and fidgeting can utilize significant amounts of energy during the day (**Figure 6.8**) (Villa blanca et al., 2014). And don't subscribe to the myth that exercising will increase appetite and food consumption. In fact, except for individuals who expend enormous amounts of energy (e.g., lumberjacks, football players), the opposite is true. Appetite and food consumption tend to decrease as physical activity increases (Thackray et al., 2016).
- *Limit mindless snacking.* Mindless snacking is the kind we do when we are ravenously hungry, stressed, surfing the web, on social media, or zoned-out watching TV. We wish that bag of chips were bottomless. TV advertisers encourage mindless snacking. They know that when you're watching TV you're in a state

---

NEAT stands for nonexercise activity thermogenesis. This is energy you use while doing regular activities such as sitting, talking on the phone, walking, and reading. While doing their daily activities, some people more than others have a propensity to move parts of their bodies. They fidget, wiggle, tap their fingers and toes, and take breaks to move and stretch. It turns out that these folks can utilize several hundred calories of energy doing these NEAT movements, and they rarely have a weight problem.

The propensity for NEATness is probably genetic, but it is something that a non-NEAT person can pick up easily. Modifying an environment is one way to force people to move rather than sit, ergo, the NEAT desk, designed by Dr. James Levine and his colleagues at the Mayo Clinic. It can be used with a treadmill, exercise bike, standing, or regular chair. It has see-through panels that let in light and allow a person to stay visually connected with the rest of the room. Using the NEAT desk at 1 mile per hour (mph) uses about 100 calories per hour. Dr. Levine recommends walking 15 minutes every hour and during all phone calls. In an average 8-hour workday, this would result in expending more than 200 calories, which, without equivalent energy intake, would produce a loss of 1 to 1.5 pounds a month.

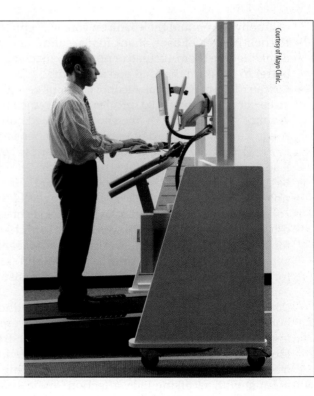

■ **Figure 6.8**

A NEAT Desk

Mindful Eating

Eating should be a relaxed, pleasurable activity but is rarely that in our hectic daily lives. We eat on the run or take only enough time to grab a bite. Most teenagers polish off a full plate of food in a couple of minutes. Just as taking time for physical activity is important for your body, so is taking time with your meals. You can begin to break the habit of wolfing down your food by practicing "mindful eating."

Practice this mindful eating exercise every day until you feel that you have become more aware of your food and the nourishment you receive from it.

Start by choosing a very small piece of food, perhaps a grape, slice of carrot, or a piece of dried fruit. Sit quietly and slowly place the food in your mouth. Pay attention to its texture and flavor.

Begin to chew it very slowly and notice the response in your mouth—how your saliva starts to flow and how your jaw is moving. Chew until you feel ready to swallow; pay attention to the process of swallowing.

When you eat a meal, focus all of your attention on the food and the satisfaction of eating. Do not read or watch TV while eating. Make eating a quiet, pleasurable occasion. Do not bring problems or arguments to the table. By eating slowly and quietly you also will hear the message from your stomach when it is full. Listen to the message and stop eating.

Mindful eating can be a powerful technique in weight control and limiting the consumption of food that your body does not need.

of autohypnosis, and they bank on your susceptibility to their images of beer, snack foods, candy, and soft drinks. Ignore them. Instead of mindless snacking, it's better to focus on the food you are eating.

- *Consume little or no alcohol.* Alcohol contains seven calories per gram (about 100 calories per 12-ounce beer, 4-ounce glass of wine, or one shot of distilled liquor). A couple of beers per day without a compensatory reduction in food intake or increase in exercise could lead to an excess of body fat rather quickly.
- *Be aware of eating triggers.* Many of us are susceptible to environmental cues that trigger eating. For example, some people cannot pass a candy or soft-drink machine without feeding it money in exchange for it feeding them. At some worksites, well-meaning supervisors and coworkers provide pastries and candy for staff members, who may have difficulty resisting, especially when stressed or fatigued.
- *Don't feed your feelings.* Stress, anxiety, loneliness, boredom, fatigue, and anger can motivate overeating. Many people derive emotional comfort from food. One possible explanation is that as children, we learn to associate eating (particularly nursing as infants) with receiving love, affection, and comfort. Another possibility is that when we consume certain foods, particularly those containing sugar and fat, they alter brain chemistry and contribute to feelings of calm.

The energy equivalent of 1 pound of body fat is 3,500 calories. If you want to adopt a weight-reducing program that results in a loss of 1 pound a month, plan your dietary and physical activities so you can produce a net daily deficit of 120 calories. Walk a little more each day or cut out a soft drink or a couple of cookies. If you want to lose 1 pound a week, plan for a net daily deficit of 500 calories that includes at least a 300-calorie expenditure per day of exercise (Table 6.4). The number of calories is not nearly as important as *making a plan to which you can realistically adhere over the long haul.* Here are some other suggestions:

- Keep a diary of your weight-loss activities and modify things in your plan that do not work.
- Keep faith with your intention to attain a healthful weight. Don't let the inevitable setbacks demoralize you.
- Don't slavishly count calories or constantly weigh yourself; focus on developing healthy behaviors and feeling good.
- Ignore weight-loss and exercise-machine advertising.

Besides being good for you, altering your lifestyle to maintain a healthy body weight is also good for the planet. Instead of driving or riding in a car for short trips, if all Americans between the ages of 10 and 64 walked or biked for 30 minutes a day, not only would they collectively shed 3 billion pounds and eliminate the current epidemic of overweight but also annual carbon dioxide emissions in the United States would be lessened by 64 million tons, and 6.5 billion gallons of gasoline would be saved (Higgins & Higgins, 2005).

Table 6.4

Approximate Energy Expenditures During Various Activities

Light exercise (4 calories per minute)		
Cycling 5 mph	Slow dancing	Table tennis
Walking 3 mph	Volleyball	Yoga
Canoeing	Softball	T'ai chi ch'uan
House cleaning	Golf	
Moderate exercise (7 calories per minute)		
Tennis	Basketball	Snowshoeing
Fast dancing	Swimming 30 m/min	Walking 4.5 mph
Cycling 9 mph	Heavy gardening	Roller skating
Heavy exercise (10 calories per minute)		
Jogging	Mountain climbing	Skiing
Climbing stairs	Cycling 12 mph	Ice skating
Football	Handball and racquetball	

Uncle Joe's Successful Weight Loss

Joe had a heart attack at age 55 and needed quadruple bypass surgery to save his life. Joe is 5 feet 7 inches, and at the time of his heart attack he weighed 225 pounds (BMI = 35). Joe wasn't always big. He says he got that way from 30 years of the near-daily ritual of meeting up with buddies after work at the local tavern for a few beers and a kielbasa (or two) before going home for dinner.

After his surgery, Joe retired from work as well as from his visits to the tavern. His wife tossed out all of the junk food in their house and put them on a healthy diet. Like a tough drill sergeant, she got Joe out of bed early each morning for a 5-mile couple walk–talk around their town—rain, sleet, or shine. In a couple of years, Joe had achieved his current weight of 155 pounds (BMI = 24). He looks and feels great, and his wife is grateful she didn't become a widow.

Joe is like a lot of people who have succeeded at healthy weight loss. He gave himself lots of time to develop new health habits, and he was diligent about adhering to them. He accepted help, encouragement, and support from his wife, children, friends, and his doctors. Not only did Joe look and feel better, he felt good about himself for accomplishing an important goal and making it possible for him and his wife to have a long, enjoyable retirement together.

Assisted Management of Overweight

Managing body weight is principally a matter of adopting healthful living habits: eating whole-grain foods and fresh fruits and vegetables, limiting consumption of fast foods and junk foods, and increasing movement. Still, some people cannot successfully manage weight on their own, and they may benefit from seeking the help of a health professional. Methods that health professionals employ to help people reduce and maintain body weight include psychological counseling, hypnotherapy, medications, liposuction, and surgery.

Counseling and Hypnosis

Counseling for weight loss involves helping individuals examine the reasons for their unhealthful eating and exercise behaviors and developing ways to behave more healthfully. Hypnosis has been shown to increase the benefits of counseling. Counseling for weight loss and maintenance focuses on the following (Wadden et al., 2014):

- Increasing one's self-awareness of the inner dialogue that contributes to the weight problem; for example, changing the thought "I've had a bad day so I deserve a treat; I'll have some fries" to "I deserve a treat; I'll take a soothing bath"
- Keeping records of eating and exercise activities in order to assess current behavior and target personal and environmental changes

- Changing the environmental factors that trigger overeating and underexercising, for example, not having a full cookie jar on the kitchen counter or not going out for fast food with friends when the goal is socializing rather than sating hunger
- Educating yourself about healthy nutrition and physical activity
- Setting realistic weight-management goals and adopting feasible plans for accomplishing them
- Teaching about "feeding one's feelings" and the tendency to eat when feeling stressed
- Providing social support for weight-management activities
- Identifying and managing mental health issues, such as depression and anxiety, that may be associated with weight issues

Psychological counseling is generally effective in facilitating weight loss of about a pound a week and a significant percentage of the initial body weight, and it promotes weight-loss maintenance for several months after treatment ends (Jones, Wilson, & Wadden, 2007).

Medications

Several medications have been approved by the FDA for medically supervised weight loss (Khera et al., 2016). These include drugs that alter the balance of certain neurotransmitters and help the pancreas secrete insulin, and a drug that blocks the absorption of fat from the intestines (orlistat). Medications can result in the loss of about 5% of initial body weight after several months. Continued use can help retain that degree of fat loss but tends not to produce further loss. Weight-loss medications carry a variety of unpleasant side effects, which often lead to discontinuing use and regaining the lost weight. This is why health professionals consider medications to be an adjunct to lifestyle modification (diet, exercise, and greater awareness of eating habits) and not to be used alone to achieve weight loss.

Weight-Reduction (Bariatric) Surgery

Weight-reduction **(bariatric) surgery** is for people with a BMI over 40 or with a BMI between 35 and 40 who have severe weight-related medical conditions, such as heart disease or type 2 diabetes, and who have not responded to supervised diet and exercise regimens or drug therapy. There are several methods of weight-loss surgery. Some involve constricting the stomach to make the person feel full after having consumed small amounts of food. Other methods involve surgically restructuring the

TERMS

(bariatric) surgery: weight loss surgery

Treating the Underlying Emotional Causes of Obesity

Mrs. Johnson made an appointment with a psychologist to discuss being overweight. She was 40 years old, 5 feet 5 inches tall, and weighed 180 pounds. She worked as a nurse at a community hospital and had no serious medical problems. She was married, but her husband had lost his job, they had three teenage children at home. Her take-home pay was modest, and the family had difficulty paying bills. She ate mostly junk food and fast-food and did not exercise.

Because appropriate weight depends on both a healthy mind and body, the psychologist helped Mrs. Johnson discover the stress and negative emotions that were contributing to the weight problem. They included job or family stress, depression, anger, loneliness, and boredom.

Social aspects of being overweight were also explored. What were the barriers to obtaining healthy food? Did her job require a lot of travel or sitting for extended periods? Together they explored how exercise could be incorporated into her daily life.

Mrs. Johnson came to see that she had a high-stress, low-paying job, an unsatisfying marriage, and children at a difficult stage of development. Her life was out of control. With the psychologist's help, Mrs. Johnson adopted a healthy, balanced diet and began walking—and later jogging—in the morning before work. Later, she added weight training to her exercise program. After a few months she obtained a better-paying job with regular hours. She and her husband went to a marriage counselor and the marriage improved. After about a year, Mrs. Johnson's weight stabilized at 130 pounds. She maintained her diet and continued to exercise.

Many overweight people have problems similar to Mrs. Johnson's. Counseling, diet changes, exercise, and social support can help most overweight people who are willing to make the effort to change their lives.

---

gastrointestinal tract so that only a fraction of the food ingested in a meal is absorbed into the body and the activities of some of the nerves and hormones that control eating and metabolism are altered.

Bariatric surgery is not cosmetic surgery to produce a particular body size and shape. Its aim is to lessen the amount of food the body processes and to alter the physiological mechanisms that manage energy balance. On average, bariatric surgery produces a long-term loss of 50% to 70% of presurgery body weight and establishes a much healthier metabolism, for example, considerably reducing the risk of type 2 diabetes (Schroeder et al., 2016). Weight reduction from bariatric surgery can last for several years. About 180,000 weight-reduction surgeries are performed in the United Stated each year. The rate of surgical complications is about 17% and the risk of death is about 1% (Chang et al., 2014).

Liposuction

Liposuction is the surgical removal by suction of fat stored under the skin and is not recommended as a substitute for proper diet, exercise, and counseling for weight loss and weight management. It is for shaping the body. Indeed, after the surgery, without attention to diet and exercise, fat may appear on other parts of the body, and in time, patients actually may gain weight. Annually, more than 200,000 liposuction procedures are performed in women and men in the United States by plastic surgeons, dermatologists, and other physicians. Liposuction is currently the most common cosmetic surgical procedure performed. Liposuction is associated with many risks; anyone considering it should investigate the procedure thoroughly. Although rare, deaths have occurred from liposuction.

Weight-Control Fads and Fallacies

"Lose weight effortlessly, even as you sleep!" "New diet discovery lets you lose excess pounds in just one week!" So claim advertisements for products and eating regimens that are directed to chronic dieters and others concerned about being overfat. Some products, such as "diet rings" and weight-loss soaps, are clearly worthless, but some overweight people are so desperate they will try anything.

Unfortunately for consumers, nearly all of the claims made by heavily advertised weight-control regimens and products are exaggerated and misleading. The U.S. Federal Trade Commission estimates that weight-loss scams are the most prevalent types of fraud, affecting nearly 5 million Americans per year. By themselves, these are not likely to produce a significant reduction in body fat over any long-term period.

> If slaughterhouses had glass walls, everyone would be a vegetarian.
> *Paul McCartney*

Although totally ineffective, these products are advertised in reputable magazines and newspapers, on TV, and on the Internet, which contributes to their credibility. Something to consider: If any of the products advertised for rapid, effortless weight loss really worked, surely every overweight person would use them and the obesity epidemic would be history. Some popular and largely ineffective weight-loss schemes include body wraps and chemicals and supplements, which are described below.

Body Wraps

Body wraps are hot linens, blankets, saran or plastic sheets, elastic or rubber waist belts, or whole-body garments that are applied in spas or at home, often in combination with herbal compounds, minerals, amino acids, and other substances. Commonly, body wraps promise to open pores to let fat and other toxins escape the body. A wrap designed for just one part of the body (such as the waist or hips) is supposed to reduce the size of just that body region ("spot reducing").

Body wraps do result in weight loss and a reduction in body size. The catch is that the weight lost is body water and not body fat. The lost body water is quickly regained and so is the lost body weight. Because these products cause a loss of body water, they make dehydration a potential danger. Some athletes have died from exercising while using body wraps.

Chemicals and Supplements

A number of products that contain drugs and "natural" substances are sold as weight-loss remedies. Often these products are used in conjunction with calorie restriction, modification in eating behavior, and exercise programs, so they appear effective to the naive consumer. However, no single product by itself has been shown to reduce weight safely and permanently. The Federal Trade Commission has warned consumers about worthless weight-loss scams, including the HCG Diet, L'Occitane skin cream, LeanSpa, and Sensa products. Several types of popular, generally ineffective weight-loss products include:

- *Appetite suppressants/energy boosters:* If they actually contain the ingredients listed on the label (because they are unregulated there is no guarantee that they do), these products contain chemicals that act as central nervous system (CNS) stimulants such as ephedra *(ma huang),* synephrine (bitter orange), and caffeine (guarana, yerba mate). Ingestion of sufficient quantities of a CNS stimulant can result in short-term loss of a couple of pounds. However, these substances

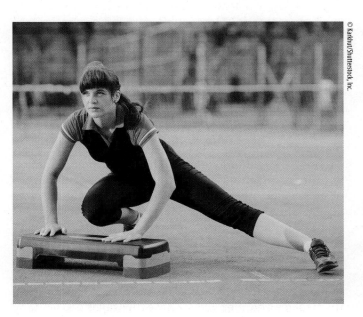

Exercise is essential to effective weight management.

Inform Yourself: Don't Buy Worthless and Sometimes Harmful Weight-Loss Products

Nearly all dietary weight-loss supplements that individuals buy in stores and on the Internet are not regulated by the U.S. Food and Drug Administration or the Federal Trade Commission. This means that consumers have no certainty that a product manufacturer's claims about a product's efficacy, safety, and even its ingredients are true. Before you buy any weight-loss product, check out what experts have to say about it. Use the Web. Don't do a general search because you are likely to be inundatd with Web sites that sell stuff rather than inform. Start with these authoritative Web sites:

- Federal Trade Commission Scam Tag: Weight Loss (https://www.consumer.ftc.gov/taxonomy/term/878)
- National Center for Complementary and Integrative Health: Weight Control (https://nccih.nih.gov/health/weightcontrol)
- Food and Drug Administration: Weight Loss Fraud (https://www.fda.gov/drugs/resourcesforyou/consumers/buyingusingmedicinesafely/medicationhealthfraud/ucm243756.htm)

have side effects, especially ephedra, which increases the risk of psychiatric, temperature-control, and gastrointestinal problems, and these products have been associated with several deaths. Do not risk your life to lose a few pounds. A related product, *hoodia gordonii,* a South African plant, is purported to be a nonstimulant appetite suppressant. It is supposed to act in the hypothalamus to produce a feeling of fullness. No scientific studies have yet found hoodia to be effective. Products containing triatricol, or "triac," a thyroid hormone–like substance, are marketed as "metabolic accelerators." Because it can cause heart attacks and strokes, the FDA has banned supplements containing "triac." However, triac-containing products are still sold on the Internet along with other thyroidlike chemicals.

- *Fat burners/fat blockers:* These products claim to oxidize ("chemically burn") stored body fat or stop the production of body fat. They contain chemicals such as hydroxycitric acid (HCA), conjugated linoleic acid (CLA), green tea, licorice, pyruvate, vitamin B, and L-carnitine. All of these are generally ineffective. Chitosan, derived from chitin found in crustaceans,

TERMS

liposuction: surgery used to remove fat under the skin to reshape parts of the body

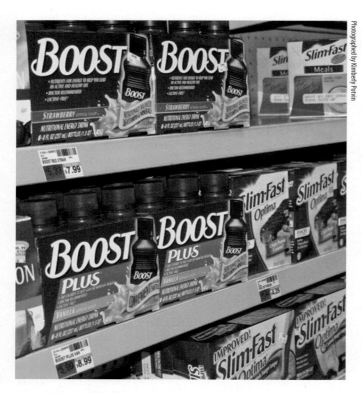

Photographed by Kimberly Potvin

People take hundreds of different herbs, supplements, and other pills to lose weight.

is supposed to bind fat in the digestive tract. Studies indicate that this also is ineffective.

- *Bulk-producing agents:* These include methylcellulose, psyllium, and agar. They are supposed to produce a sense of fullness in the gastrointestinal tract, thus suppressing appetite. These agents swell when mixed with water and are much more effective as laxatives than as weight reducers. Glucomannan, a bulk-producing starch derived from konjac tubers, is often touted by health food enthusiasts as a "natural" weight-loss method. There is no evidence that glucomannan or any other bulk producer aids weight loss.
- *Vitamins, minerals, and amino acids:* Vitamins, minerals, and some amino acids (including arginine, ornithine, tryptophan, and phenylalanine) are occasionally sold as weight-loss agents. For example, spirulina, a product made from blue-green algae, is claimed to be effective in reducing weight because it contains the amino acid phenylalanine, which supposedly regulates the body's appetite. Chromium (generally listed on product labels as chromium picolinate) is supposed to alter carbohydrate metabolism and thus result in weight loss. No studies have ever confirmed this hypothesis. Vitamins, minerals, and amino acids have not been

shown to be effective in causing weight loss. And in very high doses, some of these substances, although "natural," can be harmful.

Body Image

Body image is a person's mental picture of her or his body. Nearly everyone has a body image. Nearly everyone judges that image as good or less good by comparing her or his body image to a standard of the "ideal body" communicated to individuals by their culture and people who are important to them, such as lovers, family, and friends. The judgment a person makes about her or his body image is called *body esteem*. Individuals with a positive body image tend to have higher body esteem than do individuals with a less positive body image.

Many women are excessively concerned about their body image and tend to have low body esteem because they believe themselves to be overweight. Books, films, TV, and popular magazines (especially women's magazines) consistently send messages that our society esteems thin women and disdains heavy ones. Whereas maintaining appropriate body size is associated with good health, attempting to achieve an unrealistic ideal of one's body shape leads many women to judge themselves as unattractive and lowers their self-esteem.

Body dysmorphic disorder is a preoccupation with an imagined defect in one or more of one's body parts, which causes considerable personal and social distress and occupational impairment. Some men tend to be concerned with their muscularity (*muscle dysmorphia*, or "bigorexia") and height, genitals, and thinning hair. Females tend to be concerned about their body size, buttocks, breasts, thighs, facial features, and body hair (Bjornsson, Didie, & Phillips, 2010). The preoccupation with imagined physical defects leads to seeking medical procedures such as cosmetic ("aesthetic") surgery, cosmetic dentistry, or cosmetic dermatology (skin abrasions, Botox). Males may engage in extreme body building activities, excessive consumption of ineffectual sports supplements, abnormal eating patterns, and ingestion of various illegal drugs. Females are at high risk for anorexia nervosa (see the following section). Almost always, efforts to change the identified defect do not produce mind–body harmony. Cognitive behavioral therapy and certain medications can help individuals reduce their preoccupation with their imagined defects and help them establish a more realistic attitude about their bodies.

For the most part, standards of attractiveness and a healthful appearance are set by companies seeking to sell products and increase profits. Advertisements try to convince women that they fall short of an ideal and that by purchasing a product, dieting, or exercising to change their body size and shape, they can improve themselves and their lives. These messages cause many women to judge themselves on how they look and cause many men to judge women largely by their physical appearance. Overconcern about body image and weight can have adverse health consequences, including the following:

- Depression from low body esteem and low self-worth
- Poor nutrition from extensive dieting
- Inadequate calcium and iron intake from undernutrition
- Anorexia or bulimia
- Musculoskeletal injuries from overexercising
- Risks associated with cosmetic surgery
- Cigarette smoking to reduce body weight

Eating Disorders

Eating disorders are complex psychophysiological conditions that manifest as compulsive, unusual eating behavior. Three of the most common eating disorders are anorexia nervosa, a voluntary refusal to eat; bulimia, binge eating and immediate purging of the ingested food either by vomiting or by using laxatives or intense exercise; and binge eating disorder, episodes of binge eating without subsequent purging. Occasionally, anorexia involves purging as well. The lifetime prevalence of eating disorders among American adults is approximately 5%. About 90% of those affected with anorexia nervosa or bulimia are women; nearly half of those with binge eating disorder are men. Eating disorders are anchored in tightly held, biologically inaccurate, and perfectionistic core beliefs, such as "You can never be too thin," "Any fat is bad," "I'm too fat," and "Anything I eat immediately turns to fat that everyone else can see." Striving to adhere to these core beliefs fosters compulsive disordered eating and purging behaviors (e.g., excessive exercise). In some instances, individuals hold so tightly to these beliefs and their associated behaviors that they reject any suggestions that they are at risk and must change or face serious health consequences and even death.

Compared to the general population, eating disorders are more prevalent among athletes, particularly among those whose bodies are exposed to view (swimmers, runners, gymnasts, dancers) or those whose performance may be affected by body weight (wrestlers, swimmers, divers, gymnasts, jockeys, and crew) (Joy et al., (2016)). Among athletes, attitudes and behaviors to lessen body weight, such as overexercising, dieting, or using drugs to lessen weight, are often considered normal and are even valued. Unfortunately, "thinner is better" activities rob the body of strength and energy, so they lead to decreased performance and occasionally illness. Also, acceptance of disturbed eating behaviors, overexercising, and compulsive attempts at perfecting performance can attract people to certain sports who are vulnerable to developing an eating disorder. Women athletes who expend many more calories than they consume risk developing the **female athlete triad**: (1) cessation of menstruation (amenorrhea), (2) disordered eating, and (3) weak bones from osteoporosis. Athletes also are at risk for orthorexia, a rigid fixation with righteous and healthy eating. Orthorexia is associated with planning, buying, and preparing "proper" meals and guilt, anxiety, and self-punishment through excessive exercise for not doing so. Orthorexia is also associated with feeling safe from diseases and superior to others for one's total commitment to the eating regime.

Anorexia Nervosa

Anorexia nervosa is characterized by a relentless pursuit of thinness resulting in progressive weight loss and metabolic disturbances. Most of those affected are young women. Anorexia is not caused by any known disease-causing agent but by self-induced starvation, which can lead to serious illness and even death.

Elizabeth Barrett Browning (1806–1861), one of England's most famed poets, is thought to have had anorexia nervosa. As a teenager, Elizabeth was nagged by her parents to eat and gain weight, yet she stubbornly refused to eat much more than toast. When she met her future husband, poet Robert Browning, she weighed only 87 pounds. Apparently, the Barrett family possessed characteristics found in other families with an anorectic member: overprotectiveness, overinvolvement with each other, and inability to express or resolve intrafamilial conflict.

Persons with anorexia nervosa are likely to defend their emaciated appearance as normal and will insist that weight gain makes them feel fat. Besides distortions in normal body image, people with anorexia nervosa tend to be preoccupied with food. They may spend an inordinate amount of time planning and preparing elaborate meals for others, while they themselves eat only a few bites and claim to be full. Often they will not eat in the presence of others; when they do, they may dawdle over their food. Some anorectic persons resort

TERMS

anorexia nervosa: disorder occurring most commonly in adolescent females, characterized by abnormal body image, fear of obesity, and prolonged refusal to eat, sometimes resulting in death

body dysmorphic disorder: a preoccupation with an imagined defect in one or more of one's body parts

body image: a person's mental image of his or her body

female athlete triad: combination of disordered eating, cessation of menstruation (amenorrhea), and weakened bones (osteoporosis)

Eating Disorders Are a Worldwide Concern

Eating disorders among women have become a worldwide problem. Once common primarily in North America and Europe they now have spread to other regions of the world, including Saudi Arabia, China, Russia, Latin America, and Asia.

Experts say the growing prevalence of eating disorders is caused by young women trying to emulate advertising models and actors that they see in American and European media and on the Internet. These media present images of "ideal" women as unrealistically thin, which causes some women to lose social and psychological confidence in themselves; they attempt to regain it by disordered eating behaviors. For example, after the introduction of TV to the island of Fiji in 1995, the number of teenage girls with eating disorders rose from 3% to 15%. At the time, Fiji had only one TV station, which broadcast shows from the United States, Australia, and the United Kingdom. Whereas the increase might be attributable to something other than TV, researchers believe that the dramatic jump in the prevalence of eating disorders after the introduction of American and European images on TV is the most plausible explanation.

In Argentina, aggressive advertising by the diet and cosmetic industries was generally recognized as contributing to an epidemic of eating disorders. Major newspapers distributed discount coupons for diet and liposuction clinics. And Argentine clothing manufacturers—out of step with international standards—sized women's clothes much too small (e.g., a "medium" T-shirt that is more suitable for a preadolescent than an adult), reinforcing the idea that a woman must be extremely thin to be socially desirable. The Argentine government and health establishment instituted a large media campaign of their own to educate young women on the dangers of believing what they see on TV, in the movies, and in magazines with respect to eating, body size, and cosmetic surgery.

---

to self-induced vomiting or frequent use of diuretics or laxatives to reduce their body weight. These practices may lead to severe depletion of body minerals, which can precipitate abnormal heart rhythms and even cardiac arrest. Despite the low intake of calories, anorectic persons are remarkably energetic.

Persons with anorexia may see themselves as responding to demands of others rather than taking initiative in life. Young people with anorexia tend to be obedient, dutiful, helpful, and excellent students. Some psychologists interpret the intense preoccupation with weight loss as an expression of an underlying fear of incompetence. Control of eating and body weight becomes a way of demonstrating general control and competence.

That anorexia nervosa affects predominantly young women suggests that its roots lie in our society's preoccupation with slimness as a prerequisite to social success. Anorexia may also reflect an attempt to remain a child who is cared for and fed by others, who can be stubborn and obstinate, and who has no sexual identity or desires. Anorexia may also be a manifestation of a struggle for a sense of identity and personal effectiveness through controlling the environment; the resulting stubborn, rejecting behavior then becomes reinforced by the attention received from others. The family of the anorectic person becomes so engrossed with the symptoms that they avoid dealing with conflicts among themselves.

Three goals characterize the treatment of anorexia nervosa: (1) weight gain, (2) changed attitudes toward food and eating, and (3) resolution of underlying personal and family conflicts. Unfortunately, therapeutic intervention is not always successful and the condition may persist for years. Anorexia nervosa has a 15% to 20% mortality rate.

Bulimia

Bulimia is marked by a voluntary restriction of food intake followed by a binge–purge cycle: extreme overeating, usually of high-calorie junk foods, immediately followed by self-induced vomiting, use of diuretics or laxatives, or intense exercise. Like anorexia nervosa, bulimia occurs primarily in young women with a morbid fear of becoming fat, who pursue thinness relentlessly. Most bulimic persons are model individuals: good students, athletes, extremely sociable, and pleasant. Fearing discovery of their bulimic behavior, they frequently carry out their binge–purge episodes in private. Bulimic persons usually are aware that their binge–purge behavior is abnormal; however, they are unable to control it. Many feel guilty and depressed about their problem, which leads to a tendency to hide the behavior. Bulimia can pose a serious risk to health for many of the same reasons that anorexia does.

Several theories have been proposed to explain bulimia. One is that bulimia is a maladaptive way of dealing with anxiety, loneliness, and anger. Another suggests that bulimia is a manifestation of the drive to become the "ideal" woman, achieving the societal norm of slimness. Bulimic persons tend to have low self-esteem and a weak sense of identity.

Recovering from bulimia includes stopping binge–purge cycles and regaining control over eating behavior. Persons with bulimia must also establish more appropriate ways to handle unpleasant feelings and discomfort with close relationships, and their self-esteem must be improved. Often psychological counseling is helpful.

Binge Eating Disorder

Binge eating disorder is characterized by an uncontrolled consumption of large quantities of food in a short period of time, even if the person does not feel hungry. During binge episodes, food is consumed much faster than usual, and frequently the person is alone to avoid embarrassment about the amount of food eaten. A binge episode is often followed by feelings of disgust, depression, and guilt.

About 2% of adults in the United States (about 4 million people) have binge eating disorder, and most of them are overweight. About 10% to 15% of people who are mildly obese and who try to lose weight on their own or through commercial weight-loss programs have binge eating disorder. The disorder is even more common in people who are very overweight.

Many people with binge eating disorder have a history of depression and impulsive behavior (acting quickly without thinking). Many people who are binge eaters say that being angry, sad, bored, or worried can cause them to binge eat. People with binge eating disorder tend to be malnourished because they consume large amounts of fat and sugar, which have few essential nutrients.

Most people with binge eating disorder have tried to control it on their own, but are unable to control it for very long. People with binge eating disorder should get help from a health professional, which could include instruction in how to keep track of and change unhealthy eating behaviors, identifying social factors that contribute to the problem, psychological counseling, and medications.

It's in Your Hands

Successful weight management involves reducing intake of calories (often by recognizing the social and psychological reasons that cause overeating) and increasing the level of physical activity. Heavily advertised reducing schemes, such as body wraps, diet pills, and fad diets, are almost totally ineffective in producing permanent fat reduction and weight loss.

The primary reason that people are overfat is that their lifestyles do not include sufficient physical activity to use up the calories ingested in food. You can begin today to consciously watch what you eat and how much you exercise. When offered a cookie, decline. When you have the choice between the elevator and stairs, take the stairs. These efforts, which appear to be small, can make a difference when made daily and over an extended period of time.

TERMS

binge eating disorder: an uncontrolled consumption of large quantities of food in a short period of time, even if the person does not feel hungry

bulimia: serious disorder, especially common in adolescents and young women, marked by excessive eating, often followed by self-induced vomiting, purging, or fasting

Critical Thinking About Health

1. Jordana couldn't stand herself anymore, so she went to the campus health center's peer nutrition counseling program for help.

   "I disgust myself," she told her counselor. "I'm fat, fat, fat and no matter what I do I can't change it. I jog, I don't eat ice cream. I suck."

   Jordana's BMI calculated out to 28.4. "It's a little on the high side," said the counselor, "but you're not in the danger zone."

   "Tell that to my Dad," Jordana snapped. "And my boyfriend. When they look at me, their eyes go right to my stomach. It's like that's all I am—a stomach on legs!"

   a. What expectations regarding body size and shape do you experience as a member of your sex?

   b. How were these expectations transmitted to you and by whom (or by what social institution)?

   c. How are these expectations enforced in your peer group, and what are the social penalties for not meeting such expectations?

   d. To what lengths do people go to meet these expectations? Are any of these practices extreme or unhealthy?

2. **Sam:** Oh, man, not Roni. She's too wide!
   Mick: No, she's not. She's real nice. Call her.
   Sam: Nah.
   Mick: You're a loser, man. You didn't like Nan because her face was too round. You didn't like Carla because she was too tall. You didn't like Evy because . . . why didn't you like Evy, anyway? I forget.
   Sam: Thunder thighs.
   Mick: You're going to wind up one lonely dude.

   a. Is Sam really destined to be lonely or is he being smart to wait for someone who matches his ideal of the perfect body?

   b. In your peer group, are there examples of people being attracted to people who do not resemble the ideal? Can you explain that discrepancy?

   c. What is the social purpose of an ideal body size and shape?

3. It is likely that in the near future there will be many drugs that are moderately effective in producing weight (fat) loss. It is also likely that these drugs will carry some risks to health.

   a. Do you think that such drugs should be made available to anyone who wants them, or should such medications be restricted to people whose weight puts them at serious risk for health problems and premature death?

   b. Besides potential harm from side effects, is it appropriate for people to depend on drugs for weight maintenance instead of modifying dietary and exercise habits and learning to reduce stress?

4. How have eating disorders touched your life?

Chapter Summary and Highlights

Chapter Summary

Our ancient ancestors were physically active, having to spend most of their time and energy finding enough food to feed themselves and their families. In the past, most people were lean, often because they did not have enough food. Over thousands of years, plants and animals became domesticated, people clustered in towns and cities, and food became plentiful. The industrial revolution meant that machines began to do most of the hard work. People had leisure time and became less active physically. Today, in a computer-TV-smartphone world, people live very sedentary lives both at home and at work. Hardly anyone in America walks to school or work anymore. Thus, approximately 68% of the American population is overweight. People who are overweight and who do not exercise regularly are at higher risk for heart disease, diabetes, and cancer than are people who are lean and fit. As with all aspects of personal health, you are the one responsible for the quality and quantity of food you consume and the amount of exercise you get daily.

Weight-loss programs, drugs, and expensive advice are a multi-billion-dollar industry. None produce long-term weight loss or fitness. Maintaining a healthy weight is simply a matter of energy consumed versus energy used day after day after day. Body energy is measured in units called *calories* that are listed on all packaged and processed foods. The body's energy needs depend on height, weight, age, and degree of daily activity. Consuming fewer calories and using more calories in movement and exercise is the guaranteed method of weight loss. People who are overweight when young are usually overweight throughout life. The time to get your weight under control is when you are young and can exercise more vigorously than when you are older. To feel what your body endures when you are overweight, hold a 30- to 40-pound backpack in front of you and walk around with it all day. You *can* choose to be of a healthy weight. The time to start eating healthy and being physically active is now.

Highlights

- Approximately two-thirds of the U.S. population is overweight and at risk for a variety of illnesses, including heart disease, type 2 diabetes, hypertension, and gallbladder disease.

- Obesity is defined as having a body weight 20% (for men) and 30% (for women) over recommended weight for height or a body mass index greater than 30.

- Health problems are less likely when the waist-to-hip ratio is less than 0.8 (women) or 0.95 (men).
- Body fatness is maintained by neural and hormonal signals acting on the brain, which controls feelings of hunger and satiety. Many physiological, psychological, social, and environmental factors affect the brain and thus body weight.
- People eat for reasons other than hunger, such as social interaction, recreation, and relief from stress.
- Successful weight control involves changing eating and exercise habits.

- Healthy body weight corresponds to having a body mass index between 19 and 25. There are a variety of ways to achieve a healthy body weight. Starvation dieting is not one of them.
- Counseling, surgery, and medications can help some overweight people lose body fat and maintain a healthy body weight.
- There are three major ineffective weight-control schemes: body wraps, diet pills, and diet programs.
- Three common eating disorders are anorexia nervosa, bulimia, and binge eating disorder.

For Your Health

Fast food consumption is a major contributor to overweight. Do some "Fast-Food Restaurant Research" (Exercise 6.1, in the Workbook) to assess your consumption of fast food and how it contributes calories and saturated fat to your diet. The other exercises in Chapter 6 help with weight management also.

References

American College Health Association. (2016a). *American College Health Association-National College Health Assessment II: Canadian Reference Group Data Report Spring 2016.* Hanover, MD: American College Health Association.

American College Health Association. (2016b). *American College Health Association-National College Health Assessment II: Undergraduate Student Reference Group Data Report Spring 2016.* Hanover, MD: American College Health Association.

Benton, D. (2015). Portion size: What we know and what we need to know. *Critical Reviews in Food Science and Nutrition, 55,* 988–1004.

Bjornsson, A. S., Didie, E. R., & Phillips, K. A. (2010). Body dysmorphic disorder. *Dialogues in Clinical Neuroscience, 12,* 221–232.

Boggiano, M. M. (2016). Palatable Eating Motives Scale in a college population: Distribution of scores and scores associated with greater BMI and binge-eating. *Eating Behaviors, 21,* 95–98.

Boggiano, M. M., et al. (2015). Real-time sampling of reasons for hedonic food consumption: Further validation of the Palatable Eating Motives Scale. *Frontiers in Psychology, 6,* 744. doi: 10.3389/fpsyg.2015.00744

Boyland, E. J., & Halford, J. C. (2013). Television advertising and branding: Effects on eating behavior and food preferences in children. *Appetite, 62,* 236–241.

Burgess, E. E., et al. (2014). Profiling motives behind hedonic eating: Preliminary validation of the Palatable Eating Motives Scale. *Appetite, 72,* 66–72.

Chang, D. H., et al. (2014). The effectiveness and risks of bariatric surgery: An updated systematic review and meta-analysis, 2003–2012. *JAMA Surgery, 149,* 275–287.

Dansinger, M. I., et al. (2005). Comparison of the Atkins, Ornish, Weight Watchers, and Zone diets for weight loss and heart disease risk reduction. *Journal of the American Medical Association, 293,* 43–53.

Fleischhacker, S. E., et al. (2011). A systematic review of fast food access studies. *Obesity Reviews, 12,* e460–471.

Ford, E. S., & Dietz, W. H. (2013). Trends in energy intake among adults in the United States: findings from NHANES1–3. *American Journal of Clinical Nutrition, 97,* 848–853.

Frank, L. D., Andresen, M. A., & Schmid, T. L. (2004). Obesity relationships with community design, physical activity, and time spent in cars. *American Journal of Preventive Medicine, 27,* 87–96.

Harris, J. L., et al. (2016). *Snack FACTS 2015: Evaluating snack food nutrition and marketing to youth.* Storrs, CN: University of Connecticut Rudd Center for Food Policy and Obesity. Retrieved from http://uconnruddcenter.org/files/Pdfs/SnackFACTS_2015_Fulldraft03.pdf

Higgins, P. A. T., & Higgins, M. (2005). A healthy reduction in oil consumption and carbon emissions. *Energy Policy, 33,* 1–4.

Janesick, A., & Blumberg, B. (2011). Minireview: PPARγ as the target of obesogens. *Journal of Steroid Biochemistry and Molecular Biology, 127,* 4–8.

Jones, L. R., Wilson, C. I., & Wadden, T. A. (2007). Lifestyle modification in the treatment of obesity: An educational challenge and opportunity. *Clinical Pharmacology and Therapeutics, 81,* 776–779.

Joy, E., et al. (2016). 2016 update on eating disorders in athletes: A comprehensive narrative review with a focus on clinical assessment and management. *British Journal of Sports Medicine, 50,* 154–162.

Khera, R., et al. (2016). Association of pharmacological treatments for obesity with weight loss and adverse events. *Journal of the American Medical Association, 315,* 2424–2434.

Mokdad, A. H., et al. (2003). Prevalence of obesity, diabetes, and obesity-related health risk factors, 2001. *Journal of the American Medical Association, 289,* 76–79.

National Weight Control Registry. (2017). NWCR facts. Retrieved from http://www.nwcr.ws/Research/default.htm

Ochner, C. N., et al. (2015). Treating obesity seriously: When recommendations for lifestyle change confront biological adaptations. *The Lancet Diabetes and Endocrinology, 3,* 232–234.

Partridge, S. R., et al. (2016). Poor quality of external validity reporting limits generalizability of overweight and/or obesity lifestyle prevention interventions in young adults: A systematic review. *Obesity Reviews, 16,* 13–31.

Ramage, S., et al. (2014). Healthy strategies for successful weight loss and weight maintenance: a systematic review. *Applied Physiology, Nutrition, and Metabolism, 39,* 1–20. Retrieved from http://www.nrcresearchpress.com/doi/pdfplus/10.1139/apnm-2013-0026

Rosenheck, R. (2008). Fast food consumption and increased caloric intake: A systematic review of a trajectory towards weight gain and obesity risk. *Obesity Reviews, 9,* 535–547.

Schroeder, R., et al. (2016). Treatment of adult obesity with bariatric surgery. *American Family Physician, 93,* 31–37.

Thackray, E. E., et al. (2016). Exercise, appetite and weight control: Are there differences between men and women? *Nutrients, 8,* 583. Retrieved from https://www.ncbi.nlm.nih.gov/pmc/articles/PMC5037567/

Villablanca, P. A., et al. (2016). Nonexercise activity thermogenesis in obesity management. *Mayo Clinic Proceedings, 90,* 509–519.

Wadden, T. A. (2016). Behavioral treatment of obesity in patients encountered in primary care settings: A systematic review. *Journal of the American Medical Association, 312,* 1779–1791.

World Health Organization. (2016). Overweight and obesity fact sheet. Retrieved from http://www.who.int/mediacentre/factsheets/fs311/en/

Yu, Y.-H., et al. (2015). Metabolic vs. hedonic obesity: A conceptual distinction and its clinical implications. *Obesity Reviews, 16,* 234–247

Suggested Readings

Bays, J. C. (2009). *Mindful eating: A guide to rediscovering a healthy and joyful relationship with food.* Boston: Shambhala Publications.

Bray, G. A., & Bouchard, C. (2014). *Handbook of obesity: Clinical applications.* London, UK: Informa Healthcare. Two experts provide up-to-date coverage of the range of subjects that make up the field of obesity research.

Gudzune, K. A., et al. (2015). Efficacy of commercial weight-loss programs. *Annals of Internal Medicine, 162,* 501–512. Compares weight loss, adherence, and harms of commercial weight-loss programs versus professional behavioral and medical interventions.

Hoffman, J. (2012). *The weight of the nation: Surprising lessons about diets, food, and fat from the extraordinary series from HBO Documentary Films.* New York: St. Martins Press. Shows how our minds, our bodies, corporate America, farms, and society's overall love of food contribute to the obesity epidemic. Based on an HBO special series.

Ludwig, D. S., & Pollack, H. A. (2009). Obesity and the economy. *Journal of the American Medical Association, 301,* 533–535. Discusses how economic factors affect the prevalence of obesity in the United States.

Mitchison, D., & Hay, P. J. (2014). The epidemiology of eating disorders: Genetic, environmental, and societal factors. *Clinical Epidemiology, 17,* 89–97. Summarizes current research on the sociodemographic, environmental, and genetic correlates of eating disorders in adults.

National Eating Disorders Association. Provides programs and services for individuals and families that have encountered these illnesses. http://www.nationaleatingdisorders.org/

Ornish, D. (2002). *Eat more, weigh less: Dr. Dean Ornish's Advantage Ten program for losing weight safely while eating abundantly.* New York: Quill. You can eat more and weigh less if you know what to eat.

Power, M. L., & Schulkin, J. (2013). *The evolution of obesity.* Baltimore: Johns Hopkins University Press. Discusses the influences of evolutionary biology, history, physiology, and medical science to explain the current obesity epidemic.

Wing, R. R., & Phelan, S. (2005). Long-term weight loss maintenance. *American Journal of Clinical Nutrition, 82,* 222S–225S. Retrieved from http://ajcn.nutrition.org/content/82/1/222S.long. Describes how several thousand people lost 60 pounds or more and kept the weight off for years by engaging in high levels of physical activity (1 hour per day), eating a low-calorie, low-fat diet, eating breakfast regularly, self-monitoring weight, and maintaining a consistent eating pattern across weekdays and weekends.

World Health Organization. (2017). Report of the Commission on Ending Childhood Obesity. Retrieved from http://www.who.int/end-childhood-obesity/news/draft-implementation/en/. Proposes actions for United Nations Member States to implement the commission's recommendations to address childhood obesity.

Yu, Y.-H., et al. (2015). Metabolic vs. hedonic obesity: A conceptual distinction and its clinical implications. *Obesity Reviews, 16,* 234–247.

Zylke, J. D., & Bauchner, H. (2016). The unrelenting challenge of obesity. *Journal of the American Medical Association, 315,* 2277–2278. Retrieved from http://jamanetwork.com/journals/jama/fullarticle/2526613. Points out that the obesity epidemic is 30 years on without any sign of relenting. Suggests that the food supply is a major cause of obesity and that food manufacturers and restaurants must become part of the conversation to turn around the obesity epidemic.

Recommended Websites

American Obesity Treatment Association
Education, information, and advocacy on overweight and obesity.

Overweight and Obesity
Data and health recommendations from the Centers for Disease Control and Prevention.

Weight Control Information Network
The U.S. National Institutes of Health provides science-based information on overweight and weight control.

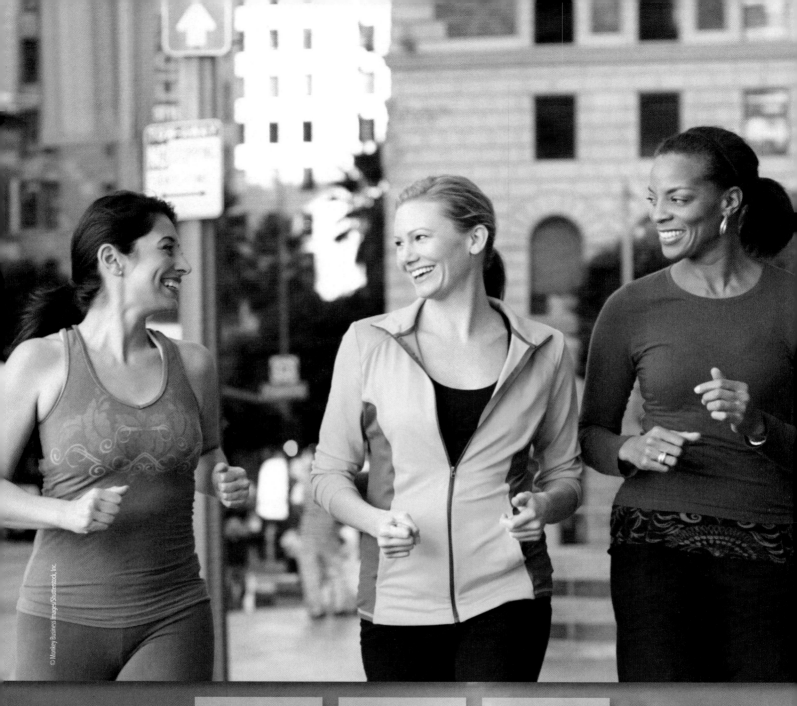

© Monkey Business Images/Shutterstock, Inc.

Health Tips

Incorporate Movement into Your Daily Activities

Weight Training Dos and Don'ts

Walking in Balance

Preventing Sports Injuries

Hydration for Sport and Recreational Physical Activity

Dollars & Health Sense

Caveat Emptor: The Business of Sports Supplements

Wellness Guide

Financial Incentives to Get Healthy

Getting into Shape

First Aid for Sports Injuries: RICE

CHAPTER 7

Movement and Physical Activity for Health

Learning Objectives

1. List reasons that individuals get too little movement and physical activity.

2. Describe the four categories of physical activity: household tasks, work-related movement, leisure-time activities, and performance-based activities.

3. Explain three different measurements of physical activity: calories per minute, METs, and PAL.

4. Describe levels of physical activity for health.

5. Explain the six components of physical activity: motivation, cardiorespiratory fitness, body strength, endurance, flexibility, and body composition.

6. Describe guidelines for integrating physical activity into one's life.

7. Discuss the types of performance-enhancing substances.

8. Define *overuse injuries*.

9. Discuss exercising in hot and cold weather.

Modern society depends on a vast array of machines (and the computers and "intelligent" software that control them) to carry out efficiently numerous industrial and economic processes. People also depend on machines to accomplish more easily the tasks of daily living.

Although it has freed people from considerable physical labor, the integration of work-saving machines into the fabric of modern life has had the inadvertent consequence of increasing risks to health from too little movement. Sedentariness and inadequate amounts of physical activity increase the risk of heart disease, overweight, type 2 diabetes, high blood pressure, osteoporosis, some forms of cancer, and premature death (Centers for Disease Control and Prevention, 2017). About 50% of U.S. adults, including college students, risk their health by being physically inactive; 60% of adults worldwide likewise put their health at risk (Ladabaum et al., 2014). Studies show that humans do best when they expend about 1,000 calories a week in movement activities of any kind, including those involved in working, carrying out the tasks of daily living, and recreation (Simon, 2015).

A physically inactive lifestyle is a new dimension in human history. For 99% of the many thousands of years that humans have inhabited the earth, adults have had to walk, run, lift, bend, and carry in order to find and raise their own food, provide themselves with shelter, raise children, and protect themselves. However, starting about 200 years ago and accelerating greatly in the twentieth century, people began using machines to carry out all manner of activities (**Table 7.1**). Now, most of the North American labor force works in occupations that involve sitting at a

desk, standing behind a counter, or occasionally walking a few steps while tending to others' needs and requests.

Regardless of the type of work, a vast majority of Americans travel to their jobs while sitting in a vehicle. Furthermore, when they get home, even if they have few household tasks to do, many people watch TV, play video games, or interact with the Internet and social media rather than move their bodies (other than to go to the refrigerator). People living in modern, industrialized societies are thought to expend almost half as much energy each day carrying out the tasks of living as ancient humans did (Booth, Chakravarthy, & Spangenburg, 2002).

About half of American adults spend a large percentage of their waking hours in **sedentary behavior** (from the Latin *sedere*, meaning "to sit"), such as sitting at a desk 8 to 10 hours a day (**Figure 7.1**). Sedentary behavior is characterized by very little energy expenditure over that needed to stay alive, even less than to fuel a brief walk every day. Independent of the amount of physical activity, sedentary behavior increases the risk of overweight, poor health, and mortality (Matthews et al., 2012). Engaging in an hour of moderate physical activity (e.g., walking) for every 8 hours of sitting can offset much of the health risk associated with many hours of sedentary behavior (Ekelund et al., 2016).

Recognizing that physical inactivity is detrimental to health, many countries, communities, health professionals, public health organizations, schools, employers, and religious organizations are seeking ways to encourage people to be more physically active, as the following illustrate:

- The U.S government, the European Union, the World Health Organization, and other governmental bodies have made engaging in physical activity national goals and are developing programs that encourage individuals to devote 30 minutes a day to some sort of movement activity.

Table 7.1

Twentieth-Century Innovations That Contribute to Reduced Physical Activity

Year	Innovation
1900	Modern escalator invented
1901	Vacuum cleaner invented
1903	Airplane invented by the Wright brothers
1904	Tractor invented
1906	First Mack trucks built
1908	Ford begins to mass produce and sell Model T automobile
1923	Frozen food invented
1923	Television invented
1950	First automatic elevators
1951	First computers sold commercially
1954	First McDonald's
1956	Establishment of U.S. Interstate Highway System
1976	Apple home computer invented
1981	First IBM PC sold
1990	World Wide Web/Internet protocol and language created

Data from Transportation Research Board, Institute of Medicine. (2005). *Does the built environment influence physical activity?* Washington, DC: National Academy of Sciences.

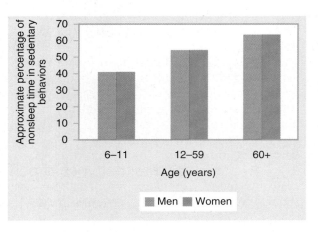

■ **Figure 7.1**

Percentage of Nonsleep Time Americans Spend in Sedentary Behaviors, by Age Group
Sedentary activities include sitting, lying, standing, or minimally walking.

Data from Mathews, C. E., et al. (2008). Amount of time spent in sedentary behaviors in the United States, 2003–2004. *American Journal of Epidemiology, 167*, 875–881.

Financial Incentives to Get Healthy

Imagine the following scenario. Your employer wants the staff to be healthier by becoming more physically active, so the company is going to pay employees to walk 7,000 steps a day. Steps are counted via a smartphone app, and the total number of steps is transmitted to the program's exercise central database for recording. Participants receive $25 to enroll. In their monthly paychecks, they receive $20 for each month of participation in the program and any earnings from walking. Your employer is offering three incentive options. Which option would you choose?

Pay4play	Double winner	Take the money (and run)
Receive $2 for each day you walk 7,000 steps.	Receive a lottery number between 00 and 99 on each day you walk 7,000 steps. One winning number is drawn each day. You receive $5 for a one-digit match and $50 for a two-digit match (and a bump in your health for walking even if you don't win any money).	Receive a $60 credit at the first of each month. Deduct $2 a day for each day you do not meet the 7,000-step requirement.

Behavioral economists and health professionals are experimenting with ways to incentivize health behavior changes. The fictitious program described here is derived from an actual experiment of similar design conducted by researchers at the University of Pennsylvania Perelman School of Medicine (Patel, et al., 2016). The results are depicted in the accompanying graph. From the data in the graph, which incentive is the most powerful? Was that the one you chose? Can you explain the results?

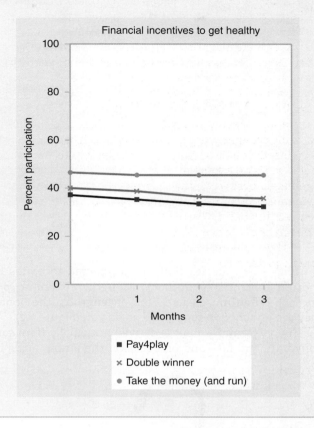

Financial incentives to get healthy

- ■ Pay4play
- × Double winner
- ● Take the money (and run)

- Employees receive company-supplied training and time at work to engage in various types of physical activities.
- New housing developments are required to include inviting public spaces, parks, walking and biking paths, and close access to public transportation and shopping to minimize driving.
- Walking during work hours is encouraged by placing parking lots some distance from buildings, giving employees pedometers or fitness apps, resetting elevators to run slowly to encourage walking stairs, and making staircases wide, carpeted, brightly painted, and with music and picture windows.
- Communities designate and maintain "safe walking" routes for schoolchildren and adult walkers.
- Colleges, universities, churches, and other organizations offer programs that encourage walking and other types of physical activity.

The Definition of Physical Activity

Physical activity is anything you do when you are not sitting or lying down, from clicking your computer's mouse to running a marathon. Among Americans and residents of developed countries, physical activity occurs in the following contexts (**Table 7.2**):

- *Doing household tasks*, such as washing the floor, being with and taking care of children, and gardening
- *Work-related movement*, for example, walking from a desk to the elevator, being a server in a restaurant, or working in construction
- *Leisure-time activities*, such as taking a walk or engaging in recreational exercise such as dancing, running, swimming, or tennis
- *Skill-based performance activities*, for example, exercising the body (or specific body regions) in order to excel at a particular activity or sport

Physical activity is scientifically defined in terms of the amount of energy expended to produce movement. Movement occurs when energy derived from food

TERMS

sedentary behavior: a pattern of living that lacks sufficient physical activity for good health

Table 7.2

Comparison of Energy Used in Various Physical Activities

Context	Moderate intensity (4–7 calories/minute, 3–6 METs)	Vigorous intensity (7+ calories/minute, 6+ METs)
Household	Gardening	Shoveling snow
	Scrubbing a floor	Pushing a lawn mower
	Carrying a child	Active play with a child
Work	Sawing with a power saw	Hand sawing hard woods
	Waiting tables	Firefighting
	Packing boxes for shipping	Loading/unloading a truck
Leisure	Walking 3–4 miles per hour	Jogging/running
	Yoga	Circuit weight training
	Dancing (most kinds)	Tennis (singles)
Performance	Weight training	Circuit weight training
	Shooting baskets	Football practice
	Skateboarding	Long-distance running

NOTE: METs = metabolic equivalents.
Modified from *General Physical Activities Defined by Level of Intensity* (2010).
U.S. Centers for Disease Control and Prevention. Retrieved from http://www
.cdc.gov/nccdphp/dnpa/physical/pdf/PA_Intensity_table_2_1.pdf

is utilized by muscles that are connected to bones to shorten (*concentric contraction*) or lengthen (*eccentric contraction*). When muscles shorten or lengthen, the bones they are attached to move, and so do you (**Figure 7.2**).

Energy for movement is derived principally from carbohydrate and fat—and on occasion the amino acids in protein, but not vitamins and minerals—which the body acquires from food and can store until needed. There are 4 calories of energy in a gram of carbohydrate and protein, and 9 calories of energy in a gram of fat. Energy can be derived from food with or without the addition of oxygen. Oxygen-absent energy production is called **anaerobic**; oxygen-present energy production is called **aerobic**. Compared with oxygen-absent, oxygen-present energy production is nearly 20 times more efficient, which is the major reason you breathe.

Oxidation is the chemical term for the process of oxygen-present energy production. *Burning* is another term for the process of oxidation. When biological material is burned in a fire, oxidation generates very little useful energy and considerable heat. When carbohydrate and fat are burned in cells, oxidation is controlled to capture the energy for useful work and to minimize energy lost as heat. So, when you hear the expression "burn calories," it means extracting energy to fuel cellular processes and not melting fat with heat.

The nervous system controls movement by signaling muscles to contract. Some movements are *reflexive*, meaning they do not require a conscious decision, for example, when quickly pulling your hand from a hot stove. A *voluntary movement*, like kicking a ball, involves both decision and movement-control centers in the brain, which send nerve signals to specific muscles, resulting in movement.

Physical activity is measured in terms of calories used per minute, metabolic equivalents, or physical activity level, as follows:

- *Calories used per minute*: A nutritional or movement calorie is scientifically defined as the energy equivalent of the amount of heat energy required to raise a kilogram of water from 15.5°C to 16.5°C. Muscles do not use heat as an energy source; energy is chemically extracted from carbohydrate and fat within muscle cells and provided directly to the tissue that creates movement. A calorie can fuel about 25 steps

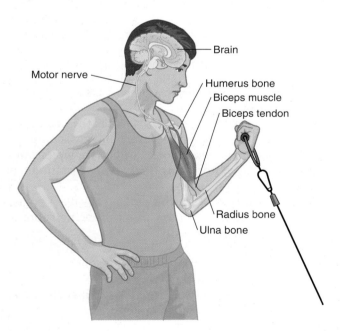

■ **Figure 7.2**

The Human Movement System
The human movement system consists of muscles, bones, tendons (which attach muscles to bones), and ligaments (which attach bones to bones). Movement occurs when the brain sends a signal via a specific nerve connecting it to a specific muscle. If the nerve signal directs a muscle to shorten, the two bones it connects move toward each other. If the nerve signal directs the muscle to lengthen, the two bones it connects move away from each other.

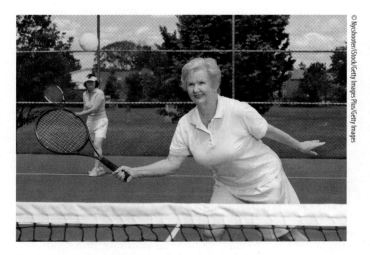

Tennis is an excellent form of exercise at any age.

Incorporate Movement into Your Daily Activities

- At school or work, take movement breaks by walking or doing desk exercises instead of taking food breaks. If you are the social type, go with a friend on a talk-walk.
- Exercise while watching TV (for example, use hand weights, a stationary bicycle, treadmill, or stair climber or stretch).

of walking. The calories utilized in various physical activities are presented in Table 7.2.

- *Metabolic equivalents (METs)*: **Metabolic equivalents, or METs,** are per-minute multiples of the amount of energy used while sitting or lying still, which is defined as 1 MET. For people of average size, 1 MET is about 1.2 calories. Moderate physical activity utilizes 3 to 6 METs; vigorous physical activity utilizes more than 6 METs (see Table 7.2).
- *Physical activity level (PAL)*: **Physical activity level (PAL)** is a measure of the amount of energy expended per day over and above that required for *basal* or *resting* metabolism, which is the energy needed to fuel basic life functions (i.e., heartbeat, breathing, kidney and brain function, etc.). A person is considered sedentary if the PAL is less than 1.4, that is, the daily energy expended to fuel all forms of movement is less than 1.4 times the energy expended in basal metabolism. PAL values between 1.4 and 1.7 indicate a moderate level of physical activity. PALs greater than 1.7 indicate a vigorous level of physical activity (**Figure 7.3**).

Any movement or activity can be discussed in terms of the following (FITT) dimensions:

- *Frequency*: how often the movement or activity occurs
- *Intensity*: the energy required to render the movement or activity
- *Time*: how long the movement or activity takes place
- *Type or mode*: the kind of movement or activity

For example, you can walk (*type*) for 10 minutes (*time*) to a particular class three times a week (*frequency*) at a pace utilizing 4 calories per minute (*intensity*). Thus, each walk to class utilizes 40 calories of energy, with a resulting expenditure of about 120 calories per week (10 minutes × 4 calories per minute).

Physical Activity for Health

In the 1950s, a pioneering study on the relationship of movement and health found that 30% fewer conductors in London's double-decker buses had heart disease compared to their coworkers who drove the buses. The reason: Conductors were more active than the drivers because they were continually moving between decks taking passengers' tickets. Since that time, thousands of studies have confirmed that movement and physical activity are good for health, irrespective of smoking status, body weight, and other health-related characteristics.

Moderate amounts of regular physical activity, whether it is household, work-related, leisure-time, or performance-enhancing, counteracts the deleterious effects of inactivity and sedentariness and contributes to health and well-being in a variety of ways (**Table 7.3**). A moderate amount of physical activity expends between 1.4 and 1.7 times the energy required for basal metabolism, which for most people amounts to 120 and 300 calories per day of activity, or a total of about 600 to 1,500 calories per week (**Figure 7.4**).

The scientifically based finding that *moderate* levels of physical activity are beneficial to health stands in stark contrast to the exhortations of the health club, exercise equipment, dietary supplement, and fashion industries, as well as the advertising, popular magazines, and infomercials that support them. These commercial interests would have people believe that movement for health requires considerable time, special equipment and clothing, excessive effort, and sweating a lot in order to attain a svelte, lean body (and for men one that is highly muscular

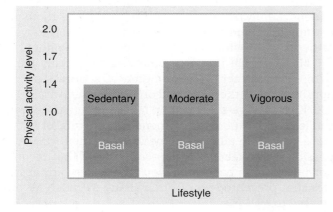

■ Figure 7.3

Physical Activity Levels
Physical activity level (PAL) is the amount of daily energy expended over and above a person's basal or resting metabolism, which is the energy required to fuel basic life functions while at rest.

TERMS

aerobic: biological energy production using oxygen

anaerobic: biological energy production without using oxygen

metabolic equivalents (METs): per-minute multiples of the amount of energy used while lying still

oxidation: the chemical term for the process of oxygen-present energy production

physical activity level (PAL): a measure of the amount of energy expended per day over and above that used for basal metabolism

Table 7.3

Health Benefits of Physical Activity

Puts into life the good feelings and enjoyment that come from body movement

Increases the ability to cope effectively with stress

Increases endurance in daily activities and lessens fatigue

Increases longevity

Strengthens the heart muscle

Decreases the heart rate

Increases blood flow to the heart

Maintains normal blood pressure and reduces high blood pressure

Increases blood levels of high-density lipoproteins (good) cholesterol

Reduces blood levels of low-density lipoproteins (bad) cholesterol

Reduces blood levels of triglycerides (fats)

Boosts the immune system, thus lessening the risk of colds and other infections

Enhances sleep

Maintains a healthy body weight

Improves food choices

Increases bone mass and reduces the risk of osteoporosis

Prevents and alleviates chronic low back pain

Lessens the desire to smoke cigarettes and consume alcohol and drugs

Lessens depression

Enhances self-image, self-esteem, and creativity

Park your car a 10- to 15-minute walk from your destination.

Walk/march in place when on your phone.

Walk/march in place during every TV commercial.

Table/desk/chair push-ups: Stand; place hands on table/desk/back of chair; perform 10 push-ups.

Set phone timer: At your desk, move/stretch at least 3 to 4 minutes every hour.

Chair on fire: Sit on edge of chair; stand; sit and then stand immediately (chair on fire!); do 10 reps.

Walk during breaks and lunch. Don't eat/sit the entire time.

Hold walking meetings. Stand during presentations/webinars.

Take the stairs, not the elevator.

Take the longest walking route feasible to the restroom, even if you have to go to another floor.

Take the longest walking route to any source of food.

Do partial squats, knee, and calf raises while waiting for the copier/microwave/fax etc.

Keep a resistance band to perform strengthening/stretching exercises at your desk/while watching TV.

Walk/jog in place for 2 minutes *whenever* you get up from your desk.

Desk dance. Move your feet, arms, and shoulders to favorites from your playlist.

Keep an exercise log to keep you focused.

Walk/talk with a buddy to keep it fun.

Listen to audiobooks to keep it interesting.

Walk a dog to be a pal.

■ **Figure 7.4**

Put a Little Movement in Your Life

Data from University of California, Riverside MoveMore. https://wellness.ucr.edu/move_more/movemore.html.

---

or "cut")—appearances more suited to computer-enhanced images than real people. You do not have to run like an Olympic athlete or look like a model in a fitness advertisement to be healthy.

An efficient way to attain a moderate level of physical activity is to walk briskly for 30 to 45 minutes on most days of the week (Figure 7.4). Your pace should be such that your heart and breathing rates increase slightly but not so much that you cannot carry on a conversation while walking; for most people, this pace is about 3 to 4 miles per hour. Also, you should experience a light to moderate increase in **relative perceived exertion**, which is awareness that you are responding to exercise (sensations of effort and muscular force, breathing rate, and body and skin temperature).

Although it seems tame in comparison to running on a treadmill, walking is nevertheless excellent for health (Kelly et al., 2014). It strengthens the heart and skeletal muscles, increases breathing ability, clears and quiets the mind, reduces stress, uses calories (weight maintenance), and causes few injuries, if any. Other than appropriate footwear, walking requires no special clothing or equipment and, with a little preplanning, can be worked into any busy schedule; you can break up the total walking time into several small parts and attain the same health benefits. Walk stairs instead of riding an elevator, park the car 10 minutes from your destination and walk the rest of the way, take a dog for a walk twice a day (Fido will be forever grateful), do a walk-talk with a friend, family member, or spouse (good for relationship maintenance and also fun), and make it a habit to walk rather than sit while you talk on your mobile phone.

Many people find that counting their daily steps with a **pedometer**, accelerometer, or a fitness phone app, helps keep them focused on walking (Bravata et al., 2007). An average-sized person takes 2,000 steps to walk a mile. Health experts recommend taking a total of 10,000 steps per day in all one's activities combined—15,000 if possible—and keeping a step-count diary that records not only the number of steps you take but also any obstacles that prevented you from walking as much as you wanted to.

People who enjoy vigorous physical activities (e.g., running, swimming, singles tennis) should do them at least 3 days a week for 20 minutes each time. Vigorous activities have PALs of between 1.7 and 2.5. They utilize 7 or more calories per minute, make you breathe hard and sweat, and

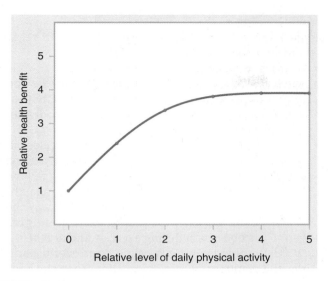

■ Figure 7.5

Relative Health Benefit of Physical Activity
The graph is a composite from many studies that demonstrate the positive effect of physical activity on health. Notice that the graph is not linear; the largest benefit comes from changing from no to little daily physical activity to low-to-moderate levels of physical activity. High levels of physical activity do not produce corresponding gains in health. Health benefits include lessened risk of morbidity and mortality from cardiovascular disease, cancer, hypertension, and type 2 diabetes. Each level of physical activity (e.g., walking, running, cycling) corresponds to between 500 and 1,000 calories per week of activity.

Modified from Bouchard, C., et al. (2015). Less sitting, more physical activity, or higher fitness? *Mayo Clinic Proceedings, 90*, 1533–1540.

are sufficiently intense that you cannot easily talk to anyone while doing them. Compared with moderate physical activity, vigorous physical activity provides slightly greater heart-health benefits and longevity (Bouchard et al., 2015) (**Figure 7.5**). However, it also carries a higher risk of physical injury and psychological burnout, either of which can curtail activity for weeks or even months.

Besides direct effects on health, both moderate and vigorous physical activity can provide time and attention for you. Many people feel overwhelmed by the demands of school, jobs, and family. Just taking a few minutes several days a week to move your body can give you a chance to relax, reflect, and indulge your imagination. Also, physical activity can reduce stress, anxiety, and depression; improve mental functioning; and contribute to enhanced work performance by inducing healthy changes in the brain (Sale et al., 2014).

Psychological Benefits of Physical Activity and Movement

In addition to many physiological benefits, physical activity and movement can also enhance mental health. Studies have shown that moderate physical activity can reduce stress, anxiety, and depression; improve sleep

and mental functioning; and contribute to enhanced work and academic performance (Chu et al., 2014). These outcomes are thought to be related to increases in metabolism, oxygenation, and blood flow in the brain; changes in neurotransmitters that are associated with alertness (norepinephrine), pleasure and reward (dopamine), euphoria, well-being, and decreased sensitivity to pain (endorphins, enkephalins, and endocannabinoids); and changes in growth factors affecting specific neurons in the brain (Portugal et al., 2013). Physical activity can also promote the experience of relaxed concentration, regular breathing rhythms, and increased self-awareness, outcomes similar to meditation and yoga.

Another mental health benefit of physical activity comes from simply setting aside time on most days from life's other activities and responsibilities in order to devote yourself to something you enjoy.

Components of Physical Activity

Although your whole being responds to movement, it is possible to identify the following six components of physical activity:

1. *Motivation:* the willingness to focus attention and energy on movement
2. *Cardiorespiratory fitness:* the body's ability to obtain and utilize fuel and oxygen efficiently during sustained, effortful physical activity
3. *Body strength:* the ability to lift or move an object (including your body, as when you walk or climb stairs)
4. *Endurance:* the ability to move an object (including yourself) without becoming quickly fatigued
5. *Flexibility:* the ability to move a joint (where two bones meet) through its anatomical range of motion
6. *Body composition:* the body's relative amounts of water, bone, fat, and tissue

These six components and activities that promote them are discussed in the following subsections.

Motivation

Your ancient ancestors did not require specific motivation to be physically active. Because they had to move their bodies to acquire food and avoid environmental dangers, hunger and fear were motivation enough for movement. Most modern humans can eat and be safe without much daily movement; indeed, many occupations require little movement. Thus, to gain the health

TERMS

pedometer: a step counter
relative perceived exertion: awareness of one's relative response to exercise

benefits from movement, other motivations must come into play, including the following:

- Being paid, such as in an employer-sponsored exercise class
- Desiring to be healthy
- Desiring to "look good"
- Enjoying socializing while engaging in a movement activity
- Accomplishing a personal goal, such as losing weight, climbing a mountain, running a distance race, or biking 50 miles

Regardless of the motivation, it is important that one's chosen physical activities be enjoyable, or at the very least not objectionable. Doing enjoyable activities promotes continuing with them. If what you do is unpleasant, however, you won't do it for very long. This might mean experimenting with several types of activities in order to find ones that you are likely to make a regular part of your life. It might mean engaging in more than one activity to break up monotony and boredom. **Cross-training** is incorporating more than one activity into your regular activity plan, for example, walking 4 days a week and doing strength training or cycling 2 days a week (and resting 1 day).

Also, it is important to realize that obstacles to accomplishing one's movement goals arise frequently. Regardless of your motivation and dedication, there may be weeks or even months when getting your desired level of physical activity is a challenge. Perhaps you get sick or injured. Perhaps your schedule is very tight and there seems to be no time for anything but work. Perhaps you lose interest in former activities. At such times it is important not to become so discouraged that you give up wanting physical activity in your life. Realize that obstacles are to be expected and that they will pass in time. When they do, you can resume your desired activities or replace them with better alternatives.

Cardiorespiratory Fitness

Cardiorespiratory fitness is the degree to which the body can supply sufficient fuel (carbohydrate, fatty acids, and oxygen) to produce sustained, effortful physical activity—in other words, the degree to which someone is "in shape." Exercise physiologists define cardiorespiratory fitness in terms of the maximum amount of oxygen the body can utilize in physical activity, called *VO$_2$ max* ("volume of oxygen maximal"). Studies show that higher fitness levels, defined by VO$_2$ max, are associated with a lower risk of death from cardiovascular disease (DeFina et al., 2015). It is not known how cardiorespiratory fitness reduces the risk of heart disease; one suggestion is that it lowers blood levels of total and bad cholesterol and triglycerides, which are progenitors of heart disease. Cardiovascular fitness also lowers the heart rate.

Because modern lifestyles do not require vigorous physical activity in the carrying out of daily life tasks, attaining high levels of cardiorespiratory fitness requires planned bouts of sustained, high-intensity, vigorous activity, called **aerobic training**, what many people call working out.

Aerobic Training

Aero is derived from Greek, meaning "air." With regard to physical activity,

- *Aerobic* means requiring oxygen.
- *Aerobic exercise* is any activity that requires the body to use more oxygen than it does in usual activities.
- *Aerobic capacity* is the extent to which an individual can perform aerobic exercise.
- *Aerobic training* is engaging in aerobic exercises *on a regular basis* to increase the amount of oxygen the body can process in a given time. Aerobic training requires that the heart and lungs work harder than usual to provide oxygen to exercising muscles. In this way, they become more efficient in acquiring and delivering oxygen to the body, both during exercise and at rest.

When aerobic training is carried out over a period of time, the resultant physiological changes in the heart, lungs, and muscles are called the **training effect**, or "in shape." You induce the training effect by exercising such that the heart rate during exercise increases to between 60% and 80% of its theoretical maximum. This is called your **target heart rate**. To determine your target heart rate:

- Calculate your theoretical maximum heart rate (MHR) by subtracting your age from 220.
- Multiply your MHR by 60% and 80% to determine the lower and upper limits of your target heart rate, called the *target zone, target heart rate zone,* or "in the zone."

For example, for a 20-year-old, the MHR is 200 (220 − 20), and the lower and upper limits of the target zone are 120 (60% × 200) and 160 (80% × 200) heartbeats per minute (see **Table 7.4**).

Three to 4 days of exercise per week are sufficient to produce a training effect. Two days per week may suffice for people already in good condition. One day a week does little to improve fitness and may increase the risk

Table 7.4

Maximum and Target Heart Rates Predicted from Age

Take your pulse for 15 seconds immediately after exercising, and multiply by 4. If heart rate is in the target range for your age, optimal training benefits have been obtained. If below target range, step up activity. If above the maximum, take it easier during workouts and gradually increase intensity.

Age (in years)	Predicted maximum heart rate (in beats per minute)	Target heart rate range (in beats per minute)
20	200	120–160
25	200	117–156
30	194	114–152
35	188	111–148
40	182	108–144
45	176	105–140
50	171	102–136
55	165	99–132
60	159	96–128
65	153	93–124

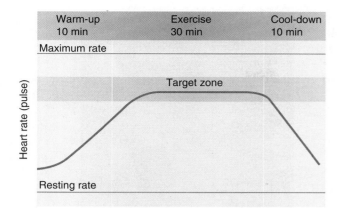

■ Figure 7.6

Heart Rate Pattern for a Typical Exercise Routine
A diagram of heart rate during warm-up, aerobic exercise, and cool-down.

of injury. Also, exercising more than 5 days a week does little to increase fitness. It does expend calories, but it also makes one susceptible to injuries.

A session of aerobic exercise should begin with about 10 minutes of warm-up activity during which heart rate gradually increases (**Figure 7.6**). As the intensity of activity increases, the target zone heart rate is attained and maintained for 20 to 30 minutes. This is followed by a cool-down period during which the heart rate returns to preexercise levels. You can obtain your heart rate with a heart rate monitor, a device you strap to your chest or wrist, or by counting your heartbeats at your wrist or carotid artery (**Figure 7.7**).

Body Strength

Body strength is the ability of a muscle or group of muscles to move an object, including your body. Whereas it often conjures up images of supermuscular body builders lifting heavy weights, body strength for health requires minimal, if any, change in body size and lifting of weights. The goal is to have sufficient strength to carry out normal tasks (work, lifting packages, walking stairs, shoveling snow) and participate in physical activities without injury. Two popular ways to increase body strength are strength training and Pilates.

Strength Training

Strength training (also called *resistance training*) involves building muscle and bone strength by repetitively moving individual muscles or muscle groups against resistance, commonly applied by weights, such as barbells, dumbbells, and exercise machines, and also by pushing against an immovable object (**isometric training**). Some of the benefits of strength training include the following:

- Enhanced ability to combat fatigue in everyday activities
- Improved fitness
- Preventing and rehabilitating orthopedic (musculoskeletal) injuries
- Reduction in body fat

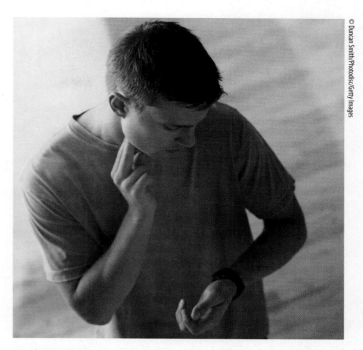

© Duncan Smith/Photodisc/Getty Images

■ Figure 7.7

Measuring Your Heart Rate
Place your index and middle finger (not your thumb) on the opposite wrist an inch below the thumb or at the side of the throat (Adam's apple). Press until you feel the pulsations. Count the beats for 15 seconds. Multiply by 4 to get heart rate in beats per minute.

- Increased basal metabolic rate
- Decreased blood pressure
- Lower risk for cardiovascular disease
- Lessen low back pain

Many people imagine that the goal of strength training is to greatly enlarge the size of the body's muscles. This is an image proffered by the media (and advertising to sell dietary supplements and exercise machines)

▮TERMS▮

aerobic training: exercise that increases the body's capacity to use oxygen

cardiorespiratory fitness: the degree to which the body can supply sufficient fuel and oxygen to produce sustained, effortful physical activity

cross-training: incorporating more than one activity into a regular activity plan

isometric training: strength training by pushing against an immovable object

strength training: the use of resistance to increase one's ability to exert or resist force for the purpose of improving performance

target heart rate: the heart rate during strenuous exercise associated with inducing the training effect

training effect: beneficial physiological changes as a result of aerobic exercise

Weight Training Dos and Don'ts

Do

- Use spotters when trying major lifts.
- Keep your back straight when lifting.
- Use proper lifting technique.
- Wear shoes with good traction.
- Use equipment that is in good condition.
- Follow safety rules.

Don't

- Hyperventilate or hold your breath—breathe out when you press.
- Continue if you feel pain; ice the painful region.
- Lift if you feel lightheaded.
- Exercise a set of muscles more than three times per week.
- Cheat on technique to lift heavier weights.

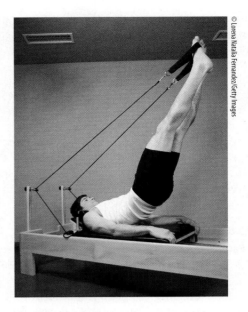

The Pilates method strengthens core muscles.

that idealizes a muscular body as a sign of attractiveness. Many men believe that a large, muscular body is the definition of masculinity. However, from a health point of view, the goal of strength training is stronger muscles, not necessarily bigger ones. Strength training for health means having the strength to participate without hindrance in activities of daily living and the ability to move muscles over a period of time (endurance). Strength training to increase muscle size is a very specialized activity (*body building*).

To engage in strength training for health and fitness, the American College of Sports Medicine recommends the following for healthy adults:

- Follow a specific activity plan (workout) two to three times a week.
- Perform 8 to 10 resistance exercises per workout.
- Exercise all major muscle groups.
- Repeat each exercise 8 to 12 times ("reps").
- Use an amount of weight that can be moved the desired number of times.
- Breathe normally while exercising.
- Move a muscle or muscle group through the full range of motion.
- Warm up prior to and cool down after an exercise session.

Whereas gyms and health clubs can supply all manner of strength training equipment, one needs only a few 5- or 10-pound dumbbells and a simple training program to derive considerable health benefits from strength training.

Strength training can involve progressive increases in the time, intensity, and amount of weight moved. Muscle strength is built by moving heavy weights a few times per set, whereas endurance is built by moving smaller weights through many repetitions. Also, in an extended training program, the repetitions, number of sets, amount of weight, and other exercise variables should

vary (called *periodization*). To avoid injury (see the Health Tip "Weight Training Dos and Don'ts"), it is imperative that one receive professional assistance in the design of a strength training program and professional instruction in strength training methods.

Compared with most aerobic exercise, strength training produces only a modest improvement in cardiovascular fitness. The time spent exercising is insufficient to increase the heart rate long enough to produce a training effect. The energy expended during strength training is about 4 calories per minute, nearly the same as for walking or swimming at a comfortable pace.

A common myth associated with strength training is that consuming high-protein foods and special vitamin supplements will increase muscle mass. This assumption is incorrect. Muscle tissue responds to the demands of work, not to food. In a progressive strength training regimen, sufficient protein to build new muscle tissue will be obtained in a well-balanced diet. Excess protein and vitamins are simply excreted.

Pilates

Pilates is a widely used method of body conditioning developed by Joseph H. Pilates (pronounced Puh-lah-tees) in the 1920s. Pilates was born in Germany in 1880 and was a frail child with asthma and rickets who was determined to be strong. He was interned in England during World War I because of his German citizenship. While in England, he became a nurse and began designing exercise apparatus for immobilized hospital patients. The devices and exercises became the foundation for his method of body conditioning and strengthening. In 1926, he moved to New York City and opened his first Pilates Studio. The body building and fitness regimen he developed became widely used all over the world by dancers, actors, sports teams, spas, and fitness enthusiasts. Dancers such as

Martha Graham and George Balanchine were among the first to adopt his fitness techniques. Today, his exercises are recommended by coaches, trainers, physical therapists, chiropractors, and others.

The Pilates method consists of hundreds of stretching and strengthening exercises that are performed on a mat with or without Pilates rings and other devices used to assist in strengthening muscles. Many of the exercises are designed to strengthen the back, abdomen, and buttocks; Pilates believed that these regions were the core of strength and the basis of good posture. Like yoga, the Pilates method emphasizes a balance of mind, body, and spirit. Rather than performing many repetitions of exercises, Pilates advocated intense mental concentration on performing each exercise with precision and awareness. Although developed many years ago, the Pilates exercises are still widely used to improve strength and performance and for overall body conditioning.

Endurance

Endurance is the ability to move an object, including yourself, without becoming quickly fatigued. Endurance is a combination of fitness, strength, and motivation. The fitness aspects of endurance relate to the body's ability to acquire and utilize oxygen, carbohydrate, and fat to fuel movement for an extended period of time. The strength aspect of endurance involves having sufficiently strong muscles to carry out an activity for an extended period without damage. The motivational aspect of endurance is the will to carry on with an activity even though you feel fatigued.

Endurance develops by extending yourself past former limits of physical activity. In this way, the anatomy and physiology of the heart, lungs, muscles, and energy-supplying and energy-utilizing systems, and your own expectations of your ability to persevere, gradually adapt to meet the challenges of extended activity. Endurance training generally involves both aerobic and strength training activities.

Flexibility

Flexibility is the degree to which you can rotate, bend, and twist a part of your body. Rotating, bending, and twisting occur where bones meet, an anatomical structure called a *joint*. For example, your elbow is a joint at which the two lower arm bones attach to the upper arm bone, allowing you to bend your arm. Imagine how difficult arm movement would be if you had no elbow joint.

Joints are held together by ligaments and tendons, which are elastic, fibrous bands of *connective tissue*. Flexibility is determined by the pliability of a joint's connective tissue and associated muscles. Every joint has a **range of motion**, which is the amount of rotating, bending, or twisting that the anatomy of the joint allows. Satisfactory flexibility is being able to move a joint through its full range of motion. Satisfactory flexibility contributes the following health benefits:

- Lessens the effort in carrying out physical tasks, such as lifting a package or bending to pick up something.
- Fosters good balance, which aids mobility and reduces the risk of falling.
- Reduces bodily and psychic tension resulting from stress.
- Lessens the risk of low back pain.
- Reduces exercise-associated soreness.
- Improves blood flow to muscles.
- Lessens the risk of activity-related injuries.

Movement at a joint can increase its flexibility; lack of movement can reduce it. That is one reason that exercisers feel "loose" after activity, whereas sedentary people tend to feel stiff and have difficulty bending. Flexibility at a particular joint can be fostered by specific stretching exercises (**Figure 7.8**). Each joint's flexibility is independent of other joints; that is, you can be more flexible at one joint than you are at another. Activities such as yoga and t'ai chi ch'uan, which are discussed next, help increase flexibility at many joints simultaneously.

Yoga

Yoga is a system of exercises formulated in India thousands of years ago to unite one's mind and body. The word *yoga* means to join or yoke together. Of the several kinds of yoga, the most common is *Hatha yoga,* which uses body postures, called poses or *asanas,* breathing techniques *(pranayama),* and meditation to bring the body, mind, and spirit into healthy harmony. In yoga practice, one pays attention to the physical, mental, and spiritual effects of doing each posture (called *observing*). Also, yoga's breathing techniques increase a sense of positive energy and minimize negative inner self-talk. About 21 million U.S. adults practice yoga each year (Cramer et al., 2016).

Yoga is best learned from an experienced practitioner. The method is generally practiced for 30 minutes at a time, two or more days a week. A combination of postures, called the Sun Salute, can be done daily to increase flexibility and bring the mind and body into harmony (**Figure 7.9**). The principal physical benefits of yoga are enhancing muscular fitness and body flexibility; the exercises are not sufficiently strenuous to produce significant cardiovascular benefit. Nevertheless, yoga can help

---

TERMS

endurance: the ability to move an object without becoming quickly fatigued

flexibility: the degree to which one can rotate, bend, and twist a part of the body

Pilates: a system of stretching and strengthening exercises

range of motion: the amount of rotating, bending, or twisting allowed by the anatomy of a joint

yoga: a system of exercises formulated in India thousands of years ago to unite one's mind and body

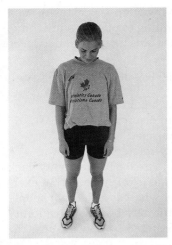
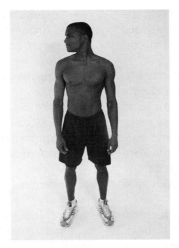
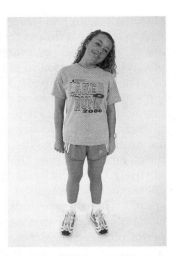

Neck   Drop your chin to your chest. Turn your head as far right as you can without moving your shoulders and hold. Repeat to the left. Tilt your head toward the left ear without bending your torso or hunching your shoulders and hold. Repeat to the right.

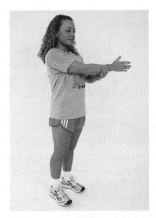

Shoulder Stretch 1   With your left hand, grasp your right elbow and pull your arm across your chest, keeping it bent at a 90° angle. Alternate arms.

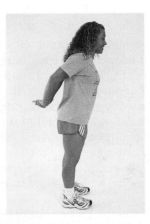

Shoulder Stretch 2   Standing, grasp both arms behind your back and raise them up as far as you can.

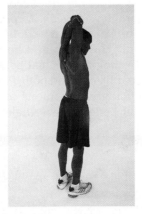

Triceps Stretch   Grasp the opposite elbow and pull the arm behind the head and down until a stretch is felt in the back of the arm. Hold and then repeat for the other arm.

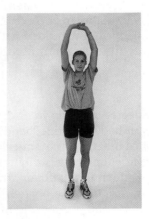

Upper-Back Stretch   Clasp your hands in front of your body, and press your palms forward.

(continued on next page)

■ **Figure 7.8**

Flexibility Exercises
It is best to do stretching exercises when the muscles are warm. You should stretch to the point of mild discomfort, but stop immediately if you experience pain—particularly in the lower back or knees. Hold all stretches for 15 to 30 seconds, rest for 30 to 60 seconds, and then repeat the stretch, trying to go a little further. For all standing stretches, legs should be hip-width apart, with knees slightly bent, back straight, and weight evenly distributed from the front to the back of the feet.

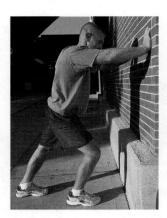

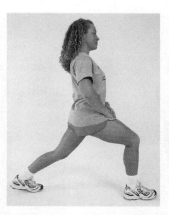

Calf Stretch   Stand approximately 2 to 3 feet away from a wall, tree, or stretching partner. Move one foot in close to the wall, while keeping the back leg straight behind you with the foot and heel flat on the ground. Slowly move your hips forward, bending the forward knee and keeping the back foot on the ground. You should feel a slight stretch in your calf muscles. Repeat with the opposite leg.

Lunge Stretch   Step forward and bend your forward knee, keeping it directly above your ankle. Stretch your other leg back behind you but don't lock your knee. Press your hips forward and down to stretch. Your arms can be at your sides, on top of your knee, or on the ground for balance. Repeat on the other side.

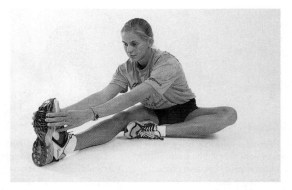

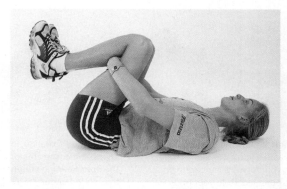

Modified Hurdler   Sit with your right leg straight out in front of you and your left leg tucked close to your body. Reach toward your right foot as far as possible. Do not curve your back. Go only as far as you can with a straight back. Repeat for the other leg.

Lower-Back Stretch   Lie on your back and pull both knees in to the chest. Keep your lower back on the floor.

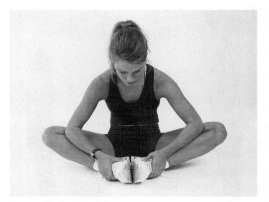

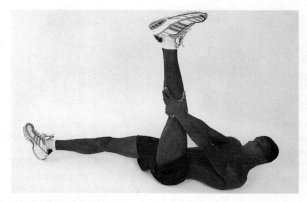

Groin Stretch Sit with your back straight (don't slouch; you may want to put your back against a wall) and bend your legs, with the soles of your feet together. Try to get your heels as close to your groin as is comfortably possible. For a passive stretch, push your knees to the floor as far as you can (you may use your hands to assist but do not resist with the knees) and hold them there. This can be hard on the knees, so please be careful. Now, keep your knees where they are, and then exhale as you bend over, trying to get your chest as close to the floor as possible.

Supine Hamstring Stretch Lie on your back and pull one leg up to a stretched position. The leg should remain as straight as possible. The opposite leg should be bent with the heel on the floor; keep your lower back on the floor. Alternate legs.

■ **Figure 7.8**

Flexibility Exercises (*continued***)**

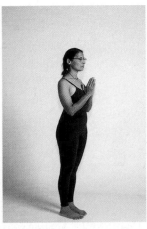

Position 1   Stand erect with your feet hip-width apart and palms together in front of your chest. Inhale and exhale slowly and calmly.

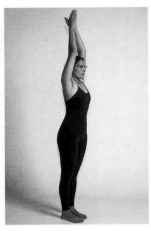

Position 2   Inhaling, raise your arms above your head, palms facing in. Lengthen through the spine, but do not arch your back.

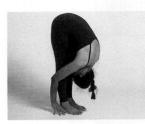

Position 3   Exhaling, bend forward from the hips, keeping your arms extended and your head hanging loosely between them. Keep your legs slightly bent and relax your neck and shoulders.

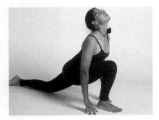

Position 4   Inhaling, bend both knees and place your palms flat on the floor by the outsides of your feet. Extend your left leg back. Stretch your chin toward the ceiling.

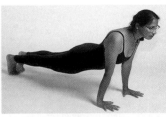

Position 5   Continue while holding the breath if you can—don't strain. Reach your forward leg back next to the other leg. Hold your body straight, supported by your hands and toes, with ankles, hips, and shoulders in a straight plane.

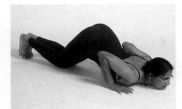

Position 6   Exhaling, lower your knees, chest, and chin or forehead to the floor, keeping your hips up and toes curled under.

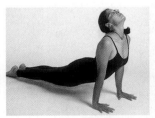

Position 7   Inhaling, bring the tops of your feet to the floor, straighten your legs, and come up to straight arms, opening the chest and stretching your chin toward the ceiling. Be careful not to overarch your lower back.

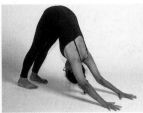

Position 8   Exhaling, curl your toes under and raise your hips into an inverted "V." Push back with your hands and lengthen your spine by reaching your hips upward. Keep your head hanging loosely.

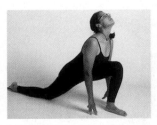

Position 9   Inhaling, lift your head and bring your left leg between your hands, keeping the right leg back. Raise your chin toward the ceiling.

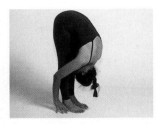

Position 10   Exhaling, bring your left foot forward so your feet are together. Bend forward from the hips, keeping your legs slightly bent and your upper body relaxed. If you can, touch your head to your knees and place your palms beside your feet.

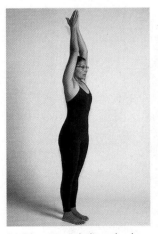

Position 11   Inhaling, slowly straighten up with your arms extended above your head. If you have any lower back pain, be sure to bend your knees.

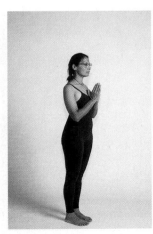

Position 12   Exhaling, bring your hands together in front of you. Close your eyes for a moment and feel the sensations in your body.

■ **Figure 7.9**

The Sun Salute
This Hatha yoga exercise is a series of 12 postures, or asanas, intended to be done in one flowing routine. Each of the 12 postures is held 3 seconds. Many good Sun Salute videos can be viewed online.

Getting into Shape

Undertake a program to increase aerobic conditioning by following these guidelines.

1. *Frequency:* You should exercise three to five times a week.
2. *Intensity:* You should exercise within 60% to 80% of your exercise target heart rate.
3. *Time:* You should exercise within your exercise target heart rate for 20 to 60 minutes each time.
4. *Type of exercise:* Appropriate exercises are rhythmic and continuous and use the large muscles of the legs and hips. Such exercises include walking, jogging, bicycling, swimming, cross-country skiing, and aerobic dancing.
5. *Warm-up and cool-down:* It is optimal to raise the body's core temperature about 1°F to 3°F by doing the warm-up and stretching activities before the aerobic workout. After the aerobic workout, you should slow

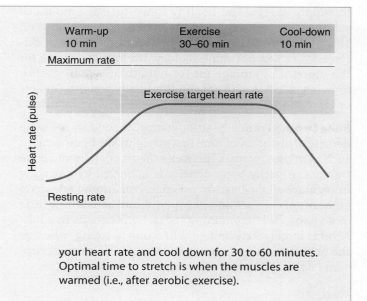

your heart rate and cool down for 30 to 60 minutes. Optimal time to stretch is when the muscles are warmed (i.e., after aerobic exercise).

reduce risk factors for cardiovascular disease, high blood pressure, and diabetes. It also helps reduce symptoms of osteoarthritis.

Besides building strength and flexibility, yoga enhances well-being, mood, attention, mental focus, and stress tolerance. It can lessen sleep problems. Yoga is a beneficial, low-risk, low-cost adjunct to the treatment of stress, anxiety, posttraumatic stress disorder (PTSD), depression, stress-related medical illnesses, substance abuse, and rehabilitation of criminal offenders (Birdee et al., 2017).

T'ai Chi Ch'uan

T'ai chi ch'uan comes from China and is based on a system of martial arts. In practicing t'ai chi, the individual concentrates on moving the joints of the body freely and developing internal energy. The practice of t'ai chi can be an ideal way of improving your health and staying in shape. There are several major styles of t'ai chi (named

after the families that founded them) and great variation within each style. All t'ai chi forms are low impact, improve balance and coordination, increase mobility, and reduce stress.

T'ai chi is best learned from a teacher because it is difficult to learn from a book or video. Some teachers practice the martial aspects of t'ai chi, which can include self-defense applications of movements from the t'ai chi form. You need not become a great fighter to benefit from practicing t'ai chi.

T'ai chi can offer immediate benefits, but it takes many years to become highly skilled. Beware of teachers who say that they have secrets or shortcuts. It is your own diligent practice that will bring you the full benefits of t'ai chi. The teacher is there to show you the way.

Body Composition

Body composition refers to the relative amounts of the body's major constituents, that is, water, protein (called the *fat-free mass*), minerals (including the calcium and phosphate in bones), and essential and storage fat. Two health concerns relating to body composition are body fat percentage and bone density.

Body Fat Percentage The body has two kinds of fat: essential fat to carry out life functions and storage fat

T'ai chi exercises help maintain physical fitness and mind–body harmony.

© kali9/E+/Getty Images

TERMS

body composition: the relative amounts of the body's major components

t'ai chi ch'uan: a Chinese martial arts system of movements that enhances freedom of movement and focus of mind

to supply energy. The healthy range for the amount of storage fat for nonathletic, young adult males is between 10% and 20% of the total body weight. Because of differences in sex hormone biology, the healthy range for the amount of storage fat for nonathletic, young adult females is 15% to 30% of the total body weight. Greater or lesser body fat percentages can be a risk to health.

Bone Density From a health perspective, one wants bone density of about 4% of total body weight; low bone density, such as in osteoporosis, increases the risk of falls and bone fracture. Healthy bone density is achieved by engaging in regular weight-bearing exercise, consuming adequate amounts of calcium and phosphate, and consuming little or no phosphate-containing sodas. Bone density in adulthood is largely determined when one is young, which is the reason young people are encouraged to exercise, consume dairy foods, and not to consume sodas.

Physical Activity Among College Students

According to the American College Health Association (2016a, 2016b), about 60% of North American college students acquire less than the recommended amounts of physical activity. Like many in the general adult population, North American college students carry out most of their daily tasks while sitting—in lectures, at libraries, and studying. Many student jobs involve sitting at desks or standing behind counters (restaurant servers who walk a lot are exceptions). During nonschool/nonwork leisure time, many students watch TV, listen to music, play video games, or involve themselves in social media and the Internet. Travel is often by car.

Most college students know they should be more physically active, but they encounter a variety of barriers to doing so. For example, many students believe that health-promoting physical activity should be vigorous, frequent, and prolonged; they mistakenly imagine that physical activity for health requires lengthy workouts at a gym or running nearly every day—a serious time investment that many cannot realistically make. Moreover, whereas many college students were active in sports while in high school, they find exercise for its own sake to be boring and even unpleasant. Furthermore, if exercise facilities are crowded or otherwise uninviting, or the campus community is perceived as unsafe, students are less likely to go out to exercise. Perceiving these barriers as insurmountable, students give up on putting physical activity in their lives altogether.

So, if you actively participate in sports or are otherwise moving your body around for at least half an hour a day on most days of the week in any way you can, keep doing it. If not, find ways to do so and not necessarily by taking up a sport or exercising vigorously. A "just do it" attitude, buying new exercise clothes and shoes, and going to a gym several times a week (especially at odd hours) are unnecessary and unlikely to be maintained for very long.

It's better to get into the habit of walking for 30 minutes almost every day. Remember, moderate amounts of physical activity are sufficient to promote health and reduce stress. Your goals are to find activities that you enjoy, that you can work into your schedule, and that you can make a regular part of your life.

Integrating Physical Activity in Your Life

Some individuals enjoy movement. Others, however, are not so inclined. In order to gain its health benefits, they must find pleasant (not distasteful) ways to integrate physical activity into their lives. This is especially true for those whose lifestyles are sedentary. Anything they can do to increase their amount of movement each day produces multiple rewards. Indeed, the greatest health gains derive from going from a sedentary to a moderate degree of daily physical activity (Figure 7.4).

Here are some guidelines for incorporating physical activity into your life.

1. *Define specific goals.* Goals can be general or specific. For example, "I want to be in shape" or "I want to lose weight" are general goals. "I want to walk 9,000 steps a day" or "I want to run a mile 4 days a week" are specific goals. Include among your goals that you want to do activities that you enjoy and that you want to make a regular part of your life for the long term. If you are unsure about your exercise goals, then set as a goal to make some more specific goals by experimenting with three kinds of activity to see what each offers.

2. *Research.* Consult books, magazines, the Internet, or teachers, coaches, and health professionals to determine ways to accomplish your goals. Be sure to assess the authoritativeness of the information you acquire; you do not want to undertake an injurious activity or set an unattainable goal and have a failure experience. Because they are not experts, consulting friends may be of limited usefulness.

3. *Make a plan.* Having defined your goals and acquired information on how to accomplish them, make a realistic and feasible plan for putting and maintaining physical activity in your life. Be sure your activity plan fits into your schedule; use a time audit to identify times of the week during which you can exercise. Also, choose activities that are interesting (or likely to be) and enjoyable. That way you are more likely to want to do them. Write down your plan; perhaps discuss it with a coach, teacher, or health professional. Even better, take a class. That way you will learn proper technique, have a built-in schedule, and will have the enjoyment of being with others.

4. *Get a physical checkup.* Consult a health professional if you have been inactive for many months or have concerns about your body's ability to perform at the level you want.

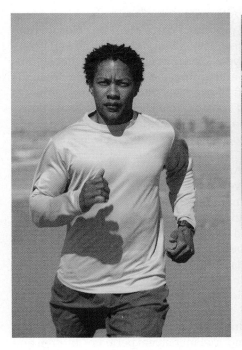
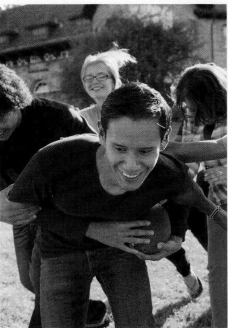
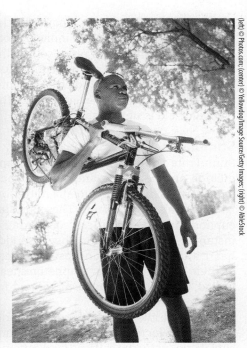

When choosing an exercise, pick one that's fun and convenient for you. (See Workbook, Chapter 7.)

5. *Progress slowly.* Deliberate progress enables you to assess the feasibility of your choices and also to integrate them into your normal life routine. Try not to let your enthusiasm for beginning a new plan stimulate you to take on too much too soon. You don't want to get sore or injure yourself.

6. *Track progress.* Keep a diary of your activity. For each activity day, record the time you spent doing the activity, what you experienced doing the activity, any obstacles that prevented you from carrying out a day's activity, and strategies for overcoming any obstacles.

7. *Evaluate.* Each week, ask yourself if your plan is working to accomplish your goals. If so, continue. If not, identify the obstacles and make course corrections, for example, by changing the choice of activities, the time devoted to them, and perhaps even your goals themselves.

Performance-Enhancing Substances

The saying "Better living through chemistry" aptly describes the intentions of those who use any of a variety of substances, called **ergogenic aids**, to increase strength and endurance, enhance athletic performance, or bulk up or "body sculpt" to feel better about their physical appearance. Performance-enhancing substances include stimulants to increase alertness and "energy" and to "burn fat," muscle enlargers, and endurance enhancers. They come in the form of dietary supplements, herbals, over-the-counter and prescription-only pharmaceuticals, and illegal drugs.

Many people mistakenly assume that because herbs and dietary supplements are marketed as "natural" they are safe. Before taking any kind of herbal or dietary supplement, keep in mind that the U.S. government does not regulate dietary supplements, so consumers cannot be certain that any product conforms to information on the

Walking in Balance

Native Americans have an expression that helps when trying to understand our place in the physical world. The expression "walking in balance" means engaging your body with your mind in the natural world, feeling a sense of connectedness with nature. Walking in balance suggests that we combine the powers of the mind and body to become more aware of ourselves in our environment.

During your next workout try this: While you dress and warm up, remind yourself that you are taking time away from your problems and worries—a mini vacation, if you will, from daily responsibilities. The mission during this exercise period (preferably walking or running) is to see where you are exercising as if you were seeing it for the first time. Notice the trees, the birds, the clouds in the sky, and so on. Try to feel that you are a part of nature by noticing as much about the natural world as you can.

TERMS

ergogenic aids: substances used to increase strength and endurance

product label. For example, frequently the actual amount per serving (dose) is not as indicated on the label. Also, although manufacturers promise to adhere to manufacturing standards, they are not compelled to, so products may contain impurities and other chemicals not listed on the label. If one eats and exercises healthfully, any kind of ergogenic aid is unnecessary.

Stimulants

Stimulants commonly used as performance enhancers include amphetamine and similar chemicals, ephedra (*ma huang*), synephrine (hoodia, bitter orange) and similar chemicals, and caffeine. These substances can induce euphoria, increase alertness, combat fatigue, and, in some instances, reduce appetite. They also increase the risk of heart attack, seizures, and psychotic episodes. Because of their harmful effects, amphetamines are legally controlled, and ephedra has been banned for sale in dietary supplements.

Energy drinks generally contain a variety of substances purported to increase alertness and endurance and to combat fatigue, including caffeine (and caffeine-like substances such as theophylline); the herb guarana, which contains caffeine; taurine; ginseng; ginkgo; creatine; carnitine; glucuronolactone; and lots of sugar. Research has shown that energy drinks can enhance endurance but they are less likely to affect muscle strength and power and neuromuscular performance (Mora-Rodriguez & Paralles, 2014).

Muscle Enlargers

Muscle enlargers include protein and amino acid dietary supplements, androgenic anabolic steroids, and human growth hormone. Although new muscle tissue is made of protein, ingesting protein or certain amino acids will not produce new muscle tissue. Muscles grow in response to work, not food. Anyone consuming a balanced diet obtains sufficient protein and amino acids to meet the demands of nearly any kind of exercise; body builders or athletes who need to build considerable strength are exceptions.

Androgenic anabolic steroids (testosterone and similar substances) are used to build muscle strength in women and men. They are legal only by prescription for medical reasons. Androstenedione ("andro") is a "prohormone" that is converted in the body to testosterone. Prior to 2005, androstenedione and similar substances could be purchased legally as dietary supplements. However, in 2005, the U.S. Food and Drug Administration banned the sale of andro and other testosterone prohormones because they are dangerous. Potential long-term consequences of testosterone use in men include infertility, erection problems, breast development (gynecomastia), heart disease, liver disease, and cancer. In women, steroids can cause male pattern baldness, deepening of the voice, increased facial hair, and abnormal menstrual periods. Children and young adults who use steroids are at risk for early onset of puberty and premature cessation of bone growth.

Human growth hormone (HGH or GH) is manufactured by the pituitary gland and secreted into the bloodstream. Although reputed to enhance athletic performance by increasing energy and/or building muscle mass, scientific evidence of any ergogenic effects is lacking (Baumann, 2012). Despite unscrupulous advertising claims to the contrary, HGH cannot be taken orally because it is broken down in the digestive system.

Caveat Emptor: The Business of Sports Supplements

Everyone has heard of professional, Olympic, and other high-level athletes who have been punished for taking banned—and often illegal—substances (e.g., steroids, hormones, and other drugs). Apparently, in a world where winning is everything, some elite athletes are willing to risk their careers and their health to gain a competitive edge.

Unfortunately, a significant number of high school athletes, college athletes, nonathletes, and people who just want to "look good" also take drugs to gain a competitive edge. Among athletes, the edge might be enhanced athletic performance. Or it may be solidifying one's identity as an athlete or gaining recognition as an athlete among one's peers. Among the "body conscious," the edge is generally sculpting the body to compete socially for friends and sexual and intimate partners.

The dietary supplement industry is masterful at catering to concerns about competing athletically and socially. Advertising of supplements supports a variety of "fitness" magazines and a host of e-commerce "sports supplement" websites that lure potential consumers with information of dubious authority, all with the intention to sell them something. For example, a body building website tells visitors about the ban on testosterone prohormones but not to worry because "we have a number of other products that work just as well." The banner of a "sports nutrition" website shows a cluster of several nearly naked, "buff" college-age men and women, offering a plethora of generally worthless products to enhance performance, increase energy, and lose weight (and look just like the models in the banner). Media depicting muscular, "fit" models influence people to view their own bodies as inferior (Hausenblas et al., 2012).

The dietary supplement industry is estimated at $15 billion a year and is largely unregulated. A federal law in 1994 made it possible for manufacturers of dietary supplements not to adhere to the same testing for safety, efficacy, and purity as required for prescription and over-the-counter medications. With over 50,000 dietary supplements on the market, U.S. government agencies cannot investigate the purity and safety of every batch of a particular supplement, nor can claims made in the advertising of every supplement be evaluated for truthfulness. In the world of dietary supplements, the watchword is *caveat emptor:* Let the buyer beware.

Endurance Enhancers

Endurance enhancers include B vitamins, creatine, and erythropoietin.

Creatine, a natural substance in muscle tissue required for muscle contraction, can be purchased as a nutritional supplement. Some, but not all, studies show that creatine supplementation might enhance short-burst activity, such as weight lifting or sprinting. It is not helpful for endurance activities. In doses commonly in use (3 to 5 grams per day), creatine is apparently not harmful. However, because herbs and other nutritional supplements are unregulated, one cannot be sure of the purity or dose of any such product.

Erythropoietin is a hormone that increases the number of red blood cells, thus increasing the body's ability to carry oxygen to tissues. Erythropoietin is a prescription medication given to people whose bodies cannot produce sufficient blood cells, such as people undergoing cancer treatment. It is used illegally by athletes to increase endurance, especially at high elevations. The drug can be very dangerous, causing heart attacks and strokes.

Sports Injuries

Regardless of type, physical activity and sports participation carry some risk of injury, whether it's working up a blister while walking in new shoes, pulling a leg muscle while cycling, or jamming a finger in a volleyball game. When an injury occurs, one should apply first aid in the form of **RICE** (rest, ice, compression, and elevation; see the Wellness Guide "First Aid for Sports Injuries: RICE"). When an injury heals, one should endeavor to prevent the injury (and others) from occurring again (see the Health Tips box).

About half of injuries in physical activity occur because some part of or the entire body is being exercised beyond its biological limits. Such injuries are referred to as **overuse injuries**. Commonly, overuse injuries affect the skin and muscles, tendons, ligaments, and joints, which are constructed of fibrous bands of protein (**Table 7.5**). These fibers can be torn if they are overworked, as when lifting a heavy weight or running farther or faster than one should, or when forced to perform when fatigued. Damage can also occur by repeated small injuries that lead over time to a more serious problem. The common causes of overuse injuries are excessive exercising, faulty technique, and poor equipment.

> Long ago when men cursed and beat the ground with sticks, it was called witchcraft. Today it's called golf.
> *Will Rogers*

All bodies are not anatomically capable of the same degree of physical exertion, especially the high performance exhibited by marathon runners or triathletes. The architecture of the body, the alignment of the legs, the capacity of the lungs, the size and strength of the bones and muscles, and other anatomical factors set limits on an individual's physical ability. Few people have the biological endowment to perform at championship levels. Physical activity can be much more enjoyable when you respect, accept, and appreciate your body's biological limits.

Don't ask your muscles to do more than they can. Relishing the pain of overexertion—"going for the burn"—is dangerous. Pain is the body's message that something is wrong, not that the exerciser is dedicated and courageous. If you want to increase your performance, progress slowly, following a supervised regimen. Injuries are more likely if equipment such as weights and other kinds of apparatus is used improperly or is in disrepair.

Most people participate in physical activity because they want to have fun, they want to gain a sense of accomplishment by doing something well, and they want to feel physically and psychologically better. While pursuing these goals, no one wants to be hurt. It turns out that maximizing the "have fun, do well, feel good" aspects of physical activity and minimizing the potential for injury go together.

Table 7.5	
Common Overuse Injuries	
Strain	Commonly referred to as "pulled muscles" or "pulled tendons." Caused by overstretching, tearing, or ripping of a muscle and/or its tendon
Tendonitis	Inflammation of a tendon caused by chronic, low-grade strain of a muscle–tendon unit
Bursitis	Inflammation of the lubricating sac that surrounds a joint (bursa) caused by repeated low-grade strain of the joint's supporting tissues
Sprain	Overstretching or tearing of ligaments
Blisters	Fluid-filled swellings on the skin caused by undue friction from the rubbing of skin against shoes, clothing, and equipment

TERMS

androgenic anabolic steroids: synthetic male hormones used to increase muscle size and strength

creatine: a natural substance in skeletal muscle tissue required for muscle contraction, which can also be purchased as a dietary supplement

erythropoietin: a hormone that increases the number of red blood cells, thus increasing the body's ability to carry oxygen to tissues

human growth hormone: a naturally occurring pituitary hormone

overuse injuries: injuries to muscles, tendons, ligaments, and joints resulting from too much exercise

RICE: an acronym for rest, ice, compression, elevation; the first aid measures for sports injuries

Hydration for Sport and Recreational Physical Activity

Are You Hydrated? Take the Pee Test

1	
2	
3	

PROPERLY HYDRATED

If your urine matches the colors 1–3 (above the red line), you are properly hydrated and should continue to consume fluids at the recommended amounts

4	
5	

DEHYDRATED

If your urine matches the colors 4–8 (below the red line), you are dehydrated and at risk for cramping and heat illness!

6	
7	
8	

**YOU NEED TO DRINK
MORE WATER OR SPORTS DRINK**

Healthy Hydration
Females: 55% of body weight (BW)
Males: 60% of body weight (BW)

Dehydration
> 2%–5% BW lost in sweat.

Severe Dehydration
> 6%–10% of BW lost in sweat.

Hydration refers to the amount of water in the body. During physical activity, muscles produce heat. Body water is lost as sweat to maintain body temperature. Because hydration also can affect the amount of body sodium, attention to proper fluid also applies to sodium.

Beware of overhydration. Drink only enough water to restore body weight lost as sweat. Too much water can result in dangerous, even life-threatening, sodium loss.

Hydration Guidelines

When	Quantity	Form
Everyday	1 mL/calorie consumed (2 L = 64 ounces)	Water in food and fluids; let thirst be your guide.
Every 2–4 hours	5–10 mL/kg BW to achieve pale yellow urine	Water, sports drinks (low carb + sodium); salted snacks or small beverages with meals to help with fluid retention. Hyperhydration with water or glycerol increases the need to pee and no performance advantage. Also can lower sodium to dangerously low levels.
During activity	0.4–0.8 L/hr.	Water, sports drinks (maximum of 8% carbs); cold fluid can help in hot environment; flavored fluid encourages consumption.
After activity	1.25–1.5 L fluid for every 1 kg BW lost	Water; sports drinks. Limit alcohol due to its diuretic effects. Caffeine OK if < 180 mg.

Data from American Dietetic Association, Dietitians of Canada, and the American College of Sports Medicine. (2016). Nutrition and athletic performance. *Medicine & Science in Sports and Exercise, 48,* 543–568. Retrieved from http://journals.lww.com/acsm-msse/Fulltext/2016/03000/Nutrition_and _Athletic_Performance.25.aspx.

Physical Activity in Cold and Hot Weather

Your body is designed to maintain its operating temperature at 37°C (about 98°F). Because heat always moves toward cold, your body loses heat in cold environments and absorbs heat in warm environments. Moreover, exercised muscles produce heat, which can elevate body temperature. Sweating is the evaporation of body water to rid the body of excess heat.

Cold Stress

Overexposure to cold, windy/wet weather may lead to an abnormally low body temperature (hypothermia).

Symptoms of hypothermia include shivering, muscle weakness, numbness, drowsiness, and occasionally unconsciousness. In instances of cold stress, get out of the cold environment and seek protection from the wind. Gently remove wet clothes and replace them with dry ones. Rewarm the body by immersion in warm (105–110°F; 41–43°C) water and wrapping in warm blankets. Do not consume alcohol "to warm up" because alcohol dilates arteries and causes heat loss. Seek medical attention as soon as possible.

Frostbite is the freezing of tissues with the formation of ice crystals in the fluid around cells and blood vessels.

First Aid for Sports Injuries: RICE

Most sports injuries involve the release of fluids and other substances from damaged tissues. Immediate treatment of a sports injury, therefore, requires limiting any swelling and internal bleeding by administering RICE—rest, ice, compression, and elevation.

Rest: Resting and possibly immobilizing an injured region prevent additional tissue damage and limit internal bleeding.

Ice: Cool an injured region immediately with crushed ice or ice cubes wrapped in a towel (to avoid frostbite), a cold pack, or a bag of frozen peas or corn. The cold reduces swelling, internal bleeding, and pain. Cool for 30 minutes. Allow the region to warm for 15 minutes, and then cool again.

Compression: Wrap the injured region with an elastic bandage to control swelling. Be careful not to wrap so tight as to turn the skin pale or cause lack of sensation.

Elevation: Raise the injured region to limit swelling and internal bleeding.

Frostbitten skin may become white or grayish-yellow. The onset of frostbite is usually painful, but pain generally diminishes and the region becomes cold and numb. Gently rewarm a frostbitten region and seek medical attention as soon as possible.

To prevent cold stress during exercise follow these recommendations:

- Dress appropriately for cold weather. Wear no more than three layers of clothing; be sure all layers can be opened if necessary to cool the body overwarmed by vigorous exercise.
- Wear mittens rather than gloves to allow the fingers to insulate each other.
- Wear appropriate thermal head covering.
- Keep the feet warm and dry.
- Be prepared to change into warm, dry clothes quickly.

Heat Stress

Heat stress results from the loss of considerable body water and minerals from sweating, from dehydration, and the unavailability of sufficient body water to cool the body through sweating. Types of heat stress include the following:

Heat cramps: painful, constant contraction of one or more muscles. Stop activity, replace water and minerals by drinking water or dilute fruit juice; massage and stretch the cramping muscle(s); and rest and cool the body before returning to activity.

Heat exhaustion: weakness, nausea, dizziness. Stop activity; lie down and elevate the legs 12 to 18 inches; replace water and minerals by drinking water or dilute fruit juice; and cool the body with wet cloths and by going to a cool room. Rest for several days before returning to activity. Consult a physician.

Heat stroke: high body temperature (105°F/41°C), disorientation, alteration in normal mental status, unconsciousness. Stop activity, remove clothes, and cool the body with cold water or ice packs. Replace water and minerals by drinking water or dilute fruit juice. Seek medical attention immediately.

To prevent heat stress during exercise follow these recommendations:

- Acclimate to exercising in hot, humid environments by gradually increasing the level of physical activity over the span of several days.
- Be wary of overexertion in hot/humid conditions. Heat stress may occur rapidly.
- Drink lots of fluid (water, dilute fruit juice, or sports drinks) before activity and regularly during extended activity. Do not rely on thirst to signal fluid loss or high body temperature.
- Wear light-fitting, light-colored clothing made of breathable fabric and a light-colored cap and sunscreen to limit sun exposure.
- Exercise during the coolest times of the day (morning and evening) and in the shade.

Preventing Sports Injuries

- Strengthen muscles.
- Be physically fit and improve endurance.
- Don't overwork the body.
- Improve body flexibility with stretching exercises before and after activity.
- Be aware of how the body is functioning.
- Be aware of hazards in the environment; use facilities designed for sports activity.
- Use state-of-the-art equipment, particularly athletic shoes, and protective gear.
- Participate only when weather conditions are safe.
- Improve running or playing form; get expert coaching.
- Rehabilitate injuries adequately before returning to activity.

Critical Thinking About Health

1. Another Christmas day at Grandma's. Well, almost. After everyone had eaten all they possibly could and all the children had ripped open their Christmas gifts, Suzanne's Uncle Ron sat next to her on the couch.

   "I understand that you're taking a health class at school," he said.

   "That's right," Suzanne replied.

   "Then tell me," Uncle Ron continued, "what's the best exercise? My New Year's resolution is to get back in shape, and I want to do it right this time. I'm joining the gym on January 2. What workouts do you recommend?"

   a. What advice should Suzanne give her uncle? Take into account that Uncle Ron has tried working out before, apparently without success. Uncle Ron is a 39-year-old telecommunications engineer who works long hours at a computer terminal when he's at his office. His job also requires him to travel, so he eats a lot of fast food. He is married and has three young children.

2. What are the effects on society and on organized sports of athletes using performance-enhancing drugs, even when such substances are legal?

3. How far? How fast? How much? How might questions such as these affect a person's attitude and approach to physical activity for health (i.e., not competition)? List a new set of questions that illustrate a noncompetitive perspective on physical activity for health.

Chapter Summary and Highlights

Chapter Summary

Many people enjoy exercising and participate in some form of regular exercise. Many more do not and live sedentary lives with little body movement other than getting off the couch and into bed. As the famous comedian W. C. Fields quipped, "Every time I think about exercise I lie down until the thought passes." To entice people to exercise more, a vast exercise/sports industry has created exercise machines of all kinds, 24-hour gyms, spas, competitions, and classes in exercise dance (zumba), yoga, t'ai chi, Pilates, and many others.

For many people, life has become so busy that there simply is no time to even think about exercising. If you are among those without time to exercise, you need to rethink your priorities. Taking an extra 30 to 60 minutes a day to walk instead of drive can constitute a major step (pun intended) toward better health. All exercise involves sustained movement to increase flexibility, strength, and endurance. The most important aspect of making the decision to exercise is commitment. Just as you devote effort to accomplishing other goals, like graduating from college, you need to make the same kind of strong commitment to move your body.

Modern society puts many obstacles in the path of daily movement activity. Work at a job; schoolwork; and time spent on social media, playing video games, watching movies, and texting friends are many ways we can use time every day—time that could be used for movement. Begin now to figure out a way to exercise. Begin with small steps, perhaps a 20-minute walk or jog around the neighborhood. Walk your dog. Go to the nearest park and do the exercises you learned in gym a long time ago. Exercise restores awareness, improves concentration, and makes you more self-assured in social interactions. Start slowly. Pay attention to your body. Loosen up before vigorous exercise. Remember to slow down and cool down when you are finished. Here we go! Enjoy.

Highlights

- Many people live sedentary lives because machines carry out most of the physical labor of living. Sedentariness is associated with a variety of risks to health, which is the reason governments and social institutions are seeking ways to help individuals increase the amount of physical activity in their lives.
- Physical activity is any kind of movement, including doing household tasks, work-related movement, leisure-time activities, and performance-based activities.
- Physical activity is measured as calories of energy expended per minute, metabolic equivalents (METs), and physical activity level (PAL).
- Moderate, rather than vigorous, amounts of physical activity are sufficient for health. Experts recommend walking briskly for 30 minutes on most days of the week.
- Physical activity has six components: motivation, cardiorespiratory fitness, body strength, endurance, flexibility, and body composition.
- Guidelines for integrating physical activity into life involve goal setting, developing and carrying out a plan, and tracking and evaluating progress.
- Performance-enhancing substances include stimulants (e.g., amphetamines, caffeine), muscle enlargers (e.g., androgenic anabolic steroids), and endurance enhancers (e.g., creatine).
- The most common cause of sports injury is exercising a body part or the entire body beyond its biological limit to the point of injury. Common injuries include strain, tendonitis, bursitis, sprain, and blisters.
- Exercising in hot or cold weather requires taking special precautions to prevent injury and illness.

For Your Health

Movement is necessary for health and well-being, yet modern life is highly sedentary. Put more movement into your life by doing Exercise 7.1 (in the Workbook, Chapter 7), "Putting Exercise into My Life." The other exercises offer additional options for movement activities.

References

American College Health Association. (2016a). *American College Health Association-National College Health Assessment II: Canadian Reference Group Data Report Spring 2016.* Hanover, MD: American College Health Association.

American College Health Association. (2016b). *American College Health Association-National College Health Assessment II: Undergraduate Student Reference Group Data Report Spring 2016.* Hanover, MD: American College Health Association.

Baumann, G. P. (2012). Growth hormone doping in sports: A critical review of use and detection strategies. *Endocrinological Reviews, 33,* 155–186.

Birdee, G. S., et al. (2017). Cross-sectional analysis of health-related quality of life and elements of yoga practice. *BMC Complementary and Alternative Medicine, 17,* 80. doi: 10.1186/s12906-017-1599-1

Booth, F. W., Chakravarthy, M. V., & Spangenburg, E. E. (2002). Exercise and gene expression: Physiological regulation of the human genome through physical activity. *Journal of Physiology, 543,* 399–411.

Bouchard, C., et al. (2015). Less sitting, more physical activity, or higher fitness? *Mayo Clinic Proceedings, 90,* 1533–1540.

Bravata, D. M., et al. (2007). Using pedometers to increase physical activity and improve health. *Journal of the American Medical Association, 298,* 2296–2304.

Centers for Disease Control and Prevention. (2017). Benefits of physical activity. Retrieved from https://www.cdc.gov/physicalactivity/basics/pa-health/index.htm

Chu, A. H. Y., et al. (2014). Do workplace physical activity interventions improve mental health outcomes? *Occupational Medicine, 64,* 235–245.

Cramer, H., et al. (2016). Prevalence, patterns, and predictors of yoga use: Results of a U.S. nationally representative survey. *American Journal of Preventive Medicine, 50,* 230–235.

DeFina, L. F., et al. (2015). Physical activity versus cardiorespiratory fitness: Two (partly) distinct components of cardiovascular health? *Progress in Cardiovascular Disease, 57,* 324–329.

Ekelund, U., et al. (2016). Does physical activity attenuate, or even eliminate the detrimental association of sitting time with mortality? *Lancet, 388,* 1302–1310.

Hausenblas, H. A., et al. (2012). Media effects of experimental presentation of the ideal physique on eating disorder symptoms: A meta-analysis of laboratory studies. *Clinical Psychology Reviews, 33,* 168–81.

Kelly, P., et al. (2014). Systematic review and meta-analysis of reduction in all-cause mortality from walking and cycling and shape of dose response relationship. *International Journal of Behavioral Nutrition and Physical Activity, 11,* 132. doi: 10.1186/s12966-014-0132-x

Matthews, C. E., et al. (2012). Amount of time spent in sedentary behaviors and cause-specific mortality in U.S. adults. *American Journal of Clinical Nutrition, 95,* 437–445.

Mora-Rodrigues, R., & Pallarés, J. G. (2015). Performance outcomes and unwanted side effects associated with energy drinks. *Nutrition Reviews, 72,* 108–120.

Patel, M. S., et al. (2016). Framing financial incentives to increase physical activity among overweight and obese adults. *Annals of Internal Medicine, 164,* 385–394.

Portugal, E. M. M., et al. (2013). Neuroscience of exercise: From neurobiology mechanisms to mental health. *Neuropsychobiology, 68,* 1–14.

Sale, A., et al. (2014). Environment and brain plasticity: towards an endogenous pharmacotherapy. *Physiological Reviews, 94,* 189–234.

Simon, H. B. (2015). Exercise and Health. *American Journal of Medicine, 128,* 1171–1177.

Tremblay, M. S., et al. (2017). Sedentary Behavior Research Network (SBRN)—Terminology Consensus Project process and outcome. *International Journal of Behavioral Nutrition and Physical Activity, 14,* 75. Retrieved from https://ijbnpa.biomedcentral.com/articles/10.1186/s12966-017-0525-8

Suggested Readings

Anderson, B. (2015). *Stretching.* New York: Shelter Publications. Easy-to-follow exercises and drawings.

Benaugh, B. (2006). *Yoga for stress relief.* Yoga-instructor Barbara Benaugh teams with the Dalai Lama on this DVD that teaches how to practice this ancient mind–body method for modern stresses.

Blake, H., & Hawley, H. (2012). Effects of t'ai chi exercise on physical and psychological health of older people. *Current Aging Science, 5,* 19–27. Discusses recent research on the many health benefits of t'ai chi exercise.

PilatesInsight.com. Retrieved from http://www.pilatesinsight.com/. All about Pilates.

Recommended

American Dietetic Association, Dietitians of Canada, and the American College of Sports Medicine. (2016). Nutrition and athletic performance. *Medicine & Science in Sports and Exercise*, 48, 543–568. Retrieved from http://journals.lww.com/acsm-msse/Fulltext/2016/03000/Nutrition_and_Athletic_Performance.25.aspx. Provides guidelines for the appropriate type, amount, and timing of intake of food, fluids, and supplements to promote optimal health and performance across different scenarios of training and competitive sport.

American Heart Association. (2017). Walking. Take the first step. Retrieved from http://www.heart.org/HEARTORG/HealthyLiving/PhysicalActivity/Walking/Walking_UCM_460870_SubHomePage.jsp. All about incorporating walking into your life for health and wellness.

American Society of Sports Medicine. (2016). Exercise as medicine. Retrieved from http://www.exerciseismedicine.org/assets/page_documents/EIM%20Fact%20Sheet%20February%202016.pdf. Describes how exercise and physical activity are integral to the prevention and treatment of chronic disease and should be regularly assessed as part of medical care when including exercise in treatment plans for patients.

Centers for Disease Control and Prevention. (2017). Physical activity. Retrieved from https://www.cdc.gov/physicalactivity/index.html. Thorough resource covering physical activity basics, data and statistics, resources and publications, and worksite and community efforts to promote physical activity.

Katz, P. P., & Pate, R. (2016). Exercise as medicine. *Annals of Internal Medicine*, 165, 880–881. Discusses the advantages of making exercise a regular part of every healthcare encounter.

Ladabaum, U., et al. (2014). Obesity, abdominal obesity, physical activity, and caloric intake in U.S. Adults: 1988–2010. *American Journal of Medicine*, 127, 717–727.

Mora-Rodrigues, R., & Pallarés, J. G. (2015). Performance outcomes and unwanted side effects associated with energy drinks. *Nutrition Reviews*, 72, 108–120. Analyzes the effects of energy drink ingredients on prolonged submaximal (endurance) exercise, short-term strength and power (neuromuscular performance), and the effects of energy drink ingredients on the fluid and electrolyte deficit during prolonged exercise.

Simon, H. B. (2015). Exercise and health: Dose and response, considering both ends of the curve. *American Journal of Internal Medicine*, 128, 1171–1177. Reviews research on the effects of moderate and vigorous exercise on health.

World Health Organization. (2017). Physical activity. Retrieved from http://www.who.int/topics/physical_activity/en/. Data, statistics, and fact sheets on physical activity and its relation to global health. Physical inactivity has been identified as the fourth-leading risk factor for global mortality, causing an estimated 3.2 million deaths globally.

Zhu, W. (2017). *Sedentary behavior and health: Concepts, assessments, and interventions*. Urbana, IL: Human Kinetics. Presents evidence on sedentary behavior, its apparent health risks, and suggestions on measuring and altering this behavior.

Recommended Websites

American Society for Sports Medicine
Information on exercise and exercise equipment.

National Center for Chronic Disease Prevention and Health Promotion
Information and education about making physical activity a part of your life.

Method Alliance (PMA)
Information about the Pilates method and its creator.

The President's Council on Physical Fitness and Sports
Information on exercise.

U.S. Department of Health and Human Services, Physical Activity Guidelines for Americans
Describes the types and amounts of physical activity that offer substantial health benefits to Americans.

PART THREE

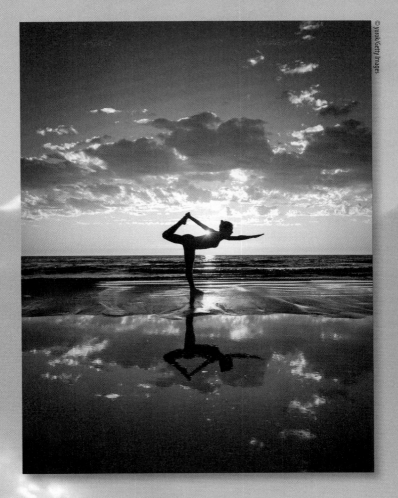

© yurok/Getty Images

Building Healthy Relationships

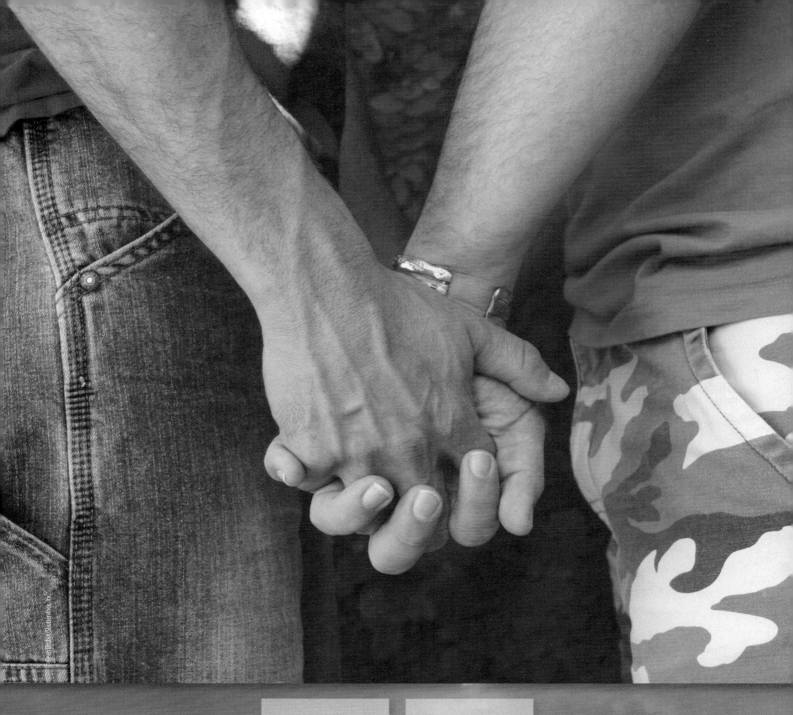

**Health
Tips**

*Alcohol: The Risky Social/
Sexual Lubricant*

*Tips for Enhancing
Sexual Experience*

*Be Good at Sexual
Communication*

**Wellness
Guide**

Attend to Your Sexual Health

*Gay (Same-Sex) Marriage:
Social and Health Issues*

CHAPTER 8

Healthy Sexuality and Intimate Relationships

Learning Objectives

1. List and define the major dimensions of human sexuality: physical, psychological, orientation, behavioral, and relationship.

2. Describe female and male sexual anatomy.

3. Describe the menstrual cycle and name three common menstrual difficulties.

4. Define *sexual orientation*.

5. List and describe the phases of the sexual response cycle.

6. Describe common sexual difficulties.

7. Describe the stages of development in intimate relationships.

8. Identify and describe the essential components of good communication.

> Love is a great exaggeration of the worth of one individual over the worth of everybody else.
>
> *George Bernard Shaw*

Sexuality represents a truly holistic aspect of living, for it involves the simultaneous expression of mind, body, and spirit—the whole self.

The World Health Organization (2015) defines healthy sexuality as

a state of physical, emotional, mental, and social well-being in relation to sexuality; it is not merely the absence of disease, dysfunction, or infirmity. Sexual health requires a positive and respectful approach to sexuality and sexual relationships, as well as the possibility of having pleasurable and safe sexual experiences, free of coercion, discrimination, and violence. For sexual health to be attained and maintained, the sexual rights of all persons must be respected, protected, and fulfilled.

To that definition we can add that healthy sexuality includes the following:

1. Accepting sex and sexuality as natural aspects of being human throughout the life span.
2. Knowing and understanding biological sexual functions and responses.
3. Possessing skills for maintaining and enhancing sexual relationships.
4. Assessing one's own sexuality education and becoming the sex educator of one's own children.
5. Having confidence in one's own values and capacity for making wise sexual decisions.
6. Knowing and accepting sexual values and practices different from one's own.
7. Increasing one's capacity for intimate relationships and communication.

Although sexuality is commonly represented in advertising and other media as having to do solely with physical gratification and social status, most people are aware that sexuality involves much more than the stimulation of the body's sex organs. Sexuality has several dimensions, including the following:

1. *The physical dimension:* those parts of the body that define a person as a female or male, contribute to sexual experiences, and are involved in reproduction
2. *The psychological dimension:* values, beliefs, attitudes, and emotions that influence a person's sexual thoughts and behaviors
3. *The orientation dimension:* the tendency to feel attracted to, and the desire to emotionally bond with, a member of the same or other sex
4. *The behavioral dimension:* physical and social activities intended to meet one's sexual wants and needs
5. *The relationship dimension:* aspects of sexuality that interface and integrate with intimate relationships

From the standpoint of personal health, sexuality is an area over which you have considerable individual control. You choose when and with whom you wish to have sex, and which feelings you wish to express in sexual ways. With some fundamental knowledge of sexual biology, you can conduct your sexual life responsibly, thus avoiding unnecessary illness and exercising a choice of whether and when to have children.

Sexuality: The Physical Dimension

One of the fundamental functions of sexuality is biological reproduction. Males produce reproductively capable sperm and deposit them in the female reproductive tract

---

Attend to Your Sexual Health

Women: Regular Gynecological Exams

The gynecological exam is a medical examination of a woman's reproductive system—the internal and external pelvic organs and the breasts. The internal exam (called a pelvic exam) includes examination of the vagina and cervix, the bladder, the ovaries, and the fallopian tubes for any abnormalty in size and shape. A urine test, a blood test for iron deficiency, a test for sexually transmitted diseases (STDs), and a Papanicolaou (Pap) test can also be part of the gynecological exam. The Pap test (or Pap smear) is a screening test for cancer of the cervix. A few cells are taken from the cervix and observed for abnormalities. The Pap test does not screen for sexually transmitted diseases. STD tests must be requested.

Women who are or have been sexually active, or have reached age 18, should have physical exams annually.

Men: Testicular Self-Examination

Because testicular cancer is the most common cancer in men aged 15 to 35 years, young men are encouraged to check their testes about once a month for the appearance of any abnormal lumps or swellings—possible signs of testicular cancer. Men who examine themselves regularly become familiar with the way their testicles normally feel.

Testicular self-examination should be performed after a warm bath or shower. The heat relaxes the scrotum, making it easier to find anything unusual.

1. Stand in front of the mirror. Look for any swelling on the skin of the scrotum.
2. Examine each testicle with both hands. The index and middle fingers should be placed under the testicle while the thumbs are placed on the top. Gently roll the testicle between the thumbs and fingers. It's normal for one testicle to be larger than the other.
3. Find the epididymis (the soft, tubelike structure at the back of the testicle that collects and carries the sperm). Do not mistake the epididymis for an abnormal lump.

If you find a lump, contact your doctor right away. Testicular cancer is highly curable, especially when treated promptly.

during sexual intercourse. Females provide reproductively capable eggs, called **ova**, and a safe, nutrient-filled environment in which the fetus develops for the nine months of pregnancy.

Male and female sexual biology is genetically determined at conception by the presence of X and/or Y chromosomes. The fusion of an X-bearing egg with the X-bearing sperm produces a female (XX); fusion with the Y-bearing sperm produces a male (XY). Once the chromosome pattern is set, the development of the sexual anatomy follows from the precise instructions of the genes contained in the chromosomes. A particular chromosome set determines whether the as yet immature sex cells that appear at about the fifth week of development will eventually produce sperm or ova. The sex chromosomes determine whether the fetus will ultimately develop the male sex organs—testes, sperm ducts, semen-producing glands, and penis—or the female organs—ovaries, fallopian tubes, uterus, vagina, and external female genitals.

The genetic determination of sexual biology also specifies the pattern of male or female steroid hormone production, which in turn affects the **secondary sex characteristics** that distinguish males and females: the extent and distribution of facial and body hair; body build and stature; and appearance of breasts (**Figure 8.1**) and some behavioral tendencies.

Female Sexual Anatomy

A woman's internal sexual organs consist of two **ovaries**, which lie on either side of the abdominal cavity, the **fallopian tubes**, the **uterus**, and the **vagina**; together these structures make up a specialized tube that goes from each ovary to the outside of the body (**Figure 8.2**). The function of the ovaries, which are about the size and

▌TERMS▐

fallopian tubes: the usual site of fertilization; a pair of tubelike structures that transport ova from the ovaries to the uterus

ova: female eggs (singular, *ovum*)

ovaries: a pair of almond-shaped organs in the female abdomen that produce egg cells (ova) and female sex hormones

secondary sex characteristics: anatomical features appearing at puberty that distinguish males from females

uterus: the female organ in which a fetus develops

vagina: a woman's organ of copulation and the exit pathway for the fetus at birth

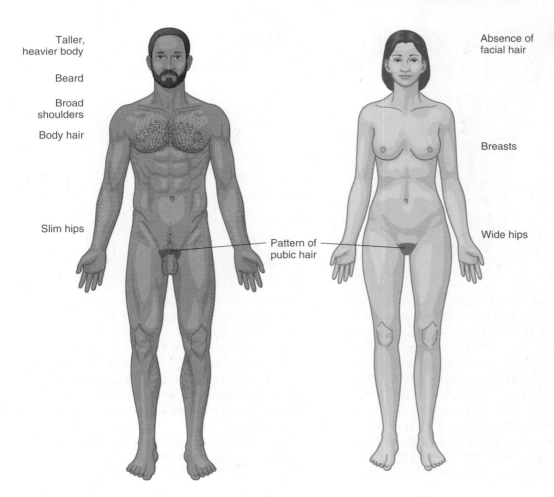

■ **Figure 8.1**

Secondary Sexual Characteristics of Men and Women

Taller, heavier body

Beard

Broad shoulders

Body hair

Slim hips

Pattern of pubic hair

Absence of facial hair

Breasts

Wide hips

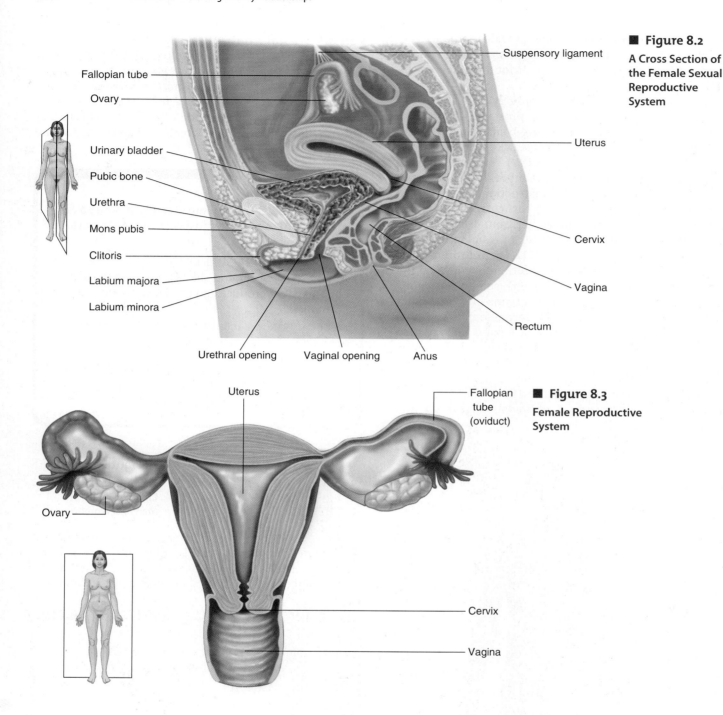

A Cross Section of the Female Sexual Reproductive System

Suspensory ligament

Fallopian tube

Ovary

Uterus

Urinary bladder

Pubic bone

Urethra

Cervix

Mons pubis

Clitoris

Labium majora

Vagina

Labium minora

Rectum

Urethral opening   Vaginal opening   Anus

Uterus

Fallopian tube (oviduct)

■ **Figure 8.3**

Female Reproductive System

Ovary

Cervix

Vagina

shape of almonds, is to produce fertilizable ova as well as sex hormones, which control the development of the female body type, maintain normal female sexual physiology, and help regulate the course of pregnancy. The fallopian tubes gather and transport the ova that are released from the ovaries (about one each month). The two fallopian tubes connect to the uterus, an organ about the size of a woman's fist, which is situated just behind the pelvic bone and the bladder (**Figure 8.3**). The uterus is part of the passageway for sperm as they move from the vagina to the fallopian tubes to effect fertilization; after fertilization, it provides the environment in which

the fetus grows. It is the inner lining of the uterus that is shed each month in menstruation.

The lower part of the uterus is the **cervix**, and the cavity of the uterus is connected to the vagina by means of a small opening called the *cervical os*. The cervix secretes mucus, which changes in consistency depending on the phase of the menstrual cycle. Some women learn to estimate the time of **ovulation** (ovum release) by examining their cervical mucus.

The vagina is a hollow tube that leads from the cervix to the outside of the body. The sexually nonaroused vagina is approximately 3 to 5 inches long. Normally,

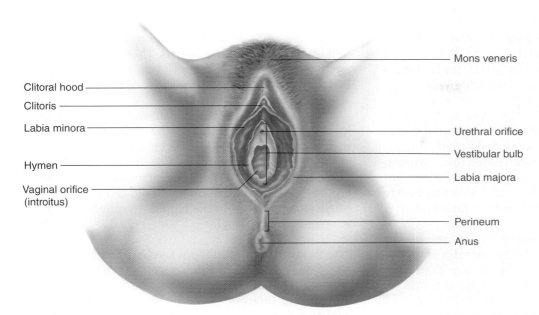

Mons veneris

Clitoral hood

Clitoris

Labia minora

Hymen

Vaginal orifice (introitus)

Urethral orifice

Vestibular bulb

Labia majora

Perineum

Anus

the vaginal tube is rather narrow, but it can readily widen to accommodate the penis during intercourse, a tampon during menstruation, the passage of a baby during childbirth, or a pelvic examination. The vagina possesses a unique physiology that is maintained by the secretions that continually emanate from the vaginal walls. These secretions help regulate the growth of microorganisms that normally inhabit the vagina, and they also help to cleanse the vagina. Because the vagina is a self-cleansing organ, it is usually unnecessary to employ any extraordinary cleansing measures, such as douching. Very often douching merely upsets the natural chemical balance of the vagina and increases the risk of developing vaginal inflammation, called **vulvovaginitis** or *vaginitis*. Symptoms of vulvovaginitis include irritation or itching, redness or swelling of the vagina and vulva, unusual discharge, discomfort or a burning sensation when urinating, and, sometimes, a disagreeable odor.

Vulvovaginitis is commonly referred to as a "yeast infection." Whereas yeast (typically *Candida albicans*) can cause vulvovaginitis, other microorganisms, such as the protozoan *Trichomonas vaginalis,* bacteria, and viruses, also cause it. Even irritation from vaginal sprays, spermicidal products, and other chemicals can produce symptoms of vulvovaginitis. Anyone with symptoms of vulvovaginitis should see a health practitioner to obtain an accurate diagnosis and treatment.

A number of factors increase susceptibility to vulvovaginitis, including the use of antibiotics, emotional stress, a diet high in carbohydrates, hormonal changes caused by pregnancy or birth control pills, chemical irritants, intercourse without adequate lubrication, and heat and moisture retained by nylon underwear and pantyhose.

The **vulva** encompasses all female external genital structures—pubic hair, the folds of skin, the **clitoris**, and

the urinary and vaginal openings (**Figure 8.4**). The smaller, inner pair of folds are called the **labia minora**, and the larger, outer pair are called the **labia majora**. The clitoris, a highly sensitive sexual organ, is situated above the vaginal opening.

The opening of the **urethra**, which is the exit tube for urine, is located at the vaginal region just below the clitoris. The fact that the urethra is only about one-half inch long and located close to the vagina makes it susceptible to irritation and infection, called **urethritis**, often characterized by a burning sensation during urination, the frequent urge to urinate, and sometimes a red-orangish hue due to blood in the urine. Occasionally, bacteria introduced into the urethra migrate the short distance to the bladder and produce a bladder infection called **cystitis**.

TERMS

cervix: the lower, narrow end of the uterus

clitoris: erotically sensitive organ located above the vaginal opening

cystitis: inflammation of the bladder

labia majora: a pair of fleshy folds that cover the labia minora

labia minora: a pair of fleshy folds that cover the vagina

ovulation: release of an egg (ovum) from the ovary

urethra: a tube that carries urine from the bladder to the outside

urethritis: an irritation or infection of the urethra caused by bacteria

vulva: the female external genital structures

vulvovaginitis: inflammation of the vaginal region

The symptoms of cystitis are similar to those of urethritis. The occurrence of urethritis or cystitis is often referred to as a **urinary tract infection**, or **UTI**.

The most frequent causes of a UTI are irritation from sexual intercourse and the introduction of bacteria (principally, *Escherichia coli*) from the anal region into the vaginal region and into the urethra. To prevent UTIs, care should be taken not to introduce anal bacteria into the vaginal region during sexual activity (manually or with the penis). It is recommended that a woman urinate immediately after having sex, wear absorbent cotton underpants or underpants with a cotton crotch, and wipe the urethra in the front-to-back direction after urinating.

The risk of urethritis or cystitis can be lessened by drinking a lot of fluids to wash the bacteria from the urinary tract and by drinking cranberry juice to prevent bacteria from clinging to the cells lining the urinary tract. If a UTI occurs, it is advisable not to drink alcohol or ingest caffeine or spices, for these substances may irritate an already inflamed urinary tract. Also, avoid vaginal sprays and douches. If pain is severe or if there is blood in the urine, consult a physician. UTIs can be successfully treated with medications.

The **breasts** consist of a network of milk glands and milk ducts embedded in fatty tissue and are affected by pregnancy, nursing, or birth control pills, as well as the different phases of the menstrual cycle. The variation in breast size among women is due to differing amounts of fatty tissue within the breasts. There is little variation among women in the amount of milk-producing tissue; thus, a woman's ability to breastfeed is unrelated to the size of her breasts.

The breasts are supplied with numerous nerve endings, which are important in the delivery of milk to a nursing baby. These nerves also make the breast highly sensitive to touch, and many women find certain forms of tactile stimulation to be sexually pleasurable. Sexual arousal, tactile stimulation, and cold temperatures can cause small muscles in the nipples to contract, resulting in erection of the nipples.

The Fertility or Menstrual Cycle

About once a month, a woman usually produces a single ovum that can be fertilized. These periods of ovum production are referred to as the woman's **fertility cycle** (**Figure 8.5**). During the fertility cycle, a woman's body undergoes several hormonally induced changes to prepare her body for pregnancy. One of these changes is the thickening of the lining of the uterus, the **endometrium**, to support the first stages of pregnancy. In addition, special blood vessels in the uterus increase in size. Their role is to bring maternal nutrients to the embryo and, later in pregnancy, to the fetus. If conception does not

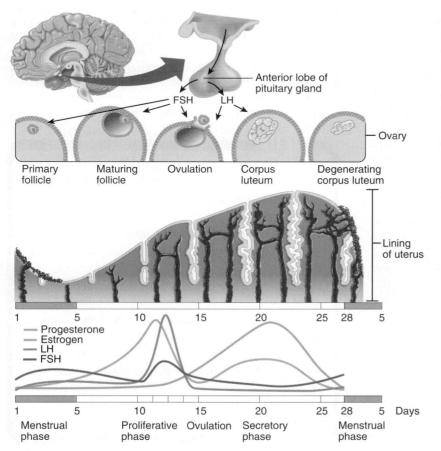

■ **Figure 8.5**

The Menstrual Cycle

Menstrual phase (days 1–5): The beginning of a cycle is marked by the first day of menstrual bleeding. Proliferative phase (days 6–14): Hormones from the hypothalamus trigger the release of follicle-stimulating hormone (FSH) from the pituitary gland, which circulates through the blood to the ovaries and stimulates the production of estrogen and the maturation of an egg. Estrogen stimulates the proliferation of the lining of the uterus and uterine blood vessels. Ovulation phase (days 14–15): The egg is released from the ovary. Secretory phase (days 16–25): Hormones from the hypothalamus trigger the release of luteinizing hormone (LH) from the pituitary gland, which circulates through the blood to the ovaries and stimulates the production of progesterone from a structure called the corpus luteum. Progesterone stimulates the development of nutrient-producing glands in the lining of the uterus. Next menstrual phase: If pregnancy does not occur, hormone levels drop, the uterine lining breaks down, and menstruation ensues.

occur, the endometrium and the special blood vessels are sloughed off and leave the body via the vagina. This is **menstruation**. Between 15 and 45 milliliters (about 2 to 3 teaspoons) of material are discharged over the span of 3 to 6 days. The length of time from one menstruation to another is the **menstrual cycle**.

The length and regularity of the menstrual cycle vary from woman to woman. Most women experience cycles of approximately 28 days, with cycle lengths between 24 and 35 days being the most common. Shorter and longer cycles are possible. Irregular cycles, in which the number of days between menstruations varies from cycle to cycle, can occur. Irregular cycles are common when females first begin to menstruate and also when they stop producing ova later in life.

The menstrual cycle is controlled by a number of hormones. Hormones from the hypothalamus in the brain influence the release of two hormones from the pituitary gland, **follicle-stimulating hormone** (FSH) and **luteinizing hormone** (LH). These hormones circulate throughout the woman's bloodstream and induce the secretion of estrogen and progesterone from the ovaries, which help prepare a woman's body for pregnancy. If fertilization does not occur, the hormonal support of the endometrium stops, and the uterine tissue is lost in a menstrual discharge.

For some women, menstruation may be accompanied by unpleasant symptoms. For example, it is estimated that half of women experience abdominal pain, commonly referred to as "cramps" and medically referred to as **dysmenorrhea**, usually during the first day or so of menstruation. Although psychological, anatomical, and hormonal factors can contribute to menstrual cramps, in most cases they occur because naturally occurring substances called prostaglandins induce strong contractions of the uterine muscle tissue. The prostaglandins are formed when the uterine lining breaks down; they likely function to promote removal of menstrual tissue from the body. In some instances dysmenorrhea is the result of medical problems such as endometriosis, pelvic inflammatory disease (PID), uterine fibroids, and tumors in the pelvic cavity.

In many instances, the severity of cramps is lessened or eliminated by taking nonsteroidal anti-inflammatory drugs (e.g., ibuprofen) or if no ovum is released, which is why women who take combination oral contraceptives ("the pill") often experience relief of cramps. Other ways to lessen menstrual cramps include having a flexible body, practicing meditation or other mental relaxation exercises, or taking medications that reduce levels of prostaglandins.

Another menstrual difficulty is changes in feelings and disposition as the time of menstruation approaches and during the first day or two of menstrual flow. As many as 70% of women report having these or other premenstrual symptoms at some time in their lives. These symptoms may include headache, backache, fatigue, feeling bloated, breast tenderness, depression, irritability, unusual aggressive feelings, and social withdrawal. With the onset of menstruation, the symptoms virtually vanish. In about 5% of women, premenstrual symptoms are severe enough to cause **premenstrual dysphoric disorder (PMDD)**, which is characterized by a combination of marked mood swings, depression, irritability, and anxiety.

Relief from premenstrual symptoms can be achieved by reducing the intake of caffeine, sugar, and salt around the time of menstruation, increasing exercise, increasing the intake of vitamin B_6 (50–100 mg), having an adequate intake of calcium (1,200 mg a day), and taking certain medications (U.S. National Library of Medicine, 2013).

Another common menstrual difficulty is **amenorrhea**, defined as the interruption or cessation of regular menstrual periods. The most common reason periods stop is pregnancy, but the list of factors that can interfere with regular menstruation is quite long. Some factors are psychological stress, depression, marital or sexual problems, fatigue, ingestion of opiate drugs, medications for depression, anxiety, hormonal imbalances, nutritional abnormalities such as severe calorie-restriction diets, anorexia nervosa, and extreme physical activity.

Menopause

Menarche is the first menstruation a young woman experiences. The average age for menarche is between 12 and 13 years, although it can occur as early as 10 years or as late as 19 years. **Menopause** is the gradual cessation of ovulation and menstruation.

TERMS

amenorrhea: cessation of menstruation

breasts: a network of milk glands and ducts in fatty tissue

dysmenorrhea: abdominal pain during menstruation ("menstrual cramps")

endometrium: the inner lining of the uterus

fertility cycle: the near-monthly production of fertilizable eggs

follicle-stimulating hormone: stimulates ovaries to develop mature follicles (with eggs); the follicle produces estrogen

luteinizing hormone: stimulates the release of the ovum (egg) by the follicle; the follicle produces progesterone

menarche: the first occurrence of menstruation

menopause: the cessation of menstruation in midlife

menstrual cycle: the period of time from one menstruation to another

menstruation: the regular sloughing of the uterine lining via the vagina

premenstrual dysphoric disorder (PMDD): premenstrual symptoms severe enough to impair personal functioning

urinary tract infection (UTI): inflammation and/or infection of the urethra and/or bladder, usually by bacteria

Menopause is a time when the ovaries stop producing ova and the ovaries' production of hormones wanes considerably. Therefore, the two principal biological consequences of menopause are that a woman no longer is capable of becoming pregnant and that her body may undergo changes from the diminished production of estrogen. Many women experience menopause between ages 50 and 52; however, it can occur as early as age 35 and as late as age 55. The age at which menopause occurs may be affected by hereditary, social, and nutritional factors. There is no relation between the age at which menopause occurs and the age at which a woman first begins to menstruate.

Because menopause signifies the end of a woman's reproductive capacity, some people believe that it necessarily means the end of her sexual interest and abilities. This belief is not supported by biological fact, nevertheless, it can have a powerful effect on a woman's (and her partner's) mind and body. Women who accept menopause as a normal part of life can continue to be sexually active.

Although menopause brings biological changes, some of which may be uncomfortable for a while, it is important that menopause not be viewed as a disease (NIH Consensus Panel, 2005). The tendency among women and their healthcare providers to medicalize menopause led to more than 30 years of replacement therapy with estrogen (hormone replacement therapy), which was thought to be safe but ultimately was shown to increase the risk of heart disease and cancer. Now, replacement therapy with hormones is intended only for women with specific symptoms related to menopause. Some women find relief of menopausal symptoms from nondrug alternatives, such as soy protein, isoflavone extract, and whole foods (Franco et al., 2016).

Male Sexual Anatomy

Male sexual anatomy consists of two **testes**, the sites of sperm and sex hormone production; a series of connected sperm ducts that originate at the testes, course through the pelvis, and terminate at the urethra of the penis; glands that produce seminal fluid; and the **penis** (**Figure 8.6**).

The testes are located in a flesh-covered sac, the **scrotum**, that hangs outside the man's body. In the embryo, the testes develop inside the body, but just before birth they descend into the scrotum. Inside the scrotum, the testes are kept at a temperature a few degrees cooler than the internal body temperature, a condition necessary for the production of reproductively capable sperm. Normally, the scrotum hangs loosely from the body wall, although cold temperatures, fear, excitement, or sexual stimulation may cause it to move closer to the body. One testis is usually a little higher than the other.

When a man ejaculates, sperm are propelled through the sperm ducts and out of the penis by contractions of the smooth muscle that lines the sperm ducts and the muscles of the pelvis. As they move out of the body, the sperm mix with secretions of seminal fluid from the

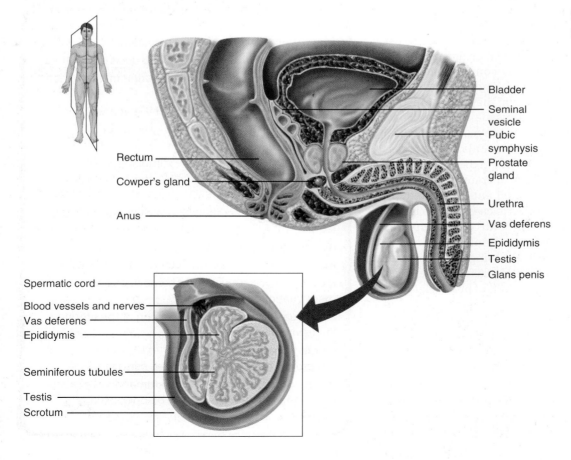

■ **Figure 8.6**
Male Reproductive Organs

Bladder
Seminal vesicle
Pubic symphysis
Prostate gland
Urethra
Vas deferens
Epididymis
Testis
Glans penis

Rectum
Cowper's gland
Anus

Spermatic cord
Blood vessels and nerves
Vas deferens
Epididymis
Seminiferous tubules
Testis
Scrotum

seminal vesicles, **prostate gland**, and **Cowper's glands** to form **semen**. The semen, which is the gelatinous milky fluid emitted at ejaculation, contains a mixture of about 300 million sperm cells and about 3 to 6 milliliters of seminal fluid. The seminal fluid contributes 95% or more of the entire volume of semen.

The penis is normally soft, but when a man becomes sexually aroused, its internal tissues fill with blood and the penis enlarges and becomes erect. All men are born with a fold of skin, the **foreskin**, that covers the end of the penis. In the United States today, parents of male infants can elect to have the foreskin removed surgically within hours after a child's birth. Removal of the foreskin is called **circumcision**. Muslim and Jewish traditions call for the circumcision of all males. Although circumcision may lessen the risk of adult penile cancer and the transmission of sexual infections to sex partners, the American Academy of Pediatrics does not recommend routine neonatal circumcision (American Academy of Pediatrics, 2012). Removal of the foreskin does eliminate the buildup of **smegma**, a white, cheesy substance that can accumulate under the foreskin. The belief that circumcision leads to an increase in sexual arousal because it exposes the glans and the related belief that circumcision produces an inability to delay ejaculation are myths. For most men, circumcision has no effect on sexual arousal and sexual activity.

Sexuality: The Psychological Dimension

The psychological dimension of sexuality consists of one's emotions—most frequently joy, excitement, pleasure, love, and affection—and the conscious and unconscious beliefs that guide the interpretation of experience and generate behaviors designed to meet one's sexual and relationship needs. These include assessments of one's social and sexual attractiveness, self-worth, and appropriate attitudes and behaviors.

They also include beliefs about what is "natural," beautiful, and good, the behaviors considered "proper" for sexual activity, when and where sexual activity may take place, and who may legitimately have sex with whom. Some beliefs are specific to an individual and others are shared among a group. Occasionally a society's shared beliefs are codified into law, such as the prohibition of prostitution.

Beliefs are acquired through **socialization**, the process by which a social group confers attitudes and behavioral expectations upon individuals. It is through socialization that individuals learn what sexuality means for members of their group. Socializing influences include parents, family, school, peer groups, religion, employment setting, and mass media.

Gender

Gender (derived from the Latin *genus*, meaning "type," "kind," or "sort") refers to the tendency for individuals to classify themselves and be classified by their social group—socially, psychologically, behaviorally, and even morally—according to their biological sex. Gender is a complex attribute encompassing beliefs about the presumed basic nature of members of each biological sex (*gender stereotypes*), social expectations based on biological sex (*gender roles*), and a fundamental part of one's sense of self (*gender identity*).

Gender stereotypes are beliefs about the "natural" or "typical" characteristics of males and females; for example, believing men to be aggressive, logical, independent, and unemotional or women be cooperative, intuitive, dependent, and emotional. Gender stereotypes often are enforced by negative attitudes about and consequent shaming of individuals who do not conform to the accepted stereotype. For example, a boy who plays with dolls may be derided as a sissy; a girl who plays football and climbs trees may be teased as a tomboy. Nearly all social groups possess gender stereotypes.

The gender role consists of socially desirable behavioral expectations for males and females; for example, expecting males to do physical labor or be institutional leaders and women to marry, see to the emotional and physical needs of spouses and children, and maintain the household, even if working outside the home in the paid workforce.

Gender identity is the psychological sense of oneself as being a male, female, or nongendered. Gender identity is highly likely to be principally determined prenatally by the action of sex steroid hormones and other neurological factors acting on core structures in the brain. Postnatal parental and social environmental factors may also play a role. Gender identity develops in most individuals by the age of two, and it tends not to change, although

> ## ▎TERMS▎
>
> circumcision: a surgical procedure to remove the foreskin from the penis
>
> Cowper's glands: small glands secreting drops of alkalinizing fluid into the urethra
>
> foreskin: a fold of skin over the end of the penis
>
> gender: social classification based on biological sex
>
> penis: the male's organ of copulation and urination
>
> prostate gland: gland at the base of the bladder providing seminal fluid
>
> scrotum: the sac of skin that contains the testes
>
> semen: a whitish, creamy fluid containing sperm
>
> seminal vesicles: glands that secrete a fluid that is a component of semen
>
> smegma: a white, cheesy substance that accumulates under the foreskin of the penis
>
> socialization: the process by which social groups confer attitudes and expectations upon individuals
>
> testes: a pair of male reproductive organs that produce sperm cells and male sex hormones

individuals may play-act as someone of the other or neither sex from time to time.

Most of the time, one's gender identity is consistent with one's sexual biology referred to as *cis gender*. However, in a few individuals, gender identity is in part or wholly incongruent with the biological sex, a situation referred to as *transgender*. These individuals, even as children, fundamentally and sincerely believe themselves to be men or women "trapped" in the body of the other biological sex. They often dress like, play with toys characteristic of, and prefer playmates of the other sex. As teenagers and adults, they may reject their own biological sexuality and dress and behave as the other biological sex. As adults, transgender individuals may take hormones and/or undergo surgery to attain a body that is congruent with their gender identity. Transgender individuals are not mentally ill, although they may experience anxiety and depression in environments that are not accepting and hostile (Dhejne et al., 2016).

Some individuals refer to their gender as "Q," meaning "Questioning" or "Genderqueer." *Questioning* refers to being unsure of one's gender identity. *Genderqueer* refers to not accepting the traditional binary definition of gender identity (male or female) in favor of a more flexible, nonbinary definition. *Gender nonconforming, bi-gender, nonbinary*, or *being fluid* are other terms for someone who does not self-identify solely and uniquely as the sex assigned at birth or the other traditionally defined sex.

Sexuality: The Orientation Dimension

Sexual orientation is the propensity to be sexually and romantically attracted to members of a particular sex. People with a same-sex orientation are referred to as *homosexual;* people with an other-sex orientation are referred to as *heterosexual*. People whose orientation is for either sex are referred to as *bisexual*. It is estimated that 5% to 10% of adults are exclusively homosexual. Some surveys indicate that about 50% of the population have had some same-sex sexual experience, often occurring in childhood and adolescence when sexual experimentation is common. Many people say they are erotically aroused by individuals of their sex but have no desire to act on those feelings.

Traditionally, American culture has forbidden same-sex sexual and intimate relationships, asserting that they are wrong, immoral, unnatural, or indicative of psychological illness. Neither the American Psychological

Gay (Same-Sex) Marriage: Social and Health Issues

An essential component of health depends on living in society without fear and with confidence that the basic rights of all persons are protected. In many countries, however, individuals with same-sex orientation face imprisonment and even legal execution for living in accordance with their biological nature. Although the United States does not imprison homosexual persons for their desire to romantically bond to and engage in sexual activity with individuals of their same biological sex, these individuals still face ostracism and verbal and physical abuse in many locales. Living in constant fear of being attacked can create significant health problems.

Since marriage is a fundamental social institution, those who are married enjoy a variety of legal and social benefits that can contribute to their health and well-being (see boxed text for a list of benefits provided). Historically in America, however, partners of the same sex who wished to receive the benefits of legal marriage and the companionship, intimacy, healthy sexual expression, and the security and joys of family life, were denied the legal right to marry. In June 2015, the U. S. Supreme Court ruled marriage between same-sex individuals to be legal throughout the country, affirming the legal right of same-sex couples to marry regardless of jurisdiction. With the 2015 decision the Supreme Court brought the United States in line with many other countries that had legally approved same-sex marriage.

Obtaining the legal rights and benefits of marriage has not been easy for many Americans. Objections to same-sex marriage derived, in no small measure, from both homophobia and criminalization of homosexuality. For many decades in many U. S. jurisdictions, sexual activity between same-sex individuals was a crime under "Sodomy Laws." These laws also criminalized certain, arbitrarily defined as "unnatural," sex acts between heterosexual individuals. Sodomy laws were in effect in many states until 2003 when the U. S. Supreme Court declared them unconstitutional. Besides sodomy laws, laws banning same-sex marriage have historical counterparts in miscegenation laws. These laws banned marriage between Caucasians and non-white persons such as Asians, Africans, or Native Americans. Miscegenation laws were based solely on discrimination and exclusion of non-white persons. Over time, states recognized and rejected the racism on which miscegenation laws were based, and they were repealed. California was the last state to decriminalize interracial marriage when it repealed its miscegenation laws in 1967.

The legal status of same-sex marriage shows that most Americans accept the principle that denying basic rights to others because of sexual orientation, skin color, or religious beliefs is unacceptable.

Benefits provided by legal marriage:

- Companionship, emotional security, and care when ill.
- Legal social inclusion.
- Hospital visitation rights when a spouse is sick.
- Being eligible to receive the tax benefits accorded to the married.
- Access to spousal/family health insurance.
- The right to inherit money and property from a deceased spouse.

Association nor the American Psychiatric Association considers same-sex orientation to be a mental illness. Scientific studies have failed to uncover any inherited, hormonal, or metabolic abnormalities that account for same-sex orientation. The neuropsychological mechanisms underlying the development and patterning of sexual orientation are unknown. One thing that is certain is that sexual orientation is rarely a choice; to each individual, it seems "natural."

By and large, same-sex intimate relationships are similar to other-sex ones, with the possible exception that they involve less gender-specific stereotypical behaviors. Some same-sex relationships are casual and do not involve long-term commitments, whereas others involve a deep and lasting emotional commitment and sexual exclusivity. Sexual orientation in itself does not affect the desire to love and be loved and to be involved in committed, caring relationships.

In recent years, lesbian, gay, bisexual, and transgender individuals have organized into a social-political group referred to as the *LGBTQ community*. This group and its supporters advocate for the same legal rights and social acceptance promised to all citizens by the Declaration of Independence and the U.S. Constitution.

People sometimes confuse transgender, transvestism, and homosexuality:

- Transgender refers strictly to gender identity and whether this sense of oneself is consistent with one's sexual anatomy.
- Transvestism is adopting the appearance of the other sex. Societies tend to dictate how men and women should dress, whether or not or which kind of jewelry to wear, the type of body art, and the length of the hair. For example, a human sexuality instructor may wear a man's business suit, have short hair, speak in a baritone voice, and insist on being addressed as "Mr. so-and-so," and may even tell personal stories suggesting a male's typical history, but none of this can assure students that their instructor is a biological male and/or self-identifies as such.
- Homosexuality is the propensity to be sexually attracted to and generally desirous of emotional attachment to members of one's same biological sex. Nearly always, a homosexual individual's gender identity is consistent with her or his biological sex. Homosexual men and women do not imagine themselves to be members of the other sex, and they do not wish to be so.

Sexuality: The Behavioral Dimension

The behavioral dimension of sexuality includes activities intended to produce a sexual experience. Although sexual activity is generally thought of in terms of genital stimulation, genital responses, and orgasm, in reality sexual experience also involves feelings of affection, love, joy, intimacy, sexual interest, and desire; being able

Table 8.1

Reasons for Sexual Activity Given by American College Students

Reason	Examples
Reproduction	To have children
Curiosity and adventure	How will this feel?
	What's that person like?
	What would it be like to ___ with _____?
Sexual release	Feeling "horny"
	Relief of sexual tension
Love/intimacy	To communicate as a couple
	To express love
	To feel emotionally close
Other reasons	To prove one's femininity/masculinity
	To maintain the relationship
	Duty
	To control another
	To abuse another
	To make money
	To relieve stress
	To relieve boredom
	To relieve loneliness
	To have fun
	To give/receive comfort
	To gain a sense of accomplishment
	To prove one's attractiveness
	To prove adult status
	To gain/maintain acceptance in a social group (peer pressure)

to discover and create sexual pleasure in oneself and a partner; and evaluating and interpreting the effect of sexual experience on oneself, one's partner, and one's relationship with the partner. In should be noted that sexual activity can be motivated by wants not related to creating erotic pleasure or interpersonal intimacy (**Table 8.1**).

Generally, sexual activity requires that a person be interested in creating a sexual experience. In North America, adults are expected to be highly and frequently interested in sex, in reality the desire for sexual activity varies among individuals and couples, changes over time, and is influenced by interpersonal and psychological factors. Various physical and psychological situations can affect sexual interest as well. For example, many women report a transient loss of sexual interest during the first few weeks after childbirth. Depression and physical illness are also often associated with loss of interest in sex.

TERMS

sexual orientation: the propensity to be sexually and romantically attracted to a particular sex

Alcohol: The Risky Social/Sexual Lubricant

How many people do you know say they need to drink to have a good time? Probably lots. Many students say they use alcohol to quell their nervousness about going to parties or other social gatherings, or that they need alcohol to feel less nervous or inhibited about sex. The problem with using alcohol to reduce anxiety is that it reduces other physical processes and inhibitions that often protect us from danger. So if you need to get tipsy or drunk before you can say "yes" to sex, consider the following:

- Alcohol can suppress the body's ability to respond sexually, thus impairing erection, lubrication, and orgasm.
- Being drunk can impair your ability to feel pleasure or even be aware of what you are doing.
- You might have sex with someone you would not otherwise be involved with ("beer goggles").
- You create a situation for sexual assault.
- It's easy to get unintentionally pregnant.
- You may forget to practice safer sex and thereby increase the risk of HIV/AIDS or another sexually transmitted disease.

Having sexual desire does not necessarily mean that a person will behave sexually. Human sexual behavior is not "reflexive"; sexual activity does not occur automatically whenever one feels "horny" or one is presented with a sexual opportunity. Instead, sexual activity is the result of a decision (except in instances of sexual coercion and assault).

Consenting to a sexual experience involves consideration of the social situation in which sexual activity takes place. Societies have rules and norms that govern sexual activity. Individuals are not permitted to have sex with just anyone or in any social setting. Even in a situation or relationship in which sexual activity is socially permitted and opportunities to have sex are present, a person can decide "yes," "no," "not yet," or "maybe" by evaluating physical and emotional feelings at the time, personal criteria for being sexual within the presenting situation, and the expectation of how having sex at that time will affect oneself and the relationship.

Sexual Arousal and Response

There is no formula for creating sexual arousal. Everyone has preferences. In situations and circumstances that they deem appropriate for sex, most people respond sexually to being touched in certain ways. Some regions of the body are highly sexually sensitive in nearly all people. These are the erogenous zones—the genitals, the breasts, the anus, the lips, the inner thighs, and the mouth.

When a person becomes sexually aroused, the brain and nervous system respond by preparing the body for sexual activity. Impulses from the brain are transmitted by the spinal nerves to various parts of the body that cause the tightening of many skeletal muscles (**myotonia**); changes in the pattern of blood flow (**vasocongestion**), especially in the pelvis; increases in heart rate, blood pressure, and respiratory rate; increases in the general level of excitement and erotic feelings.

Increased pelvic blood flow in the male produces erection of the penis. The penis enlarges because the spongy tissues within it fill with blood. In the female, increased pelvic blood flow produces lubrication of the vagina and swelling of the clitoris and vaginal lips. Vaginal lubrication is produced by the release of fluids from the walls of the vagina. Swelling of the clitoris and vaginal lips is caused by the filling with blood of spongy tissues within them. In some women the changes in blood flow caused by sexual arousal also produce a swelling of the breasts.

Regardless of the type of sexual stimulation, the physiological response in both men and women is similar and follows a pattern called the **sexual response cycle**, which consists of four phases (**Figure 8.7**):

- *Phase 1:* Excitement, in which the person experiences sexual arousal from any source and the body responds with specific changes, including erection of the penis in males and vaginal lubrication and swelling of the clitoris and genitalia in females.
- *Phase 2:* Plateau, in which the physiological changes of the excitement phase level off, although subjective feelings of sexual arousal tend to increase.
- *Phase 3:* Orgasm, in which the tensions that build during excitement and plateau are released.
- *Phase 4:* Resolution, in which the body returns to the physiologically nonstimulated state. Resolution may include a *refractory period,* a period of time (from minutes to days) during which orgasm and ejaculation cannot occur.

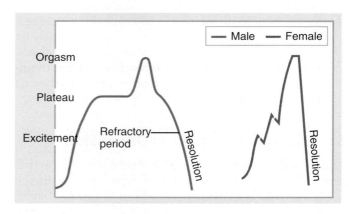

■ **Figure 8.7**
Sexual Response Cycle

There is considerable variation in the extent and duration of the sexual response cycle among individuals of either sex. The nature of the response can even vary in the same person because each sexual episode is different.

Orgasm

When sexual arousal builds to a certain point, the associated sexual tensions are released in an **orgasm**. The orgasmic response in both women and men frequently is associated with rhythmic contractions of the pelvic muscles; tightening of the muscles of the face, hands, and feet; and feelings of pleasure. Most commonly, men ejaculate during orgasm, although it is possible for males to experience orgasm without ejaculation and vice versa. The media have perpetuated the myth that during male or female orgasm, bells ring, the earth shakes, lights flash, and moans and groans are elicited, but often orgasms are quiet.

Orgasmic experiences vary greatly from person to person and from one encounter to another. For all persons there are "big orgasms" and "little orgasms" depending on the level of arousal. Sometimes, if a person is not sufficiently aroused, or too tired, tense, or ill, there may be no orgasm.

Our society is oriented toward achievement, and it has become common to apply measures of success to sex, especially orgasm. For example, many people believe that "success" is determined by the number of orgasms a woman has during a sexual episode. By this standard, a successful male is someone who can delay ejaculation until his partner has experienced at least one orgasm and preferably more, whereas a successful female is someone who can have more than one orgasm in every sexual encounter. Men and women who cannot "manufacture" the appropriate number of orgasms may be erroneously labeled "inadequate" by themselves and others. When people become overly concerned with "succeeding" or "performing well," they can become psychologically detached from the activity. Rather than abandon themselves completely to sexual experience, they withdraw their attention and observe their actions. This is called **spectatoring**.

Masturbation

Masturbation is self-stimulation to produce erotic arousal, usually to the point of orgasm. Although social and religious attitudes in many cultures consider it improper, immoral, or perverse, masturbation is nevertheless practiced widely throughout the world and even among other animal species.

Many people find masturbation a rewarding variation in their sex lives. People masturbate for many of the same reasons that they have partner sex: to experience erotic pleasure; to relieve physical tensions; to produce a sense of relaxation; to induce sleep; and, when done with a partner, to create feelings of intimacy and bonding.

Tips for Enhancing Sexual Experience

- Create pleasure by stimulating the whole body, not just the genitals.
- Vary the manner and intensity of stimulation. Allow sensations to build and wane.
- Try not to make sex = work.
- Set aside time that is free of intrusions and distractions. Disconnect the phone; lock the door to ensure privacy.
- Make yourself an open, effective channel for sexual arousal before sexual activity begins. Satisfying sex is not a mechanical activity involving only bodies, but a blending of mind–body energies. Remove sex-negative energies such as hunger, fatigue, and anger, and focus your energy on sex through deep breathing or other relaxing activity.
- Be aware of differences between you and your partner in the state of readiness for sexual activity. Try to synchronize both partners' states of sexual arousal through talking, light touching, dance, massage, and so on, before sexual activity begins.
- Address concerns about birth control and STDs prior to sexual experience.
- Take your time. Go slowly.
- Communicate likes and dislikes to your partner either verbally or nonverbally.
- Do not focus just on orgasms. Learn to appreciate the many sexual sensations from touching all parts of the body.
- Either partner may reach orgasm through manual, oral, or other means of stimulation before or after intercourse.
- Sexual activity need not stop after one partner reaches orgasm. If a couple chooses, lovemaking can continue until both wish to stop.
- Neither individual may desire an orgasm during a particular sexual episode. Physically expressing love and caring does not require orgasm.

Often, people find masturbation to be a way to understand what pleases them sexually.

A number of personal harmful effects have long been rumored to result from masturbation. Among them are

TERMS

masturbation: self-induced sexual stimulation

myotonia: muscle tension

orgasm: the climax of sexual responses and the release of physiological and sexual tensions

sexual response cycle: the four-phase physiological response to sexual arousal in both men and women

spectatoring: observing one's own sexual experience rather than fully taking part in it

vasocongestion: the engorgement of blood in particular body regions in response to sexual arousal

Be Good at Sexual Communication

Even though sex can be a very important part of an emotionally close relationship, communicating about sex can be difficult. Many people believe that sex is private or "dirty" and not a proper topic for discussion. Some people don't have a sexual vocabulary other than sexual slang, and they don't feel comfortable using those kinds of words with an intimate other. Also, a common romantic myth is that people in love intuitively know each other's feelings and desires, and so talking about sex is unnecessary.

Sometimes gestures, touches, and glances can communicate sexual messages, but such nonverbal cues run the risk of being missed or misunderstood. Verbal communication lessens the risk of misunderstandings and hurt feelings. Talking about sex in the early part of a relationship can prevent the development of negative patterns, especially the unspoken assumption that it's not OK to talk about sex.

If talking about sex is difficult for you, it might help to share with your partner your unease: "The sexual aspects of our relationship are important to me, but I'm nervous [uncomfortable, shy, etc.] about talking about this subject" or "There's something I want to talk about, but it's hard for me. I'd like to try, but before I do I'd like to be sure that at first you'll just listen and not comment."

Then, you can share your personal and family history about sexuality and sex talk. You can describe how sexual topics were dealt with in your family and peer group, how you learned sexual words, and your current attitudes about talking about sex. Eventually you will develop sufficient comfort to talk about specific sexual aspects of your relationship.

hair loss, insanity, pimples, warts, unhappy personal relations, and the inability to have children. There is no evidence that any of these claims are true. Physically, masturbation is harmless as long as it is not injurious to the stimulated organs.

Sexual Abstinence

Although someone may have interest in and desire for sex, he or she may choose to abstain from sexual activity.

> It's been so long since I made love, I can't remember who gets tied up.
>
> *Joan Rivers*

For religious reasons, certain people practice lifelong sexual abstinence (sometimes called celibacy, which literally means remaining unmarried). Individuals may also refrain from sexual intercourse until they marry, to avoid unintended pregnancy or sexually transmitted infection, because they do not feel emotionally ready for sex or intimacy, have negative attitudes about sexual relations, have difficulties with sexual activity because of prior sexual abuse or assault, and/or wish to avoid the negative consequences of hooking up (Napper, 2016). For those who are sexually experienced, a measured abstinence from sexual intercourse can provide a healthful "time out"; for example, when recovering from a physical or emotional illness or a deep loss, such as the death of a loved one or the breakup of a love relationship.

Some people find abstaining helpful while recovering from the breakup of a love relationship. The healing of the emotional wound seems to proceed more smoothly without the emotional intensity that often accompanies sexual interaction.

Sexual abstinence can also provide an opportunity to develop a new set of personal and relational experiences. By avoiding the intimacy that often accompanies sex, abstinence provides a way to discover new dimensions in interpersonal relationships. Without the diversion of sex (or the search for sex partners) an individual can focus on self-development, career, or school and put energy into friendships. New romantic relationships can develop without the pressure for sex early in the relationship, thus permitting the partners to develop trust and caring before becoming sexual.

Sexual Difficulties

Many individuals expect sex always to be exciting and satisfying; and anything less is cause for concern. Life is full of changes, however, and the demands of career or parenting or occasional illness can sometimes produce a temporary loss in interest in sex or the ability to engage in sex (**Table 8.2**). Such changes in sexual interest and ability are normal and usually resolve in time. Persistent difficulties with sex may signal that consulting a health professional would be helpful.

Lack of Interest Therapists and counselors refer to the lack of interest in sex as hypoactive sexual desire or sexual aversion, and note that it can result from the following:

1. *Underlying sexual difficulty:* One or both partners may have some physical difficulty engaging in sex: A man may be unable to gain or maintain an erection, or a woman may experience pain during intercourse. Such problems can make sexual activity unpleasant for either or both partners, and they eventually lose interest in sexual activity.
2. *Failure to communicate likes and dislikes:* One partner may find some aspects of sex unsatisfying and not communicate this information to the other partner. Resentment and displeasure may subsequently build up to the point that interest in sex is lost.
3. *Boredom:* Like anything else that becomes predictable and routine, sex can become boring if it is always done in the same way and at the same time. As with other activities, the old cliché is true: "Variety is the spice of life."

Table 8.2

Factors Contributing to Sexual Difficulties

Types of factors	Examples
Organic factors	Illness of any kind
	Hormonal, vascular, and neurological illness
	Fatigue or psychoendocrine stress
	Medications and recreational drugs
Values, beliefs, and attitudes	Negative values about sex
	Sex is dirty; sex is sinful
	Genitals (especially female) are dirty
	Women are not supposed to enjoy sex
	Men are supposed to always be interested in sex
	Men are supposed to always be capable of sex
	Narrow definition of sex
	Sex = penis-in-vagina intercourse
	Goal orientation (sex = orgasm)
	Performance expectations
Personality and experiences	Low self-esteem
	Emotional difficulties (anxiety, depression, grief)
	Prior incidence of sexual abuse
	Poor body image
Relationship factors	Discomfort with intimacy
	Relationship problems
	Fear of pregnancy or sexually transmitted disease
	Sexual orientation

4. *Stress, fatigue, and depression:* Being emotionally drained by work or other responsibilities or being "low" or "blue" can interfere with sexual desire.

5. *Alcohol and other drugs:* Frequent ingestion of alcohol and other drugs can lower sexual desire. Drug use can also turn off a partner who does not want to make love to someone who is drunk or on drugs. Some medications can also lessen interest in sex.

6. *Pregnancy and children:* During pregnancy and child raising, the increase in responsibilities and the decrease in private time can lower interest in sex. Busy couples must make an effort to schedule time to be together (for sex and other activities).

7. *Hostility and anger:* Unresolved conflicts are a common cause of lost sexual interest. It may be difficult to feel intimate with someone with whom you are angry.

8. *Change in physical appearance:* Once they are in a relationship, some people stop caring about their appearance, which may lessen a partner's sexual interest.

9. *Physical illness:* Physical illnesses can cause some people to believe they shouldn't have sex. For example, the man who has a heart attack may be afraid to have sex because he fears another heart attack.

Erection Problems Difficulty in attaining or maintaining an erection can result from vascular disease in the pelvic region, being sick or injured, and being stressed or depressed. It can also result from smoking and the use of alcohol, marijuana, opiates, other recreational drugs, and some medications, including those for neurological disease and high blood pressure. Erection problems also result from fear of sexual performance (including anxiety about one's ability to get an erection), fear of pregnancy or contracting an STD, or the wish not to be sexual with a particular partner. Counseling and/or drugs that increase blood volume in the penis (e.g., Viagra; Cialis) are common treatments.

Rapid Ejaculation Rapid or "premature" ejaculation is persistent or recurrent ejaculation before a man or his sexual partner wishes it. Rapid ejaculation is reported to occur in 25% of American men, most commonly between the ages of 20 and 40. Because it is a reflex activity, with practice a man can learn to control ejaculation voluntarily just as he does with bladder function. The key to controlling ejaculation is awareness of the bodily sensations that signal the onset of ejaculation, followed by modulation of sexual arousal according to one's desires. A variety of counseling techniques can help men learn to control ejaculation. Other methods include lessening penile sensations (condoms, topical anesthetics) or using selective serotonin reuptake inhibitors (SSRIs), which cause ejaculatory delay (McMahon et al., 2013).

Painful Intercourse In women, painful intercourse can be caused by vaginal infections, insufficient vaginal lubrication before intercourse (usually the result of not being sufficiently sexually aroused), and anxiety-produced spasms of the muscles surrounding the vagina, which makes vaginal penetration painful. Another source of pain associated with intercourse is a deep, aching sensation in the pelvis for women or in the scrotum ("blue balls") for men. This condition is caused by the congestion of blood in the pelvic region brought about by sexual arousal. Orgasm often reverses the congestion, but lack of orgasm can cause blood to remain and cause discomfort and pain.

Orgasm Difficulties Both men and women can have difficulty experiencing orgasm. Most often this difficulty is the result of insufficient sexual arousal, perhaps because of aversion to a particular partner, fear of pregnancy or sexually transmitted diseases, fear of letting go emotionally, lack of trust, or negative attitudes about sexual pleasure.

Sexuality: The Relationship Dimension

Most people find that sexual activity influences—and is influenced by—interpersonal relationships characterized by feelings of love, intimacy, and emotional closeness. Sexually relating individuals share themselves with each other in special ways that they do not share with friends,

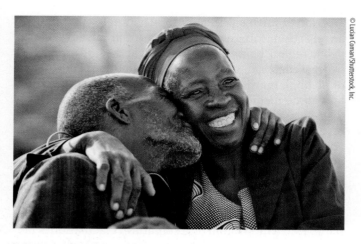

Intimacy is a basic human need at every age.

even close ones. They expose their bodies to each other; they touch each other; they create powerful emotions; their bodies join physically.

Intimacy is a feeling of closeness, trust, and openness with another person that tells us that our innermost self can be shared without fear of attack or emotional hurt and that we are understood in the deepest sense possible.

Intimate relationships can have an enormous impact on one's sense of vitality and well-being. When an intimate relationship is flowing smoothly, it can produce rich emotional satisfaction unparalleled by almost any other experience. Those who are involved in genuinely supportive and caring relationships tend to feel confident about the potential of life to be harmonious and beautiful. On the other hand, when an intimate relationship is not going well, those involved can be overwhelmed by moroseness and unable to think of anything but their misery. They can be angry, depressed, anxious, or distraught, sometimes to the point of being unable to function at work or at school.

Many people mistakenly equate genuine intimacy with sexual intercourse. This happens because love and affection are feelings associated with intimacy. But intimacy is a feeling, not an act. It is the *quality* of a relationship between two people—a shared experiencing of their personal lives. People who have an intimate relationship may or may not choose to express their intimate feelings with sex.

The Life Cycle of Intimate Relationships

Intimate relationships tend to develop through the stages of (1) selecting a partner, (2) developing intimacy, and (3) establishing commitment. Before an intimate relationship can develop, however, the partners have to be psychologically open to entering and maintaining it. Some individuals choose not to be involved in an intimate relationship, perhaps because they wish to devote energies to school, work, or self-development, or they find intimate relationships to be distracting or psychologically threatening. In some instances, previous life experiences can leave an individual fearful of emotional closeness,

which can block the establishment of intimacy. In some of these instances, there are repeated attempts to form relationships; however, without the element of intimacy, these relationships can fail.

Factors that influence the choice of intimate partners include the following:

- *Proximity:* People are most likely to become intimate with someone with whom they are in physical proximity.
- *Similarity:* Similar age, religion, race, education, social background, attitudes, values, and interests affect the possibility for intimacy in two ways: They influence proximity, and they reflect social norms for permissible peer intimacies. Note, for example, biases against interracial and older–younger intimacies. Colleges and universities provide students with relatively easy access to a "pool of eligibles" because they bring together individuals of similar age, intelligence, expectations, and values.
- *Physical appearance:* Physical appearance provides cues that indicate who among the pool of eligibles is a desirable intimate partner. Those who are judged "attractive" tend to be thought of as kind, understanding, and affectionate ("what is beautiful is good"). Pairing with someone who is considered physically attractive enhances one's social status and self-esteem.

Developing Intimacy

Most people want their intimate relationships to develop feelings of closeness, positive regard, warmth, and familiarity with the other's innermost thoughts and feelings. This deep knowledge of each other comes from sharing the most important and often secret aspects of one's personality—one's goals, aspirations, strengths, weaknesses, and physical and sexual desires. The sharing of such private information is called **self-disclosure**.

When relationships among college students begin, little intimate information is usually disclosed. People talk about the weather, sports, TV, celebrities or politics. They gossip about professors, students, or other people they know. And they ask each other the classic leading questions: Where are you from? What do you do? What's your major? People face these questions so many times that they become adept at revealing as much or as little about themselves as feels comfortable. It is when they begin to talk about their personal history, current life problems, hopes and aspirations, and fears and personal failures that they begin to disclose important information—important because disclosing it makes them feel vulnerable. Most people discuss their deepest feelings only with those in whom they have developed considerable trust.

Intimacy develops through a progressive, mutual revealing of innermost thoughts. Psychologists compare people's personalities to onions—having many layers, from an outer surface to an inner core. As acquaintances gain more and more knowledge about each other, they

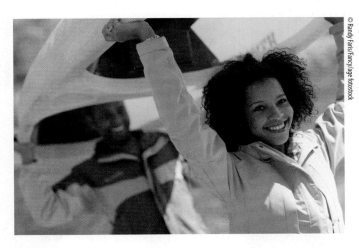

Intimacy begins by doing fun things together.

> The question that women casually shopping for perfume ask more than any other is this: "What scent drives men wild?" After years of intense research we know the definitive answer. It is bacon.
>
> *John Lanchester, The New Yorker*

penetrate deeper and deeper through the layers of the other's personality, which establishes their intimacy. Another view compares intimate development to the peeling of an artichoke. Resistance and barriers to sharing information about oneself are like the leaves of the artichoke; as intimacy progresses, intimates peel away the leaves to get to the other's "heart."

Self-disclosure leads to the development of intimacy in two ways. First, you tend to be affected either positively or negatively by the information that is disclosed. If you make a positive judgment, you are likely to want to continue interacting with that person, for you believe that future interactions will be equally or even more positive. The same logic applies to negative assessments. If your reaction is unfavorable, you are likely to terminate the relationship, or perhaps maintain it on a lesser level of intimacy.

The second way that self-disclosure leads to intimacy is the *act* of self-disclosure, which, regardless of the information offered, often leads to reciprocal self-disclosure. By sharing important information, you communicate that you trust the other person, and usually that person accepts your trust and becomes more willing to disclose information. In this way, intimacy progresses by a cycle of self-disclosure leading to trust, which brings about self-disclosure, which leads to more trust, and so on.

Establishing Commitment

After a period of self-disclosure, individuals may sense that their relationship has progressed to a state of "us-ness," that it has become a special friendship, a love relationship, or a marital-type relationship. This state of "us-ness" is one of commitment, which has three aspects:

- *An action, pledge, or promise:* One makes a promise and thus announces one's intention explicitly, even if it is only to the partner. Various social values and norms regarding keeping promises and the guilt and loss of self-esteem that come with breaking promises are among the "push" factors that keep a person committed. If the promise involves a social ritual (i.e., marriage ceremony, getting pinned), then family, friends, and the state become additional "push" factors.
- *A state of being obligated or emotionally compelled:* This state involves a cluster of emotions such as love, comfort, caring, and relief from separation anxiety and loneliness.
- *An unwillingness to consider any partner other than the current one:* The rewards of the current relationship outweigh the costs of exploring other opportunities for intimacy.

Endings

Everything in the universe (even the universe itself!) has a beginning and an end. Close relationships have a beginning and an end also. Sometimes a relationship lasts for only a few minutes; sometimes it lasts until one of the partners dies (and even then the relationship may still be "alive" in the imagination of the surviving partner). Sometimes the structure of a close relationship persists, but the closeness and the dynamism wane, creating a "shell" relationship without vitality. Sometimes a relationship goes through cycles of birth and death within the structure of its ongoingness. When a close relationship ends, some or all of its structure, exchange of resources (e.g., love, caring, financial support), and feelings of attachment and emotional bondedness end also.

Endings occur for a variety of reasons. Partners' feelings of attachment and bondedness may be absent or weak. Life goals, values, or interests may no longer be shared. One or both partners may be unwilling or unable to invest personal resources such as greater time shared with the partner or to commit to an emotionally or sexually exclusive relationship. Whether partners continue in a relationship also is affected by their assessment of other options, such as another potential partner or singlehood. Without suitable alternatives, leaving a relationship may seem difficult, unwise, or impossible.

Another reason ongoingness stops is that the partners, either individually or as a dyadic unit, are unable to move the relationship into its next stage. For example, some couples cannot navigate the transition from being idealistic,

---

TERMS

self-disclosure: sharing personal experiences and feelings with someone

passionate lovers to realistic, companionate lovers. In non-marital close relationships, a partner may not be considered suitable as a potential marital partner, even in the presence of considerable love, attachment, and liking.

Another factor associated with endings is lack of support, or even hostility, from the partners' social network. Families may not accept a son's or daughter's choice of a dating or marital partner. Interracial, disabled, and same-sex relationships are still heavily stigmatized in our society.

Occasionally the seeds of an ending are sown into a relationship at its beginning. For example, partners may seek emotional closeness as a way to cope with or avoid personal problems. They may feel rejected and lonely because of the breakup of a previous relationship. They may feel that they cannot take care of themselves. They may be afraid of leaving home or school. If, as often happens, a partner or relationship does not turn out to be the solution to a personal problem, a disappointed, angry, or frustrated partner may seek alternative ways of coping. These alternatives, such as drug or alcohol abuse, extra-relationship affairs, or physically or emotionally abusing the partner (or other family members), may destroy the relationship.

When a breakup does occur, individuals may feel tired, lethargic, lonely, sad, depressed, angry, resentful, and guilty. They may be unable to sleep or eat, may miss class, or be unable to work. They may withdraw from friends. They may find concentrating difficult because they are continually thinking about the partner and what happened in the relationship. They may feel helpless ("What will become of me?") and hopeless ("I'll never find a true love") or skeptical and cynical ("Love can never work out").

Some partners feel relaxed, hopeful, and relieved that what they identify as a bad or going-nowhere relationship has ended and they are free to pursue personal goals or find a relationship partner who is better suited to them. Sometimes individuals feel euphoric and self-confident. They say that the separation was for the best, and they become more active and outgoing. This positive outlook may alternate with feelings of loss and emotional distress.

When a person is emotionally (and sometimes physically) wracked with the pain of an ending, he or she may have difficulty seeing any good in that experience, but endings often mark the start of a new and better future. A study of remarried people showed that many had learned a lot about themselves and the nature of close relationships from a previous marriage(s) and found that their current marriage was much more satisfying. Guiding principles for enhanced relationships are patience and experience.

Communicating in Intimate Relationships

Communication is a symbolic process of creating and sharing meaning. At the heart of communication is an individual act that involves imparting a message to

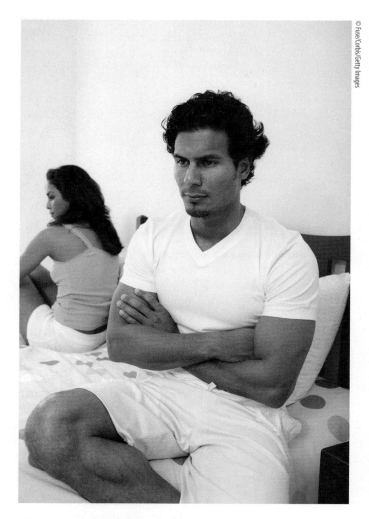

When communication breaks down, stress and tension can occur.

another person to signify that an interpersonal relationship exists, share information or feelings, to coordinate behavior with another, or to persuade someone to do something.

A communication act begins as a mental image; an idea, a wish, or a feeling (or some combination of these). If humans were capable of mind reading, people could impart mental images directly to each other. Few people can read minds, however, so communication requires that thoughts be transformed into symbols that can carry information. Those symbols make up the message. The most common symbols in communication are

- *Words:* spoken or printed
- *Visual images:* paintings, sculpture, photos
- *Posture or body language:* gaze, touch, smile, physical proximity, folding arms, frowning, turning away
- *Objects:* flowers, gifts, food
- *Behaviors:* doing a favor, giving a kiss, making eye-contact, ignoring an appointment

Encoding a mental process into the symbols that make up a message is only half of a communication act. The other half is taking in the symbols that make up the message and decoding them into meaningful mental processes. Thus, a communication act requires two transformations: in the sender, the transformation of mental images into symbols; in the receiver, the transformation of symbols into mental images.

Consider this example of a communication act between Beth and Ron one rainy morning. Beth doesn't want Ron to get wet in the rain, so she decides to use spoken words as the symbols to encode her thoughts. Beth says, "Ron, it's raining." Ron hears Beth's words and decodes them into a mental image of the weather that day, and he picks up his umbrella.

> Start every day with a smile and get it over with.
>
> *W. C. Fields*

In this communication act Beth accomplished her goal. But a different outcome could have occurred if one or more of the steps in the communication act had been distorted, weakened, or blocked completely. For example, if Beth had said "it's raining" in a tone of voice that Ron didn't appreciate, or if her words had been misunderstood, the communication process would have been distorted.

Every communication act carries two types of messages or potential meanings. The first is the **literal message**, which is the message conveyed by the symbols themselves, as in the words "it's raining." The second is the **metamessage** (*meta* is the Greek word for "beyond," "additional," or "transcendent"), which carries implicit messages about the reason for the communication, how the message is to be interpreted, and the nature of the relationship between the sender and receiver.

When Beth said to Ron, "it's raining," not only did she send a literal message about the weather but she also sent several metamessages, including "I care about you" and "an expectation in our relationship is that we help each other out."

After Beth had told Ron that it was raining, if Ron had kissed Beth and said, "Thanks, honey, for looking out for me," he would have been responding to one of the metamessages in the communication. If Ron had interpreted the metamessage as "Ron, you're terribly childlike and I have to make decisions for you"—even though Beth didn't intend to impart that message—Ron might have responded angrily with something like "Beth, I can look out for myself!" Her feelings may then have been hurt and possibly they would have had an argument. Acknowledging and responding to metamessages can sometimes be much more significant than dealing with the literal ones.

Sending Clear Messages

A clear message is one in which the symbols represent as closely as possible the sender's intent. Clear messages are best delivered with **I-statements**; these are sentences that begin with (or have as the subject) the pronoun "I." I-statements clearly identify the sender as the source of a thought, emotion, desire, or act: I think…I feel…I want (need)…I did (will do)….

You-statements, which begin with (or have as the subject) the pronoun "you," as in "You always…," "You never…," "You are…," or the interrogatives "Why don't you…?" or "How could you…?" often are put-downs or character assassinations. They imply that the receiver is not OK. Very often the not-OK message is explicit, as in "You're incompetent" or "You're stupid"—just about any negative adjective will do. People often respond to the metamessage in a you-statement, which is "I think you're no good," by feeling attacked, which can lead to hurt feelings and counterattacks or withdrawal.

Effective Listening

Effective communication requires both talking and listening. Effective listening is important because the listener not only takes in the speaker's message but also helps establish the physical and emotional context for the communication. The listener also must communicate to the speaker that the message was received. This is called **feedback**. Some techniques for effective listening are giving the sender your full attention, making eye contact, listening, being empathic, being open for receiving the message, giving verbal feedback, acknowledging the sender's feelings, praising the sender's efforts, and being unconditional.

Give the Speaker Your Full Attention Don't fake it. If you can't pay attention because you are tired, hungry, distracted, angry, or whatever, tell the speaker how you feel and ask if it's OK to talk after you rest, or eat, or go to the bathroom, or just talk at another time. The speaker is likely to grant your request if immediacy is not an issue, because he or she wants your full attention.

Make Eye Contact Try to assume similar postures (i.e., both sitting or both standing) to create a sense of equal status. Making eye-to-eye contact allows the speaker to feel comfortable as well as conveys that you are listening to him or her and taking in the complete message.

Just Listen Don't interrupt until you have a signal that the speaker is finished or the speaker has asked for a response, unless you don't understand what is being

---

TERMS

feedback: response of the receiver of a message to let the sender know the message was received

I-statements: statements beginning with "I"; positive communication skill

literal message: a message that is conveyed by symbols

metamessage: how the message is interpreted between sender and receiver

you-statements: statements beginning with "you"; negative communication skill

communicated. You can acknowledge that you are actively listening with gestures, nods, and vocalizations like "uh-huh," "yes," "go on," "I see," and so forth.

Be Empathic Try to "hear" the speaker's feelings as well as the words. Be open to the speaker's intentions and motivations as well as her or his ideas. Ask yourself, "What is this person feeling right now?"

Be an Open Channel for Receiving a Message Don't judge or evaluate the speaker or the message while the speaker is talking. Try not to correct the speaker or, if the speaker is being critical of you, to think of a defense.

Give Verbal Feedback Don't mind read. Summarize in your own words your understanding of the speaker's thoughts and emotions. This way the speaker can find out if the message that was intended was actually received. If so, then you can respond. If not, then the speaker can try again. Ask for clarification if there's something you don't understand. You can say something like, "I don't think I understand everything you were saying about your mother. Can you tell me again, maybe in a different way?"

Acknowledge the Speaker's Emotions "It seems to me that you're feeling…" and if you're not sure, add "Do I have that right?" By acknowledging or providing feedback, you are sharing what you believe are the speaker's emotions. If you are incorrect, the speaker can relay that to you.

Praise the Speaker's Effort Acknowledge the speaker's efforts for investing the time, energy, and caring to communicate with you, especially if the communication was a difficult one.

Be Unconditional Let the speaker know that you respect him or her even if you are uncomfortable with the messages that are being communicated. Assure the speaker that even though things may be difficult, you are willing to continue talking and working through difficult feelings.

Expressing Anger Constructively

Disagreements and conflicts are inevitable in any close relationship. The notion that people in intimate relationships shouldn't fight because love makes them see eye to eye on everything and the idea that you can't possibly be angry with someone you love are romantic myths. By expressing anger constructively, intimates fight for the success of their relationship as well as for their individual needs.

In constructive fighting, there should be no "winner" and no "loser." Good fights are efforts of individuals to be heard and to improve the relationship. The best fights occur when the people involved feel that they have gained something.

Here are some suggestions for expressing anger constructively:

- Try not to let anger and resentment build up over time. Express feelings when you become aware of them.
- Agree on a time, a place, and the content for fights. It is certainly acceptable to get mad spontaneously if that is how you feel, but it is better to set aside a specific time for the resolution of an issue rather than trying to deal with it when you or your partner may not be psychologically or physically ready to argue. Be sure that the person you are angry with knows what the issue is before the fight.
- Be specific as to what you are angry about and stick to the issue. Don't bring up old hurts. Try not to discuss second and third topics, especially as a means of retaliation.
- Attack the problem, not each other. Don't denigrate the other's personal qualities. Use I-statements to communicate resentments. I-statements tell how you feel. You-statements are often received as personal attacks. At the same time, express appreciation for your partner as a person. This acknowledges that we can be angered by our partners' behaviors and feel loving toward them as people at the same time.
- Try to resolve the issue with an air of compromise and respect. Try to understand the other's point of view.
- Know when it is time to stop. Sometimes you can sense that the argument isn't getting resolved. It is okay to acknowledge that and to take a few hours or days to reconsider things and to discuss the issue again. Sometimes emotions are too high and it is not possible to think clearly. That may be the time to stop the fight until tempers cool.
- Engaging in sex or any other affectionate behavior before an issue is resolved should not be taken as a sign that everything is forgotten. Such behavior shows that the fight fits into what is believed to be a healthy relationship.
- Don't hold grudges.

Critical Thinking About Health

1. Set aside some time to reflect on (and write down) your earliest learning experiences about sexuality. Were they open and positive or shrouded with secrecy and shame? How have these experiences shaped your adult sexual attitudes and behaviors? What, if anything, would you like to change?

2. Make a list of situations and relationships in which sexual activity is permissible for you personally. Would your list be different for your son or daughter's? Explain.

3. In the United States when a boy is born, the parents are faced with the decision of whether to have him circumcised. Proponents of circumcision have any number of reasons for supporting it: religion, culture, health, or hygiene. Opponents of circumcision say that it is unnecessary surgery that brings with it unnecessary risk and pain to the child. What are your beliefs on circumcision? On what do you base your beliefs? Talk to someone who disagrees with you and see if your beliefs change or soften.

4. Communication is critical to negotiating condom use, whether for birth control or prevention of sexually transmitted diseases. There are many reasons why men and women do not want to use a condom, but you must be prepared in advance to respond thoughtfully and respectfully to ensure a condom will be used. Describe how you would respond to the following statements:

   Condoms are too expensive.
   Sex isn't pleasurable with a condom.
   I'm Catholic; I'm not allowed to use a condom.
   I can't believe that you think I have an STD.
   If you really loved me, you wouldn't ask me to use a condom.

5. List all the people (e.g., parents, siblings, friends, boyfriends or girlfriends, spouses) that you are currently "intimate" with. (Remember that "being intimate" does not mean "having sex.") Describe what each of those relationships means to you and discuss how they all contribute to your health and happiness.

Chapter Summary and Highlights

Chapter Summary

Awareness of sex and sexuality arises in childhood when we become aware of our biological sex and that there are two sexes. Which one am I? Then we learn to establish our social sexual identity, the gender identity. Even as a child we develop our sexual orientation, the sense of the sex to which we are attracted. People display a spectrum of sexual orientations just as people have a range of intellectual abilities. If everyone realized that sexual orientation is a complex trait like intelligence, perhaps there would be much less prejudice and violence against people whose sexual orientation and preferences differ from the majority. As we grow and mature both physically and sexually, we feel the need to explore our sexuality with ourselves and with others of the opposite sex or with those of the same sex.

Intimacy is a basic human need. Infants bond to mothers (or a substitute caretaker) shortly after birth. As we grow older we share intimate thoughts and feelings with family and friends. Some thoughts and feelings are easily shared; others are not. Becoming physically intimate with another person for the first time is scary. Because the outcome of intimate interactions can have a profound effect on one's sexual and psychological development, relationships should be developed slowly, with trust and understanding the primary goals. In our fast-paced world, taking time to develop a relationship is often ignored. Today, people often consider instant sexual gratification as a major goal of interpersonal interaction. Learn to treasure your intimate moments with others and take the time needed to allow trust to develop fully.

Highlights

- Sexuality has several dimensions: the physical (biological), psychological, orientation, behavioral, and relationship dimensions.
- One's sexual biology is determined by genetic makeup, which in turn determines the nature of sex organs: the testes, sperm ducts, semen-producing glands, and penis in the male; and the ovaries, fallopian tubes, uterus, vagina, and external genitalia in the female.
- One's sexual psychology is rooted in emotions and beliefs about sexuality.
- Sexual orientation is the tendency to feel attracted to, and the desire to emotionally bond with, a member of the same or other sex.
- Sexual arousal and response involves four phases: excitement, plateau, orgasm, and resolution.
- Sexual difficulties include lack of interest in sex, inability to attain or maintain an erection, lack of ejaculatory control, painful intercourse, and difficulties with orgasm.
- Intimate relationships involve sharing one's innermost self. They develop through three stages: selecting a partner, developing intimacy through self-disclosure, and commitment.
- Effective communication is crucial for developing and maintaining relationships.

For Your Health

Communication is an integral part of healthy relationships. Do the Listening Exercise (in the Workbook, Chapter 8) to enhance your ability to communicate with important others. The other exercises offer enhancements to relationships.

References

American Academy of Pediatrics. (2012). Newborn male circumcision. Retrieved from https://www.aap.org/en-us/about-the-aap/aap-press-room/pages/newborn-male-circumcision.aspx

Dhejne, C., et al. (2016). Mental health and gender dysphoria: A review of the literature. *International Review of Psychiatry, 28,* 44–57.

Franco, O. H., et al. (2016). Use of plant-based therapies and menopausal symptoms: A systematic review and meta-analysis. *Journal of the American Medical Association, 315,* 2554–2563.

McMahon, C. G., et al. (2013). Standard operating procedures in the disorders of orgasm and ejaculation. *Journal of Sexual Medicine, 10,* 204–229.

Napper, L. E., et al. (2016). Assessing the personal negative impacts of hooking up experienced by college students: Gender differences and mental health. *Journal of Sex Research, 53,* 766–775.

NIH Consensus Panel. (2005). Demedicalization of menopause. Retrieved from http://consensus.nih.gov/2005/menopausestatement.htm

U.S. National Library of Medicine. (2013). Treating PMS symptoms. Retrieved from http://www.ncbi.nlm.nih.gov/pubmedhealth/PMH0057412/

World Health Organization. (2015). Defining sexual health. Retrieved from http://www.who.int/reproductivehealth/topics/sexual_health/sh_definitions/en/

Suggested Readings

The Boston Women's Health Book Collective. (2011). *Our bodies, ourselves: A book by and for women.* New York: Touchstone. This book reflects the vital health concerns of women of diverse ages, ethnic and racial backgrounds, and sexual orientation—a must-read for every woman. Companion website is https://www.ourbodiesourselves.org.

Golanty, E., & Edlin, G. (2011). *Human sexuality: The basics.* Sudbury, MA: Jones & Bartlett Learning. A basic college-level text.

Gottman, J. M. (2004). *The seven principles for making marriage work.* New York: Orion. A renowned couples researcher and professor of marital therapy shows how to maintain healthy intimate relationships.

Harvard Medical School. (2017). Men's sexual health. Retrieved from http://www.health.harvard.edu/topics/mens-sexual-health. Numerous authoritative articles on a range of physical, psychological, interpersonal, and social factors influence a man's sexual health.

McCarthy, B. M., & Metz, M. E. (2007). *Men's sexual health: Fitness for satisfying sex.* New York: Routledge. Focuses on an integration of mind and body, helping men and women understand how to pursue sexual and relational health and overcome sexual problems, with the goal of greater acceptance and satisfaction.

Satcher, D., et al. (2015). Sexual health in America. *Journal of the American Medical Association, 314,* 765–766. The former U.S. Surgeon General and colleagues discuss the elements of sexual health in the United States based on wellness and prevention of sexuality-related illness.

University of Texas at Austin Counseling and Mental Health Center. (2017). Building a healthy relationship from the start. Retrieved from https://www.cmhc.utexas.edu/vav/vav_healthyrelationships.html. Concise information on all aspects of building and maintaining healthy intimate relationships.

Recommended Websites

Daily Reproductive Health Report
Daily news stories on human sexuality and reproduction, from the Kaiser Family Foundation.

Go Ask Alice!
A health (including sexuality, sexual health, and relationships) question-and-answer Internet service produced by the Columbia University Health Education Program.

MayoClinic.com
Sexual health basics by the Mayo Clinic staff.

Sex Information and Education Council of the United States (SIECUS)
Information and education about sexuality and responsible sexual choices.

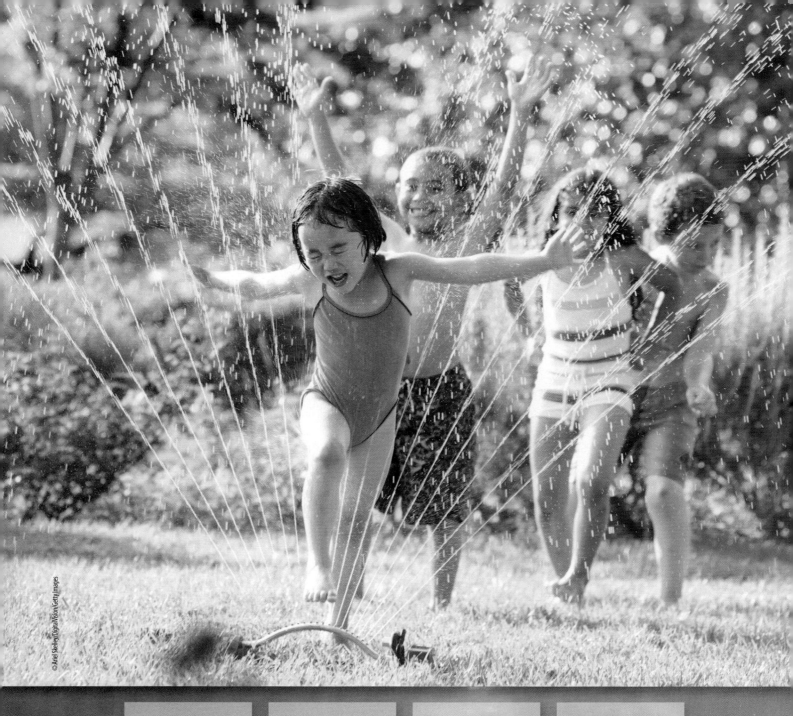

Health Tips

Pregnancy and Childbirth: Belly-Breathing Exercise

Dollars & Health Sense

Buying At-Home Pregnancy (and Other) Health Products on the Internet

Global Wellness

Infant Mortality

Wellness Guide

Home Pregnancy Testing

Boy or Girl: Should Parents Have the Right to Choose?

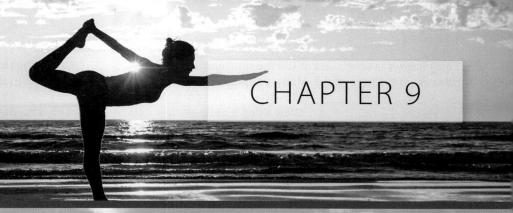

CHAPTER 9

Understanding Pregnancy and Parenthood

Learning Objectives

1. List and discuss reasons for becoming or not becoming a parent.

2. Describe the processes of fertilization and implantation.

3. Explain how pregnancy tests work.

4. Describe the major health habits in pregnancy.

5. Describe amniocentesis and chorionic villus sampling.

6. Describe the three stages of labor.

7. List the benefits of breastfeeding.

8. Discuss infertility and pregnancy options for infertile people.

This chapter is about one of the most profound life experiences: creating a child. Many people are awed by the idea that the union of one of their body's cells with a cell from their mate can bring forth a unique human being whose well-being is highly dependent on the physical and emotional foundations they provide. There is a tremendous responsibility in being the best kind of parent so that both the child and society benefit.

> You know what I did before I got married? Anything I wanted to.
>
> *Henry Youngman*

People want children for a variety of reasons, including the following:

- To create a social structure (family) to which one can belong
- To manifest a couple's sense of love and emotional bonding
- To improve a marriage
- To leave a legacy to the world
- To carry on the family name
- To accede to social and family pressure to have children
- To feel important, needed, loved, and proud
- To feel more feminine or masculine
- To add fun, excitement, love, and companionship to one's life

Choosing Whether to Be a Parent

Not everyone chooses to become a parent. Some see parenthood as infringing on their career goals or as an unnecessary or unwanted addition to their intimate partnership. Some may have doubts about their psychological or economic abilities to nurture or support children. Others may know or suspect that their children might inherit a genetic disease. Still others may feel that they do not want to contribute more children to an already overpopulated world.

Giving birth to and raising a child requires major adjustments in the parents' lives. The career plans of one or both parents and the distribution of family resources—time, energy, physical space, and money—may change. First-time parents may feel overwhelmed by their responsibilities. The decision to parent should not be taken lightly. The years of parenting are often intense. However, you will never experience such responsibility, hard work, and intimacy as that involved in the growth and development of another human being.

Children do not ask to be born. Parents make that decision. Therefore, before committing to this decision, potential parents must be as certain as they can that their decision is appropriate for their life goals and that they have the means to care for their children.

Becoming Pregnant

For most people, becoming a parent involves pregnancy—a 40-week period during which a fetus grows inside the mother's uterus and the mother's body undergoes changes to nurture the developing child. Every pregnancy begins with **fertilization**, which is the fusion of a father's sperm cell with a mother's ovum to form the first cell of their child, called the fertilized egg, or **zygote**. When a man ejaculates during sexual intercourse, hundreds of millions of sperm cells are released into the vagina. Propelled by the swimming motion of their long tails, these tadpole-like cells make their way through the uterus and into the fallopian tubes, the usual site of fertilization (**Figure 9.1**). Only one sperm cell fertilizes the egg. After fertilization, the zygote moves to the uterus, where it implants into the inner lining of the uterus and develops as an **embryo**.

During each of a woman's menstrual cycles, usually one ovum, but sometimes two or more, is readied for fertilization. Once freed from the ovary at ovulation, an egg can survive for about 24 hours.

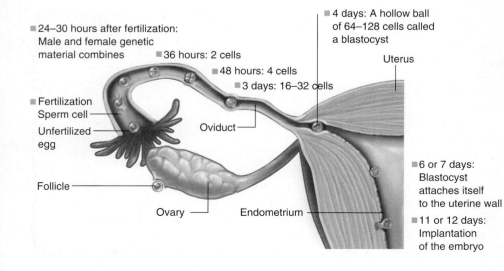

■ 24–30 hours after fertilization: Male and female genetic material combines

■ 36 hours: 2 cells

■ 48 hours: 4 cells

■ 3 days: 16–32 cells

■ 4 days: A hollow ball of 64–128 cells called a blastocyst

Uterus

■ Fertilization Sperm cell

Unfertilized egg

Oviduct

Follicle

Ovary

Endometrium

■ 6 or 7 days: Blastocyst attaches itself to the uterine wall

■ 11 or 12 days: Implantation of the embryo

■ **Figure 9.1**

Fertilization and Early Development of the Embryo

Joining of sperm and egg in fertilization. After fertilization, the zygote travels down the fallopian tube to the uterus. Implantation of the zygote begins approximately 6 days after fertilization.

Sperm are produced in the testes in narrow, highly coiled, tubelike structures called **seminiferous tubules**. It takes about 70 days for an immature sperm cell to develop into a mature sperm. Once in the vagina, sperm can survive up to 7 days.

The cervix is the gateway for passage from the vagina to the uterus. For most of the menstrual month, fluid produced by glands in the cervix is dense. This thick cervical mucus is a barrier to sperm and microorganisms. Near the time of ovulation, the cervical mucus becomes more fluid and has the consistency of an egg white, and it becomes organized into channels that orient sperm movement toward the uterus.

Within seconds following ejaculation in the vagina, some sperm move through the cervix and uterus and into the fallopian tubes. The majority of sperm, however, become trapped in coagulated semen in the upper portion of the vagina. After about 20 minutes, the coagulated semen liquefies and sperm move into microscopic folds in the cervix. Weak or abnormal sperm are unlikely to move beyond the cervix. Healthy, motile sperm tend to be released into the uterus continuously throughout the ensuing 48 hours. Several hundred sperm capable of fertilization approach an ovum, but only one succeeds in penetrating the ovum's outer membrane.

During the first 3 days after fertilization, the cells of the embryo replicate at about daily intervals, and the embryo moves along the fallopian tube toward the uterus. By about the fourth day after fertilization, the embryo, now composed of between 50 and 100 cells, arranged as a fluid-filled sphere, enters the uterus. On about the sixth day after fertilization, the embryo attaches to the lining of the uterus; shortly thereafter, it implants in the uterus by eroding the uterine lining.

Pregnancy

Soon after the embryo implants in the uterus, it secretes a hormone unique to pregnancy, called **human chorionic gonadotropin (HCG)**, into the maternal bloodstream (**Figure 9.2**). Under the influence of HCG, the mother's ovaries are stimulated to increase the production of estrogen and progesterone, which in turn forestalls the next menstrual period and permits the pregnancy to continue. Increases in the levels of estrogen and progesterone bring about the first noticeable signs of pregnancy: absence of the next menstrual period, occasional nausea and vomiting referred to as "morning sickness," enlarged and tender breasts, increased frequency of urination, fatigue, and enlargement of the uterus. Both clinical and home pregnancy tests are based on analyzing a woman's urine for the presence of HCG.

On rare occasions, the fertilized egg implants outside the uterus, usually in a fallopian tube where its passage is blocked by tubal malformation or scarring or twisting from a prior infection, often gonorrhea or chlamydia.

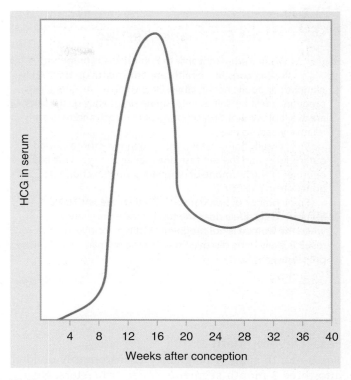

■ **Figure 9.2**

Pattern of Human Chorionic Gonadotropin (HCG) Secretion During Pregnancy

A pregnancy in which the fertilized egg implants somewhere other than in the uterus is called an **ectopic pregnancy**. Implantation in a fallopian tube also is called a tubal pregnancy. If a tubal pregnancy remains undiscovered, the embryo will become too large for the fallopian tube sometime between the eighth and twelfth weeks of pregnancy and the tube will burst, creating internal bleeding and a critical situation that requires immediate medical intervention.

TERMS

ectopic pregnancy: a pregnancy occurring outside the uterus, usually in a fallopian tube

embryo: the developing infant during the first two months of conception

fertilization: the fusion of a sperm cell and an ovum

human chorionic gonadotropin (HCG): a hormone produced during the first stages of pregnancy; it is used as a basis for pregnancy tests

seminiferous tubules: convoluted tubules in the testicles that produce sperm

zygote: the first cell of a new person, formed at fertilization

Home Pregnancy Testing

When a woman wants to know if she is pregnant, she can consult a healthcare provider or go to a family planning or public health clinic. Or she can administer a pregnancy test herself. Several home pregnancy testing kits are available without prescription at low cost, and they are relatively easy to use.

Virtually all chemical tests for pregnancy—those carried out in clinics and the self-test kind—analyze a woman's blood or urine for the hormone of pregnancy, human chorionic gonadotropin (HCG).

Some brands of home pregnancy tests are not 100% accurate. Only rarely does the test indicate pregnancy when the woman is not pregnant. A "false-positive" result is likely to be discovered when the woman seeks prenatal care.

Home tests for pregnancy can be wrong about 20% of the time, indicating that a woman is not pregnant when in fact she is. About half of these "false-negative" results occur because the test has been administered too early in the pregnancy; the other half are corrected if the test is readministered in about a week. However, about 10% of women who are pregnant still get the inaccurate test result that they are not pregnant. This is one of the most serious drawbacks of home pregnancy tests because the risks of complications in pregnancy and abortion rise the longer a pregnant woman waits to obtain professional care.

In spite of the possibility of inaccuracy, many physicians and family planning consultants believe home pregnancy testing to be useful. It enables women to take a more active part in their own health care, and it may help women who "would rather not think about it" confront the possibility that they are pregnant.

Fetal Development

The 9-month span of pregnancy is customarily divided into three 3-month segments called trimesters. Nearly all of the fetal body forms by the tenth week after fertilization. During the rest of pregnancy, the fetal body grows and many of the organs become functional; at birth the average fetus weighs about 3,000 grams (almost 7 pounds).

Fetal development and growth take place with the fetus enclosed in a fluid-filled membranous sac called the **amnion**, which forms during the second week of development. As it develops in the **amniotic fluid**, the fetus is able to grow unimpeded by the mother's internal organs. The amniotic fluid also protects the fetus from potentially damaging jolts when the mother changes her body position. The amnion ruptures just before birth, sometimes called "breaking of the bag of waters."

The growth and development of the fetus are supported by the placenta, an organ unique to pregnancy. The **placenta** manufactures many hormones needed to sustain pregnancy and is responsible for transporting oxygen and nutrients from the mother to the fetus and waste products from the fetus to the mother.

A number of changes occur in a pregnant woman's physiology (**Figure 9.3**). For example, the blood plasma increases in volume as much as 50% over her nonpregnant levels, the heart beats 10% faster and with 20% to 30% greater output per minute, the number of red blood cells increases, and breathing becomes deeper and slightly faster. One of the most striking changes during pregnancy is the growth of the uterus. The nonpregnant uterus is approximately 7 to 8 centimeters long (2¾ to 3½ inches) and weighs about 60 to 100 grams (2 to 3½ ounces). By the end of pregnancy, the uterus is approximately 30 centimeters long (12 inches) and weighs nearly 1,000 grams (2.2 pounds).

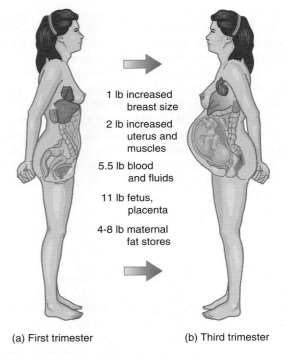

1 lb increased breast size

2 lb increased uterus and muscles

5.5 lb blood and fluids

11 lb fetus, placenta

4-8 lb maternal fat stores

(a) First trimester   (b) Third trimester

■ **Figure 9.3**

Changes in a Woman's Body During Pregnancy
Through a pregnancy, the shape of the pregnant woman's body changes dramatically.

Sexual Interaction During Pregnancy

A woman's sexual interest and responsiveness may change throughout the course of her pregnancy because of the many psychological, emotional, and physical changes that influence her attitude toward and enjoyment of sex. In some pregnancies, sexual interest increases. In others, it decreases. Some of the most common reasons women give for decreasing sexual activity during pregnancy include physical discomfort, feelings of physical unattractiveness, and fear of injuring the unborn child.

It is now generally accepted that in pregnancies where there are no risk factors, sexual activity and orgasm may be continued, as desired, until the onset of labor. Unless her healthcare provider counsels a pregnant woman to the contrary, there is no physical reason to forgo sex during pregnancy.

Some couples find that pregnancy is a good time to explore new lovemaking positions—side by side, rear entry, or woman above are generally more comfortable at this time. Even if intercourse is not desired, pregnancy can also be a time to try other sensual and sexual pleasures, such as oral sex, mutual masturbation, massage, or just total body touching and holding.

Health Habits During Pregnancy

Every child deserves to be born as healthy as possible. It is only fair to the unborn child—who did not ask to be conceived—that all the genetic potential to develop a healthy body and mind be given the opportunity to be fully expressed. Few of us are as careful about maintaining proper health habits as we could be. Most people live with whatever risk might be associated with nonhealthy behaviors and are presumably willing to accept the consequences of those behaviors. But when a woman is pregnant, disregarding fundamental health practices endangers her child as well as herself, and perhaps more so, because the developing baby's body and mind are extremely vulnerable to damage. A mother-to-be must make every effort to practice good health habits. If her developing baby could talk, he or she might say, "Mom,

my lifelong health and well-being are in your hands now. I know 9 months is a long time to have to be concerned about what you eat and drink, but it's important to me that you do the right things for both of us. Not only will that give me the chance to become the best person I can be but will also keep you healthy so we can share a lot of good times after I'm born." The factors that deserve a pregnant woman's attention to ensure her own health and that of her baby are proper nutrition, obtaining professional prenatal care, getting enough exercise, refraining from smoking and consuming alcohol or other drugs while pregnant, and accepting and dealing with emotional and sexual feelings that may be different from those experienced when not pregnant.

Nutrition

Throughout pregnancy, the fetus's cells and physiological capacities are developing. Perhaps more than at any other time of life, an ample supply of nutrients is required so that the formation of new cells and the development of organs proceed optimally. All fetal nutrients come from the mother by way of the placenta. Therefore, a pregnant woman directly influences the nutritional status

> ▌**TERMS**▐
>
> **amnion:** the inner membrane that forms a fluid-filled sac surrounding and protecting the embryo and fetus
> **amniotic fluid:** fluid in the amniotic sac
> **placenta:** the flat, circular vascular structure within the pregnant uterus that provides nourishment to and eliminates wastes from the developing embryo and fetus and is passed as afterbirth after the baby is born

---

Buying At-Home Pregnancy (and Other) Health Products on the Internet

Shopping on the Internet is a marvel. You can buy anything, including unapproved at-home pregnancy test kits. The Food and Drug Administration (FDA) approves some at-home diagnostic kits, but not all. Some test kits are approved only for health clinics and not for home use. Ads for some at-home pregnancy test kits promise in-home results, but most tests should be followed with a second, more sophisticated laboratory test to confirm the results.

If you want to buy a test kit over the Internet, avoid products that claim to test for more than one thing, such as pregnancy and HIV infection, are made in a country other than the United States, or are made by only one laboratory and sold directly to the public. If you have any doubts, check whether the FDA has

approved the product for use at home (1-888-INFO-FDA [1-888-463-6332]). The FDA offers these general precautions for buying healthcare items on the Internet:

- Don't be fooled by a professional-looking website. Anyone can hire a webpage designer to create an appealing site.
- Avoid websites with only a post office box number and no telephone number.
- Avoid websites that use the words "new cure" or "miracle cure."
- Avoid products with impressive-sounding terminology, language often used to deceive.
- Avoid products that claim the government, medical profession, or research scientists have conspired to suppress the product.
- Beware of claims that the test complies with all regulatory agencies.
- Beware of tests labeled for export only. This usually means that the test is not cleared or approved for sale in the United States.

Table 9.1

Recommended Daily Dietary Reference Intakes (DRI) for Nonpregnant, Pregnant, and Lactating Women, Ages 25–50

	Nonpregnant	Pregnant	Lactating
Protein (g)	46	71	71
Carbohydrate	130	175	210
Vitamin A (μg)	700	770	1,300
Vitamin D (μg)	5	5	5
Vitamin C (mg)	75	85	120
Thiamin (mg)	1.2	1.1	1.4
Riboflavin (mg)	1.1	1.4	1.6
Niacin (mg)	14	18	17
Vitamin B$_6$ (mg)	1.3	1.9	2.0
Folate (mg)	400	600	500
Vitamin B$_{12}$ (mg)	2.4	2.6	2.8
Calcium (mg)	1,000	1,000	1,000
Phosphorus (mg)	700	700	700
Iron (mg)	18	27	9
Zinc (mg)	8	11	12
Iodine (mg)	150	220	290

Data from Suitor, C. W., & Meyers, L. D. (2007). *Dietary Reference Intakes Research Synthesis*: Workshop summary. Washington, DC: National Academies Press. Retrieved from http://nap.edu/11767

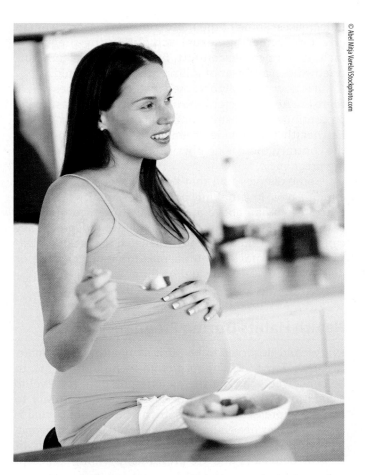

Nutritious, healthy foods are especially important when feeding two.

of her baby, and she must be aware that she has to "eat for two," meaning that her diet should contain adequate nutrients for herself and for her baby. Mothers-to-be who eat highly nutritious diets during pregnancy are more likely to give birth to healthy babies than are mothers whose diets are nutritionally poor. Pregnant women should increase their intake of essential nutrients and calories (**Table 9.1**). For some women it is advisable to supplement a generally well-balanced diet with extra iron and folic acid.

Many pregnant women are concerned with the amount of weight they gain. Although it is never healthy to weigh too much, current obstetric practice allows a mother-to-be to gain about 28 to 30 pounds by the end of pregnancy, most of which comes in the last two-thirds of pregnancy. About 7 of these pounds are contributed by the fetus. The enlarged uterus accounts for another 2 pounds, and the placenta and amniotic fluid contribute 1 pound each. About 4 to 8 pounds of fluid are added to the maternal system as extra blood and extracellular fluid, and the mother may gain about 4 pounds of body fat.

Physical Activity and Exercise

There are benefits to being physically active during pregnancy. Some women feel lethargic during pregnancy. In just a few weeks, their bodies take on unfamiliar proportions and they have to carry up to 20% more weight than when they are not pregnant. They may feel uncomfortable, unattractive, and clumsy. Through movement and exercise, a pregnant woman can become accustomed to the temporary changes in her body and accept pregnancy as a positive and fulfilling time of her life. Physical activity also helps prepare the mother's body for childbirth, which is often physically demanding. By keeping active, a pregnant woman can improve her circulation and thereby reduce swelling and formation of varicose veins in the lower legs, which can be common in pregnancy. As a group, well-conditioned women who engage in aerobics or run regularly tend to have shorter labors and fewer cesarean deliveries. Exercise during pregnancy can tone a woman's muscles so that after delivery her body returns more quickly to its pre-pregnant shape. Perhaps the greatest benefit from physical activity during pregnancy is maintaining the habit of being active.

The degree of physical activity a pregnant woman engages in depends on her desires and abilities (**Table 9.2**). Some athletic women engage in sports almost to the day of delivery. Women who are not routinely athletic are wise to begin a program early in pregnancy that involves exercises to maintain correct posture, strengthen abdominal muscles, and improve their breathing and ability to relax.

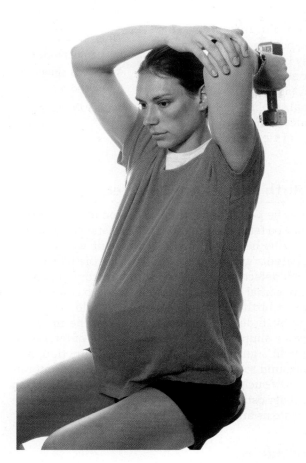

Staying physically active during pregnancy has many benefits.

Table 9.2

Safe Physical Activity During Pregnancy

Safe even for beginners	Safe for experienced exercisers	Unsafe*
Walking	Running	Downhill snow skiing
Swimming	Racquet sports	Contact sports
Cycling	Strength training	Scuba diving
Low-impact aerobics		
Prenatal yoga		

*Avoid exercises that increase the risk of falling, involve extra weight bearing, and, after the first 3 months of pregnancy, involve lying on the back.

Modified from American College of Obstetricians and Gynecologists. (2015). Exercise during pregnancy. Retrieved from http://www.acog.org/~/media/For%20Patients/faq119.pdf?dmc=1&ts=20120322T1318238628

Emotional Well-Being

Pregnancy can be a time of intense feelings, not only for the mother-to-be but also for her partner and others who are close to her. Enthusiasm, excitement, anticipation, fear about the baby's condition, uncertainties about one's suitability as a parent, and a desire for more (or less) love, affection, and sex are all natural. Recognizing that intense feelings are normal in pregnancy and accepting them with patience and understanding are the keys to a rewarding experience.

Perhaps the best way to deal with intense feelings at any time in life, including pregnancy, is to take time each day to quiet the mind and body with meditation, yoga, or other relaxation methods. Massage is also beneficial, and it fulfills some of the desires of those who feel more sensual during pregnancy.

Prenatal Care

Pregnancy involves several profound biological changes. Not only does the fetus develop from a single cell to a 7-or 8-pound newborn infant (composed of many millions of cells) but the mother's body also undergoes a number of anatomical and physiological changes to support fetal development. Moreover, the fetal–maternal relationship is maintained by the placenta, an organ that develops only during pregnancy and is expelled from the mother's uterus after the baby is born. Any rapidly changing system is vulnerable to errors and problems, and so it is with pregnancy and fetal development. That is why it is recommended that mothers-to-be receive professional prenatal care. A number of studies have shown that the more prenatal care a woman receives, the fewer problems she will have during pregnancy and childbirth and the more likely that her infant will be born healthy. Professional prenatal care can help a mother-to-be avoid the consequences of a number of pregnancy-specific illnesses, such as high blood pressure (preeclampsia), pregnancy-induced diabetes, and infection. These illnesses can threaten both the mother's health and the proper development and delivery of her baby. Professional prenatal care can also help manage problems resulting from a malfunctioning placenta and can educate a mother about proper nutrition and advise her on how smoking or consuming alcohol at any time during pregnancy can adversely affect her baby's development. Maternal infections that are harmful to the fetus, such as rubella (German measles), syphilis, gonorrhea, toxoplasmosis, herpes, and HIV, can be detected and managed. Another reason for prenatal care is to be sure the maternal and fetal blood cells are immunologically (Rh factor) compatible.

Risks to Fetal Development

A variety of factors can adversely affect an embryo or fetus during development, causing what are commonly referred to as **birth defects**. About 3% of all babies born in the United States each year (about 120,000) have birth defects (Centers for Disease Control and Prevention,

TERMS

birth defect: an anatomical or functional abnormality present at birth that is inherited or caused by the effects of a chemical, such as alcohol

2016a). Birth defects can mildly or severely affect the structure and/or function of almost any part of the fetal body. Depending on the severity, a birth defect can significantly hamper one or more life functions and even shorten the affected person's life span. About 20% of all infant deaths are due to birth defects.

Most birth defects occur in the first 3 months of pregnancy when the fetal tissues and organs are forming. However, because tissues and organs develop during the entire pregnancy, a fetus can be susceptible to birth defects for the entire period of intrauterine life. The principal causes of birth defects include heredity, the mother being older than 34 years, the mother's health (such as exposure to certain viruses and bacteria, diabetes, obesity, and medication use), the mother's lifestyle (smoking, alcohol and drug ingestion, poor nutrition), and exposure during pregnancy to environmental pollutants and industrial chemicals.

Drugs

Any drug or medicine ingested by a pregnant woman potentially can harm her fetus, resulting in birth defects or possibly even fetal death. All illegal psychoactive drugs, such as heroin, methamphetamine, and cocaine, pose dangers to a developing fetus because they may cause neurological abnormalities and addiction. Alcohol and tobacco also are dangerous (see the following sections), as are prescription and over-the-counter medicines and many dietary supplements. For her own health and the health of her child, a woman should avoid all drugs during pregnancy except those deemed necessary by a healthcare provider.

Alcohol

When alcohol crosses the placenta, it reaches a level in the fetus equal to that in the body of the mother. Because the body of the fetus is small and its detoxification system immature, alcohol remains in fetal blood long after it has disappeared in the mother's blood. Thus, drinking alcohol can harm the fetus, and the risk of damage increases as the quantity and frequency of maternal alcohol consumption increase. The fetus is at risk of developing fetal alcohol syndrome (FAS) if the mother drinks six or more drinks per day during her pregnancy. The symptoms of FAS include growth retardation, facial malformations, and central nervous system dysfunctions, including mental retardation and behavioral dysfunctions. FAS is the third most common cause of mental retardation in the Western world, after Down syndrome and malformations of the nervous system. This is particularly distressing because FAS is totally preventable.

Cigarette Smoking

Maternal smoking increases the chances of spontaneous abortion and of complications that can result in fetal or infant death. Smoking reduces the amount of oxygen in the bloodstream, which can adversely affect the fetus by slowing its growth. Infants of mothers who smoked during pregnancy often weigh less and are in poorer general health than are infants of nonsmoking mothers. Smoking may be teratogenic, causing cardiac abnormalities and anencephaly (absence of a cerebrum). Maternal smoking appears to be a significant factor in the development of cleft lip and palate.

> When I was a kid my parents moved a lot…but I always found them.
> *Rodney Dangerfield*

How Birth Defects Are Detected

Tests may be performed if there is reason to suspect that there may be fetal abnormalities. Circumstances in which tests may be beneficial include pregnant women over age 35, parents who have previously given birth to a child with birth defects, and parents with a history of genetic or chromosomal disorders who may want to confirm the absence of birth defects in an unborn child. Common tests for birth defects include examining the mother's blood (via a simple blood test) for evidence of fetal birth defects and signs of abnormal placental function, and an ultrasound to check the fetus for abnormal anatomical issues. If such tests are suggestive of a problem, then further diagnostic tests can be conducted. These include amniocentesis and chorionic villus sampling.

Amniocentesis

A reliable and accurate test, known as an **amniocentesis**, can be performed between the 14th and 18th week of pregnancy. The procedure captures fetal cells that have been sloughed off in the normal course of development by inserting a hollow needle with the assistance of ultrasonographic imagery through the woman's abdominal wall and into the uterine cavity to draw out a sample of the amniotic fluid (fluid surrounding the fetus). The procedure can detect several hundred fetal hormonal abnormalities and biochemical defects.

The test can be performed during any trimester if enough fluid is present. If done during the first trimester, it is usually for genetic studies; in the second trimester, for Rh isoimmunization studies; and in the third trimester, for assessing fetal lung maturity.

Chorionic Villus Sampling

Chorionic villus sampling (CVS) is used during the first trimester of pregnancy to detect biochemical disorders and chromosomal abnormalities. Chorionic villi are threadlike protrusions on a membrane surrounding the fetus that are composed of fetal cells. This test involves inserting a thin catheter with the assistance of ultrasonographic imagery through the abdomen or vagina and cervix into the uterus, where a small sample of chorionic villi is removed for analysis. This procedure has an advantage over amniocentesis because it can be done as early as the 8th week after the last menstrual period.

Childbirth

For the parents, the moment of childbirth can bring a mixture of feelings that might include great joy, relief that the 9 months of waiting are over, and surprise at the baby's appearance. All in attendance may experience concern for the condition of the mother and baby and awe and wonder at the miracle of new life.

Childbirth Preparation

A variety of programs and organizations provide education for parents-to-be in preparation for the childbirth experience and parenthood. These are usually 6- to 8-week courses, sometimes called "natural childbirth," "Lamaze," or simply childbirth preparation. Childbirth preparation classes can enhance the intimate relationship of the expectant couple and increase their confidence and self-esteem. In addition, women who participate in childbirth preparation are likely to have less pain and discomfort in childbirth, to require less medication, and to have fewer complications. Prepared parents are also more likely to have positive attitudes toward childbirth and parenting. Fathers who attend childbirth preparation classes tend to feel more comfortable about sharing the birth experience with their partners and about helping them during it. They are also more likely to be interested and involved in parenting after the baby is born.

Almost all childbirth preparation courses teach prospective parents the basic biology of pregnancy and childbirth. They also teach breathing and relaxation exercises, and some teach imagery and affirmations, all intended to make the delivery of the baby proceed smoothly and comfortably. While attending these courses, parents-to-be meet other expectant couples with whom they can share their feelings and experiences. The classes also address birthing options. Because childbirth preparation courses reflect the biases of those who teach them, prospective parents are likely to gain more complete information about birthing options by consulting additional sources (e.g., books, websites, and other parents).

Studies have shown that continuous emotional support during childbirth can shorten labor time, give the woman in labor greater perception of control, decrease her need for pain medication, and, overall, lead to fewer complications that affect the baby. On the other hand, labor can be slowed or stopped if the woman feels uncomfortable, anxious, frightened, or experiences performance pressure because of others' expectations about how the labor should be proceeding.

Giving Birth

A few weeks before the onset of childbirth, or **labor**, the fetus becomes positioned for birth by descending in the uterus, a process called **lightening**. When this happens the pressure on some of the mother's internal organs is relieved and she may find it easier to breathe, stand, and digest food. In about 95% of all births the fetus is in a

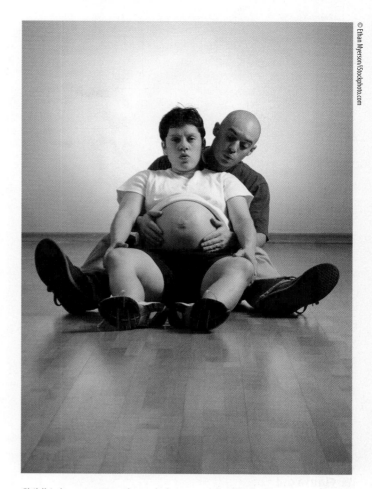

Childbirth preparation classes help ensure a healthy baby.

head-down or horizontal position. When not head-down, the fetus may be head-up, referred to as a *breech position*. In nearly all instances, the fetus's legs are tucked up against its abdomen in the "fetal position."

Throughout much of pregnancy, the uterus contracts intermittently, tightening in waves that sometimes are so gentle that the woman is unaware of them. During the last half of pregnancy, a woman may at times feel her abdomen becoming hard or otherwise perceive the uterine contractions as they prepare her body for the true

---

TERMS

amniocentesis: a procedure that involves aspiration of amniotic fluid from the uterus to detect certain abnormalities in the fetus

chorionic villus sampling (CVS): a method to detect biochemical disorders and chromosomal abnormalities in the fetus

labor: the process of childbirth

lightening: the positioning of the fetus for birth by descent in the uterus

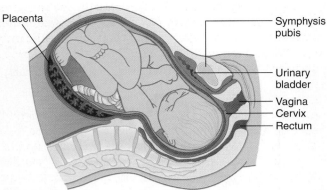

A Early first-stage labor

Placenta

Symphysis pubis

Urinary bladder

Vagina

Cervix

Rectum

B Later first-stage labor: the transition

Ruptured amniotic sac

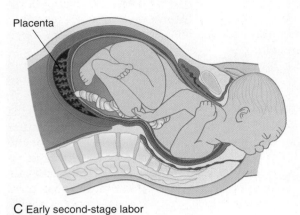

C Early second-stage labor

Placenta

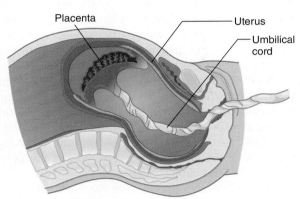

D Third-stage labor: delivery of placenta

Placenta

Uterus

Umbilical cord

■ **Figure 9.4**

Childbirth

The stages of labor. (a) Early first stage: The cervix is dilating. (b) Late first stage (transition stage): The cervix is fully dilated, and the amniotic sac has ruptured, releasing amniotic fluid. (c) Second stage: The birth of the baby. (d) Third stage: Delivery of the placenta (afterbirth).

labor. Health professionals refer to these as **Braxton-Hicks contractions**. They can be distinguished from true labor by their occurrence at irregular intervals and their rather short duration.

There are three generally recognizable stages in the process of childbirth (**Figure 9.4**). Before the first stage begins, the cervix has already effaced (flattened and thinned) and dilated slightly. The **first stage** of labor starts with the beginning of uterine contractions and lasts until the cervix is fully dilated. Another indication of first-stage labor may be the "bloody show," the discharge of the mucus plug from the cervix. The first stage is the longest of the three stages, usually lasting 10 to 16 hours for the first childbirth and 4 to 8 hours in subsequent deliveries. This stage lasts until the cervix is dilated about 10 centimeters.

The **second stage** of labor begins when the cervix is fully dilated and the infant descends farther into the birth canal (normally, head first). This stage lasts from 30 minutes to 2 hours. During this time, the woman can

actively push with each contraction until the fetus is expelled. The remaining amniotic fluid gushes out. The infant is cleaned and its vital signs, such as breathing and color, are quickly checked. The umbilical cord is clamped several inches from the navel, and the baby soon begins to breathe.

The **third stage** of labor lasts from the time of birth until the delivery of the placenta, or **afterbirth**. With one or two more uterine contractions, the placenta usually separates from the uterine wall and is expelled from the vagina, generally within 30 minutes after the baby is born.

Medical Interventions

Options for Controlling Discomfort

Intense discomfort or pain can accompany labor, especially in the later phases of the first stage and the early stages of the second. The intensity of feeling is caused by stretches and strains on the uterine muscle tissue, effacement of the cervix, and stretching of the perineum. Pain relief methods include relaxation techniques, deep breathing, acupuncture, hypnosis, massaging and supporting of the perineum by the birth attendant, medications that block pain awareness (analgesia), and medications that block the pain sensations (anesthesia). The most common anesthesia used during labor is a regional anesthetic to diminish sensation only in the pelvic region. This leaves the mother conscious during labor so that she can actively "bear down" to help push the baby out. General anesthesia (complete unconsciousness) is used only in cases of difficult births and interventions, such as cesarean sections.

Social and psychological support also contribute to lessening labor pain and discomfort. Women who expect to be able to manage childbirth successfully generally have less discomfort and require less pain medication than those who are fearful (American Society of Anesthesiologists, 2016). This is one reason pregnant women are encouraged to take childbirth preparation classes. Also, women who have continuous emotional support during childbirth generally need less pain medication. Support can come from a husband or other family member, a trained labor assistant called a *doula,* a nurse, or other obstetric professional. Giving birth in a home-like setting and with caregivers in attendance who the mother knows also contribute to a more successful birthing experience.

Induction of Labor

Induction of labor involves medically stimulating uterine contractions and, hence, the onset of labor. Induction of labor now occurs in about 20% of American childbirths, a doubling in percentage since 1990. The main reasons for labor induction include extended pregnancy (41–42 weeks), toxemia (elevated maternal blood pressure), premature rupture of the amniotic sac, and an excessively large baby (macrosomia).

The most common methods of inducing labor are administering prostaglandins to the cervix, breaking the amnionic sac, and giving the hormone oxytocin (Pitocin). A centuries-old method of labor induction involves a birth attendant stimulating a laboring woman's breasts to produce the release of oxytocin from the mother's posterior pituitary gland, as would occur when the mother later nurses her infant. Other nonmedical methods for labor induction include herbal compounds, castor oil, hot baths, enemas, acupuncture, acupressure, and sexual intercourse.

Episiotomy

Episiotomy is an incision in the perineum from the vagina to the anus, which can be performed during the first stage of labor to enlarge the vaginal opening. Not long ago, episiotomies were routine obstetrical procedures because it was believed they lessened tearing of the vaginal tissues and aided postbirth healing after delivery. It is now known, however, that episiotomies increase the risk of injury and do not aid significantly in postbirth healing. Episiotomies should be performed only when medically necessary and not routinely.

Cesarean Birth

When a normal vaginal delivery is considered dangerous, impossible, or undesirable for a variety of reasons a fetus can be removed from the mother's body through an incision made in the abdominal wall and uterus, in a surgical procedure called a **cesarean section**, or **C-section**. Cesarean births may be recommended in a variety of health situations, including a fetal head that is too large for the mother's pelvic structure, maternal illness, active herpes infection in the vagina, fetal distress during labor, birth complications such as breech fetal presentation (feet or bottom coming out of the uterus first), or previous C-section.

For both mother and baby, cesareans are less safe than uncomplicated vaginal deliveries, and they cost more. In the United States today, nearly 30% of births are cesarean. In 1970, only 5% of births were cesarean. Among the reasons offered for this increase are the parents and/or physician wanting a convenient labor, and the doctor and hospital not wanting to risk a difficult labor to avoid an expensive lawsuit. Obstetrical malpractice judgments are the largest among medical subspecialties, and obstetrical liability insurance is the highest among primary care practitioners. Thus, it is in the doctor's, the hospital's, and the malpractice insurance company's interests to encourage a mother to have a cesarean rather than risk difficulties during childbirth.

> ### TERMS
>
> **afterbirth:** placenta and fetal membranes
>
> **Braxton-Hicks contractions:** normal uterine contractions that occur periodically throughout pregnancy
>
> **cesarean section (C-section):** delivery of the fetus through a surgical opening in the abdomen and uterus
>
> **episiotomy:** an incision in the perineum to facilitate passage of the baby's head during childbirth, while minimizing injury to the woman
>
> **first-stage labor:** the beginning of labor during which there are regular contractions of the uterus
>
> **second-stage labor:** the stage during which the baby moves out through the vagina and is delivered
>
> **third-stage labor:** the stage during which the afterbirth is expelled

Pregnancy and Childbirth: Belly-Breathing Exercise

In Lamaze classes, expectant mothers (and fathers) are taught to place the emphasis of their breathing on the lower stomach or diaphragm. During the several hours of labor and the actual delivery, this breathing skill is employed to ease the pain of childbirth. What is taught and practiced in the stressful event of childbirth is now taught and practiced in several other stressful situations as well.

Each breathing cycle is composed of four distinct phases:

Phase I: Inspiration, taking the air into your lungs through the passage of your nose or mouth

Phase II: A very slight pause before exhaling the air out of your lungs

Phase III: Exhalation, releasing the air from your lungs and through the passage it entered

Phase IV: A very slight pause after exhalation before the next inhalation is initiated

These phases can be enhanced when the breathing cycle is exaggerated by taking a very slow and comfortable deep breath. When trying this technique, try to isolate and recognize these four phases by identifying them as they occur. Remember not to hold your breath at any one time during each phase. Rather, learn to regulate your breathing by controlling the pace of each phase in the breathing cycle. Remember that diaphragmatic breathing is not the same as hyperventilation: This style of breathing is slow, relaxed, and as deep as feels comfortable. The most relaxing phase of breathing is the third phase, exhalation. In this phase the chest and abdominal areas relax, producing a relaxing effect throughout the body. When focusing on your breathing, feel how relaxed your whole body becomes during exhalation, especially your chest, shoulders, and abdominal region.

An Energy Breathing Exercise

There are three phases to this exercise, and you can use this technique either sitting or lying down.

1. First get comfortable, allowing your shoulders to relax. If you choose to sit, try to keep your legs straight. As you breathe in, imagine that there is a circular hole at the top of your head. As the air enters your lungs, visualize energy in the form of a beam of light entering the top of your head. Bring the energy down from the crown of your head to your abdomen as you inhale. As you exhale, allow the energy to leave through the top of your head. Repeat this 5 to 10 times, trying to coordinate your breathing with the visual flow of energy. As you continue to bring the energy down to your stomach area, allow the light to reach all the inner parts of your upper body. When you feel comfortable with this first phase, you are ready to move on to the second phase.

2. Now, imagine that in the center of each foot there is a circular hole through which energy can flow in and out. Again think of energy as a beam of light. Concentrating on only your lower extremities, allow the flow of energy to move up from your feet into your abdomen as you inhale from your diaphragm. Repeat this 5 to 10 times, trying to coordinate your breathing with the flow of energy. As you continue to bring the energy up into your stomach area, allow the light to reach all the inner parts of your lower body.

3. Once you have coordinated your breathing with the visual flow of energy through your lower extremities, begin to combine the movement of energy from the top of your head and your feet, bringing the energy to the center of your body as you inhale air from your diaphragm. Then, as you exhale, allow the flow of energy to reverse. Repeat this 10 to 20 times. Each time you move the energy through your body, feel each body region—each muscle, organ, and cell—become energized. At first it may be difficult to visually coordinate the movement of energy coming from opposite ends of your body, but this will become very easy with practice.

The Postpartum Transition

After the child is born, the mother goes through several weeks of postpartum transition called the **puerperium**. During this time, the physiological changes of pregnancy slowly reverse and the vagina and the surrounding structures recuperate from labor. Uterine tissue that is no longer needed is discharged for the first month or so after childbirth. The discharge, called *lochia*, at first resembles a heavy menstrual flow, then typically tapers off after a week or two. Following delivery, estrogen and progesterone levels, which were high during pregnancy, drop rapidly, reaching almost zero about 72 hours after birth.

During this period, the mother and her partner begin to adjust to their often demanding new life situation. Childbirth and infant care are exhausting. Many women experience the "baby blues," which are transitory mood changes involving tiredness, depression, loneliness, or fear. These feelings usually abate in the weeks following childbirth, but about 13% of women experience postpartum depression severe enough to be disabling and to require professional help (Ko et al., 2017). Postpartum mood changes are so common that experts suggest they may be related to the massive changes in hormone levels that accompany childbirth. Others, although not denying the effects of hormonal changes, point out that childbirth is a life transition that brings many changes and psychological adjustments for the woman, her partner, and other family and household members.

It is recommended that couples refrain from intercourse for several weeks following childbirth to allow the uterus and vagina to return to prepregnancy states. Intercourse is usually physically safe within 3 to 4 weeks after delivery, but this all depends on the mother's desire and comfort.

Breastfeeding

The preparation of the breasts for nursing begins in the early weeks of pregnancy with an increase in the number of milk ducts and the deposit of fat in the breast tissue. This growth causes breast tenderness early in pregnancy.

In addition to the increase in breast size, the nipples enlarge and often deepen in color. About midway into pregnancy, the breasts begin to manufacture **colostrum**, a yellowish precursor to actual mother's milk. For the first few days after birth, colostrum is the major substance emitted from the breasts. As the newborn nurses, colostrum is drained from the breasts and is replaced by mother's milk. Colostrum contains nutrients and is especially high in antibodies that protect the infant against infection. Mother's milk contains specific milk proteins, antibodies, lactose, fat, and water. The synthesis of milk is controlled by the pituitary hormone **prolactin**, the levels of which rise tremendously during pregnancy and are maintained as long as the mother continues to nurse.

Milk is delivered from the breast through the coordinated activity of the mother and infant. Inserting the nipple into the baby's mouth activates the baby's sucking reflex. When the baby sucks, nerve impulses that stimulate the release of the hormone oxytocin are transmitted from the breast to the mother's brain. Oxytocin circulates through the mother's bloodstream to the breasts, where it causes the muscle cells that line the milk ducts to contract and eject milk from the nipple. Oxytocin also stimulates contractions of the uterus, so breastfeeding helps return the uterus to its prepregnant size.

A mother can nurse for many months. As long as the baby is sucking and the breasts are regularly drained of milk, the hormonal stimulation of milk production will continue. Without such stimuli, milk production stops. The many advantages of breastfeeding include the following:

- It is economical, readily available, and eliminates the effort involved in purchasing, preparing, and heating bottles and formula.
- It transfers immunity (protection against infections) from the mother to the infant, and breast milk itself and the act of nursing stimulate the development of the infant's own immune defenses.
- Breast milk promotes development of the infant's digestive system.
- Breastfed babies have fewer allergies, less diarrhea, fewer dental problems, and less colic (stomachache).
- Breast milk is nutritionally balanced for human infants; formulas containing cow's milk are not nutritionally identical to human milk, although they are nutritionally adequate.
- Breastfeeding may increase the psychological attachment between mother and infant.
- The hormones involved in the production and release of milk cause uterine contractions, which help the uterus return to its normal size. During the first week or so after childbirth these contractions may be intense and even painful. Thereafter some women describe them as pleasurable, sensual, or erotic.

Many women find that breastfeeding offers them a relaxing, pleasurable experience with their babies. Often the pleasurable feelings of breastfeeding will have an

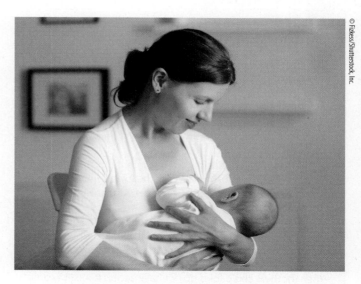

Breast milk provides a baby with essential nutrients and helps prevent infections.

erotic tone, possibly producing genital sensations and even occasionally orgasm. These feelings and responses are normal and natural, and a woman need not feel guilty or distressed by them.

The many advantages of breastfeeding do not mean that bottlefeeding is not wholesome. Many healthy, well-adjusted people were bottlefed infants. Some women are physically unable to breastfeed. Some mothers choose not to breastfeed because work, family, and other responsibilities make it inconvenient. Breastfeeding in public or at work is, unfortunately, still not acceptable in many communities or places of employment. Some women choose not to breastfeed because they fear that changes in the shape of their breasts will decrease their sexual attractiveness.

Some women breastfeed their infants for several weeks or months and then gradually substitute bottle feedings for breast feedings until the child is completely **weaned**, that is, has stopped nursing altogether. More important than whether the milk comes from the breast or a bottle is the physical contact and loving the infant receives while being fed.

TERMS

colostrum: yellowish precursor liquid to actual mother's milk contains antibodies and protein

prolactin: a hormone produced by the anterior lobe of the pituitary gland that stimulates milk production

puerperium: the six weeks after childbirth, also called postpartum period

wean: to discontinue breastfeeding, using other means to provide nutrients

Infant Mortality

The first year of any infant's life can be risky, especially if there is an insufficient healthcare system to intervene when a pregnant woman, an infant, or an infant's mother gets sick. The worldwide infant mortality rate (the rate at which babies die before their first birthday) is 42 deaths per 1,000 live births. This means that worldwide, 7.1 million infants die each year.

There is an enormous disparity in infant mortality among countries (**Table 9.3**). Monaco has the lowest infant mortality rate, at 1.80 deaths per 1,000 live births; Afghanistan is among the highest, at 112.8 deaths per 1,000 live births.

When mothers and babies have access to good health care, infant mortality is caused by serious birth defects, preterm delivery and low birth weight, automobile accidents, sudden infant death syndrome (SIDS), and infections, including HIV. When mothers and babies do not have access to health care, infants die because of complications surrounding childbirth, malnutrition, infection (e.g., HIV and malaria), unsanitary conditions, and absence of the mother or other caretaker.

The overall U.S. infant mortality rate is 5.8 deaths per 1,000 live births. The infant mortality rate in Canada is 4.60 deaths per 1,000 live births. The U.S. rate is higher than in other industrialized countries because many Americans do not have access to quality health care. The U.S. infant mortality rate varies by race. The rate for non-Hispanic Caucasians is 5.76 deaths per 1,000 live births; African Americans, 13.63; Hispanics, 5.8; American Indians and Alaskan Natives, 4.9; and Asian/Pacific Islanders, 8.06.

To reduce the rate of infant mortality in the world, the World Health Organization wants to increase the availability of health services to all mothers. To reduce the rate of infant mortality in the United States, the Department of Health and Human Services wants to increase the proportion of mothers getting early prenatal care; decrease the incidence of SIDS; lessen the percentage of pregnant women who smoke cigarettes, drink alcohol, and take other drugs; and reduce the number of low-birth-weight infants.

Table 9.3

Infant Mortality Rate (Deaths per 1,000 Live Births) in Various Countries*

Country	Rate	Country	Rate
Afghanistan	112	China	12
Somalia	97	Mexico	12
Chad	87	Panama	10
Uganda	58	Sri Lanka	9
Pakistan	54	Russia	7
Senegal	50	Qatar	6
Haiti	48	United States	6
Gabon	45	Cuba	5
India	40	Canada	5
Kenya	38	Denmark	4
Bolivia	36	Ireland	4
Azerbaijan	25	France	3
North Korea	23	Sweden	3
Brazil	18	Japan	2
Jordan	15		

Modified from U.S. Central Intelligence Agency. (2013). Country comparison: Infant mortality rate. *World Fact Book*. https://www.cia.gov/library/publications/the-world-fact-book /rankorder/2091rank.html

* Values rounded to nearest whole number.

Infertility

Approximately one in five of all American married couples of childbearing age is **infertile**, which means that they are unable to become pregnant after a year of trying. Male factors are responsible for infertility in about 40% of infertile couples; female factors are responsible in another 40% to 50%. In about 10% of infertile couples, no cause can be determined. With professional help, about half of all infertile couples can eventually have children. A significant percentage of couples medically determined to be infertile eventually have children without medical interventions. Permanent infertility is called **sterility**.

In both sexes, infertility can be caused by a variety of conditions that adversely affect the functioning of an otherwise normal reproductive system. For example, ill health, cigarette smoking, chronic alcohol use, marijuana and other drug abuse, exposure to radiation or toxic chemicals, malnutrition, anxiety, stress, and fatigue can lessen a person's reproductive capabilities. Medical treatments or changes in lifestyle can often restore fertility. Age also plays a role. Women in their 20s conceive more readily than women in their late 30s and early 40s.

Because sperm and ovum production and the functions of the male and female reproductive tracts are absolutely dependent on adequate hormone production, hormonal problems are a common cause of infertility in both men and women. Infertility can result from undersecretion of the hypothalamic hormone gonadotropin-releasing factor (GnRF) and from the pituitary hormones follicle-stimulating hormone (FSH) and luteinizing hormone (LH). Infertility also can be caused by abnormal synthesis or release of testosterone from the testes and estrogen and progesterone from the ovaries. Fertility often can be restored by augmenting low levels of hormones

> The reason grandparents and grandchildren get along so well is that they have a common enemy.
>
> *Sam Levenson*

with either natural or synthetic hormones such as clomiphene or pergonal. Use of such "fertility drugs," however, increases the chance of multiple births.

Infertility can also be caused by anatomical abnormalities or damage to the male or female reproductive systems. A common cause of damage is scarring and subsequent blocking of the fallopian tubes and, less frequently, the epididymis by gonorrhea or chlamydia infections. The scar tissue from such diseases blocks the tubes and prevents the passage of sperm and ova. Growths and tumors in the reproductive tract can also block the passage of sperm and ova. Sometimes surgical repair of blocked or damaged tubes can restore fertility.

Problems with insemination and sperm delivery and transport can also cause infertility. For example, a man may have difficulty getting and maintaining an erection or ejaculating into the vagina. A woman may produce very thick or voluminous cervical mucus, which can block entry of sperm into the uterus. Sometimes a couple has trouble conceiving because they are not having intercourse near the time of ovulation.

Enhancing Fertility Options

A variety of medical interventions are available to help infertile couples become pregnant. For example, conception is unlikely if fewer than 20 million healthy sperm are deposited in the vagina. If a man produces too few healthy sperm in a single ejaculate, sperm from several ejaculates may be combined and introduced into the woman's reproductive tract with a syringe; this procedure is called **artificial insemination**. If the male partner cannot produce sufficient numbers of healthy sperm even for artificial insemination, the couple may become pregnant by artificial insemination with semen from a donor. Each year in the United States, several thousand babies are conceived by artificial insemination.

Another way to try to overcome infertility is **in vitro fertilization (IVF)**, which is employed when a woman's fallopian tubes do not function properly and for other reasons, for example, to avoid passing an inherited disorder to a child.

In vitro fertilization involves the following steps:
- A doctor removing several ova (usually 2–12) that are ready for fertilization
- Obtaining healthy sperm from the male partner or male donor
- Fertilizing the eggs in a laboratory dish until at least one embryo develops to the 4- to 8-cell stage
- Administering hormones to the woman to prepare her body for pregnancy
- Inserting several embryos into the woman's uterus (several are implanted to increase the chance of pregnancy; remaining embryos are frozen and stored for future use if necessary)

The first baby to be conceived by IVF was born in England in 1978. Since then, more than 1 million babies worldwide have been conceived using IVF. Despite the widespread use of IVF, the procedure is not without risk, and it fails more often than it succeeds. The success rate for IVF as determined by resulting in a live birth ranges between 20% and 40% depending on many factors such as the woman's age, the experience of the medical professionals conducting the procedure, and the number of embryos inserted into the uterus (Centers for Disease Control and Prevention, 2016b). Even when only a single child is conceived by using IVF, the chance of delivering a low-birth-weight baby or one with congenital defects is about twice that for a baby conceived through sexual intercourse.

GIFT (gamete intrafallopian transfer) and ZIFT (zygote intrafallopian transfer) are similar to *in vitro* fertilization. With GIFT, the ova are placed in equal numbers in each of the fallopian tubes, and semen is introduced directly into the tubes. With ZIFT, eggs are fertilized *in vitro* and an embryo is placed in the fallopian tube. These procedures are successful between 10% and 20% of the time.

For some couples, the prospect of not being able to have a child is devastating. Many of these couples embark on lengthy efforts, which may cost many thousands of dollars and consume much of their emotional energy, to become pregnant and have a healthy baby. Such couples may be asked to keep careful records of the woman's fertility cycle and to time intercourse for maximum likelihood of conception. They may be counseled to have intercourse at certain times after hormone treatments. They may make repeated visits to fertility clinics to undergo IVF or other medical interventions.

About 40,000 infertile couples in the United States attempt to have a child using IVF techniques each year. However, for most of these couples repeated attempts to conceive end in failure. For women under age 35, the success rate, that is, giving birth to a healthy baby, is approximately 20%; for women over age 40, the success rate is under 10%. In addition to the poor success rate, couples can pay several thousand dollars for each attempt to become pregnant, and health insurance generally does not cover any IVF costs.

▌TERMS▐

artificial insemination: introduction of semen into the uterus or oviduct by other than natural means

infertile: unable to become pregnant or to impregnate

in vitro **fertilization (IVF):** a procedure in which an egg is removed from a ripe follicle and fertilized by a sperm cell outside the human body; the fertilized egg is allowed to divide in a protected environment for about 2 days and then is inserted into the uterus

sterility: the state of permanent infertility

Boy or Girl: Should Parents Have the Right to Choose?

American parents can opt for "family balancing" by choosing the sex of their next child. Although controversial, sex selection is regarded as an ethical decision by the American Society for Reproductive Medicine. Techniques currently available that allow parents to have a child of a desired sex are *in vitro* fertilization (IVF) and sperm sorting.

IVF: In vitro fertilization can guarantee the birth of a baby of the chosen sex. Several eggs are medically collected from the prospective mother and fertilized in a laboratory dish with the father's sperm. A single cell is removed from the developing embryo and analyzed to see if the chromosomes are XX (girl) or XY (boy). One or two embryos of the desired sex are then implanted into the uterus of the mother (or surrogate), who has been hormonally prepared for pregnancy. If the pregnancy is successful, one (or two) babies of the desired sex will be born. IVF is most commonly used to prevent a couple with known genetic defects from having a genetically handicapped child. In addition to sex, the embryo can be tested for the presence of specific genetic defects and only embryos without abnormal genes are implanted. IVF is particularly useful for preventing sex-linked traits, such as hemophilia and some forms of muscular dystrophy, from being inherited.

Sperm sorting: Sperm sorting separates sperm carrying an X chromosome from those carrying a Y chromosome. A woman can be artificially inseminated with sperm that will produce an embryo of the desired sex. This technique is far simpler and less traumatic to the woman than IVF, but its success rate is only about 90% for females and 75% for males. So, a couple has to be prepared to accept a child that is not of the desired sex if the sperm sorting method is used.

Sex selection has been condemned partly because in countries such as India and China, sex selection has been used to abort female fetuses because male offspring are more desirable. In India, mobile ultrasound scanners go from village to village, and, for a small fee, a woman can have the sex of her fetus determined. If it were a girl, the fetus often would be aborted. In India, this practice skewed the normal male-to-female ratio at birth of 106:100 to 130:100. Both India and China have banned the use of ultrasound scans for purposes of sex selection. In the United States, there is no evidence that ultrasound scans are used for sex selection and abortion of an undesired fetus.

Sex selection can be seen as a form of sexism—that people regard one sex as being inferior to the other. But, so far, in the United States sex selection has been used for family balancing: A couple with one or more children of one sex want to have a child of the opposite sex.

It's possible that sex selection will lead to selection of traits other than sex as more genetic tests become available. A couple might want their child to be tall, intelligent, muscular, or musical. Opponents of the new reproductive technologies argue that they open the door to "designer babies" in which parents choose the traits they desire in their children. This concept raises the specter of eugenics (selective breeding for "good" genes) as practiced by the Nazis, who introduced reproductive policies in the 1930s in which people with certain traits were encouraged to reproduce and others, such as Jews, Gypsies, and persons with disabilities, were exterminated.

Controversy over the use of new reproductive technologies and genetic testing for desired traits is certain to increase in the future.

Adoption

There are many reasons why adults may want to raise children who are not biologically their own. They may be partially motivated by a concern with overpopulation and a desire to give homeless children love and security. Another common reason is that a couple is unable to have children because of infertility. One alternative for couples, or even single people and gay couples, is adoption. Many adoptions bring the anticipated happiness to otherwise childless couples.

There are three avenues to pursue when couples would like to adopt a child. Most commonly, adoptions are handled through state-licensed *private* or *public adoption agencies,* usually nonprofit social services, which handle approximately 70% of all adoptions. An agency adoption may be the best option for adopting an older child or a child with special needs, although agencies also help in the adoption of infants and children from other countries.

Signing up with an adoption agency can be a lengthy process, often lasting several years.

Another way to adopt a child is through an *independent* or *private adoption.* The individuals wishing to adopt a child make arrangements with a woman who wants to give up custody of her child, often with an attorney, physician, or cleric serving as an intermediary. Every state has its own laws concerning independent adoption, and the prospective parents should know the laws in their state as well as the state of the birth mother. In all independent adoptions, the birth parents can give consent for adoption only after the birth of the child.

A third avenue to pursue is an *international adoption.* This is becoming an increasingly popular avenue for prospective parents. Both state and federal requirements must be met in international adoptions; however, the waiting period is not as lengthy as it is in private or public adoptions.

Critical Thinking About Health

1. "Hmmmm," muttered Dr. Johnson, the hospital's new chief of medicine, as he pored over the hospital's recent birthing statistics. Dr. Johnson's curiosity and concern were piqued by data showing a wide variation in the rates of labor induction among the medical practitioners at the hospital: Dr. Smith, 7%; Dr. Anderson, 12%; Dr. Tompkins, 45%; and Dr. Hastings, 74%. Dr. Johnson knew that the U.S. national rate was 20%, and at the hospital he managed prior to this assignment the rate was 12%.

   Following a hunch, Dr. Johnson checked the hospital's computerized records to determine the days and times of the births at the hospital for the previous 4 months. He discovered that Dr. Tomkins had only one weekend delivery during that time period, and Dr. Hastings had no weekend deliveries and only two after 2 A.M.

   Dr. Johnson investigated the medical records further and discovered that Dr. Hastings had noted in several patients' medical records that the women had requested labor induction for reasons of personal convenience. Although Dr. Johnson personally disagreed with the practice of inducing labor for reasons of convenience, he nevertheless believed that if something went wrong, compared to nights and weekends when the hospital was not fully staffed, weekday births were financially less risky for the hospital.

   Should Dr. Johnson do anything to change the labor induction practices at the hospital? If so, what should he do? If not, why not?

2. We know that drugs, alcohol, and smoking are dangerous to a developing fetus. Imagine that you are working as a server in a restaurant.
   a. What would you say or do if a customer who was pregnant ordered a glass of wine?
   b. What would you say or do if a customer who was pregnant was smoking a cigarette?

3. Comment on this point of view: People have been having babies for thousands of years. Nowadays, the entire process is way too medicalized with birthing classes, hospital delivery rooms, anesthesia, fetal monitoring, episiotomy, labor induction, cesareans, circumcision of male infants, and bottlefeeding.

Chapter Summary and Highlights

Chapter Summary

Becoming pregnant and giving life to a new human being is one of the most awe-inspiring and rewarding experiences in life. Becoming parents changes peoples' lives forever. Whereas many couples plan and strive to become pregnant, many others become pregnant unintentionally and are unprepared to take on the role of parent. People who are uncertain or who do not wish to be a parent should use one of the many available methods of contraception. Discussing pregnancy risks with a prospective partner should be undertaken early in a relationship. Having such a discussion can foster trust and understanding. Some couples who desire to become pregnant and have a child may find that one partner is infertile. Modern reproductive technologies now make it possible for many infertile couples to still have a child. Because of circumstances beyond their control, many babies and young children find themselves without parents. Adoption by persons and couples eager to take on the challenges of parenting gives orphaned children new lives and new hope.

   Good health habits during pregnancy are especially important. The pregnant mother-to-be is responsible for two lives, hers and her unborn child's. All tobacco smoking and consumption of alcohol should be stopped during pregnancy and when a woman is trying to become pregnant. No medicines should be taken without consulting a physician. Many medicines and exposure to many chemicals in the environment can cause developmental defects in the brain and/or body of a fetus. Pregnant couples want to give birth to a healthy child. The more couples learn about how to maintain a healthy pregnancy and the birthing process, the more likely the outcome will be joyful for all involved.

Highlights

- Conception, pregnancy, and childbirth are important and meaningful life experiences. The decision to become a parent requires psychological and physical preparation so every child can have parents prepared to meet its needs.

- Fertilization is followed by cleavages of the embryo as it moves into the uterus. About the sixth day after fertilization, the embryo implants in the lining of the uterus, and for the next 266 days or so the fetus develops. After 40 weeks of pregnancy a baby is born.

- Healthy habits during pregnancy such as good nutrition, seeking prenatal care, exercise and physical activity, and emotional well-being contribute to a successful pregnancy.

- Taking drugs, consuming alcohol, and smoking cigarettes during pregnancy can cause fetal damage or birth defects. Tests, such as amniocentesis or chorionic villus sampling, are available to determine whether birth defects are present.

- Optimal childbirth can be achieved by attending childbirth preparation classes, ensuring emotional support for the mother during childbirth, and

- making wise choices about medical interventions, such as episiotomy and pain management.
- Childbirth is divided into three stages. The first stage starts with the beginning of labor and lasts until the cervix is fully dilated. The second stage is the birth of the baby. The third stage is the delivery of the placenta.
- The period after childbirth may involve breastfeeding and resumption of sexual activities.

- Approximately 20% of American married couples are infertile. Some of these couples can be medically assisted to become pregnant; pregnancy also may occur with *in vitro* fertilization or artificial insemination.
- Adoption is an alternative for couples. Children can be adopted through a private or public adoption agency, in an independent or private adoption, or an international adoption.

For Your Health

Perhaps not now but some day you may consider becoming a parent. Use the "Parenthood and Me" questionnaire (see Workbook Chapter 9) to help clarify your motivations for possibly becoming a parent.

References

American College of Obstetricians and Gynecologists. (2015). Exercise during pregnancy. http://www .acog.org/Resources-And-Publications/Committee -Opinions/Committee-on-Obstetric-Practice /Physical-Activity-and-Exercise-During-Pregnancy -and-the-Postpartum-Period

American Society of Anesthesiologists. (2016). Practice guidelines for obstetric anesthesia: An updated report by the American Society of Anesthesiologists Task Force on Obstetric Anesthesia and the Society for Obstetric Anesthesia and Perinatology. *Anesthesiology, 124*, 270–300.

Centers for Disease Control and Prevention. (2016a). Birth defects: Data and statistics. Retrieved from https:// www.cdc.gov/ncbddd/birthdefects/data.html

Centers for Disease Control and Prevention. (2016b). 2014 *Assisted Reproductive Technology National Summary Report*. Atlanta, GA: U.S. Department of Health and Human Services.

Ko, J. Y., et al. (2017). Trends in postpartum depressive symptoms. *Morbidity and Mortality Weekly Report, 66*, 153–158. Retrieved from https://www .cdc.gov/mmwr/volumes/66/wr/mm6606a1 .htm?s_cid=mm6606a1_w#F1_down

Suggested Readings

Boston Women's Health Book Collective. (2011). *Our bodies, ourselves: Pregnancy and birth*. New York: Touchstone. A comprehensive, accessible, up-to-date book for expectant mothers.

Knoepfler, P. (2015). *GMO sapiens: The life-changing science of designer babies*. Singapore: World Scientific Publishing. Discusses cutting-edge biotech discoveries, including bioengineering, genomics, synthetic biology, and stem cells, that have made genetically modified people possible.

Murkoff, H., & Mazel, S. (2011). *What to expect when you're expecting*. New York: Workman Publishing. This popular guide to pregnancy covers every aspect of the prenatal period, from developmental stages to nutrition.

Recommended Websites

American Academy of Family Physicians

Provides information on a variety of topics related to pregnancy, childbirth, and caring for a newborn.

American Academy of Pediatrics

Information about immunizations, childhood illnesses, and child safety.

KidsHealth

Provides doctor-approved health information about children, from before birth to adolescence.

Motherisk Program at the Hospital for Sick Children, Toronto, Canada

Up-to-date information on the risk of medications on fetal development.

Parenthood.com

Tons of information about becoming pregnant, pregnancy, and parenthood.

Parents Place

Lots of information about pregnancy, including a detailed week-by-week pregnancy guide.

Design Credits: Sky image © yurok/Getty Images; Icon background: © jiris/Shutterstock, Inc.; Heart icon: © Olegro/Shutterstock, Inc.; Caduceus icon: © LarryRains/Shutterstock, Inc.; Globe icon: © Leone_V/Shutterstock, Inc.; Yoga icon: © jiris/Shutterstock, Inc.; Couple icon: © Nath Srikhajon/Shutterstock, Inc.

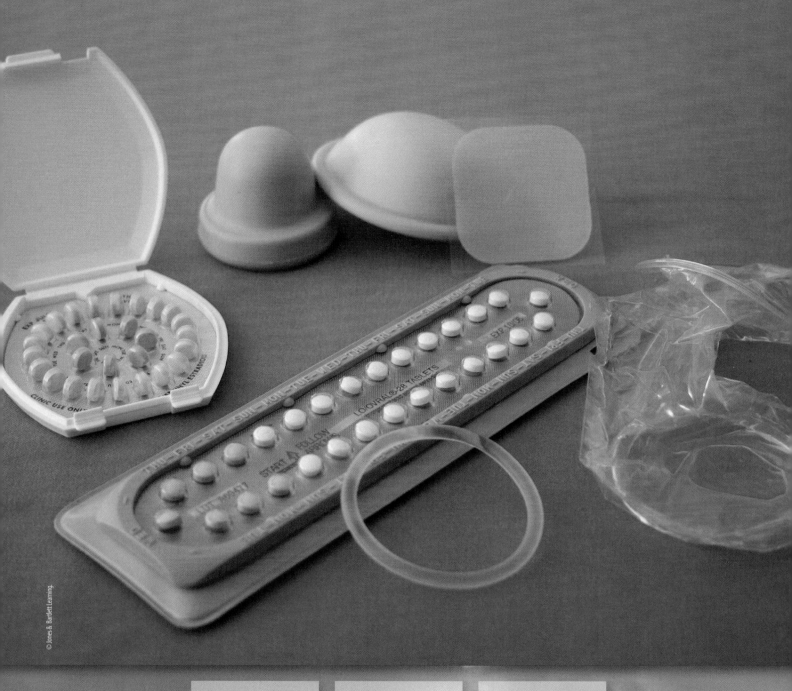

Health Tips

If You Missed Taking Your Hormonal Contraceptive

Global Wellness

Fertility Control Around the World

Wellness Guide

A Comparison of Contraceptive Methods

CHAPTER 10

Fertility Control

Learning Objectives

1. List five reasons for using fertility control.

2. State the typical and lowest observed failure rates for several fertility control methods.

3. List and describe four methods of combined hormonal contraception.

4. Describe two types of progestin-only contraception.

5. Explain how an IUD is used to prevent pregnancy.

6. List and describe five barrier methods of contraception.

7. Describe four fertility awareness methods of contraception.

8. Explain why many people do not use fertility control methods.

9. Describe male and female sterilization techniques.

10. Identify factors affecting fertility control decision making.

11. Describe methods of medical and surgical abortion.

Most North American women are fertile for almost 29 years (age 15 to 44). During that period of their lives, those in stable sexual relationships may have sexual intercourse many, many times. Yet, on average, North American women of childbearing age want only two children. This means that, for a variety of reasons (Table 10.1), most sexually active fertile North American women do not want to risk becoming pregnant unintentionally.

Fortunately, knowledge of human reproductive biology and modern biotechnology have produced an array of relatively safe, reliable methods to help reduce the risk of unintended pregnancy. (see the Wellness box, "A Comparison of Contraceptive Methods"). Some fertility control techniques are pre-conception methods (contraceptives). They work by preventing the development

> Whenever I hear people discussing birth control, I always remember I was the fifth.
>
> *Clarence Darrow*

or union of sperm and ova. Other techniques are post-conception methods. They inhibit the development of the fertilized ovum or embryo.

In the United States, there are about 61 million sexually active women in the most fertile stage of their lives (Daniels et al., 2015). Of this group, about 62% use some form of contraception (Table 10.2). About 19% are not sexually active or regularly sexually active, 5% are pregnant or just had a baby, 5% want to get pregnant, and 10% cannot get pregnant or are sexually active and do not take steps to avoid pregnancy. North American college students are frequent users of contraception (Table 10.3).

As you consider the topic of fertility control discussed in this chapter, keep in mind that sex without intercourse is a highly effective way to prevent pregnancy. Genital (penis-in-vagina) intercourse is not the only way to give and receive sexual pleasure. Touching, kissing, and stroking can bring intense sexual enjoyment and even orgasm to both partners.

A Comparison of Contraceptive Methods

Low effectiveness*

Method	Advantages	Disadvantages
Withdrawal	No health problems	Requires considerable ejaculatory control
Spermicides	No health problems; no prescription required	Must be used with each incidence of intercourse; messy
Fertility awareness	No health problems	Difficult to predict "safe" days; several days of abstinence may be required
Female condom	No prescription required	Vaginal irritation; must be used prior to intercourse

Moderate effectiveness†

Method	Advantages	Disadvantages
Male latex condom	No health problems; no prescription required	May break or tear
Diaphragm	No health problems	Must be used before intercourse; must be fitted by a clinician
Cervical cap	Can remain in place for up to 24 hours	Must be fitted by a clinician; cervical irritation

High effectiveness‡

Method	Advantages	Disadvantages
Combination hormonal methods (pills, patch, ring, injection)	Easy to use; not intercourse dependent	Side effects; serious risks to health in some users
Progestin-only methods (mini-pill, injection)	Easy to use; not intercourse dependent	Side effects
IUD	Not intercourse dependent	Side effects; irregular bleeding, heavy menstrual bleeding and cramps; increased risk of pelvic infection
Surgical sterilization (tubal ligation; vasectomy)	One-time procedure	Some postsurgical discomfort

*Low effectiveness: Failure rate greater than 20%.
†Moderate effectiveness: Failure rate between 6% and 19%.
‡High effectiveness: Failure rate between 0% and 5%.

Table 10.1

Some Common Reasons for Fertility Control

Reason	Explanation
Enhancing sexual pleasure	Anxiety about the possibility of pregnancy can divert a person's attention from the sexual experience and interfere with the flow of sexual feelings. Also, worry during intercourse can cause difficulties with erection and ejaculation in men and with vaginal lubrication and orgasm in women.
Family planning	Safe, reliable fertility control affords couples the opportunity to plan the size of their family and the timing of their children's births. Couples can have children when the family's financial, personal, and social resources are sound and the parents' relationship is ready for raising a child or children.
Increasing women's life choices	Fertility control allows women to choose when to devote time and energy to various life pursuits, including parenthood. In the not-too-distant past, when fertility control methods were unreliable, it was difficult for a woman to integrate her personal goals with parenthood because she had little control over the timing of the births of her children.
Health considerations	Fertility control helps couples reduce the risk of passing a hereditary disease to children. Fertility control also is advantageous to women for whom pregnancy and childbirth may be a significant health risk. Fertility control can prevent pregnancy in teenagers, who experience more pregnancy-related problems than older women.
World overpopulation	Some couples keep their families small because they want to take some responsibility for limiting the growth of the human population. Some people fear that overpopulation will create pressures for food, water, living space, energy, and other resources.

Table 10.2

Contraceptive Choices of Sexually Active U.S. Women: 2011–2013

Contraceptive Choice	Percent (%)
Birth control pill	16.0
Female sterilization	15.5
Condom	9.4
Intrauterine device (IUD)	6.4
Male sterilization	5.1
Withdrawal	3.0
Injectable (Depo-Provera)	2.8
Contraceptive ring or patch	1.6
Rhythm methods	0.8
Implant	0.8
Other methods	0.4

Data from Daniels, K. et al. (2015, November 10). Current contraceptive use and variation by selected characteristics among women aged 15–44: United States, 2011–2013. *National Health Statistics Reports, Number 86*, 1–14.

Table 10.3

Contraceptive Behavior of North American College Students

	Male (%)	Female (%)
Had vaginal intercourse in past 30 days	41	49
Used protection last time had vaginal intercourse	49	54
Method		
Pill	62	58
"Shot"	5	7
Implant	7	6
Patch	2	1
Ring	3	3
IUD	8	9
Male condom	69	61
Female barrier	0	0
Spermicide	5	3
Rhythm	6	8
Withdrawal	29	33
Sterilization	2	2
Used emergency contraception in last 12 months	9	13
Unintentionally pregnant	1	1

Data from American College Health Association (2016a). *American College Health Association-National College Health Assessment II, Canadian Reference Group Data Report, Spring 2016*. Hanover, MD: American College Health Association, 2016. American College Health Association (2016b). *American College Health Association-National College Health Assessment II, Undergraduate Student Reference Group Data Report Spring 2016*. Hanover, MD: American College Health Association.

Choosing Fertility Control

No fertility control method is perfect for everyone. Except for total abstinence from sexual activity, no single method is 100% effective, 100% free of side effects, absolutely safe, financially available to everyone, and 100% reversible. Without a perfect contraceptive, avoiding an unintended pregnancy requires weighing the benefits and drawbacks of the various methods and choosing the one(s) that both partners are comfortable using and that they will use properly each time sexual intercourse takes place. Even the most technologically perfect contraceptive would fail if it were not used properly and consistently.

Most users of fertility control are principally concerned with two questions: How well does the method work? Is it safe? A fertility control method's effectiveness is measured in terms of its **failure rate**, which is the percentage of women who, on average, are likely to

TERMS

failure rate: likelihood of becoming pregnant if using a birth control method for one year

Table 10.4

Effectiveness Rates of Common Birth Control Methods

Method	Typical use failure rate (%)	Lowest observed failure rate (%)
No method (chance)	85	85
Withdrawal	22	4
Combination birth control pill	9	0.3
Contraceptive patch	9	0.3
Vaginal ring	9	0.3
Hormonal injection	3	0.3
Progestin-only pill	6	0.5
Hormonal implants	0.05	0.05
Copper-T IUD	0.8	0.6
Hormonal IUD	0.2	0.2
Male latex condom	18	2
Female latex condom	21	5
Diaphragm	12	6
Sponge		
No prior births	12	9
Prior births	24	20
Spermicides	28	18
Fertility awareness	24	3–5
Tubal ligation	0.5	0.05
Vasectomy	0.15	0.1

Data are percentage of women becoming pregnant using a method for one year. Typical use failure rate means the method was not always used correctly. Lowest observed failure rate means the method was nearly always used correctly and with every act of sexual intercourse.

Adapted from Trussell, J. (2011). Contraceptive failure in the United States. *Contraception, 83*, 397–404.

become pregnant using a particular method for a year. Each method has two failure rates: the **lowest observed** or "perfect" **failure rate**, a measure of how a method performs when used consistently and as intended, and the **typical use failure rate**, a measure of how a method performs allowing for all of the errors and problems typically associated with a method (**Table 10.4**).

Considerations about the safety of fertility control methods must take into account the health risks of a particular method, such as serious illness, the possibility of infection and its consequences, the risk of death, the risk of being unable to have children in the future, any effects on unborn children, and undesirable and unhealthful changes in the body.

Evaluation of a fertility control method's safety should also assess the physical and psychological consequences of an unintended pregnancy. These include the risks associated with terminating the pregnancy by abortion and the risks associated with carrying the pregnancy to term. Factors such as a woman's age, her physical health, whether she has had previous children, and her capacity to care for another child also need to be evaluated. Of course, the most serious risk associated with the use of any contraceptive is the risk of death, which is rare.

Withdrawal

The **withdrawal method** of fertility control (coitus interruptus) requires that the man withdraw his penis from the vagina before ejaculation. In theory, withdrawal prevents sperm from being deposited in the vagina and subsequently fertilizing an ovum. The male must exercise great control and restraint to withdraw the penis in time. Withdrawal is risky because a small emission may occur before ejaculation (pre-ejaculate), which may contain sperm, HIV, or other sexually transmitted bacteria or viruses. Even if no sperm are actually deposited in the vagina, pregnancy is possible if sperm are released near the vagina and enter later, perhaps inadvertently, through body-to-body contact.

Withdrawal can diminish a couple's sexual pleasure. When the man must concentrate on withdrawing and the woman is concerned about whether he will withdraw in time, neither is free to fully experience the pleasure of sexual intercourse.

Douching

Douching (rinsing of the vagina with fluid) after sexual intercourse is a method of birth control that is almost totally ineffective. After ejaculation in the vagina, thousands of sperm move through the cervix and enter the uterus within a few seconds. There simply isn't time to flush out sperm from the vagina before a significant number enter the uterus. Furthermore, the force from the spray of the douche may propel sperm into the uterus, aiding conception rather than preventing it.

Hormonal Contraceptives

In 1960, the U.S. Food and Drug Administration approved the use of hormonal contraceptives for women. Since that time, millions of American women and hundreds of millions of women worldwide have adopted this form of fertility control because of its high effectiveness, reversibility, tolerable side effects, ease of use, and low cost.

Combined Hormonal Contraceptives

Combined hormonal contraceptives contain two kinds of synthetic hormones that are chemically similar to a woman's natural ovarian hormones, estrogen and progesterone. The ways these agents prevent pregnancy are shown in **Table 10.5**. Combined hormonal contraceptives are available as pills, a skin patch, a vaginal insert, and by injection.

Combined contraceptive pills (birth control pills) generally come in packets of 21, 24, or 28 pills. A 90-day, extended-use pill is also available, which has the advantages of fewer menstrual cycles per year and less opportunity to forget starting up a new packet of pills after a menstrual period. A 365-day pill is also available. In the 21-pill packet, all the pills contain specific amounts of hormone. In the

Table 10.5

Mechanisms of Action of Estrogens and Progestogens Used in Oral Contraceptives

Hormone	Mechanisms of action
Estrogens	1. Inhibition of ovulation by suppressing the release of pituitary hormones FSH and LH
	2. Inhibition of implantation of the fertilized egg
	3. Acceleration of transport of the ovum in the fallopian tube
	4. Accelerated degeneration of the corpus luteum, which secretes progesterone, and consequent prevention of normal implantation of the fertilized ovum
Progestogens	1. Production of thick cervical mucus, which blocks sperm transport from the vagina to the uterus
	2. Change in the character of cervical mucus such that sperm are less able to effect fertilization
	3. Deceleration of ovum transport in the fallopian tubes
	4. Inhibition of implantation
	5. Interruption of the hormonal regulation of ovulation

FSH, follicle-stimulating hormone; LH, luteinizing hormone.

24- and 28-pill packets, 21 of the pills contain hormones; the others (called "reminder pills") are inert or contain iron to help prevent iron-deficiency anemia. The first pill in a packet is taken on a predetermined day, and one pill is taken each day thereafter. Approximately 2 days after the last active pill is taken, a menstrual period occurs.

A pill should be taken at the same time each day to increase its effectiveness. It is recommended that pill taking be associated with a routine activity, such as going to bed or tooth brushing, to lessen the risk of forgetting. Forgetting near midcycle, when an egg is available for fertilization, can result in a pregnancy.

The effectiveness of combined pills may be lessened when they are taken simultaneously with St. John's wort and possibly other herbs or certain other medications, such as antibiotics, anticonvulsants, and a variety of pain relievers and anti-inflammatory drugs. Pill users should consult a health professional about this possibility.

Approximately half the women using combined oral contraceptives experience unwanted and unintended side effects. Most of the time the side effects present little long-term risk to health, and often they disappear after several cycles on the pill. The more common of the less serious side effects are nausea, weight gain, breast tenderness, mild headaches, spotty bleeding between periods, decreased menstrual flow, increased frequency of vaginitis, increased depression, and lowering of the sex drive. Some other frequent side effects are considered beneficial by many women. Among these are lessening of acne, diminution and even absence of menstrual cramps, decreased number of menstrual bleeding days, and absolute regulation of the menstrual cycle, which can be important for travelers and athletes.

Studies indicate that pill use may help prevent certain diseases. Compared with other women, women who take combined birth control pills have about one-third the chance of developing pelvic inflammatory disease, one-half the chance of developing benign (noncancerous) breast disease and ovarian cysts, nearly complete protection against ectopic pregnancy, and one-half the risk of developing iron-deficiency anemia. Data also indicate that combination birth control pills may protect against rheumatoid arthritis, endometrial cancer, and ovarian cancer.

There is no evidence that long-term fertility is lessened by using combined hormonal contraceptive pills, even after many years of use. Some women, however, experience menstrual irregularities in the first few months after discontinuing the method. Even so, they can still become pregnant soon after discontinuing the pill. There is no association between pill use and subsequent birth defects in children born to pill users, unless a woman ingests pills while she is pregnant (e.g., becomes unintentionally pregnant while taking the pill). In this case, birth defects are possible because the hormones in the pills may damage the embryo and fetus.

For a small percentage of women, combined oral contraceptives present a risk of fatal blood clots and heart attack. Women most at risk are those who are over age 35 and those who smoke cigarettes. These women should consider using a birth control method other than the pill. Any pill user who experiences severe abdominal pain, chest pain, headaches, unusual eye problems (blurred vision, flashing lights, temporary blindness), or severe calf and thigh pain should consult a physician or family planning agency immediately. The risk of developing liver disease, gallbladder disease,

TERMS

combined hormonal contraceptives: pills, a skin patch, a vaginal insert, and injections that contain two kinds of synthetic hormones that are chemically similar to a woman's natural ovarian hormones, estrogen and progesterone

douching: rinsing the vaginal canal with a liquid; not an effective means of birth control or STD prevention

lowest observed failure rate: likelihood of becoming pregnant if using a birth control method consistently and as intended

typical use failure rate: likelihood of becoming pregnant considering all the potential problems associated with a birth control method

withdrawal method: removing the penis from the vagina just prior to ejaculation; also called coitus interruptus or pulling out

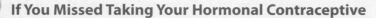

If You Missed Taking Your Hormonal Contraceptive

Being late or not taking a hormonal contraceptive can increase the risk of pregnancy. No matter what type of oral contraceptive you take, if you take it late or miss taking it:

1. Contact your healthcare provider to ask what to do. You can also check the patient package insert, and the pill manufacturer's website.
2. Use a backup birth control method (e.g., diaphragm; sponge plus condom) for the rest of that pill cycle.

General rules for late pill taking
- More than 12 hours late: Take the "late" pill and use a condom for the next week.
- Between 12 to 24 hours late: Take the "late" pill as soon as you remember, and take the regular pill for that day at the scheduled time. Use condoms for the next week.

Combination pills
- Take the missed pill as soon as you remember, and take the next pill at the regular time, even if you take two pills in one day.
- If you miss any of pills 15 to 21, ask your doctor or pharmacist for special instructions. She or he may ask you to continue taking your pills but to start a new pack instead of taking the remaining pills.
- If you forget to take two or more pills, contact your healthcare provider for instructions. Depending on the type of pill, you may need to start a new pack or double up on pills for a while.

Progestin-only pill
- Take the missed pill as soon as you remember, and take the next pill at the regular time, even if you take two pills in one day. Use a backup method for the next 2 days.

Contraceptive patch
- The patch contains 2 days of extra hormone. If left on for more than 9 days, use a backup method for the remainder of the cycle.

Contraceptive ring
- The ring contains a week's worth of extra hormone. Women should check the ring periodically to be sure it is in place and removed when required.

high blood pressure, and stroke is also slightly greater for pill users.

An alternative to hormonal contraceptive pills is a hormone-containing *skin patch,* which is applied to the lower abdomen, buttocks, or upper body (not the breasts) and which releases hormones slowly. Each patch is worn continuously for 1 week and then replaced with a new patch on the same day of the week for a total of 3 weeks. The fourth week is patch free. This is when menstruation occurs. In general, the patch is similar to the pill in effectiveness, side effects, and risks. Occasionally, the patch does not stay attached to the skin and contraceptive effectiveness is lost. Also, some women experience skin irritation and discontinue the patch. The product may be less effective in women whose bodies are large.

Another combined hormonal method is the *vaginal contraceptive ring,* a flexible device about 2 inches in diameter containing hormones that are similar to the active ingredients in combined contraceptive pills. A woman inserts the ring herself. After the ring is inserted, the hormones are continuously released. A ring is used for 3 weeks, then removed. After 7 days, during which time a menstrual period occurs, a new ring is inserted. The ring is highly effective and has the same side effects and risks as hormonal contraceptive pills. One additional caution is that the ring can be expelled before the 3 weeks are over. If the ring has been out of the vagina for more than 3 hours, an additional method of contraception (generally a barrier method) must be used until the ring has been back in place for 7 days. Other side effects of the vaginal ring include vaginal discharge, vulvovaginitis, and irritation.

Progestin-Only Contraceptives

Progestin-only contraceptives are available as pills, implants, and injectables. Progestin-only contraceptives work by inhibiting ovulation and thickening the cervical mucus, making it more difficult for sperm to reach the egg. They also cause changes in the lining of the uterus that damage sperm and make implantation less likely to occur. Side effects may include menstrual irregularities, weight gain, depression, fatigue, decreased sex drive, acne or oily skin, and headaches. Progestin-only contraceptives are completely reversible. A woman returns to her previous level of fertility when she stops using any of the progestin-only methods.

The **mini-pill** is a progestin-only pill containing 0.35 milligrams of progestogen or less. Twenty-one pills are taken one a day, and then pill taking stops for a week to allow for a menstrual period.

Progestin-only implantation methods (e.g., *Nexim-planon*) involve inserting a 1.5-inch hormone-containing plastic rod under the skin, where it remains for 4 years. During this time the hormone continuously seeps into the user's bloodstream and brings about its contraceptive effects. Implantable methods are very effective, but their common side effects (irregular bleeding, prolonged bleeding, frequent bleeding, and absence of menstruation) are responsible for frequent discontinuation of the method.

Progestin-only injectable methods (e.g., *Depo-Provera*) involve injecting a 12-week supply of a hormone intramuscularly. The hormone is released at a steady rate. At the end of the 12 weeks, a replacement injection or another contraceptive must be obtained.

To stop using Depo-Provera, the woman does not get the next injection. Most women who get pregnant do so within 12 to 18 months of the last injection. This method can be used while breastfeeding, starting 6 weeks after delivery. The FDA warns that prolonged use of Depo-Provera can increase the risk of bone loss.

The Intrauterine Device

The **intrauterine device (IUD)** is a small device, containing copper or the hormone progesterone, inserted by a healthcare professional into a woman's uterus (**Figure 10.1**). A short string hangs into the vagina where it cannot be seen but where a woman can reach up and feel for its

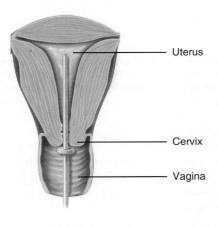

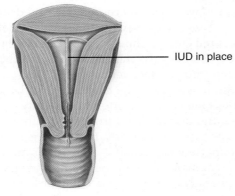

Uterus

Cervix

Vagina

IUD in place

■ **Figure 10.1**

The IUD

The IUD is inserted past the cervix into the uterus. Prior to insertion, the length of the uterus is measured with an instrument called a sound. Upon insertion the arms of the IUD gradually unfold. Once the inserter is removed, the threads attached to the IUD will be clipped to extend into the vagina through the cervical opening.

placement once a month. The most likely mechanisms by which IUDs work include killing or weakening sperm and altering the timing of the ovum's or embryo's movement through the fallopian tube.

IUDs available in the United States are flexible plastic devices shaped like a T. One type is impregnated with hormone (progesterone or a synthetic progestin). Another type is wrapped with fine copper wire, which slowly dissolves and releases copper ions. Both the hormone and copper augment an IUD's effectiveness by damaging sperm and slowing sperm migration in the woman. Some IUD users experience heavier menstrual flow or menstrual cramps. IUD use is associated with an increased risk of pelvic inflammatory disease and uterine perforations with insertion, and ectopic pregnancy.

Barrier Methods

Barrier methods of fertility control involve devices that physically block the path of sperm movement in the female reproductive tract and usually bring sperm in contact with a sperm-killing (spermicidal) chemical, most often nonoxynol-9. Several contraceptive methods work on this principle, including the diaphragm; the cervical cap; the contraceptive sponge; spermicidal foams, jellies, and creams; and the condom.

The Diaphragm

The **diaphragm** is a dome-shaped latex cup, which is placed in the vagina to cover the cervix (**Figure 10.2**). A metal spring in the rim of the diaphragm holds the device snugly in place between the back wall of the vagina and the pubic bone in the front of the pelvis. In this position the diaphragm blocks the movement of sperm from the vagina to the uterus, although it does not fit snugly enough to keep all of the sperm out. Its primary purpose

▌T E R M S▐

diaphragm: a soft, rubber, dome-shaped contraceptive device worn over the cervix and used with spermicidal jelly or cream

intrauterine device (IUD): a flexible, usually plastic, device inserted into the uterus to prevent pregnancy

mini-pill: a progestin-only contraceptive pill

progestin-only contraceptives: work by inhibiting ovulation and thickening the cervical mucus; completely reversible

progestin-only implantation methods: inserting a 1.5-inch hormone-containing plastic rod under the skin, where it remains for three years

progestin-only injectable methods: injection of a 12-week supply of hormone, which is released at a steady rate

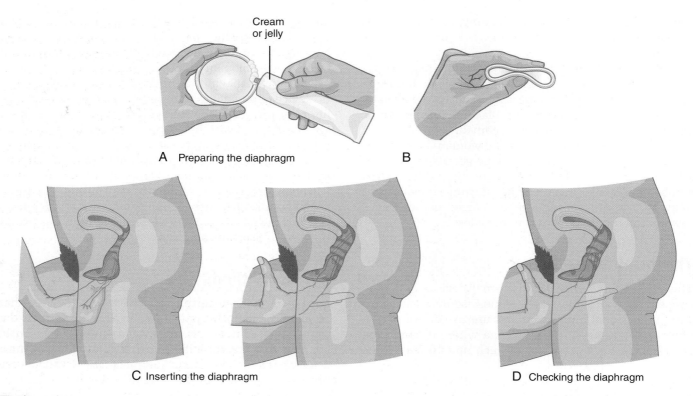

A   Preparing the diaphragm   B

C   Inserting the diaphragm   D   Checking the diaphragm

■ **Figure 10.2**

Procedure for Inserting a Diaphragm

(a) Before inserting the diaphragm, coat the rim and cup with a spermicidal cream or jelly. (b) Squeeze the rim of the diaphragm together between your thumb and index finger. (c) Insert the diaphragm into the vagina with the rim facing up and push it toward the small of your back. As you let go of the diaphragm, it will spring open; continue to guide it to your cervix with the tips of your fingers. (d) Be sure to check that the diaphragm completely covers the cervix.

is to hold a spermicide in place next to the cervix. Correct usage requires that the rim and cup of the diaphragm be coated with a tablespoon or two of a spermicidal jelly or cream. The diaphragm should be left in place 6 to 8 hours after intercourse. The spermicides used with the diaphragm also help prevent the transmission of some microorganisms responsible for genital infections.

One major advantage of the diaphragm is the absence of major medical problems associated with its use. A very few women or their partners may be allergic to the latex or the spermicide, and some develop urinary tract infections. Some women may experience discomfort with the diaphragm in place. Changing brands or getting a better-fitting diaphragm often solves these problems.

Another advantage is that the diaphragm can be inserted up to 6 hours before intercourse, so a couple does not have to interrupt sexual pleasuring to insert the device. If a diaphragm is inserted several hours before sexual activity, however, it is advisable to put an additional amount of spermicidal jelly or cream into the vagina before intercourse. The diaphragm must be left in place 6 to 8 hours after last intercourse, but should not be left in place longer than 24 hours because of the possible risk of toxic shock syndrome.

Each woman must be fitted (by a family planning professional or a physician) with a diaphragm that is the correct size for her. The need for proper fitting is one reason that

diaphragms are available only by prescription. Any change in a woman's body size—a gain or loss of several pounds, pregnancy, or pelvic surgery—is reason to check the fit and have a new diaphragm prescribed if necessary. A woman should not use another woman's diaphragm because the fit might be wrong, lowering the device's effectiveness.

After each use the diaphragm should be washed with mild soap and water, rinsed thoroughly, and dried in the air or with a towel. Perfumed talcum powders, petroleum jelly, or scented creams should not be used with the diaphragm. Occasionally the rubber darkens, but this generally does not impair effectiveness.

One disadvantage of the diaphragm is the possibility of dislodgment during intercourse. Only rarely will a man feel the diaphragm during sexual intercourse if the device is inserted properly. If either the man or the woman experiences unusual sensations or discomfort during intercourse, then the diaphragm may not be inserted correctly, it may have become dislodged during intercourse, or it may be the wrong size. Another disadvantage of the diaphragm is an increased risk of toxic shock syndrome. Women with a history of toxic shock syndrome are advised to use a different method.

Periodically the diaphragm should be held against a light to check for tiny holes and weak spots (where the rubber buckles). With proper care a diaphragm will last a year or two.

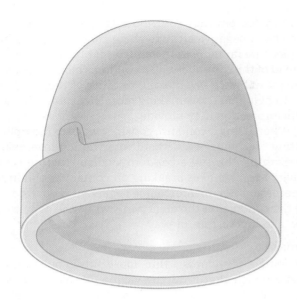

■ **Figure 10.3**
Cervical Cap

The Cervical Cap

The **cervical cap** is a cup-shaped rubber device that snugly covers the cervix similar to the way a thimble fits on a finger (**Figure 10.3**). Like a diaphragm, a cervical cap needs to be coated with spermicide to be as effective as possible and remain in place for 8 hours after last intercourse. Cervical caps come in several sizes and must be fitted for each woman. One difference between the diaphragm and the cervical cap is the fact that the cervical cap can be inserted up to 24 hours before intercourse.

The major disadvantages of the cervical cap are difficulty with insertion and removal, occasional discomfort during intercourse, dislodgment during intercourse, and possibly irritation of the cervix. The cervical cap should not be left in place for more than 48 hours.

The Contraceptive Sponge

The **contraceptive sponge** is a dome-shaped device made of a compressible, spongy material, which is inserted in the vagina to cover the cervix. The sponge contains **spermicide**, so it prevents pregnancy by blocking, absorbing, and destroying sperm. Once inserted, the sponge can be left in place for 24 hours. After use, it is discarded. The sponge is less effective than the diaphragm or cervical cap but more effective than spermicides alone. If left in the vagina longer than 24 hours, the risk of toxic shock syndrome increases. Information about toxic shock syndrome is included with product information. The sponge is available without a doctor's prescription.

Vaginal Spermicides

When used alone, spermicidal chemicals, such as nonoxynol-9 or octoxynol-9, can provide some degree of contraception. The chemicals are available as foams, creams, jellies, and suppositories without a doctor's prescription. Spermicides are placed in the vagina immediately before intercourse and before every subsequent intercourse in a sexual episode. Although often displayed in stores with feminine hygiene products, vaginal spermicides are not to be confused with douches, deodorants, or vaginal lubricants, none of which are effective as contraceptives.

The effectiveness of all of the vaginal spermicides depends on a sufficient quantity of sperm-killing chemical bathing the cervix at the time of ejaculation. Users must put the spermicide in the vagina immediately before every act of intercourse and before each subsequent intercourse in the same sexual encounter.

Users of foam should be sure that the foam is frothy and bubbly, which is achieved by shaking the container about 20 times before filling the applicator. Because there is no way to know how much foam remains in a container, a spare container should be kept on hand.

Vaginal spermicides tend to be slippery, which occasionally can be a nuisance, but the moisture can augment a woman's natural vaginal lubrication and enhance sensation. In rare instances, someone may be allergic to a particular product. Changing brands may alleviate this problem. Some women experience irritation if a suppository has not dissolved completely before intercourse takes place. Spermicides do not cause birth defects.

Male Condoms

The male **condom**, or rubber, is a membranous sheath that covers the erect penis and catches semen before it enters the vagina. About 99% of male condoms are made of latex or polyurethane; the rest, so-called skin condoms, which are not effective against STDs, are manufactured from lamb intestines.

When stored in a cool, dry place, condoms retain their effectiveness for up to 5 years. Kept in a warm environment, such as in a wallet, in the back pocket of one's pants, or in the glove compartment of a car, the latex will deteriorate. To be most effective, condoms must be used with water-based lubricants, such as K-Y Jelly, because petroleum-based lubricants, such as Vaseline, destroy the latex.

A primary reason for condom failure in preventing pregnancy is error in use. Used in conjunction with

---

TERMS

cervical cap: small latex cap that covers the cervix, used with spermicidal jelly or cream inside the cap

condom: a latex or polyurethane sheath worn over the penis (male condom) or inside the vagina (female condom); can be both a barrier method of contraception and act as a prophylactic against sexually transmitted diseases

contraceptive sponge: a dome-shaped device coated with spermicide

spermicide: a chemical that kills sperm; particularly foams, creams, gels, and suppositories used for contraception

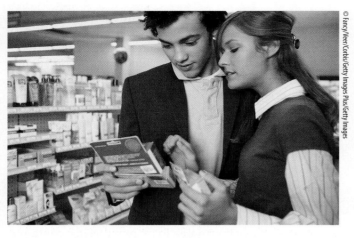

Condoms are an effective form of fertility control and provide protection against STDs. It's important that both partners take responsibility for using condoms.

another barrier method, such as a diaphragm or spermicidal foam, condoms are nearly 100% effective. Another advantage is that condoms help prevent the transmission of chlamydia, gonorrhea, herpes, HIV infection, and other kinds of infections.

Some people complain that the condom diminishes pleasurable sensations, but the device does not totally block genital feeling, which, in any event, is only one

of many factors that contribute to sexual arousal and pleasure. A negative attitude about condoms may diminish pleasure far more than a thin layer of latex ever could. Instead of thinking about how condoms block sensations, it might enhance lovemaking to think of them as a fun way to help make lovemaking more pleasurable because of the protection they provide.

When using a condom, consider ways to incorporate putting on the device without interrupting lovemaking. For example, having a condom available before sexual activity begins makes breaking off contact to obtain one unnecessary. Before intercourse begins, either partner can put the condom on the erect penis while the couple continues to fondle, talk, or play.

Female Condoms

The female condom is a thin, loose-fitting polyurethane plastic pouch that lines the vagina. It has two flexible rings: an inner ring at the closed end, used to insert the device inside the vagina and hold it in place, and an outer ring that remains outside the vagina and covers the external genitalia. **Figure 10.4** shows the insertion and positioning of the female condom. Because the device is made from polyurethane, which is 40% stronger than latex, the female condom can be used with any type of lubricant without compromising the integrity of the device.

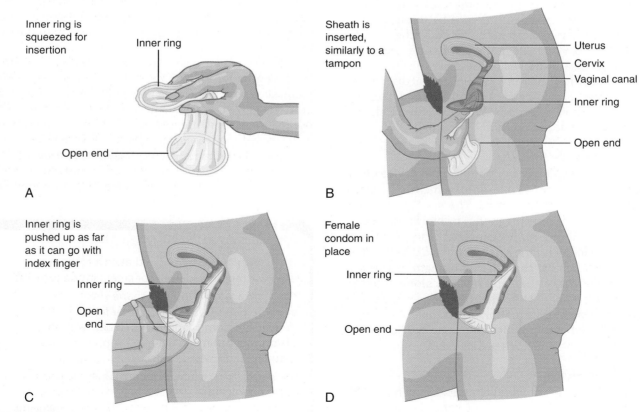

■ Figure 10.4
Female Condom Insertion and Positioning

Two advantages of the female condom are that it warms up instantly to body temperature once it is inserted, thus enhancing sensation for both partners, and it provides protection from STDs (by covering both internal and external genitalia), including HIV, and prevents pregnancy. The female condom can be obtained in drugstores and supermarkets, and it can be used by people allergic to latex or spermicide.

A disadvantage of the female condom is that occasionally the outer ring may be pushed inside the vagina. Other problems include difficulties in insertion and removal; minor irritation; discomfort or breakage, which can be decreased by using enough lubrication; and that it costs more than male condoms.

Fertility Awareness Methods

Fertility awareness methods (also called natural family planning, the rhythm method, or periodic abstinence) attempt to determine when an ovum has been released from the ovary and is capable of being fertilized. In general, the time when a woman is most fertile occurs 14 days before her next menstrual period, or midcycle in a woman with a regular 28-day cycle.

Fertility awareness methods of birth control either estimate when ovulation is most likely to occur or indicate when ovulation has already taken place, thereby telling a couple the days in the menstrual cycle not to have unprotected intercourse. Those are referred to as "unsafe days." The days when a woman is not likely to be fertile are referred to as "safe days." On unsafe days, a couple should use an alternative method of birth control, such as condoms, a diaphragm, or spermicidal foam. Other options include enjoying ways of sexual pleasuring other than genital intercourse or practicing complete sexual abstinence.

Couples using fertility awareness methods should realize that, even on safe days, fertilization is still possible because of natural variations in a woman's reproductive processes. Therefore, safe days are really *relatively* safe days.

Fertility awareness offers the advantages of posing no health risks; furthermore, some people's religious convictions make fertility awareness the only acceptable method of birth control. The effectiveness of fertility awareness is among the lowest of the common methods, about 25 pregnancies per 100 women per year. Failures occur because people do not keep careful records, they find the intervals of abstinence during the unsafe days too long, and they find having to plan sex only for the safe days a hindrance to spontaneous lovemaking.

Calendar Rhythm

Calendar rhythm is a way to estimate the most likely fertile, or unsafe, days in a woman's menstrual cycle by assuming that

1. Ovulation usually takes place 14 days (plus or minus 2 days) before the onset of the next menstrual flow.

2. An ovum is capable of being fertilized for 24 hours.
3. Sperm deposited in the vagina remain capable of fertilization for up to 3 days.

Using calendar rhythm effectively requires knowledge of the female fertility cycle and instruction in doing the calculations correctly (**Figure 10.5**). Family planning agencies, women's health clinics, books, and websites on fertility awareness methods can be helpful in learning the method.

The Temperature Method

The **basal body temperature (BBT)** is the lowest temperature in a healthy person during waking hours. In 70% to 90% of women, the BBT rises approximately 1°F after ovulation, presumably because of changes in hormone levels. By keeping a daily record of the BBT, a woman can determine when ovulation has occurred and therefore the unsafe and safe days for intercourse between ovulation and the beginning of the next menstrual cycle. Because the BBT method cannot predict when ovulation will occur, a woman must still estimate with another fertility awareness method (calendar method, mucus method) the safe and unsafe days before ovulation.

Temperature measurements should take at least 5 minutes. Temperature measurements should be taken at the same time each day, and a record should be kept on a graph (**Figure 10.6**). Once the BBT has risen for 3 consecutive days, a woman can assume that ovulation has taken place and that the rest of the days in that menstrual cycle are safe for unprotected intercourse.

The Mucus Method

Certain hormone-sensitive glands in the cervix produce mucus that changes in amount, color, and consistency during different phases of the menstrual cycle. Learning to recognize the changes in cervical mucus can help determine when ovulation occurs, and safe and unsafe days for intercourse can be planned accordingly.

The mucus method requires that cervical mucus be examined frequently during the cycle. Samples of mucus may be obtained with a finger, on toilet tissue, or from

TERMS

basal body temperature (BBT) method: uses daily body temperature readings taken immediately after waking to identify the time of ovulation; approximately 24 hours after ovulation, the BBT increases

calendar rhythm: estimation of fertile, or unsafe, days to have intercourse

fertility awareness methods: methods of birth control in which a couple charts the cyclic signs of the woman's fertility and ovulation and/or uses basal body temperature, mucus changes, and other signs to determine fertile periods

■ **Figure 10.5**

Calendar Rhythm Method
The calendar rhythm method is based on avoiding intercourse when sperm can fertilize an ovum. Unsafe days for intercourse in this chart are days 12 to 16.

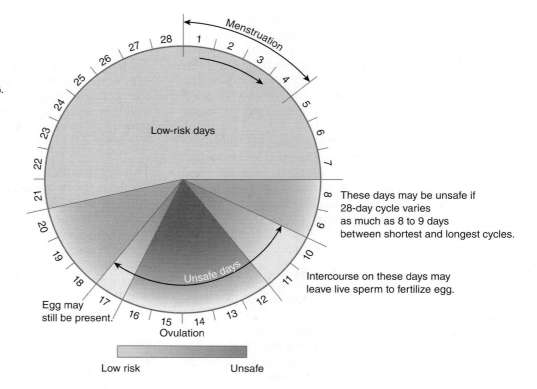

discharge on underpants. Collection with a finger is best because it permits direct determination of the amount and consistency of mucus.

Because douching, vaginal infections, semen, contraceptive foams and jellies, vaginal lubricants, medications, and vaginal lubrication from sexual arousal can interfere with the recognition of mucus patterns, women wishing to use the mucus method should obtain instructions from someone experienced with the method, a family planning

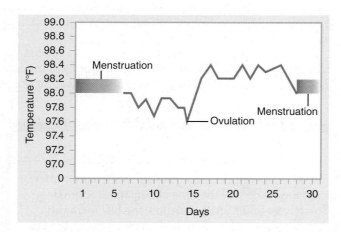

■ **Figure 10.6**

Basal Body Temperature Method of Contraception
A woman's body temperature rises about one degree during the days following ovulation. Once the BBT has risen for 3 consecutive days, assume that ovulation has taken place and that the rest of the days in that menstrual cycle are safe for unprotected intercourse. To use the BBT method, a woman must record her basal body temperature each morning before engaging in any activity. Temperature measurement should last at least 5 minutes.

clinic, or a health center. A woman should plan on charting her cervical mucus for at least a month to learn her individual pattern of mucus changes before relying on the method for fertility control.

The **sympto-thermal method** involves using the temperature and mucus methods simultaneously.

Chemical Methods

Two chemical methods of fertility awareness are available. Each estimates with considerable accuracy the expected time of ovulation. These products are usually marketed to couples who wish to become pregnant by knowing when an ovum is most likely to be available for fertilization. The same knowledge can be used to avoid intercourse and thereby lessen the risk of pregnancy. One method uses an at-home urine test to measure the amount of **luteinizing hormone (LH)** in a woman's urine, which sharply increases about 2 days prior to the time of ovulation. The other method uses a small device called a *fertility monitor* to test for changes in the composition of a woman's saliva around the time of ovulation.

Sterilization

Sterility is being permanently unable to have children. For people who are certain that they do not want children or, as is more often the case, no more children, surgical methods that render a person sterile but have no effect on sexual arousal or activities may be the most desirable form of birth control. Indeed, for American married couples over age 30, "permanent fertility control" (sterilization of

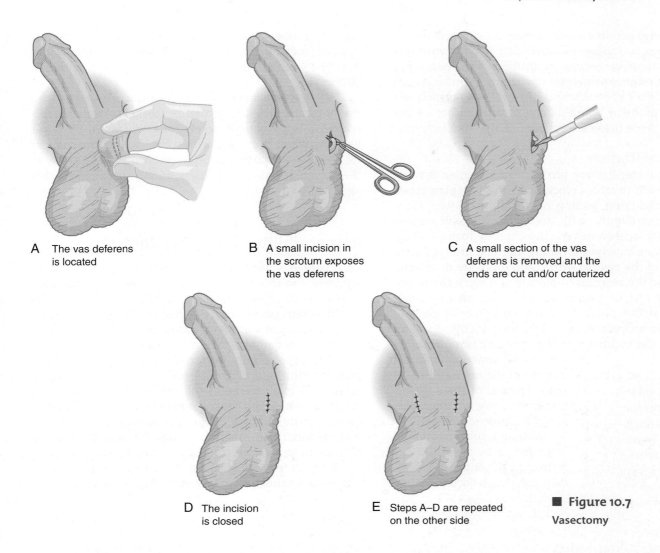

A   The vas deferens is located

B   A small incision in the scrotum exposes the vas deferens

C   A small section of the vas deferens is removed and the ends are cut and/or cauterized

D   The incision is closed

E   Steps A–D are repeated on the other side

■ **Figure 10.7**
Vasectomy

either the male or female partner) has become the most frequently chosen method of fertility control. The popularity of sterilization as a method of fertility control stems from its nearly 100% effectiveness, the relative safety of the procedure, and its relatively low one-time cost.

Male Sterilization

The sterilization of a man is called **vasectomy**. Approximately 500,000 men in the United States choose vasectomy every year. This procedure involves the cutting and tying of each of the two vasa deferentia, the sperm-transporting tubes between the testes (where sperm are made) to the penis (**Figure 10.7**). When these tubes are cut, sperm are no longer emitted upon ejaculation because their passage is blocked. Because the cut is made "upstream" from the organs that produce seminal fluid, a man still ejaculates, but the fluid contains no sperm. And because sperm make up only a small percentage of the total volume of the semen, neither a man nor his partner is aware of any change in their sex life, except that no other form of contraception is needed.

Although vasectomy should be considered a permanent form of contraception, it is sometimes possible to reverse the condition by rejoining the cut ends of the vasa deferentia. The success of vasectomy reversal as measured by the ability to have children again is about 50%, although some surgeons claim much higher reversal rates.

One of the reasons vasectomy is such a popular method of contraception is that it is uncomplicated and causes few problems. The procedure is usually carried out in a doctor's office with a local anesthetic in about 15 to 30 minutes. The incidence of postoperative complications

TERMS

luteinizing hormone (LH): anterior pituitary hormone that causes a follicle to release a ripened ovum and become a corpus luteum; in the male, it stimulates testosterone production and the production of sperm cells

sympto-thermal method: using both the basal body temperature and the mucus methods at the same time

vasectomy: a surgical procedure in men in which segments of the vasa deferentia are removed and the ends tied to prevent the passage of sperm

is very low, and within a week most men can return to regular activities, including sex. About one-half to two-thirds of vasectomized men develop antibodies to sperm, but there is no evidence to suggest that this is harmful. A man can be fertile for several weeks after vasectomy, because the sperm pathway contains sperm present before the vasectomy. Once these are ejaculated, the man is sterile.

Female Sterilization

The principal sterilization procedure for women is **tubal ligation**, which involves blocking of the fallopian tubes by cutting and tying, sealing, or closing them with clips, bands, or rings (**Figure 10.8**). Most tubal ligations are performed under local anesthesia in a clinic or doctor's office. The procedure involves entering the abdominal cavity and inflating the cavity (with carbon dioxide or nitrous oxide gas) so the surgeon can locate and block the tubes.

Usually one or two incisions about an inch long are made at the pubic hair line and/or belly button. Alternatively, an incision is made in the back of the vagina (*culpotomy*). The incidence of postoperative complications is very low; any complications that do occur are more to do with the skill of the surgeon rather than any inherent danger in the procedure itself.

Although tubal ligation is intended to be a permanent form of birth control, accidental pregnancies occur because a blocked tube spontaneously reopens. Surgical reversal of tubal blocking may be possible if a woman later decides that she wants to have children, with a success rate of 50% to 70%.

Another female sterilization technique is **hysterectomy**, the surgical removal of the uterus. Most experts do not recommend hysterectomy solely for sterilization purposes because, when compared with tubal ligation, the chances for postoperative complications are 10 to 100 times greater, the operation is more expensive, and the negative psychological effect may be greater.

Responsibility for Fertility Control

Most people engage in sexual activity because they want a joyous, rewarding experience. Because an unintended pregnancy can cause enormous hardship, birth control is an important part of every sexual relationship. Denying the possibility of pregnancy by assuming "it can't happen to me" is just gambling against the odds.

The responsibility for fertility control has two components. First, a fertility control method must be chosen, taking into consideration the nature of an individual's sexual activities or a couple's sexual relationship, the frequency of intercourse, future plans regarding children, and personal and religious values. Second, the chosen method must be used consistently and correctly.

For both technological and sociological reasons, there has been a tendency to associate the responsibility for

> If only one could tell true love from false love as one can tell mushrooms from toadstools.
>
> *Katherine Mansfield*

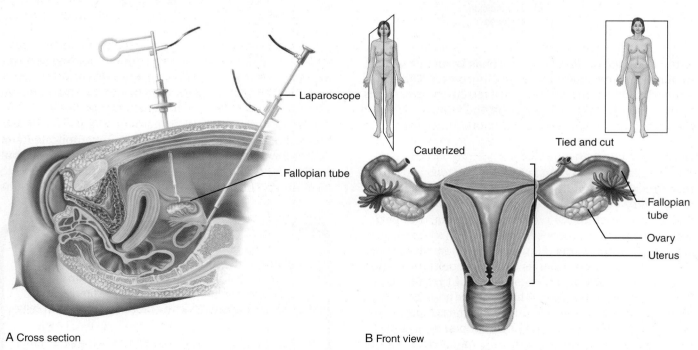

A Cross section

B Front view

■ **Figure 10.8**

Tubal Ligation

Female sterilization by laparoscopic ligation. (a) Side view: The tubes are located using a laparoscope and cut, tied, or cauterized through a second incision. (b) Front view: The tubes after ligation.

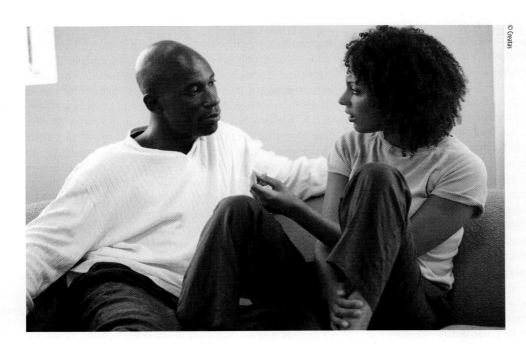

© Creatas

Choosing a fertility control method should be a decision made by both sexual partners and should be discussed before having sex.

fertility control with the partner for whose body a particular method is designed. For example, in the late nineteenth century, when withdrawal and the condom were the principal methods of fertility control, and women were not supposed to be interested in sex, men were considered to be the ones responsible for fertility control (when it was used at all). In the late 1960s, when the pill and IUD were heralded as "perfect" contraceptives and women began to assert themselves socially and politically, the responsibility for fertility control shifted almost totally to women.

Today, a large percentage of sexually active people believe that both partners in a sexual relationship should share the responsibility for fertility control. Yet, because so many methods are intended for use by the woman, in actual practice many women are left to manage fertility control on their own. Having to take total responsibility for fertility control can create resentment that blocks the feelings that many people wish to express with sex.

The responsibility for fertility control can be shared in a number of ways. The most important is to discuss it. In an ongoing relationship, there are many opportunities to talk about fertility control. Couples can go to fertility control clinics together, they can read and discuss information about the advantages and disadvantages of the different methods, and they can try out various methods to find out which are best suited for them. They can share the time and the financial costs of their chosen method, or they can divide responsibilities. For example, if a woman has to take time to go to a clinic or doctor, her partner could pay for the clinic visit and the contraceptives.

Partners can also share in using their chosen method. They can discuss any difficulties or concerns they have with their method of fertility control. Partners can even

remind each other to use their chosen fertility control method. A man can learn how a diaphragm is used, a woman can learn about the condom, and they can incorporate into their lovemaking preparing to use these and other barrier methods. Furthermore, partners can share the responsibility of inserting, removing, and cleaning the woman's diaphragm or cervical cap. If a woman is using fertility awareness methods, a man can share the responsibility by helping to determine the safe and unsafe days and by sharing the responsibility for abstaining from sexual intercourse when necessary.

Partners who share the responsibility for fertility control are more likely to use their chosen method(s) properly, which makes fertility control more effective. And reducing the fear of pregnancy makes sex more enjoyable. Another benefit of sharing this responsibility is that it tends to enhance intimacy in a relationship. The discussion of fertility control and the mutual decision making involved in choosing and using a method lead to better communication.

It is always a good idea for you to have some method of fertility control with you if you anticipate that sexual intercourse might occur. For example, both men and women can carry a condom or spermicides with them on dates or to parties if they think that sexual activity is a possibility.

TERMS

hysterectomy: surgical removal of the uterus

tubal ligation: a surgical procedure in women in which the fallopian tubes are cut, tied, or cauterized to prevent pregnancy; a form of sterilization

Talking About Fertility Control

A couple shares the responsibility for fertility control because both partners are responsible if an unintended pregnancy occurs. This fact alone is the most important reason for discussing fertility control. Although it is important to discuss fertility control before having sex, many individuals are embarrassed to do so. Talking about contraception implies that sex is going to take place, which may force an individual to face internal conflicts about engaging in sex. Many individuals subscribe to the myth that good sex should be spontaneous rather than planned. Therefore, sex and fertility control remain undiscussed. First-time partners may not discuss fertility control before sex because they fear spoiling a romantic mood.

Still, the best time to discuss fertility control is *before* sexual intercourse. A partner might say, "I would really like to make love (have sex) with you, and I want to be sure we're protected." That kind of introduction can be followed by a statement of preference and personal responsibility, such as, "I prefer to use condoms" or "I'm on the pill" or using a question such as "What birth control method do you prefer?" or "What are we going to do about control?"

In some cases, even if a man is concerned about an unintended pregnancy and sexual diseases, he may not feel comfortable bringing up the topic, fearing embarrassment or appearing ignorant or weak. Many women, however, appreciate a man who initiates a discussion of birth control. Communication about birth control and other sexual matters, such as the role of sex in a relationship, likes and dislikes, and preventing STDs, is vital to a healthy sexual relationship.

Why People Do Not Use Fertility Control

About 15% of sexually active, fertile American women do not regularly use birth control despite being at risk for an unintended pregnancy (Daniels et al., 2015). Contraceptive nonuse is responsible for half of the 3.1 million unintended pregnancies that occur each year in the United States. Some of the major reasons that people do not use fertility control, even if they wish to avoid pregnancy, include the following:

- *Low motivation:* People who have mixed feelings about avoiding pregnancy are less motivated to use fertility control. For example, a couple that has decided that they want to have a child "sometime in the near future" is less likely to be motivated to use fertility control than is a couple that is absolutely certain they do not want a child until some specified time, or at all.
- *Lack of knowledge:* Lack of knowledge about the process of conception and how to use fertility control effectively can lead to an incorrect perception of the risk of becoming pregnant. For example, some people

believe the myths that pregnancy is not possible if a woman has an orgasm, if she urinates after intercourse, or if she is having sexual intercourse for the first time. Sometimes a method is believed to be more effective than it really is, or the chosen method is used incorrectly. For example, some people erroneously believe that a woman is most fertile during the bleeding days of the menstrual cycle and thus practice fertility awareness at the wrong time. Some couples lose, misplace, or run out of their primary method and do not have a backup method available.

- *Negative attitudes about fertility control:* Some people believe that fertility control is immoral, a hassle, unromantic, or harmful. One's own negative attitudes or the perceived negative attitudes of others, such as peers or parents, can inhibit one from obtaining contraceptives. People use these as excuses not to visit doctors or clinics, or they may shy away from obtaining over-the-counter contraceptives.
- *Relationship issues:* Individuals in committed relationships are better contraceptors than individuals who are not in such relationships. Involvement with a committed partner tends to lessen guilt associated with sexual activity and hence improves attitudes about contraceptive practice. People in a committed relationship tend to have sexual intercourse more often and regularly, which gives the couple opportunities to talk about contraception and to become adept at using method(s). Individuals with irregular sexual contact, either because of geographical separation or relationship problems, may have difficulties in establishing a birth control regimen. In new or casual sexual relationships, there is a tendency to use no method or a poor method at first.

Emergency Contraception

Emergency contraception ("the morning-after pill") is designed to prevent pregnancy if fertilization might have occurred. Situations that warrant emergency contraception include having unprotected intercourse, misusing a contraceptive (e.g., forgetting to take birth control pills; condom slipping off), or sexual assault. Emergency contraception is not intended to be a primary birth control method.

There are two forms of emergency contraception, chemical and IUD insertion. The chemical form involves taking orally either levonorgestrel, a synthetic hormone present in oral contraceptives (sold as *Plan B One-Step* or *Next Choice*), or the drug ulipristal acetate (sold by prescription as *Ella*). Plan B One-Step and Next Choice are available for women and men over the age of 17 from a licensed pharmacy or clinic without a prescription; persons under age 17 can obtain them with a doctor's prescription. Both types of chemical emergency contraception are highly effective.

Emergency contraception with an IUD involves inserting a copper-T IUD up to 5 days after unprotected intercourse. This method is more effective than the chemical methods, reducing the risk of pregnancy following unprotected intercourse by more than 99%.

The World Health Organization recommends that women obtain an advance supply of emergency contraception pills because they must be taken soon after unprotected intercourse. Having emergency contraceptive pills on hand does not affect a woman's contraceptive use, does not increase her frequency of unprotected sex, and does not increase the frequency of emergency contraceptive use.

Abortion

Abortion is the intentional, premature termination of pregnancy. It is one of the oldest and most widely practiced methods of fertility control. Chinese medical writings from 2700 B.C. recommended abortion. In the United States each year, 6.1 million pregnancies occur. About 45% of these pregnancies are unintended, and about half of these unintended pregnancies end in **abortion** (Finer & Zolna, 2016).

Consider the following statistics on unintended pregnancies:

- 68% of women who use contraceptives consistently and correctly account for 5% of all unintended pregnancies.
- 18% of women who use contraceptives inconsistently or incorrectly account for 41% of all unintended pregnancies.
- 14% of women who do not practice contraception at all or who have contraceptive gaps of a month or more during the year account for 54% of all unintended pregnancies (Sonfield et al., 2014).

Currently, almost all developed countries permit abortions without restriction completely or with a few grounds, such as socioeconomic reasons. Less developed countries are more likely to restrict abortion (World Health Organization, 2012).

Two methods of safe, legal abortion are available: surgical and medication. **Surgical abortion**, also called *vacuum* or *aspiration abortion*, involves removing the postfertilization contents of the uterus with a vacuum instrument. **Medication abortion**, also called *chemical abortion*, involves the pregnant woman taking medications that stop pregnancy and force expulsion of the uterine contents. Surgical abortion is the more common of the two methods. It involves a local anesthetic, gradual widening of the cervix, and emptying of the uterus with gentle suction. It can be performed from as soon as pregnancy is confirmed up to the 10th week after fertilization. The procedure takes about 10 minutes.

Abortion between the 6th and 14th weeks of pregnancy is carried out by dilation and suction curettage, called D&C or vacuum aspiration. Anesthetic is used and the cervix is dilated. The uterus is then emptied with gentle, machine-operated suction. A curette (narrow metal loop) may be used to clean the walls of the uterus.

Dilation and evacuation (D&E) is performed after the 15th week of pregnancy. The cervix is dilated and the uterus is emptied with medical instruments, suction, and curettage. After the 20th week, abortion is very rare.

Medication abortion is carried out prior to the 7th or 8th week after fertilization. *Methotrexate* or *mifepristone* (also called *RU 486*) is given to a pregnant woman to block the action of the naturally occurring hormone progesterone, which is essential for successful implantation and pregnancy. Blocking progesterone's actions in the early phases of pregnancy causes a miscarriage. After the progesterone blockers, *misoprostol* (a type of hormone called a *prostaglandin*) is given to induce contractions of the uterus and expel the uterine contents within hours or days.

Medication abortion can be carried out as soon as pregnancy is confirmed and is effective up to 63 days after the last menstrual period. Medical abortion with methotrexate is about 90% effective; with mifepristone (RU 486), between 92% and 95% effective. RU 486 should not be confused with Plan B. RU 486 is used to discontinue a pregnancy. Plan B is used to prevent a pregnancy from occurring.

The procedure is overseen by trained medical personnel in a clinic over the course of a week, after which time a menstrual period occurs, which ends the pregnancy. Methotrexate and misoprostol can cause serious birth defects. The procedure carries a very small risk of toxic shock, which can be fatal. If a medication abortion is unsuccessful, a follow-up surgical abortion is usually performed.

A different form of medication abortion can be carried out after the 12th week of pregnancy. This method involves infusing saline (salty water), urea, or prostaglandin into the uterus. Saline and urea kill the fetus, and prostaglandin-induced uterine contractions empty the uterus.

> Tolerance implies no lack of commitment to one's own beliefs; rather, it condemns the oppression or persecution of others.
>
> *John F. Kennedy*

TERMS

abortion: the expulsion or extraction of the products of conception from the uterus before the embryo or fetus is capable of independent life; abortions may be spontaneous or induced

medication abortion: nonsurgical abortion using specific medications to stop pregnancy

surgical abortion: the most common abortion method, in which the uterus is emptied with the gentle suction of a manual syringe

Fertility Control Around the World

The World Health Organization estimates that 64% of married or in-union women aged 15 to 49 years in almost all regions of the world use some method of fertility control (World Health Organization, 2012). Contraceptive use is about 70% among women in highly developed regions, such as North America and Northern Europe, and about 34% in less developed regions, such as Central Africa.

About 17% of women in the world who do not want to become pregnant within the upcoming 2 years, or at all, do not use any method of contraception, and another 9% use methods with low effectiveness. This means that, globally, 215 million women have an unmet need for modern contraception. The main reasons for unmet needs for contraception include poor access to quality health services, limited availability of a variety of contraceptive methods, lack of birth control information, concerns about safety or side effects, and cultural factors such as social, religious, or partner disapproval.

Because so many women lack access to modern contraceptives, about 40% of all pregnancies worldwide are unintended, and about 56% of these result in an induced abortion. Moreover, about 20 million of these abortions are unsafe, that is, carried out by persons lacking the necessary skills or in an environment lacking the minimum medical standards, or both. Lacking quality care, about 70,000 women die of an unsafe abortion every year.

The mortality rate from abortion is highest among developing nations; for example, 680 women die per 100,000 abortions in Africa, compared with 0.7 per 100,000 in developed regions. Obviously, when women have access to family planning services, the number of women both seeking abortions and dying as a result of them is low.

The World Health Organization and the World Bank estimate that a contribution of between $6 and $9 per person per year would provide basic family planning and maternal and neonatal health care to women in developing countries. Choosing when to become pregnant (and avoiding abortion) enhances a woman's health and well-being, which, in turn, enhances the health and well-being of her family and community.

Unmarried women in their 20s account for the majority of abortions, and about 90% of abortions are performed prior to the 13th week of pregnancy (Jatlaoui et al., 2016). The main complications of surgical abortion include incomplete abortion requiring repeat procedure and excessive bleeding during the procedure. Complications associated with medication abortion include failed procedure (ongoing pregnancy), incomplete abortion, and bleeding. The rate of complications from abortion prior to 10 weeks is less than 2% (Upadhyay et al., 2015). The risk of death from abortion is about 0.6 per 100,000 abortions; the risk of death from pregnancy and childbirth is about 8.8 per 100,000 live births (Raymond & Grimes, 2012).

Psychological Aftereffects of Abortion

Despite the fact that abortion in the United States and Canada is legal and over 1 million North American women annually receive one, the decision to terminate a pregnancy voluntarily is rarely an easy one. Most women are ambivalent about abortion, as are many men.

Whereas it is not unexpected that some unintentionally pregnant women and often their male partners (Altshuler et al., 2016) experience sadness, grief, and feelings of loss following elective abortion, some also experience depression and anxiety. Factors that increase the risk of negative psychological responses to abortion include the need for secrecy, low anticipated social support for the abortion decision, low self-esteem, using avoidance and denial as coping strategies, and characteristics of the particular pregnancy, including the extent to which the woman wanted and felt committed to it (Kimport et al., 2011). A variety of studies indicate that a woman's postabortion mental health reflects her mental health status prior to the abortion (Major et al., 2009). A study of nearly 1,000 pregnant American women who sought an abortion showed that the long-term psychological well-being among women who had an abortion was similar to women who sought an abortion but did not undergo the procedure (Biggs et al., 2017).

The Legal and Moral Aspects of Abortion

The propriety of abortion as a socially sanctioned method of fertility control has been debated for centuries. More than 2,000 years ago, the Greek philosophers Aristotle and Plato recommended abortion, whereas Hippocrates, the founder of modern medicine, forbade it. Throughout the Middle Ages and the Renaissance, abortion was common, although various religious leaders objected to the practice on ethical grounds.

When the U.S. Constitution was ratified, and for several decades after, abortion was legal if it took place before the time of quickening—when a woman could feel fetal movements. Quickening usually occurs near the 16th week of pregnancy. The first statutes regulating abortion were enacted in the 1820s in Connecticut and New York. These laws prohibited abortion before the time of quickening, principally to protect women from what by modern standards were primitive and dangerous surgical techniques. By the end of the Civil War, more states had enacted restrictive abortion legislation, not only to preserve the health and life of a pregnant woman but also to encourage American-born women to have children and to discourage nonreproductive sex. By 1900, abortion was illegal in all U.S. jurisdictions, and it remained so for more than 60 years.

Restrictive abortion laws did not stop women from having abortions, however. In the first decades of the twentieth century, millions of women obtained illegal

U.S. Abortion Facts

African-American 28%

Hispanic 25%

Caucasian 39%

Other races and ethnicities, 9%

Fifty-one percent of abortion patients in **2008** were using a *contraceptive method* in the month they became pregnant, most commonly condoms (27%) or a hormonal method (17%)

- 23% of currently married pregnant women obtain abortions
- Never-married women obtained 46% of all abortions (31% were cohabiting)
- Women who had at least one birth obtained 59% of all abortions

Of women with incomes of 100% to 199% of the federal poverty level, 26% obtained abortions

Of women with incomes less than 100% of the federal poverty level ($15,730 for a family of two), 49% obtained abortions

- Women aged 20–24 obtained 34% of all abortions
- Women aged 25–29 obtained 27% of all abortions
- Women aged 18–19 obtained 8% of all abortions
- Women aged 15–17 obtained 3% of all abortions
- Girls younger than 15 obtained 0.2% of all abortions

Reasons for having an abortion:

- Concern for or responsibility to other individuals
- The inability to afford raising a child
- Belief that having a baby would interfere with work, school, or the ability to care for dependents
- Not wanting to be a single parent
- Having problems with their husband or partner

Women identifying as...

- Mainline Protestant obtained 13% of all abortions
- Evangelical Protestant obtained 24% of all abortions
- Catholic obtained 38% of all abortions
- Some other or no religious affiliation obtained 8% of all abortions

Data from Finer, L. B., & Zolna, M. R. (2016). Declines in unintended pregnancy in the United States, 2008–2011. *New England Journal of Medicine, 374*, 843–852.

abortions. Those with money could travel to other countries where abortion was legal and performed in a hospital with trained personnel, or they could obtain a clandestine abortion performed by an American physician who accepted the risk of prosecution in return for a high fee. Most women, however, had to obtain abortions from nonmedical people who often performed the procedure using coat hangers, spoons, disinfectant, or lye. Many women were maimed or killed by such procedures. The psychological trauma even of successful procedures was enormous. By the 1950s, an estimated 200,000 to 1 million women were getting illegal abortions annually.

By the 1960s, people began to take into account the social and psychological costs of illegal abortion, and on January 22, 1973, the U.S. Supreme Court declared that states could not make laws prohibiting abortion on the ground that they violated a woman's right to privacy, in this case, the right to decide about the outcome of a pregnancy. This decision, known as *Roe v. Wade,* declared (1) that the decision to have an abortion during the first trimester (12 weeks) of pregnancy should be left entirely to the woman and her physician, and (2) during the second trimester, individual states could regulate the abortion procedure for only one purpose—to protect the woman's health.

Many people have mixed feelings about abortion. Because there is no universally accepted scientific definition of when a life begins, some individuals view abortion as murder. Some opponents of abortion believe that its availability encourages irresponsible sexual behavior. Some see abortion as a threat to family life. Even the staunchest proponents of abortion rights would prefer that abortions never occur, but they argue that women must have the right to control their bodies. They believe that abortion is a necessary last resort if contraception fails, if a woman becomes pregnant because of rape or incest, if the child may suffer a serious birth defect, or if the woman's life and health are jeopardized by pregnancy or childbirth.

Critical Thinking About Health

1. "Oh, not again," said a disgusted Janet Haley, chief of research at Leeward Pharmaceuticals, as she waved the hard copy of an email in the air at her group's weekly staff meeting. "Every 5 years someone gets the bright idea that we need to develop a high-tech contraceptive for men. They just don't get it."

   "It could be done, you know," said Richard Duval, one of the company's newest and brightest researchers. "Sure, hormonal methods are no good, but there's lots more we can do with metabolic inhibitors, sperm viability, semen composition…"

   "No offense, Richard, but you aren't getting it either. Even if we had a method for men, who'd buy it? Can't you just see a woman asking, 'Did you take your pill today, honey?'"

   a. Do you agree that developing a contraceptive pill for men would be an unsound business decision? Explain your reasoning.

2. When choosing a method of contraception, a couple decided to base their decision on a method's lowest observed/theoretical failure rate. Explain why it would be better for them to use the typical use/actual failure rate.

3. The placard read "Not paying for your playing." Students from the Committee for Fairness took turns holding the placard on the steps of the Student Health Center, talking to anyone who would stop, especially reporters from the campus newspaper and the local TV station. The CFF students were objecting to the fact that contraceptives were available at the Student Health Center. "They're not medicines," they argued. "We don't think our health center fees should pay for sexual partying."

   a. Do you agree or disagree with this point of view?

   b. What are the advantages and disadvantages to any institution or community of making fertility control methods available to anyone who wants them?

Chapter Summary and Highlights

Chapter Summary

A wide variety of fertility control methods are available to individuals and couples who want to have sexual intercourse but who do not want to become pregnant or to become a parent. These include many kinds of hormonal contraceptives, male and female condoms, fertility awareness methods, IUDs, spermicides, and sterilizations methods—vasectomy for men and tubal ligation for women—and others. Couples who engage in sexual intercourse and who do not want a child should discuss various fertility control methods and decide whether one partner or both will be responsible for making sure a contraceptive method is used.

About half of all pregnancies in the United States are classified as unintended or unplanned, and the majority occur among young couples who are not prepared for a pregnancy because of age, life circumstances, finances, or emotional maturity. These unintended pregnancies can be terminated with medical assistance. However, although abortion is legal in the United States, abortion is still extremely controversial and difficult to obtain in many states. Proponents of abortion believe a woman has the right to choose what is best for her health and her body; opponents of abortion believe that a fetus has rights equal to or more important than the potential mother's rights and that all abortions are immoral and wrong. More than 4 million pregnancies are confirmed in the United States each year. Of these, 30% to 40% end in the first

trimester because of a miscarriage (spontaneous abortion). About 20,000 to 30,000 more are stillborn (die at birth or late in pregnancy). The majority of miscarriages result from genetic defects that prevent normal human development.

Highlights

- A variety of safe, reliable, and effective fertility control methods are available. These include combination and progestin-only hormonal contraception, barrier methods (condom, diaphragm, cervical cap, and spermicides), fertility awareness methods, the IUD, and sterilization.
- A contraceptive's effectiveness is measured in terms of lowest observed and typical use failure rates.
- Although most fertility control methods are designed for use in the woman's body, both partners share the responsibility for fertility control. Communication and cooperation are keys to shared responsibility.
- People who say they do not want to have a baby, yet do not practice fertility control, tend to have low motivation, lack of knowledge of human reproduction and fertility control methods, negative attitudes toward fertility control, or are in relationships that hinder correct fertility control practice.
- Medical and surgical abortions are available.
- Abortion became legal in the United States in 1973 with the Supreme Court's *Roe v. Wade* decision.

For Your Health

If you are considering using a particular method of contraception, use the checklist in Exercise 10.1 (in the Workbook) to assess its suitability for you and your partner.

Look at Exercise 10.2, also, to rate the suitability of various contraceptives for you and your partner.

References

Altshuler, A. L., et al. (2016). Male partners' involvement in abortion care: A mixed-methods systematic review. *Perspectives in Sex and Reproductive Health, 48,* 209–219.

Biggs, M. A., et al. (2017). Women's mental health and well-being 5 years after receiving or being denied an abortion: A prospective, longitudinal cohort study. *JAMA Psychiatry, 74,* 169–178.

Daniels, K., et al. (2015, November 10). Current contraceptive use and variation by selected characteristics among women aged 15–44: United States, 2011–2013. *National Health Statistics Reports, 86,* 1–14.

Finer, L. B., & Zolna, M. R. (2016). Declines in unintended pregnancy in the United States, 2008–2011. *New England Journal of Medicine, 374,* 843–852.

Jatlaoui, T. C., et al. (2016). Abortion surveillance–United States, 2013. *Morbidity Mortality Weekly Report, 65,* 1–44. Retrieved from https://www.cdc.gov/mmwr/volumes/65/ss/ss6512a1.htm

Kimport, K., et al. (2011). Social sources of women's emotional difficulty after abortion: Lessons from women's abortion narratives. *Perspectives in Sex and Reproductive Health, 43,* 103–109.

Major, B., et al. (2009). Abortion and mental health: Evaluating the evidence. *American Psychologist, 64,* 863–890.

Raymond, E. G., & Grimes, D. A. (2012). The comparative safety of legal induced abortion and childbirth in the United States. *Obstetrics and Gynecology, 119,* 215–219.

Singh, S., Darroch, J. E., & Ashford, L. S. (2014). *Adding it up: Costs and benefits of investing in sexual and reproductive health.* New York: Guttmacher Institute and United Nations Population Fund (UNFPA). Retrieved from www.guttmacher.org/sites/default/files/report_pdf/addingitup2014.pdf

Sonfield, A., Hasstedt, K., & Gold, R. B. (2014). *Moving forward: Family planning in the era of health reform.* New York: Guttmacher Institute.

Trussell, J. (2011). Contraceptive failure in the United States. *Contraception, 83,* 397–404.

Upadhyay, U. D., et al. (2015). Incidence of emergency department visits and complications after abortion. *Obstetrics and Gynecology, 125,* 175–183.

World Health Organization. (2012). Facts on induced abortion worldwide. Retrieved from http://www.who.int/reproductivehealth/publications/unsafe_abortion/abortion_facts/en/

Suggested Readings

Hatcher, R. A., et al. (2011). *Contraceptive technology* (19th ed.). New York: Thompson Reuters. The most comprehensive discussion of contraception and abortion available, written by world-renowned experts in the field.

Planned Parenthood. (n.d.). All about birth control methods. Retrieved from https://www.plannedparenthood.org/learn/birth-control. Comprehensive birth control education website with video.

Trussell, J., et al. (2014). Emergency contraception. Retrieved from http://ec.princeton.edu/questions/ec-review.pdf. Provides a detailed academic review of the medical and social science literature about emergency contraception.

United Nations, Department of Economic and Social Affairs, Population Division. (2015). *Trends in contraceptive use worldwide, 2015* (ST/ESA/SER.A/349). Comprehensive and timely estimates on global trends in family planning, assessing current and future contraceptive demand and setting policy priorities to ensure universal access to sexual and reproductive health and the realization of reproductive rights.

Recommended Websites

Birth Control Guide
The U.S. Food and Drug Administration's descriptions of the major birth control methods.

The Emergency Contraception Website
All about emergency contraception, from Princeton University.

Family Planning Information
Compiled by the Emory University School of Medicine.

Planned Parenthood
All there is to learn about family planning.

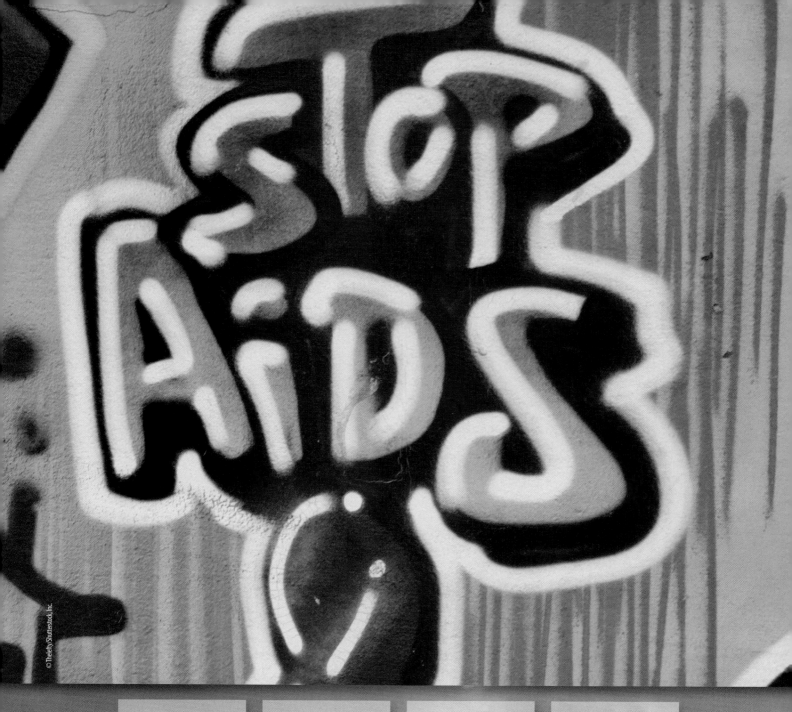

Health Tips

Condom Sense

Dollars & Health Sense

Can the Worldwide HIV/AIDS Epidemic Be Stopped?

Global Wellness

HIV/AIDS Covers the Globe

Managing Stress

Why It Is Vital to Stay HIV Free

CHAPTER 11

Protecting Against Sexually Transmitted Diseases and AIDS

Learning Objectives

1. Describe the impact of sexually transmitted diseases (STDs) on society.

2. List the risk factors for contracting an STD.

3. Identify the causative agent, symptoms, and treatment for the following diseases: trichomoniasis, chlamydia, gonorrhea, syphilis, genital herpes, genital warts, pubic lice, scabies, and HIV/AIDS.

4. Describe the importance of testing for HIV infection and common testing procedures.

5. Identify several "safer sex" practices.

6. Describe the importance of effective communication in reducing the risk of STDs and AIDS.

> Women need a reason to have sex. Men just need a place.
>
> *Billy Crystal*

Throughout the world, about 30 different infectious diseases can be passed from person to person through sexual contact; 11 are common in North America (**Table 11.1**). These infections are called **sexually transmitted diseases (STDs)** or sexually transmitted infections (STIs). The World Health Organization estimates that 370 million people in the world acquire an STD each year; in the United States, the number is more than 7 million (**Figure 11.1**). About 40% of these infections occur in people under age 25 (U.S. Centers for Disease Control and Prevention, 2016).

Sexually transmitted diseases have been afflicting humans for thousands of years. Ancient Chinese medical

Table 11.1

Common Sexually Transmitted Diseases (STDs)

STD	Symptoms	Treatment
HIV/AIDS	Flulike symptoms followed by any of a number of diseases characteristic of immunodeficiency	New drugs may retard viral reproduction temporarily; opportunistic infections can be treated to some degree
Chlamydia	Usually occur within 3 weeks: men have a discharge from the penis and painful urination; women may have a vaginal discharge but often are asymptomatic	Antibiotics
Genital warts	Usually occur within 1 to 3 months: small, dry growths on the genitals, anus, cervix, and possibly mouth	Podophyllin
Gonorrhea	Usually occur within 2 weeks: discharge from the penis, vagina, or anus; pain on urination or defecation or during sexual intercourse; pain and swelling in the pelvic region; genital and oral infections may be asymptomatic	Antibiotics
Hepatitis B	Low-grade fever, fatigue, headaches, loss of appetite, nausea, dark urine, jaundice	Rest, proper nutrition; vaccination for hepatitis B
Genital herpes	Usually occur within 2 weeks: painful blisters on site(s) of infection (genitals, anus, cervix); occasionally itching, painful urination, and fever	None; acyclovir relieves symptoms
Molluscum contagiosum	Smooth, rounded, shiny, whitish growths on the skin of the trunk and anogenital region	Surgical
Pubic lice	Usually occur within 5 weeks: intense itching in the genital region; lice may be visible in pubic hair; small white eggs may be visible on pubic hair	Gamma benzene hexachloride
Scabies	Tiny, itchy lesions caused by mites burrowing into the skin	Topical insecticides
Syphilis	Usually occur within 3 weeks: a chancre (painless sore) on the genitals, anus, or mouth; secondary stage, skin rash (if left untreated); tertiary stage includes diseases of several body organs	Antibiotics
Trichomoniasis	Yellowish-green vaginal discharge with an unpleasant odor; vaginal itching; occasionally painful intercourse	Metronidazole

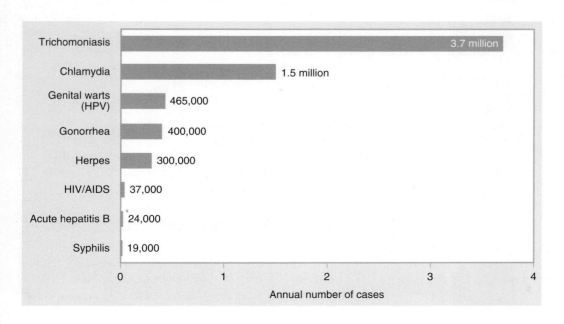

■ **Figure 11.1**

Estimated Yearly Number of STDs in the United States

Data from: U.S. Centers for Disease Control and Prevention. Retrieved from www.cdc.gov/std/stats/sti-estimates-fact-sheet-feb-2013.pdf and www.cdc.gov/std/statsis/tables/44.htm

Table 11.2

Famous People with an STD

No one knows for sure, but historians say these famous people were infected with an STD.

Abraham	Job	Dürer	Gauguin
Sarah	King David	Schubert	Boswell
Julius Caesar	Cleopatra	Molière	Goethe
Charlemagne	Napoleon	Van Gogh	Oscar Wilde
Henry VIII	Columbus	Nietzsche	Goya

The Greats: Peter and Catherine

writings describe diseases of the genitalia that were probably syphilis. The ancient Egyptians described genital diseases that were probably gonorrhea. Old Testament and Talmudic writings describe a condition called "ziba," which was associated with the emission of fluid, referred to then as "issue," from the nonerect penis or the vagina. "Ziba" was probably gonorrhea, and "issue" was probably the discharge associated with gonorrhea. Many famous historical figures are thought to have had sexually transmitted diseases (**Table 11.2**).

The human and social costs of STDs are enormous. In the United States, the direct and indirect economic costs of the major STDs and their complications total $20 billion a year. The human suffering and economic costs wrought by AIDS are also well known. Less well known are the disappointment and suffering of thousands of women who are left infertile after a serious STD-related pelvic infection. Women who acquire a human papillomavirus (HPV) infection (genital warts) are predisposed to cervical cancer. And the million people who acquire genital herpes each year will be potentially infectious for their entire lives.

What Is an STD?

An STD is an infection that is transmitted by sexual behavior. An infection occurs when one or more biological agents inhabit parts of the body they are not supposed to and acquire nutrients from the body so they can survive and reproduce. Human STDs are caused by viruses, bacteria, protozoa, worms, and insects.

STD-causing agents can get into the body through (1) breaks in the skin; (2) the mucous membranes of the body's orifices—nose and mouth, penis, vagina, urethra, and anus; and (3) the blood, either by injection or during sexual activity by means of tiny microscopic abrasions on the penis or in the vagina, anus, or mouth. Some STD-causing agents enter body cells by attaching to specific sites, called *receptors*, on a body cell's surface. Once inside the body, the infectious agents reproduce and their population grows in numbers.

In general, STDs are not transferred by air, water, or contact with doorknobs, toilet seats, and other inanimate objects. In the case of insects, however, contact with any surface on which the organisms, their larvae, or eggs might be present may cause an infection.

A certain number of STD-causing agents must be transferred to cause an infection. This number varies according to how well the recipient's body can defend itself and a variety of specific host–parasite factors. For chlamydia and gonorrhea, the transfer of about 1,000 organisms is sufficient to cause an infection, and the risk of becoming infected with one exposure is about 60% to 90% in men and 20% to 35% in women. With syphilis, the requisite number of infecting organisms is about 100.

STD Risk Factors

Several factors increase the risk of contracting an STD. Being aware of these factors can help you decrease your risk of infection and help you to support STD prevention efforts in your community.

Multiple Sexual Partners

About 16% of unmarried adults have more than one sex partner in a year (England & Brown, 2016). About 24% of North American college students have more than one sexual partner in a year (American College Health Association, 2016). Also, many people in supposed sexually exclusive relationships have sex outside the relationship, generally without the "exclusive" partner's knowledge. Individuals who are unaware that their partners are sexually active with other people have higher rates of STDs than do individuals who do know their partners are sexually active with others (Drumright, Gorbach, & Holmes, 2004).

False Sense of Safety

Using hormonal contraceptives tends to decrease the use of condoms, which help prevent transmission of STDs. The availability of antibiotics and HIV medicines makes many people less afraid of sexually transmitted diseases. They erroneously believe that there is a cure for every STD.

Absence of Signs and Symptoms

Some STDs have very mild or no symptoms, so the infection can worsen and may be unknowingly passed on to others. One study showed that approximately 8% of college students were infected with chlamydia and did not know it. Another 1.5% were infected with gonorrhea and did not know it. People infected with HIV can have mild or no symptoms for years, yet still be infectious.

TERMS

sexually transmitted diseases (STDs): infections passed from person to person by sexual contact

Untreated Conditions

Some individuals lack sufficient knowledge of the signs and symptoms of STDs to know that they are infected. Those who are not accustomed to seeking health care, or who financially cannot afford it, are less likely to seek treatment for an infection. Furthermore, many individuals with STDs do not comply with treatment regimens. When medications are not taken for the required length of time, an infection may not be completely eradicated even though symptoms may disappear. People who do not complete treatment may still be infectious.

Impaired Judgment

The use of drugs, including alcohol, can increase the risk of transmitting STDs because people with drug-impaired judgment are less likely to use condoms. Also, people in a drugged condition may be more likely to have sex with someone they do not know; they may know nothing of their partner's past sexual and drug history.

Lack of Immunity

Some STD-causing organisms, such as HIV and herpesvirus, can escape the body's immune defenses, causing individuals to remain infected and transmit the infection. This may permit reinfection and also makes the development of effective vaccines difficult or impossible.

Body Piercing

Piercing of the body, particularly the genitals, increases the risk of transmission of STDs. The wound from piercing gives organisms direct access to the bloodstream, and pierced genitals may impede proper use of condoms. Moreover, people with nipple, tongue, and lip jewelry may have a higher risk of infection via oral sex. People who have their bodies pierced should follow after-care instructions faithfully to prevent infection and should abstain from sexual contact in the pierced region until the hole is completely healed, which usually takes 3 to 6 months.

Value Judgments

Unlike nearly all other kinds of infections, STDs are associated with sinfulness, dirtiness, condemnation, shame, guilt, and disgust. These negative attitudes keep people from getting checkups, contacting partners when an STD has been diagnosed, and talking to new partners about previous exposures. In the nineteenth century, when syphilis was a scourge of Europe, rather than trying to prevent its spread (effective treatments had not yet been invented), countries blamed the disease on the weak character or immorality of their neighbors: The English referred to syphilis as the "French disease," and the French called it the "Spanish disease." Prejudice and scapegoating helped spread the disease.

> If love is the answer, could you please rephrase the question?
>
> *Lily Tomlin*

Denial

With respect to contracting an STD, many people think, "It can't happen to me," or "He is too nice to have an STD," or "She isn't the type of person who would have an STD." Because there are no vaccinations against most of the infectious agents that cause STDs, the only way to prevent them is for sexually active individuals who are not in lifelong single-partner (monogamous) sexual relationships to assume responsibility for protecting themselves and their partners. This means becoming aware of the signs and symptoms of the common STDs and seeking treatment when such signs occur. It means that sexually active people who have more than one partner within a year should obtain periodic (about every 6 months) STD checkups. It also means knowing about and practicing "safer sex."

Common STDs

The most common STDs in the United States and Canada can be categorized according to the type of organism causing them (**Table 11.3**). Organisms that cause STDs are viruses, bacteria, protozoa, and insects.

Trichomoniasis

Although not commonly thought of as sexually transmitted diseases, vaginal infections caused by the protozoan *Trichomonas vaginalis* can be transmitted during intercourse. Symptoms tend to occur only in women (vaginal itching and a cheesy, odorous discharge from the vagina), but the organisms can survive in the urethra of the penis and under the penile foreskin. A man who harbors these organisms can infect other partners or even reinfect the partner who transmitted the organisms to him.

Table 11.3	
Agents That Cause Common STDs	
Infectious agent	Disease
Bacteria	
Chlamydia trachomatis	Chlamydia
Neisseria gonorrhoeae	Gonorrhea
Treponema pallidum	Syphilis
Viruses	
Herpes simplex virus, types 1 and 2	Genital herpes
Human papillomavirus	Anogenital warts
Human immunodeficiency virus (HIV)	AIDS
Hepatitis virus B	Hepatitis
Molluscum contagiosum virus	Molluscum contagiosum
Protozoa	
Trichomonas vaginalis	Trichomoniasis (vaginitis)
Insects	
Phthirus pubis	Lice ("crabs")
Sarcoptes scabiei	Mites ("scabies")

About 4 million new cases of trichomoniasis are diagnosed each year. Clinically, a diagnosis is made by collecting fluid from the vagina and testing for the presence of *Trichomonas* organisms. Medications are effective in treating these infections. An infected woman's male partner(s) should also undergo treatment.

Bacterial Vaginosis

The vagina normally contains a variety of bacteria that support a healthy vaginal environment. However, overgrowth of certain types of bacteria (generally *Gardnerella vaginalis*) can cause an infection called **bacterial vaginosis (BV)**, which can be sexually transmissible through intercourse. Symptoms of BV include vaginal discharge, which may have a "fishy" smell, particularly after intercourse. Sometimes BV has no symptoms.

Chlamydia

Chlamydia is caused by the microorganism *Chlamydia trachomatis,* which specifically infects certain cells lining the mucous membranes of the genitals, mouth, anus, rectum, the conjunctiva of the eyes, and occasionally the lungs. The chlamydial microorganisms bind to surfaces and induce the host cells to engulf them. After gaining entrance to the cell, these organisms resist a host cell's defenses and eventually "steal" from the host cell the biochemical compounds required for their own survival. The chlamydial organisms use the stolen nutrients to reproduce and multiply, and ultimately the host cell dies.

In the United States and other Western countries, chlamydia is the most commonly reported bacterial STD. Each year approximately 1.5 million Americans contract chlamydia. In as many as one-third of all cases, chlamydia occurs simultaneously with gonorrhea. Newborns also are susceptible to chlamydial infection if their mothers are infected at the time of delivery. The most common complications of chlamydial infection in newborns are conjunctivitis (eye infection) and pneumonia.

One reason that chlamydial infections are so common is that a large percentage of infected individuals often have extremely mild or no symptoms. Thus, infected individuals can unknowingly transmit the infection to new sex partners. When symptoms do occur, they include pain during urination (dysuria) in both men and women and a whitish discharge from the penis or vagina. Symptoms generally appear within 7 to 21 days after infection.

Chlamydia can be treated with antibiotics. Left untreated, the chlamydial bacteria can multiply and cause inflammation and damage to the reproductive organs in both sexes. In men, untreated chlamydia can result in inflammation of the epididymis (*epididymitis*), characterized by pain, swelling, and tenderness in the scrotum and sometimes by a mild fever. Damage to the tissues in the epididymis can eventually lead to sterility. In women, chlamydial infections affect the cervix, uterus, fallopian tubes, and peritoneum. Often, chlamydial infections of the reproductive tract produce no symptoms until the infection is advanced. A woman may then experience chronic pelvic pain, vaginal discharge, intermittent vaginal bleeding, and pain during intercourse. Infection of the fallopian tubes can produce scar tissue that damages the tubes' lining and partially or completely blocks the tubes. These effects may increase the risk of ectopic pregnancy or render a woman infertile; thousands of cases of female infertility per year result from fallopian tube damage from chlamydia.

Chlamydial infections induce an immune response in the host, but for unknown reasons infected individuals do not gain immunity to future chlamydial infections. This means that treated individuals can be reinfected upon exposure to chlamydia.

Gonorrhea

Gonorrhea, also known as "the clap," is caused by the bacterium *Neisseria gonorrhoeae.* Gonorrheal organisms specifically infect the mucous membranes of the body, most often the genitals, reproductive organs, mouth and throat, anus, and eyes. *N. gonorrhoeae* cannot survive on toilet seats, doorknobs, bedsheets, clothes, or towels. Transmission in adults almost always occurs by genital, oral, or anal sexual contact; infection of the eyes occurs by hand (often through self-infection). Each year, about 300,000 American adults are infected with gonorrhea.

Newborn babies exposed to gonorrheal organisms in the mother's birth canal may develop gonorrhea of the eyes. Most states require that antibiotics or a few drops of silver nitrate be put into the eyes of babies immediately after birth to kill the gonorrhea bacteria and prevent possible blindness.

Although the bacteria causing them are different, the symptoms of gonorrheal and chlamydial infections are very similar. Like chlamydia, many people infected with gonorrheal organisms do not develop symptoms and their infections go unnoticed. If the infection progresses, men may develop epididymitis and women may develop infections of the uterus, fallopian tubes, and pelvic region. Such infections may cause sterility. When symptoms appear, they include painful urination in both sexes and a yellowish discharge from the penis or vagina. Occasionally there is pain in the groin, testes, or lower abdomen. The first symptoms of gonorrhea usually appear within 7 to 10 days after exposure.

TERMS

bacterial vaginosis (BV): a bacterial infection of the vagina

chlamydia: a sexually transmitted disease caused by the bacterium *Chlamydia trachomatis*

gonorrhea: a sexually transmitted disease caused by gonococcal bacteria (*Neisseria gonorrhoeae*)

Gonorrhea can be treated with antibiotics. However, new antibiotic-resistant strains of the organism constantly emerge. In nearly half of all cases of gonorrhea, chlamydia also is present. Individuals undergoing diagnosis for gonorrhea should also be tested for chlamydia.

Syphilis

Syphilis is caused by a spiral-shaped bacterium called *Treponema pallidum*. These organisms are transmitted from person to person through genital, oral, and anal contact, as well as are acquired from infected blood. Syphilis can also be transmitted from a mother to her unborn fetus, perhaps as early as the ninth week of pregnancy.

The first noticeable sign of syphilis is a painless open sore called a **chancre** ("shanker"), which can appear any time between the first week and third month after infection. If the infection is not treated within that period, the chancre will heal and the disease will enter a secondary stage, characterized by a skin rash, hair loss, and the appearance of round, flat-topped growths on most areas of the body. Left untreated, the signs of the secondary stage also disappear, and the infection enters a symptomless (latency) period, during which the syphilis organisms multiply in many other regions of the body. In the final, tertiary stage, the disease eventually damages vital organs, such as the heart or brain, and can cause severe symptoms or death. Syphilis can be treated with antibiotics at any stage of the infection.

Genital Herpes

Herpes infections of the genital region are caused by either of two strains of herpes simplex virus (HSV): HSV-1, which is associated primarily with cold sores on the mouth ("fever blisters"), and HSV-2, associated primarily with lesions on the penis, vagina, or rectum. As many as 50 million American adults have been infected with HSV-1 or HSV-2. Each year up to 1 million American adults acquire a genital herpes infection.

Infections with HSV-2 are often asymptomatic. Indeed, 90% of people infected with HSV-2 do not know it. Nevertheless, they are infectious and may contribute to the spread of the disease by having unprotected sex. If they appear, symptoms of a genital herpes infection are evident within 2 to 20 days after contact with the virus.

The major symptoms of a genital herpes infection are the presence of one or more blisters, which eventually break to become wet, painful sores that last about 2 or 3 weeks; fever; and occasionally pain in the lower abdomen. Eventually these initial symptoms disappear, but the herpes virus remains dormant in certain of the body's nerve cells, permitting periodic recurrences of symptoms at or near the site(s) of the initial infection. Stress, anxiety, poor nutrition, sunlight, and skin irritation can bring on recurrences.

Recurrences are usually mild and last only about a week. They may be telegraphed by a tingling feeling or itching in the genital area, or pain in the buttocks or down

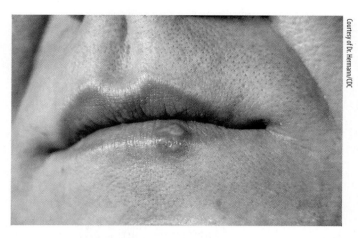

"Cold sores" on the lip or inside the mouth are a common occurrence in people who are infected by the herpes simplex virus. The sores usually heal in a week or so but can flare up again because the viral infection is permanent.

the leg. For some people, these early symptoms can be the most painful and annoying part of an episode. Sometimes, only the tingling and itching are present, and no visible sores develop. At other times, blisters appear that may be very small and barely noticeable, or they may break into open sores that crust over and then disappear. Herpes is extremely contagious when a sore is present. People with open lesions should avoid sex with others until the lesions disappear. Even if no sore is present, transmission is possible, although much less likely, through the "shedding" of virus particles from the skin.

Whereas genital herpes infections are caused most frequently by HSV-2 and oral herpes infections are caused most frequently by HSV-1, both HSV-2 and HSV-1 can cause genital and oral infections with identical symptoms. Thus, people with oral herpes can transmit the infection to partners via oral sex. They can also transmit it to themselves through masturbation. Occasionally, sores also appear on other parts of the body where the virus has entered through broken skin.

Herpes simplex also can infect the eyes, leading to impaired vision and even blindness. If the virus is present in the birth canal, newborn babies can be infected, often resulting in brain damage and abnormal development. In the United States, about 500 babies are born each year with herpes, and two-thirds of infected babies who are not treated die. Pregnant women who have had a prior genital herpes infection should tell their physicians in order to prevent transmission of HSV to their babies.

There is no cure for herpes, and individuals remain infected for life. Drugs such as acyclovir can minimize the duration and severity of the symptoms of an initial infection or a recurrence.

Human Papillomavirus and Anogenital Warts

Human papillomaviruses (HPV) are a group of more than 100 types of viruses, about 40 of which can be passed from

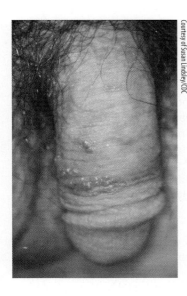

Genital warts on the penis are caused by infection of the skin by papilloma viruses. Genital warts can be removed by a variety of treatments but sometimes recur.

Courtesy of Susan Lindsley/CDC

person to person through sexual contact. About 6 million Americans are infected with HPV each year. Approximately 20 million Americans are currently infected with HPV. HPV is so common that nearly all sexually active men and women will be infected with HPV at some point in their lives. The majority of HPV infections are symptomless and go away on their own. However, persistent infections with one or more of 10 types of HPV can cause cervical cancer in women.

Men are susceptible to HPV infection also. Several HPV types can infect the genital area, including the skin on and around the penis or anus. They can also infect the mouth and throat. Most men who are infected with any type of HPV never develop any symptoms or health problems, but each year several thousand men develop HPV-caused cancers of the penis, the anal region, or the back of the throat including the base of the tongue and tonsils. Compared to men who have sex exclusively with women, men who have sex with men are 17 times more likely to acquire an HPV infection.

Some types of HPV may cause visible warts (*Condylomata acuminata*) on or around the genitals or anus within 3 months of contact with an infected person. Other types of HPV do not cause visible **anogenital warts**, although they infect the vagina, cervix, penis, and the mouth and larynx (as a result of oral sex with an infected person). The types of HPV that cause visible warts on hands and feet are different from those that cause growths in the genital region.

Visible anogenital warts usually are raised or flat, single or multiple, small or large, sometimes cauliflower shaped, soft, moist, pink, or flesh-colored swellings. They can appear on the vulva, in or around the vagina or anus, on the cervix, and on the penis, scrotum, groin, or thigh. The warts are contagious. Anogenital warts can be removed by self-applied medications (imiquimod cream, podophyllin or podofilox solutions). Also, they can be removed by a healthcare provider. Clinician-applied treatments include applying 10% to 25% podophyllum resin,

trichloroacetic acid, or bichloroacetic acid; physically excising the wart; and cryosurgery (freezing), electrocautery (burning), or exposure to laser. Treatments remove the warts but not HPV in cells, so warts can reappear after treatment. Without treatment, warts may disappear or they may grow more numerous, or larger.

Many genital HPV infections do not cause visible warts. The virus lives in the skin or mucous membranes and usually causes no symptoms. A health practitioner can detect invisible infections in either of several ways: (1) applying vinegar (acetic acid) to suspected infected regions and looking for infected cells to whiten; (2) viewing the vagina and cervix with a magnifying instrument (culposcopy); (3) removing a small amount of tissue (biopsy) for analysis of HPV DNA; and (4) performing a Pap smear to look for abnormalities in cervical cells associated with HPV infection.

High-risk HPV infections are invisible; they are associated with cancer of the cervix, vulva, vagina, anus, penis, or larynx. Low-risk HPV infections cause visible warts and may cause minor Pap test abnormalities, but not cancer. Because the Pap smear is such a common procedure, cervical cancer has decreased. Nevertheless, about 12,000 American women develop cervical cancer each year; about 4,000 die each year of the disease.

The types of HPV that infect the genital area are spread primarily through genital contact. Because most HPV infections have no signs or symptoms, most infected persons are unaware they are infected, yet they can transmit the virus to a sex partner. Rarely, a pregnant woman can pass HPV to her baby during vaginal delivery.

There is a vaccine against two types of HPV that cause about 70% of cervical cancers and two types of HPV that cause about 90% of genital warts. The vaccine is given in a series of three injections over a 6-month period. The vaccine is highly effective in preventing HPV infection in young women who have not yet been exposed to HPV.

TERMS

anogenital warts: hard growths caused by an infection with human papillomavirus (HPV) that appear on the skin of the genitals or anus

chancre: the primary lesion of syphilis, which appears as a hard, painless sore or ulcer, often on the penis or vaginal tissue

herpes: a sexually transmitted disease caused by herpes simplex virus (HSV)

human papillomavirus (HPV): a genus of viruses including those causing papillomas (small nipplelike protrusions of the skin or mucous membrane) and warts

syphilis: a sexually transmitted disease caused by spirochete bacteria (*Treponema pallidum*)

Indeed, it is recommended that all young persons be vaccinated against HPV before they reach the age at which they are likely to become sexually active. Other ways to prevent HPV infection are to avoid skin-to-skin contact with an infected person, avoid sexual contact if warts are visible, and male use of latex condoms.

Hepatitis B

Hepatitis B is a disease of the liver caused by infection by hepatitis B virus (HBV), one of several types of hepatitis viruses. Compared with other hepatitis viruses, which tend to be transmitted in fecally contaminated food, HBV is transmitted sexually and by blood, in a manner similar to HIV, the AIDS virus. Hepatitis B virus is sexually transmitted 100 times more effectively than HIV.

The symptoms of hepatitis B infection include low-grade fever, tiredness, headaches, loss of appetite, nausea, dark urine, and jaundice (i.e., yellowing of the white of the eyes and the skin). The first symptoms, which are flulike, tend to occur 14 to 100 days after infection. Signs of liver disease (e.g., dark urine, jaundice) appear later. No specific therapy exists for HBV infection. Rest, proper nutrition, and avoidance of substances harmful to the liver (e.g., alcohol and drugs) are required for recovery, which may take many months. Long-term liver damage is possible, including liver cancer and death.

> Sex is like air....It's not important unless you aren't getting any.
>
> *Anonymous*

A vaccine against HBV exists and everyone is advised to be vaccinated, especially children, health workers, and others who are at high risk of exposure.

Molluscum Contagiosum

Molluscum contagiosum is caused by a virus of the same name. Fewer than 100,000 infections occur in the United States each year. The infection is characterized by the appearance of freckle-sized, smooth, rounded, shiny, whitish growths on the skin of the trunk and anogenital region. Generally, there are no associated symptoms. The lesions may resolve spontaneously, but it is best to have them removed by a healthcare provider; otherwise, they may be transmitted to others or reoccur.

Pubic Lice

Pubic lice (*Phthirus pubis*), also known as "crabs," are barely visible insects that live on hair shafts primarily in the genital–rectal region and occasionally on hair in the armpits, beard, and eyelashes. Thus, pubic lice are not usually found on the head. Scalp hair is the ecological niche of the head louse, *Pediculus humanus capitis*.

Lice feed on blood taken from tiny blood vessels in the skin, which they pierce with their mouth. Some people are sensitive to the bites and may experience itching, which is often the main symptom of infestation. The lice can also be seen; they look like small freckles. The eggs of lice are enclosed in small white pods (called nits), which attach to hair shafts. The presence of nits is also a sign of infestation.

Transfer of lice is through physical—usually sexual—contact. They can also be transmitted through contact with objects on which eggs might have been laid, such as towels, bed linens, and clothes. An infestation of pubic lice can be eliminated by washing the pubic hair with liquids or shampoos containing agents that specifically kill lice (e.g., pyrethrins, piperonyl butoxide, and gamma benzene hydrochloride). All of an infected person's clothes, towels, and bed linens should also be washed with cleaning agents made specifically for killing lice.

Scabies

Scabies is an infestation of certain regions of the skin by extremely small (invisible to the naked eye) mites, *Sarcoptes scabiei*. The mites burrow into the skin, where they live and lay eggs. The tiny lesions produced by the mites often cause intense itching, which is the major sign of a scabies infection. The mites produce tiny burrows across skin lines, which often go unnoticed. Occasionally, an infestation will produce small round nodules. The mites tend to live in the webs between the fingers, on the sides of fingers, and on the wrists, elbows, breasts, abdomen, penis, and buttocks. Rarely do mites live on the face, neck, upper back, palms, and soles.

Scabies can be transmitted both sexually and nonsexually. All that is required is close personal contact. The itching and physical symptoms often take several weeks to appear. Scabies can be treated with topical agents that kill the mites and their eggs.

Acquired Immune Deficiency Syndrome (AIDS)

AIDS is caused by **human immunodeficiency virus**, or **HIV**. HIV infection causes the disease by destroying immune system cells and weakening the body's immune system. Destruction of the body's immune system makes HIV-infected individuals susceptible to a variety of bacterial, viral, and fungal infections that a person with an intact immune system could readily ward off. HIV infection in the brain leads to loss of mental faculties (AIDS dementia).

HIV is mainly transmitted by blood, semen, or vaginal fluids of infected people. When individuals become infected with HIV, their immune systems are still intact and they produce copious antibodies to HIV. The mounting of an immune response in the early phases of an HIV infection provides the basis for HIV testing. Nearly all of the tests for HIV infection detect antibodies to HIV. A positive result (seropositive) indicates that a person has been exposed to sufficient quantities of HIV particles to mount an immune response. Some tests measure the RNA or DNA of HIV itself. This test is used to screen blood supplies and the level of HIV in an infected individual (called the *viral load*).

An HIV-infected individual may not manifest symptoms of AIDS for as many as 15 or 20 years after the initial infection. During this latency period, the infected person is contagious and can spread the infection to others, even

HIV/AIDS Covers the Globe

Since the worldwide HIV/AIDS pandemic began in the early 1980s, the prevalence of HIV/AIDS has increased dramatically such that, in 2016, 36.7 million people in the world were living with HIV (see figure), and 35 million people had died of AIDS. About 2 million people become infected with HIV each year. About 19 million people living with HIV are accessing anti-HIV medications. It is estimated that by 2020, the number of people worldwide with HIV/AIDS will exceed 40 million.

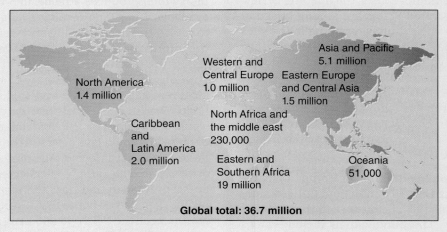

North America
1.4 million

Western and Central Europe
1.0 million

Eastern Europe and Central Asia
1.5 million

Asia and Pacific
5.1 million

Caribbean and Latin America
2.0 million

North Africa and the middle east
230,000

Eastern and Southern Africa
19 million

Oceania
51,000

Global total: 36.7 million

Number of People Living with HIV/AIDS.

Data from United Nations Programme on HIV and AIDS (UNAIDS), 2016. Retrieved from http://www.unaids.org

though she or he is symptomless. The first signs of AIDS are usually mononucleosis-like symptoms (e.g., swollen lymph glands, fever, night sweats) and possibly headaches and impaired mental functioning caused by HIV infection of the brain. As the disease progresses, individuals most often suffer weight loss, infections on the skin (shingles) or in the throat (thrush), one or more opportunistic infections, and cancer.

Because there is no way to rid the body of HIV and hence cure AIDS, treatment of the disease relies on (1) medically managing the opportunistic infections that result from immune suppression, and (2) attempting to suppress HIV infection within the affected person's body. Treating HIV infection involves administering combinations of different drugs, but unfortunately, the combination therapies are not a cure and not all HIV-infected individuals respond. Also, because the drugs only suppress HIV, even those who do respond must take the drugs for life lest the virus begin multiplying again. Because HIV mutates rapidly, in many cases drug resistance develops. Finally, combination drug treatments cost about $10,000 per person per year, so they are unavailable for the economically disadvantaged, who make up 90% of the more than 37 million HIV-infected people in the world.

Because many viral diseases have been conquered by vaccination, much effort has gone into developing vaccines against HIV, but without success so far. The only effective way to control the spread of AIDS is to prevent the transfer of HIV from person to person. This is accomplished by using condoms, reducing exposure to infected individuals, and avoiding casual sex.

Reducing the Risk of HIV/AIDS Because the first reported cases of AIDS in the United States were among male homosexuals, and because many thousands of men in that group have died from AIDS, some people mistakenly believe that only homosexual men can get AIDS. This is not so. Anyone can get AIDS. The reasons that so many homosexual males acquired AIDS include the following:

- Without knowledge of the infectious agent HIV, it was impossible to take precautions.
- In the late 1970s and early 1980s, sexual mores among young people, including male homosexuals, permitted multiple sexual partners, affording HIV rapid access to a large population.
- Anal intercourse provides HIV a highly efficient route of infection because microscopic tears in the rectum give the virus access to the recipient's blood. Microscopic tears in the penis also allow blood transmission, and blood in semen provides a further avenue of infection.

December 1 of each year is World AIDS Day.

TERMS

human immunodeficiency virus (HIV): the virus that causes AIDS; it causes a defect in the body's immune system by invading and then multiplying within certain white blood cells

pubic lice: small insects that live primarily in hair in the genital and rectal regions

scabies: infestation of the skin by microscopic mites (insects)

After it was determined that HIV caused AIDS, and once strategies were developed to stop its transmission, the frequency of new HIV infections among homosexual males declined dramatically. This decline demonstrated that educational efforts and motivation can prevent the transmission of HIV/AIDS and other STDs. Although AIDS is still a threat to male homosexuals, the majority of new cases of AIDS in the United States are among injection drug users who share their drug paraphernalia (needles and syringes) with others and among persons who engage in sexual intercourse with these individuals. Worldwide, most of the transmission of HIV/AIDS is through heterosexual intercourse. This being the case, researchers have found that adult males who undergo circumcision are much less likely to contract HIV/AIDS from an HIV-infected female sex partner than are uncircumcised males (Morris et al., 2017).

Testing for HIV Infection Health officials do not advocate that everyone be tested for HIV infection. But certainly those with a reasonable risk of exposure to the virus are candidates for testing. These individuals include males who have had unprotected sex with other males and anyone who has

- Had unprotected sex with someone who is known or suspected to be infected with HIV
- Had a sexually transmitted disease
- Had unprotected sex with someone while drunk
- Had sex with someone whose AIDS-risky behaviors are unknown
- Had several sexual partners
- Shared needles or syringes to inject drugs of any kind

Testing begins with a counseling session. You will be given materials to read before the session with a counselor or doctor. In the session, you'll be asked why you want to be tested and about your behavior and that of your sex partner(s). This will help your counselor and you to determine whether testing is appropriate. If testing is appropriate, your counselor or doctor will describe the test and how it is done, provide basic AIDS education, explain confidentiality issues, discuss the meaning of possible test results and what impact you think the test result will have on you, and talk about whom you might tell about your result.

The most common HIV tests involve taking a small sample of blood from the arm or a drop of blood from a finger-stick. Less common are urine and oral-fluid tests. The blood, urine, or oral fluid is sent to a laboratory, where it is analyzed for antibodies to HIV. Commonly, the results are returned in a week or two. A rapid HIV test, which produces a result in 5 to 30 minutes, is also available. When your result is available, you will be asked to return to the counseling and testing center to receive the information. This is true for everyone tested regardless of the results.

Consumers should be wary of at-home HIV test kits. Most test kits advertised and sold over the Internet are faulty. The kits show a negative test result on samples that would test positive for HIV by standard methods. Using one of these kits could give a person the false impression that he or she is not infected. At-home *collection* kits are less error-prone. The sample is collected in private at home and sent to a lab that does the analysis and returns the results. Reliable at-home HIV testing kits are in development. Check the U.S. Food and Drug Administration (FDA) website (https://www.fda.gov/BiologicsBloodVaccines/SafetyAvailability/HIVHomeTestKits/ucm126460.htm) for up-to-date information on at-home test kits.

HIV tests can be obtained from physicians and a variety of health agencies. There are two kinds of HIV testing: anonymous and confidential. In the anonymous system, individuals are identified only by a self-selected number or alias, so the true identity is never recorded. In the confidential system, one's name is part of the medical record, which is supposed to be confidential.

Before HIV tests became available, thousands of people were inadvertently infected with HIV as a result of receiving HIV-tainted products derived from blood or blood transfusions (for example, tennis star Arthur Ashe). In the 1980s, thousands of people with **hemophilia** (a hereditary blood disease) received clotting factor derived from pooled blood that was contaminated with HIV, and many have since been stricken with AIDS. In France, a national scandal erupted when it was learned that French health officials knowingly continued to allow hemophiliacs to receive contaminated

---

Why It Is Vital to Stay HIV Free

It's hard for me to remember the seemingly carefree life that I led in Los Angeles, San Francisco, and New York City before my AIDS diagnosis. It's been so long that I can barely remember what it felt like. I don't wish for anyone to have to lose that feeling. I take 37 pills every day: 14 drugs with breakfast, 9 vitamins and herbs with lunch (to help counteract and balance the drugs), and 14 more drugs with dinner. Doing this leads, of course, to the dreadful bouts of diarrhea, irritability, nausea, and fatigue that accompany these medications

and take place at times, it seems, without any rhyme or reason. Yet I take them religiously because they appear to enhance the quality of my life, but not without paying a price: the constant anxiety and doubt that goes along with swallowing toxic chemicals that no one really knows for sure what the long-term physical and mental effects may be. I don't wish this on anyone either.

Mark W. Baker
Provincetown Positive (newsletter)
Fall/Winter, 1997

blood products. All clotting factor products used today are manufactured by biotechnology companies and are free of viral contamination. In addition, all blood donations in the United States today are tested for HIV and other viral contamination. However, new strains of HIV continually arise, and tests are not available for all of them. For any elective surgery, patients often are advised to donate their own blood beforehand should a transfusion be required.

Reducing the STD Epidemic in the United States

STDs are an ongoing major health problem for both individuals and for all countries, including the United States. Recognizing this, the U.S. government made reducing the prevalence of STDs a major goal in Healthy People 2020.

The STDs of greatest concern are HPV, HIV/AIDS, chlamydia, and gonorrhea because they affect millions of Americans and are treatable. Current medical practice calls for treatment of people who seek treatment. These patients are instructed to tell their sexual partners about the infection and to encourage them to seek treatment also. This advice is rarely followed. So, for every person who is treated, many others go untreated and continue to pass the infection to others.

An approach that appears to be more successful involves having the person undergoing treatment distribute antibiotics to known sexual partners so they can treat themselves anonymously. Public health officials hope this approach will reduce the rate of transmission of the more common, treatable STDs.

If the goal of reducing STDs in the United States is to be accomplished, all sexually active individuals need to practice safer sex and take all possible measures to avoid contracting an STD. Equally important is to avoid transmitting infections to others.

Preventing STDs

Preventing STDs requires that societies provide continuous, widespread public health programs and services for STD education and treatment. It is also crucial that infected individuals seek prompt treatment, take responsibility for not infecting other individuals, and practice safer sex to lower their risk of infection.

The stigma associated with STDs is a great hindrance to prevention efforts. Thinking about STDs in moral terms, that is, associating them with dirtiness and immorality, makes people reluctant to think and talk about them. It also makes society want to ignore STD epidemics. During World Wars I and II, American society supported massive gonorrhea and syphilis control programs; as a result, the incidence of these infections dropped tremendously.

When the threat of a postwar STD epidemic seemed to wane, moralistic concerns thwarted the continuation of control efforts, and the incidence of STDs increased. Public health officials realize that ongoing efforts are the only way to control STDs.

Judgmental attitudes also make talking about STDs difficult. To have to tell a partner that you have an STD, or even to say that you once had an infection and are now perfectly okay, can bring feelings of guilt and shame, which can lead to the avoidance of discussion altogether. Similarly, to ask about a partner's previous STDs may be interpreted as an accusation that the person is "loose" or immoral. To avoid feeling embarrassed or risk offending a sexual partner, people are likely to avoid the topic of STDs. Prevention would be enhanced if sexually active individuals developed an open attitude about talking about STDs (and other aspects of sex) and acquired the necessary communication skills.

Practicing Safer Sex

The surest way to reduce the risk of acquiring a sexually transmitted disease is to abstain from sexual intercourse. This does not mean that one has to give up sexual interaction. There are many ways of giving and receiving sexual pleasure without engaging in sexual intercourse: touching, kissing, exchanging a massage, even sleeping together without intercourse.

Another way to reduce risk is to know a partner's sexual history, including all high-risk activities in which a partner may have engaged. Often this kind of information is difficult to gain early in a relationship because exchanging information about sexual histories requires a certain level of trust, which takes some time to develop.

Until you have this knowledge, it is essential to protect yourself by using condoms together with spermicides when having sex. Women and men who are sexually active should come to accept as standard practice with new partners the use of condoms together with spermicides because birth control pills offer no protection against STDs. Sexually active women and men should carry condoms and spermicides whenever the possibility of sex exists and use them. This requires overcoming the gender role stereotypes that women who admit to being sexual are "sluts" and men who behave the same way are "studs." The female condom, a polyurethane plastic sheath that a woman inserts into her vagina, has been shown to prevent the transmission of STDs.

> **TERMS**
>
> **hemophilia:** a hereditary disease (primarily in men) caused by lack of an essential blood clotting factor; results in excessive bleeding in response to any scratch or injury

Can the Worldwide HIV/AIDS Epidemic Be Stopped?

More than 37 million people in the world have HIV/AIDS, and since the beginning of the worldwide epidemic over 40 years ago, more than 30 million people have died from AIDS. One reason the AIDS epidemic has persisted is that HIV, the virus that causes AIDS, has withstood the efforts of hundreds of scientists to create a vaccine against it. Until there is a vaccine, the world's human population must continue to combat HIV/AIDS with other, less effective tools. With currently available prevention and treatment strategies and effort, the United Nations estimates that the number of people living with HIV and the number of people who will die of AIDS will increase significantly by 2030.

To avert this occurrence, UNAIDS, a division of the United Nations, has launched the "90-90-90 Program." Its goal is an ambitious, immediate increase in worldwide efforts to stop the spread of HIV/AIDS such that, by 2020, 90% of all people living with HIV will know their HIV status (so as to seek treatment and not infect others), 90% of all people with diagnosed HIV infection will receive anti-HIV medications, and 90% of all people receiving anti-HIV medications will respond successfully (UNAIDS, 2017). This reduction in HIV prevalence by 2020 is predicted to lead to eventual control of the epidemic, if not complete eradication.

About 95% of people with HIV/AIDS live in developing countries, where poverty is endemic and healthcare systems are inadequate. These countries lack the financial resources to increase screening for HIV infections, supply anti-HIV drugs to treat HIV-infected individuals, and provide medical support for those who are sick. In order to accomplish the 90-90-90≈Program goals, investments are required from wealthier countries, nongovernmental organizations, and individuals. In 2012, the world spent $19 billion for HIV/AIDS prevention and health care, principally anti-AIDS drugs; the United Nations estimated that $24 billion was needed. In 2012, the United States and Canada combined contributed more than $6 billion for anti-HIV/AIDS programs. Wealthy countries contribute money to anti-HIV/AIDS programs for both humanitarian reasons and for economic, security, and health ones.

The World Bank estimates per capita economic growth declines in poor countries hit by HIV/AIDS. That's because when a poor country's meager financial resources are devoted to dealing with HIV/AIDS, insufficient money is available to build schools, roads, electricity generating plants, and other necessary infrastructure. This can create a humanitarian crisis and a failed state, which drains resources from the rest of the world and impedes attaining world peace and prosperity.

Some barriers to safer sex include the following:

- *Denying that there is a risk.* Many people assume that STDs happen only to "dirty," "promiscuous," and "immoral" people, and because they themselves have sex only with people who are "clean" and "nice," getting an STD is impossible. Another form of denial is to tell oneself, "I eat right. I exercise. I can't get an STD."
- *Believing that the campus community is insulated from STDs.* The truth is that about half of college students are sexually active before they enter college. As a result, students can arrive on campus with an infection. Also, on many campuses, students in the same living groups and student organizations have sex with one another. One infected person could lead to a whole chain of infections.
- *Feeling guilty and uncomfortable about being sexual.* This prevents individuals from planning sex, carrying condoms and spermicides, and talking about possible risks with new partners.
- *Succumbing to social and peer pressure to be sexual.* These pressures encourage people to be sexual in situations that are potentially risky, such as one-night stands and brief relationships that are sexual virtually from the beginning. The risk of infection is lessened when individuals resist peer pressure to have sex with a relative stranger and ask themselves instead, "Is this the right relationship?" "Is this the right partner?" "Am I going to feel OK about this afterward?"

STD Communication Skills

The pressure to be sexual early in a relationship, before the partners know each other well enough to talk about their past sexual experiences, may force partners to deny there may be a risk. A less risky strategy would be to postpone sexual interaction by saying, "I'd like to be close to you, but I'm not ready to have sex until we get to know each other better." "Not yet" and "maybe" are options when weighing an invitation to be sexual.

Even if a person is ready to talk about the sexual aspects of a new relationship, including birth control and possible exposure to STDs, it can be difficult because of fear of being rejected, offending the partner, or just spoiling the mood. Disclosing one's discomfort about talking about the subject is one way to relieve anxiety about it. A conversation could begin with one partner saying, "There's something I want us to talk about and I feel sort of uncomfortable about it, but I think it's important to both of us, so here goes."

After that introduction, the individual can offer information by saying something like, "We don't know each other very well; I'm concerned about sexual diseases. I want you to know this about me." That person should offer all of the information that he or she would like to be told. After hearing the disclosure, the other person is more likely to respond in kind. And if more information is desired, one could say something like, "Thanks for telling me all of that. I'd feel more comfortable if I knew a little more about…" whatever it is.

What if the other person gets offended or won't talk about this subject? Or what if the other person can't be trusted? If partners cannot discuss something as serious as STDs, it is prudent to postpone sexual interaction until the relationship has progressed to a greater level of trust. Potential sexual partners should remember that being under the influence of alcohol or other drugs can affect judgment in making decisions about what is and is not safe. Also, being drunk or stoned can impair using condoms effectively—or using them at all!

Safer sex does not mean no sex. It does not mean that sex is dangerous. It does not mean that sex cannot be fun. It does mean that sex is cooperative. It means that partners are making choices together.

Condom Sense

Latex condoms are effective in preventing the transfer of organisms that cause HIV/AIDS and other STDs. Natural or skin condoms, which are somewhat effective as contraceptives, are too porous to block the transmission of infectious agents. The FDA tests both domestic and international condoms for cracks and other defects in the rubber, leaks, and resistance to breakage. Tested and approved European condoms carry the CE Mark; in the United Kingdom, approval is indicated with the Kitemark. Elsewhere in the world, condoms are also ISO approved.

Putting on a Male Condom

- Use a fresh condom to lessen the possibility of leakage or breakage. Condoms that have been in a wallet, purse, drawer, or auto glove compartment may have been weakened by the heat. Store condoms in a cool, dry place. Don't use a condom past its expiration date.
- Take the condom out of its package carefully so as not to damage it (no teeth, no fingernails). If there are holes or breaks, or if it's sticky or brittle, toss it out and use another.
- Put the condom on the erect penis before intercourse begins (see figure). Interrupting intercourse to put on a condom increases the chances of pregnancy and HIV transmission because the man might not be able to control ejaculation. Also, putting on the condom at the beginning offers the best protection against skin-to-skin transmission of STDs.
- Unroll the condom onto the erect penis (pull back the foreskin). Leave about one-half inch at the tip to catch semen. Some condoms have specially designed (reservoir) tips for semen collection. The tip of the condom should be pressed free of air to prevent breakage after ejaculation.
- Do not use Vaseline or mineral oil as a lubricant. They will destroy the latex. If a lubricant is desired, use a water-based lubricant such as K-Y Jelly or Astroglide.
- After ejaculation, withdraw the penis before it becomes soft. Otherwise, the condom might slip off. When removing the penis, hold the condom on the penis to be sure it does not slip off.
- Check the condom for holes or breaks. If any appear, spermicidal foam or jelly should be put into the vagina immediately, and possible emergency contraception ("the morning-after pill") should be sought.
- Condoms should be used only once and then discarded.

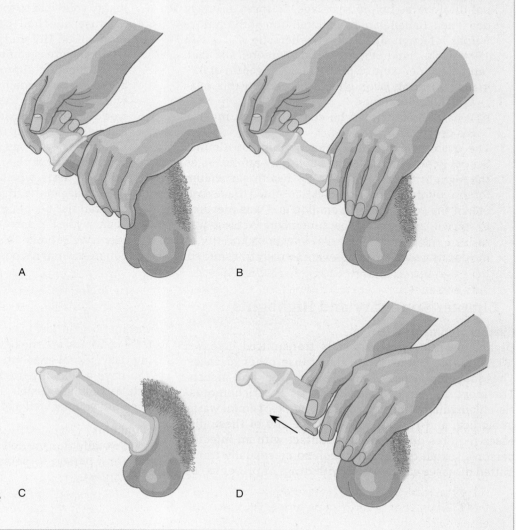

A   B

C   D

Critical Thinking About Health

1. Research has consistently shown that a vast majority of college students know a lot about STDs and AIDS, and yet only 50% of students whose behavior puts them at risk for acquiring an STD or AIDS practice safer sex techniques. To many observers, such risk taking seems illogical, not to mention dangerous. One could postulate, however, that college students are behaving rationally (from their point of view) when they do not practice safer sex.
   a. Looking at your behavior and the attitudes of those of the people in your peer group, can you explain why some college students do not protect themselves from STDs and HIV?
   b. From your knowledge of your peer group's attitudes, how would you advise your college's administration to lessen the risk of STDs and HIV among its students?

2. From their first moments together it was obvious that Ilana and Jason were going to make a great couple. Every one of their friends said so. Yet Jason was troubled. Although they had agreed not to have sexual intercourse before marriage, as their intimacy deepened, Ilana felt obliged to tell him of the genital herpes infection she acquired when she was a wild 15-year-old. "I'm not that person anymore," she said, "and it's under control. Still, you never get rid of it."
   a. Do you think Jason should proceed in this relationship with Ilana?
   b. What factors should he consider when making his decision?

3. The monthly meeting of the Washington County School Board had never had so many attendees as the night of the vote on the new health curriculum for the county's middle schools. It seemed that everyone in the county had an opinion and was prepared to voice it to the seven board members. At issue was revising the module on sexual infections and HIV to include *how* such infections were actually transmitted.

Some parents objected to including any discussion of STDs and HIV in the health curriculum, arguing that doing so only makes the students curious about sex and drugs and encourages experimentation. A second group of parents, while supporting a discussion of the diseases and the organisms that cause them, nevertheless objected to any discussion of behaviors involved in their transmission. They believed that the children ought to know about the biological aspects of the issue as a foundation for their own efforts at dissuading their children from any experimentation with unsafe sexual practices and experimentation with drugs. A third group of parents argued that the only way to ensure prevention was to discuss the behaviors involved. They claimed that the children would not take the discussion seriously unless all aspects of the issue were covered, and hence would be tempted either to disregard the information altogether or to become curious about what was not covered and put themselves at risk. If you were one of the school board members, how would you vote and how would you justify your vote to the parents in your district?

4. Because she had consistently voted to support research on HIV and AIDS, it shocked many people when Congresswoman Harmas refused to vote for the $7.8 billion appropriations bill to pay for protease inhibitor medicines for the medically indigent with AIDS both in the United States and around the world. "I have total compassion for these people," said Harmas, "but at $10,000 a year, we cannot afford to take care of everyone who is sick. Furthermore, in our country, most of the money will go to treating injection drug users, who ought to know better than to get the disease in the first place. And for all the poverty-stricken sick people, principally in Asia and Africa, all I can say is, I'm sorry, complain to your own government. We're broke." Do you agree or disagree with the congresswoman's position?

Chapter Summary and Highlights

Chapter Summary

Organisms that cause sexually transmitted diseases (STDs) are the same kinds that cause other diseases. These include viruses, bacteria, protozoa, and insects. The most frequently diagnosed STDs are trichomoniasis, chlamydia, gonorrhea, syphilis, herpes, genital warts, pubic lice, and HIV/AIDS. To acquire one of these diseases requires direct physical contact with an infected person's sexual organs. Although some sexually transmitted diseases can be cured with drugs or prevented by

vaccination, the key to controlling all STDs is prevention. Male condoms are the best defense against STDs; avoiding risky sexual encounters is another. If you think that you have a sexually transmitted disease, seek medical help as soon as possible. Do not engage in sexual activities until you are well and no longer infectious.

Highlights

- Sexually transmitted diseases are infections passed from person to person, most frequently by sexual contact.

- Millions of sexually transmitted infections occur each year in the United States.
- STDs are epidemic in the United States because people are uninformed about them, because they engage in high-risk behaviors, and because vaccines and cures (for several) are unavailable.
- The most common STDs in the United States are trichomoniasis, chlamydia, gonorrhea, syphilis, herpes, genital warts, pubic lice, and AIDS.

- Preventing STDs involves supporting public health efforts to inform the populace about STDs and their prevention and treatment. It also requires individuals to practice safer sex and to comply with treatment when they are infected.
- *Prevention is the key!*

For Your Health

It is likely that HIV/AIDS has affected your life even if you have no personal contact with someone with the disease. Examine this issue more closely and personally in "AIDS and Me" (Exercise 11.1 in the Workbook). Also check out one of the best HIV/AIDS movies ever, *And the Band Played On* (Exercise 11.2, in the Workbook).

References

American College Health Association. (2016). National College Health Assessment. Retrieved from http://www.acha-ncha.org/

Centers for Disease Control and Prevention. (2016). Reported STDs in the United States. Retrieved from https://www.cdc.gov/std/stats15/default.htm

Drumright, L. N., Gorbach, P. M., & Holmes, K. K. (2004). Do people really know their sex partners? Concurrency, knowledge of partner behavior, and sexually transmitted infections within partnerships. *Sexually Transmitted Diseases, 31,* 437–442.

England, P., & Brown, E. (2016, Fall). Who has how many sexual partners? *Contexts.* Retrieved from https://contexts.org/blog/who-has-how-many-sexual-partners/

Morris, B. J., et al. (2017). CDC's male circumcision recommendations represent a key public health measure. *Global Health: Science and Practice, 5,* 15–27.

United Nations Programmed on HIV/AIDS (UNAIDS). (2017). 90-90-90: An ambitious treatment target to help end the AIDS epidemic. Retrieved from http://www.unaids.org/sites/default/files/media_asset/90-90-90_en.pdf

United Nations Programme on HIV and AIDS (UNAIDS). (2016). UNAIDS report on the global AIDS epidemic. Retrieved from http://www.unaids.org/

Suggested Readings

Centers for Disease Control and Prevention. Division of Sexually Transmitted Diseases. Statistics, health information, and treatment guidelines. Retrieved from www.cdc.gov/std

Hayden, D. (2003). *Pox: Genius, madness, and the mysteries of syphilis.* New York: Basic Books. A discussion of the impact of syphilis on many of history's famous figures and the culture they created, including Oscar Wilde, Abraham Lincoln, and Hitler.

Holmes, K. K., et al. (2007). *Sexually transmitted diseases.* New York: McGraw-Hill. The most comprehensive medical text in the field.

Malani, P. N. (2017). Visions for an AIDS-free generation. *Journal of the American Medical Association, 316,* 154–155. Discusses the current state of HIV/AIDS progress and suggests strategies to bring about an end to the HIV/AIDS epidemic.

Marr, L. (2007). *Sexually transmitted diseases: A physician tells you what you need to know.* Baltimore: Johns Hopkins Press. Detailed information on all STDs.

World Health Organization. Sexually transmitted infections. Retrieved from http://www.who.int/topics/sexually_transmitted_infections/en/. A global view of activities, reports, news, and WHO programs.

Recommended Websites

American Social Health Association
Dedicated to stopping sexually transmitted diseases and their harmful consequences to individuals, families, and communities.

HIVInsite
All about HIV/AIDS—medical issues, prevention, statistics, and policy analysis—from the University of California, San Francisco Medical Center.

Joint United Nations Programme on HIV/AIDS
International views of the AIDS epidemic.

National Center for HIV, STD, and TB Prevention
Public health surveillance, prevention research, and programs to prevent and control human immunodeficiency virus (HIV) infection and acquired immune deficiency syndrome (AIDS), other sexually transmitted diseases (STDs), and tuberculosis (TB).

U.S. Centers for Disease Control and Prevention, Division of STDs
Up-to-date information on all aspects of STDs.

PART FOUR

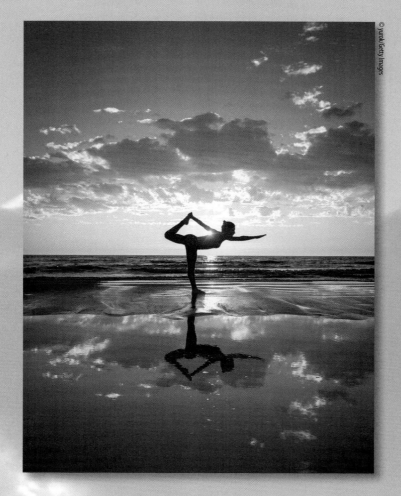

©yurok/Getty Images

Understanding and Preventing Disease

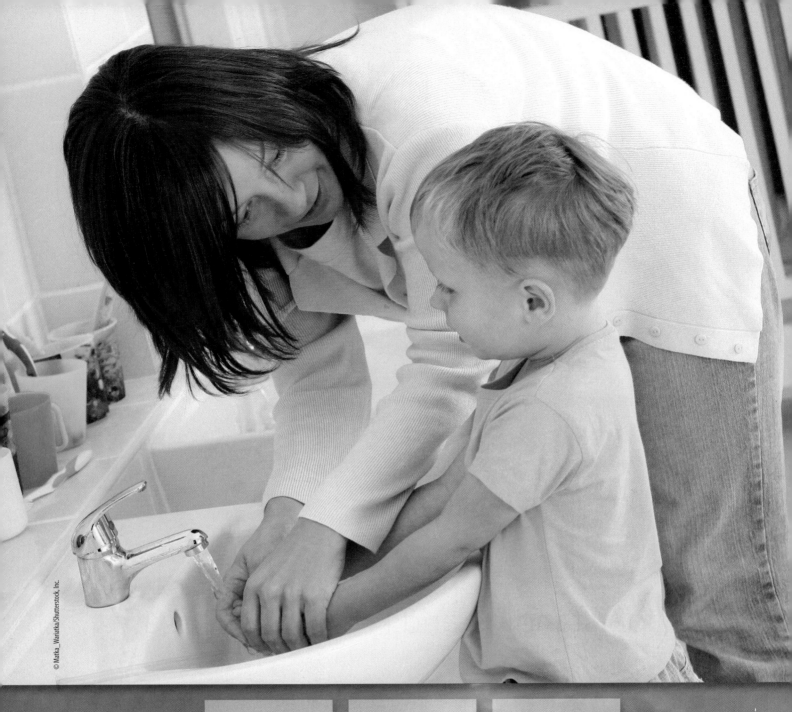

© Matka_Wariatka/Shutterstock, Inc.

Health Tips

Stuffy Sinuses?

HPV Vaccine Prevents Cervical Cancer. So Get Vaccinated!

Getting Rid of Dust Mites May Help Allergies

Global Wellness

Prevent Sickness While Traveling

Worldwide Infectious Disease Eradication Programs

Wellness Guide

The Human Microbiome at Birth

Getting Rid of Head Lice Safely

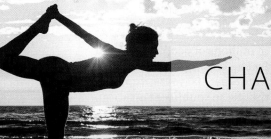

CHAPTER 12

Reducing Infections and Building Immunity: Knowledge Encourages Prevention

Learning Objectives

1. Define *pathogen, communicable disease, vector, immunizations, opportunistic infections, nosocomial disease, immune system, antibodies, antigens,* and *autoimmune diseases.*

2. Describe the human microbiome.

3. Identify and explain how infectious diseases are prevented and treated.

4. Discuss the importance of antibiotics with regard to bacterial infections and the implications of antibiotic-resistant strains of bacteria.

5. Discuss how immunizations prevent infections.

6. Discuss the etiology, symptoms, and treatments for cold and flu, Lyme disease, mononucleosis, and ulcers.

7. Explain how antibodies battle infectious diseases.

8. Describe how unwanted activities of the immune system cause allergies.

9. Discuss organ transplants, blood transfusions, and the Rh factor.

10. Describe how HIV causes AIDS and ways to prevent HIV/AIDS infections.

In past centuries, hundreds of millions of people died from infectious diseases caused by bacteria, viruses, protozoa, and other microorganisms. In the last 100 years, improvements in public sanitation, personal hygiene, nutrition, immunizations, and antimicrobial drugs have greatly reduced the amount of sickness and number of deaths

> Life is what happens when you're making other plans.
>
> *Tom Smothers*

from infectious diseases. However, infectious diseases such as malaria, tuberculosis, HIV/AIDS, and diarrhea from bacterial and viral infections still cause millions of deaths each year, primarily in poor, underdeveloped countries where poverty, undernutrition, and inadequate sanitation create conditions that foster infectious diseases. Globally, infectious disease is among the 10 most common causes of death.

Even the healthiest person can contract an infectious disease. We all have occasional colds, flu, or stomach upsets from food-borne infections. Usually these infections are self-limiting, and we become well in a few days or weeks. Other infectious diseases, such as pneumonia, tuberculosis, or "staph" infections, can be serious enough to require medical intervention to forestall disability and even death. Understanding how infectious microorganisms cause disease and how your immune system and modern medicine battle infections is essential for maintaining wellness.

Most microorganisms are not harmful when they are present in or on the body. In fact, the human body contains as many as 10 times the number of bacteria cells as it does its own human cells, and most of these trillions of bacteria perform many essential functions in many parts of the body. But there are also areas of the body that must remain totally free of bacteria, or sterile (**Table 12.1**). If normally sterile areas of the body become infected by microorganisms, an infectious disease results. Any microorganism that infects the body and causes disease is called a **pathogen**.

Although it is possible to prevent and treat infections by microorganisms through modern sanitation, hygiene, vaccinations, and medicines such as antibiotic drugs, there is growing concern over potential harmful effects of the overuse of antimicrobial chemicals. For example, widespread use of antibiotics in commercially raised animals such as cattle, pigs, and poultry has created "super" strains of pathogenic bacteria that are not killed by antibiotic drugs.

The overuse of antibiotics to treat infections that are not caused by bacteria (viruses are not killed by antibiotics) also encourages the development of antibiotic-resistant strains of pathogenic bacteria, especially in hospitals. In addition, the growing use of antibacterial soaps, cosmetics, toothpaste, and other products encourages the emergence of antibiotic resistance among bacteria and may be counterproductive to promoting health. The development of immune system responses depends

---

Table 12.1

Bacteria in the Body

Some areas of the body harbor millions of bacteria, most of which are beneficial; other areas of the body are sterile (no bacteria).

Sterile body areas
Respiratory tract (below the vocal chords)
Sinuses and middle ear
Liver and gallbladder
Urinary tract above the urethra
Bones, joints, muscles, and blood
Cerebrospinal fluid (the brain and spinal column)
The linings around the lungs (pleura) and abdominal cavity (peritoneum)

Body areas that are colonized with bacteria
Skin: Contains thousands of bacteria per square centimeter and some fungi. The microorganisms are beneficial or harmless unless the skin is damaged or a person is already sick.

Nasopharynx and oropharynx: May contain billions of bacteria per milliliter of fluid, including pathogenic bacteria that can cause disease, but only in people whose immune systems are weak.

Esophagus and stomach: Thousands of bacteria are ingested with food. Most people have been infected with bacteria that cause ulcers (*Helicobacter pylori*) but do not have any symptoms of ulcers.

Small intestine: Low concentration of bacteria; species of *Lactobacillus* are common.

Large intestine: Billions of bacteria per milliliter of fluid are present; almost all are anaerobic species (bacteria that only grow in the absence of oxygen). All fecal matter contains billions of bacteria.

Vagina: Contains millions of bacteria, including species of *Lactobacillus* and *Escherichia coli* as well as other anaerobic bacteria.

---

on early exposure to a wide range of environmental stimuli, including exposure to bacteria. When children play in the dirt, for example, they are getting valuable exposure to microorganisms that help their immune systems develop. Too much hygiene can be as detrimental to health as too little hygiene.

Many studies have indicated that children raised on farms have far fewer allergies, hay fever, or asthma compared to children raised in urban environments. The immune systems of children growing up on farms also possess cells that help prevent allergic responses (Schuijs et al., 2015). These observations suggest that farm dust, which contains animal microorganisms not found in cities, stimulates the immune system so as to lessen the risk of allergic reactions later in life. This is called the *hygiene hypothesis*. It was proposed about 30 years ago to explain why children raised in hyper-clean environments are more susceptible to asthma and allergies. To adults, it advises against the overzealous pursuit of cleanliness and admonishment of children not to touch anything "dirty," because doing so increases the risk of developing allergies. The desire of young children to touch and taste objects in their environments is important for the development of an immune system that is not prone to allergic responses.

The Human Microbiome

The human body contains 10 to 100 times more microorganisms than it does its own human cells. The vast majority of these microorganisms are bacteria; microorganisms classified as archaea, eukaryotes, and viruses also are present in smaller numbers. The overall composition of microorganisms inhabiting a human body is referred to as the **human microbiome**. Most of the organisms of the human microbiome inhabit the intestines (gut), the part of the digestive system that extends from the mouth to the anus. They are also found in the nose, vagina, and on the skin.

In 2007, the U.S. National Institutes of Health, a part of the federal government that sponsors much of the biological and medical research in the United States, authorized a long-term initiative to discover and understand the role of the human microbiome in human health and disease. Scientists began by taking thousands of samples of the overall human microbiome from hundreds of volunteers in rural and urban areas across the country. More than 10,000 different species of bacteria were identified from many sites on the human body (**Figure 12.1**), and were present in different amounts in each individual. Overall, the microorganisms in the human microbiome produced more than 60,000 different proteins, which is 300 times the number of proteins that all the cells of the human body produce.

This enormous diversity of microbial proteins in the human body can affect human metabolism and overall health (Glasner, 2017). For example, the community of microbes in an individual may influence the person's susceptibility to certain infectious diseases; contribute to the onset of obesity, diabetes (types 1 and 2), allergies, asthma, autism, some cancers, and chronic gastrointestinal

---

TERMS

human microbiome: the total composition of bacteria, fungi, viruses, and other microorganisms that inhabit a human body

pathogen: a disease-causing organism

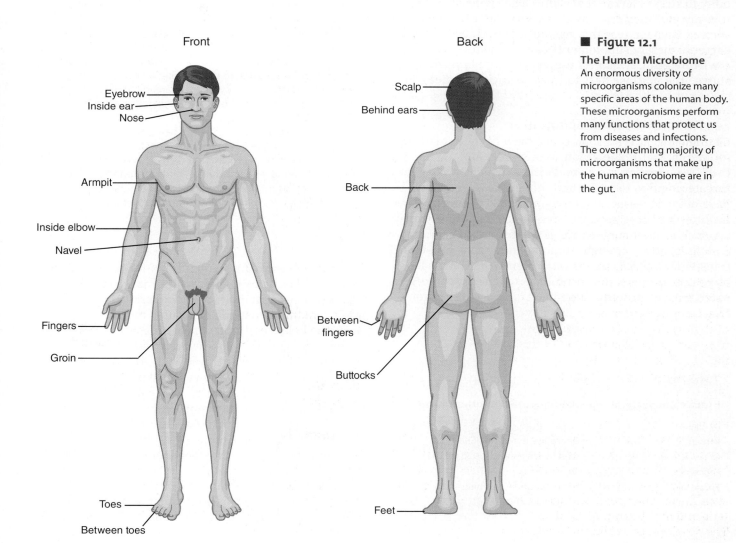

Front

Eyebrow
Inside ear
Nose

Armpit

Inside elbow

Navel

Fingers

Groin

Toes

Between toes

Back

Scalp
Behind ears

Back

Between fingers

Buttocks

Feet

■ **Figure 12.1**

The Human Microbiome
An enormous diversity of microorganisms colonize many specific areas of the human body. These microorganisms perform many functions that protect us from diseases and infections. The overwhelming majority of microorganisms that make up the human microbiome are in the gut.

disorders such as Crohn's disease and irritable bowel syndrome; and impact the person's response to certain medicines. The microbiome of the mother may even affect the health of her children (see the Wellness Guide, "The Human Microbiome at Birth").

Whereas it may not be surprising that the billions of microorganisms in the gut could affect the health of the body, it is surprising that these microorganisms might also affect the brain and play a significant role in anxiety, depression, and other mental afflictions. Many species of gut bacteria produce neurotransmitters that are chemically identical to those in the brain (Table 12.2). The bacterial neurotransmitters can move through the bloodstream to the brain, just as psychiatric medications taken by mouth do, or they can stimulate the vagus nerve, which is an information channel between the gut and the brain. Laboratory animals born under sterile conditions so they do not have a microbiome exhibit reckless behaviors, memory difficulties, and antisocial behaviors as adults (Sanders, 2016). A number of human studies suggest that alterations in the composition of the human microbiome can affect mood and susceptibility to stress (Sarkar et al., 2016). The expression "I feel it in my gut" may one day be shown scientifically to be correct. Because research has not determined if taking bacterial dietary supplements can safely mitigate anxiety, depression, sleeplessness, or other troubling mental states, it is perhaps best for now to stick to a diet consisting of healthy foods.

Fecal Microbiota Transplantation

Clostridium difficile (*C. difficile*) is a bacterium that causes inflammation of the colon (*colitis*). A major result of *C. difficile* infection is severe diarrhea, which can be life-threatening due to water and mineral loss. People who have other illnesses, elderly who live in long-term care facilities, or those requiring prolonged use of antibiotics, such as after surgery, are at greater risk of acquiring *C. difficile*, often through unintended person-to-person transfer of *C. difficile* spores via unsterile/ungloved hands of healthcare personnel who have touched a contaminated surface or item. *Clostridium difficile* can live for a long time on surfaces.

The Human Microbiome at Birth

During intrauterine development, the fetus is in a sterile environment. But that changes during birth because the vagina is naturally laden with bacteria, viruses, fungi, and other microorganisms. As the baby enters the vagina, its head becomes covered with vaginal fluid and millions of microorganisms enter the ears, nose, and mouth. The baby's entire digestive tract becomes flooded with microorganisms that are characteristic of the mother's vaginal microbiome. These microorganisms become the baby's first microbiome and begin to affect development of the immune system. A healthy vaginal microbiome initiates a healthy microbiome in the baby. However, disease-causing microorganisms also can be acquired by the baby if the vaginal fluid contains pathogens such as the human immunodeficiency virus (HIV). If the baby is infected with HIV during birth, without postnatal treatment with anti-HIV medications it is likely to develop AIDS.

Childbirth by Cesarean section is sterile, so a baby's first encounter with microorganisms is from the hands of hospital personnel. Thus, the microbiome of a Cesarean baby is very different from one delivered vaginally. One indication that Cesarean babies may have different immune systems than vaginally delivered babies is that they are twice as likely to develop asthma as vaginal babies. Some doctors now consider exposure to vaginal fluid to be so essential to establishing a healthy microbiome in a baby that they treat Cesarean babies with vaginal fluid from the mother immediately after delivery. Sterile cotton swabs are dipped in the mother's vaginal fluid and used to swab the baby's head, ears, nose, and lips. In this way, the Cesarean baby can start its own microbiome with the microorganisms it would have received during a vaginal birth. This is just one example of how important the microbiome is now regarded in promoting development of the immune system.

Antibiotics are the standard treatment for *C. difficile* infection, but often the disease returns again and again. One likely reason for this is that long-term antibiotic exposure or multiple unsterile exposures to bacterial spores upset the balance of microorganisms in the gut microbiome, thus giving *C. difficile* a survival advantage. An experimental method approved by the U.S. Food and Drug Administration (FDA) that shows great promise in treating *C. difficile* infection in patients who had previously failed to recover with antibiotic therapy, but which not everyone can stomach, is **fecal microbiota transplantation (FMT)**. This method involves obtaining a fecal preparation from a carefully screened, healthy stool donor and transplanting it into the colon of a patient via oral capsules, nasal tube, or colonoscopy. In a number of patients, FMT has completely eradicated *C. difficile* infection, sometimes in less than a day. Besides *C. difficile* infection, FMT shows promise in treating a serious autoimmune disease of the gut

Table 12.2

Human Gut Bacteria That Manufacture Neurotransmitters

Organism	Neurotransmitters
Bacillus	Dopamine; norepinephrine
Bifidobacterium	Gamma-aminobutyric acid (GABA)
Enterococcus	Serotonin
Escherichia	Norepinephrine; serotonin
Lactobacillus	Acetylcholine; GABA
Streptococcus	Serotonin

called Crohn's disease, which affects as many as 700,000 Americans (Eakin, 2014).

Most of the research on fecal transplants thus far has been carried out in laboratory animals that have been bred with conditions mimicking those of people. For example, mice bred to become obese on a standard diet lost weight when given fecal transplants from lean mice. The reverse was also true. When lean mice were given fecal transplants from obese mice, they gained weight and their microbiomes changed to resemble that of obese mice. These experiments show that microbiomes could play an import role in weight management in humans irrespective of diet or genetic makeup (Marotza & Zarrinparb, 2016). Evidence for a similar effect in people comes from studying the microbiomes of very obese individuals who undergo gastric bypass surgery in order to lose weight. After the surgery, the microbiome of obese patients begins to resemble the microbiome of healthy persons of normal weight.

A Healthy Microbiome

As evidence gathers pointing to the important roles that the human microbiome plays in health and disease, a question to consider is "How can one acquire a healthy microbiome?" The likely answer, as with so many facets of healthful living, is to consume a healthy diet consisting of fresh fruits and vegetables, nuts, seeds, and fiber, and free of too much sugar, manufactured food additives, pesticides, and alcohol; limit exposure to cigarette smoke and other pollutants, antibiotics, and antiseptics; manage stress; and to reinvigorate the microbiome after taking medications, particularly antibiotics.

Agents of Infectious Disease

A remarkable variety of microorganisms, including bacteria, viruses, protozoa, yeast, and small worms, can infect the human body, causing disease, sickness, and death (**Figure 12.2**). All microorganisms except viruses are considered alive because they can grows and reproduce on their own. Viruses, however, are not considered alive because they only grow and reproduce after they infect a cell and usurp its cellular machinery to make more viruses. Some common human diseases caused by viruses are colds, flu, polio, hepatitis, chicken pox, mumps, measles, herpes, and HIV/AIDS. Each of the viruses that cause these diseases is different and infects a specific tissue or organ in the body.

Other infectious diseases, such as pneumonia, tuberculosis, cholera, plague, typhoid fever, and gonorrhea, are caused by specific pathogenic bacteria. Often pathogenic

> **TERMS**
>
> fecal microbiota transplantation (FMT): transplanting fecal material from a healthy donor to the colon of an unwell person to create a healthful change in the patient's intestinal micrombiome

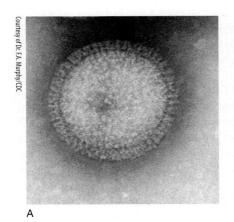

A

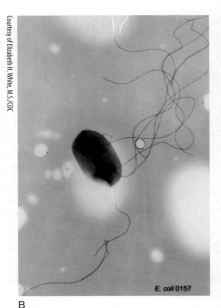

B

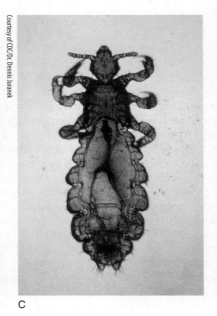

C

■ **Figure 12.2**

Infectious Organisms
Electron micrographs of (a) an influenza virus that causes flu, (b) *Salmonella* bacteria that cause food poisoning, and (c) head louse. Both the "flu" virus and the bacteria are easily passed from person to person and cause widespread epidemics.

bacteria and viruses cause disease only if the individual is already in a weakened state, particularly if the immune system is not functioning optimally.

If an infectious disease is shown to be caused by a specific microorganism, that cause is called its **etiology**. For example, tuberculosis usually is caused by a specific bacterium called *Mycobacterium tuberculosis,* infectious mononucleosis is caused by the Epstein-Barr virus, and giardiasis (an infection of the small intestine) is caused by the protozoan *Giardia lamblia.*

Infectious agents enter the body in a variety of ways. If the infectious organism is passed from person to person, the disease is called a **communicable disease**. Colds, measles, chicken pox, AIDS, and gonorrhea are all communicable diseases.

Infectious organisms also can be transferred to people from animals, especially insects. In these instances, the animal or insect is said to be the **vector**, or carrier, of the disease-causing microorganism. For example, **malaria** is usually caused by a microscopic protozoan called *Plasmodium falciparum.* When a person with malaria is bitten by a mosquito, blood (and the malaria parasite) is taken up by the mosquito and transferred into another person by a bite from the same mosquito. Thus, mosquitoes are the vectors for malaria. (Only a few species of mosquitoes carry the malarial parasite.)

Rabies is a disease of the nervous system caused by the rabies virus present in infected dogs, cats, bats,

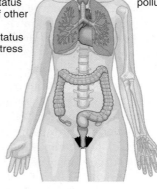

Internal
- Age
- Sex
- Immunological competence
- Previous infections
- Hormonal status
- Presence of other diseases
- Nutritional status
- Emotional stress level
- Heredity

External
- Infection in the community
- Season of year
- Hygiene and sanitation
- Drugs and medications
- Environmental pollutants or toxins

■ **Figure 12.3**

Factors Affecting the Risk of an Infectious Disease
Various internal and external factors determine whether disease will result from infections by viruses, bacteria, or other kinds of infectious agents.

skunks, and other animals. An infected animal is a vector for rabies, and the virus is transmitted to another person through the saliva of the rabid animal.

Whether a person gets an infectious disease depends on a wide range of factors, including the competence of the immune system, nutritional status, stress, the presence of other diseases, and environmental conditions (**Figure 12.3**). For example, many people are exposed to bacteria that can cause pneumonia. However, pneumonia usually develops in older people whose immune systems are weak or in younger people who are susceptible to infections for many reasons. Some people are more resistant to infectious organisms than others because of genes that they inherited.

Tuberculosis (TB) is not simply caused by infection with the bacterium *Mycobacterium tuberculosis.* Robert Koch, a famous nineteenth-century microbiologist, called TB the "disease of poverty" because it was associated with squalor, overcrowding, poor nutrition, and poor sanitation. Today, many people have small tubercular lesions in their lungs but have no symptoms of disease because they enjoy good nutrition, good living conditions, and are in good general health. However, in some urban areas where people live in squalor and poverty, TB is once again emerging as a problem.

In many regions of the world, millions of people still die from infectious diseases (**Table 12.3**). Various kinds of worms (roundworm, pinworm, hookworm, and tapeworm) infect over 1.5 billion people worldwide. Another 200 million people are debilitated by the waterborne parasite that causes the disease schistosomiasis. Malarial parasites infect over 200 million people each year and cause nearly 500 million deaths annually around the globe. About 1.7 billion children in Asia, Africa, and Latin

Getting Rid of Head Lice Safely

Nature constantly evolves new species of organisms that are resistant to toxic chemicals in their environments. For example, the mosquitoes that carry the microorganism that cause malaria in humans were reasonably controlled for decades by the pesticide DDT. But over years of exposure, many mosquito populations developed resistance to DDT, and so malaria is still a major problem, principally in tropical regions where the mosquitoes abound.

Head lice are no different. They have now evolved so that many infestations can no longer be controlled with previously effective treatments. The tiny head louse (*Pediculus humanus capitis*) does not cause serious disease but does carry considerable social stigma, is socially disruptive, and is costly to society in terms of lost work and school time. Children with head lice quickly pass them on to other children during close contact while playing. All members of a family may become infected. Sometimes schools must shut down to halt the epidemic.

Fortunately, highly effective treatments for head lice infections are available. A single, 10-minute application of ivermectin lotion kills head lice and stops the infection of other persons. The new treatment is more effective than older treatments and is simple for parents to use. At the first sign of head lice on yourself or others, apply this lotion.

Prevent Sickness While Traveling

The Centers for Disease Control and Prevention (CDC) provides travelers to other countries with the latest information of disease outbreaks and health risks around the world. The CDC advisory system consists of four categories of warnings.

The lowest category of risk is called "In the News." This describes outbreaks or health risks that are newsworthy but which present little or no health risk to travelers who take standard precautions such as drinking bottled water and not eating contaminated fresh fruits and vegetables.

The next category, called "Outbreak Notice," also does not restrict travel but advises travelers of disease outbreaks in localized areas. Travelers are advised to make sure their vaccinations are up to date.

The third category is called "Travel Health Precaution." This category also does not restrict travel but usually advises travelers to avoid specific areas or to take additional health precautions. Outbreaks of infectious diseases occurring over a large geographic area usually fall into this category.

The category of highest risk is called "Travel Health Warning" and advises travelers not to travel to the area unless absolutely necessary. Vacationers should cancel their plans. The severe acute respiratory syndrome (SARS) epidemic in Asia in 2002–2003 fell into this category.

Anyone traveling outside the United States should check the CDC travel advisory website at http://www.cdc.gov /travel or call (877) 394-8747 for the latest information on disease outbreaks and health information. If you want a list of English-speaking physicians in the area you are traveling to, contact the International Association for Medical Assistance to Travellers (http://www.iamat.org).

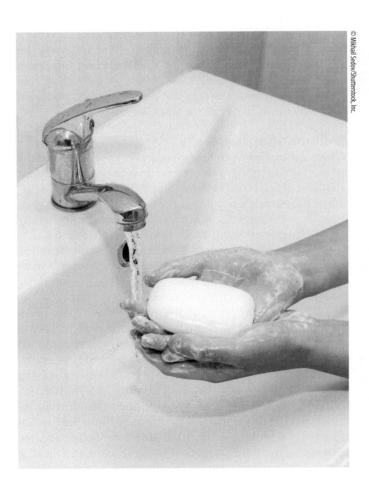

© Mikhail Sedov/Shutterstock, Inc.

Table 12.3

Estimated Annual Deaths Worldwide from Infectious Diseases

Acute respiratory infections	3.2 million
Diarrheal diseases	1.4 million
Tuberculosis	1.4 million
HIV/AIDS	1.1 million
Malaria	439,000
Meningitis	315,000
Hepatitis (A, B, C, D)	145,000
Pertussis (whooping cough)	273,000
Leishmaniasis	140,000

Data from World Health Organization. (2016). Disease burden and mortality estimates. Retrieved from http://www.who.int/healthinfo/global_burden_disease/estimates/en/index1.html

Fighting Infectious Diseases

Infectious diseases are fought in four ways: (1) sanitation, (2) treatment with antibiotics and other drugs, (3) vaccinations, and (4) healthful living. Stopping the spread of infectious organisms requires that they be destroyed both in infected people and in the environment.

America contract severe diarrhea caused by infectious organisms, and half a million children die from diarrhea each year. Many countries lack the resources to ensure safe water supplies, public sanitation, safe waste disposal, and adequate health care—factors that can control the spread of most infectious diseases.

TERMS

communicable disease: an infectious disease that is usually transmitted from person to person

etiology: specific cause of disease

malaria: a disease of red blood cells that produces fever, anemia, and death

vector: the carrier of infectious organisms from animals to people or from person to person

Thus, reducing the burden of infectious diseases is the responsibility both of individuals and of communities. Individuals need to practice good hygiene, avoid unsafe sex, and make sure required immunizations are up-to-date, especially for children. Communities have a responsibility to make sure water is safe to drink, the food supply is not contaminated, garbage and wastes do not pollute the environment, and people receive education and counseling on how to avoid sexually transmitted diseases.

Scientific understanding of the causes of infectious diseases first began in the late nineteenth century with the research of the French scientist Louis Pasteur, who established the germ theory of disease by showing that microscopic organisms could cause infections and disease. Pasteur discovered that these microorganisms could be rendered harmless by heat or by treatment with antiseptic chemicals. Like many radically new scientific ideas, Pasteur's were ignored at first. Today, pasteurization, the process of warming raw foods such as milk and other dairy products to make them safe to consume, is common practice.

The use of antiseptic (sterile) techniques to reduce the number of infections and deaths after surgery was adopted slowly in the United States, despite the fact that a famous American physician, Joseph Lister, had successfully implemented Pasteur's advice in his hospital. (The antiseptic mouthwash Listerine is named in his honor.) Before antiseptic techniques were introduced in hospitals, surgery or childbirth in a hospital often led to death from subsequent infection.

Today, dozens of over-the-counter wash products, including liquid, foam, and gel hand soaps; bar soaps; and body washes, contain antibacterial ingredients. According to the FDA (2016), scientific evidence showing that these products are better at preventing illness than washing with plain soap and water is inconclusive. Moreover, the wide use of these products has raised the question of potential negative effects of the antibacterial chemicals within them on human health, which is the reason that 19 such chemicals, including the widely used *triclosan* and *triclocarban*, have been banned for use in over-the-counter soaps. Also, the wide use of these antibacterial agents increases the risk of organisms developing resistance to antibacterial chemicals, including antibiotic drugs. The FDA's best advice for cleaning hands is to wash your hands with plain soap and water for about 20 seconds each time (the length of time to sing the ABC song) (see Infographic).

Sanitation, sterile techniques, and public health programs were not actively implemented in the United States until the beginning of the twentieth century. Only then did the incidence of many infectious diseases, such as tuberculosis, plague, pneumonia, and diphtheria, begin to decline dramatically. Many medical historians claim that sanitation is the most significant medical advance of all time because it contributed to preventing millions of cases of infectious disease caused by contaminated water and food.

Understanding Antibiotics

In the late 1940s, another highly effective tool was discovered for combating infectious diseases caused by bacteria. The antibiotic **penicillin**, which is produced by a species of mold, was able to cure many kinds of bacterial infections. Today, hundreds of antibiotic drugs are available for treating infectious diseases caused by bacteria. Many other drugs are now available for treating diseases caused by viruses, protozoa, worms, and other microorganisms. These drugs either destroy the microorganisms or hold their numbers in check so the risk of infection and disease is greatly reduced.

Antibiotics block essential biochemical reactions of microorganisms that infect the body, thereby preventing them from growing. The most useful antibiotics selectively interfere with the growth of bacteria without affecting the functions of body cells. Antibiotics kill both harmful and helpful bacteria in the body; however, once the harmful bacteria have been killed, the helpful bacteria quickly repopulate their normal sites.

Antibiotics do not prevent the growth of viruses because viruses are not living cells. Viruses infect and take over the cellular functions of body cells, thus ensuring their own growth and propagation. Finding a drug that will specifically kill a virus but not also kill body cells is very difficult but many antiviral drugs are now available.

Antibiotic Resistance

When antibiotics were first discovered, they were greeted as wonder drugs capable of curing some of the most deadly bacterial infectious diseases, such as plague, tuberculosis, pneumonia, syphilis, and a slew of less serious diseases. Indeed, antibiotics have been exceptionally useful drugs over the past 70 years, but we are now witnessing a decline in their general effectiveness. One of the primary reasons is that many pathogenic bacteria have acquired new genes that make them resistant to one or several of the most effective antibiotics.

Within a few years of the discovery of penicillin, penicillin-resistant bacteria began appearing in patients with bacterial infections. Bacteria also rapidly acquired resistance to other antibiotics, such as tetracycline, erythromycin, and chloramphenicol. Antibiotic resistance can be transferred among bacteria in nature in a small piece of **deoxyribonucleic acid (DNA)** that carries antibiotic-resistance genes. Harmless bacteria of one species can transfer antibiotic-resistance genes to many other species of bacteria, including ones that cause disease. In this way, bacteria that cause gonorrhea, pneumonia, tuberculosis, and "staph" infections have become resistant to many previously effective antibiotics.

For example, tuberculosis (TB) is a lung infection caused by a bacterium called *Mycobacterium tuberculosis*. It is one of the top 10 causes of death worldwide. Many different strains of *M. tuberculosis* cause tuberculosis; one strain causes XDR-TB (extensively drug-resistant TB). According to the World Health Organization, in 2017 this deadly strain of bacteria was detected in patients in 117 countries. XDR-TB is resistant to all of the antibiotics usually prescribed to cure ordinary tuberculosis infections. The only treatment now available for XDR-TB patients consists of 2 years of treatment with several highly toxic drugs; 50% to 80% of patients die from the treatment. Those who survive often suffer from permanent nerve damage and other serious symptoms caused by the drugs. What makes XDR-TB infection particularly worrisome is that it is transmitted by close personal contact; all family members may become infected. Besides TB, many sexually transmitted diseases, such as chlamydia and gonorrhea, are now resistant to most of the antibiotics that have been effective previously. The antibiotics rifampin and isoniazid had been very effective in treating TB, but now these drugs are sometimes ineffective because the TB bacteria have acquired multiple antibiotic resistance.

The antibiotic methicillin had been used for years as a very effective treatment for skin and soft tissue infections caused by the bacterium *Staphylococcus aureus*. Over the years, bacteria of this species mutated until a very virulent strain, *methicillin-resistant Staphylococcus aureus (MRSA)*, emerged. These virulent "staph" infections are often found among patients in hospitals. In 2016, Daniel Fells, a 10-year veteran tight end for the New York Giants, had to retire from football because of a MRSA foot infection thought to be contracted from treatment of an ankle injury with MRSA-contaminated medical equipment. Fells underwent 10 surgeries to save his foot and his life.

Antibiotic resistance results from practices in two areas: agriculture and health care. In agriculture, about 50% of all antibiotic chemicals used in the United States (about 3 million pounds a year) are routinely given to farm animals to prevent them from getting infections, which would make them sick and lessen their weight and marketability. Some of the bacteria that the antibiotics are supposed to kill are resistant, and after a while the property of resistance is passed from animal to animal and even to soil bacteria via animal feces. If the animal flesh or the water runoff from an animal production facility is contaminated with resistant bacteria, the property of resistance can be transferred to bacteria that infect people.

In health care, because professionals use antibiotics extensively, hospitals, and particularly intensive care units, can give rise to antibiotic resistant bacteria through inadvertent transmission via healthcare staff. Among community-based doctors, it is estimated that more than half of the prescriptions that are written for antibiotics are unnecessary, as they are generally written for people with colds and flu. Colds and flu are caused by viruses, which cannot be killed by antibiotics. So why do doctors prescribe them when they are useless? One reason is that the doctor has made a diagnostic or treatment error. Another reason is that the patient, or a patient's parent

in the case of a child, demands an antibiotic to treat some symptoms, and the doctor complies. Either way, antibiotics unnecessarily enter the environment and contribute to the problem of antibiotic resistance.

Scientists around the world have been warning about the increase in antibiotic resistance for decades. Since the discovery of the first antibiotic, penicillin, in the 1940s, these "wonder drugs" have been used indiscriminately in many industries. The beef, poultry, and pork industries feed their animals thousands of tons of antibiotics annually to enhance growth and prevent infections. Antibacterials are added to soaps, deodorants, hand wipes, sprays—almost any product used to fight "germs." Most bacteria that humans encounter in the environment pose little or no health danger. In fact, most bacteria on the skin and in the digestive system are beneficial and protect people in countless ways. Increasingly, countries are banning the unnecessary and indiscriminate use of antibiotics and insisting that these essential drugs be reserved for the treatment of serious human diseases (Margalida et al., 2014).

A battle to abolish the use of antibiotics in animal feed has been going on for decades in the United States. In 2003, the World Health Organization (WHO) released a report concluding that the use of antibiotics endangered human health and was of little benefit to livestock. The European Union (EU) has ordered member countries to completely stop using antibiotics in feed for pigs and poultry. Even McDonald's, which buys more than a billion pounds of beef a year, has pledged to buy only antibiotic-free beef. In 2014, the FDA implemented a voluntary plan with industry to phase out the use of certain antibiotics for enhanced food production. Whether this plan will actually reduce antibiotic use in animal production remains to be seen. Many believe that not totally banning the use of antibiotics in animal feed is another example in which profit and politics supercede scientific advice and human health.

In the 1990s, the FDA approved two drugs, Baytril and SaraFlox, that could be added routinely to poultry feed. These two drugs belong to a class of extremely effective antibiotics called fluoroquinolones; members of this family of drugs are used to treat the bacteria that cause anthrax and foodborne infections. Scientists and the American Medical Association warned that such use in animal feed would lead to the emergence of antibiotic-resistant strains. After several years of use, this is exactly what happened, and the FDA tried to ban the use of the

TERMS

deoxyribonucleic acid (DNA): a chemical substance that carries genetic information in all cells of all organisms

penicillin: an antibiotic produced by mold and capable of curing many bacterial infections

drugs in livestock. Drug companies fought the FDA, and it was years before the drugs were finally withdrawn from the market. But it was too late; resistance had already occurred. Fluoroquinolone drugs are now much less effective in treating staph infections.

In 2007, the FDA again succumbed to drug company pressures and approved the use of a powerful antibiotic, cefquinome, for use in animal feed. Again the American Medical Association and many other health organizations warned that adding this drug to animal feed would, within a few years, lead to antibiotic-resistant strains of pathogenic bacteria and render this powerful class of drugs much less effective. Despite the overwhelming evidence of the health peril from overuse of antibiotics in animals and people, the U.S. government still has not restricted the unnecessary use of antibiotics as most other countries have done (Woolhouse & Ward, 2013). Every year in the United States, drug companies sell thousands of tons of antibiotics for use in livestock and people. Time after time over the last several decades, the FDA has bowed to industry pressures and has failed to perform its primary mission to protect the health of Americans.

How the Body Protects Itself

The best way to avoid infectious diseases caused by pathogenic microorganisms is to keep them out of the body. The skin and mucous membranes prevent the entry of most microorganisms into the body by functioning as physical barriers. That is why a wound often exposes the body to infection (**Figure 12.4**). The skin is mildly acidic and provides a poor habitat for most harmful microorganisms, although the skin is covered with beneficial bacteria.

The eyes, nose, throat, and breathing passages are protected by mucous membranes that continuously produce secretions that flush away harmful organisms and particles. Mucous membranes also secrete enzymes that can destroy toxic substances. The mouth, digestive system, and excretory organs also are protected by membranes that guard the internal organs.

Tears keep the surface of the eyes moist and serve to wash away foreign particles. Wax secreted from the ears protects the delicate hearing apparatus. The mucous coating of the respiratory tract is sticky and provides a trap for irritating particles and microorganisms in the air; microscopic hairs called **cilia** keep the mucus moving out of the bronchial tubes. Coughing and spitting are mechanisms that remove foreign material from the breathing passages. Sneezing and blowing the nose eliminate irritating particles that are inhaled.

Cells and enzymes in the blood quickly form clots that seal off any break in the skin, thereby preventing the entry of harmful substances and infectious organisms. If some bacteria do enter the wound before it is sealed off,

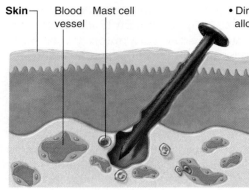

Skin — Blood vessel   Mast cell

- Dirty nail penetrates skin, allowing bacteria to enter
- Blood vessels dilate, causing area to become red and hot
- Histamine released
- White blood cells rush to area to attack bacteria

■ **Figure 12.4**

Inflammation Response
Penetration of the skin by any unsterile sharp object often produces an inflammation response, the normal response of the body to injury or infection.

other special cells that are part of the immune system attack and destroy the invaders.

If microorganisms or foreign particles penetrate the skin and enter the blood, they soon encounter specialized cells called **leukocytes**, the colorless white blood cells that can be distinguished from the red blood cells that transport oxygen. Only about 1 in 700 cells in the blood is a leukocyte, but their number can increase dramatically if an acute infection occurs. That is why blood is tested for the number of white blood cells when an infection is suspected.

Specialized white blood cells called **macrophages** are associated with specific organs and are vital to the body's internal defense mechanisms. Macrophages are able to engulf and digest foreign cells and particles that invade the body. Organ-specific macrophages protect the lungs, stomach, and other organs from damage by foreign substances.

Common Infectious Diseases

Infectious diseases, depending on their cause and consequences, present special public health problems and personal concerns for many people. To better understand how to cope with infectious disease, we'll review colds and flu, Lyme disease, mononucleosis, ulcers, and hepatitis. HIV/AIDS is discussed later in this chapter.

Colds

Most people, especially children, contract several colds and possibly flu every year. Both diseases are caused by viruses that infect cells of the respiratory tract. Up to 80% of common colds are caused by *human rhinovirus* (HRV), but many other viruses also infect the respiratory tract and cause colds. Because HRV is so diverse genetically, it has been impossible to construct an effective vaccine.

It may be hard to believe, but the average American spends about 5 years of his or her life suffering from colds. A cold caused by one virus does not protect a person from catching a cold caused by a different strain, which explains why colds can occur one after another or several times a year.

Although cold symptoms may be quite discomforting, colds generally do not result in long-term illness or death. Billions of dollars are spent by Americans every year on medications that are supposed to alleviate cold symptoms, such as sore throat, cough, congestion, runny nose, and pain. Physicians joke that a cold will go away in about a week with rest and medications or in about 7 days if nothing is done. It takes the immune system about a week to produce the specific proteins (antibodies) that inactivate the viruses and for tissues to heal.

High-tech modern medicine has nothing to offer that can prevent a cold, although enormous research efforts have been expended to find a drug that would reduce the risk of catching a cold. Although many of the "discoveries" of cold research were announced with great fanfare, none has worked.

Americans suffer an estimated 500 million colds a year. Anyone with a cold is caught between a rock and a hard place. Staying at home means lost income and possibly causing a major disruption at work. For example, if a physician with a cold stays away from work, all the appointments must be canceled or switched to other doctors whose schedules already are full. If a person decides to go to work despite being sick, sneezing, and coughing, other workers are likely to become infected and face the same problem of whether to stay at home or go to work. In the end, each sick person must decide how bad he or she feels. Is it worth going to work and infecting others? Are you really too sick to go to work? The choice is never easy.

Influenza

Influenza, or flu, is caused by a different kind of virus than the ones that cause colds. Flu is a much more serious disease. The symptoms of flu are body aches, high fever, loss of appetite, and other complications. Infections of the respiratory system by a flu virus can so weaken people that they contract pneumonia, a bacterial infection, and die.

There are many different strains of flu virus, and new strains arise continually. Because flu is so debilitating and serious, vaccines are prepared each year that are supposed to be specific to the expected viral types for that year. The problem is that scientists have to guess which flu strain will be the cause of the next epidemic, because it takes about a year to prepare and distribute the vaccine.

In some years, the flu vaccine is quite effective, but in others, it is not. People with respiratory problems such as asthma, people with immune system deficiencies, and the elderly, who are most susceptible to pneumonia, are advised to get a flu shot each year to help prevent infection.

Never getting a cold or flu is probably impossible. However, certain precautions can help reduce the risk. During seasons when colds and flu are present, try to

> **TERMS**
>
> cilia: microscopic hairs in the lining of the bronchial tubes
> leukocytes: white blood cells that fight infections
> macrophages: specialized cells that destroy and eliminate foreign particles and microorganisms from the body

Stuffy Sinuses?

When your nose is stuffed up from a cold or allergies, instead of taking a decongestant pill or using a nasal spray, try soothing your swollen nasal passages with a dilute saline (salt water) solution. Research shows that this method, called *nasal sinus irrigation*, really works (Harvey et al., 2007). Saline irrigation washes the mucus, bacteria, allergens, and other debris from your nose, and it shrinks swollen membranes and improves the flow of air. Although you can buy prepared nasal solutions, it is easy to make your own using the following method.

1. Fill a clean 1-quart glass jar with tap or bottled water.
2. Add 2 to 3 heaping teaspoons of either pickling/canning or kosher salt. Do not use table salt, because it contains a large number of additives. If you prefer a weaker solution, use about half the amount of salt (best for kids).
3. Add 1 teaspoon baking soda (sodium bicarbonate).

4. Mix well and store at room temperature. Make fresh weekly.
5. Pour the amount of solution you plan to use into a clean bowl to avoid contaminating the entire jar. The solution can be warmed slightly in a microwave, but be sure the solution is only warm, not hot.
6. Fill an ear-cleaning rubber bulb or Water Pic with an irrigation tip with the salt solution. Stand over the sink (or in the shower) and squirt liquid into each nostril, aiming the stream toward the back of your head, not the top. This will allow the solution to flow from your nose into your mouth so you can spit out the salty water. It does not matter if you swallow some of the liquid.
7. You can irrigate your nose two to three times a day. After a few days the stuffiness should disappear and you should breathe more freely.
8. Consult with a health professional before using this nasal irrigation procedure to be sure it is safe for your symptoms.

stay away from crowds as much as possible. The viruses are easily transmitted in droplets from people who are coughing or sneezing. Being in a classroom, theater, bus, subway, or any crowded place increases the risk of being infected. The viruses also are easily transmitted by bodily contact, such as shaking hands with someone with a cold who has recently wiped his or her nose or mouth. So it's a good idea to wash your hands frequently during cold and flu season.

Structure of Influenza Viruses Hundreds of different strains of the flu virus can be constructed by reassortment of its eight segments of genetic [ribonucleic acid (RNA)] information (**Figure 12.5**). Two proteins on the surface of the virus determine which cells it can attach to and its lethality to specific species. The hemagglutinin (H) protein binds to specific receptors on cells. Usually, the particular H protein restricts the infection to one or several species of animals. For example, avian flu viruses readily attach to receptors on bird cells but usually are unable to attach effectively to human cells. The neuraminidase (N) protein helps the viruses escape from infected cells so that they can infect other cells. There are 15 different H proteins and about 9 different N proteins; the combinations of the two proteins characterize the particular strain of flu. For example, for the 2017–2018 flu season, vaccines were prepared for the H1N1 and H3N2 strains of virus.

Defining an Influenza Pandemic The World Health Organization defines an influenza pandemic in six phases; in the final phase, the virus has spread to many countries in at least two distinct regions of the world. During the last century there were three major influenza pandemics: one in 1918 and smaller ones in 1957 and 1968.

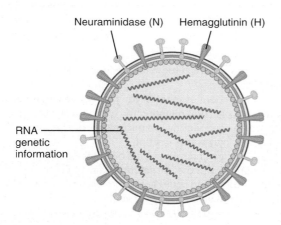

Neuraminidase (N)   Hemagglutinin (H)

RNA
genetic
information

■ **Figure 12.5**

Diagram of an Influenza Virus
The genetic information is contained in eight segments of ribonucleic acid (RNA). These can reassort and mutate to give rise to many different strains of viruses. Two proteins on the surface of each virus determine which species of animals it can infect. The hemagglutinin (H) protein recognizes specific cell receptors and allows the virus to infect those cells. The neuraminidase (N) protein helps new viruses to escape from infected cells.

The 1918 influenza pandemic was the worst in recorded history—estimates range up to 40 million deaths over a period of less than 2 years. The number of influenza deaths was greater than all the deaths in World War I or in the 30 years of the current HIV/AIDS pandemic.

On September 7, 1918, during World War I, a soldier at a training camp near Boston became very ill with a high fever. By September 16, several dozen new cases of influenza were admitted to the army hospital. By September 23, 12,604 cases of flu were reported among the 45,000 soldiers stationed in the camp (Taubenberger, 2005). By November, one-third of the U.S. population was infected. These numbers show how swiftly a deadly strain of flu virus can spread in a population.

In a remarkable bit of scientific detective work, the strain that caused the 1918 flu pandemic has been reconstructed by recovering flu genetic material from victims who died and were buried in the arctic permafrost. The 1918 virus was an H1N1 strain, the 1957 virus was an H2N2 strain, and the 1968 virus was an H3N2 strain.

The 2009 Influenza Pandemic

In April 2009, hundreds of cases of influenza were reported in Mexico. These infections were caused by a strain of virus that normally infects swine and so initially it was called "swine flu." Further analysis of the virus revealed that it contained genetic material from swine, bird, and human flu viruses. The virus was quickly identified as an H1N1 strain similar to the 1918 virus. This immediately raised fears of a serious worldwide flu pandemic.

Within a month, confirmed cases of H1N1 flu had spread from Mexico to 47 U.S. states and almost 40 countries around the world. Fortunately, the new H1N1 strain lacked the virulence that made the 1918 flu strain so deadly. Most cases of the H1N1 flu were relatively mild, and infected people recovered quickly. Also, the new strain was susceptible to two antiviral drugs, oseltamivir phosphate (Tamiflu) and zanamivir (Relenza). These drugs interfere with the neuraminidase viral protein and prevent the release of new viruses from cells, thus slowing the spread of the infection in the body.

Avian Influenza

The strain of avian flu that is circulating among birds in Southeast Asia, Europe, and Africa is a strain called H5N1. Millions of domestic fowl in Thailand, Vietnam, Singapore, and elsewhere were destroyed to try to stop the spread of the deadly strain of bird flu. However, because millions of wild birds also carry the virus, it is unlikely to be eradicated. Although the virus mainly infects and kills birds, about 300 people have been infected by this H5N1 strain of bird flu, about half of whom have died.

It is thought that almost all of the people who have been infected by the H5N1 avian flu strain acquired the infection from handling or eating birds that carried the virus. However, in a few cases, person-to-person transmission of the virus may have occurred. Because of the enormous number of infected birds in the world, it is expected that the virus eventually will mutate and be capable of person-to-person transmission. Fortunately, this has not occurred yet.

Lyme Disease

Lyme disease was first recognized in 1975, when a number of children were diagnosed with an arthritis-like disease in Lyme, Connecticut. The disease was soon recognized as a distinct tickborne disease caused by pathogenic bacteria (*Borrella burgdorferi*) transmitted in a tick bite; the disease is called Lyme disease after the place where it was first discovered. In 1982, the first year of surveillance, 491 cases were reported. The number swelled to 17,029 in 2001. Since 2007, the Centers for Disease Control and Prevention estimates that 28,000 cases of Lyme disease occur annually in the United States. At least 96% of all Lyme disease cases occur in just 14 states: Connecticut, Delaware, Maine, Maryland, Massachusetts, Minnesota, New Hampshire, New Jersey, New York, Pennsylvania, Rhode Island, Vermont, Virginia, and Wisconsin.

The most common place to get Lyme disease is in woods during warm months when ticks are abundant and are feeding on deer and small mammals, including household pets that can bring the ticks into the home. The bacterium *Borrelia burgdorferi* is carried by a few species of tick (mainly, *Ixodes scapularis*). When this tick attaches to the skin and bites, the bacteria are injected into the blood.

If unrecognized and left untreated, Lyme disease progresses through three stages.

Stage 1: This stage begins a few days after the tick bite and lasts about a month. A red rash appears around the tick bite and gradually spreads out on the skin. A person may not recognize the rash as stemming from a tick bite, but the rash is quite distinctive to an experienced physician's eye. The person may also feel tired, have headaches, and notice some joint pain.

Stage 2: After a month or two, if left untreated, about 15% of those persons bitten experience severe neurological symptoms such a meningitis and encephalitis. A few people will develop heart problems, and most will notice pain in the joints, muscles, tendons, and bones.

Stage 3: Within weeks and up to 2 years after the tick bite, about 60% of people develop arthritis characterized by pain and swelling of joints, especially the knees.

Because the symptoms of Lyme disease are similar to many other diseases, it is difficult to diagnose, especially if the patient does not report being bitten by a tick. Blood tests are helpful in making the diagnosis but are not completely reliable. Lyme disease is treated with antibiotics at all stages, and treatment is most effective if taken soon after the appearance of the characteristic rash.

No vaccine is currently available to protect against Lyme disease, although several laboratories are working to develop one.

To avoid contracting Lyme disease, it is important to be completely covered with clothing—especially when hiking—in tick-infested areas. Pants should be tucked into boots. Proper dress alone can reduce the risk of contracting Lyme disease from a tick bite by at least 40% (Vazquez et al., 2008). Use light-colored clothing so that ticks can be seen more easily. If pets hike with you, examine them carefully afterward for ticks. Ticks embedded in the skin can be removed by pulling on them carefully with tweezers, making sure that the head is removed.

Even after several rounds of treatment with antibiotics, as many as 20% of Lyme disease patients experience pain, fatigue, and other symptoms for years. It is thought that neither antibiotics nor the immune system completely eliminate all Lyme disease bacteria. A tiny fraction of the bacteria (called *persister cells*) become dormant and cannot be killed. Eventually, after antibiotics have been eliminated from the body, the bacteria revive, grow, and produce disease symptoms anew. Newer treatments use pulsed administration of antibiotics to try to kill the persister cells.

New genetic engineering techniques offer hope of eliminating Lyme disease from environments in which mice are a reservoir of the pathogenic bacteria (Specter, 2017). In the laboratory, genes for antibodies to Lyme bacteria are transplanted into uninfected mice. When these mice reproduce, the anti-Lyme–antibody genes are inherited by the new generation of mice and are available to destroy any Lyme bacteria that enter the mouse from a tick bite. Releasing the antibody-carrying mice into a native environment where they can mate with wild mice will eventually create a population of mice immune to Lyme disease and eliminate the reservoir for the bacteria.

Mononucleosis

Mononucleosis (commonly called "mono") is an infectious disease caused by the Epstein-Barr virus (EBV) that is ubiquitous in all human populations. It is spread easily from person to person, especially in crowded conditions. It sometimes is called the "kissing disease" because the virus is present in saliva and readily transferred by

---

▌TERMS▐

Lyme disease: a serious, difficult-to-diagnose infectious disease caused by bacteria deposited by ticks when they bite

mononucleosis: an infectious disease caused by the Epstein-Barr virus, common among college-age adults

Table 12.4

Viruses That Remain in the Body for Life After Infection

Virus	Symptoms	Spread by	Remains in
Herpes simplex 1	Cold sores on lips or in mouth	Direct contact; most infectious when lesions are present	Nerve cells
Herpes simplex 2	Painful blisters on genital organs	Direct contact; oral–genital sex can transmit type 1 or 2 to mouth or genital area	Nerve cells
Cytomegalovirus (CMV)	No symptoms in most children and adults; CMV can cause stillbirth and intellectual disabilities in fetuses	Body fluids: blood, urine, saliva	White blood cells
Varicella zoster virus	Chicken pox in children; shingles in adults	Person to person	Nerve cells
Epstein-Barr virus (EBV)	Mononucleosis	Saliva (kissing)	Lymph glands
Human immunodeficiency virus (HIV)	From none to full symptoms of AIDS	Sexual intercourse (homosexual or heterosexual), blood transfusions, contaminated needles of injection drug users, mother-to-child transmission before or after birth	T cells of the immune system and other body cells

mouth-to-mouth contact. About half of all children in the United States are infected by EBV by age 5, but in most children, the infection goes unnoticed because there are no symptoms. Once someone has been infected by EBV, he or she usually carries the virus for life without having symptoms or signs of disease. EBV and a number of other viruses can become permanently established in the body (**Table 12.4**).

If a teenager or young adult becomes infected by EBV, symptoms develop but usually clear up in several weeks without further illness. Symptoms of mononucleosis include swollen glands, sore throat, fever, chills, and, above all, complete exhaustion and loss of energy. About half of those infected develop an enlarged spleen, and a small percentage develop jaundice (yellow coloration of the skin and eyes). Fortunately, these symptoms resolve in 2 to 4 weeks in a healthy young adult.

> There are two ways of being disappointed in life. One is to not get what you want and the other is to get it.
>
> *George Bernard Shaw*

There is no specific treatment for mononucleosis, but there are precautions that can facilitate recovery. The primary focus is rest and more rest. For the first 2 weeks, you may hardly be able to drag yourself out of bed. When you start to feel stronger, however, it is important to continue to rest. Trying to resume normal activities too soon can cause a relapse and extend the illness. Fluid intake is also important; drink as much water, juice, soup, or tea as you can. Some people find that taking herbs that act as immune system boosters (echinacea and astragalus) can speed recovery.

The primary reason to avoid strenuous activities, especially contact sports, for a month or more after a diagnosis of mononucleosis is to protect the spleen. If the spleen is enlarged, an injury could rupture it and create a serious medical problem that may necessitate surgery and removal of the spleen. Because mono affects young people who may be involved in competitive athletics, it is important that they understand why they must continue to be relatively inactive even when they no longer feel sick. Also, because EBV infection affects the liver, it is important not to drink alcohol or take other drugs that may further injure the liver.

The incubation time for EBV is quite long. Children may show symptoms in 1 to 2 weeks after infection; however, adults may not develop symptoms for 1 to 2 months. Thus, it is often difficult to know from whom you received the virus. Once you know that you have mononucleosis, it is important to try not to spread it among family and friends. Do not kiss anyone, and avoid sharing drinks or food. Try not to sneeze or cough when others are close by, and carry tissues to cover your mouth and nose. Even after all symptoms of mono have disappeared, active virus particles remain in the saliva for many months—up to 6 months in some studies—so you still need to exert caution so as not to spread EBV to close associates and loved ones.

Ulcers

For most of the last century, it was thought that **gastric ulcers** (sores or holes in the lining of the stomach) or duodenal ulcers that occur in the first part of the small intestine were caused by stress, anxiety, smoking, and alcohol consumption. However, in 1983, two medical researchers in Australia shocked the medical world by announcing that most stomach ulcers were caused by a bacterial infection in the lining of the stomach of susceptible persons. For several years this view was treated with skepticism, but now it has been established unequivocally that as many as 90% of these ulcers are caused by particular stomach bacteria (*Helicobacter pylori*). Without the presence of these bacteria in the stomach, ulcers hardly ever occur.

Approximately 50% of the U.S. population is infected with *H. pylori,* and in developing nations the incidence of infections is estimated at 70% or higher. Most people become infected as children and do not experience any symptoms at the time. However, later in life some of those carrying the bacteria will develop ulcers. People get ulcers at any age, and men and women are affected equally. In addition to causing ulcers, *H. pylori* is associated with an increased risk of stomach cancer. About 1% to 3% of infected persons eventually will develop stomach cancer. That rate is six times greater than the rate for uninfected persons.

The most common ulcer symptom is a gnawing or burning pain in the abdomen between the breastbone and the belly button. The pain often occurs when the stomach is empty, between meals, and in the early morning hours, but it can occur at any other time. It may last from minutes to hours and may be relieved by eating food or taking antacids. Less common symptoms include nausea, vomiting, or loss of appetite. Sometimes ulcers bleed. If bleeding continues for a long time, it may lead to anemia with weakness and fatigue.

A physician can determine if an ulcer is caused by *H. pylori* infection by the following tests:

- *Blood:* A blood test can confirm if you have *H. pylori.*
- *Breath:* A breath test can determine if you are infected with *H. pylori.* In this test, you drink a harmless liquid and, in less than 1 hour, a sample of your breath is tested for *H. pylori.*
- *Endoscopy:* Your healthcare provider may decide to perform an endoscopy. This is a test in which a small tube containing a camera is inserted through the mouth and into the stomach to look for ulcers. During the endoscopy, small samples of the stomach lining can be obtained by biopsy and tested for *H. pylori.*

Antibiotics cure ulcers; therapy is 1 to 2 weeks of an antibiotic and a medicine that will reduce the acid in the stomach. This treatment is extremely effective in eliminating *H. pylori* and means that there is a greater than 90% chance that the ulcer can be cured (Garza-González et al., 2014).

Hepatitis

Hepatitis is a serious liver disease caused by excess alcohol consumption, exposure to pesticides, certain drugs, and any one of several different viruses that infect liver cells. The most common infections are caused by hepatitis A, hepatitis B, and hepatitis C viruses. The sources of infection and liver disease severity vary for each of the viruses.

Hepatitis A This virus (HAV) causes liver disease in approximately 200,000 Americans each year but is fatal in less than 100 persons. At least one-third of Americans have been infected with hepatitis A at some time in their lives, and most suffer only mild symptoms and recover

completely. The primary source of HAV infection is fecal–oral transmission; one can become infected from contaminated water or from eating food that has been handled by an infected person. Not washing hands after going to the toilet and subsequently handling food is the primary means of transmitting HAV. The symptoms of being infected include jaundice, fatigue, loss of appetite, abdominal pain, and intermittent diarrhea. The symptoms usually clear up within a few weeks, and there is no persistent liver infection. A very effective vaccine is available for those individuals who are at high risk of exposure to HAV or who travel to areas of the world where hepatitis A disease is widespread.

Hepatitis B Infection of the liver by hepatitis B virus (HBV) causes serious liver disease; it persists as a chronic infection and may eventually cause liver failure or liver cancer and death. Worldwide, as many as 250 million people are thought to have a chronic HBV infection; about 600,000 HBV-infected people die each year from liver failure. Not all infections by HBV produce symptoms, but when they do the symptoms include jaundice, fatigue, abdominal pain, loss of appetite, nausea, and vomiting.

HBV is transmitted by blood; infection can result from blood transfusions, use of contaminated needles by injection drug users, sexual intercourse (heterosexual or homosexual) in which minute amounts of blood are exchanged, and by perinatal transmission, in which an infected pregnant woman passes the virus to her fetus. The incidence of hepatitis B disease has been decreasing as a result of the availability of a highly effective vaccine and prevention programs aimed at high-risk groups of people such as injection drug users and sexually active individuals. The blood used for transfusions now is screened routinely for the presence of HBV, and infection by this means is no longer a danger.

A vaccine against HBV is available, and it is recommended that all children be vaccinated for hepatitis B. In addition, all persons who are at high risk of exposure to hepatitis B—healthcare workers, hemodialysis patients, sexually active individuals, and injection drug users—should obtain the HBV vaccination.

Hepatitis C Hepatitis C (HCV) is sometimes called the silent epidemic because until recently relatively little was known or publicized regarding this infection. However, HCV infection is now the most common reason for liver transplantation. It is estimated that 4 million people in

TERMS

gastric ulcers: open sores in the stomach from infection by the bacterium *H. pylori*

hepatitis: serious disease of the liver caused by hepatitis virus A, B, C, D, or E; also caused by chemicals and alcohol

the United States are chronically infected by HCV and that many eventually will develop serious liver disease. Worldwide, it is estimated that 71 million people are infected with HCV and about 400,000 die from complications of the infection each year.

Hepatitis C virus has been well characterized only since 1989; prior to that time millions of people became infected from contaminated blood without knowing it. HCV is not a single viral strain but consists of many related viruses. Like the flu virus, HCV can change its genetic information easily, which is one of the reasons that it is difficult to treat and why no vaccine has been developed. HCV is transmitted exclusively in blood and blood products; it is not transmitted by casual contact.

Americans who are infected with HCV generally were infected many years ago, before the virus was identified. Most do not even know they carry the virus until symptoms develop. A sensitive antibody test can detect if a person has been infected with HCV, and another test can detect the level of the viruses in the blood.

Until recently, HCV infections were treated with two antiviral drugs that had to be taken for almost a year and that produced serious side effects. These treatments were successful only in a small fraction of people who stuck to the arduous regimen. Now, two new drugs, Sovaldi (sofosbuvir), and olysio (simeprevir) have been approved for treating HCV. These drugs cure more than 90% of patients and are effective against several of the most common strains of HCV. The side effects are minimal and the treatment requires taking one pill a day for 12 weeks.

In 2015, the cost of being treated with sofosbuvir was $84,000; the cost for simeprevir was $66,000. Obviously, the cost of being cured of HCV is out of reach for all but the very wealthy. Most of the people who are able to get the drugs are on Medicare or Medicaid, so the U.S. government picks up the cost. It is estimated that the actual cost of producing the pills needed for the 12-week treatment is less than $200. Drug companies argue that the high prices are necessary to recoup the costs of developing the drugs and money lost on drugs that are unsuccessful. Eventually, the drugs will become affordable when their patents expire around 2025.

The risk of HCV infection in the United States today is quite low, except for intravenous drug users who share needles and healthcare workers who get an accidental needle puncture while treating a patient. The blood supply is screened for HCV, so transfusions are safe. However, HCV infections are still a risk in other parts of the world, especially from blood transfusions.

Hepatitis D This virus (HDV) is defective, is unable to grow by itself, and is only detected in the presence of HBV infection.

Hepatitis E This virus (HEV) is similar to HAV in that it is transmitted by a fecal–oral route in contaminated food and water. It causes the same symptoms as hepatitis

A and does not result in chronic infection. Hepatitis E occurs primarily in underdeveloped countries where sanitation is poor. Travelers should avoid drinking unbottled water, using ice, or eating fresh fruits and vegetables that may be contaminated. No vaccine currently is available for hepatitis E.

Although viruses are the primary cause of hepatitis, remember the golfer in Ireland who suffered from nonviral hepatitis. It turned out that at each hole he licked his golf balls to clean them before teeing off. The herbicide residue on the balls eventually damaged his liver and caused hepatitis. The herbicide was used heavily on the golf course to control weeds, and the chemicals were picked up by the golf balls as they rolled in the grass.

Emerging Infectious Diseases

Emerging infectious diseases are infections that newly appear, or reemerge, within a vulnerable population of people or known infections that are suddenly spreading rapidly. Emerging infections can be caused by previously known, undetected, or newly evolved infectious agents.

Many factors contribute to the emergence of new infectious diseases. They include the increasing growth and mobility (e.g., international air travel) of the world's population, overcrowding in cities with poor sanitation, mass-produced food and its international distribution, unsanitary food preparation, new or increased exposure of humans to disease vectors such as mosquitoes (see Infogaphic), people living in close contact with animals that can host infectious organisms, overuse of antibiotics, poverty, wars, and destructive ecological changes due to economic development, land use, and climate change.

Zika Virus Zika virus (ZIKV) was identified in 1947 in the Zika forest in Uganda, Africa. It is transmitted to people by several species of mosquitoes, primarily female *Aedes aegypti* mosquitoes. Over the years, people infected by Zika viruses in Africa and Asia had no symptoms or very mild ones, such as a slight fever and headache. However, by 2015, Zika viruses migrated to South and Central America, causing a very dangerous infection in pregnant women whose babies were then born with *microcephaly*, a birth defect characterized by a small head and defective brain development. The severity of birth defects varies widely; some Zika-infected babies appear normal at birth, whereas others have severe birth defects. *Congenital Zika syndrome* is a condition in which babies and fetuses exhibit one or more of the following: severe microcephaly;

TERMS

emerging infectious diseases: infections that newly appear, or re-emerge, within a vulnerable population of people or known infections that are suddenly spreading rapidly

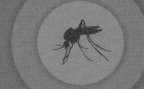

CDC's Response to **Zika**
HOW TO PROTECT AGAINST MOSQUITO BITES

Accessible Version: https://www.cdc.gov/zika/prevention/prevent-mosquito-bites.html

Zika virus is spread to people mainly through the bite of an infected mosquito. Mosquitoes that spread Zika virus bite mostly during the day, but they can also bite at night. The best way to prevent Zika is to protect yourself from mosquito bites.

Use insect repellent

Use Environmental Protection Agency (EPA)-registered insect repellents with one of the following active ingredients: DEET, picaridin, IR3535, oil of lemon eucalyptus or para-menthane-diol, or 2-undecanone. Always follow the product label instructions.

- When used as directed, these insect repellents are proven safe and effective, even for women who are pregnant or breastfeeding.
- Reapply insect repellent as directed.
- Do not spray repellent on the skin under clothing.
- If you are also using sunscreen, apply sunscreen first.
- The effectiveness of non-EPA registered insect repellents, including some natural repellents, is not known.

If you have a baby or child

- Do not use insect repellent on babies younger than 2 months old.
- Do not use products containing oil of lemon eucalyptus or para-menthane-diol on children younger than 3 years old.
- Dress your child in clothing that covers arms and legs.
- Cover crib, stroller, and baby carrier with mosquito netting.
- Do not apply insect repellent onto a child's hands, eyes, mouth, and any cut or irritated skin.
  - » Adults: Spray insect repellent onto your hands and then apply to a child's face.

Treat clothes and gear

- Treat items such as clothing and gear with permethrin or buy permethrin-treated clothes and gear.
  - » See product information to find out the number of washings or length of time the protection will last.
  - » If treating items yourself, follow the product instructions.
  - » Do not use permethrin products directly on skin.

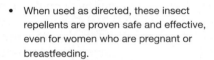

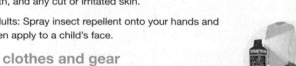

Active ingredient
Higher percentages of active ingredient provide longer protection

DEET

Picaridin (known as KBR 3023 and icaridin outside the US)

IR3535

Oil of lemon eucalyptus (OLE) or para-menthane-diol (PMD)

2-undecanone

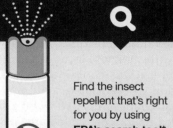

Find the insect repellent that's right for you by using **EPA's search tool***.

* The EPA's search tool is available at: www.epa.gov/insect-repellents/find-insect-repellent-right-you

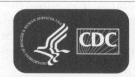

U.S. Department of Health and Human Services
Centers for Disease Control and Prevention

www.cdc.gov/zika

CS265864A   September 15, 2017

brain damage or diminished brain tissue; defects at the back of the eyes; limited range of joint motion; or excess muscle tone that restricts body movements.

West Nile Virus West Nile virus (WNV) is found throughout much of the world—Africa, the Middle East, India, Indonesia, and some areas of Europe. West Nile virus was first reported in the United States in 1999, when a large number of crows at the Bronx Zoo were found dead on the zoo grounds; this was followed by the death of a number of other birds in the zoo's collection. Soon afterward, several people in the New York area were hospitalized with symptoms of encephalitis. Blood samples were analyzed, and it was found that the RNA of the virus matched that of a West Nile virus strain previously isolated in Israel.

Mosquitoes that bite infected birds or other animals can transmit WNV to people. After about 2 weeks of incubation in a person, WNV may cross the blood–brain barrier (which restricts many infectious agents from reaching the brain) and infect the nervous system. In a few people, once the virus has infected the brain and nervous system, symptoms such as tremors, convulsions, paralysis, coma, and death may follow. The good news is that most people who are bitten by a WNV-infected mosquito will *not* develop serious symptoms and will recover completely without any lasting effects.

In addition to mosquito bites, people also can become infected with WNV through blood transfusions and organ transplants. Blood can be tested with an antibody test that can show whether a person has been infected by WNV. However, because it takes a week or longer for antibodies to develop after a WNV infection, an infected person may donate blood or an organ and the virus can go undetected.

Ebola Ebola is a deadly virus named for a small river in the Peoples' Republic of Congo, where it was first detected by scientists in 1976. Since its initial discovery in a remote village in the Congo, Ebola infections have appeared and disappeared numerous times in villages in the Congo as well as in other remote locations in sub-Saharan Africa. Each outbreak was contained by being confined to a small region where people could not easily move in or out. That all changed in 2014, when a single infected person showed up in a populated area of West Africa. Many people became infected and the infection quickly spread through Sierra Leone, Guinea, Liberia, and Mali.

Ebola viruses are among the smallest viruses. Each virus particle contains only seven genes whose genetic information is carried in a tiny RNA molecule. The seven genes produce seven proteins that allow the virus to attach to human cells, penetrate the cells, replicate the RNA, and produce new virus particles. Ebola belongs to a class of viruses called *hemorrhagic viruses* because they produce extensive bleeding. The death rate from Ebola varies widely but averages more than 50% of people infected. Marburg, Lassa, and Rift Valley fever are other types of hemorrhagic fevers. Ebola was first transmitted to people when people ate or came in contact with fruit bats in Africa. The bats serve as a reservoir for Ebola but are not harmed by the virus. Testing of thousands of animals in Africa over the years showed that only certain species of bats normally carry the Ebola virus without being harmed by it.

After becoming infected with Ebola, a person may develop symptoms within a few days or as long as 21 days or more in a few instances. The symptoms are similar to most viral infections—fever, headache, and body pain. Vomiting and diarrhea follow. As of 2014, there were no specific medicines for treating Ebola; patients received supportive therapy, primarily fluids to replace the body fluids that were lost. Death occurs from failure of the kidneys, liver, or loss of blood. All body fluids of an Ebola patient carry infectious viruses including tears, sweat, and semen. Caring for Ebola patients is extremely hazardous as evidenced by the high rate of healthcare worker deaths in West Africa. A number of infected doctors and nurses who were flown to specially outfitted U.S. hospitals were successfully treated and recovered. By the end of 2014, more than 5,000 Ebola deaths were recorded in West Africa.

An Ebola vaccine that provides almost complete protection against the virus has been produced. In the event of an Ebola outbreak, the vaccine will first be used to protect healthcare workers who are in close contact with patients, then susceptible individuals and populations in the region of the outbreak will be vaccinated. The Ebola vaccine should prevent any future Ebola outbreaks from causing an epidemic or spreading to remote areas of the world.

The Immune System Battles Infections

The world teems with infectious viruses, bacteria, and other microorganisms that can cause disease if they invade the body. Most people stay well most of the time because the body contains a remarkable array of defense mechanisms that help keep disease-causing microorganisms out or that can destroy them if they invade the body. We only occasionally have an infectious disease because the **immune system** acts to protect the body from infectious organisms and foreign substances.

The immune system takes time to develop. At birth, a baby is protected from infectious diseases by antibodies that were present in the mother's blood and passed on to the newborn. **Antibodies** are proteins that recognize and inactivate viruses, bacteria, and harmful substances that can cause disease. Babies also receive antibodies in breast milk, which helps to protect them while their own immune systems mature during the first year or so of life.

Many factors can adversely affect the development and functioning of the immune system. Perhaps the most important factor is poor nutrition, especially early in life.

Without a healthy diet, a child is extremely susceptible to infections that a weak immune system cannot fight. Immunity is also strengthened when bacteria that constitute the mother's microbiome also are transferred to the baby as it passes through the birth canal. Inadequate nutrition and infectious diseases are the principal reasons that children die in many undeveloped and impoverished countries of the world. Other factors that affect the development or functions of the immune system are hereditary disorders, viral infections, stress, and many drugs and chemicals, including alcohol and tobacco.

Severe combined immune deficiency (SCID) is a rare genetic disease that renders the immune system inoperable. Babies with SCID must be protected from any exposure to germs. However, because germs are everywhere, without protection and treatment, the affected child will usually contract a fatal infection within a few years. The only cure for SCID is a complete bone marrow transplant if a suitable donor can be found. In 1971, David was born with SCID and no suitable donor could be located. He was immediately placed in a large sterile chamber (the bubble chamber) where he was raised in sterile conditions until he was about 11 years old, at which point he decided to leave the hospital bubble chamber. His home was equipped with a sterile, portable bubble chamber. To get around outside he used a sterile spacesuit supplied by NASA. Despite these precautions, David acquired an infection that could not be treated. He died in 1984, at age 13. In January 2015, Levi was born with SCID. As with David, no suitable bone marrow transplant donor could be found. But a few months after birth, Levi received an injection of DNA containing a normal copy of the defective gene he had inherited (Mullin, 2017), which overcame his disease and allowed him to survive. After 50 years of mostly failures, this was a major success for the technique of gene therapy.

The Lymphatic System

The immune system, which is part of a larger and more complex system called the **lymphatic system**, has many organs and cells that must act in concert to protect people from infectious diseases (**Figure 12.6**). The lymphatic vessels contain fluid called lymph. At various intervals along the lymphatic vessels are nodules called **lymph nodes**. The "swollen glands" that people experience in the neck, under the arms, in the groin, or in other areas of the body are caused by enlarged lymph nodes that are engaged in filtering out infectious organisms or foreign particles capable of causing disease. Thus, swollen and sore lymph nodes are a sign that the body is fighting an infection.

Bone marrow, tonsils, adenoids, the spleen, and the thymus all produce cells that allow the body to mount an immune response against infectious microorganisms. When bacteria or viruses infect the body, the immune system produces diverse kinds of white blood cells that function in different ways to destroy them (**Table 12.5**).

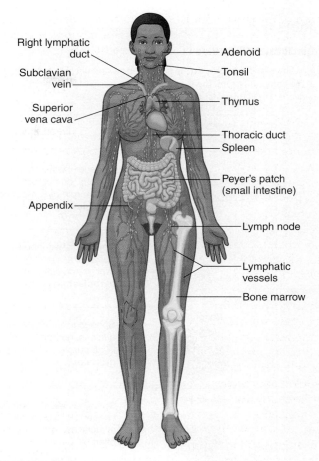

■ Figure 12.6

The Lymphatic and Immune Systems
Bone marrow, lymph nodes, and other organs of the immune system are shown. The lymphatic system performs many functions in protecting the body from infectious diseases.

The **T cells** (also called *T lymphocytes*) circulating in the blood are ready to attack infectious organisms immediately, because T cells recognize the "foreignness"

TERMS

antibodies: proteins that recognize and inactivate viruses, bacteria, and other organisms and toxic substances that enter the body

immune system: an interacting system of organs and cells that protect the body from infectious organisms and harmful substances

lymph nodes: nodules spaced along the lymphatic vessels that trap infectious organisms or foreign particles

lymphatic system: a system of vessels in the body that trap foreign organisms and particles; the immune system is part of the lymphatic system

T cells: cells of the immune system that attack foreign organisms that infect the body

Table 12.5

Specialized White Blood Cells

All white blood cells originate in bone marrow and become specialized as they mature in different organs. Specialized cells carry out different functions of the immune system. The B cells and T cells recognize foreign proteins on infectious bacteria, viruses, and other organisms and substances. B cells are converted to plasma cells that manufacture antibodies.

White Blood Cell Type	Description	Function	Life Span
Neutrophil	Spherical; with many-lobed nucleus, no hemoglobin, pink-purple **cytoplasmic granules**	Cellular defense—phagocytosis of small microorganisms.	Hours to 3 days
Eosinophil	Spherical; two-lobed nucleus, no hemoglobin, orange-red staining **cytoplasmic granules**	Cellular defense—phagocytosis of large microorganisms such as parasitic worms; releases anti-inflammatory substances in allergic reactions.	8 to 12 days
Basophil	Spherical; generally two-lobed nucleus, no hemoglobin, large purple-staining **cytoplasmic granules**	Inflammatory response—contain granules that rupture and release chemicals enhancing inflammatory response.	Hours to 3 days
Monocyte	Spherical; **single nucleus** shaped like kidney bean, no cytoplasmic granules, cytoplasm often blue in color	Converted to macrophages, which are large cells that entrap microorganisms and other foreign matter.	Days to months
B lymphocyte	Spherical; round **singular nucleus**, no cytoplasmic granules	Immune system response and regulation; antibody production sometimes causes allergic response.	Days to years
T lymphocyte	Spherical; round **singular nucleus**, no cytoplasmic granules	Immune system response and regulation; cellular immune response.	Days to years

of specific proteins on the surface of bacteria, viruses, and other pathogens. The response of the T cells is called **cell-mediated immunity** because the T cells attach directly to the infectious organisms and inactivate them. Once cells have been identified as foreign by the T cells, the macrophages and other immune system cells complete the process of their destruction and elimination from the body.

The **B cells** (also called *B lymphocytes*) comprise the final and most effective immune system defense; the response of the B cells is called **humoral immunity**. The B cells function by producing antibodies, which recognize all proteins and other substances that are foreign and potentially harmful to the human body.

All mammals have similar immune systems and manufacture antibodies; these immune systems evolved with the earliest animals on earth. Without a functional immune system, people and animals would quickly succumb to the countless infectious microorganisms in the environment. Because the immune systems of all mammals are quite similar, researchers use rats, mice, and other small animals to study how cells of the immune system are synthesized and how they function.

The foreign proteins on viruses, bacteria, and other infectious organisms are called **antigens** (*antibody generators*). Every person has a collection of B cells circulating in the blood that can recognize any foreign protein on any infectious organism in the world that may be encountered during their lifetime.

A particular B cell can recognize a foreign antigen on a virus or bacterium and begin to make more B cells just like itself. Eventually, these B cells (at this stage called *plasma cells*) manufacture vast amounts of one specific antibody that attaches to all of the specific pathogens in the body. Once the antibodies have recognized and inactivated them, other white blood cells finish the job of destruction. To produce the correct antibodies in large amounts takes about a week after an infection, which is why other quicker-acting immune system defense mechanisms are also needed.

The B cells and T cells interact among themselves in complex ways to produce a full-fledged immune response. Small molecules called **cytokines** coordinate the activities of the B cells and T cells. Many of the natural cytokines, such as interferons and interleukins, that regulate functions of the immune system are now also manufactured by biotechnology companies. Some of these products are used in the treatment of cancer and other diseases in which the functions of the immune system are impaired.

T cells are also divided into different classes according to their specific functions. Helper T cells increase the proliferation of B cells, killer T cells destroy cancer cells and other pathogenic organisms, and suppressor T cells retard the growth of other immune system cells. A special class of T cells called CD4 cells are important indicators in the diagnosis and development of AIDS. When the level of CD4 cells in the blood falls, a person becomes extremely susceptible to infection by many different microorganisms, causing one of the more than two dozen infectious diseases that characterize AIDS.

Immunizations

One of the great achievements of modern medicine has been the development of **immunizations** (vaccinations) to prevent many serious infectious diseases caused by bacteria and, more important, by viruses. Viral diseases include whooping cough, measles, mumps, hepatitis, smallpox, and polio. Smallpox has been eliminated throughout the world. Polio has almost been eliminated. Other bacterial and viral diseases have been markedly reduced in the United States as a result of vaccinations.

Vaccination is the administration, usually by injection (hence the name "shot"), of substances called **vaccines**. When you are vaccinated, inactivated viruses or bacteria and other substances are injected into the body. The body's immune system responds by producing antibodies (proteins) that can inactivate the infectious microorganisms. If you later encounter the active, disease-causing organisms, you are protected by "memory cells" that quickly produce the antibodies needed to destroy the infectious agents.

For example, the crippling disease poliomyelitis has been virtually eradicated in the United States as a result of the widespread use of the polio virus vaccine. The first polio vaccine was developed in 1954 by Jonas Salk, using chemically inactivated viruses. The polio vaccine now used is derived from a genetically inactivated virus developed in 1957 by Albert Sabin. Both methods of viral inactivation prevent the dead virus from causing disease and confer long-lasting immunity. However, a handful of polio cases occur each year as a result of the genetically inactivated polio vaccine now in use.

In general, vaccination is safe and effective in preventing a number of infectious diseases. Vaccinations are recommended for both children and adults, but vaccinations are crucial for young children and adolescents (**Figure 12.7**). Other vaccinations are recommended only for people at particular risk of exposure to a certain disease. For example, travelers to a country where cholera, typhoid fever, or hepatitis A is prevalent should be vaccinated for these diseases. Vaccination for influenza is recommended for people susceptible to lung infections, such as children and those who are elderly or have asthma.

New Vaccines

In 2005, an improved vaccination for bacterial meningitis was approved in the United States. Each year, about 3,000 Americans contract meningococcal disease, which infects the brain, spinal fluid, and blood. About 300 people die from this infection each year and others are seriously disabled. The new vaccine, called Menactra, is recommended for all adolescents aged 11 to 18, the group that is most at risk. The vaccine is not approved for children younger than 11.

In 2006, a vaccine against several strains of human papillomavirus (HPV) was approved in order to protect women from developing cancer of the cervix. HPV is

---

TERMS

antigens: foreign proteins on infectious organisms that stimulate an antibody response

B cells: cells of the immune system that produce antibodies

cell-mediated immunity: the response of T cells to infections

cytokines: small molecules that coordinate the activities of B cells and T cells

humoral immunity: the response of B cells to infections

immunizations: vaccinations to prevent a variety of serious diseases caused by both bacteria and viruses

vaccines: inactivated bacteria or viruses that are injected or taken orally; the body responds by producing antibodies and cells that provide lasting immunity

Vaccine ▼ Age ▶	Birth	1 month	2 months	4 months	6 months	9 months	12 months	15 months	18 months	19-23 months	2-3 years	4-6 years
Hepatitis B[1] (HepB)	1st dose	←2nd dose→				←3rd dose→						
Rotavirus[2] (RV) RV1 (2-dose series); RV5 (3-dose series)			1st dose	2nd dose								
Diphtheria, tetanus, & acellular pertussis[3] (DTaP: <7 yrs)			1st dose	2nd dose	3rd dose			←4th dose→				5th dose
Haemophilus influenzae type b[4] (Hib)			1st dose	2nd dose			←3rd or 4th dose→					
Pneumococcal conjugate[5] (PCV13)			1st dose	2nd dose	3rd dose		←4th dose→					
Inactivated poliovirus[6] (IPV:<18 yrs)			1St dose	2nd dose			←3rd dose→					4th dose
Influenza[7] (IIV)					Annual vaccination (IIV) 1 or 2 doses							
Measles, mumps, rubella[8] (MMR)							←1st dose→					2nd dose
Varicella[9] (VAR)							←1st dose→					2nd dose
Hepatitis A[10] (HepA)							←2 dose series→					

Range of recommended ages for all children

Range of recommended ages for catch-up immunizations

Range of recommended ages for certain high-risk groups

■ Figure 12.7

Recommended Vaccination Schedule for Children Ages 0 to 6

Data from Centers for Disease Control and Prevention. (2017). Child and adolescent immunization schedules. Retrieved from http://www.cdc.gov/vaccines/schedules/hcp/imz/child-adolescent.html

the most common sexually transmitted disease in the United States. About 10,000 American women are diagnosed with cervical cancer each year. For these reasons, the HPV vaccine (called Gardasil) is recommended for all young persons before they become sexually active. Several states and many schools require HPV vaccinations for girls and boys as a public health measure, much as other vaccinations and tests for TB are required to protect public health. However, mandatory HPV vaccination is not acceptable to everyone (Colgrove et al., 2010). Some parents think that HPV vaccination encourages sexual promiscuity. Others argue that forcing people to be vaccinated for any reason is wrong.

In 2007, a vaccine against herpes zoster was approved for use in adults older than 60 years. Herpes zoster viral infection causes chicken pox in children. In adults, it causes *shingles,* an extremely painful outbreak of sores on the trunk of the body. However, the vaccine provides only partial protection against shingles in adults. The vaccine is only recommended for older people who may be at high risk for shingles; many physicians do not recommend it to their patients.

Worldwide, more than 2 million children under the age of 5 are hospitalized annually for severe diarrhea and its complications; more than half a million die. These children have been infected by a strain of rotovirus.

HPV Vaccine Prevents Cervical Cancer. So Get Vaccinated!

Human papillomavirus (HPV) is the most common sexually transmitted disease in the United States, accounting for approximately 14 million new infections each year. The Centers for Disease Control and Prevention (2017) estimates that 79 million Americans are currently infected with HPV, and that almost all Americans will become infected with HPV at some time in their lives. Most HPV infections are acquired via vaginal, anal, or oral sex with an HPV-infected partner.

There are dozens of types of HPV. Infections with most types cause no or only mild symptoms and resolve within a couple of years. However, infection with HPV types 16 and 18 account for approximately 70% of cervical cancers, which is diagnosed in about 30,000 American women each year. HPV types 6 and 11 are responsible for approximately 90% of cases of genital warts.

A very effective vaccine that prevents HPV infection is available (Markowitz et al., 2016). Health authorities recommend that all females aged 11 through 26 years be vaccinated. Vaccination is also recommended for men who have sex with men (MSM) through age 26 and other males ages 22 to 26 years. Vaccination is also recommended through age 26 years for immunocompromised persons (including those infected with HIV) who have not been vaccinated previously. Currently, among 13- to 17-year-olds, only about 50% of girls and 30% of boys have been vaccinated. About 70% of female and 30% of male U.S. college students have been vaccinated (Lanning et al., 2017). The Healthy People 2020 goal is that 80% of the U.S. population be vaccinated.

Increasing the number of young people who are vaccinated against HPV requires overcoming some obstacles. For example, parents of preteens and teens may object to having their children vaccinated for religious reasons, believing that abstinence from sexual intercourse is the only way to prevent sexually transmitted diseases, or believing that vaccinations of any kind are unsafe. Most college students, particularly males, want to be vaccinated against HPV, but they face barriers to HPV vaccination, including finding an available provider and overcoming the cost of the vaccine (Brunk, 2016).

Cancer of the cervix is not benign. It's a boon to humankind that a vaccine has been developed to protect women from this disease. It's up to parents and potential sexual partners to be sure that the young people they care about are vaccinated while young to prevent cervical and any other HPV-related cancers later in life.

Almost all children in the world are infected by rotovirus at some point, and most of them have only mild symptoms that usually disappear without treatment. However, children who are malnourished or otherwise unhealthy can die from a rotovirus infection. Two safe and effective oral vaccines are available. Most of the children who die from rotovirus infections live in poor, tropical countries. Rotovirus vaccines must be kept refrigerated, and the countries where the vaccine is most needed cannot afford to keep the vaccine refrigerated until it is delivered to poor villages. In 2017, a new rotovirus vaccine was developed that does not require refrigeration. If this vaccine becomes widely used, it will have an enormous impact on reducing serious disease and death from rotovirus infections worldwide.

Vaccination Risks

Vaccination is widely regarded as one of the greatest public health achievements of all time and the principal cause of the dramatic global decrease in sickness and death from infectious diseases. Smallpox has been eradicated from the world by vaccination, and polio is on the verge of being eradicated. Since 1912, the Centers for Disease Control and Prevention has kept records of disease incidence before and after the introduction of a vaccine. In addition to the diseases just mentioned, there has been a 99% reduction in cases of measles, diphtheria, mumps, and rubella and a 97% reduction in whooping cough (pertussis) in the United States as a result of vaccinations.

Vaccination is not 100% risk free. There are often mild reactions that generally disappear in a few days. Roughly speaking, about one per million vaccinations results in serious neurological damage or death. These cases are indeed tragic, but when counterbalanced by the hundreds of millions of lives saved, vaccination is safer than taking an aspirin. In recent years, however, a vocal minority has attacked vaccination, in general, as being unsafe and unnecessary despite firm scientific evidence to the contrary (Poland & Jacobson, 2011). False claims about specific vaccines and adverse effects include the following:

Vaccine	Adverse Effect
Measles	Autism
Diphtheria, pertussis, and tetanus (DPT)	Sudden infant death syndrome
Haemophilus influenzae type B	Diabetes
Hepatitis B	Multiple sclerosis

Given the frequency and number of childhood vaccinations, it is not surprising that a condition occurs in rare cases shortly after a child is vaccinated. It also is not surprising that distraught parents, looking for a cause, blame the vaccination.

Controversy over vaccinations has arisen from the claim that a mercury-based preservative (thimerosal) in vaccines is the cause of the marked increase in autism among young children. The preservative has been used for years to prevent deterioration of the vaccines, particularly where refrigeration is not available. Because of parents' concerns, thimerosal was removed from all U.S. vaccines in 1999. A number of studies have concluded that there is no causal association between thimerosal-containing

Worldwide Infectious Disease Eradication Programs

The World Health Organization (WHO) identifies, directs, and funds infectious disease eradication programs around the world. In 1959, WHO began a program to eradicate smallpox from the entire world. Smallpox had been a scourge for centuries, killing an estimated 2 million people a year. In 1978, the last smallpox victim was reported; since then, no smallpox cases have been reported anywhere in the world.

Eradicating smallpox is regarded as one of the greatest accomplishments of the twentieth century. Since that time, WHO has embarked on other eradication programs, including the eradication of polio. Several times it was thought that the end of polio was in sight, but every year a few cases occur. To eliminate a disease completely, all people in an infected region must be vaccinated. In some regions of the world, political, religious, and cultural beliefs make this difficult. Despite these difficulties, WHO continues to work on eradicating a number of infectious diseases around the world (Enserink, 2010) (see accompanying table).

WHO Infection Eradication Programs

Disease	Eradication status
Smallpox	Eradicated in 1978, after a 20-year effort. No cases have been reported anywhere in the world since then. The eradication of smallpox from the world is regarded as one of the greatest accomplishments of the twentieth century.
Rinderpest	A deadly viral disease of cattle that rapidly spreads through a herd once a single animal is infected. Outbreaks in Africa kill millions of cattle. In 1990, a vaccine was developed that did not require refrigeration. In 2010, no rinderpest cases were reported anywhere in the world. Although not given the wide attention that smallpox eradication received, the eradication of rinderpest virus is a magnificent accomplishment.
Polio	After a 20-year effort, the incidence of polio has been reduced by 99%. Despite the effort, 1,604 cases of polio were reported in 2009 in Asia and Africa. No cases were reported in the Western hemisphere.
Guinea worm disease	This is another human disease that is on the brink of total eradication. In 1986, an estimated 3.5 million cases occurred in Africa and Asia. In 2013, a mere 148 cases were recorded, mostly in Sudan. People become infected by drinking larvae-contaminated water. The eradication program did not use vaccines or medicines but an intense effort to provide clean water to at-risk communities.
Lymphatic filariasis	A mosquito carries a microscopic worm that infects over 120 million persons in Asia, Africa, and South America. The infection produces horribly swollen limbs (elephantiasis). The disease is treated with drugs donated by the drug companies Merck and SmithKlineGlaxo. WHO hopes to markedly reduce the disease by 2020.
Measles	About 10 million cases of measles occur worldwide each year. The measles vaccine eliminated all cases of measles in the Americas in 2002, but new outbreaks have occurred in most countries in recent years. WHO is making new efforts toward eradication.
River blindness	This is a problem in Africa and South America. It is caused by roundworms transmitted by black flies. About 18 million people are affected worldwide. WHO is formulating an eradication program.
Malaria	In 2009, it was estimated that 225 million people had malaria, primarily in tropical countries. New technologies are being used to develop malaria vaccines; these are funded primarily by the Bill and Melinda Gates Foundation. Eradication of malaria remains a hope but is decades away.

Adapted from Enserink, M. (2010). What's next for disease eradication? *Science, 330*, 1736–1739.

vaccines and childhood autism (U.S. Food and Drug Administration, 2017a).

Despite scientific evidence that supports the remarkable safety record of vaccinations, parents whose children acquired debilitating conditions after being vaccinated began to sue pharmaceutical companies that manufactured vaccines. Some of these suits were successful, and companies began to discontinue the manufacture of essential vaccines. To protect the nation's supply, the U.S. government passed the National Childhood Vaccine Injury Act in the late 1980s, which included establishment of a panel called the Vaccine Injury Compensation Program (VICP). This panel is empowered to award damages to parents who present evidence that their child's health was severely damaged by administration of a vaccine. However, the existence of the VICP has provided the safeguards that encourage pharmaceutical companies to develop new

and improved vaccines. In 2011, the U.S. Supreme Court ruled that vaccine manufacturers cannot be sued on grounds that a vaccine is defective. This decision should help maintain the supply of essential vaccines and spur the development of new ones.

Understanding Allergies

Allergies are the immune system's response to foreign substances called **allergens** that the body perceives as being harmful but which usually are not. Pollens, molds, house dust, animal hair, foods, drugs, chemicals, and many other substances can act as allergens. The body responds to allergens by manufacturing a particular class of antibodies (immunoglobulin E, or IgE) that triggers the allergic reaction (**Figure 12.8**). No one knows why allergic responses evolved or what benefit they might have

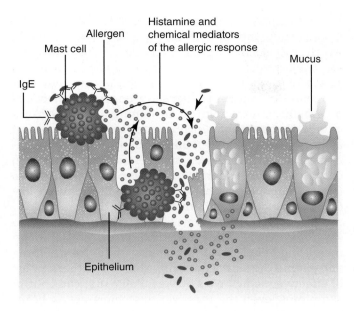

■ **Figure 12.8**

Chemistry of an Allergic Reaction
An allergen (a substance from a plant, insect, or other organism) binds to antibody proteins (IgE) on mast cells. This triggers the release of histamines and other inflammatory substances that characterize the allergic response. These reactions occur mainly in the nose, lungs, skin, and digestive tract.

Getting Rid of Dust Mites May Help Allergies

Dust mites are a major contributor to peoples' allergies. Strictly speaking, it is not the mites but their feces that are highly allergenic. Mites live by the millions in bedding, clothing, carpets, drapes, wall coverings, and upholstered furniture. They are particularly abundant in mattresses, pillows, blankets, quilts, and fuzzy animals.

Getting rid of dust mites is difficult. Because they burrow deeply into objects and are so tiny, vacuum cleaners usually do not remove them. Removal of such items as carpets, plush furniture, drapes, and other cloth from rooms is recommended. Encasing mattresses and pillows with hypoallergenic covers may help. Frequent washing of pillows, bedding, and clothes is recommended. Soaking bedding and clothes in one part liquid detergent to three parts eucalyptus oil for 30 minutes before washing removes 95% of mites and their debris. Try these steps if your allergies are severe.

provided, but millions of people today can attest to the misery caused by allergic responses.

The allergic reaction is usually accompanied by the secretion of mucus and the release of **histamine**, an inflammatory chemical that is abundant in cells of the skin, respiratory passages, and digestive tract. That is why most allergic reactions are associated with the skin (eczema, hives, contact dermatitis), the respiratory passages (asthma, hay fever), and the digestive tract (swelling, vomiting, diarrhea).

Contact Dermatitis

Contact dermatitis is an inflammation of the skin that affects millions of people because many of the things we touch or put on our skin can cause allergic reactions that manifest as rashes, blisters, or hives. Walking in the woods where poison ivy or poison oak grows can produce serious rashes in susceptible persons. Peeling a mango can cause people who are allergic to the skin of this fruit to break out in a rash; however, they usually can eat the flesh of the fruit without experiencing a reaction.

Contact dermatitis actually arises by two distinct mechanisms: *allergic contact dermatitis* involves reactions of the body's immune system cells with specific proteins that contact the skin, resulting in redness, itching, and inflammation. In contrast, *irritant contact dermatitis* does not involve an allergic response but rather is caused by cell damage and inflammation as a direct result of substances that contact the skin. Diaper rash is a common form of irritant dermatitis in babies. The hands also are frequently affected by irritant dermatitis arising from

frequent contact with hard surface cleansers. Cosmetics also may cause irritant dermatitis, especially scented soaps and skin creams. When allergy tests are all negative and a skin condition persists, the condition is diagnosed as irritant dermatitis.

One increasingly common form of allergic contact dermatitis is latex allergy. It is estimated that latex allergies range from 1% to 6% in the general population, and among people who work in hospitals, such as nurses, the frequency is as high as 8%.

Latex is a form of sap extracted from rubber trees and is used in tires and rubber products of all kinds, especially protective gloves, which are used throughout the healthcare industry and other industries where materials must not be contaminated by touch. In the 1980s, the epidemics of AIDS and hepatitis B, both of which are caused by viruses transmitted in blood, created an unprecedented increase in the use of protective latex gloves.

The milky latex sap extracted from rubber trees contains hundreds of different proteins; more than 50 have been purified and have been found to be allergenic. (Most allergies are caused by some kind of protein.) When these latex proteins interact with the skin, they can cause blisters and rashes. When they interact with sensitive mucous membranes in the vagina, rectum, or urethra

TERMS

allergens: foreign substances that trigger an allergic response by the immune system

contact dermatitis: an allergic reaction of the skin to something that is touched

histamine: a chemical released by cells in an allergic response; causes inflammation

from using condoms or other contraceptive devices, or during medical exams, the latex proteins may occasionally cause **anaphylactic shock** and death. Surgical instruments containing latex coverings or surgical gloves can cause severe reactions in sensitive patients.

The proteins in latex are similar to many proteins found in such fruits as banana, mango, papaya, cherry, peach, and avocado. Latex-related proteins also are found in milk, potatoes, and tomatoes. People who notice that they have become allergic to certain foods may, in fact, have become sensitive to latex. Physicians can test for latex allergies and can advise latex-sensitive people on what foods to avoid.

Asthma

Asthma is a chronic disease involving inflammation and narrowing of the airways of the respiratory system, rendering breathing difficult and occasionally nearly impossible. The inflammation and narrowing are caused by the tightening of muscles that surround the airways, the swelling of cells that line the airways, and the production of mucus. Asthma is often a reaction to inhaling a respiratory irritant, such as cigarette smoke or cold air, or a substance to which someone is allergic. In susceptible individuals, exercise and stress also can trigger an *asthma attack*. Asthma sufferers are counseled to avoid situations and substances that trigger attacks. They also can use inhalers that contain drugs that alleviate an asthma attack or drugs that help prevent attacks from occurring. Very severe asthma attacks may require emergency medical intervention. Asthma affects people of all ages, but it most often starts in childhood. In the United States, 18.4 million people have asthma.

Although asthma attacks can be caused by both biological and environmental factors, they can also arise or be made worse by emotional upset and stress. For example, an asthmatic person who gets into a violent argument with a husband, wife, or parent may begin to experience breathing difficulties. Some asthmatic children often improve dramatically when separated from family situations that are stressful and emotionally upsetting. Adult asthmatics often notice that their attacks occur more frequently or become worse when they are upset or under stress that cannot be managed. Thus, asthmatics have an immunological makeup that makes them sensitive to allergens, but they also respond physically to emotions and stress in ways that other people do not.

The prevalence of asthma is increasing in the United States and worldwide. Scientists are unsure of the reasons for this increase, but certain risk factors have been identified, including a family history of allergy, low socioeconomic status, non-Caucasian ethnicity, male gender, age greater than 5 years, and exposure to tobacco smoke, dust, or cockroaches. The roles of maternal diet, breastfeeding, the time of introduction of baby foods, and the use of formulas in developing allergies have also been examined. There is no evidence that maternal diet or breastfeeding affects the risk of asthma.

One explanation for the increase in asthma is the hygiene hypothesis, discussed earlier in the chapter, which suggests that an extremely clean household environment can fail to provide the necessary exposure to germs required to "educate" the immune system so it can learn to launch its defense responses to infectious organisms. Instead, immune defense responses are altered in ways that contribute to the development of asthma. The hygiene hypothesis is supported by observations that allergic diseases and asthma are more likely to occur when the incidence and levels of certain allergens (bacterial lipopolysaccharide, or LPS) in the home are low (U.S. Food and Drug Administration, 2017b).

Although the symptoms of asthma vary from mild to severe, deaths resulting from asthma are rare, although increasing. People no longer need to suffer from asthma and endure the fear of not being able to breathe. A range of effective medicines is now available that can control symptoms, even the most serious. Short-acting bronchodilators that are inhaled at the onset of symptoms can provide immediate relief. For persistent asthma, short-term and long-term corticosteroid inhalers are available. With daily use, these can effectively suppress wheezing symptoms and breathing difficulties. Cromolyn inhalers also suppress symptoms in many people, and oral corticosteroids prevent asthma in the most severe cases. The goal of asthma treatment is to find the right medication at the lowest dose that leaves an asthmatic free of symptoms. And, of course, it is still important to eliminate as many allergens as possible from the home environment.

Food Allergies

Food allergies (not to be confused with *food intolerance*) are allergic responses to a particular food. The reaction can be local (such as vomiting, diarrhea, or abdominal cramps; pain and tightening of the throat; and trouble breathing) or it can involve the whole body (such as hives occurring over the entire body). Food allergies are most common in children but can occur in anyone at any age.

When people are tested for food allergies, six substances account for 90% of the allergic reactions—eggs, peanuts, milk, fish, soy, and wheat. Severe allergic reactions produce anaphylactic shock, a systemic reaction that can quickly cause death. Anaphylactic shock can be brought on by an immediate, strong allergic reaction to food, a bee sting, or a drug. Approximately 400 deaths occur in the United States each year from anaphylactic shock.

Children are at particular risk of developing allergies to nuts, particularly peanuts. (Strictly speaking, the peanut is a legume, not a nut.) Children tend to outgrow most of their childhood allergies, but this is not true for an allergy to Brazil nuts, almonds, hazelnuts, and walnuts. Because the reactions in nut allergies can be quite serious, including anaphylactic shock, most people with nut allergies including peanuts, have to be extremely careful about what foods they eat because many manufactured products may contain trace amounts of nut residues.

Peanut allergies are especially common and dangerous—some people suffer to such a serious degree that even a minuscule amount of peanut protein can lead to anaphylactic shock and death. For years, people with peanut allergies had to learn how to live with them and avoid peanuts—something that is almost impossible to do all of the time. Now the health dangers of peanut allergies are widely recognized, and a number of steps can be taken to reduce potential exposure. Many airlines no longer serve peanuts, and many school lunch programs have eliminated peanuts or post warnings when they are served.

Eating in restaurants is always hazardous for those with peanut allergies, especially in Thai, Indonesian, or Vietnamese restaurants. If a pan has had peanut oil in it, enough remains to cause a reaction, even if it is cleaned before being used again. A 50-pound bag of dried molé from which the sauce is made has a handful of peanuts in it, more than enough to cause a reaction for someone eating in a Mexican restaurant.

A cutting board that has been used to cut peanuts a week ago still has enough peanut protein and oil on it to produce a reaction if it is used to cut something that goes into your dinner. A jelly jar also is very dangerous. If a spoon or knife that touched peanut butter is used to scoop out jelly, that jar is potentially harmful to someone with severe peanut allergies.

Buying foods in bulk can be risky; for instance, when there are scoops used in bins. Suppose someone uses a scoop to get some trail mix that has peanuts in it. That scoop is now contaminated. If it is used to scoop food out of other bins, they all become contaminated with enough peanut protein to cause a reaction. Today, most stores have a separate scoop for each bin, and the scoop is wired down so it cannot be moved.

About 20% of people report food intolerance of one sort or another at some time in their lives, yet studies show that the actual number of people who are physiologically allergic to foods actually is less. About 6% to 8% of children test positive for food allergies and only about 3% of adults. The discrepancy between what people report as an allergic reaction and what is demonstrated by allergy tests probably results from the power of suggestion. If someone reads or is told that many people are allergic to eggs, he or she may begin to experience a reaction when eggs are eaten. Also, vomiting after eating a particular food can produce a subsequent aversion or apparent allergic reaction to that food.

The power of suggestion in causing food allergies has been demonstrated by experiment (Jewett et al., 1990). In this study, patients who reported that they had a food allergy were given a series of injections to desensitize them to the food causing the allergy. One group was desensitized with a placebo (saline) injection; another group was desensitized with an injection of the allergen.

Neither the patients nor the doctors knew which injections contained saline and which contained the allergen. Seven of 18 patients reported that their food allergies were prevented by the placebo shots. Others reported that their symptoms worsened when they received the saline placebo. Thus, placebo effects can cure food allergies or they can make them worse, as in this experiment. How we view food in our minds has a powerful effect on how it is received by the body.

The FDA requires that all food labels list the presence of any of the eight most common food allergens. If even a trace amount of the allergen could be present, the food allergen still must be listed on the label. The eight most common food allergens, listed in order according to the number of people affected, are: milk, egg, peanut, tree nut, wheat, soy, fish, and shellfish. More than 90% of all persons with food allergies test positive for one of more of these eight foods. Occasionally, people are also allergic to certain fruits and vegetables.

Recognition of "Self"

The immune system is able to recognize and destroy almost any foreign material, which is how it protects the body from infectious diseases. To prevent it from attacking the body's own cells, the immune system distinguishes cells of the body as "self" from foreign substances and other cells (even those of another person) that are "nonself."

During fetal development, as the body's tissues are being formed, all of the antibody-producing cells that could attack the body's own cells are destroyed. It is not yet known how these particular antibody-producing cells are selected out of the millions of different cells and destroyed, but such a mechanism is vital to protect the organs and tissues of the body from destruction.

Autoimmune Diseases

The immune system must function without mistakes to distinguish "self" from "nonself" because any error that caused antibodies to attack the body's own cells could result in serious disease or death. Unfortunately, mistakes in the functioning of the immune system do occur

---

TERMS

anaphylactic shock: a severe allergic reaction involving the whole body that can cause death

asthma: a chronic disease involving inflammation and narrowing of the airways that makes it difficult to breathe

food allergies: allergic responses to something that is eaten

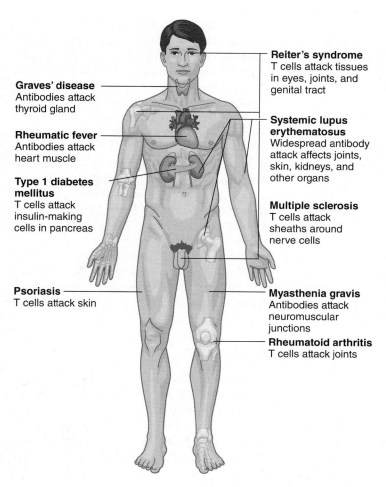

Graves' disease
Antibodies attack
thyroid gland

Rheumatic fever
Antibodies attack
heart muscle

**Type 1 diabetes
mellitus**
T cells attack
insulin-making
cells in pancreas

Psoriasis
T cells attack skin

Reiter's syndrome
T cells attack tissues
in eyes, joints, and
genital tract

**Systemic lupus
erythematosus**
Widespread antibody
attack affects joints,
skin, kidneys, and
other organs

Multiple sclerosis
T cells attack
sheaths around
nerve cells

Myasthenia gravis
Antibodies attack
neuromuscular
junctions

Rheumatoid arthritis
T cells attack joints

■ **Figure 12.9**

Autoimmune Diseases
These occur when the body's immune system goes awry and cells of
the immune system begin attacking the body's own cells because they
are mistakenly recognized as foreign.

and produce **autoimmune diseases** (**Figure 12.9**). Some inherited disorders, fortunately quite rare, can result in the loss of the immune system's ability to distinguish "self" from "nonself." Environmental factors, such as viral infections, nutritional problems, and other unknown agents, may also cause the immune system to make mistakes that lead to autoimmune diseases.

Lupus erythematosus is an autoimmune disease that most frequently affects women between the ages of 18 and 35. In this disease, for reasons still unknown, antibodies are synthesized that attack the genetic information in cells (DNA), especially in cells of the blood vessels, skin, and kidneys. Many organs of the body are affected, and the symptoms—rashes, pain, and anemia—flare up and wane throughout life, which usually is shortened. In general, autoimmune diseases affect women more often than men.

Arthritis is one of the most common chronic diseases; approximately one in seven Americans has some form of arthritis. There are about 100 forms of arthritis and arthritis-related conditions, but the common denominator is pain and stiffness in joints throughout the body (**Figure 12.10**). The causes of arthritis vary widely, but many forms are the result of autoimmune disease in which the body's immune system mistakenly attacks cartilage and bone. Drugs can relieve many of the

symptoms of autoimmune diseases, such as pain and inflammation, but the diseases themselves have no cure.

As with most chronic diseases of unknown etiology, the mind can exert a powerful role in controlling the symptoms of arthritis or in aggravating them. Relaxation and visualization exercises that emphasize mobility and comfort can be of great benefit in relieving the pain, stiffness, and inflammation associated with arthritis.

An autoimmune disease that affects the central nervous system is **multiple sclerosis (MS)**. Recent research suggests that MS may be initiated by a viral infection that somehow causes the immune system to produce antibodies that attack **myelin**, a substance that sheaths and insulates nerve fibers in the brain and spinal cord.

Although drugs can help reduce the symptoms of autoimmune diseases, these diseases are caused by complex malfunctions of the immune system. Because the mind also affects the functions of the immune system, many people who suffer from autoimmune diseases find relief in alternative therapies, mental relaxation techniques, and nutritional changes.

Organ Transplants

Like blood cells, all body cells have antigens on their surfaces that are different for everyone except identical

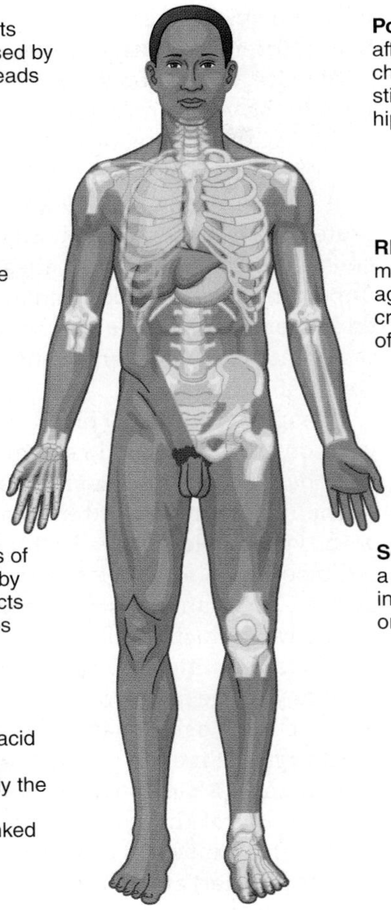

Ankylosing spondylitis affects mostly younger men. It is caused by a spinal inflammation that spreads to other areas of the body.

Fibromyalgia affects mostly women. The symptoms include fatigue, pain, insomnia, and stiffness but usually no inflammation of the joints.

Osteoarthritis affects millions of older Americans. It is caused by the erosion of cartilage that acts as a shock absorber at the tips of bones.

Gout affects mostly men. It is caused by the buildup of uric acid in the blood, crystals of which accumulate in joints, especially the big toe for unknown reasons. Overeating and alcohol are linked to the condition.

Polymyalgia rheumatica affects mostly older women. It is characterized by muscle pain and stiffness in the neck, shoulder, and hip.

Rheumatoid arthritis affects mostly women. It strikes at any age and can eventually be crippling as a result of destruction of joints.

Scleroderma is characterized by a thickening of the skin and inflammation of joints and internal organs.

■ **Figure 12.10**

Common Forms of Arthritis and Arthritis-Related Diseases and Their Symptoms

twins. If tissue or organs from one person are grafted onto another, the immune system produces antibodies to the foreign cell antigens, causing destruction of the cells and rejection of the transplanted organ.

The more alike two persons are genetically, the more likely it is that the transplanted tissue will be accepted by the recipients body. Identical twins are genetically identical; this is why tissue transplants between identical twins have the greatest chance of success. To minimize the rejection of transplanted organs, the **histocompatibility** (similarity of cell surface antigens) between the donor and recipient is determined by immunological tests. Just as red blood cells have particular groups of strongly antigenic proteins on their cell surfaces, so other cells in the body have antigenic proteins called **HLA (human leukocyte antigens)** that are crucial in determining whether a transplanted organ is accepted or rejected (**Figure 12.11**). The greater the similarity in HLA between donor and recipient, the greater the chance that the tissue will be accepted and function normally in its new host. From the number of HLAs already determined, calculations show that there are so many different HLA combinations that each unrelated person is immunologically unique.

Today, the transplantation of hearts, kidneys, livers, and other organs has become a relatively common procedure in many hospitals. However, organ transplants are extremely costly, complicated procedures and are not always successful. Many more people are waiting for suitable organs than can be supplied from living or deceased donors. Patients

TERMS

autoimmune diseases: mistakes in the functioning of the immune system that cause it to attack tissues in the body

arthritis: a variety of chronic diseases involving inflammation, stiffness, and pain in joints of the body

lupus erythematosus: an autoimmune disease that mostly affects women

multiple sclerosis (MS): an autoimmune disease that affects the central nervous system

myelin: a substance that sheathes and insulates nerve fibers in the brain and spinal cord

histocompatibility: the degree to which the antigens on cells of different persons are similar

HLA (human leukocyte antigens): antigens that are measured to determine the suitability of an organ for transplantation from donor to recipient

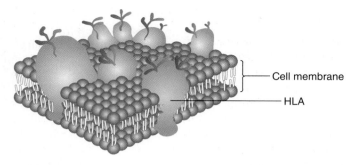

Cell membrane

HLA

■ **Figure 12.11**

Antigens and the Immune System
A vast array of different HLAs is embedded in the outer membranes of cells, projecting beyond their surfaces. These antigens can be recognized by the body's immune cells and antibodies. Because every person's antigens are different, tissue transplanted from one person to another is usually rejected because the donor's HLAs are recognized as foreign and destroyed by the immune response of the recipient.

whose survival depends on the availability of a suitably matched organ often wait months to receive one, and often no organ becomes available before the patient dies.

The organ most often transplanted is the kidney. Because people have two kidneys, relatives sometimes donate one of their healthy kidneys to another close relative if their HLA genes are well matched. If the match is perfect for HLAs and ABO blood type, the success rate is 90% survival at 1 year for the recipient. Brothers and sisters have one chance in four of inheriting the same HLA genes from their parents, which is why close relatives are examined first as possible donors. Bone marrow transplants also are used as a last resort in cases of aplastic anemia, acute leukemia, and radiation sickness.

The rejection of transplanted organs can be controlled to some degree with **immunosuppressive drugs** (corticosteroids, cyclosporine); however, treatment with these drugs lessens resistance to infections and sometimes enhances development of other diseases. Long-term immunosuppressive drug therapy itself results in increased susceptibility to cancer. It makes more sense to prevent kidney and heart diseases than to rely on surgical transplants.

Blood Transfusions: ABO and Rh Factors

In the early part of the twentieth century, a blood transfusion often led to the patient's death. Because the patient's

immune system recognized the donor's blood cells as being "foreign," it attacked them with both T cells and antibodies. The antibodies caused clumps of blood cells to form in the veins and arteries, impeding the flow of blood and oxygen and causing death.

The two most important human red blood cell surface antigens are the ABO and Rh-positive/Rh-negative proteins. There are actually many other groups of antigens on red blood cells, but these two are by far the most important ones in evoking an immune response that can endanger health. **Table 12.6** shows the pattern of donor–recipient ABO blood types that must be matched for a successful transfusion.

People with type O blood have neither A nor B antigens on their red blood cells and are **universal donors**; their blood cells will not stimulate an antibody response in the recipient, no matter what the blood type. People with type AB blood have both antigens present on their red blood cells and do not synthesize A or B antibodies because these antigens are recognized as "self" and those antibody-producing cells are destroyed. People with type AB blood are **universal recipients** and can accept blood from any of the four groups.

The Rh-positive antigen and the antibody that reacts against it cause problems primarily in pregnancy. A woman is Rh-negative if her red blood cells do not contain any of this antigen. If the red blood cells of a developing fetus have the Rh-positive antigen (inherited from the father) and if some of the fetus's red blood cells enter the mother's blood supply, production of anti-Rh antibodies can be stimulated by her immune system, which recognizes the fetal cells as foreign. This usually does not cause any difficulty during the first pregnancy and might even go unnoticed until the woman becomes pregnant again.

Now, if the second fetus is also Rh-positive, the Rh-positive antibodies (synthesized during the first pregnancy) in the mother's blood attack the developing infant's red blood cells, resulting in anemia, brain damage, or even death. Fortunately, doctors can manage this problem safely and effectively. At the time the first child is delivered, the mother is given an injection of anti-Rh antibodies that destroys any Rh-positive antibodies in her blood. In this way, any danger to the fetus during a subsequent pregnancy is avoided.

Table 12.6

Permissible Transfusions Determined by ABO Blood Group

Blood group	Genotype	Antigens on red blood cells	Transfusions cannot be accepted from	Transfusions are accepted from
O (universal donor)	OO	None	A, B, AB	O
A	AA, AO	A	B, AB	A, O
B	BB, BO	B	A, AB	B, O
AB (universal recipient)	AB	A, B	None	A, B, AB, O

AIDS and HIV

Acquired immune deficiency syndrome, or **AIDS**, is a fatal infection caused by the **human immunodeficiency virus (HIV)**. Infection with HIV gradually weakens the body's immune system, exposing it to **opportunistic infections** caused by any of a wide variety of microorganisms. AIDS patients become progressively weaker with each infection and eventually die. The course of HIV infection is unpredictable; some individuals progress to full-blown AIDS and die within months. Others have no symptoms even after 10 years or more of HIV infection (**Figure 12.12**).

Long-term HIV-infected survivors have three genes that keep the HIV level low enough to maintain immune function and prevent development of AIDS.

For the majority of HIV-infected patients, powerful drugs must be taken to keep HIV in check and prevent progression to AIDS. These drugs fall into several different classes: nucleoside reverse transcriptase inhibitors (NRTIs), nonnucleoside reverse transcriptase inhibitors (NNRTIs), protease inhibitors (PIs), fusion inhibitors, entry inhibitors, and HIV integrase and transfer inhibitors. Drugs usually are given in combinations to maximize effectiveness and reduce the chance that the patient will develop a drug-resistant strain of HIV.

Many antiretroviral drugs are so effective that they can reduce the detectable amount of HIV in the blood to almost zero for long periods of time. When the drugs are stopped, however, HIV reemerges from immune system cells where it has been unaffected by antiretroviral drugs. In 2015, it was estimated that 17 million people worldwide were infected with HIV and being treated with antiretroviral drugs. Another 6,000 were becoming newly infected every day (Haynes & Burton, 2017).

After almost 40 years of intense scientific research and billions of dollars spent, there still is no vaccine to prevent HIV/AIDS or any drug that will eliminate the HIV virus from the body and actually cure the disease. Until such time that a vaccine is developed, sexually active individuals must practice *safe sex* during homosexual or heterosexual intercourse.

AIDS was first recognized as a distinct disease in the early 1980s in the United States. The disease quickly spread worldwide. More than half of the world's current AIDS victims live in Africa, and most have no access to drugs that can retard the spread of HIV in the body. Left untreated, AIDS eventually develops in most HIV-infected individuals.

TERMS

acquired immune deficiency syndrome (AIDS): a syndrome of more than two dozen diseases caused by HIV

human immunodeficiency virus (HIV): the virus that causes AIDS

immunosuppressive drugs: drugs to suppress the functions of the immune system (e.g., after organ transplants)

opportunistic infection: any infectious disease in a patient with a weakened immune system; often occurs in AIDS patients

universal donors: people whose blood is accepted by everyone during transfusion

universal recipients: people whose blood type is compatible with anyone else's blood

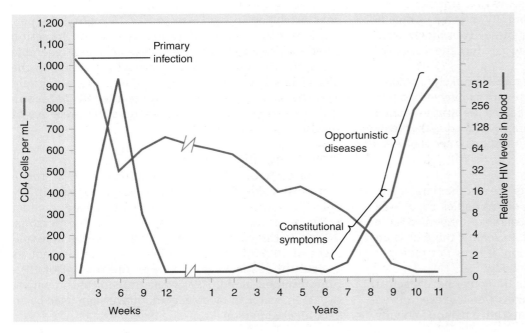

■ **Figure 12.12**

HIV and the Immune System
After infection with HIV, levels of the virus in the blood rise sharply as the body's immune system attacks the virus, as it should. Within 3 months, the virus is undetectable. During this time, however, HIV is multiplying in lymph nodes and infecting CD4 T cells, which gradually decrease in number. As the number of CD4 T cells decrease, the immune system weakens, and the infected person becomes susceptible to opportunistic diseases. Without treatment, in time the opportunistic diseases progress to cause severe illness and death.

Scientists have traced the ancestors of HIV to monkeys that lived in Africa thousands of years ago. These monkeys carried a mild form of a *simian immunodeficiency virus* (SIV). These monkey viruses did not cause disease and were transmitted from one generation of monkeys to the next. Because humans consume monkey meat, they must have been exposed to SIV many times over the centuries without ill effects. However, in the twentieth century, monkey and chimpanzee SIV transmitted to people became both contagious and deadly. In the time since HIV/AIDS was first identified in the 1980s, more than 70 million people worldwide have died. Approximately 36.7 million people worldwide are infected with HIV and at least half of them are women of reproductive age. HIV usually is transmitted from a pregnant woman to the newborn unless antiviral drugs are administered to both mother and child.

AIDS is called a syndrome because it is defined by the appearance of any one of several different infectious diseases. It also is characterized by a very low level of a particular immune system cell called the CD4 T cell. In an uninfected person, the CD4 T cell level is 800 to 1,200 cells/milliliter; in an AIDS patient, the level can be 100 cells/milliliter or less. Once HIV infects CD4 T cells, it replicates and releases viruses that infect additional cells.

HIV is a very small virus with little genetic information; however, it is very effective at infecting cells (**Figure 12.13**). One reason for the efficiency is HIV's ability to take control of an infected cell's normal biochemical activities and utilize them during infection. The elements of a cell that HIV takes over are called *dependency factors*. Dozens of cellular HIV dependency factors have been identified that play some role in the infection and continued virus production. The importance of identifying these HIV dependency factors is that some are targets for drugs that can prevent growth of HIV.

Anti-HIV drugs also prevent sexual transmission of HIV and transmission of the virus from HIV-infected women to their babies during birth. Making these drugs widely available in all countries is a major way to reduce the number of new HIV infections worldwide.

Men who are circumcised are much less likely to become infected by HIV during intercourse with an infected woman and also are much less likely to transmit the virus to women partners. The World Health Organization reports that male circumcision reduces the risk of infection by about 60%.

The HIV Antibody Test

Upon infecting a person, HIV acts like all other viral infections by stimulating synthesis of antibodies capable of inactivating the virus. Detection of these antibodies is the basis of the **HIV antibody test**. In reality, the test is an indirect measure of HIV infection; it does not measure the actual amount of HIV in the body.

The test is positive only after antibodies have reached a detectable level, which can take several weeks or even months after infection. In the interim, a person is highly

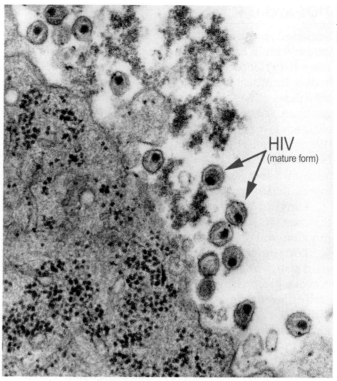

HIV
(mature form)

■ **Figure 12.13**

The AIDS virus as seen under the electron microscope. The arrows point to human immunodeficiency viruses being released from infected cells.

infectious but will show negative results on the HIV antibody test. Thus, even a recent negative test may not mean that a person is uninfected.

Another problem with HIV antibody tests is false-positive results that create unnecessary anxiety. A false positive means that the test shows that the person has antibodies in his or her blood that resemble ones produced in response to HIV. In reality, the person is not infected and the test is in error. Infection by other viruses or bacteria whose antigens resemble those of HIV can lead to a false-positive result on the HIV antibody test. Any positive AIDS test result should be rechecked. The most accurate test for HIV infection is the **Western blot**, which measures the presence of specific HIV proteins.

Preventing HIV Infection

Compared with other viral infections, such as those that cause colds, flu, or hepatitis, HIV is not very infectious. The virus is *never* transmitted by casual contact between an infected person and uninfected persons. "Never," in this context, means that no well-documented cases of HIV infection have been reported except as a result of sexual intercourse or the receipt of HIV-contaminated blood. HIV is not transmitted in saliva, sweat, air, water, or by objects that have been used by an HIV-infected person.

Preventing Infections

Infections are, to some degree, unavoidable. However, the elements of healthy living that we have been emphasizing can both reduce the risk of contracting an infectious disease and also hasten recovery. Foremost is maintaining health by proper nutrition and a reasonable amount of exercise. These factors, as well as sufficient rest and sleep, increase the ability of the immune system to fight infectious organisms.

Vaccinations against certain infections can provide almost complete protection. Check your record of immunizations with your family physician and update any that have not been received on schedule or that you are not sure that you received as a child (See "My Vaccination Record" in the Workbook, Chapter 12). Many infections, such as mumps or measles, that are usually mild in childhood can be serious if acquired as an adult.

Never forget that the mind interacts with the immune system and also contributes to the body's propensity to ward off or to succumb to infections. Stressful situations and emotional upsets lower the body's defenses and make it more vulnerable to infectious microorganisms. Finally, use common sense and stay away from people and situations that are known to carry a high risk of infection. For example, do not travel to an area that is having a cholera epidemic. Do not expose yourself unnecessarily to people with colds, flu, chicken pox, or other highly contagious diseases. With reasonable precautions many infectious diseases are preventable. And by maintaining good health, the body will quickly and completely recover from most infections when they do occur.

TERMS

HIV antibody test: detects antibodies in blood that are produced in response to infection by HIV

Western blot: a test that measures the level of specific HIV proteins in blood

Critical Thinking About Health

1. Describe one infectious disease you have had in the past few years (other than a cold). Discuss the following: (a) how you think you caught the disease, (b) what kind of microorganism caused it, (c) what the symptoms were, (d) how the disease was treated, and (e) any advice you were given on how to avoid contracting the disease in the future. Have you made any changes in your lifestyle to reduce the risk of contracting an infectious disease as a result of this experience?

2. What kind of infectious disease worries you the most: Lyme disease, AIDS, hepatitis, tuberculosis, sexually transmitted diseases in general, or others? Explain your concerns over contracting this disease, including any circumstances in your life that might have given rise to your concerns. Describe all that you know about this particular disease and how your concerns have altered your lifestyle or behaviors.

3. Find out all that you can on foodborne infectious diseases. Describe the kinds of microorganisms in foods that cause disease and ways that people can protect themselves from becoming infected. Do you have any concerns about the foods that you eat? Can you reduce or eliminate these concerns by making changes in your diet?

4. A variety of mind–body exercises are effective in controlling the symptoms of allergies, asthma, arthritis, and other immune system diseases. Learn as much as you can about how the immune system works. Discuss how you think the mind affects the immune system and how it can affect symptoms of the diseases just mentioned. Have you had any personal experience in using your mind to change the symptoms of a disease that has its roots in some form of immune system malfunction?

Chapter Summary and Highlights

Chapter Summary

The human body contains trillions of microorganisms, mostly bacteria, that are essential to normal body function and good health. The complete catalog of different microorganisms in and on a person's body is called the *human microbiome*. Everyone's microbiome has a different composition, and it plays a vital role in maintaining a person's health and resistance to disease. However, if microorganisms grow in regions of the body where they do not belong or if foreign microorganisms invade the body, disease may result. Viruses, bacteria, protozoa, fungi, worms, and insects can all infect the human body and cause disease. Some disease-causing organisms are passed from person to person and can spread rapidly in a population, causing an epidemic or a pandemic if the infection spreads worldwide. Fortunately, the body has several lines of defense against diseases-causing organisms. The immune system produces a variety of cells and proteins that recognize foreign organisms and foreign cells that enter the body and destroy them. But some microorganisms have evolved mechanisms that help them avoid attack by the immune system's defenses. Human immunodeficiency virus (HIV), the virus that causes AIDS, is one such virus that can avoid eradication by the immune system.

Immunization refers to injection of substances that prime the immune system to immediately attack specific disease-causing viruses and bacteria should a person encounter them. Immunizations are the safest and most effective way to prevent serious diseases such as mumps, measles, polio, flu, pneumonia, cervical cancer, hepatitis, and others. Sometimes the body's immune system recognizes certain proteins as harmful when they are, in fact, harmless. This produces symptoms of allergy—sneezing, coughing, headache, vomiting, diarrhea, even death from shock. Every person carries a unique set of proteins on their cells that distinguishes one person from another. Transplant of organs or blood transfusions from one person to another depend on matching certain key proteins between donors and recipients of blood or tissues. Long-term use of drugs helps prevent rejection of a transplanted organ by the recipient's immune system.

Highlights

- Infectious diseases are caused by a myriad of pathogenic organisms: viruses, bacteria, fungi, protozoa, and worms. Growth of certain microorganisms in the body can cause a wide range of diseases and sickness; some produce only mild symptoms, but others produce serious disease and death.
- Some pathogenic microorganisms are easily passed from one person to another and cause communicable diseases.
- Some infectious diseases are caused by a vector, such as an insect or other animal, that transmits the pathogenic microorganism to an uninfected person.
- Hepatitis B and C infections are transmitted in blood and affect millions of people worldwide.
- In the United States, emerging infectious diseases are of concern: West Nile virus that causes encephalitis is one. In 2016, a mosquito-borne virus called Zika emerged as a major threat to pregnant women. Becoming infected by Zika during pregnancy often

caused women to give birth to babies with under-developed brains and heads, a birth defect called *microcephaly*. Zika infections are most common in warm, tropical areas such as Central and South America, but the Zika virus has also been detected in southern states such as Florida.

- Many pathogenic bacteria are becoming resistant to antibiotics, making treatment of serious infectious diseases difficult.
- Antibiotics kill microorganisms but do not kill viruses, which are not alive in the sense that cells are.
- Infectious disease is fought in four ways: sanitation, antibiotics, vaccination, and healthful living.
- Vaccinations are vital to preventing serious infections. Approved vaccines are safe except in rare cases of adverse reactions.
- The skin and mucous membranes keep harmful substances from entering the body.
- Specialized white blood cells circulate in the body, attacking and destroying invading foreign organisms.

- The immune system produces cells that make antibodies, which are proteins that recognize any foreign substance or organism.
- Malfunctioning of the immune system causes auto-immune diseases and allergies.
- Each person carries a unique set of antigens on cells of the body that make tissues and organs unique to each individual.
- Transplantation of organs or blood requires that the donor and recipient be matched with respect to histocompatibility, which is the matching of HLA or ABO antigens.
- AIDS results from infection by HIV, which destroys CD4 cells of the immune system. Immunodeficiency leads to opportunistic infections that eventually cause death.
- Long-term survivors of HIV infection have genes that make them resistant to infection by HIV and to development of AIDS.
- Many drugs help to keep HIV in check in persons infected with AIDS.

For Your Health

Everyone should have a copy of their health records, including "My Vaccination Record" (Exercise 12.1, in the Workbook).

References

Brunk, D. (2016, April 1). College students report perceived barriers to HPV vaccine. *Family Practice News*. Retrieved from https://www.mdedge.com/familypracticenews/article/107754/gynecologic-cancer/college-students-report-perceived-barriers-hpv

Centers for Disease Control and Prevention. (2017). Human papillomavirus. Retrieved from https://www.cdc.gov/hpv/index.html

Colgrove, J., et al. (2010). HPV vaccination mandates—lawmaking amid political and scientific controversy. *New England Journal of Medicine, 363,* 785–791.

Eakin, E. (2014, December 1). The excrement experiment. *The New Yorker,* 64–71.

Enserink, M. (2010). What's next for disease eradication? *Science, 330,* 1736–1739.

Garza-González, E., et al. (2014). A review of *Helicobacter pylori* diagnosis, treatment, and methods to detect eradication. *World Journal of Gastroenterology, 20,* 1438–1349.

Glasner, M. E. (2017). Finding enzymes in the human gut microbiome, *Science, 355,* 577–578.

Harvey, R., et al. (2007). Nasal saline irrigations for the symptoms of chronic rhinosinusitis. *Cochrane Database of Systematic Reviews*. Retrieved from http://www.cochrane.org/reviews/en/ab006394.html

Haynes, B., & Burton, D. R. (2017). Developing an HIV vaccine. *Science, 355,* 1129–1130.

Jewett, D. L., et al. (1990). A double-blind study of symptom provocation to determine food sensitivity. *New England Journal of Medicine, 323,* 429–433.

Lanning, B., et al. (2017). Improving human papillomavirus vaccination uptake in college students: A socioecological perspective. *American Journal of Health Education, 48,* 116–128.

Margalida, A., et al. (2014). One health approach to use of veterinary pharmaceuticals. *Science, 346,* 1296–1298.

Markowitz, L. E., et al. (2016). Prevalence of HPV after introduction of the vaccination program in the United States. *Pediatrics, 137,* e20151968

Marotza, C. A., & Zarrinparb, A. (2016). Treating obesity and metabolic syndrome with fecal microbiota transplantation. *Yale Journal of Biology and Medicine, 89,* 383–388.

Mullin, E. (2017). Gene therapy 2.0. *MIT Technology Review*, 120, 49–51.

Poland, G. A., & Jacobson, R. M. (2011). The age-old struggle against the antivaccinationists. *New England Journal of Medicine*, 364, 97–99.

Sanders, L. (2016, April 2). Microbes and the mind. *Science News*, 23–25.

Sarkar, A., et al. (2016). Psychobiotics and the manipulation of bacteria–gut–brain signals. *Trends in Neurosciences*, 39(11), 763–781. http://doi.org/10.1016/j.tins.2016.09.002

Schuijs, M. J., et al. (2015). Farm dust and endotoxin protect against allergy through A20 interaction in lung epithelial cells. *Science*, 349, 1105–1110.

Specter, M. (2017, January 2). Rewiring the code of life. *The New Yorker*, 34–44.

Taubenberger, J. K. (2005, January). Capturing a killer flu virus. *Scientific American*, 63–71.

U.S. Food and Drug Administration. (2016). Antibacterial soap? You can skip it—use plain soap and water. Retrieved from https://www.fda.gov/ForConsumers/ConsumerUpdates/ucm378393.htm

U.S. Food and Drug Administration. (2017a). Thimerosal and vaccines. Retrieved from https://www.fda.gov/biologicsbloodvaccines/safetyavailability/vaccinesafety/ucm096228

U.S. Food and Drug Administration. (2017b). Asthma: The hygiene hypothesis. Retrieved from https://www.fda.gov/biologicsbloodvaccines/resourcesforyou/consumers/ucm167471.htm

Vazquez, M., et al. (2008). Effectiveness of personal proactive measures to prevent Lyme disease. *Emerging Infectious Diseases*, 142, 210–216.

Woolhouse, M. E. J., & Ward, M. J. (2013). Sources of antimicrobial resistance. *Science*, 341, 1460–1461.

Suggested Readings

Bakalar, N. (2003). *Where the germs are: A scientific safari.* New York: Wiley. If you are curious about germs, both healthy and unhealthy, this is a fun book for information.

Blaser, M. J. (2014). *Missing microbes—how the overuse of antibiotics is fueling our modern plagues.* New York: Holt. This book describes the problems the United States now faces in treating bacterial diseases because it failed to regulate the overuse of antibiotics years ago when it was urged to do so by scientists.

Cohen, J. (2010, July/August). Can AIDS be cured? *Technology Review*, 44–51. Explores the possible answers to this question.

Eakin, E. (2014, December 1). The excrement experiment. *The New Yorker.* 64–71. Inside and out our bodies are covered with trillions of microorganisms. They play crucial roles in health and sickness. Some diseases (Crohn's disease) are now being treated with fecal transplants from healthy donors to unhealthy patients.

Eaton, E. S. (2017, June 24). Prescribing a predator. *Science News*, 22–26. Some human pathogenic bacteria are now resistant to as many as 26 different antibiotics. This article describes how researchers are looking for alternatives to destroy antibiotic resistant bacteria that infect us.

Finlay, B. B. (2010, February). The art of bacterial warfare. *Scientific American*, 56–63. Discusses the properties of beneficial and harmful bacteria and how bacterial infections are treated.

Finley, D. B., & Arrieta, M. C. (2016). *Let them eat dirt.* New York: Workman Publishing. This book explains how microorganisms in the human microbiome keep us alive and healthy. It is important for young children to be exposed to many microorganisms in many different environments for their immune systems to develop. Hence, don't worry when toddlers touch dirty objects or put things in their mouths. The microorganisms they ingest actually help their immune systems develop normally. Of course, as every parent knows, there is a limit to what you allow your toddler to put into his or her mouth.

Gaidos, S. (2014, June 14). T-force. *Science News*, 22–25. Describes how scientists are manipulating immune system cells to help the body fight cancer and other diseases.

Groopman, J. (2011, February 7). The peanut puzzle. *The New Yorker*, 26–30. Every year thousands of Americans are rushed to hospitals after being exposed to peanuts in food; dozens die. This article explains what we know and what we do not know about peanut allergy. Scientists still do not know why food allergies are on the rise in children, but new treatments can desensitize many affected children by exposing them to allergy-causing proteins that have been chemically modified.

Kupferschmidt, K. (2017). The science of persuasion. *Science*, 356, 366–373. An important series of scientific articles debunking each of the myths regarding the dangers of vaccination, including studies showing that the schedule of vaccinations for children is safe.

McKenna, M. (2011, April). The enemy within. *Scientific American*, 47–53. Describes how bacteria around the world are rapidly becoming resistant to our most effective antibiotics and what the consequences to health will be.

Mitman, G. (2007). *Breathing space: How allergies shape our lives and landscapes*. New Haven, CT: Yale University Press. An excellent discussion of all aspects of allergies, including their history, treatment, desensitization, and ways to avoid allergens.

National Center for Infectious Diseases. (2003). Health information for international travel, 2003–2004. Available: http://bookstore.phf.org. Contains a wealth of information on specific countries, diseases likely to be encountered, and drugs and vaccinations recommended.

Schardt, D. (2016, December). Microbiome. *Nutrition Action*, 9–11. An excellent introduction to the human microbiome in all its many functions and how microorganisms in the body keep us healthy.

Specter, M. (2003, February 3). The vaccine. *The New Yorker*, 54–65. A devastating account of the AIDS epidemic and the efforts scientists are making to find a vaccine to prevent HIV infection.

Specter, M. (2007, December 3). Darwin's surprise. *The New Yorker*, 64–73. Explains how human health and evolution actually depend on viruses and bacteria within us. If you read no other science article, read this one.

Specter, M. (2012, October 22). Germs are us. *The New Yorker*, 32–39. Each of us harbors a unique mix of beneficial and harmful microbes. Healthy people often harbor different populations of microbes than sick people. If scientists can decipher which microbes are beneficial, doctors, in the future, may treat patients with microbial mixtures; this new form of treatment is called probiotics.

Specter, M. (2017, January 2). Rewiring the code of life. *The New Yorker*, 34–44. A truly amazing story about how a scientist plans to eliminate Lyme disease from two islands, Martha's Vineyard and Nantucket, off the coast of Massachusetts. More than a quarter of the inhabitants of these islands have had Lyme disease. He and his team plan to use the latest genetic engineering techniques. His problem: convincing the residents that it's safe.

Recommended Websites

Allergy Newswire
A good site for current information and advice on allergic conditions.

Centers for Disease Control and Prevention
The CDC is the research and education division of the U.S. Public Health Service.

Emerging Infectious Diseases
An online journal from the Centers for Disease Control and Prevention (CDC).

Food Allergy Network
Information and education on food allergies.

MedlinePlus on Infectious Diseases
From the U.S. National Library of Medicine.

World Health Organization Report on Infectious Diseases
Updates on outbreaks of infectious diseases around the world.

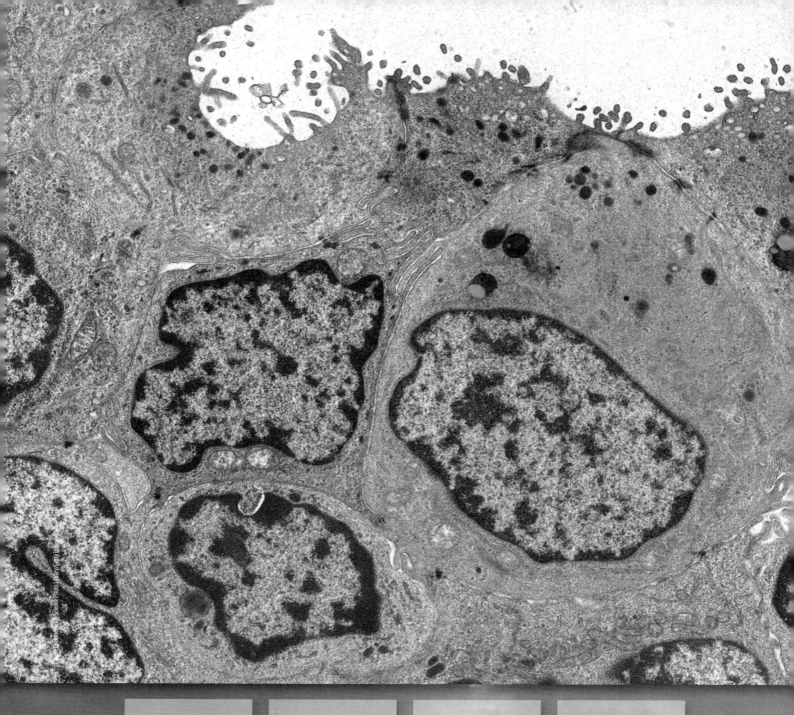

Health Tips

Abortion Does Not Increase Risk of Breast Cancer

Signs of Melanoma

Don't Be Fooled by "Miraculous" Cancer Cures

Dollars & Health Sense

The Cost of Extending Life Among Terminally Ill Cancer Patients

Managing Stress

Visualization Helps Healing

Wellness Guide

Breast Cancer and Mastectomy

Breast Self-Examination

Testicular Cancer: Self-Exam

What Do Indoor Tanning Lamps and Cigarettes Have in Common?

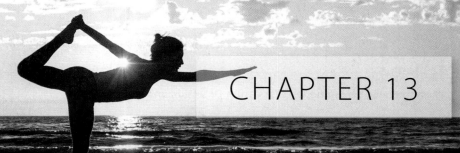

CHAPTER 13

Cancer: Understanding Risks and Means of Prevention

Learning Objectives

1. Identify and describe the most important ways to prevent cancer.

2. Briefly discuss the incidence of cancer today and why mortality has not fallen.

3. Define the following terms: *cancer*, *tumor*, *benign tumor*, *malignant tumor*, *metastasis*, and *xenoestrogen*.

4. Explain the difference between inherited diseases and genetic diseases.

5. Describe the kinds of environmental agents that cause cancer.

6. Explain ways to prevent skin cancer.

7. Discuss some risk factors associated with breast cancer.

8. Describe how to do a breast self-exam (BSE).

9. Discuss how cigarette smoke contributes to cancer.

10. Discuss the association between diet and cancer.

11. Briefly describe the three medical treatments for cancer.

12. Describe several coping mechanisms for someone with cancer.

13. Explain the risks and benefits of being tested for a cancer susceptibility gene.

Table 13.1

Recommended Screening Tests for Cancer Detection and Prevention

Test	Sex	Age	Frequency of testing
Colonoscopy[1]	M & F	50 and over	Every 10 years
Flexible sigmoidoscopy[1]	M & F	50 and over	Every 5 years
Double-contrast barium enema[1]	M & F	50 and over	Every 5 years
Fecal occult blood test (FOBT)[1]	M & F	50 and over	Every year
Fecal immuno chemical test (FIT)	M & F	50 and over	Every year
FIT-DNA test	M & F	50 and over	Every year
Digital (finger) rectal examination[2]	M	50 and over	Every year
Prostate-specific antigen[2]	M	50 and over	Every year
Pap test[3]	F	18 and over	Women should begin getting a Pap test with the start of sexual activity, but no later than at 21 years of age, and repeat the test at least every 3 years
Breast self-examination[4]	F	20 and over	Every month
Breast clinical examination[4]	F	20–40	Every 3 years
		40 and over	Every year
Mammography[4]	F	40 and over	Every 1–2 years

Note: The CDC reports that clinical and breast self-exams have not been shown to reduce the incidence of breast cancer death and that women should rely on mammogram for adequate screening.

Adapted from the following sources:

[1] Centers for Disease Control and Prevention. (2017). *Colorectal cancer screening*. Retrieved from http://www.cdc.gov/cancer/colorectal/basic_info/screening/index.htm

[2] Centers for Disease Control and Prevention. (2017). *Prostate cancer*. Retrieved from http://www.cdc.gov/cancer/prostate/basic_info/get-screened.htm

[3] Centers for Disease Control and Prevention. (2017). *Cervical cancer*. Retrieved from http://www.cdc.gov/cancer/cervical/basic_info/screening.htm

[4] Centers for Disease Control and Prevention. (2017). *Breast cancer*. Retrieved from http://www.cdc.gov/cancer/breast/.

On the basis of recent statistics, one of two men and one of three women in the United States will develop some type of cancer during their lifetime. Each year nearly 600,000 Americans die from cancer. Despite the dismal statistics, the news about cancer is not all bad. Many cancers *are* preventable if people adopt healthy lifestyles. Avoiding cigarette smoke and tobacco in *any* form is the most important action anyone can take to prevent cancer, especially lung and pancreatic cancers, which are most often incurable. Cigarette smoke is estimated to be the primary cause in the development of at least 30% of all cancers. Overweight and obesity, low levels of physical activity, and poor nutrition also increase the risk of cancer.

> Pain has an element of blank:
> it cannot recollect
> when it began, or if
> there were a day when
> it was not.
>
> *Emily Dickinson*

A healthy diet that includes low levels of beef and high levels of fresh fruits, vegetables, and fiber will markedly reduce the risk of cancer. Avoiding excess exposure to ultraviolet (UV) radiation in sunshine and tanning booths is essential to lessen the risk of skin cancer later in life. Finally, knowing what chemicals in the environment are cancer-causing can help you avoid dangerous substances. Overall, if everything known about cancer prevention were practiced by everyone, up to two-thirds of *all* cancers could be prevented.

Another positive note is that about half of all cancer patients can be cured if their cancer is detected at an early stage before cancer cells have spread. Being "cured" of cancer means that a person's life expectancy is the same as for a person who never had cancer. It is important to have cancer screening tests as indicated for your age and risk group (**Table 13.1**). You should also watch for early warning signs in functions of the body that may indicate that a cancer is developing.

Understanding Cancer

Incidence of Various Cancers

The annual number of new cases of cancer at various body sites is shown in **Figure 13.1**. Although the incidence of some cancers has decreased somewhat since 2000, the incidence of other cancers, such as non-Hodgkin lymphoma and melanoma, has increased. Thus, overall, cancer rates have not changed much since the 1980s, despite the introduction of sophisticated medical screening methods. That the incidence of cancer has not changed suggests that medical science and society at large must turn more attention to prevention if cancer rates are to decline significantly.

What Is Cancer?

The term *cancer* comes from the Latin word meaning "crab." Cancer was characterized as a crablike disease by the Greek physician Hippocrates, who observed that cancers spread throughout the body, eventually cutting off life. Now **cancer** generally is defined as the unregulated

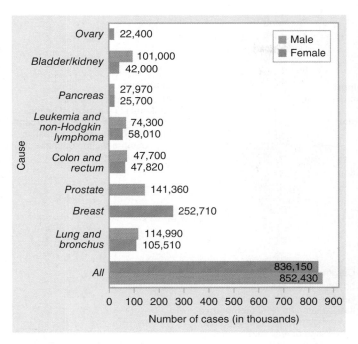

■ Figure 13.1

Estimated Number of New Cancer Cases, United States, 2017
Data from American Cancer Society. (2017). *Cancer facts and figures*, 2017. Retrieved from http://www.cancer.org/research/cancer-facts-statistics/all-cancer-facts-figures/cancer-facts-figures-2017.html

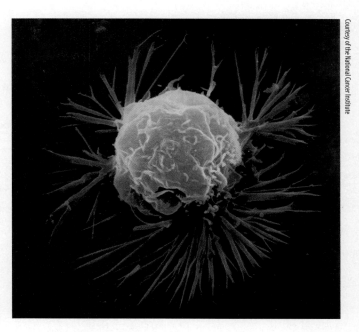

Electron micrograph of a breast cancer cell.

multiplication of specific cells in the body. The word *cancer* actually refers to more than 200 different diseases, but in all cases, certain body cells multiply in an abnormal, unregulated manner.

Normally, the growth and reproduction of every cell in the body are regulated; this regulation, in turn, determines the size and functions of tissues and organs. If a normal body cell begins to grow abnormally and reproduces too rapidly, a mass of abnormal cells eventually develops what is called a **tumor**. A tumor usually contains millions of abnormal cells before it can be detected or diagnosed.

If the cells of the tumor remain localized at the site of origin in the body and if they multiply relatively slowly, the tumor is said to be benign. **Benign tumors**, such as cysts, warts, moles, and polyps, do not spread to other parts of the body. Benign tumors usually can be removed and generally are not a threat to life; in fact, a benign tumor weighing several hundred pounds was surgically removed from a woman who recovered fully. Benign tumors cannot regrow if all of the abnormal cells are removed by surgical excision of the tumor.

Malignant tumors are composed of cells that multiply rapidly, have other abnormal properties that distinguish them from normal cells, and invade other normal tissues. In particular, malignant cells may have altered shapes and cell-surface characteristics that contribute to their rapid proliferation. Many malignant cells also have abnormal chromosomes or altered

genes, and they manufacture abnormal proteins. The numerous altered properties of malignant cells enable a **pathologist**, a physician who specializes in the causes of diseases, to determine whether the cells removed from a tumor are malignant and to what degree, a process called "staging" the tumor.

The cells of most malignant tumors also undergo **metastasis**, a process in which cells detach from the original tumor, enter the lymphatic system and bloodstream, and are carried to other organs. Once the malignant cells spread to other organs, they develop into new tumors that often grow more rapidly than cells in the original tumor. Metastases and the growth of new tumors in many organs of the body eventually disrupt a vital body function, which is the cause of death.

Cancers are medically classified according to the organ or kind of tissue in which the tumor originates. The four major categories of cancers are *carcinomas*,

> **TERMS**
>
> benign tumors: tumors whose cells do not spread to other parts of the body
>
> cancer: unregulated multiplication of cells in the body
>
> malignant tumors: tumors whose cells spread throughout the body
>
> metastasis: the process by which cancer cells spread throughout the body
>
> pathologist: a physician who specializes in the causes of diseases
>
> tumor: a mass of abnormal cells

■ **Figure 13.2**

Four Major Categories of Cancers and Approximate Frequencies of Occurrence

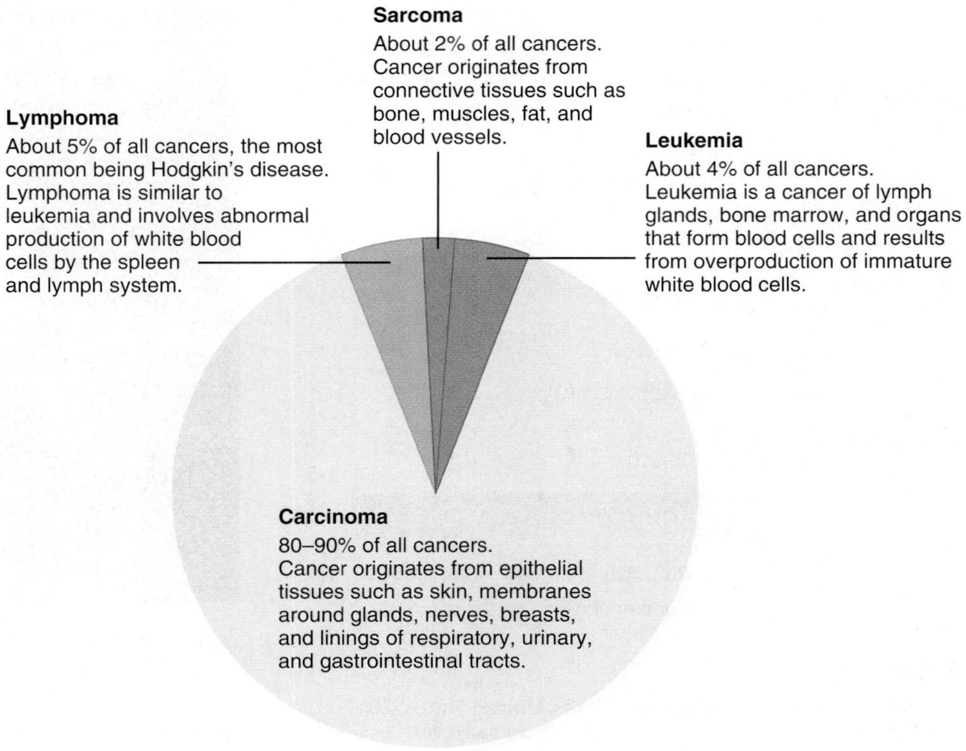

Sarcoma
About 2% of all cancers. Cancer originates from connective tissues such as bone, muscles, fat, and blood vessels.

Lymphoma
About 5% of all cancers, the most common being Hodgkin's disease. Lymphoma is similar to leukemia and involves abnormal production of white blood cells by the spleen and lymph system.

Leukemia
About 4% of all cancers. Leukemia is a cancer of lymph glands, bone marrow, and organs that form blood cells and results from overproduction of immature white blood cells.

Carcinoma
80–90% of all cancers. Cancer originates from epithelial tissues such as skin, membranes around glands, nerves, breasts, and linings of respiratory, urinary, and gastrointestinal tracts.

sarcomas, leukemias, and *lymphomas* (**Figure 13.2**). Within these major categories are numerous subgroups that generally describe the organ in which the cancer originates, such as adenocarcinoma of the stomach or small cell carcinoma of the lung. About half of all human cancers originate in one of four organs: the lung, breast, prostate, or colon, which is why so much research is devoted to these particular forms.

Cancer does not develop all at once in a cell. Several changes must occur in the genetic information (i.e., DNA) carried in a single cell before it can become a cancer cell and multiply into a tumor. Cells change their abnormal growth properties one step at a time; each genetic change pushes the cell further along the spectrum of abnormal growth. Not all cells acquire the same genetic changes, nor can anyone predict when the changes will occur. That explains why some cancers develop and grow rapidly and cause death in months, whereas other cancers grow so slowly that the person eventually dies from a cause other than cancer.

Once a tumor has been detected, cells can be removed from it in a procedure called a **biopsy**; the cells are then examined under the microscope by a pathologist. In stage I, cancer cells can be distinguished from normal cells. The cancer cells are still localized (usually referred to as cancer *in situ*) and removal of the tumor usually results in a cure. In stage II, the cancer cells have begun to metastasize and may have migrated to nearby lymph nodes. That is why lymph nodes near the tumor are removed and examined to determine whether cancer

cells have spread. By stage III, the cancer cells have spread throughout the body, and tumors may have begun to grow in other organs. In stage IV, tumors are found throughout the body and often are resistant to treatment.

The number of deaths from cancer by organ and by sex are shown in **Figure 13.3**. Lung cancer is now the leading cause of death in both women and men. Cancer of the colon and rectum, the third leading cause of death for both men and women, is believed to be strongly associated with fat-rich diets, low fiber, and overweight and obesity.

Causes of Cancer

Most Cancers Are Not Inherited

Many people live in fear of cancer, often because one or more closely related family members have died from some type of cancer. They may believe that cancer is passed on in the genes or that, at least, the susceptibility to cancer is inherited. Neither of these beliefs is correct for the vast majority of cancers. However, a persistent fear of developing cancer can generate stress that may weaken the immune system and contribute to the development of disease, including cancer.

Scientific studies indicate that 90% to 95% of *all* cancers, including breast, lung, stomach, colon, skin, or prostate, are *not* inherited from parents except in a few rare families in which members do inherit one or more cancer susceptibility genes.

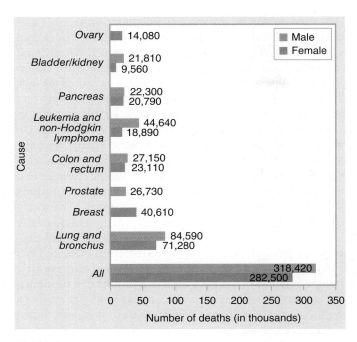

■ Figure 13.3

Estimated Deaths from Common Cancers, United States, 2017
Data from American Cancer Society. (2017). *Cancer Facts and Figures*, 2017. Retrieved from http://www.cancer.org/research/cancer-facts-statistics/all-cancer-facts-figures/cancer-facts-figures-2017.html

Confusion about genes often stems from misunderstanding the meanings of the words "genetic" and "inherited." The two are not synonymous. All of your cells (except for red blood cells) contain exact copies of the chromosomes and genes that were in the fertilized egg from which you developed. The genes in the chromosomes of any cell of your body, such as skin, lung, or stomach cells, can be chemically changed by environmental agents such as chemicals and radiation. These genetic changes in skin, lung, or stomach cells may transform them into cancer cells. Thus, cancer is a genetic disease in that genes are changed in a person's body cells; however, it is *not* an inherited disease because defective genes are not usually passed on from parents. Thus, a parent who acquires cancer cannot pass it on to his or her child.

Even if several close family members have died of cancer, it does not mean that cancer "runs in the family" and is an inherited disease. Currently, about 1 of every 4 deaths each year in the United States is due to cancer. If your grandparents and 8 aunts or uncles have died, probably 2 or 3 of them died of cancer simply by chance. If they all smoked cigarettes, it would not be surprising if more than 3 of 10 close relatives died of cancer.

One of the best pieces of evidence showing that most cancers are *not* inherited comes from a study of World War II veterans. The health of 15,000 pairs of identical or nonidentical (fraternal) twin brothers was followed for many years after World War II. No difference was observed in the different twin pairs in the development of cancer. That is, if one identical twin contracted cancer, the other identical twin was no more likely to get cancer than the average person.

Because identical twins share identical genes (i.e., they are natural clones that developed from the same fertilized egg that split into separate embryos), they should carry identical cancer-causing genes. The fact that identical twins do not *both* develop cancer at significantly higher rates than the average person means that most cancers are *not* caused by inherited genes. For most people, lifestyle (e.g., diet, weight, smoking, drinking alcohol) plays a far greater role in causing cancer than any genes that are passed on from parents.

Cancer Susceptibility Genes

Although only a small fraction (estimates range between 5% and 10%) of all cancers are strongly influenced by heredity, some families do transmit cancer susceptibility genes to children. A **cancer susceptibility gene** does not cause cancer directly; however, it makes a person carrying such a gene more vulnerable to environmental factors that contribute to the risk of developing cancer.

Cancer susceptibility genes show a small statistical association with cancer development in a large population of patients with cancer. However, they do not specifically cause cancer. It is thought that most cancer susceptibility genes have little effect in the vast majority of people, although some play significant roles in the development of specific cancers, most notably breast cancer. *BRCA1* and *BRCA2* genes are susceptibility genes for breast or ovarian cancer; *APC*, *MSH2*, and *MLH1*, for colorectal cancer. People who carry these abnormal genes are at higher risk for certain cancers compared to people without these genes.

A large-scale effort is currently underway in research laboratories worldwide to evaluate and understand all genes that are causally related to the development of cancer in people. As of 2016, 29 cancer-causing genes had been identified that play a direct role in the development of a human cancer. These cancer-causing genes are different from the hundreds of cancer susceptibility genes described previously, and are relatively rare compared to cancer susceptibility genes (**Table 13.2**).

Many genes that increase the risk of colorectal cancer have been identified, and some of their biological functions in cells also are understood (**Figure 13.4**). If a person inherits an abnormal form of any one of three

TERMS

biopsy: removal of cells from a tumor for examination under a microscope

cancer susceptibility gene: gene responsible for familial breast cancer and genes that cause susceptibility to colorectal cancer; increases the risk of a person developing cancer in his or her lifetime

Table 13.2

Cancer Susceptibility Genes

Abnormalities (mutations) in these genes can be inherited. Each abnormal gene may contribute to the development of cancer in a specific organ.

Gene	Organ affected
Breast cancer	
BRCA1	Breast, ovary
BRCA2	Breast
p53	Breast, brain
Colorectal cancer	
MSH2	Colon, uterus
MLH1	Colon, uterus
PMS1, PMS2	Colon, other
APC	Colon
Melanoma	
MTS1 (CDKN2)	Skin, pancreas
CDK4	Skin
Prostate cancer	
HPC1	Prostate
MSR1	Prostate
AR	Prostate
CYP1	Prostate
SRD5A2	Prostate

suppose a person inherited an *MSH2* mutation and 20 years later a colon cell acquired an *APC* mutation. Those two mutations make that colon cell begin to reproduce itself at a faster rate; at some point, one cell among the faster-growing ones acquires a third mutation in either a *K-ras*, *DDC*, or *p53* gene. That cell now has three mutations and may develop into cancer of the colon. Along the way to tumor formation, other mutations also may occur. On average, when colon cancer cells are examined, they have at least three of the mutations described in Figure 13.4. Now you can understand why chance genetic changes and exposure to environmental agents that cause mutations play such important roles in the development of cancer.

We now understand that every cancer is biologically unique, which is the reason that many hospitals and clinics offer personalized cancer treatments. With today's techniques for rapid sequencing of DNA, the specific abnormal genes in a cancer patient's tumors can be identified and treatments tailored for precise biological targets. For those cancer patients who can afford it, personalized cancer treatments may be of significant benefit. The most effective and least harmful treatment for a specific kind of tumor may be identified by personalized tests. In addition to more targeted and safer chemotherapy, a variety of revolutionary immunotherapy treatments are becoming available to treat even advanced cases of some cancers.

genes, *APC*, *MSH2*, or *MLH1*, the risk of colorectal cancer is increased. However, fewer than 5% of all colorectal cancer patients inherit any of these colorectal cancer susceptibility genes.

During a person's lifetime, mutations continue to arise and accumulate in cells lining the colon. For example,

Environmental Factors That Cause Cancer

The causes of cancer or, more correctly, the risk factors associated with the development of cancer are numerous and complex. It often is difficult to point to a single cause of a cancer, but certain environmental factors

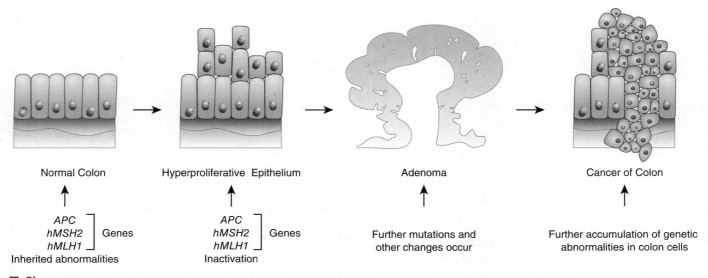

Normal Colon	Hyperproliferative Epithelium	Adenoma	Cancer of Colon
APC hMSH2 hMLH1] Genes Inherited abnormalities	APC hMSH2 hMLH1] Genes Inactivation	Further mutations and other changes occur	Further accumulation of genetic abnormalities in colon cells

■ **Figure 13.4**

Mutant Genes Contribute to Development of Cancer Cells

Changes in several genes can lead to increased risk of colorectal cancer. Abnormalities in *APC*, *MSH2*, or *MLH1* genes can be inherited from parents. Other changes may occur in genes of colon cells during the course of a person's life before development of a cancer. Examination of colorectal cancer cells indicates that most of them have accumulated several genetic changes, either inherited or acquired.

Table 13.3

Environmental and Lifestyle Risk Factors That Contribute to Cancer

Factor	Amount of risk	Types of cancer
Nutrition	About *half* of cancer deaths are caused by nutritional problems: Excess calories Excess fat consumption Obesity Nutritional deficiencies, especially fiber and vitamin A	Cancers of the colon, rectum, stomach, breast, and ovaries
Cigarettes and alcohol	About *one-third* of cancer deaths are caused by smoking cigarettes and excessive alcohol consumption	Cancers of the lung, pancreas, mouth, larynx, liver, esophagus, and bladder
Occupation	About 5% of cancer deaths are caused by substances in the workplace, such as asbestos, benzene, and vinyl chloride	Cancers of the bladder, lung, stomach, blood, liver, bones, and skin
Radiation	About 3% of cancer deaths are caused by ionizing radiation, such as x-rays and ultraviolet light	Blood, skin
Other	Other cancer deaths result from heredity, chronic disease, drugs, and infections	Various cancers

are strongly correlated with the occurrence of particular cancers. Two examples are the strong correlation between cigarette smoking and lung cancer and exposure to ultraviolet light and skin cancer. Even in these examples, not everyone who smokes heavily or stays in the sun day after day will get lung or skin cancer.

Epidemiology is the branch of science that investigates the causes and frequencies of diseases in human populations. Many epidemiological studies show that as many as 80% to 90% of all cancers are caused by exposure to environmental agents that are known to increase the risk of cancer (**Table 13.3**). For example, smoking cigarettes while young puts a person at 10 to 20 times higher risk of developing cancer later in life than persons who do not smoke. Eating fat-laden fast food frequently may be convenient, but it is ultimately unhealthy and may contribute to the development of certain cancers. Because each of us can change our diets, stop smoking, and avoid other cancer-causing risks in the environment, preventing cancer is a realistic and attainable goal.

Three classes of environmental agents—ionizing radiation, infectious microorganisms (viruses and bacteria), and cancer-causing chemicals (carcinogens)—have been shown to increase the risk of cancer in both laboratory animals and people. Each of these agents increases the risk of cancer by producing chemical changes (**mutations**)

in genes in any cell in the body and causing it to multiply abnormally. If a cell undergoes one or more mutations in genes that regulate its growth, it may begin to multiply rapidly and develop into a tumor. Environmental factors cause mutations and also affect the rate of abnormal cell growth (**Figure 13.5**).

Ionizing Radiation

Ionizing radiation consists of x-rays, ultraviolet (UV) light, and radioactivity whose energy can damage cells and chromosomes. The high rate of leukemia among survivors of the Hiroshima and Nagasaki atomic bomb

TERMS

epidemiology: a branch of science that studies the causes and frequencies of diseases in human populations

ionizing radiation: radiation, such as x-rays, that can damage cells and cause cancer; also used to treat cancer

mutations: permanent changes in the genetic information in a cell; only mutations in sperm and eggs are inherited

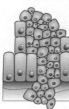

Factors that change genes in cells	Tumor	Factors that promote growth of genetically abnormal cells
Ionizing radiation Infectious microorganisms (viruses and bacteria) Carcinogenic chemicals		Hormones Nutritional deficiencies Reduced immune system Aging Immunosuppressive drugs

■ **Figure 13.5**

Environmental Factors That Cause Cancer

Environmental factors change both genes and the growth properties of cells that may lead to the development of cancer.

blasts in 1945 leaves no doubt that radioactivity increases the risk of cancer.

In the United States, among children born in southern Utah in the 1950s who were exposed to radioactive fall-out from nearby tests of atomic bombs, the number of leukemia deaths was two to three times greater than among children born in southern Utah before and after the atomic tests. In a landmark legal decision in 1984, a federal court ruled that the U.S. government was negligent in conducting atomic bomb tests in southern Utah in the 1950s because the tests released radioactive material into the atmosphere. The court ruled that the families who were exposed to radioactivity as a result of these tests, and whose members died as a result of exposure to the radioactivity, were entitled to compensation.

The nuclear reactor accident at Chernobyl in Ukraine in 1986 also released large amounts of radioactivity, particularly radioactive iodine, strontium, and cesium, into the atmosphere. Not only was the region around the reactor affected but radioactive fallout occurred over much of Europe. In some countries, milk and crops were so contaminated that they had to be destroyed. Some of the radioactivity was detected in countries as distant as the United States and Japan.

In 2011, a catastrophic earthquake and tsunami caused major damage to several nuclear power plants in Fukushima, Japan. Considerable amounts of radioactivity were released over several weeks that resulted in the evacuation of thousands of people from the area because it was thought to be unsafe. It is evident that living near nuclear power plants, especially ones at risk from earthquakes or floods, has become a major health concern for people around the world. Germany and Switzerland have decided to phase out all nuclear power plants.

The most common source of ionizing radiation in nature is ultraviolet (UV) radiation in sunlight. Because children and young people spend long hours in the sun, people acquire as much as 80% of their lifetime UV exposure by age 20.

Ultraviolet radiation in sunlight is characterized by two different wavelengths, called UVA and UVB. Until recently, it was thought that only UVB was dangerous, but now it appears that both forms of UV radiation are harmful. Reducing the time of exposure to intense sunlight and using sunscreen creams to protect exposed areas of the body reduce the risk of skin cancer.

In recent years, there has been a growing concern over increased risk of developing cancer from diagnostic medical imaging, especially CT (computerized tomography) scans (McCollough, et al., 2015). The use of CT scans has skyrocketed in the past decade, especially in asymptomatic patients to rule out the possibility of any disease. One thing driving the rapid rise in the use of CT scans is the cost of the scanning machines. Hospitals need to perform many CT scans to pay for the expensive machines, which encourages physicians to order CT scans even for conditions that previously were easily diagnosed without them.

The amount of ionizing radiation received by a patient undergoing a CT scan varies greatly depending on the area of the body being imaged. It is helpful to understand the dose of radiation received if it is expressed in terms of the average background radiation to which we are all exposed. A chest CT scan requires the equivalent of 2 years' worth of natural background radiation; a CT scan of the head uses about 8 months' worth of background radiation (Lin, 2010). If a person receives several CT scans for a variety of medical conditions, the overall radiation dose is quite high and increases the risk of cancer. The annual number of CT scans performed in the United States is estimated at 80 million and is increasing by 10% each year (Brenner & Hricak, 2010). Of particular concern is the growing use of CT scans on children. A child's cells are still growing and reproducing and are at greater risk from exposure to radiation than are adult cells; thus, they are at greater risk of developing cancer later in life.

Patients need to be aware of the perils of unnecessary CT and other x-ray scans recommended for themselves and their children. Discuss with your physician the rationale for any recommended imaging procedure and ask if it is crucial to the diagnosis. Of course, in emergency situations, imaging procedures are essential to know how to best help the patient. To become better informed about medical imaging technologies and cancer risk, go to www.xrayrisk.com.

Infectious Microorganisms

In 1911, Peyton Rous, a scientist working at the Rockefeller Institute in New York, showed that cancer could be produced in chickens by injecting them with a virus isolated from chicken tumors. Since then, other viruses, called **tumor viruses**, have been found in animals such as mice, cats, and monkeys.

A few viruses are associated with an increased risk of cancer in humans. They are hepatitis B and C viruses (liver cancer), papillomavirus (genital and cervical cancer), human T-cell leukemia-lymphoma virus (leukemia and lymphoma), and Epstein-Barr virus (cancer of the nose or pharynx). Infection by HIV, the virus that causes AIDS, is associated with the development of a particular cancer called Kaposi's sarcoma. And a bacterium that is found in the stomach and causes ulcers (*Helicobacter pylori*) is associated with an increased risk of gastric cancer, one form of lymphoma, and possibly pancreatic cancer.

Chemical Carcinogens

A **chemical carcinogen** is an environmental substance that can interact with cells to initiate cancer, usually by chemically altering the chromosomes or genes in cells. Genes are responsible for manufacturing the enzymes and other proteins a cell needs to function properly. An altered gene usually makes an abnormal protein that may change the growth properties of a cell and cause it to become a cancer cell.

Table 13.4

Examples of Occupational Cancers

Chemical/physical agent	Cancer type	Exposure of general population	Examples of workers frequently exposed or exposure sources
Arsenic	Lung, skin	Rare	Insecticide and herbicide sprayers; tanners; oil refinery workers
Asbestos	Mesothelioma, lung	Uncommon	Brake-lining, shipyard, insulation, and demolition workers
Benzene	Myelogenous leukemia	Common	Painters; distillers and petrochemical workers; dye users; furniture finishers; rubber workers
Diesel exhaust	Lung	Common	Railroad and bus-garage workers; truck operators; miners
Formaldehyde	Nose, nasopharynx	Rare	Hospital and laboratory workers; manufacture of wood products, paper, textiles, garments, and metal products
Hair dyes	Bladder	Uncommon	Hairdressers and barbers (inadequate evidence for customers)
Ionizing radiation	Bone marrow, several others	Common	Nuclear materials; medicinal products and procedures
Mineral oils	Skin	Common	Metal machining
Nonarsenic pesticides	Lung	Common	Sprayers; agricultural workers
Painting materials	Lung	Uncommon	Professional painters
Polychlorinated biphenyls	Liver, skin	Uncommon	Heat-transfer and hydraulic fluids and lubricants; inks; adhesives; insecticides
Radon (alpha particles)	Lung	Uncommon	Mines; underground structures; homes
Soot	Skin	Uncommon	Chimney sweeps and cleaners; bricklayers; insulators; firefighters; heating-unit service workers
Synthetic mineral fibers	Lung	Uncommon	Wall and pipe insulation; duct wrapping

Some industrial and agricultural chemicals are tested to determine their cancer-causing potential. Unfortunately, many thousands more chemical substances already in use have not been adequately tested. Of the thousands of chemical substances that have been tested, many have been found to be carcinogenic and should be avoided if at all possible. Carcinogens include cigarette smoke, pesticides, asbestos, heavy metals (lead, mercury, cadmium), benzene, and nitrosamines.

Despite the long list of carcinogenic substances, some scientists and public health officials argue that tobacco is the only substance of consequence with respect to the numbers of cancers caused. Although the argument has some basis, it is of small consolation to persons who acquire cancer from exposure, often without their knowledge, to carcinogenic substances in the environment or workplace (**Table 13.4**).

In some industries, workers have cancers that almost never arise in the general population. For example, **mesothelioma** is a rare form of lung cancer that only occurs among persons exposed to asbestos fibers. Long-term exposure to the heavy metals beryllium and cadmium increases workers' risk of prostate cancer. Workers exposed to vinyl chloride, the starting material for polyvinyl chloride (PVC) pipes and other products, develop a rare form of liver cancer not found in the general population. Fortunately, with current occupational and safety regulations, these types of occupational cancers occur infrequently.

The total number of cancers attributable to industrial chemicals is small compared with those caused by tobacco and diet; however, cancers caused by industrial chemicals are preventable or avoidable. Before you accept a job it might be wise to determine what chemicals you will be exposed to for long periods.

Do Xenoestrogens Cause Cancer?

Estrogens are hormones that regulate a variety of biological functions in women, including the growth and development of breast tissue. Many chemicals that we are exposed to in the environment mimic the action of normal estrogen to some degree; such chemicals are called **xenoestrogens** (literally, foreign estrogens).

Substances that contain xenoestrogens include the pesticides DDT (banned in the United States but still used elsewhere), methoxyclor, kepone, chlordane, atrazine, and endosulfan. Polychlorinated biphenyls (PCBs), which were used in electrical transformers for many years, also

TERMS

chemical carcinogen: a chemical that damages cells and causes cancer

mesothelioma: a form of lung cancer caused by asbestos

tumor viruses: viruses that infect cells, change their growth properties, and cause cancer

xenoestrogens: environmental chemicals that mimic the effects of natural estrogen; may cause cancer

are xenoestrogens. Bisphenol-A, a component of polycarbonate plastics that are widely used in water bottles, baby bottles, food cans, and many other plastics, also is a xenoestrogen.

Considerable evidence points to environmental xenoestrogens as agents in the development of some cancers, particularly breast cancer. In the 1960s and 1970s, Israel had one of the highest incidences of breast cancer in the world. In 1976, Israel banned all chlorinated pesticides and made it illegal for milk products to have any detectable pesticide residues. In the years following the pesticide ban, rates of breast cancer declined dramatically. These findings support the theory that pesticides acting as xenoestrogens are a major contributor to breast cancer.

It is impossible to avoid all exposure to xenoestrogens because they are everywhere in the environment. Eating broccoli, cabbage, and soy products may help counteract the effects of xenoestrogens. This advice comes from the observation that Asian women have much lower rates of breast cancer in comparison with Caucasian or African American women. Asian diets are richer in these vegetables, which may contain chemicals that block the biological activities of the xenoestrogens.

Facts About Common Cancers

Lung Cancer

Lung cancer is the deadliest of all cancers worldwide. In the United States, lung cancer is the number one cause of cancer deaths for both men and women. About 225,000 new lung and bronchus cancers are diagnosed in the United States every year, which accounts for about 13% of all cancers. More women die each year from lung cancer than from breast cancer. Smoking cigarettes is the primary cause of nearly 90% of all lung cancers.

The survival rate of lung cancer patients is dismal; among all patients, after being diagnosed only 7% live another 5 years. Medical costs of treating lung cancer are about $40 billion annually, making it the costliest of all cancers.

The risk of lung cancer varies significantly among ethnic and racial groups. African Americans and native Hawaiians are at highest risk, especially at lower levels of cigarette smoking (less than a pack a day). White Americans, Japanese Americans, and Latinos are about half as likely to get lung cancer as the other two groups at comparable levels of smoking. The reasons for racial and ethnic differences are not clear but may have to do with inherited lung cancer susceptibility genes that vary among groups of people.

The rate of lung cancer in other nations is rising rapidly as more and more people take up cigarette smoking. Women in developing countries begin to smoke at early ages to appear sophisticated and because of peer pressure. International efforts are under way to reduce smoking around the world among young people, especially among young girls. China and other developing nations will have to cope with epidemics of lung cancer soon. The concerted effort in the United States to get people to stop smoking and to prevent access of young people to cigarettes is an attempt to reverse the epidemic of lung cancer in this country.

Breast Cancer

Both men and women can develop breast cancer, but it occurs very rarely among men. Although more women die from lung cancer than breast cancer, more than twice as many women contract breast cancer.

Increased weight, lack of exercise, and alcohol consumption contribute to an increased risk of breast cancer. Research does not support the view that the amount of fat in the diet increases the risk of breast cancer. Other factors that increase the risk of breast cancer among women to varying degrees are the following:

- Mother who had breast cancer before age 60
- First menstruation before age 14
- First child born after age 30
- No biological children
- Menopause after age 55
- Benign breast disease
- Estrogen replacement therapy after age 55
- Consuming more than 3 ounces of alcohol a day
- Inheritance of *BRCA1*, *BRCA2*, and other susceptibility genes
- Exposure to xenoestrogens

The Controversy over Mammograms A mammogram is an x-ray image of the breasts that is used to detect the presence of any abnormal breast tissue. For years it was recommended that all women over 40 years of age get mammograms to help detect an abnormal growth that might indicate development of breast cancer. But there has been ongoing scientific controversy over whether women who are not at high risk for breast cancer should be getting yearly mammograms at a relatively young age. In 2008, the controversy intensified when the U.S.

Abortion Does *Not* Increase Risk of Breast Cancer

In 2002, the National Cancer Institute (NCI) website announced that scientists had found no association between abortion and subsequent risk of breast cancer. Some members of Congress raised a hue and cry, and the information was removed from the NCI website.

NCI then assembled more than a hundred scientific experts from various fields to review the data. Only one member disagreed with the otherwise unanimous conclusion: "There is no association between abortion and the risk of breast cancer" (Couzin, 2003).

Breast Cancer and Mastectomy

A diagnosis of breast cancer is devastating news for any woman, but it is especially difficult for younger women who may not have decided yet about motherhood and nursing. Treatments for breast cancer have increased the likelihood of a cure but still usually require removal of part or all of the affected breast. Then there is the question of what to do about the healthy breast. Because the risk of developing cancer eventually in the healthy breast is significantly increased, many younger women elect to have both breasts removed even though one is healthy.

In 2012, one out of three women younger than age 45 elected to remove both breasts even though only one had cancer. This number is up dramatically from earlier years when the ratio was 1 woman in 10. Why are so many young women choosing to have a bilateral mastectomy when cancer is present only in one breast? More puzzling is the fact that half the women making the choice to remove both breasts live in five states—Colorado, Iowa, Missouri, Nebraska, and South Dakota. No explanation has been found for this clustering. Many women cite the reason for their decision as not having to worry about the return of breast cancer later in life. But these women may not be making the best decision.

At present, no evidence suggest that the removal of a healthy breast has any effect on longevity. Several medical organizations, including the Society of Breast Surgeons and the Board of Internal Medicine, recommend not removing a healthy breast unless certain genetic factors are present. Two genes, *BRCA1* and *BRCA2*, increase the risk of breast cancer. If a woman with one or both of these genes is diagnosed with breast cancer, it usually is recommended that a double mastectomy be performed even if one breast is unaffected. But ways to silence these genes or counteract their effects with drugs are currently under investigation. Younger women who are diagnosed with breast cancer should carefully evaluate all the information before electing to have a healthy breast removed.

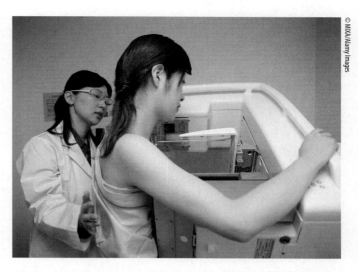

Mammograms can detect breast cancer at an early stage and improve chances for successful treatment.

preventive benefits of routine mammograms are modest (Welch, 2010). Mammograms turn up many breast abnormalities that are not cancer. These false positives subject women to additional medical procedures that are costly, worrisome, and sometimes harmful. Often surgical biopsies are performed that are unnecessary and that leave the breast disfigured. Thus, it seems prudent for all women, particularly those at low risk, to evaluate their own concerns and needs with the help of a knowledgeable health professional. Despite the controversy, the American Cancer Society still recommends that all women 40 to 50 years of age get a mammogram every 1 to 2 years.

Lifestyle Changes Help Prevent Breast Cancer Among women in industrialized countries, the lifetime risk of developing breast cancer is about 10%, and breast cancer remains a leading cause of death among women in these countries. In the United States, breast cancer is diagnosed in about 200,000 women each year; about 40,000 women die annually. The incidence of breast cancer among African American women is higher than for white American woman. Also, breast cancer deaths among African American women are higher than for white women. For women with *BRCA1* or *BRCA2* mutations, the lifetime risk of breast cancer is as high as 80% to 90%—considerably higher.

Living healthfully—for example, maintaining a normal body weight—is effective in reducing a woman's risk of breast and other cancers. Other ways that help prevent breast cancer include maintaining a low-fat diet,

Preventive Services Task Force released new guidelines that recommended against routine mammograms for women between the ages of 40 and 50 (Woolf, 2010). The American Cancer Society and many women's groups strongly opposed the recommendation. The controversy mainly revolved around the word "routine." The task force did not say that women under age 50 should not get mammograms; the task force recommended that women under 50 should decide, in consultation with their physicians, whether or not a mammogram was helpful. The task force said that routinely screening every woman under 50 years of age was not a useful public health policy. One fact that was mostly lost in the debate was that the majority of breast cancers detected early were the result of periodic breast exams that women performed themselves.

More than a half century of using mammograms and dozens of comprehensive studies indicate that the

TERMS

mammogram: x-ray picture used to detect tumors in the breast

Breast Self-Examination

Breast self-examination (BSE) should be done once a month so you become familiar with the usual appearance and feel of your breasts. Familiarity makes it easier to notice any changes in the breast from month to month. Early discovery of a change from what is "normal" is the main idea behind BSE. The outlook is much better if you detect cancer in an early stage. If you menstruate, the best time to do BSE is 2 or 3 days after your period ends, when your breasts are least likely to be tender or swollen. If you no longer menstruate, pick a day such as the first day of the month, to remind yourself it is time to do BSE. Here is one way to do BSE:

1. Stand before a mirror. Inspect both breasts for anything unusual such as any discharge from the nipples or puckering, dimpling, or scaling of the skin.

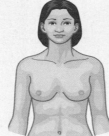

The next two steps are designed to emphasize any change in the shape or contour of your breasts. As you do them, you should be able to feel your chest muscles tighten.

2. Watching closely in the mirror, clasp your hands behind your head and press your hands forward.

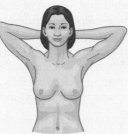

3. Next, press your hands firmly on your hips and bow slightly toward your mirror as you pull your shoulders and elbows forward.

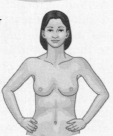

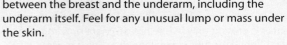
Some women do the next part of the exam in the shower because fingers glide over soapy skin, making it easy to concentrate on the texture underneath.

4. Raise your left arm. Use three or four fingers of your right hand to explore your left breast firmly, carefully, and thoroughly. Beginning at the outer edge, press the flat part of your fingers in small circles, moving the circles slowly around the breast. Gradually work toward the nipple. Be sure to cover the entire breast. Pay special attention to the area between the breast and the underarm, including the underarm itself. Feel for any unusual lump or mass under the skin.

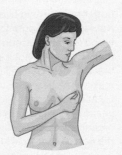

5. Gently squeeze the nipple and look for discharge. (If you have any discharge during the month—whether or not it is during BSE—see your doctor.) Repeat steps 4 and 5 on your right breast.

6. Steps 4 and 5 should be repeated lying down. Lie flat on your back with your left arm over your head and a pillow or folded towel under your left shoulder. This position flattens the breast and makes it easier to examine. Use the same circular motion described earlier. Repeat the exam on your right breast.

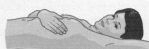

consuming adequate amounts of fresh fruits and vegetables, engaging in physical activity, and limiting alcohol consumption.

Women with a diagnosis of breast cancer can increase their chances of survival by engaging in physical activities such as walking briskly for 3 to 5 hours a week.

Treating Breast Cancer For too many years, surgical removal of one or both breasts along with underlying tissue—a procedure called a *radical mastectomy*—was the recommended treatment for women with a diagnosis of breast cancer. In recent years, a surgical procedure called a *lumpectomy*, in which only the tumor itself is removed, has been shown to be as effective as a mastectomy in terms of long-term survival among most women with early-stage breast cancer. However, if cancer cells were found in underarm lymph nodes, these also were removed, usually resulting in a painful, often complicated recovery. For more than a century, it had been assumed that if cancer cells were present in lymph

Testicular Cancer: Self-Exam

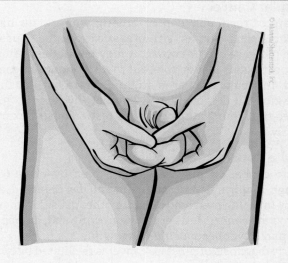

The testicles (also called testes or gonads) are located behind the penis in a pouch of skin called the scrotum. The testicles produce and store sperm, and they are also the body's main source of male hormones. These hormones control the development of the reproductive organs and other male characteristics, such as body and facial hair, low voice, and wide shoulders.

Testicular cancer is rare. It accounts for only about 1% of all cancers in American men. However, cancer of the testicle is the most common cancer in men 15 to 35 years old. Men who have an undescended testicle (a testicle that has never moved down into the scrotum) are at higher risk of developing cancer of the testicle than other men whose testicles have moved down into the scrotum. This is true even if surgery has been done to place the testicle in the appropriate place in the scrotum. The symptoms of testicular cancer include the following:

- A lump in either testicle
- Any enlargement of a testicle
- A feeling of heaviness in the scrotum
- A dull ache in the lower abdomen or the groin
- A sudden collection of fluid in the scrotum
- Pain or discomfort in a testicle or in the scrotum
- Enlargement or tenderness of the breasts

These symptoms are not sure signs of cancer. They can also be caused by other conditions. However, it is important to see a doctor if any of these symptoms lasts as long as 2 weeks. Any illness should be diagnosed and treated as soon as possible. Early diagnosis of testicular cancer is especially important because the sooner testicular cancer is found and treated, the better a man's chance for complete recovery.

Most testicular cancers are found by men themselves, by accident or when doing testicular self-examination (TSE). The testicles are smooth, oval-shaped, and rather firm. Men who examine themselves regularly become familiar with the way their testicles normally feel. Any changes in the way they feel from month to month should be reported to a doctor. Men can improve their chance of finding a tumor by performing a testicular self-examination once a month (see the accompanying figure). TSE should be performed after a warm bath or shower. The heat relaxes the scrotum, making it easier to find anything unusual. To perform a self-exam follow these suggestions:

- Stand in front of the mirror. Look for any swelling on the skin of the scrotum.
- Examine each testicle with both hands. The index and middle fingers should be placed under the testicle while the thumbs are placed on the top.
- Gently roll the testicle between the thumbs and fingers. It's normal for one testicle to be larger than the other.
- Find the epididymis (the soft, tubelike structure at the back of the testicle that collects and carries the sperm). Do not mistake the epididymis for an abnormal lump.
- If you find a lump, contact your doctor right away. Most lumps are found on the sides of the testicle, but some appear on the front. Remember that testicular cancer is highly curable, especially when treated promptly.

nodes, the cancer would spread to other parts of the body and survival would be reduced. But now, chemotherapy or radiation therapy are recognized as sufficient to prevent recurrence of the cancer.

New DNA tests also can help determine the optimal treatments for each woman's breast cancer. By determining the cancer cells' particular molecular markers, the chemotherapy regime most likely to succeed can be administered. However, some DNA tests that detect specific breast cancer genes can bring disheartening news. Women who have BRCA1 and/or BRCA2 genes have an exceptionally high risk of getting breast or ovarian cancer at an early age. These women have two poor options. They can get frequent tests and watch for early signs of cancer, or they can choose to preemptively remove their breasts and ovaries to increase the possibility of long-term survival.

Research supports the use of integrative therapies for specific clinical indications during and after breast cancer treatment (Greenlee et al., 2017). For example, music therapy, meditation, stress management, and yoga are recommended for reducing anxiety, stress, and depression and other mood disorders and improving overall quality of life. Acupressure and acupuncture are recommended for reducing chemotherapy-induced nausea and vomiting. No strong evidence supports the use of ingested dietary supplements to manage breast cancer treatment–related side effects.

Testicular Cancer

The rate of testicular cancer among young men has been increasing, but, as with breast cancer, the causes for the increase are unknown. It may be that exposure to xenoestrogens plays a role, but that has not been confirmed. Testicular cancer is still quite rare but usually can be cured if detected early. That is why it is recommended that young men perform a testicular self-exam regularly.

Prostate Cancer

Prostate cancer occurs primarily in men over age 65, although abnormal prostate cells can be detected at autopsy in young men who die from other causes. Generally, prostate cancers are very slow-growing and, in many cases, may never become life-threatening.

Early diagnosis of prostate cancer is facilitated by two tests. One is the finger rectal exam, in which a trained person can detect if the prostate is enlarged or otherwise feels abnormal. The **prostate-specific antigen (PSA) test** detects a protein in blood that is associated with abnormal growth of the prostate gland. A high PSA level may indicate prostate cancer but also occurs with many other noncancerous conditions. Only additional tests can confirm the meaning of a high PSA level in blood.

The primary risk factor for prostate cancer is being elderly; about 80% of cases and 90% of deaths occur in men over age 65. An estimated 25 million American men over age 50 have some detectable abnormal prostate cells; however, the vast majority never develop prostate cancer because most prostate cancers grow extremely slowly. Even among those who do, most eventually die from causes other than prostate cancer. Thus, the first question is whether it is worth screening for prostate cancer, and second, whether slow-growing prostate cancers should even be treated. Because the PSA test is a weak predictor of prostate cancer, recommendations regarding its use are controversial and have changed several times over recent years. The main problem with the PSA test is that it often indicates a man has prostate cancer when he does not, a false-positive result. This leads to further expensive, painful tests that can themselves cause problems. For most of this century, the PSA test was not recommended for men but was optional. In 2016, a panel of experts again recommended that physicians advise their patients to undergo PSA testing. As with any recommended test, patients should discuss their concerns with a trusted healthcare professional.

Skin Cancer

The skin (epidermis) consists of several layers and kinds of cells. The upper layer consists of flat squamous cells, and the bottom layer contains basal cells. Interspersed among the squamous and basal cells are melanocytes, cells that give skin its characteristic pigmentation. People with more melanocytes are less susceptible to skin cancer than are light-skinned people.

Exposure to sunlight is the primary cause of all forms of skin cancer. The degree of exposure to sunlight during childhood largely determines the risk of skin cancer later in life. Two factors contribute to the risk of skin cancers. First, sun bathing and booth-tanning. Second, the continuing depletion of the ozone layer, resulting in more ultraviolet (UV) radiation reaching the earth's surface; it is the UV radiation in sunlight that causes mutations in skin cells that may lead to cancer. To reduce the risk of skin cancer, you must reduce your exposure to sunlight.

Sunlight contains ultraviolet radiation (UVR) along with visible light that we detect with our eyes (UVR is invisible). UVR is an energetic form of radiation that can penetrate skin cells, damage DNA, and initiate genetic changes that may eventually develop into a skin cancer. The two most dangerous forms of ultraviolet radiation in sunlight are UVA and UVB. Sunlight consists of about 95% UVA and 5% UVB; tanning lamps emit mostly UVB.

The three kinds of skin cancer are **basal cell carcinoma**, **squamous cell carcinoma**, and **melanoma**. Each of the three kinds of skin cancer originate from different kinds of skin cells. In the United States, about 1 million cases of skin cancer are diagnosed every year; about 2.5 million cases are diagnosed annually

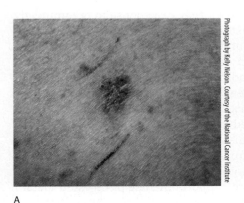
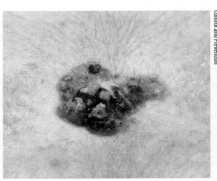
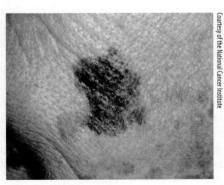

A

B

C

Any unusual growth on the skin should be checked by a health professional to determine whether it is a form of skin cancer. (a) Basal cell. (b) Squamous cell. (c) Melanoma.

What Do Indoor Tanning Lamps and Cigarettes Have in Common?

The answer to the question is that both cause cancers and premature death. Cigarettes are the primary cause of lung cancer, and tanning lamps cause skin cancers including melanomas. Tanning lamps and tanning beds of any kind cause more cancers overall than does cigarette smoking. Over the past several decades as tans have become a symbol of health and vitality, skin cancers caused by the ultraviolet light (UVB) from tanning lamps has soared. The principal component of sunlight that causes cancer is UVA, which has a wavelength of 180 to 240 nanometers. Another component of sunlight is UVB, which has a longer wavelength (250 to 280 nanometers) and is less energetic than UVA. Tanning lamps emit mostly UVB and were initially thought to be safe to use for individuals that wanted to acquire a tan. Many studies have shown that UVB radiation causes all forms of skin cancer in people and that tanning lamps are as dangerous to health as cigarettes.

Consider the following facts:

- More than half of the persons who use tanning lamps regularly will develop a basal cell carcinoma before age 40.
- Tanning lamps greatly increase the overall risk of melanoma, the most deadly form of skin cancer.
- Many states have passed laws banning persons younger than age 18 from tanning salons or from purchasing tanning lamps.
- Using tanning beds/lamps to increase vitamin D in the body is extremely dangerous.
- About 7.8 million women and 1.9 million men in the United States use tanning lamps.

Despite the proven cancer risks associated with indoor tanning devices, 59% of college students report using tanning lamps and 35% of all Americans use tanning lamps to some degree. The U. S. Department of Health and Human Services and the World Health Organization have both issued warnings about the use of artificial tanning devices. Despite all the warnings, tanning salons and tanning lamps/beds remain a multibillion-dollar business. Tanning lamps are like cigarettes; both cause cancer and death. Yet both industries are too powerful to be prevented from selling lethal products. To prevent skin cancers, do not use tanning lamps and use sunscreen or protective clothing whenever you are exposed to bright sunlight.

---

worldwide. Basal cell carcinoma and squamous cell carcinoma are usually not life-threatening, and the abnormal cells can be removed surgically or by freezing. Melanoma is a very dangerous form of skin cancer, and once it has spread the cancer is difficult to cure. About one death every hour in the United States is due to melanoma; the incidence of melanoma today is about 20 times greater than it was in the previous century, largely due to people increasing their exposure to sunlight and indoor tanning lamps/beds.

Medical treatment of melanoma includes surgical removal of the cancer in the early stages; chemotherapeutic drugs to stop the growth of cancer cells; radiation therapy, which uses high-energy x-rays or other types of radiation to kill cancer cells or keep them from growing; and immunotherapy, which uses patient's immune system to fight cancer.

Most Skin Cancers Are Preventable

The number of people in the United States with various types of skin cancer, especially melanoma, is increasing. This need not be since skin cancers are among the most preventable of all cancers. The primary cause of most skin cancers is excessive exposure to sunlight, and tanning lamps. The best way to prevent skin cancer caused by sunlight is to follow the **WAR** rule:

- **W**ear protective clothing.
- **A**void the sun between 10 A.M. and 3 P.M.

- **R**egularly apply sunscreen with an SPF greater than 15 when outdoors, even on cloudy days. Sunscreen should be reapplied every few hours, and more often if swimming or exercising.

Protecting children from sunburn and overexposure is especially important because it is the lifetime exposure to UV that is associated with skin cancers in later life. By age 65, about one American in two has had some form of skin cancer. The ozone layer in Earth's upper atmosphere filters out much of the sun's UV light; thinning of the ozone layer in recent years markedly increases the danger of overexposure to sunlight. Unless more people follow the WAR rule, the incidence of skin cancers is expected to continue to rise in the years ahead.

TERMS

basal cell carcinoma: a form of skin cancer that usually can be removed surgically

melanoma: a particularly dangerous form of skin cancer

prostate-specific antigen (PSA) test: a blood test that detects a protein associated with abnormal growth of the prostate gland

squamous cell carcinoma: cancer of the top layer of skin; most are curable if removed early

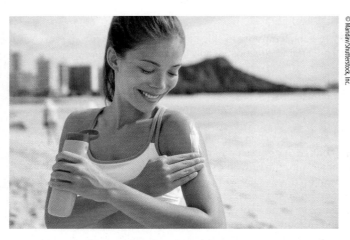

© Maridav/Shutterstock, Inc.

Signs of Melanoma

To protect yourself from melanoma, remember these "ABCD" rules when examining moles on your body for any changes. If you suspect anything, consult a physician immediately.
- Asymmetry—one half of a mole looks different from the other half.
- Border irregular—the edges of a mole are ragged or indistinct.
- Color—the pigmentation in the mole is uneven.
- Diameter—any mole that is larger than the diameter of a pencil or that has increased in size.

Wearing sunglasses that block at least 99% of all UV light is important for protecting eyes. Polarized lenses block glare but do not necessarily block UV unless the label says so. "Photochromic" lenses that darken in bright light also may not block UV light; always read the label. Over time, eye exposure to UV can cause cataracts.

The Environmental Protection Agency and the National Weather Service offer a daily email advisory to anyone wanting to know the UV levels in their area. UV intensity is rated on a point scale of 1 to 11; 6 or higher means that the UV intensity is high for the area and that exposure should be limited. The UV advisory can be accessed at epa.gov/sunsafety/uv-index-1.

Colorectal Cancer

Mortality from colorectal cancer is exceeded in the United States only by that from lung cancer, prostate cancer, and breast cancer. Colorectal cancer affects men and women equally and causes about 50,000 total deaths annually in the United States. As with many cancers, if discovered in the earliest stages, many cases of colorectal cancer can be cured surgically.

Colorectal cancer is rarely diagnosed in persons under age 40 but begins to appear more frequently in persons over age 50. The primary screening tests for it are occult blood tests, flexible sigmoidoscopy, and colonoscopy. In the occult blood test, stool samples are analyzed for the presence of blood, which may be a sign of colorectal cancer. In sigmoidoscopy, a flexible instrument is inserted via the rectum into the lower part of the colon to allow the health provider to visually examine the lining of the colon. If any abnormal tissue is observed, a complete examination of the colon (colonoscopy) is recommended.

Occult blood tests for colorectal cancer are accurate. A positive sign from an occult blood test in a stool is usually cause for additional tests. Some risk is involved with sigmoidoscopy and colonoscopy because they are invasive.

In a colonoscopy, death occurs in approximately 1 of 10,000 procedures. However, the rate of death from colorectal cancer in persons aged 50 to 54 is only about 1.8 per 10,000, so deciding to have a colonoscopy is not a simple decision. Each person needs to weigh the risks and benefits for his or her particular situation.

Certain inherited genes (see Table 13.2 and Figure 13.4) are known to increase a person's risk for colorectal cancer. Persons from families known to be at high risk can be genetically tested to see if they have inherited a colorectal cancer susceptibility gene. They may benefit from the genetic information by more frequent examination of their colon, but they also must be willing to accept the lifelong stress that comes with knowing that they are at higher than average risk for colorectal cancer.

Diet and Cancer Risk

Many epidemiological studies show that the risk of certain cancers is strongly influenced by diet. For example, consumption of alcohol and processed meats such as bacon, sausage, lunch meats, and hot dogs increases the risk of cancer. Stomach cancer is common in Japan but uncommon among white Americans in Hawaii. Japanese Americans in Hawaii have stomach cancer rates that are almost as low as the white American population. Excessive consumption of smoked and pickled foods may contribute to the higher rates of stomach cancer in Japan.

Despite the scientific uncertainty over what specific foods increase the risk of cancer, certain dietary choices may help in preventing cancer (Table 13.5). Most of these dietary recommendations also help boost the immune system, which is the body's main defense against foreign cells. B vitamins, vitamin C, and folic acid have been shown to boost the immune system and, as a consequence, may also help destroy cancer cells. These substances can be taken as supplements but also are readily available in fresh fruits and vegetables.

Our ancestors foraged for their food. They collected and ate seeds, roots, fruits, and vegetables and rarely ate

Table 13.5

Dietary Recommendations to Help Prevent Cancer

About 50% of all cancers are thought to derive from poor nutrition.

Substance or foods that help prevent cancer	Effect on cancer risk	Advice
Fiber	Helps decrease colon and rectal cancer	Obtain fiber from vegetables, fruits, whole grains
Cruciferous vegetables (broccoli, cauliflower, brussels sprouts)	Phytochemicals in these vegetables may detoxify cancer-causing chemicals	Eat more; raw or undercooked is best
Allium vegetables (onion, garlic, chives)	Sulfur-containing chemicals in allium vegetables may help prevent cancer	Eat more
Beta-carotene (15 mg), vitamin E (400 IU), and selenium (50 µg)	A daily supplement reduced cancer (mainly stomach and esophagus) in a large Chinese population	Use supplements in moderation; selenium in high doses is toxic
Folic acid	Deficiency in this vitamin increases genetic damage that may contribute to cancer	Supplement if diet is deficient
Green tea	Reduced esophageal cancer in Chinese population	Most tea drunk in United States is black tea; try green tea
Shiitake mushrooms	Extracts of shiitake mushrooms reduced tumors in laboratory animals; also reduces blood cholesterol	Add to diet

meat. Thus, the diet we consume today, filled with excess sugar, salt, fat, and meat, may be incompatible with the body chemistry we have inherited from our ancestors. The modern diet, heavy with processed foods, may result in the accumulation of toxic chemicals or an insufficient amount of some essential nutrients found in fresh fruits and vegetables, nuts, and grains.

Cancer Treatments

Treatments for cancer are surgery, **radiation therapy**, **chemotherapy**, and **immunotherapy**. Surgical removal of all or as much of a tumor as possible is considered the standard treatment for cancer, particularly if the tumor is small and cells have not spread throughout the body. If even a few cancer cells remain, however, they may grow into new tumors, which is the reason that surgery, such as mastectomy, often removes a great deal of tissue in addition to the tumor.

If there is evidence that tumor cells have spread, or if some of the tumor could not be removed surgically, then radiation or chemotherapy, or both, are used to try to destroy the remaining cancer cells. Because radiation therapy and chemotherapy destroy normal cells as well as cancer cells, only limited amounts of each treatment can be administered.

Hundreds of cancer drugs are available, many of which are quite effective for treating a specific cancer. However, many of the chemotherapeutic drugs that have been created by innovative technologies are extremely expensive. Many cancer drugs cost tens of thousands of dollars annually, and cancer treatments can end up costing hundreds of thousands of dollars, far more than most cancer patients and their families can afford without comprehensive or government health insurance.

Cancer patients often become desperate and depressed about their condition, the pain of treatments, and the prospect of death. In this state, some patients turn to unconventional therapies and

Don't Be Fooled by "Miraculous" Cancer Cures

Most people who are diagnosed with cancer become depressed or angry, especially if their doctor is pessimistic about the outcome or cannot offer hope of a cure. People who cannot be helped by conventional medicine (and many who can) often turn to an alternative medicine that offers hope of cures for untreatable, advanced cancer. Alternative medicines run the gamut from nutritional therapies, immune therapies, and light therapies to spiritual cures.

Most of the alternative cancer therapies are designed to take money from desperate patients. If you would like information on any alternative therapy you or a loved one is contemplating using, a good place to look for information is quackwatch.com. This site has links to many other sources of reliable information. If it is too good to be true, it usually is not true.

TERMS

chemotherapy: use of toxic chemicals to kill cancer cells and treat some forms of cancer

immunotherapy: medically enhancing the body's immune system to fight cancer

radiation therapy: use of high-energy radiation, such as x-rays, to kill cancer cells and treat some forms of cancer

Table 13.6

Unproven Cancer Therapies

Many cancer patients who are desperate or who have exhausted all medical treatments turn to unconventional therapies for which benefits are scientifically unproven.

Therapy	Rationale
Metabolic therapy	Toxins and wastes in the body cause cancer.
	Treatments remove cellular poisons and detoxify the body.
Herbal remedies	Herbs have natural, sacred, curative properties not known to science.
Megavitamins	High doses of vitamins kill cancer cells and rejuvenate the body.
Diet therapy	Special diets (grape, macrobiotic, shark cartilage) restore balance to the body and cure the cancer.
Electronic devices	Electrical or magnetic energy harmonizes the life forces and kills the cancer cells.

promises of "miracle" cures (**Table 13.6**). Many cancer patients choose alternative therapies in hope of a cure when conventional medicine has nothing to offer. Although unconventional therapies may be helpful or at least produce more peace of mind, patients and their families need to be wary of practitioners who make unfounded claims for unlicensed drugs and unproven therapies.

Cancer Immunotherapies

The body's own immune system can attack cancer cells growing anywhere in the body. Methods to enable the immune system to work better against cancer are called **immunotherapies**. For example, the currently available HPV vaccine induces the immune system to manufacture antibodies against HPV, thus providing protection against cervical cancer. Scientists are working on a more targeted immunotherapy in which immune system T cells are induced to recognize and attack a patient's specific cancer cells.

In 2011, the drug Yervoy was approved for treating patients with advanced melanoma. In about 20% of those treated, tumors disappeared, and the cures seem permanent (Piore, 2017). Yervoy was the first approved immunotherapy that uses *checkpoint inhibition*. Some cancers grow and spread by blocking the immune system. Checkpoint inhibition drugs remove a cancer's ability to block the immune system, allowing an effective anticancer immune response to proceed. Several other checkpoint inhibitor drugs are now available and more are in development.

Other immunotherapies use drugs to "mark" cancer cells to make it easier for the immune system to find and destroy them. Another kind of cancer immunotherapy (called *CAR-T therapy*) involves removing T cells from the blood of a person with cancer, modifying them in a laboratory or clinic so they are better able to find and destroy cancer cells, and then placing the modified cells back into the body.

Cancer immunotherapy took a positive turn in 2017, with the approval of a checkpoint inhibitor that can treat cancers caused by a specific genetic defect that results in a wide range of cancers. The genetic defect hampers the cell's ability to repair DNA that has been damaged by radiation or chemicals. Failure to repair DNA damage causes the accumulation of mutations, some of which turn normal cells into cancer cells. Prior to this, drugs were approved to treat only a specific cancer. In this case, the drug was approved to treat *any* cancer that is caused by the same genetic defect. In tests, the drug was effective against 12 different types of cancer in 77% of patients with defects in DNA repair. As many as 60,000 cancer patients a year may benefit from this new approach to cancer treatment (Saey, 2017).

Curing Childhood Cancers

Each year in the United States, about 20,000 children younger than 21 years receive a diagnosis of cancer. Because of advancements in treating these childhood cancers, about 80% of these children are cured and enter adulthood with no signs of cancer. Curing many forms of childhood cancer has been hailed as a great success story in the fight against cancer. However, studies of thousands of childhood cancer survivors have revealed that a majority of the survivors had serious chronic health problems and were more likely to die prematurely. They suffered from other cancers, heart disease, musculoskeletal disorders, and other serious conditions. The study emphasizes that survivors of childhood cancers must receive ongoing medical attention throughout their lives to detect and treat new health problems.

For cancer survivors of any age, a healthy lifestyle is crucial to help reduce the damaging effects of the toxic treatments used to cure their cancer. Childhood cancer survivors should concentrate on eating the healthiest diet possible. They should avoid smoking and try to live in areas where the environment, especially the air, is not polluted. They should exercise regularly and avoid excess weight gain. Finally, they should regularly consult a physician who is knowledgeable about the subsequent health problems of childhood cancer survivors.

Cancer Vaccines

When abnormal cells arise in the body, in most instances they are recognized and destroyed by the body's immune system. Only when abnormal cells fail

> More harm is done by fools through foolishness than is done by evildoers through wickedness.
>
> *Sufi proverb*

to be eliminated and continue to grow and reproduce does a tumor develop. Medical researchers are currently looking for ways to develop cancer vaccines and ways to boost the body's immune system so that it is better able to fend off cancer.

A vaccine is approved that, if widely used, would eliminate cervical cancer in women. This vaccine is safe and 100% effective in blocking infection by the strains of human papillomavirus (HPV) that cause cervical cancer. Vaccines against hepatitis B and C viruses, which can cause liver cancer, also are available.

Coping with Cancer

A diagnosis of cancer raises serious problems for the patient and for family and friends. Often the patient enters a state of disbelief or shock. The family has to cope with new problems. The patient must face surgery or other treatment. Along with treatment, the patient usually must deal with fear of death, anger at the disease, loss of income, changes in living habits, and, above all, the uncertainty of the outcome, which may last for months or years. These are some of the reasons why coping with cancer can be difficult. Stress and emotional upset can depress the normal functions of the immune system. There also is evidence that hostile feelings, resentment, deeply felt personal loss, and feelings of hopelessness may be important factors in coping with cancer.

The coping strategies for dealing with the emotional distress resulting from cancer, AIDS, and other serious diseases are similar. They all depend on using the mind in positive ways. The effectiveness of any therapy and the ability to cope with a life-threatening illness depend on focusing the mind on ways to enhance the healing process. Meditation and relaxation techniques are important in reducing stress. Learning how to use visual imagery can help with the effectiveness of treatments. Along with mental relaxation techniques, the mind can focus on images and suggestions that may help the immune system fight and destroy cancer cells.

A dramatic illustration of the power of belief in altering the course of cancer is the case of Mr. Wright, a patient in the 1950s. At that time, a drug called krebiozen was touted by some as a "miracle drug" that could cure cancer. Mr. Wright, who had terminal lymphosarcoma, was given a life expectancy of 2 weeks by his physician. However, Mr. Wright had enormous faith in the miracle drug and insisted that he be treated with it. After a single injection, his doctor noted that "the

The Cost of Extending Life Among Terminally Ill Cancer Patients

In many instances, cancer is a chronic illness for which a cure is not available and, unfortunately, death may be months away. In recent years, biotechnology and pharmaceutical companies have developed ways to treat advanced stages of various cancers so that those who are expected to die relatively soon from their incurable disease can have a few more months of life. Because it costs many millions of dollars to develop a new drug, these treatments are very expensive.

For example, in 2010, the Food and Drug Administration (FDA) approved a new drug, Provenge (sipuleucel-T), for treating advanced prostate cancer. Tests showed that men treated with Provenge lived an average of 4 months longer than a control group of men who did not receive the drug. The cost of treating one man with Provenge was $93,000. Treating chronic myeloid leukemia with the drug Gleevec (imatinib) costs $4,500 per month, and the drug Avastin (bevacizumab), which is used to treat advanced colorectal cancer, costs $100,000 per year.

Many people are appalled by the rising costs of medical care, but when they or a loved one is terminally ill with cancer or another disease, the cost of extending life, even for a few months, may not be considered—which is understandable. Facing death is emotionally difficult. Nevertheless, financial resources are not unlimited, and so our society faces difficult decisions about how to finance care for the terminally ill.

tumor masses had melted like snowballs on a hot stove, and in only these few days, they were half their original size" (Klopfer, 1957).

Mr. Wright was symptom free for 2 months until he read in the newspaper that krebiozen was worthless in treating cancer, whereupon he relapsed and was readmitted to the hospital. With nothing to lose, his doctor assured him that a fresh, double-strength injection of krebiozen would cure him. In actuality, Mr. Wright received an injection of salt water. Once again he was symptom free for 2 months. Then headlines again proclaimed "nationwide tests show krebiozen to be a worthless drug in treatment of cancer." Mr. Wright relapsed and died in 2 days.

Coping with cancer requires courage and conviction. A cancer patient must not give up hope, despite what the statistics predict or what physicians say about the prognosis. The patient must believe that a cure is possible and work toward that end. For many people, coping with cancer is a transforming experience and gives renewed meaning to life.

Visualization Helps Healing

As director of Biofeedback Research at the Menninger Clinic in Topeka, Kansas, Dr. Patricia Norris has documented several cases where mental imagery and visualization were used successfully to complement traditional medical treatment. Dr. Norris cites eight specific characteristics that help to make mental imagery and visualization effective as a healing tool, specifically with regard to cancer:

1. **Make the visualization personal.** The images must be self-generated. Images that are created by the practitioner and not the patient appear to be ineffective.
2. **Make the imagery "egosyntonic."** Egosyntonic means that the image must fit the values and ideals of that person. If, for example, the individual is pacifistic, then combative or warlike imagery will undermine the effectiveness of this type of treatment.
3. **Make the imagery positive.** Negative imagery reinforces negative thoughts, which are not conducive to healing. As an example, Norris notes that sharks, as a healing image, are not a good idea.
4. **Take an active role in the imagery.** Rather than imagining watching the imagery on a movie screen, you must feel the sensations of your images in the first person. You must have a sense that what you are seeing is happening inside your body, not "out there somewhere."
5. **Make the image anatomically correct and accurate.** Knowing exactly what body region and physiological system are in a disease state will dictate the type of imagery used. Consequently, you need to know whether to access the central nervous system or the immune system. Norris states that more than one image can be used in the healing process.
6. **Be constant, use dialogue.** Constancy means to be regular in generating your imagery. Norris suggests three 15-minute sessions per day, with intermittent shorter sessions throughout the day. When you feel pain, your body is communicating to you. She suggests making pain your friend. In the dialogue style of self-talk, she suggests thanking the pain for making you aware of the problem so that you may be able to fix it. Finally, she suggests "destroying" a tumor with its permission. Respond with love. Make peace with your body.
7. **Create a blueprint.** The concept of the blueprint is a strategy. A blueprint visualization is like time-lapse photography where a flower (symbolizing a tumor) is shown to bloom within seconds, and then closes up again and fades away. An example would be to see the construction of a building, starting from the hole in the earth to opening day, where you are cutting the ribbon at the front entrance.
8. **Include the treatment in the imagery.** Norris has found that patients who use mental imagery with chemotherapy treatment and radiation do better than those who "fight" these medical procedures. She notes that it helps to have benevolent feelings versus ambivalent feelings toward the treatment. She suggests one mentally "welcome the treatment into the body." Consider the treatment as a guest in your house. Based on her patient research, she offers these examples:
   (a) *Chemotherapy*—a gold-colored fluid that healthy cells, acting as a bucket brigade, pass along to the cancer cells, who in turn drink up the chemotherapy.
   (b) *Radiation treatment*—a stream of silver energy aimed at the cancerous tumor(s). Ask the white blood cells to move away or to shield themselves and act like mirrors to reflect the radiation toward the cancer cells, and then watch the cancer cells die.

Critical Thinking About Health

1. Consider this hypothetical case of a female college student. Several women in her family, including her grandmother and an aunt, died of breast cancer before they reached 65 years of age. She is only 21 years old but is very concerned about her own risk of developing breast cancer. She decides to be tested for the breast cancer susceptibility genes BRCA1 and BRCA2, even though her physician explains that no medical treatment short of prophylactic mastectomy is available. The genetic test is positive for gene BRCA1, and her risk of breast cancer is significantly higher than for other women who do not have this gene. Discuss, from your own perspective, what this woman should now do to preserve her health. Gather as many facts as you can on breast cancer and the effects of these susceptibility genes.

2. Make a list of all the factors you can think of that increase the risk of developing cancer. Order the items in your list from highest risk to lowest in your judgment. Are any of the risk factors relevant to your life?

If so, describe how you could modify your lifestyle or behaviors to reduce the risk of developing cancer.

3. A number of strategies are presented in this chapter that can help prevent cancers of various types. List and discuss ways to help prevent lung cancer, skin cancer, breast cancer, and colorectal cancer.

4. The "war against cancer" is fought by physicians and scientists in two fundamentally different ways. On the one hand, medical research tries to discover better treatments for all forms of cancer. On the other hand, epidemiologists and other researchers believe that we need to shift the scientific emphasis from seeking cures to prevention because we understand many of the environmental factors that cause cancer. Reducing exposure to risk factors could prevent as many as half of all human cancers. In your judgment, which of these positions is correct? Or do you believe both positions are equally valid? Develop facts and arguments that substantiate your views and write a report of your conclusions.

Chapter Summary and Highlights

Chapter Summary

Cancer is actually many different diseases that share the property of abnormal and unregulated cell multiplication. Although some cancers are caused by inheriting harmful variants of specific genes, about 80% to 90% of all cancers are due to environmental factors—smoking cigarettes or breathing polluted air, exposure to ionizing radiation such as sunlight or nuclear waste, infection by certain viruses, exposure to pesticides, heavy metals, petrochemicals, and certain drugs. As with other chronic diseases, maintaining proper body weight, eating a variety of fresh foods, and exercising will help prevent cancer cells from developing in the body. Although fashionable among young and old, acquiring a tan by exposure to the sun or from tanning lamps can greatly increase the risk of skin cancers. Many cancers can be treated successfully with modern drugs, but the risk of cancer recurrence is always present.

Breast cancer is of great concern to women of all ages. Regular mammograms can help women detect breast cancers at early stages, thus making more treatment options available. Certain groups of women, particularly those of Jewish ancestry, are at much higher-than-average risk of developing breast cancer because of susceptibility genes that they may have inherited. Hispanic women, on the other hand, may be of lower-than-average risk. Genetic tests are available for numerous cancer susceptibility genes, including two that are specific for breast cancer. Prevention is the best way to avoid a diagnosis of cancer. Avoid eating foods that may cause cancer such as charbroiled meats, smoked meats

and fish, and fruits and vegetables that may contain pesticide residues. Avoid chemical fumes and polluted air if possible. Do not breathe smoke from tobacco, outdoor grills, or forest fires.

Highlights

- *Cancer* refers to a number of different diseases, all of which share the common property of abnormal, unregulated cell growth in the body.
- Dietary factors and environmental agents, such as smoking and sunlight, act on the genetic material in cells to cause chemical changes that may initiate a tumor, which is a mass of abnormal cells.
- Cigarette smoking is responsible for about one-third of all cancers, especially lung cancer.
- The principal environmental agents that cause cancer are ionizing radiation, tumor viruses, carcinogenic chemicals, and, possibly, xenoestrogens.
- If everything known about cancer prevention were practiced, up to one-half of cancers would not occur; thus, cancer is largely a preventable disease.
- Only 5% to 10% of cancers are caused by genes that have been inherited. The genetic changes in body cells that result in cancer are not passed on to children because these genetic changes have not occurred in sperm or eggs.
- The treatments for cancer include surgery, radiation, chemotherapy, and immunotherapy. The goal of all three cancer treatments is the removal or destruction of as many cancer cells as possible.

- Recovery from cancer depends on good nutrition, positive attitudes, healing mental images, and medical treatment appropriate for the particular cancer. A healthy, active immune system also is an essential component in cancer prevention and recovery.
- Both breast and testicular self-examinations are positive means of early cancer detection.
- Dietary deficiencies or excesses are responsible for about one-half of all cancers.

- Overexposure to sunlight causes skin cancer, which is on the increase.
- Significantly reducing cancer requires major changes in people's lifestyles, including more attention to a healthy diet, elimination of tobacco use, limiting alcohol consumption, and reducing exposure to intense sunlight and chemical carcinogens.

For Your Health

You may not want to think about cancer, but it may serve you to estimate your risks (or the cancer risks of someone you care about) so you can take steps to lessen the chances of developing the disease. Do Exercise 13.1, "My Cancer Risks," in the Workbook. Also do "My Environmental Cancer Risks" (see Exercise 13.2 in the Workbook).

References

Brenner, D. J., & Hricak, H. (2010). Radiation exposure from medical imaging—time to regulate? *Journal of the American Medical Association, 304*, 208–209.

Couzin, J. (2003). Review rules out abortion cancer link. *Science, 299*, 1498.

Greenlee, H., et al. (2017). Clinical practice guidelines on the evidence-based use of integrative therapies during and after breast cancer treatment. *CA: Cancer Journal for Clinicians, 6*, 194–232.

Klopfer, B. (1957). Psychological variables in human cancer. *Journal of Prospective Techniques, 21*, 331–340.

Lin, E. C. (2010). Radiation risk from medical imaging. *Mayo Clinic Proceedings, 85*, 1142–1146.

McCollough, C. H., et al. (2015). Answers to common questions about the use and safety of CT scans. *Mayo Clinic Proceedings, 90*, 1380–1392.

Piore, A. (2017). Immunotherapy pioneer James Allison has unfinished business with cancer. *Technology Review, 120*, 75–85.

Saey, T. H. (2017). Therapy flags DNA typos to rev cancer-fighting T cells. *Science News, 191*, 7.

Welch, H. G. (2010). Screening mammography—a long run for a short slide? *Journal of the American Medical Association, 363*, 1276–1278.

Woolf, S. H. (2010). The 2009 breast cancer screening recommendations of the U.S. Preventive Services Task Force. *Journal of the American Medical Association, 303*, 162–165.

Suggested Readings

Collins, F. S., & Barker, A. D. (2007, March). Mapping the cancer genome. Scientific American, 50–57. Describes the project to map all of the variant human genes that may contribute to the development of cancer.

Esteva, F. J., & Hortobagyi, G. N. (2008, June). Gaining ground on breast cancer. *Scientific American*, 58–65. An update on the new treatments for breast cancer.

Groopman, J. (2012, April 28). The T-cell army. *The New Yorker*, 24–30. A fascinating tale of almost a century of research on the immune system that finally led to the first successful immunotherapy for melanoma, a deadly form of skin cancer.

Marshall, E. (2010). Brawling over mammography. *Science, 327*, 936–938. A good source to understand the controversy over mammography screening.

Mukherjee, S. (2011). *The emperor of all maladies: A biography of cancer*. New York: Scribner. A physician, medical researcher, and renowned author explains the origins or cancer and the gradual development of effective treatments. Dr. Siddhartha Mukherjee writes about cancer with great knowledge and from personal experience.

Piore, A. (2017). Immunotherapy pioneer James Allison has unfinished business with cancer. *Technology Review. 120*, 75–85. A fascinating tale of how new immunotherapies for cancer are being developed.

Rados, C. (2005, March/April). Teen tanning hazards. *FDA Consumer*, 8–9. Explains why using indoor tanning lamps increases skin cancer risks. Young people are the biggest users of indoor tanning lamps.

Schaffer, A. (2011, May/June). The cost of life. *Technology Review*, 82–84. Discusses the issue of administering life-extending, high-cost drugs and procedures to terminally ill people.

Welch, H. G. (2006). *Should I be tested for cancer? Maybe not—and here's why*. Berkeley: University of California Press. Many tests for various cancers exist, but they often are not helpful. This book explains why.

Recommended Websites

American Cancer Society
Information on types of cancer, prevention, treatment options, and medical issues.

CancerNet
The U.S. National Cancer Institute's database of cancer information.

National Breast Cancer Foundation, Inc.
Information and educational resources.

National Toxicology Program, Department of Health and Human Services
This website contains a list of all carcinogenic substances that have been tested by the government. The list is updated every two years.

Oncolink
Comprehensive cancer information from the University of Pennsylvania School of Medicine.

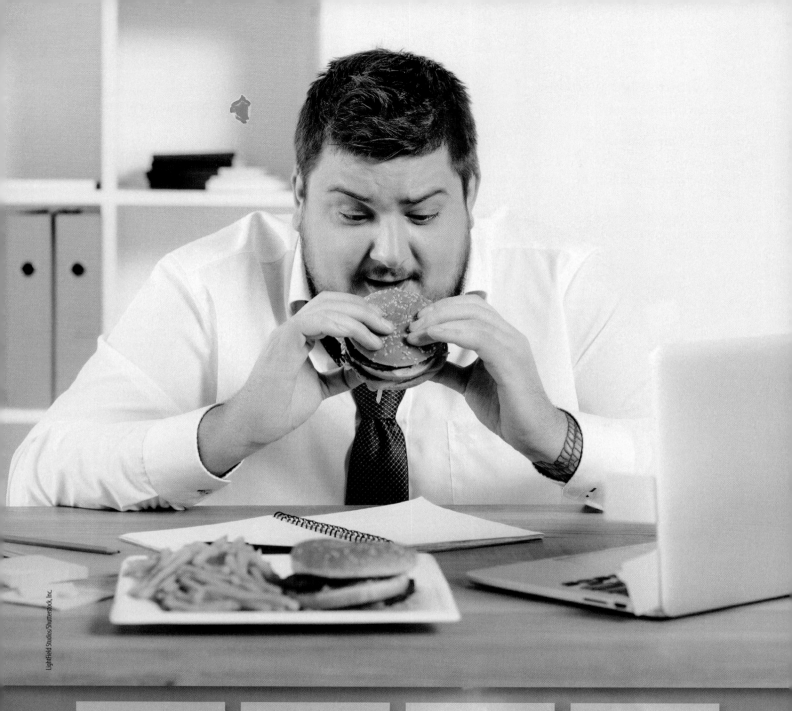

Health Tips

Infected Gums Contribute to Heart Disease

Breathing Exercise to Reduce Hypertension

Cardiovascular Fitness: Exercise Your Heart

Dollars & Health Sense

Coronary Artery Bypass Graft

Global Wellness

It's Not Too Late to Have a Healthy Heart

Wellness Guide

How to Interpret Blood Cholesterol and Lipid Measurements

Concussion to the Heart

Home Blood Pressure Monitors and Internet Consultations to Help Patients Reduce Hypertension

Genes May, or May Not, Increase the Risk of Heart Disease

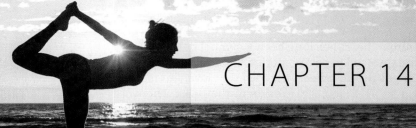

CHAPTER 14

Cardiovascular Diseases: Understanding Risks and Measures of Prevention

Learning Objectives

1. Define *cardiovascular disease* and provide three examples.

2. Describe how blood flows through the heart and blood vessels.

3. Describe two types of cardiac arrhythmia.

4. Describe how the direction of blood flow in the body is regulated.

5. Define *atherosclerosis* and explain its treatment with statins.

6. Describe coronary heart disease and the available treatments.

7. Define *stroke*, *hypertension*, and *metabolic syndrome*.

8. List three lifestyle factors that increase the risk of cardiovascular disease.

The human heart has long been a symbol of human love as it is expressed in poetry, stories, and everyday customs. Our language still reflects the idea that love and feelings reside in the heart. The word "heartfelt" implies deep feelings of caring and sincerity; "heartless," however, implies being cold and uncaring. When love relationships collapse, people refer to their "broken hearts" or the "heartlessness" of the former lover. People are described by the nature of their hearts—cruel, kind, warm, or cold; some are even referred to as having a heart of stone. When people refer to distressing experiences in life, they talk of "heartache," and when they are happy, their hearts may "leap with joy."

> Have a heart that never hardens
> A temper that never tires
> A touch that never hurts.
>
> *Charles Dickens*

Today we know that emotions, thoughts, and feelings of every kind originate in the brain, not the heart. The heart's only function is to pump blood and circulate it throughout the body. The heart is an extraordinarily effective pump; it pumps slightly more than a gallon of blood per minute through approximately 60,000 miles of blood vessels in the body. In this gallon of blood are about 25 trillion red blood cells that carry oxygen from the lungs to all the body's cells and remove the carbon dioxide that is exhaled as waste. Each day about 200 billion new red blood cells are synthesized in bone marrow (the soft material at the center of large bones) and released into the circulation. Each day the heart expands and contracts (beats) 100,000 times and pumps about 2,000 gallons of blood. A healthy heart and blood vessels are essential for survival.

That the heart works so hard it's a wonder that it can do so for so long in so many people. However, the heart is not invincible. It can be weakened by infection, injury, birth malformations, and damage resulting from its owner's behavior, such as a consuming a poor diet, not engaging in enough physical activity, and tobacco smoking.

The American Heart Association (AHA), in conjunction with the Centers for Disease Control and Prevention, the National Institutes of Health, and other government agencies has identified core behaviors, which, when implemented, can greatly enhance heart health (**Figure 14.1**). Discussion of these and other facets of cardiovascular health is the purpose of this chapter.

Cardiovascular Diseases

Cardiovascular disease (CVD) refers to any number of conditions that damage the heart (*cardio*) and blood vessels (*vascular*) (**Table 14.1**). According to the World Health Organization (2017), cardiovascular disease is the number one cause of death worldwide, accounting for about 31% of all deaths; about 18 million people die of cardiovascular disease annually. In the United States, cardiovascular disease

- Eat healthy especially fruits, vegetables, legumes, nuts, seeds, and whole grains
- Sit less, move your body, take a walk
- No tobacco smoking
- Maintain healthy blood pressure
- Go easy on fats and cholesterol
- Go easy on sugar
- Go easy on alcohol
- Maintain a healthy body weight
- Take time outs to ease your mind
- Relax, have fun, be social

■ Figure 14.1

Core Behaviors for a Healthy Heart
Data from:
* American Heart Association (http://www.heart.org/HEARTORG/Conditions/My-Life-Check—Lifes-Simple-7_UCM_471453_Article.jsp#.Wc6NRGJSzfY)
* U.S. Centers for Disease control (https://www.cdc.gov/heartdisease/what_you_can_do.htm):
* Harvard Medical School (https://www.health.harvard.edu/topics/heart-health)
* University of Wisconsin (http://www.uwhealth.org/heart-cardiovascular/health-psychology-for-healthy-hearts/38645)

is the leading cause of death, accounting for over 800,000 annual deaths (American Heart Association, 2017b). Some cardiovascular diseases stem from biological malformations present at birth (*congenital heart disease*), bacterial infections of the heart (*rheumatic heart disease*) and its

Table 14.1

Categories of Cardiovascular Disease

Disease	Description
Cerebrovascular disease	Disease of the blood vessels supplying the brain; common cause of stroke
Congenital heart disease	malformations of heart structure existing at birth
Congestive heart failure	Weakening of the heart muscle making it unable to pump blood efficiently or at all
Coronary heart disease	Disease of the blood vessels supplying the heart muscle
Deep Vein Thrombosis	Blood clots in the leg veins, which can dislodge and move to the heart, lungs, and brain
High blood pressure	Weakens the heart and damages blood vessels
Peripheral arterial disease	Disease of blood vessels supplying the arms and legs
Pulmonary embolism	Blood clots that lodge in the lungs and block blood flow to the heart
Rheumatic heart disease	Damage to the heart muscle and heart valves from rheumatic fever, caused by streptococcal bacteria

surrounding tissues (*pericarditis*), and injury. Others occur in association with other diseases (e.g., high blood pressure and type 2 diabetes). But by far, the most prevalent cardiovascular disease in the United States, and the one that is most amenable to prevention, is **coronary heart disease (CHD)**, the result of fatty deposits (called *plaque*) in the heart's **coronary arteries** that impede or completely block the transport of oxygen and nutrients to the heart muscle cells, resulting in a **heart attack**. **Stroke**, or **brain attack**, is the second most frequent cardiovascular disease. A stroke occurs when sufficient blood does not reach brain cells and they die.

The incidence of death from cardiovascular diseases among Americans has been declining steadily in recent decades (**Figure 14.2**). One major reason for this trend is that more and more people have become aware that most cardiovascular disease is preventable by adopting healthy living habits such as eating healthfully, engaging in moderate physical activity on most days of the week, not smoking tobacco, and maintaining a normal blood pressure and body weight. Another major reason for the decrease in the incidence of death from cardiovascular disease is the recent and continued development of effective surgical, medical, and psychological treatments for several of these diseases.

The Heart and Blood Vessels

The human cardiovascular system consists of the heart (the pump) and the various blood vessels (**Figure 14.3**). **Arteries** carry oxygenated blood from the heart to all organs and tissues in the body. **Veins** return blood to the heart after oxygen and nutrients have been exchanged for carbon dioxide and waste products. **Capillaries** are tiny blood vessels that branch out from arteries to circulate blood to all of the cells in the body. Blood vessels can be damaged by injury or by disease; this damage may obstruct the flow of blood carrying oxygen and nutrients.

The organ that keeps the blood circulating throughout the body is the heart, a highly specialized muscle about

the size of an adult fist that pumps blood (**Figure 14.4**). The muscular wall of the heart is called the **myocardium**. When the blood supply to heart cells is blocked, they begin to die and a heart attack results.

The heart consists of four separate chambers: The upper two chambers are called the left atrium and the right atrium; the lower two chambers are the right ventricle and the left ventricle. Blood that is depleted of oxygen enters the heart via the right atrium and then flows to the right ventricle. From there blood is pumped to the lungs, where it is reoxygenated and returned via the pulmonary veins to the left atrium. Finally, the oxygen-rich blood is pumped throughout the body's tissues from the left ventricle through the large artery called the **aorta**.

The Heart Beat

The heart contracts from 60 to 100 times a minute, depending on the body's level of activity or excitement. The entire volume of blood in the body is recirculated almost once every minute. During an average lifetime of 70 years, the heart will pump between 30 million and 40 million gallons of blood, and it will beat 2.5 billion times!

The beat of a healthy heart is characterized by its rate and its pattern, or *rhythm*. The heart rate is the number of times per minute the lower chambers of the heart (the ventricles) contract to move blood out of the heart.

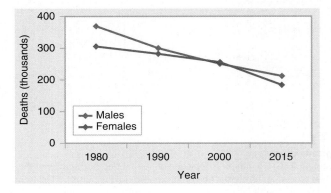

■ **Figure 14.2**

Mortality from Cardiovascular Disease in the United States (1980–2015)

Adapted from Centers for Disease Control and Prevention. (2017). Health, United States, 2016. Retrieved from http://www.cdc.gov/nchs/data/hus/hus16.pdf

> **TERMS**
>
> **aorta:** the large artery that transports blood from the heart to the body
>
> **arteries:** any of a series of blood vessels that carry blood from the heart to all parts of the body
>
> **capillaries:** extremely small blood vessels that carry oxygenated blood to tissues
>
> **cardiovascular disease (CVD):** any disease that causes damage to the heart or the body's blood vessels
>
> **coronary arteries:** two arteries arising from the aorta that supply blood vessels to the heart muscle
>
> **coronary heart disease (CHD):** disease caused by fatty deposits in the heart's coronary arteries that impede or completely block the transport of oxygen and nutrients to the heart muscle cells
>
> **heart attack:** death of, or damage to, part of the heart muscle caused by an insufficient blood supply
>
> **myocardium:** muscular wall of the heart that contracts and relaxes
>
> **stroke (brain attack):** death of brain cells due to an insufficient supply of blood to the brain, resulting in loss of muscle function, loss of speech, or other symptoms
>
> **veins:** blood vessels that return blood from tissues to the heart

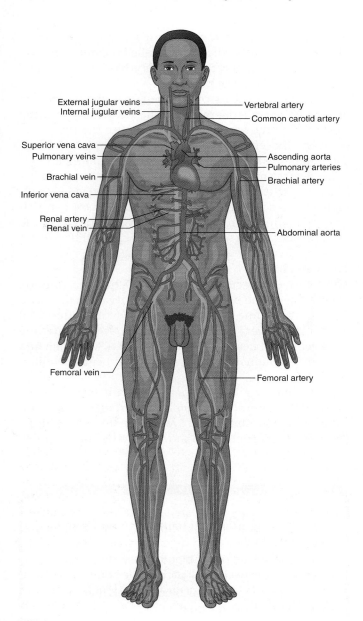

■ **Figure 14.3**

Cardiovascular System
Includes the heart, arteries, and veins. The heart receives oxygenated blood from the lungs and pumps it to all tissues in the body.

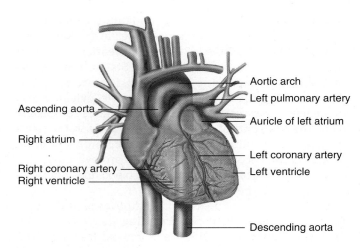

■ **Figure 14.4**

Heart and Major Arteries
Oxygenated blood is pumped through the arteries (red), and oxygen-depleted blood is returned to the heart via the veins (blue).

The heart rate is controlled by a region in the right atrium called the **sinoatrial node**. This region sends electrical signals across the surface of the heart, which causes heart muscle fibers to contract as a group so blood moves smoothly through the heart. The sinoatrial node's control of the heart rate is also influenced by electrical signals from the brain via the autonomic nervous system, and certain hormones (e.g., adrenalin) in response to varying conditions such as exercise, warm body temperature, excitement, stress, and fear.

A biological anomaly, injury, or disease can cause the heartbeat to lose its normal rhythmic pattern. An irregular heartbeat is called an *arrhythmia*. Symptoms of arrhythmias include a fast or slow heartbeat, skipping beats, shortness of breath, chest pain, lightheadedness,

The heart rhythm is a sequence of coordinated biological events that create ventricular contractions strong enough to move blood.

An **electrocardiogram**, also called an ECG or EKG, is a simple, painless test that can show how fast the heart is beating and whether the rhythm of the heartbeats is steady or irregular (**Figure 14.5**). An EKG is often part of a routine exam to screen for heart disease, and is also used to detect and assess heart problems such as heart attacks, arrhythmias (i.e., irregular heartbeat), and heart failure. Results from this test also may suggest other heart disorders.

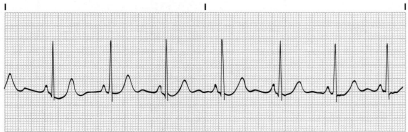

■ **Figure 14.5**

Electrocardiogram (EKG)
This electrocardiogram (EKG) is a graphical depiction of normal electrical activity of the heart. The tall spikes represent the contraction of the ventricles ("the pulse"), which send blood out of the heart into the circulation. Notice how the pulses occur at regular intervals, about 41 small squares per heart beat. The smaller bump at the left of the ventricle-spike represents the contractions of the atria. The small bump at the right of the ventricle-spike represents the ventricles preparing to contract. Each large square represents 0.2 seconds, so this heart is beating once just about every 0.8 seconds. Can you calculate the heart rate per minute?

Table 14.2

Types of Irregular Heart Rhythms

Type	Description
Premature (extra) beats	A sensation of fluttering in the chest or a skipped beat. Very common; most of the time requires no treatment, especially in healthy people. Premature beats in the atria are called premature atrial contractions, or PACs. Premature beats in the ventricles are called premature ventricular contractions, or PVCs.
Atrial fibrillation (AF)	A rapid, irregular contraction of the atria resulting from abnormal electrical signals coursing in a disorganized way through the heart tissue. This causes the walls of the atria to quiver (fibrillate) so that blood is not pumped in the normal way. Stroke and heart failure are serious complications of ongoing, untreated AF.
Atrial flutter	Similar to atrial fibrillation; the spread of electrical signals through the atria is too fast and regular (as opposed to irregular). Similar symptoms and complications as atrial fibrillation.
Paroxysmal supraventricular tachycardia (PSVT)	A very fast heart rate that begins and ends suddenly. It occurs due to problems with the electrical connection between the atria and the ventricles. Not usually dangerous, and tends to occur in young people. It can happen during vigorous exercise.
Ventricular tachycardia	A fast, regular beating of the ventricles. A few beats of ventricular tachycardia often do not cause problems, but episodes lasting for more than a few seconds can be dangerous.
Ventricular fibrillation	Disorganized electrical signals make the ventricles quiver instead of pump normally. When ventricles do not pump blood out of the heart, a person will lose consciousness within seconds and may die. To prevent death, the condition must be treated immediately with defibrillation, an electric shock to the heart.
Bradyarrhythmias	The heart rate is much slower than normal. A very slow heart rate may result in not enough blood reaching the brain.

dizziness, and sweating. Types of arrhythmias are presented in **Table 14.2**.

In addition to the sinoatrial node, the heartbeat also can be affected by nerve impulses that originate in various areas of the heart. If these signals interfere with the normal heartbeat, different areas of the heart beat independently of one another. The result is **atrial fibrillation ("a-fib")**, which are rapid, disorganized contractions of the upper chambers of the heart. This can cause blood to pool in the atria instead of being pumped into the heart's two lower chambers, the ventricles. Thus, the heart's upper and lower chambers don't work in a coordinated fashion and blood flow throughout the body is impaired.

Atrial fibrillation ("a-fib") usually develops as people age; it is estimated that nearly 3 million Americans experience atrial fibrillation to some degree. Usually the episodes are brief and no ill effects are noticed. In some instances, however, atrial fibrillation can cause a stroke. This can occur when irregular heartbeats slow the flow of blood in the heart to the extent that clots form. A blood clot that travels through the bloodstream to the brain can cause a stroke.

Atrial fibrillation can be managed with various drugs, and anyone who experiences an irregular heartbeat (usually noticed as a palpitation in the chest) should see a physician. If the fibrillation cannot be controlled with drugs, a **pacemaker** can be implanted in a person's chest. This is a small electrical device that supplies a steadying electrical signal to the heart.

Ventricular fibrillation ("v-fib") is a type of cardiac arrhythmia in which the ventricles (the lower chambers of the heart) quiver very rapidly and irregularly instead of contracting forcefully, resulting in the heart pumping little or no blood to the body. Ventricular fibrillation can be fatal if the heartbeat is not restored within a few minutes (*sudden cardiac arrest*). Certain diseases and conditions can cause problems with the ventricular heart rhythm, including coronary heart disease, physical stress, certain inherited disorders, and structural changes in the heart from high blood pressure. About 300,000 out-of-hospital cardiac arrests occur in the United States each year.

A **defibrillator** is an electrical device that can restore normal heart rhythm by delivering electrical shocks through the chest to the heart. For a heart attack victim

TERMS

atrial fibrillation ("a-fib"): rapid, erratic contraction of the upper chambers of the heart

defibrillator: an electrical device that can restart a heart that has stopped beating by delivering electrical shocks to it

electrocardiogram (EKG): a test that shows the rate and rhythm of the heart beat

sinoatrial node: the region of the heart that produces an electrical signal that causes the heart to contract

pacemaker: an electrical device implanted in the chest to control irregular heartbeats

ventricular fibrillation (v-fib): irregular quivering of the lower chambers of the heart

to survive, defibrillation should be initiated within a short period (a few minutes) after the beginning of the heart attack. By the time a patient reaches an emergency room, it is often too late for defibrillation.

For these reasons, automated external defibrillators (AEDs) have been developed and are now placed in many public areas where people congregate, such as shopping malls, sports arenas, stadiums, and airplanes. AEDs also can be purchased by individuals and kept in the home, where about 80% of heart attacks occur.

People who experience frequent abnormal heart rhythms (cardiac arrhythmias) may be candidates for an implantable cardioverter defibrillator (ICD) **Figure 14.6**. A small unit is implanted in the chest with wires attached to the heart. If the heart begins to beat irregularly, the defibrillator will deliver a pulse of electricity to the heart to restore normal heartbeats. Each year in the United States, about 100,000 patients receive an ICD at a cost of $30,000 to $50,000 per patient. The batteries last about 5 years; then, the surgery must be repeated. Most patients with ICDs will not experience an arrhythmia

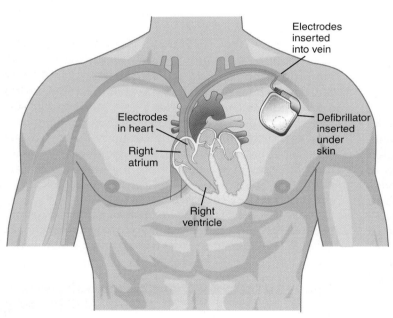

■ Figure 14.6

A defibrillator is a small metal box containing a battery, a computerized generator, and wires with sensors at their tips. The sensors detect the heart rate and rhythm and send data through the wires to the computer in the generator. If the heart rhythm is abnormal, the computer will direct the generator to send electrical pulses through the wires to regulate the heart. Pacemakers have one to three wires that are each placed in different chambers of the heart. The wires in a single-chamber pacemaker usually carry pulses from the generator to the right ventricle (the lower right chamber of your heart). The wires in a dual-chamber pacemaker carry pulses from the generator to the right atrium (the upper right chamber of your heart) and the right ventricle. The pulses help coordinate the timing of these two chambers' contractions. The wires in a biventricular pacemaker carry pulses from the generator to an atrium and both ventricles. The pulses help coordinate electrical signaling between the two ventricles. This type of pacemaker also is called a cardiac resynchronization therapy (CRT) device.

U.S. National Heart, Lung, and Blood Institute (https://www.nhlbi.nih.gov/health/health-topics/topics/pace/howdoes)

severe enough to trigger an electrical shock. But doctors still cannot distinguish with certainty those patients who definitely need an ICD from those who probably do not need one.

Regulating Blood Flow

To maintain uniform blood flow in the correct direction, the cardiovascular system is equipped with one-way valves both in the chambers of the heart and in blood vessels (**Figure 14.7**). With every heartbeat, the valves in the heart open and close to allow blood to move in one direction. In rare cases, one or more of the heart valves may be defective at birth because of developmental abnormalities. With modern techniques of open-heart surgery, defective heart valves can be repaired or replaced with artificial valves that allow the heart to function normally.

Rheumatic Heart Disease Heart valves can also be damaged by childhood throat infections caused by *Streptococcus* bacteria. Repeated streptococcal infections can cause **rheumatic heart disease** (formerly called rheumatic fever), a serious inflammatory disease of the heart valves. In susceptible people, the immune system overreacts to the presence of the bacteria. Some proteins on the heart cells are similar in structure to proteins on the bacteria, so the immune system attacks heart valve cells as well as the infectious bacteria.

The mitral and aortic valves are particularly susceptible to damage by infections. Scar tissue forms and prevents the valves from opening and closing correctly. By listening to the heartbeat, a **cardiologist**, a physician who specializes in heart diseases, can detect abnormalities in the heart's valves. Because of potential heart problems, it is important that all "strep throat" in children be treated with antibiotics to reduce the risk of developing rheumatic heart disease.

Varicose Veins Another common, but less serious, condition affecting the valves in the veins is **varicose veins**. These appear as bluish bulges in veins, usually in the legs. Blood returning to the heart from the legs has to flow against the pull of gravity, and one-way valves in the veins normally prevent the blood from draining downward. If the valves in the veins of the legs become weakened, blood tends to accumulate, distending the veins and producing visible varicose veins. The valve failures in the veins are not life-threatening and often can be corrected by surgical removal of the damaged areas.

Heart Failure

Heart failure (sometimes called *congestive heart failure*) is a condition of a heart too weakened by arrhythmia or other heart disease to pump

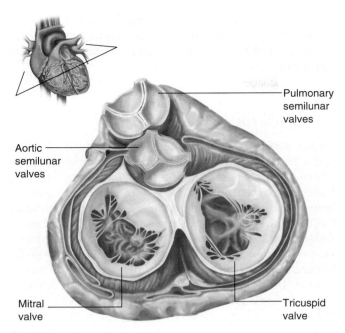

Pulmonary semilunar valves

Aortic semilunar valves

Mitral valve

Tricuspid valve

■ **Figure 14.7**

Heart Valves
The heart's valves keep the blood flowing in one direction into and out of the chambers of the heart.

sufficient blood throughout the body, even after the application of surgical and medical interventions. In this case a person experiences fatigue, diminished movement capacity, shortness of breath, and swelling (edema). The treatment for heart failure is a heart transplant. This involves being put on a waiting list and hoping that a suitable donor can be found among people who have died suddenly, such as victims of car accidents. The person with a failing heart must live and wait near a hospital where heart transplant surgeries are performed. If a suitable heart becomes available following a person's death, the donor's heart is removed and rushed to the recipient's hospital by a special medical team. Heart transplants are complex, costly, and not always successful. Still, about 2,000 heart transplants are performed in the United States each year. About 50% of heart recipients experience rejection of the new heart within the first year. All recipients must take immune-suppressive drugs for life to help prevent rejection of the transplanted heart by their own body's defenses.

Cardiopulmonary Resuscitation

Cardiopulmonary resuscitation (CPR) is hands-on emergency procedure administered to a person who has stopped breathing (e.g., near drowning), whose heart has suddenly stopped beating (sudden cardiac arrest), or who has had a heart attack and whose heart stops beating. Note that sudden cardiac arrest and heart attack

are not the same. A sudden heart attack occurs because the heart chambers are not beating in rhythm; heart attack is due to death of heart muscle. In either case, the heart become unable to pump blood throughout the body. Signs of cardiac arrest include an absence of heartbeats, blood flow, and pulse. When blood stops flowing to the brain, the person becomes unconscious and stops regular breathing.

CPR involves two actions by the person administering it: (1) mouth-to-mouth breathing, and (2) repeated, rapid, and vigorous compression of the chest. Automated external defibrillators (AEDs) are portable electronic devices that can administer a small electric shock to someone whose heart has stopped. AEDs are increasingly found in public places such as shopping malls, airports, police cars, theaters, sports arenas, public buildings, business offices, and on commercial airplanes.

Chest compressions force blood to circulate, which is critical to supplying vital organs and the brain with the oxygen remaining in the blood. Studies have shown that people who take a CPR training course can learn how to use a defibrillator in about 5 minutes and CPR in about 20 minutes.

The American Academy of Emergency Physicians (2015) recommends the following steps for administering CPR to adults. The steps are organized into "The ABCs of CPR"—Airway, Breathing, and Circulation—to help people remember the order in which to administer the steps.

Airway
Step 1: Check for responsiveness. Shake or tap the person gently. See if the person moves or makes a noise. Shout, "Are you OK?" No response: Call 911. Shout for help and send someone to call 911. If you are alone, call 911 and retrieve an AED (if available), even if you have to leave the person.

TERMS

cardiologist: a physician who specializes in diseases of the heart

cardiopulmonary resuscitation (CPR): an emergency lifesaving procedure used to revive someone who has stopped breathing or suffered cardiac arrest

heart failure: when the heart is weakened to the degree it cannot pump blood throughout the body

rheumatic heart disease: damage to heart valves from bacterial infection

varicose veins: swelling of veins (usually in the legs) resulting from defective valves

Step 2: Carefully place the person on their back. If there is a chance the person has a spinal injury, two people should move the person to prevent the head and neck from twisting. Once the airway is open, check to see if the person is breathing.

Breathing
Step 3: Place the person carefully on his or her back. Tilt the head back and lift the chin until the teeth almost touch. Look for signs of breathing.
Step 4: If the person is not breathing, pinch the nose and give the person two full breaths about two seconds long to produce a visible chest rise.

Circulation (Chest Compressions)
After giving two full breaths, immediately begin chest compressions (and cycles of compressions and rescue breaths). Do not take the time to locate the person's pulse to check for signs of blood circulation.
Step 5: Kneel at the person's side, near the chest. Place your hands in the center of the person's chest between the nipples. Place one hand on top of the other and with elbows locked press the heel of your hand into the chest.
Step 6: Give 30 hard, rapid compressions (about 100 per minute) for every two full breaths; repeat until medical help arrives or until the person starts breathing.

Immediate administration of CPR can double the chance of a person surviving sudden cardiac arrest. By making CPR rules simpler and easier to learn, it is hoped that more people will become proficient in the technique. For more information about CPR rules or to enroll in a CPR course, contact the American Heart Association at www.americanheart.org.

Infected Gums Contribute to Heart Disease

We all know that cleaning your teeth and gums prevents dental caries. Here is another strong reason for oral cleanliness. Some research has shown an association between infected gums and risk of heart disease. Bacteria found in the mouth have also been detected in the plaques that block arteries.

About one-half of all Americans over age 30 have gingivitis, a mild inflammation of the gums caused by oral bacteria; about one-third over age 30 have periodontitis, acute gum inflammation, and gum disease. (Smoking is a primary cause of this condition.) If your gums bleed when you brush or floss, see your dentist for treatment for gum disease. Maintaining oral health when you are young may also prevent heart disease later in life.

By performing Hands-Only CPR to the beat of the classic disco song "Stayin' Alive," you can double or even triple a victim's chance of survival. Learn the two easy steps to save a life at heart.org/handsonlycpr.

Atherosclerosis

Cardiovascular disease is the leading cause of death in the United States and many other countries. About 50% of those deaths are the result of **atherosclerosis**, a disease in which fibrous, fatty deposits, called **plaque**, form in the walls of one or more arteries (**Figure 14.8**). Plaques enlarge over time and ultimately slow or completely block the flow of blood in an artery, thereby harming the health of the tissues that the artery feeds. Atherosclerosis is most critical when it occurs in one or more of the four coronary arteries that carry blood in the heart itself and any artery that distributes blood in any part of the brain. Depriving heart tissue of blood can lead to death of the affected heart muscle, resulting in a heart attack. Depriving brain tissue of blood can lead to loss of neurological function (e.g., paralysis) or death from a stroke. Atherosclerosis is type of **arteriosclerosis** ("artery narrowing"), which refers to a thickening and stiffening of an artery's wall that results in a retardation of blood flow.

The development of atherosclerotic plaques in an artery is the result of three interconnected processes: (1) prior damage to an artery's wall from nicks and tears due to the force of blood flowing through it or from prior disease; (2) the deposition of excess cholesterol into the arterial wall, usually at the site of prior damage; and (3) inflammation, the process by which the immune system copes with the damage in the artery wall and the deposition of excess cholesterol.

Cholesterol is a waxy substance that has a number of vital functions in the body, including being a necessary structural component of cell membranes, a building block of several different hormones, and a precursor of bile salts. In one way or another, the body's cholesterol comes from food; about 20% from what is consumed in meals and about 80% that is manufactured primarily in the liver from dietary carbohydrates and fats. That the formation of atherosclerotic plaque involves the deposition of excess cholesterol in arteries is the reason that heathy diet recommendations include limiting foods high in cholesterol, saturated fat, trans fat, and sugar.

The liver determines the manufacture of much of the body's cholesterol and its distribution through the blood to tissues and organs when they need it. To facilitate the distribution process, cholesterol and another fat manufactured from dietary carbohydrate and fat, called triglyceride (TG), are packaged into small spherical particles called **lipoproteins**, which are able to transport them in the blood. Two types of lipoprotein particles are

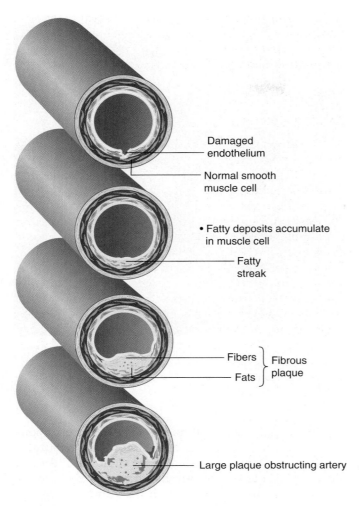

Damaged endothelium

Normal smooth muscle cell

• Fatty deposits accumulate in muscle cell

Fatty streak

Fibers ⎫ Fibrous
Fats ⎬ plaque

Large plaque obstructing artery

■ **Figure 14.8**

Development of an Atherosclerotic Lesion (Plaque) Inside an Artery
Plaque can eventually block blood flow, causing a heart attack or stroke. Many factors are involved in the formation of a plaque, including cholesterol and lipid levels, immune system cells, and inflammation.

fundamentally involved in the development of atherosclerosis: **high-density lipoproteins (HDL)** and **low-density lipoproteins (LDL)**. They have different functions that, in some sense, are opposite to one another. Other kinds of cholesterol-carrying particles also are found in the blood, but these are ultimately converted into LDL particles.

LDL Particles The cholesterol that becomes deposited in plaques that block arteries comes mainly from LDL particles. The LDL particles circulate in the blood to deliver cholesterol to tissues to build new cells or as building blocks for other biological chemicals. Any excess cholesterol is processed by the liver to maintain normal cholesterol levels in the blood. LDL receptors on the surface of liver cells bind LDL particles and remove them and the unused cholesterol from the blood. If the liver is overwhelmed with

LDL particles, however, it may not be able to process all of them. When that occurs, those LDL particles and their associated cholesterol circulate in the blood and may be deposited in the walls of arteries.

Furthermore, some LDL particles can get trapped in an arterial wall, at which point they can become chemically modified through a process called *oxidation*, and they also contribute to the formation of plaque. As the plaque grows in size, it can dislodge from the artery and block blood flow. Or, the plaque can break apart and cause a blood clot to form, which also can block the flow of blood in the artery. This is the reason LDL is called "bad cholesterol." This is one reason that LDL-lowering medications are employed to lower the risk of atherosclerosis.

HDL Particles. HDL particles are produced in the liver and intestines and are released into the bloodstream. As HDL particles circulate through the body, they pick up cholesterol and return it to the liver for removal. Thus, HDL particles in cells and arteries scavenge excess cholesterol from the blood and arteries, thereby reducing the buildup of plaques. This is the reason HDL is called "good cholesterol."

An example of the body's inability to process cholesterol are persons with an inherited disease called **familial hyperlipidemia (FH)**, which results in markedly elevated levels of cholesterol in the blood. People with this disease have two defective genes, one inherited from each unaffected parent. The normal forms of these genes are responsible for synthesizing LDL receptor proteins on liver cells that bind LDL particles and remove cholesterol from the blood. As a result of their defective genes, people with FH cannot synthesize these essential LDL receptor proteins. Cholesterol cannot be

TERMS

arteriosclerosis: hardening of the arteries

atherosclerosis: a disease process in which fatty deposits (plaques) build up in the arteries and block the flow of blood

familial hyperlipidemia (FH): an inherited disease causing extremely high levels of cholesterol in the blood

high-density lipoprotein (HDL): the carrier of cholesterol from tissues to the liver for removal from the circulation; carrier of "good" cholesterol

lipoproteins: spherical particles that transport cholesterol and fat (TG) in the blood

low-density lipoprotein (LDL): the carrier of "bad" cholesterol in blood

plaque: deposit of fatty substances in the inner lining of arteries

removed and processed in the liver, and it accumulates to exceptionally high levels in the blood. This leads to the formation of plaque that blocks arteries. People with this disease usually have heart attacks at an early age. In a few cases, transplant of a normal liver has successfully reversed the effects of FH.

Measuring Cholesterol Levels One way doctors assess a person's risk for heart and blood vessel disease due to atherosclerosis is to measure the levels of total cholesterol, LDL cholesterol, HDL cholesterol, and triglyceride (TG) in the blood from a standard blood test. These measurements are reported as milligrams per deciliter (1/10th of a liter) of blood. The interpretations of the results of a cholesterol blood test are presented in the Wellness Guide "How to Interpret Blood Cholesterol and Lipid Measurements." Often a physician will counsel someone with high blood cholesterol, high LDL-cholesterol, and/or low HDL cholesterol to adopt lifestyle habits to lessen the risk of heart disease posed by those results or suggest medication, such as statins.

Cholesterol and lipid levels in the blood are measured in various ways. Total cholesterol levels are measured in milligrams per deciliter (mg/dl) of blood. Generally, a cholesterol level below 200 mg/dl indicates a relatively low risk of coronary heart disease (CHD); 240 mg/dl or higher doubles the risk of CHD. Blood cholesterol values between 200 and 239 mg/dl indicate moderate and increasing risk of CHD. However, the total cholesterol level may not be a reliable indicator of cardiovascular disease risk because the level of HDL in the blood is also important and can modify the risk inherent in high cholesterol levels.

For example, a cholesterol level of 240 might not be considered dangerous when the HDL level is also high. Generally, if the ratio of the total cholesterol divided by the HDL level is about 4.5, the risk is said to be average. A ratio above 4.5 increases the risk of heart disease; a ratio below 4.5 reduces it. The various numbers used to establish the risk of heart disease are quite confusing, but the general rules are explained in the Wellness Guide feature on interpreting blood cholesterol and lipid measurements.

Extensive research has shown a strong association between blood cholesterol levels and coronary heart disease: The higher the blood cholesterol level, the greater the risk of all forms of cardiovascular disease. However, the amount of cholesterol in the diet is not always a good predictor of heart disease. For example, the French enjoy a diet laden with eggs, meats, and fats. They have cholesterol levels that, on average, are much higher than those of Americans. Yet the French die of heart disease at less than half the rate observed in the United States (sometimes called the "French paradox"). A dramatic example of cholesterol metabolism is that of an 88-year-old man who had eaten 25 eggs a day for more than 15 years and yet had completely normal blood cholesterol levels (Kern, 1991).

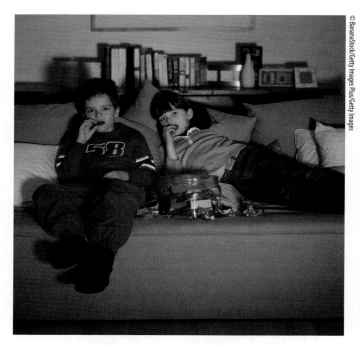

Risk factors for cardiovascular disease include cigarette smoking, high blood pressure, high blood cholesterol, sedentary lifestyle, overweight, and excessive alcohol consumption.

Other epidemiological studies show that populations vary greatly in the level of cholesterol that constitutes a risk for CHD. People with a blood cholesterol level of 200 in the United States are five times as likely to die of CHD as people in Japan with the same cholesterol levels. People in southern Europe are also at a relatively low risk for a heart attack, even when their cholesterol level is above 250 mg/dl. Atherosclerosis is primarily a disease of modern, industrialized societies. Tribal people in New Guinea, Kung tribes in Africa, and Inuit in Greenland have a low incidence of cardiovascular disease. Tarahumara Indians in Mexico have virtually no heart disease or high blood pressure as long as they consume their native diet. However, when researchers switched a group of Tarahumara Indian volunteers to a typical American diet, they gained weight and had dramatic increases in lipid and cholesterol levels in their blood (McMurry et al., 1991).

Cholesterol, Statins, and Inflammation

Statins are types of drugs that dramatically reduce the level of blood cholesterol. Statins are among the top-selling prescription drugs in the world. Statins act by inhibiting an enzyme (HMG-CoA reductase) in liver cells that manufactures cholesterol, so production of cholesterol by the body is markedly reduced. Another benefit of statins is that, by blocking the production of cholesterol, they force the liver to increase production of the receptors on liver cells that bind LDL cholesterol. This aids the removal of excess cholesterol

How to Interpret Blood Cholesterol and Lipid Measurements

In evaluating your risk of heart and artery disease, the level of four different "fat" molecules are measured: cholesterol, high-density lipoprotein (HDL), triglycerides, and low-density lipoprotein (LDL). The range of values for each is indicated below.

Cholesterol

- Below 200 mg/dl: Safe, unless the HDL level is below 35 mg/dl.
- 200 to 239 mg/dl: Borderline high. If you have other risk factors for heart disease, such as high blood pressure or an HDL level below 35 mg/dl, then you are at risk and some corrective action is needed.
- Above 240 mg/dl: High. Further tests are needed; dietary changes, as well as drugs to lower the level, may be recommended.

High-Density Lipoprotein

- 35 mg/dl: Low. Exercise and other steps may be needed to raise the level. Women generally have higher levels of HDL than men do.
- 35 to 60 mg/dl: Considered protective, especially if cholesterol levels are below 240.

Triglycerides

- Below 200 mg/dl: Considered normal range.
- 200 to 400 mg/dl: Borderline high.
- Above 400 mg/dl: High. Dietary changes recommended.

Low-Density Lipoprotein

LDL is not measured directly, but levels are calculated according to the following formula:

$$LDL = \text{Total cholesterol} - HDL - (\text{Triglycerides}/5)$$

Using this formula, an LDL value below 130 is considered safe; a value above 160 is considered high, and lipid-lowering drugs may be prescribed. However, even this formula does not satisfy all the experts, some of whom believe that the ratio of LDL to HDL is the really significant measure of risk for heart disease.

---

from the circulation. People with high cholesterol levels (hypercholesterolemia) respond to treatment with statins by a marked reduction in their blood cholesterol levels. First introduced in 1987, statin drugs are among the most prescribed drugs in the world; in the United States alone, drug companies earn more than $20 billion annually from statin sales. More than 40 million Americans over age 18 now take a statin drug to reduce the risk of dying from a heart attack (Beil, 2017). Once you have been prescribed a statin drug to reduce your cholesterol and triglyceride blood levels, it is assumed that you will take them for the remainder of your life. But the benefits and risks of taking a statin differ for each patient, and many physicians are much more cautious about prescribing a statin, especially for a young adult.

Although most people taking a statin drug experience relatively minor and manageable side effects, a significant number suffer severe and permanent liver or muscle damage. Another significant side effect of statins is neurological impairment; many users report symptoms of memory loss and reduced cognitive functioning, a kind of fuzzy thinking that affects a person's ability to concentrate on an idea or task. Cholesterol levels rise with age, so a majority of people using statins are elderly and may already have some problems with memory loss and thinking clearly and quickly. Given the uncertainty about what level of blood cholesterol actually increases the risk of heart disease, each person who is prescribed a statin drug needs to carefully weigh the benefits and risks. Because taking a statin often is for life, caution is advised, especially if cholesterol levels are not excessively high.

Besides high cholesterol, plaques in arteries can cause inflammation, an immune system response to tissue injury and damage. Studies show that a particular protein in blood (**C-reactive protein, CRP**) rises when inflammation is present. Some studies show that people with more advanced coronary artery disease have higher levels of CRP. However, many factors affect the level of CRP in the circulation (e.g., smoking, infections, inflammatory diseases) so it is not a perfect indicator for the risk of heart disease or a heart attack. Nevertheless, statins reduce the level of C-reactive protein in the blood, an indication of their therapeutic activity is anti-inflammatory.

According to the U.S. National Heart, Lung, and Blood Institute (2017), several lifestyle habits and biological conditions constitute risk factors for developing atherosclerosis and its high risk of heart attack and stroke. Many of these risk factors can be modified by adopting healthy behaviors and others can be modified by adhering to competent medical preventive treatment (**Table 14.3**).

TERMS

statins: a class of drugs that block synthesis of cholesterol in the liver and reduce the amount of cholesterol in the blood

C-reactive protein (CRP): a protein in blood that is a measure of chronic inflammation and risk of a heart attack

Table 14.3

Risk Factors for Atherosclerosis

Risk Factor	Reason
High LDL cholesterol ("bad" cholesterol)	Increased plaque development and plaque inflammation
Low HDL cholesterol ("good" cholesterol)	Decreased plaque removal
High blood triglycerides (TG)	Increased blood LDL-cholesterol
High blood pressure	Damages blood vessels
Tobacco smoking	Damages and narrows blood vessels, raises cholesterol levels, raises blood pressure
Prediabetes/diabetes	Unable to regulate the body's blood sugar level resulting in impaired fat metabolism
Overweight or obesity	Contributes to high levels of LDL ("bad cholesterol") and triglycerides
Lack of physical activity	Lowers HDL and contributes to high LDL cholesterol, high triglycerides, high blood pressure, overweight, and diabetes
Unhealthy diet	Foods that are high in saturated and *trans* fats, cholesterol, sodium (salt), and sugar can worsen other atherosclerosis risk factors
Older age	Over time, arteries undergo damage; plaque can increase over time
Genetics	Certain genetic diseases can cause high cholesterol or high TG
High C-reactive protein	Sign of inflammation in the body due to damage to blood vessels, a risk for plaque formation
Sleep apnea	A risk for high blood pressure
Stress	Increases bodily inflammation
Heavy drinking	Damages the heart muscle

U.S. National Heart, Lung, and Blood Institute. (2015). Atherosclerosis. https://www.nhlbi.nih.gov/health-topics/atherosclerosis

Coronary Heart Disease and Heart Attack

Despite its relatively small size among the body's organs, the heart utilizes about 20% of the oxygenated blood circulated throughout the body. This is because the heart continually works, day and night, and needs considerable energy and nutrients to do so.

Oxygen and nutrients are supplied to the heart through the four small coronary arteries that branch off the aorta, the body's main, and largest, artery. If one or more of the coronary arteries becomes blocked by plaque, heart muscle cells may not get enough oxygen and nutrients to function properly, and those cells may die. The death of a large number of cells can cause the heart to stop functioning—a heart attack. A mild to moderate heart attack may not be fatal, unlike a massive heart attack, which usually is.

If a heart attack has occurred, the levels of certain proteins in the blood, such as creatine kinase, troponin, myoglobin, and myosin, begin to change. Measuring the levels of these proteins allows physicians in emergency rooms (ERs) to determine quickly whether a heart attack has occurred and to initiate appropriate treatment.

If the coronary arteries become partially blocked and the heart cells do not get enough oxygen, chest pain called **angina pectoris** results. The drug nitroglycerin dilates blood vessels and is used to relieve the pain of angina. If a plaque ruptures and a coronary artery becomes completely blocked, the person may have a fatal heart attack.

Each year in the United States about a million people are admitted to hospitals because of possible heart attacks. Tests eventually rule out a heart attack in about 50% of those admitted. Chest pains that mimic those of a heart attack can be brought on by severe indigestion (heartburn), panic, and stress.

Repairing Blocked Coronary Arteries

To determine whether, or to what extent coronary arteries are blocked by plaque or blood clots, a precise image of the flow of blood through the coronary arteries that supply blood to the heart can be obtained by a procedure called **cardiac catheterization**. A thin tube is threaded from an artery in a leg or arm up into the heart's coronary arteries. A dye is injected, and high-speed x-ray film records the flow of the dye in the arteries to visualize any blockage. Several million cardiac

Concussion to the Heart

Most everyone knows what a brain concussion is—a blow to the head that may cause unconsciousness, problems in mental functioning, and headaches for weeks or months after the concussion. Concussions are frequent in contact sports such as football, and NFL quarterbacks Troy Aikman and Steve Young were forced to retire after each suffered a series of concussions.

A blow to the left side of the chest caused by a punch, thrown baseball, hockey puck, or other object may cause a concussion to the heart that is medically known as *commotio cordis*. Such a blow, even a light blow, if delivered at a very precise moment during the rhythmic beating of the heart, can induce instant fibrillation (irregular heartbeat) and sudden death. Cases of *commotio cordis* are rare. Only about 130 cases have been reported in the United States (Maron et al., 2005), but sports medicine experts suspect that many more go unreported. Unfortunately, only about 15% of affected persons—most of whom are children—survive. Sports carrying the highest risk of sudden death from *commotio cordis* are baseball, softball, and hockey.

Use of chest protectors and softer balls can reduce the risk of *commotio cordis* in some sports, especially among children and young athletes. Also, never punch or poke anyone in the chest.

Coronary Artery Bypass Graft

High-tech surgical procedures, such as coronary artery bypass graft (CABG, pronounced "cabbage"), angioplasty, and pacemaker implantation, have revolutionized the treatment of coronary heart disease (CHD). Although these surgeries prevent some heart attacks and save lives, in many instances they are performed for heart conditions such as angina (chest pain) that can be controlled with medications.

In the 1950s, angina from partially blocked coronary arteries was relieved by an operation in which a chest artery was tied off in the hope that more blood would be supplied to the patient's heart. About 40% of the patients had reduced pain following this operation. To determine whether the relief of angina pain was a placebo

Block in left coronary artery

• Once bypass is performed, this blocked section is removed

Saphenous vein graft to right coronary artery

Aorta

Pulmonary artery

Saphenous vein graft to left coronary artery

Diagram of the coronary arteries showing where grafts are made to correct blockages.

effect or actually resulted from the surgery, a number of mock operations were performed. (In the 1950s, informed consent was not mandatory in most hospitals.) Patients were given anesthesia, the chest was cut open, but nothing else was done to correct blood flow to the heart. Patients who underwent mock surgeries had just as much relief from angina as patients who had the chest artery tied off (Frank, 1973). As a result, this operation was abandoned.

In a similar fashion, coronary artery bypass operations may relieve angina as a result of the long period of rest and recuperation that patients undergo; lifestyle changes that people make also may contribute to their relief. A large part of the success of bypass surgery may be a result of a placebo effect.

catheterizations are performed each year in the United States on patients with suspected partial blockage of their coronary arteries.

When medical tests show that one or more coronary arteries are blocked, several medical procedures are available to remove the blockage. Two effective procedures are **coronary artery bypass graft (CABG)** and **percutaneous transluminal coronary angioplasty (PTCA)**.

Coronary Artery Bypass Graft Coronary artery bypass graft (CABG) is **open heart surgery**. The patient is fully anesthetized and the chest is surgically opened to expose the heart. Tubes are connected to the blood vessels leading to and from the heart so that blood can be diverted around the heart and through a mechanical pump. A part of a healthy artery or vein is removed from its normal site in the body and its ends are connected, or grafted, to the blocked coronary artery. When in place, the graft allows blood to flow around (bypass) the blocked portion of the coronary artery, creating a new path for oxygen-rich blood to flow to the heart muscle. Usually CABG is performed if three or all four of the coronary arteries are blocked ("triple" or "quadruple" bypass). About 250,000 CABG procedures are performed each year in the United States.

Although effective in restoring normal blood flow to the heart, coronary artery bypass surgery carries the risk of brain damage and cognitive loss. Stroke is the most serious complication, occurring in 1% to 6% of patients undergoing bypass surgery. Many patients also notice some loss of both short- and long-term memory.

Percutaneous Transluminal Coronary Angioplasty (PTCA) In contrast to CABG, which is an open-heart surgical procedure, percutaneous transluminal coronary angioplasty (PTCA), or simply *angioplasty*, is nonsurgical and much less invasive.

In this procedure, a thin wire is threaded from the femoral artery in the thigh up to the point of blockage in a coronary artery. Another thin tube containing a deflated balloon is then slipped over the wire and threaded up to the area of the arterial plaque. The balloon is inflated and

TERMS

angina pectoris: medical term for chest pain caused by coronary heart disease; a condition in which the heart muscle doesn't receive enough blood, resulting in chest pain

cardiac catheterization: visualization of blocked coronary arteries by using a catheter and monitoring blood flow in coronary arteries; a dye is injected through the catheter

coronary artery bypass graft (CABG): surgery to improve blood supply to the heart muscle by replacing the damaged portion of the blocked artery with a graft

open-heart surgery: surgery performed on the opened heart while the blood supply is diverted through a heart–lung machine

percutaneous transluminal coronary angioplasty (PTCA): a procedure to open blocked arteries

pushes the plaque back into the wall of the artery, thereby opening it up. Angioplasty costs about half as much as a bypass operation, but the frequency with which the blockage recurs is higher, making a repeat procedure more likely.

An alternative to balloon angioplasty for clogged coronary arteries is a procedure called *stenting*. This procedure also involves inserting a catheter into a blood vessel in an arm or leg and threading it to the point of blockage in either a coronary artery or the carotid artery in the neck. If a blockage is found, an object called a stent is inserted that props the artery open.

Stenting has become widely used because it is simpler, cheaper, and safer than bypass surgery. However, there are still questions as to whether bypass surgery or stenting is better for long-term survival. The original stents inserted into arteries consisted of bare metal. In a large number of patients, the stents and arteries often became blocked again within months or years, and the procedure had to be repeated. Now, drug-eluting stents are used that slowly release a drug that helps prevent the artery from becoming blocked again. Life-threatening blood clots can develop in some patients with drug-eluting stents implanted in one or more arteries. Some studies indicate that for partial arterial blockage, drugs alone are safer and more effective than surgical insertion of drug-eluting stents.

All procedures for opening blocked heart and carotid arteries have similar rates of success and long-term survival. The particular procedure that is recommended for an individual patient depends on many factors, including the number of arteries blocked, the age of the patient, other complicating diseases, and economic circumstances. Also, recent major technological advances in surgical procedures have increased survival rates and reduced complications. A large study published in 2016 showed that long-term survival was better with bypass surgery compared to angioplasty or stenting in comparable groups of patients (Alexander & Smith, 2016). Largely due to this finding, it is predicted that bypass surgeries will increase in the United States in the coming years, reaching 8 million annually by the year 2030. Unless Americans reduce their exposure to known heart disease risk factors, this prediction will likely be accurate.

Some American physicians question whether every coronary artery bypass and other surgeries really are always necessary. In Canada and Great Britain, where far fewer of these surgeries are performed, patients with cardiovascular disease live just as long. While not as profitable for hospitals and surgeons, in many instances lifestyle changes and appropriate medicines may be as effective, safer, and less costly than surgery in treating cardiovascular disease.

Until recently, it was medical dogma that atherosclerosis was a progressive and irreversible disease. However, clinical studies involving patients with partially blocked arteries have shown that the blockages can be improved through lifestyle changes and that this entrenched medical view is incorrect (Ornish et al., 1998). Patients who are motivated and who change their lifestyle can improve the health of their arteries and avoid surgery. However, most patients with blocked arteries still opt for the quick fix of surgery, even though, for many, it is only a temporary solution to their cardiovascular problems because arteries often become blocked again within a few years after surgery. Many physicians still feel obligated to perform bypass surgery or stenting for fear of being sued for not recommending the standard and accepted medical treatment. Thus, heart and artery surgeries probably will continue to be performed excessively in our society until views change.

Stroke

Stroke, also called *brain attack*, is the third leading cause of death in the United States, after heart disease and cancer. As with the latter two diseases, stroke is, in many cases, a preventable disease. High blood pressure is the greatest risk factor and plays a role in at least 70% of all strokes.

Stroke is a form of cardiovascular disease that affects arteries supplying blood to the brain. If a brain artery becomes blocked or ruptures, brain cells die within minutes from lack of oxygen. Parts of the body whose functions depend on these damaged areas in the brain consequently are affected. Thus, a person who has a stroke can lose the ability to speak or to see, become paralyzed in an arm or leg, or lose the use of one whole side of the body. Strokes can result from injuries to the head or from weak spots in the arteries called **aneurysms** that balloon out and rupture. Strokes also can result when the heartbeat is weak and the heart does not pump enough blood through the arteries to the brain. The effects of strokes vary greatly, ranging from mild or unnoticed symptoms to sudden death.

Two main classes of stroke are ischemic stroke and hemorrhagic stroke. *Ischemic stroke* results when one or more blood vessels in the brain become blocked due to a clot in an artery in the brain or in one leading to the brain. *Hemorrhagic stroke* results when a blood vessel in the brain ruptures, which also deprives brain cells of oxygen.

The warning signs of a stroke are any of the following conditions that occur suddenly. Immediate medical attention is needed if any of these symptoms of stroke occur:

- Sudden weakness or numbness of the face, arm, or leg on one side of the body
- Sudden dimness or loss of vision, especially in one eye
- Loss of speech, difficulty understanding speech, or trouble talking
- Sudden, severe headaches with no known cause
- Unexplained unsteadiness, dizziness, or sudden falls, especially with one of the other symptoms

Some patients at risk for strokes may benefit from a surgical procedure called **carotid endarterectomy** that removes fatty deposits by inserting a stent in a clogged artery in the neck. These arteries supply blood to the brain and, if they become blocked, may cause a stroke. Blocked neck arteries can be detected by listening to the blood flow with a stethoscope and can be confirmed by an ultrasound scan. The principal danger of the surgery is that it may precipitate a stroke—the very thing that it is designed to prevent.

The best way to prevent a stroke is to reduce the risk factors. There are five controllable risk factors for a stroke: (1) high blood pressure; (2) heart disease; (3) cigarette smoking; (4) transient ischemic attacks; and (5) high red blood cell count, which thickens the blood and facilitates formation of a clot. These risk factors can, for the most part, be controlled by lifestyle changes or medications or both. Risk factors for a stroke that cannot be changed include (1) increasing age, (2) being male, (3) race, (4) diabetes mellitus, (5) prior stroke, and (6) heredity.

High Blood Pressure (Hypertension)

Approximately 32% of Americans 18 years of age or older have high blood pressure (**hypertension**); among African American men and women the rate is more than 45%, among the highest in the world. In the United States and all industrialized countries, the risk of high blood pressure increases with age. About 7% of people 30 years old have high blood pressure; this rises to 50% among people 50 years old. However, hypertension is not inevitable. People who are strict vegetarians and who have low-salt diets are hardly ever diagnosed with high blood pressure as they age. About a third of individuals with high blood pressure are unaware that their blood pressure is high. Consequently, they also are unaware that they are at risk for heart disease, kidney disease, and stroke.

This is why hypertension is often called the "silent killer." When the cause of high blood pressure cannot be determined medically, it is referred to as **essential (primary) hypertension**. Essential hypertension accounts for more than 90% of cases of high blood pressure. The remaining cases of high blood pressure are associated with of a recognizable problem, such as a kidney abnormality, congenital defect of the aorta, or adrenal gland tumor. This type of high blood pressure is called **secondary hypertension**. Generally, when the cause of secondary hypertension is determined and corrected, blood pressure returns to normal.

High blood pressure may be caused by psychosocial factors, although the mechanisms by which these factors could cause it are not understood. For example, people with low income and poor education are at higher risk for high blood pressure. Being poor or jobless may generate stress and raise blood pressure. African and Hispanic Americans have a higher prevalence of high blood pressure than white Americans. The stress of being a member of a minority group may also increase the risk of high blood pressure and heart disease (Dolezsan, 2014). Hypertension is a disease of modern societies; even today remote tribes in New Guinea or in the forests of Brazil do not develop hypertension.

Blood pressure is a measurement of the force with which the heart pushes blood through the circulatory system. Blood pressure is a very important indicator of the health of the cardiovascular system, which is the reason doctors measure it often. A person's blood pressure is measured using an instrument that records how high in millimeters, abbreviated mm, the blood pressure can lift a column of liquid mercury, abbreviated Hg. Thus, blood pressure is measured and recorded in terms of millimeters of mercury, or mm Hg.

Each time the heart contracts, blood is pumped through the arteries and exerts pressure on the arterial walls (**Figure 14.9**). In fact, there are two pressures that are measured. The maximum pressure in the arteries occurs when the heart contracts (**systole**), pumping blood from the heart to the lungs and body. Between contractions, the blood pressure falls (**diastole**) as blood flows from one chamber of the heart to another. Healthy blood pressure is 120/80 mm Hg (systole/diastole). People with a systolic pressure of 120 to 129 mm Hg and a diastolic pressure of 80 mm Hg or less have *elevated blood pressure*. People with a systolic pressure between 130 and 139 mm Hg or diastolic between 80 and 89 mm Hg have *stage 1 hypertension*. Most of these individuals will have further increases in blood pressure until eventually they will need to be treated for high blood pressure, which is systolic blood pressure higher than 130 mm Hg and/or diastolic blood pressure higher than 80 mm Hg.

High blood pressure can be lowered by making certain changes in lifestyle. Overweight and overeating are major risk factors that can be changed; increasing physical exercise also is required to reduce hypertension. Moderating salt and alcohol consumption also is beneficial. And ensuring that you are obtaining an adequate amount of potassium (eat more bananas) will also reduce blood pressure.

Tiny receptors in the walls of the arteries respond to changes in blood pressure. If blood pressure rises, these receptors send nerve signals to relax the arteries and to

---

TERMS

aneurysm: a ballooning out of a vein or artery

blood pressure: measurement of the force with which the heart pushes blood through the circulatory system

carotid endarterectomy: removal of fatty deposits in arteries in the neck to prevent a stroke

diastole: the pressure in the arteries when the heart relaxes (the lower number)

essential (primary) hypertension: high blood pressure that is not caused by any observable disease

hypertension: high blood pressure

secondary hypertension: high blood pressure caused by a recognizable disease

systole: the pressure in the arteries when the heart contracts (the higher number)

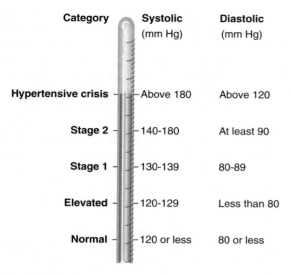

■ **Figure 14.9**

Stages of High Blood Pressure

According to current guidelines, normal blood pressure is less than 120/80 mm Hg (systole/diastole). High blood pressure (hypertension) is defined in four stages, the risk of heart disease being greater the higher the blood pressure. Weight loss, exercise, not smoking, and stress reduction are recommended ways to control hypertension at earlier stages; drugs may also be necessary at later stages.

Breathing Exercise to Reduce Hypertension

Breathing exercises are often the most efficient way to reduce stress and lower blood pressure. There are many forms of breathing exercises, ranging from simple to complicated. The following breathing exercise is a simple and effective way to reduce stress and lower blood pressure.

1. Sit comfortably upright in a chair.
2. Exhale through your mouth as completely as possible.
3. Close your mouth and breathe in through your nose slowly to a count of four. Use abdominal breathing.
4. Hold your breath for a count of seven or as long as you can.
5. Exhale slowly through your mouth to a count of eight.
6. Repeat this cycle three more times, and then stop and breathe normally.

Practice at least twice a day every day. The cycle can be increased slightly as the exercise becomes easier over time.

slow the heartbeat, thus returning blood pressure to normal levels. However, these regulatory mechanisms can be overcome by signals from the brain. Arteries can be constricted and blood pressure raised by thoughts and emotions. Fear, tension, anger, and anxiety activate the sympathetic nervous system, which sends signals to the arteries, causing them to constrict. If one's life is overly stressful or full of anger and frustration, arteries may stay constricted and blood pressure remains elevated.

Although drugs are the most effective means of controlling hypertension, mental relaxation techniques are also effective. By using biofeedback equipment that displays blood pressure values, some people learned how to develop mental relaxation states that lowered their blood pressure. In fact, some studies suggest that a variety of relaxation techniques are effective in lowering blood pressure in hypertensive patients.

Hypertension is a serious cardiovascular disease, responsible for many deaths. It can damage the heart muscle such that the heart cannot function properly or at all (heart failure). It also can cause the heart muscle to thicken, making it difficult for the heart to fill with enough blood to supply the body's organs, especially during exercise. And it can cause atherosclerosis in the coronary arteries, resulting in diminished blood flow to the heart muscle. High blood pressure can damage blood vessels, causing bulges that may burst (aneurysms), and diseases of the kidneys, brain (stroke and cognitive decline), eyes, and legs (peripheral artery disease).

Healthy lifestyle habits can help prevent high blood pressure and reduce it once it has begun. These habits include healthy eating, such as following the Dietary

Approaches to Stop Hypertension (DASH) diet, decreasing salt intake, increasing potassium intake, eating foods that are heart healthy, being physically active, maintaining a healthy body weight, limiting alcohol consumption, and managing and coping with stress. To develop a health habit, make one healthy lifestyle change at a time and add another change when you feel that you have successfully adopted the earlier changes.

Blood pressure medicines work in different ways. Some flush excess sodium from the body, which reduces the amount of fluid in the blood and helps to lower blood pressure. Others lower blood pressure by helping the heart beat slower and with less force. Still others relax the walls of blood vessels. To lower and control blood pressure, many people take two or more medicines. If you have side effects from your medicines, don't stop taking your medicines. Instead, talk with your healthcare provider about the side effects to see if the dose can be changed or a new medicine prescribed.

Hypertension is responsible for more deaths worldwide than any other condition, including tobacco use, obesity, and atherosclerosis. Researchers have hypothesized that psychological stress is an important risk factor for essential hypertension, primarily daily stress, such as that experienced at work, in family relationships, and through racial discrimination.

The Metabolic Syndrome

A model that pulls together many of the factors that are shared by people at risk for diabetes, cardiovascular disease, and heart attacks is called the **metabolic syndrome**. A person with three or more of the following risk factors is defined as having metabolic syndrome:

- Waist circumference greater than 40 inches for men and 35 inches for women
- Elevated triglyceride level of 150 mg/dl or greater

Home Blood Pressure Monitors and Internet Consultations to Help Patients Reduce Hypertension

High blood pressure is the leading reversible risk factor for heart attacks and brain attacks. For people with high blood pressure, a 10-mm reduction in systolic blood pressure means a 30% to 40% reduced risk of dying from a heart attack or brain attack. Despite effective therapies for reducing high blood pressure, efforts to do so are largely unsuccessful. Physicians who diagnose high blood pressure in patients usually recommend lifestyle changes if people smoke, are overweight, or do not exercise. Medications are also prescribed that are very effective in lowering blood pressure to more acceptable levels. Yet, fewer than a third of patients with high blood pressure achieve goals for lower blood pressure. A new strategy is to supply patients with a home blood pressure monitor with which to take frequent measurements. They also are supplied with an Internet site where their progress is monitored and questions answered by a health professional.

It is hoped that increased patient involvement with controlling their high blood pressure will increase the number of patients who successfully lower their blood pressure and thus their risk of cardiovascular disease.

- High-density lipoprotein (HDL) level of 40 mg/dl or lower for men and 50 mg/dl or lower for women
- Fasting blood glucose level of 100 mg/dl or higher (hyperglycemia)
- High blood pressure (130/85 mm Hg or higher)

A national survey indicated that 6.7% of participants between the ages of 20 and 29 met the criteria for metabolic syndrome. The prevalence increased to 43.5% for participants aged 60 to 69 years. Because of the enormous number of people with metabolic syndrome in the United States who are at high risk of diabetes, cardiovascular disease, and premature death, metabolic syndrome is regarded as a pressing public health problem. Despite the fancy techno name, metabolic syndrome is really the result of poor lifestyles—smoking, overeating and overweight, lack of exercise, and poor diet.

Lifestyle Factors and Cardiovascular Disease

About 37% of the 2.6 million American deaths each year are due to cardiovascular disease (CVD), principally coronary heart disease (CHD) and stroke, both of which are manifestations of atherosclerosis. About 50% of those deaths are preventable by adopting healthy behaviors that not only enrich life but also reduce the risk of debilitation and suffering from a preventable chronic illness (Patel, 2015).

Researchers studied the effect of seven lifestyle factors on the risk of death from cardiovascular disease in nearly 45,000 Americans (Yang et al., 2012). The healthy lifestyle factors were ones that had been previously identified as being heart-healthy. They included not smoking tobacco, engaging in more than 150 minutes a week of movement activity, not being overweight, consuming a healthy diet, having healthy levels of total blood cholesterol, and maintaining normal blood pressure and blood sugar levels. Analysis of the research determined that only 25% of the people in the study population exhibited five or more healthy lifestyle factors; 8% exhibited none or only one. The study also found that those who lived most healthfully had less cardiovascular disease and lived the longest (**Figure 14.10**).

Tobacco Smoking

Principally through the process of oxidation and the inflammation that follows, the chemicals in tobacco smoke can damage blood cells, blood vessels, and the heart itself. Damage to cardiovascular tissue increases the risk of atherosclerosis, a major contributor to coronary heart disease, chest pain, heart attack, arrhythmias, heart failure, and even death. Smoking is also a major risk factor for peripheral artery disease and subsequent risk of stroke and clogging of blood vessels in other organs and the limbs.

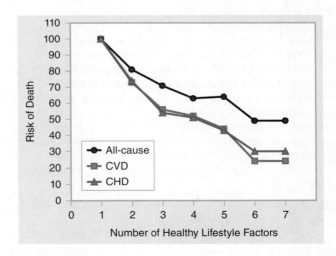

■ Figure 14.10

Association of Maintaining Healthy Lifestyle Factors on the Risk of Cardiovascular Disease

Living healthfully lessens the risk of death from all cardiovascular disease, coronary heart disease, and all causes. The healthy lifestyle factors include not smoking tobacco, more than 150 minutes a week of movement activity, not being overweight, consuming a healthy diet, healthy levels of total blood cholesterol, normal blood pressure, and a normal blood sugar level.

Yang et al., 2012.

TERMS

metabolic syndrome: a model embracing five risk factors that puts people who have at least three risk factors at risk for cardiovascular disease, diabetes, and premature death

Cardiovascular Fitness: Exercise Your Heart

The heart is a large bundle of muscle fibers that coordinate to act as a highly efficient pump. With every contraction and relaxation cycle, the heart pumps oxygen-laden blood to every organ in the body. You never have to think about it—the heart does its job automatically, day after day, year after year, until life ends.

We hear a lot about the need for physical activity but not much about exercising the heart itself. Of course, when you engage in vigorous physical exercise ("breathe hard and sweat") you also exercise your heart muscle because your heart rate increases and the heart muscle works harder to provide oxygen to exercising body muscles. However, it's possible to be physically active without working the heart very much. This is especially true for people who are busy with work, family, and other obligations, and for whom time for recreational exercise all but disappears. Also, as people approach old age many simply slow down, although many have more time to exercise after retirement.

It is well documented that cardiovascular fitness is essential to reducing the risk of cardiovascular disease. To attain cardiovascular fitness, one should exercise several times a week to the point of increasing the heart rate close to the maximum for one's age. This can be accomplished by biking, jogging (road or treadmill), or walking vigorously. It may also be helpful to create an image visualization for exercise:

See the blood leave your heart and flow rapidly through your arteries and veins. The blood is moving so forcefully and fast that it scours the linings of the blood vessels, cleansing them of any debris and deposits that might clog them.

Think of it as "power washing" the cardiovascular system, especially the heart muscle and coronary and pulmonary arteries. Go! Then slow down for a bit to let your heart rate return to normal, and then go again to increase your heart rate.

Stopping smoking at any time can reverse many of the harmful physiological effects of tobacco on the cardiovascular system. After several years of not smoking, ex-smokers have about the same risk of cardiovascular disease as nonsmokers. One key to protecting your heart is not smoking and not living or working in a smoke-filled environment.

Physical Activity

Moving the body regularly—even for just a few minutes a day—makes people feel better, gives them more energy, reduces anxiety and depression, and lessens cravings for alcohol, cigarettes, and junk food.

Moreover, 150 minutes per week of movement activity, be it recreational exercise, work-related movement, housework, or active transportation (walking, biking), can significantly reduce the risk of cardiovascular disease and death from heart attack, stroke, heart failure, and all-cause mortality (Lear et al., 2017).

Regular physical activity strengthens the heart's ability to pump blood to the lungs and throughout the body and helps maintain healthy blood pressure, normal blood sugar and fat levels, increase blood levels of HDL cholesterol ("good cholesterol"), reduce inflammation, and help reduce overweight and tobacco smoking, two lifestyle factors associated with higher CVD risk.

Diet

Diets high in processed foods, natural sugar and high fructose corn sugar, and meats containing considerable saturated fat can have a major impact on several risk factors for cardiovascular disease, including elevated LDL cholesterol, low HDL cholesterol, high blood levels of total cholesterol and triglycerides, high blood pressure, overweight, and type 2 diabetes (Rakel, 2017). Diets that lessen the risk of CVD, such as the DASH and Mediterranean diets, emphasize daily consumption of four to five cups of fruits and vegetables and three to six servings of whole-grain foods and low intake of saturated and trans fats, cholesterol, sugar, and salt (American Heart Association, 2017c). However, other dietary factors may offer additional benefits.

Soy Products

Soybeans have been cultivated around the world for thousands of years; the Chinese name for soybean is *tatou*, which means "greater bean." Soy boosts the activity of LDL receptors in the liver, and thereby helps to remove cholesterol from the blood (Lehrman et al., 2010). Soy is a rich source of isoflavones, phytochemical that block oxidation of the LDL particles, which prevents them from sticking to the walls of arteries (Gils-Izquilro et al., 2012).

Studies in which people ate 1 to 2 ounces of soy daily showed that both cholesterol and LDL levels dropped about 10%. Other studies indicate that soy is especially effective among people with cholesterol levels above 240 mg/dl. Soy is available in a multitude of products, such as soy milk, soft and firm tofu, and tofu burgers.

Fish Oils

Populations that consume large amounts of fish in their diets—Greenland Inuit and Japanese islanders—have lower rates of CHD than others. Americans who consume fish regularly in their diets also have healthier hearts. The protective effects of dietary fish have been ascribed to fish oils, in particular those containing omega-3 polyunsaturated fatty acids (omega-3 PuFAs). In some studies, supplements of fish oil have reduced levels of cholesterol and blood pressure. A summary of research on the role of omega-3 polyunsaturated oils in treatment and prevention of CVD concluded that they are most beneficial in people who are at high risk for CVD and have already experienced a heart attack or heart failure with reduced left ventricular function (Siskovick et al., 2017).

The beneficial effect of dietary fish on CVD is illustrated by observations of Bantu villagers in Tanzania. One group of Bantu lived on the shores of a lake, and people consumed about a pound of fish a day. The other Bantu population lived in nearby hills and had a diet that consisted primarily of vegetables. The Bantu people who ate fish had high levels of omega-3-polyunsaturated oils in their blood. They also had lower levels of cholesterol and lipoproteins (Pauletto et al., 1996). Sardines, salmon, and mackerel have high levels of omega-3-polyunsaturated oils, but all fish have some.

Salt (Sodium)

For decades, people have been urged to reduce their consumption of salt from an average of 10 grams per person per day to 6 grams per day or less. Many people find it difficult to reduce their salt intake because 80% of the salt consumed comes from processed foods and not from cooking or the salt shaker on the table. Because the taste of foods is enhanced by salt, food manufacturers are reluctant to reduce the amount of salt in their products. The major reason for recommending reducing salt intake to 3 grams per day is the possible increased risk of high blood pressure from consuming too much salt (Graudal et al., 2017). In people with normal blood pressure, reducing salt intake has no effect on blood pressure. However, in people with high blood pressure or whose bodies have a high sensitivity to salt, consuming less salt is associated with a drop in blood pressure.

Eliminating most processed foods from your diet will automatically reduce your daily salt intake by the currently recommended 3 grams per day. And substituting fresh foods for processed foods is one of the healthiest things you can do for yourself overall.

Trans Fats

Trans fats are chemicals (called *polyhydrogenated vegetable oils*, or PHVOs) that are manufactured from natural vegetable oils to be used in the production of commercial bakery products and for frying in restaurants and fast-food outlets. Dietary trans fats raise the level of LDL ("bad") cholesterol in the blood, which increases the risk of atherosclerosis and subsequent heart and vascular disease. Because removing trans fats from processed and restaurant foods could prevent thousands of heart attacks and deaths each year, use of trans fats was restricted nationally from the U.S. food supply in 2018. Many companies have complied with the restriction and have removed PHVOs from their products. However, trans fats cannot be completely eliminated from foods because they occur naturally in small amounts in meat and dairy products, are present at very low levels in some edible oils, and may be present in imported foods. This is a reason to check product labels.

Aspirin

A commonly used drug can significantly reduce the risk of CHD and heart attacks. Aspirin lessens the risk of blood clots and also combats inflammation. For this reason, physicians generally prescribe daily low-dose aspirin (81 milligrams, a "baby aspirin") to people who have had a heart attack or stroke, with the intention of preventing another occurrence of a life-threatening cardiovascular event. This is also the reason that some cardiologists recommend that those who might be having a heart attack or stroke *first* call 911 *and then* take a limited dose of aspirin. Medical research regarding use of aspirin to prevent a first heart attack or stroke is mixed. In general, aspirin may be recommended only to people who have known risk factors for heart attack. The anti-blood-clotting action of aspirin is dangerous, and people with low risk of heart disease should not expose themselves to that risk (U.S. Food and Drug Administration, 2016).

Alcohol

Many studies have confirmed that light to moderate alcohol consumption (up to one drink per day for women and up to two drinks per day for men) is associated with a lower risk of cardiovascular disease (Bell et al., 2017). Much of the decreased risk is due to a reduction in LDL cholesterol and an increase in HDL cholesterol, and hence a lessening of risk of death from coronary heart disease.

At moderate intake, alcohol reduces LDL cholesterol, increases HDL cholesterol, and reduces inflammation. However, at higher levels of regular consumption, alcohol is associated with high blood pressure and a weakened heart muscle. That moderate alcohol consumption is associated with a lower risk of cardiovascular disease should not be taken to mean that alcohol consumption—particularly heavy or binge alcohol consumption—is healthy. Alcohol consumption still presents many noncardiovascular health risks.

Although moderate alcohol may protect from a heart attack, many dietary and lifestyle changes are much more beneficial to your heart than drinking alcohol. On the other hand, persons who enjoy a drink occasionally need not feel guilty that they are damaging their health.

Psychosocial Factors

Psychosocial factors are associated with both the development and progression of cardiovascular disease (Smith & Blumenthal, 2011). For example, many people cope with stress by smoking or overeating (especially high-fat and high-sugar "comfort foods"), two potent risk factors for cardiovascular disease. Other psychological factors that may increase the risk for cardiovascular disease include unpleasant emotional states, such as depression, anxiety, anger, and distress; personality factors, such as hostility (Chida & Steptoe, 2009; Tindle et al., 2009); stressful social factors, including perceived racial discrimination (Doleszar et al., 2014); and low socioeconomic status and low social support (Steptoe & Kivimaki, 2012). The biological relationships between psychosocial factors and cardiovascular disease include chronic changes in the stress-hormone system (hypothalamo-pituitary-adrenal axis) and inflammation.

Both immediate and long-term stressors are related to the risk of cardiovascular disease. Immediate mental stress, such as catastrophic events (war, earthquakes) and intense sporting events (World Cup soccer), increase the risk for arrhythmias, decrease the flow of blood to the heart, and can cause a heart attack. Following the collapse of the World Trade Center on September 11, 2001, the number of cases of arrhythmia doubled compared to the weeks preceding the attack at the same time the prior year. This relationship is likely related to a sudden upsurge in excitatory nerve activity and secretion of adrenalin. Long-term stressors may be associated with cardiovascular disease through prior CVD, such as high blood pressure. Chronic stressors include work-related stress, marital dissatisfaction, financial stress, and stressful major life events (Rosengren et al., 2004).

> A man's worst enemies can't wish on him what he can think up himself.
>
> *Yiddish proverb*

Coffee, Tea, and Cocoa

Because it is widely consumed throughout the world, coffee's possible association with cardiovascular disease has been studied extensively for many years, and as yet, no remarkable findings have been noted. The sum total of evidence suggests that drinking moderate amounts of coffee (up to five cups per day) poses little or no risk for cardiovascular disease and may even be slightly helpful in certain people. Long-term heavy coffee consumption could possibly be associated with a slightly elevated risk of hypertension (Ding et al., 2014). For now, the American Heart Association (2017a) notes that moderate coffee consumption (one to two cups per day) does not seem to be harmful.

Both green and black tea contain antioxidant chemicals that help block oxidation of LDL particles in the blood vessels. Herb teas do not contain antioxidants. Studies point to the fact that regular drinkers of green tea have less cardiovascular disease than people who do not drink green tea. All tea comes from the same leaves; differences in processing produce white, green,

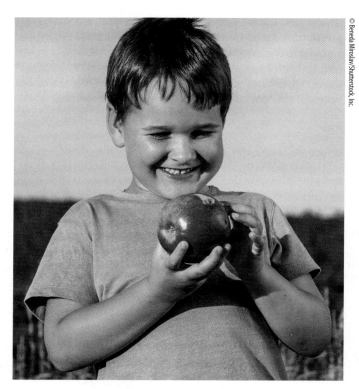

It's important to encourage children to eat heart-healthy snacks so they won't have to break bad eating habits later in life.

or black tea. Chemicals called *polyphenols* in tea are credited with providing the cardiovascular protective effects.

Cocoa also has been implicated in promoting cardiovascular health (Vlachojannis et al., 2014). The Kuna are a native people who live on sparsely inhabited islands in the Caribbean. Researchers observed that these island people have a very low incidence of high blood pressure, which seems to be associated with drinking several cups of relatively unprocessed cocoa a day. Kuna who move away from the islands usually stop drinking cocoa and also develop high blood pressure. Chemicals called *flavonoids* that are present in cocoa seem to increase blood flow and reduce the development of high blood pressure.

Genes May, or May Not, Increase the Risk of Heart Disease

In humans, inheriting any of about 50 genes is associated with an increased risk of heart disease and heart attack, and the more heart disease risk genes a person inherits, the greater the risk of developing heart disease. To what degree heart disease genes confer risk, however, is largely affected by the extent of a person's heart-healthy lifestyle. Specifically, lifestyle factors can reduce genetic risks of heart disease and heart attack by 50%.

A study by Khera and colleagues (2016) of more than 50,000 people identified each participant's number of heart disease risk genes and heart-healthy lifestyle factors, consisting of no current smoking, no obesity (body mass index less than 30), physical activity (at least once a week), and a heart-healthy diet. As might be expected, the more heart disease risk genes, the greater the risk for heart disease. However, no matter how many heart disease genes a study participant had, the risk of heart disease was lessened by 50% by adhering to a heart-healthy lifestyle.

Unhealthy habits can erode a person's health over time. While young, it is vital to take charge of your health and choose a healthy lifestyle. Your life depends on it!

Unfortunately, most of the cocoa sold in the United States is highly processed and sweetened to make it palatable. The cocoa the Kuna drink is unprocessed and quite bitter.

Preventing Cardiovascular Disease

With the increased attention given to risk factors that cause cardiovascular disease, people are now armed with knowledge that can reduce their chances of heart attacks and brain attacks. People should maintain normal weight and avoid consumption of foods containing large amounts of saturated fats, trans fats, and cholesterol. A diet rich in fresh fruits and vegetables helps protect your heart and arteries. Understanding the adverse consequences of cigarette smoking should encourage smokers to quit. Also, consuming green tea and a glass of wine with dinner might be helpful. However, nothing is better for the heart than a healthy diet and plenty of exercise.

It's Not Too Late to Have a Healthy Heart

In 1985, about 5,000 American young adults aged 18 to 30 were recruited to participate in the CARDIA (Coronary Artery Risk Development in Young Adults) study to explore the development and prevention of heart disease (Spring et al., 2014). For the next 20 years, researchers followed five lifestyle behaviors for each participant: (1) not being overweight/obese, (2) low alcohol intake, (3) healthy diet, (4) physically active, and (5) nonsmoker. The researchers also measured a variety of known heart disease risk factors and conducted two tests to identify any signs of developing heart disease. Over the 20-year study, the participants were not coached in any way to change their lifestyle; any changes during that time were by personal choice.

At the beginning of the study, 8% of the participants had all five healthy lifestyle factors and 36% had three. By the end of the study 20 years later, 25% of the participants had increased their number of healthy lifestyle factors, 40% had decreased their number of healthy lifestyle factors, and 35% had the same number as when the study began. Each lifestyle factor that changed from unhealthy to healthy resulted in a 15% reduction in risk for heart disease. And each lifestyle factor that changed from healthy to unhealthy resulted in a 15% increased risk of heart disease. For example, heavier smoking and/or being overweight at the time the study began increased the risk of showing signs of heart disease 20 years later. Never smoking or quitting smoking and not being overweight were associated with reduced risk.

These results show that no matter what your current lifestyle, it is never too late to benefit from making healthy lifestyle changes to reverse or change the progression of cardiovascular disease.

Spring, B. et al. (2014). Healthy Lifestyle Change and Subclinical Atherosclerosis in Young Adults: Coronary Artery Risk Development in Young Adults (CARDIA) Study. *Circulation*, http://circ.ahajournals.org/content/early/2014/04/28/CIRCULATIONAHA.113.005445.

Critical Thinking About Health

1. African Americans as a group have higher blood pressure, on average, than white Americans. Various hypotheses have been advanced to explain the differences in blood pressure between the races, including genetic differences, social factors, economic factors, diet, and behavioral differences. Imagine that you are a consultant to a medical charity that has been asked by a group of scientists at a medical school for $100,000 to fund a research project to explain the observed racial differences in blood pressure. The charity realizes that $100,000 is not sufficient to fund a thorough examination of this issue, so they ask you to list what you consider the three most important factors for the scientists to examine and your reasoning for your choices. The charity also asks you to propose a study for research of the factor you deem most important.

2. For yourself or anyone whom you care about, use the Mayo Clinic online tool for assessing of the risk for heart disease (https://www.mayoclinic.org/diseases -conditions/heart-disease/in-depth/heart-disease -risk/itt-20084942). Among the risk factors that can be changed, discuss how you would reduce them to improve your cardiovascular health now and for the future.

3. People in Japan or southern European countries have one-half to one-third the risk of dying from heart disease in comparison with people from the United States or northern Europe, even when their cholesterol levels, on average, are the same. A person with a cholesterol level of 250 mg/dl in Denmark has a two to three times greater risk of a fatal heart attack compared with an Italian with the same cholesterol level. Develop arguments to explain this difference that seem reasonable to you and organize your facts and ideas in the form of a hypothesis.

Chapter Summary and Highlights

Chapter Summary

The heart is the hardest working muscle in the human body. Day after day, year after year, the heart beats about 60 to 80 times a minute to pump blood continuously to every organ and cell in the body and supply the nutrients and oxygen that keep us alive. The heart pumps freshly oxygenated blood through arteries to all parts of the body; veins return oxygen-depleted blood to the lungs. The veins also carry carbon dioxide, a by-product of chemical reactions in cells, back to the lungs where it is expelled with each exhalation.

We almost never think about our heart until it fails to function properly. In a healthy person, the heart can function flawlessly for more than a hundred years, but heart disease and heart attacks are still the leading cause of death in the United States and many countries throughout the world. Many lifestyle and environmental factors can diminish or destroy the functions of the heart and circulatory system. Among the factors most destructive to the circulatory system are tobacco smoke, high levels of cholesterol and lipids, high blood pressure, and obesity. High levels of stress over prolonged periods also are unhealthy.

You can help ensure a healthy heart and circulatory system by maintaining proper weight, exercising on a regular basis, and eating a variety of fresh foods, particularly fruits and vegetables. Avoid processed foods as much as possible, especially ones high in fat, sugar, and salt. The time to protect your heart is when you are still young and healthy. Think about how you would care for a treasured possession that you want to last for a hundred years. If you have a choice of where to live, pick a place where the air you breathe and the water you drink are still relatively unpolluted. Toxic environments are not conducive to a healthy lifestyle or to the long-term health of your heart.

Highlights

- The heart is a pump that maintains blood circulation in the arteries and veins. The arteries carry oxygen and nutrients to cells, and the veins carry carbon dioxide back to the lungs.
- Damage to the heart or arteries is called cardiovascular disease, which is the leading cause of death in the United States.
- Major risk factors of heart disease that cannot be changed are heredity, gender, and age.
- Major risk factors for cardiovascular disease that can be changed are tobacco use, high blood cholesterol, high blood pressure, physical inactivity, and poor diet.
- Other factors that contribute to heart disease are diabetes, obesity, and stress.
- Various surgeries are performed to repair clogged arteries: coronary artery bypass surgery, angioplasty (stenting), and endarterectomy.
- One baby (81-mg) aspirin each day may reduce the possibility of a heart attack for someone at risk.
- Soy products, fish oils, cocoa, and green tea can keep the heart healthy.
- Heart disease is caused by modern lifestyles and can be prevented. Making changes in your diet, not smoking, and increasing exercise while you are young can help keep the heart, arteries, and brain healthy throughout life.

For Your Health

Cardiovascular diseases are the number one cause of death among Americans. Do "My Risk for Heart Disease" (Exercise 14.1 in the Workbook) so you can begin making lifestyle changes to reduce your risk for heart disease.

References

Alexander, J. H., & Smith, P. K. (2016). Coronary bypass grafting. *New England Journal of Medicine, 374,* 1954–1964.

American College of Emergency Physicians. (2015). How to Perform CPR. Retrieved from http://www.emergency careforyou.org/EmergencyManual/HowToPerformCPR /Default.aspx

American Heart Association. (2017a). Caffeine and heart disease. Retrieved from http://www.heart.org /HEARTORG/HealthyLiving/HealthyEating/Nutrition /Caffeine-and-Heart-Disease_UCM_305888_Article .jsp#.WdlAxGJSzfY

American Heart Association. (2017b). Heart disease and stroke statistics at a glance. Retrieved from https:// www.heart.org/idc/groups/ahamah-public/@wcm/@ sop/@smd/documents/downloadable/ucm_491265 .pdf.

American Heart Association. (2017c). Diet and lifestyle recommendations. Retrieved from http://www.heart .org/HEARTORG/HealthyLiving/HealthyEating /Nutrition/The-American-Heart-Associations-Diet -and-Lifestyle-Recommendations_UCM_305855 _Article.jsp.

Beil, L. (2017, May 13). The statin umbrella. *Science News,* 23–26.

Bell, S., et al. (2017). Association between clinically recorded alcohol consumption and initial presentation of 12 cardiovascular diseases: population-based cohort study using linked health records. *BMJ, 356:*j909. doi: 10.1136/bmj.j909.

Centers for Disease Control and Prevention. (2014). Vital Statistics data available online. Retrieved from http:// www.cdc.gov/nchs/data_access/Vitalstatsonline.htm

Chida, Y., & Steptoe, A. (2009). The association of anger and hostility with future coronary heart disease: A meta-analytic review of prospective evidence. *Journal of the American College of Cardiology, 53,* 936–946.

Ding, M. (2014). Long-term coffee consumption and risk of cardiovascular disease. *Circulation, 129,* 643–659.

Dolezsar, C. M., et al. (2014). Perceived racial discrimination and hypertension: A comprehensive review. *Health Psychology, 33,* 20–34.

Frank, J. D. (1973). *Persuasion and healing.* Baltimore: Johns Hopkins University Press.

Gil-Izquierdo, J. L. (2012). Soy isoflavones and cardiovascular disease. *Current Pharmaceutical Biotechnology, 13,* 624–631.

Kern, F. (1991). Normal plasma cholesterol in an 88-year-old man who eats 25 eggs per day. *New England Journal of Medicine, 324,* 13.

Khera, A. V., et al. (2016). Genetic risk, adherence to a healthy lifestyle, and coronary disease. *New England Journal of Medicine, 375,* 2349–2358.

Lear, S. A., et al. (2017). The effect of physical activity on mortality and cardiovascular disease in 130,000 people from 17 high-income, middle-income, and low-income countries: the PURE study. *Lancet, 390,* 2643–2654.

Lehrman, R. H., et al. (2010). Subjects with elevated LDL cholesterol and metabolic syndrome benefit from supplementation with soy protein, phytosterols, hops, iso-alpha acids, and Acacia nilotica proanthocyanidins. *Journal of Clinical Lipidology, 4,* 59–68.

Lv, X., et al. (2015). Risk of all-cause mortality and cardiovascular disease associated with secondhand smoke exposure: A systematic review and meta-analysis. *International Journal of Cardiology, 199,* 106–115.

Maron, B. J., et al. (2005). Task Force II: *Commotio cordis. Journal of the American College of Cardiology, 45,* 1371–1373.

McMurry, M. P., et al. (1991). Changes in lipid and lipoprotein levels and body weight in Tarahumara Indians after consumption of an affluent diet. *New England Journal of Medicine, 325,* 1704–1708.

Ornish, D., et al. (1998). Intensive lifestyle changes for reversal of coronary heart disease. *Journal of the American Medical Association, 280,* 2001–2007.

Patel, S. A., et al. (2015). Cardiovascular mortality associated with 5 leading risk factors: National and state preventable fractions estimated from survey data. *Annals of Internal Medicine, 163,* 245–253.

Pauletto, P., et al. (1996). Blood pressure and atherogenic lipoprotein profiles of fish-diet and vegetarian villagers in Tanzania: The Lugalawa study. *Lancet, 348,* 784–788.

Rakel, D. (2017, September 7). The pendulum has swung: The PURE study. *Primary Care.* Retrieved from http:// www.practiceupdate.com/content/fruit-vegetable -and-legume-intake-and-cardiovascular-disease -and-deaths/57602

Rosengren, A., et al. (2004). Association of psychosocial risk factors with risk of acute myocardial infarction in 11,119 cases and 13,648 controls from 52 countries (the INTERHEART study): Case-control study. *Lancet, 364,* 953–962.

Siskovick, D. S., et al. (2017). Omega-3 polyunsaturated fatty acid (fish oil) supplementation and the prevention of clinical cardiovascular disease. *Circulation, 135,* e867–e884.

Smith, P., & Blumenthal, J. (2011). Psychiatric and behavioral aspects of cardiovascular disease: Epidemiology, mechanisms, and treatment. *Revista española de cardiología, 64,* 924–933. doi: 10.1016/j.rec.2011.06.003

Spring, B., et al. (2014). Healthy lifestyle change and subclinical atherosclerosis in young adults: Coronary Artery Risk Development in Young Adults (CARDIA) study. *Circulation, 130,* 10–17. Retrieved from http://circ.ahajournals.org/content/early/2014/04/28/CIRCULATIONAHA.113.005445

Steptoe, A., & Kivimaki, M. (2012). Stress and cardiovascular disease: An update on current knowledge. *Annual Review of Public Health, 34,* 337–354.

Tindle, H. A., et al. (2009). Optimism, cynical hostility, and incident coronary heart disease and mortality in the Women's Health Initiative. *Circulation, 120,* 656–662.

U.S. Food and Drug Administration. (2016). Use of aspirin for primary prevention of heart attack and stroke. Retrieved from https://www.fda.gov/drugs/resourcesforyou/consumers/ucm390574.htm

U.S. National Heart, Lung, and Blood Institute (2017). What are the risk factors for heart disease? Retrieved from https://www.nhlbi.nih.gov/health/educational/hearttruth/lower-risk/risk-factors.htm

Vlachojannis, J., et al. (2016). The impact of cocoa flavanols on cardiovascular health. *Phytotherapy Research, 10,* 1641–1657.

World Health Organization. (2017). Cardiovascular diseases. Retrieved February 6, 2015 from http://www.who.int/mediacentre/factsheets/fs317/en/

Yang, Q., et al. (2012). Trends in cardiovascular health metrics and associations with all-cause and CVD mortality among U.S. adults. *Journal of the American Medical Association, 307,* 1273–1283.

Suggested Readings

Beil, L. (2017, May 13). The statin umbrella. *Science News,* 23–26. For decades statin drugs were regarded as "wonder drugs" for reducing the risk of a heart attack in people with high cholesterol. Now it is not so clear, and the risks may outweigh the benefits for many people with only moderate to low risk of a heart attack. This article explains the turnaround regarding the routine use of statins.

Meadows, M. (2003, November/December). How to keep your heart healthy. *FDA Consumer,* 18–25. Suggestions on how to make dietary and other lifestyle changes that will help keep your heart healthy.

Ornish, D., et al. (1998). Intensive lifestyle changes for reversal of coronary heart disease. *Journal of the American Medical Association, 280,* 2001–2007. A report documenting that the blockages in arteries can be reversed by changes in lifestyle and that the beneficial changes persist for years.

Rubanyi, G. (2017, January). Heart therapy. *Scientific American,* 40–43. Describes how gene therapy technology may soon be able to repair regions of the heart damaged by a heart attack or other heart diseases.

Willett, W. C., & Underwood, A. (2010, February 15). Crimes of the heart. *Newsweek,* 42–43. A renowned health expert explains why prevention of heart disease and heart attacks must be vigorously pursued. If people do not change their dietary and lifestyle choices, medical costs for heart disease will bankrupt the U.S. economy.

Recommended Websites

American Heart Association
Information and education on all aspects of cardiovascular disease.

MedlinePlus on Heart Disease
From the U.S. National Library of Medicine. General information.

National Heart, Lung, and Blood Institute
Information on heart disease and high blood pressure.

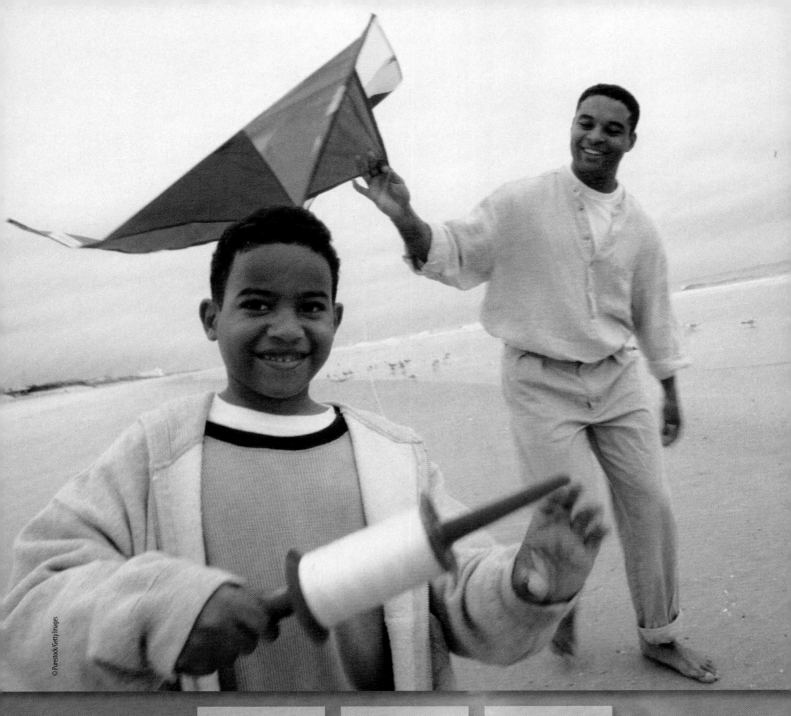

© Purestock/Getty Images

Dollars & Health Sense

The Cost of Treating Cystic Fibrosis

Global Wellness

Lactose Intolerance: A Mutation That Influenced Human Evolution

Gene Therapy Cures Sickle Cell Disease

Wellness Guide

Is There a Gay Gene?

Determining If You Are at Risk for Bearing a Child with Genetic Abnormalities

Saving a Life with a Life

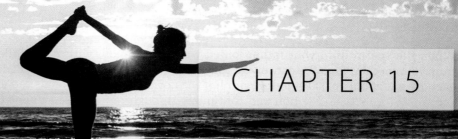

CHAPTER 15

Heredity and Disease

Learning Objectives

1. Describe the functions of DNA, genes, and chromosomes.

2. Describe several inherited diseases caused by chromosomal abnormalities.

3. List several chemicals that cause birth defects and what they were used for.

4. Explain how a familial pattern of disease differs from a hereditary (genetic) disease.

5. Describe the symptoms of fetal alcohol syndrome and how the syndrome can be prevented.

6. Explain the role of genetic counseling in preventing hereditary diseases.

7. Explain the procedure of amniocentesis.

8. Define *genetic discrimination*, and describe its consequences for people.

9. Discuss how gene therapy and embryonic stem cells may be used to treat and cure disease.

When the sperm from your father joined with the egg from your mother, you were conceived. You inherited from each parent about 20,000 genes. Beginning with conception and continuing throughout life, those genes direct and control the development and repair of your body's tissues and organs. The genes control the chemistry that keeps you alive, your particular disease susceptibilities, and, to a large extent, your overall health and life expectancy.

> People through finding something beautiful, think something else unbeautiful. Through finding one man fit, judge another unfit.
>
> *Lao Tzu,* The Way of Life

Genes are arranged in a linear array along threadlike structures called **chromosomes**, which are present in almost all cells of the body. Each person carries 23 pairs of chromosomes (a total of 46) in virtually every cell of the body. (The only major exception is red blood cells, which lose their chromosomes before they enter the blood circulation.) Males and females differ only in one pair of chromosomes, called the sex chromosomes. Men have an XY pair and women have an XX pair. The original parental chromosomes present in the fertilized egg are replicated into every cell of the fetus during development; skin, liver, heart, lung, and brain cells all contain identical sets of chromosomes. Only half of each parent's set of chromosomes is passed on in the fertilized egg, thus keeping the chromosome number the same from generation to generation.

Cells and organs differ in the body because different genes are expressed in different tissues. The orchestrated turning on and off of genes in cells is the key to development and correct functioning of the body throughout life. The flow of information from DNA in chromosomes to functional proteins in cells is the same in all living organisms, attesting to a common cellular evolutionary history (**Figure 15.1**).

Human chromosomes have a characteristic shape, size, and banding pattern that can be seen when they are stained with dyes and examined under the light microscope. Each of the 23 different human chromosome pairs can be distinguished and identified. Human chromosomes are viewed under the microscope and then photographed and arranged in pairs in a standard display called a **karyotype**.

The information carried in genes arranged along the chromosomes is contained in a chemical substance called **DNA (deoxyribonucleic acid)**. Each chromosome, depending on its size, contains thousands of different genes whose information is encoded in the chemistry of the DNA. Together, these genes determine the uniqueness of each human being. (Identical twins share identical sets of genes but differ in their traits to some extent because of environmental effects on the expression of their genes.) Because chromosomes occur in pairs, each person carries two copies of each gene; these may be identical in information or differ slightly from one another.

Most American babies are born healthy. However, about 3% to 4% of newborns have an observable **congenital (birth) defect**—an anomaly in some aspect of the body's structure or functioning that occurred during

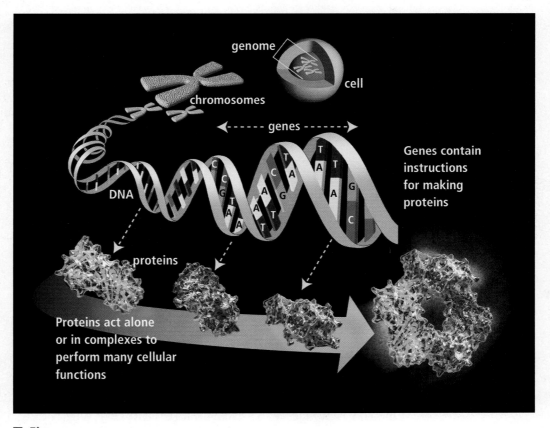

■ **Figure 15.1**

DNA—The Molecule of Life
The diagram shows the relation among DNA, genes, chromosomes, and proteins in all cells of the body. Chromosomes contain the hereditary chemical DNA. Specific short segments of DNA contain genes, most of which carry information for the synthesis of specific proteins. The information in each gene is copied into a molecule of RNA (ribonucleic acid), which is then translated into a specific protein that the cell needs.

Courtesy of the U.S. Department of Energy Genomic Science program, http://genomicscience.energy.gov.

Table 15.1

Chromosomal Abnormalities

Some genetic diseases are associated with an extra or missing chromosome. Most abnormalities in chromosome number (more or less than the normal 46) are incompatible with survival; in most cases, affected babies die before birth. However, abnormalities in chromosomes 21, X, or Y are compatible with survival but usually produce physical and mental abnormalities.

Genetic disease/disorder	Chromosomal defect	Incidence per live births	Symptoms
Turner's syndrome (female)	Missing X	1/1,000	Absence of ovaries, short stature, underdeveloped breasts
Klinefelter's syndrome (male)	Extra X	1/1,000	Small, undeveloped testes, sterility, intellectual disabilities
Down syndrome (male or female)	Extra chromosome 21	1/700	Physical abnormalities, intellectual disabilities, heart defects
XXX syndrome (female)	Extra X	1/1,000	No clinical abnormalities, height above average, possible intellectual disabilities
XYY (male)	Extra Y	1/1,000	No clinical abnormalities, height above average, controversy over "criminal" tendency

development in the mother's uterus. Congenital defects are caused by one or more of the following factors:

- Presence of an abnormal chromosome or abnormal number of chromosomes

- A chemical error in one or more genes inherited from parents; the abnormal gene alters body structure or functions
- The effect of toxins, drugs, or other environmental factors on normal fetal development

In this chapter, we discuss the origin, prevention, and treatment of common birth defects and inherited diseases.

Chromosomal Abnormalities

Errors may occur when chromosomes are distributed to sperm or egg. The distribution may result in too few or too many chromosomes being transmitted (other forms of physical chromosomal abnormalities also occur). These chromosomal abnormalities often result in hereditary diseases (**Table 15.1**). About 20% of all human conceptions have a chromosomal abnormality of some kind. The majority of fetuses with chromosomal abnormalities abort spontaneously, ending the pregnancy.

Viewing cells removed from a fetus, child, or adult can identify chromosomal abnormalities, such as the extra chromosome 21 that causes *Down syndrome* (**Figure 15.2**).

This serious inherited birth defect occurs in about 1 in every 700 babies born in the United States. However,

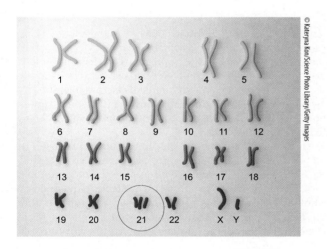

© Kateryna Kon/Science Photo Library/Getty Images

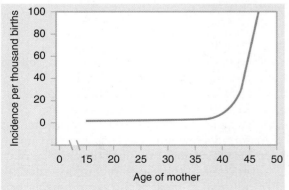

■ **Figure 15.2**

Karyotype of Individual with Down Syndrome

Note three copies of chromosome 21. Frequencies of children born with Down syndrome are shown in relation to the age of the mother. At age 35, the risk of this particular chromosomal abnormality begins to rise sharply.

Adapted from Hook, E. B. (1984). Chromosomal Abnormality Rates at Amniocentesis and in Live-Born Infants. *Journal of the American Medical Association, 249*, 2034–2038.

TERMS

chromosomes: threadlike structures in the nuclei of cells that carry an individual's genetic information

congenital (birth) defect: any abnormality observed in a newborn that occurred during development

deoxyribonucleic acid (DNA): the chemical substance that carries all of a person's genetic information in chromosomes in cells

karyotype: visual display of all of a person's chromosomes that can detect chromosomal abnormalities characteristic of inherited diseases

Lactose Intolerance: A Mutation That Influenced Human Evolution

The sugar *lactose* is present in mother's milk and is the primary source of energy for all babies when breastfed. Digestion of the sugar lactose is accomplished by an enzyme—called *lactase*—that is present in the digestive system of all newborns. The gene for producing the enzyme that digests lactose is situated on chromosome 2, and almost all babies are born with this gene activated so that they can digest breast milk or cow's milk. Very infrequently, a baby is born with an inactive gene that causes a condition known as *alactasia*. These infants cannot digest lactose in breast milk or in any milk product. If they are breastfed or given cow's milk, these infants have watery diarrhea, which can be life-threatening due to dehydration and nutrient depletion.

A much more common condition involving inability to digest the sugar lactose occurs later in life and is called *lactose intolerance*. The extent of lactose intolerance varies widely among the world's adult population (see accompanying figure).

Lactose intolerance occurs in the following way. As mentioned previously, the gene that allows babies to digest lactose is switched on in all newborns so that they can thrive on breast milk. In a majority of the world's children, the gene is switched off sometime between 2 and 5 of age. This corresponds to the normal time of weaning in most cultures. The explanation for the switching off of the gene is that, until quite recently in human evolution, people did not consume milk after weaning. The body could conserve energy for other uses by not producing an unnecessary enzyme.

About 10,000 years ago, people in northern Europe and a few tribes in Africa began to raise cows, goats, sheep, and other animals for their milk, which became an important part of the diet. Mutations in the lactase genes arose among these milk drinkers that permitted continued lactase enzyme production for life, and this genetic change was passed on from one generation to the next.

Modern genetic research has now shown that two mutations account for all the lactose-tolerant people in the world

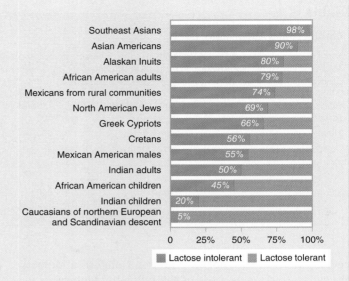

Adapted from Itan, Y., et al. (2010). A worldwide correlation of lactase persistence phenotype and genotypes. *BMC Evolutionary Biology*, 10:36. Retrieved from http://www.ncbi.nlm.nih.gov/pmc/articles/PMC2834688/?tool=pubmed/

(Enattah, et al., 2002; Gibbons, 2006). All of the adults who can drink milk without any ill effects have one or the other of these two mutations. Today, populations around the world vary from being almost completely lactose intolerant (Southeast Asians) to being almost completely lactose tolerant (Scandinavians). In the thousands of years since these mutations arose, people have carried the lactose-tolerance genes to all parts of the world.

Until recently, it has been difficult to diagnose lactose intolerance. Generally, the diagnosis is made by stopping the ingestion of milk products to see if the symptoms disappear. Now, however, a genetic test is available to determine whether a person with symptoms actually lacks the genes to produce lactase. (*Note:* Lactose intolerance is not a true milk allergy; milk allergy is an immune response to milk proteins).

---

the rate begins to increase in women around age 35 and increases dramatically after age 40. Because of the increase in Down syndrome with increased maternal age, all pregnant women over age 35 are advised to undergo genetic tests of fetal cells (see section on prenatal testing) to determine whether they are carrying a fetus with Down syndrome. If the tests are positive, women can elect to have an abortion or continue the pregnancy, knowing that they will deliver a child with Down syndrome.

The extra chromosome 21 carried in all cells of individuals with Down syndrome causes heart defects, altered facial features, and intellectual disabilities. With modern medical care, the life expectancy of a person with Down syndrome is 40 to 50 years. However, caring for a Down syndrome person beyond childhood is taxing on families both emotionally and financially. Eventually,

most individuals with Down syndrome are placed in special living situations with trained caregivers.

Chromosome 21 is one of the smallest of all human chromosomes; it contains about 450 genes. To understand which genes contribute to Down syndrome, scientists transferred a few human genes at a time into mice to determine which ones produced the characteristics of the disease. Three of the genes in chromosome 21 were found to cause all or most of the symptoms associated with Down syndrome, and it seems that only one particular gene may be the primary cause of this inherited disorder.

Hereditary Diseases

A **hereditary (genetic) disease** results from the following sequence of events. An abnormal gene (one whose chemistry has been altered) is passed on to a child from one or both parents. As a result of inheriting the defective gene (or genes), a protein is produced that is abnormal or even missing completely. For example, if an essential muscle protein is defective or missing during fetal development, muscle tissues develop abnormally. Several forms of *muscular dystrophy* are inherited in this way. If a protein necessary for bone formation is defective, short stature, or *dwarfism*, results.

If the defective protein is an enzyme, an essential chemical reaction in the body will be affected and some aspect of metabolism will be abnormal. For example, in hemophilia, a chemical called factor VIII, required for normal blood clotting, is defective as a result of an altered gene on an X chromosome. *Phenylketonuria* (PKU) is an inherited disease caused by a defect in an enzyme that is needed to digest the amino acid phenylalanine, which is present in food. If excess phenylalanine in the blood is not broken down, it accumulates in tissues and causes abnormal brain development and intellectual disabilities.

> Life is not a matter of holding good cards, but of playing a poor hand well.
>
> *Robert Louis Stevenson*

Newborn screening began in the United States in the 1960s with tests for phenylketonuria (PKU). Over the years, many additional reliable tests were developed for relatively common inherited diseases. However, it was not economically practical to screen for very rare inherited diseases; also, false-positive results would cause great emotional distress to parents who were told that they had a child with an inherited disease when, in fact, their baby was healthy. Newer tests make newborn screening much more accurate and reliable. The American College of Medical Genetics now says that newborns can be screened for more than 50 inherited disorders, some of which are

---

TERMS

hereditary (genetic) disease: any disease resulting from the inheritance of defective genes or chromosomes from one or both parents

---

Is There a Gay Gene?

In modern society, the word *gay* is used to refer to a homosexual male. Historically, the word meant "mirthful, high spirited"; later, it began to be associated with sexual conduct as in "gay blade." But how the term *gay* came to be associated with male homosexuals is still uncertain.

In 1993, a scientific research team claimed to have discovered the biological basis of male homosexuality by identifying a "gay gene." However, their methods involved statistical associations, and no actual gene was ever identified. Furthermore, genetic studies by other researchers failed to confirm the original observations or analysis. Although researchers presume that homosexuality has a basis in biology and genes, there is still no convincing evidence to support this presumption. Perhaps the best evidence is that many gay persons report that they were aware at a very early age of their attraction to other males. But this is not scientific evidence for a gay gene.

Should future research uncover specific genetic influences on sexual orientation, and given its complex nature, it seems highly unlikely that a single gene (or even a few genes) can account for homosexuality. Sexual orientation is most likely determined by hundreds of genes and numerous environmental factors that affect brain development *in utero* as well as after birth. The factors underlying sexual orientation are probably at least as complex as the ones that affect intelligence.

Research on the genetic basis of homosexuality is extremely controversial for many reasons. In the past, and even now, most homosexual men would have chosen to hide their sexual orientation because of the dire consequences of "coming out."

In the United States, prior to the 1970s, homosexuality was medically classified as a disease and homosexual men were often forced to undergo painful psychological or physical treatments to "cure" their homosexuality. Until recently, in China, shock therapy was used to "treat" homosexuals. Although gay men are well integrated in most aspects of American society today, strong prejudice still exists in many areas of the United States and in other countries. Extreme prejudice or hatred of homosexuals is called *homophobia* and is still a problem in the United States and elsewhere in the world.

Anthropological evidence indicates that homosexuality has existed in all human cultures past and present and that, in general, male homosexuals constitute between 2% and 4% of any human population. Thus, homosexuality is a typical variation among people, just like genetic variation in height or intelligence. For example, only a few percent of people are over seven feet tall or have the mind of a genius, but they are not stigmatized.

In recent years, many countries, including the United States, have passed laws recognizing the rights of gay and lesbian couples to be legally married and to have all the legal benefits granted to heterosexual couples. This is not only an advance in social equality for same-sex couples, but also a recognition that nonheterosexual orientation is as "natural" as other aspects of a person's biology. This opens the way for more tolerance. Hating someone because of the color of their skin or sexual orientation is hating them for the biology they inherited at birth. Making judgments of good/bad or normal/abnormal behavior without consideration of biological factors is shortsighted.

In the end, biology dictates much of one's sexuality, despite social norms.

extremely rare. The number of inherited disorders for which newborns are tested varies widely by state. Some states test for as few as 3 inherited disorders; other states test for as many as 40. Prospective parents can get more information on what tests are available in their state at a website maintained by the National Newborn Screening & Global Resource Center (genes-r-us.uthscsa.edu).

One of the most important newborn screening tests is for abnormalities in a gene on the X chromosome called *FMR1* (fragile X mental retardation). Because males carry only one X chromosome inherited from their mothers, only boys are affected by *fragile X syndrome*, the most common form of intellectual disability in the general population (Hagerman & Hagerman, 2008). Females carry two X chromosomes, so they usually carry one normal *FMR1* gene, which negates most of the effects of a defective gene on the other X chromosome. Because so many different mutations occur in the *FMR1* gene, the impairment of mental functions also varies widely.

Sickle cell disease is caused by a defect in hemoglobin proteins present in all red blood cells. Hemoglobin molecules pick up oxygen as blood circulates through the lungs. In sickle cell disease, the defective hemoglobin proteins change the shape of red blood cells so that they tend to clog small blood vessels. As a result, essential oxygen cannot reach tissues and organs. In 2017, the first successful cure of sickle cell disease was announced (see the Global Wellness box, "Gene Therapy Cures Sickle Cell Disease").

Familial Diseases Hereditary diseases are *always* caused by abnormal chromosomes or genes that change body structure or chemistry in some way. However, determining whether a disease or physical abnormality is inherited is not a simple matter. Many birth defects are caused by infections, teratogens, or other environmental factors, as well as by defective genes.

Sometimes a disease is said to "run in the family," which means that several members of a family have the same disease. Children of parents who suffer from certain diseases are at higher risk of developing these diseases compared with the average risk in the general population (**Table 15.2**). Allergies, obesity, or alcoholism may run in the family, but this does not mean that these diseases are always inherited or caused solely by genes. Families share many environmental factors as well as genes. For example, families share the same water, food, and air, any one of which may contain harmful or toxic substances. When parents have a poor diet, children usually do also. To appreciate the difference between an inherited disease and one that "runs in the family," consider these examples. Being a Muslim or a Catholic runs in families, as does being a Republican or a Democrat, but these traits clearly are not determined by any genes that have been inherited. Only a physician or scientist trained in medical genetics can determine whether a biological abnormality is a result of inherited genes, environmental factors, or a combination of both.

Table 15.2

Increased Risk of Certain Diseases and Disorders Among Children When One Parent Is Affected

In the list below, genes may be involved to some degree, the number of genes conferring risk, or the extent of the genetic contribution, is basically unknown. In all cases, environmental factors also are involved.

	Lifetime risk (%)	
	General population	One parent affected
Alcoholism (men)	10	40
Alcoholism (women)	3–5	12–20
Alzheimer's	5–10	10–20
Colon cancer	6	12–18
Diabetes, type 2	3–7	10–15
Depression, bipolar	1–3	9–27
Dyslexia	5–10	30–60
Psoriasis	1–2	25
Rheumatoid arthritis	1	5
Schizophrenia	1	10

Congenital Defects

Each newborn is examined immediately after birth for any observable physical abnormalities, which are called *congenital defects*. Such defects are not necessarily inherited, although abnormal genes passed on from parents may play some role. Most congenital defects are caused by a complex interaction of genes and environmental factors. Examples of congenital defects are cleft lip, cleft palate, and spina bifida (cleft spine), which result from developmental abnormalities in the formation of the oral cavity and the spine, respectively (**Figure 15.3**).

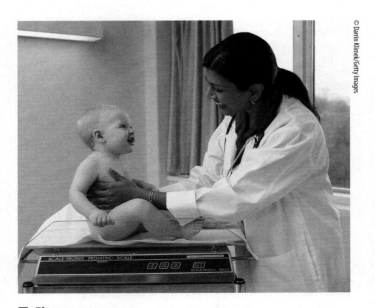

■ **Figure 15.3**

Congenital defects arise during fetal development and are detected at birth.

Cleft lip has been known to occur in only one of a pair of identical twins, so both environmental factors and genes must contribute to this abnormality. The importance of environmental factors during fetal development also is borne out by the observation that even though identical twins share identical genes, they usually are born with different birth weights. They also have different IQ scores later in life. This shows that identical twins are affected differently by environmental factors even during development.

Spina bifida is a congenital defect that affects 1 of every 1,000 newborns. It occurs when one or more spinal vertebrae fail to close and the spinal cord and nerves bulge through the cleft, forming an easily damaged, fluid-filled sac. The protruding spinal nerves are vulnerable to paralysis-causing damage and also to life-threatening infections. The most serious congenital defect of the nervous system is *anencephaly*, which refers to very abnormal brain development; affected babies are either stillborn or die soon after birth. Surgery can repair some of the damage resulting from spina bifida; however, nothing can be done for anencephaly.

Supplementing the diet of pregnant women with the vitamins folic acid and B_{12} dramatically reduces the risk of spina bifida and other birth defects. Folic acid is the most effective in preventing birth defects and should be taken before pregnancy occurs. Women who plan on becoming pregnant should take folic acid (400 micrograms per day) before and after becoming pregnant. Flour and cereals have been supplemented with folic acid for the past decade. As a result, the incidence of spina bifida birth defects has decreased significantly.

However, the number of birth defects has been increasing as fewer women supplement their diets with folate before becoming pregnant. They also are not consuming enough folate-supplemented grains, perhaps because of the fad for "low-carb" diets. The folate solution to reducing birth defects also has come under attack by some who claim that excess folate in the diet may be harmful to the elderly. The bottom line: If you are female and think you may become pregnant, take a folate supplement. It can reduce the risk of having a child with a birth defect by as much as 70%.

Any environmental agent that causes a defect in a developing fetus is called a **teratogen** (Table 15.3). Many environmental agents, such as prescription and illegal drugs, viral and bacterial infections, alcohol consumption, and cigarette smoke, act as teratogens (from the Greek, "to produce a monster") during pregnancy and may cause abnormal development in a fetus. With a little care, many teratogens can be avoided, thereby increasing the likelihood of a healthy baby. In particular, smoking cigarettes and drinking alcohol should be avoided by any woman who is pregnant or attempting to become pregnant. Alcohol is concentrated when crossing the placenta so that even one or two drinks can lead to high alcohol levels in the fetus and affect its development.

Table 15.3

Teratogens

Environmental agents (e.g., infectious viruses and other microorganisms, chemicals, medicines) can act as teratogens and cause birth defects. Many agents in addition to those listed below are suspected of causing abnormal development of the fetus.

Environmental agent	Effects
Accutane (acne drug)	Spontaneous abortion, stillbirth, malformation of the brain and heart
Alcohol	Growth deficiencies, intellectual disabilities
Antithyroid drugs	Thyroid defects
Carbamazepine	Neural tube defects
Cocaine	Fetal death, nervous system and genital abnormalities
Cytomegalovirus, herpes simplex virus, varicella zoster virus, Zika virus	Growth abnormalities, intellectual disabilities
Diethylstilbestrol (DES)	Masculinization of female, abnormalities of vagina and cervix, risk of vaginal cancer
Ionizing radiation	Growth deficiencies, intellectual disabilities, organ malformation (depending on dose)
Lithium carbonate	Heart and blood vessel defects
Methotrexate and etretinate	Prescription drugs that cause severe birth defects
Nonsteroidal anti-inflammatory drugs	Circulation defects
Phenytoin	Central nervous system defects
Polychlorinated biphenyls	Growth deficiencies, pigment abnormalities
Poor nutrition during fetal development	Growth deficiencies, intellectual disabilities
Rubella virus (German measles)	Heart and eye abnormalities, intellectual disabilities
Tetracycline (antibiotic)	Teeth and bone abnormalities
Thalidomide	Limb malformation
Tobacco smoke	Growth deficiencies, increased risk of sickness and death soon after birth
Warfarin	Central nervous system defects

Thalidomide

Thalidomide was developed by a Swiss pharmaceutical company in 1953. Originally tested as a drug for epilepsy, it was subsequently found to be an effective tranquilizer and sedative. In 1957, thalidomide was marketed in Europe and other countries around the world as the drug

TERMS

teratogen: any environmental agent that causes abnormal development of a fetus

of choice for pregnant women experiencing "morning sickness." The drug was thought to be extremely safe and had been tested in pregnant animals, where it did not act as a teratogen.

However, thalidomide is *not* safe for any woman who is pregnant. Thalidomide interferes with normal development of the bones of the arms and legs of a fetus and causes other developmental abnormalities. Between 1956 and 1961, when the teratogenic effects of the drug were finally recognized, thousands of babies in Europe and elsewhere in the world had been born with severe deformities of the arms and legs. Many thousands more were stillborn, but no one knows for sure how many pregnant women lost their fetuses or gave birth to deformed babies. The drug was never approved for sale in the United States largely because of Francis Kelsey, a physician at the Food and Drug Administration (FDA) who was responsible for new drug applications. She was concerned about the drug's side effects and delayed its approval until the devastating effects of the drug were discovered in other countries. Most countries had banned the use of thalidomide by 1961.

However, interest in the therapeutic potential of thalidomide and related drugs has not subsided. Research has continued and, in an ironic twist of fate, thalidomide (trade name, Thalomid) was approved by the FDA in 1998 for use in treating skin lesions associated with leprosy. The drug now comes with a strong warning advising doctors not to prescribe the drug for any condition for which it is not approved or for women who might become pregnant. The lesson from thalidomide is that women who may become pregnant should not take any drug—prescription, over-the-counter, or illegal—in order to protect a fetus should they become pregnant.

Fetal Alcohol Syndrome

Consumption of alcohol in any amount during pregnancy increases the risk of a *fetal alcohol spectrum disorder,* the most common form being **fetal alcohol syndrome (FAS)**. This condition is diagnosed if an infant has certain characteristic abnormal facial features, growth reduction, and neurodevelopmental abnormalities.

Although most babies with FAS are born to women who consume large amounts of alcohol during pregnancy, studies show that even moderate drinking during pregnancy increases risk.

Many women think that an occasional drink during pregnancy cannot cause any harm. They may be right, but it still is a gamble even if the risk is low. Nine months is a long time between drinks for someone who is used to drinking, even occasionally. Women who are light drinkers before becoming pregnant (about one drink per day) find it easier to give up alcohol than women who are heavy drinkers (three or more drinks per day). Despite warnings on alcoholic beverage containers, the incidence of FAS and other alcohol-related disorders in developing fetuses has remained quite high—as many as 1 in 10 newborns have been exposed to alcohol during pregnancy.

The drinking of alcohol by pregnant women who give birth to a handicapped child raises questions about individual rights. Does a mother have a right to do with her body as she sees fit even if it means harming the baby? Does society have the right to regulate the consumption of alcohol and other harmful substances by a pregnant woman? Some people argue that a pregnant woman who irresponsibly uses alcohol or drugs during pregnancy should be imprisoned while pregnant so that her use

---

The Cost of Treating Cystic Fibrosis

Each year in the United States about 30,000 babies are born with cystic fibrosis, a disease that causes severe lung and breathing problems (Kaiser, 2012). This inherited (genetic) disease occurs because an affected child inherits a defective gene from each parent. Modern medical treatments enable babies born with cystic fibrosis to survive to about age 40. Despite the improved care and therapies, there still is no cure.

In 2012, the U.S. Food and Drug Administration (FDA) and the health programs in Canada, the European Union, and other countries approved the drug Kalydeco (ivakator), which can restore lung function in a specific subtype of cystic fibrosis patients—about 4 of 100. Vertex Pharmaceuticals, the company that manufactures Kalydeco, charges $300,000 for a year's supply of pills (taken twice daily). Most cystic fibrosis patients who respond to the drug will need to take it for decades to stay alive.

Many doctors, patients and their families, and insurers, including the U.S. government, which pays for the drug through Medicare Disability and Medicaid, object to the high cost. They point out that the scientific research that discovered the drug was paid for by taxpayers and that Vertex received considerable help from the Cystic Fibrosis Association and hence spent less than the typical $1 billion to $2 billion to develop the new drug. Without some adjustment in the price, as is being demanded by the U.S. and European governments, each patient receiving the drug will produce a multi-billion-dollar profit for Vertex. In the for-profit model of drug development and sale, Vertex is doing nothing illegal to price its product as it sees fit.

The cost of Kalydeco and other new drugs approved for serious diseases—especially cancer—which is almost always more than $100,000 per treatment or annually if the drug must be given continuously, is a pressing problem facing the healthcare system. With modern genetic technologies to help produce more drugs to treat small numbers of patients, industry and drug developers will be tempted to exploit their advantage financially. Detecting and treating genetic and other serious diseases are rife with ethical and economic concerns that will become critical in the coming years.

of dangerous substances can be controlled. The ethical and legal questions surrounding pregnancy, alcohol, and drugs are unresolved.

Preventing Hereditary Diseases

Genetic Counseling

Genetic counseling is a medical specialty that helps people learn about genetic conditions, find out their chances of being affected by or having a child or other family member with a genetic condition, and make informed decisions about testing and treatment. Among the reasons for seeking genetic counseling are having a family history of a genetic condition (including a genetic condition or birth defect occurring in a previous pregnancy), to learn about genetic screening for diseases that are more common in certain ethnic groups (e.g., sickle cell disease in African Americans and Tay-Sachs disease in Ashkenazi Jews), and other genetics-related concerns. Genetic counseling professionals include *clinical geneticists*, who are doctors with expertise in genetics, and *genetic counselors*, who are non-medical professionals trained to provide counseling and support for people and families with genetic conditions. Getting a recommendation from a healthcare provider is the best way to find a genetics professional. Genetic counseling begins with objective calculations of genetic risks to a fetus, which, in some cases, guarantee that an abnormal fetus is being carried. Although genetic counselors strive to be objective, the counseling process is subtle and counselors may inadvertently interject personal opinions. For example, prospective parents who each carry a defective gene may be told that they have one chance in four of having a genetically handicapped child. Or they can be told that the odds are three to one that they will have a healthy child. Both statements express the same mathematical probabilities, but the prospective parents may well interpret the two statements quite differently. One statement emphasizes a negative outcome; the other a more positive outcome.

Giving advice or making recommendations that affect the life of another person invariably involves difficult moral decisions and many conflicting views. Ideally, the personal views of a genetic counselor should not influence the decision-making process of the couples or families involved. Clients should arrive at their own informed decisions after careful consideration of all of the medical facts and risks that have been explained to them.

Genetic Testing

Genetic testing encompasses medically supervised procedures that identify changes in chromosomes, genes, or proteins to confirm or rule out a suspected genetic condition or help determine a person's chance of developing or passing on a genetic disorder. More than 1,000 genetic tests are currently available, and more are being developed. Genetic testing can include (1) identifying single genes or short lengths of DNA to identify variations or mutations that lead to a genetic disorder, (2) analyzing entire chromosomes or long lengths of DNA to identify changes in chromosome number or shape, and (3) determining the amount or activity level of proteins, which can indicate changes to the DNA that result in a genetic disorder.

TERMS

fetal alcohol syndrome (FAS): birth defects and mental disabilities caused by ingestion of alcohol by the mother during pregnancy

genetic counseling: information to help prospective parents evaluate the risks of having or delivering a child with a genetic abnormality

genetic testing: medically supervised procedures that identify changes in chromosomes, genes, or proteins to confirm or rule out a suspected genetic condition or help determine a person's chance of developing or passing on to children a genetic disorder

---

Determining If You Are at Risk for Bearing a Child with Genetic Abnormalities

Prenatal testing and genetic counseling are advised if a person falls into any one of the following risk categories:

- Maternal age over 35 years (risk of Down syndrome)
- High or low levels of alphafetoprotein during pregnancy (risk of neural tube defect)
- Woman had a previous child with a chromosomal abnormality or neural tube defect
- Woman had a previous stillbirth or neonatal death
- Woman or mate carries a previously diagnosed chromosomal or genetic abnormality
- Woman carries a previously diagnosed defective gene
- Woman and mate carry the same previously diagnosed defective gene
- Close relatives have a child with an inherited disorder
- Woman has been exposed to a teratogenic agent during pregnancy
- Woman has recently been infected by rubella (measles) virus or cytomegalovirus

Saving a Life with a Life

Once in a while all the futuristic medical and genetic technologies work as scientists envision they will and an imagined remarkable cure becomes a reality. Several medical technologies came together for Molly Nash, an extremely sick 6-year-old who had inherited Fanconi's anemia. This is a severe blood disease that usually kills children before age 10 unless a bone marrow transplant is performed successfully. To be successful, the donor's bone marrow cells must be very closely matched to the recipient's human leukocyte antigen (HLA) cell type to prevent rejection of the transplanted tissue.

In 2000, Molly Nash's parents were offered a never-before-tried solution to their daughter's fatal condition: Her parents would have another child whose genes would closely match Molly's so a successful transplant would be possible. On August 29, 2000, Adam Nash was born and Molly received her bone marrow transplant and it worked. Here's what happened.

Doctors removed eggs from Molly's mother's ovaries. They were then fertilized in a laboratory dish using sperm from Molly's father and grown for a while *in vitro* (in glass dishes in the laboratory). When the embryos were ready to be implanted into Molly's mother's uterus, each one was genetically tested; only an embryo with precisely the right combination of HLA genes would lead to a cure for Molly. An embryo with the matching HLA genes was obtained and successfully implanted. At its birth, the umbilical cord blood was saved and later used in a bone marrow transplant for Molly. The cells in her sibling's blood were so closely matched to Molly's cells they were not rejected. Her new bone marrow cells flourished and Molly's blood disease was cured. Many things had to go just right for this procedure to work, and they did.

In 2010, Molly received her 10-year checkup. She was 16 years old and healthy. So is her 10-year-old brother Adam. Since this pioneering medical success, the procedures have been successfully performed on other children with fatal blood diseases. Today, all the major *in vitro* fertility (IVF) clinics can perform genetic testing of laboratory embryos. Most of the testing is now done to ensure that the implanted embryo does not carry genes that cause serious inherited diseases. But some scientists and others worry that the time may come when parents may want to have embryos tested for genes that confer talents, such as athletic or musical ability, eliminate susceptibility for cancer or heart disease, or prolong life. The list is endless, as are speculations about abuses. As the great Yankee baseball catcher Yogi Berra supposedly said: "Prediction is very difficult—especially if it's about the future."

Genetic testing is voluntary. Because testing has benefits as well as limitations and risks, the decision about whether to be tested is a personal and complex one. A geneticist or genetic counselor can help by providing information about the pros and cons of the test and discussing the social and emotional aspects of testing.

Genetic tests are most useful when they are used to prevent passing on genes that cause serious inherited disorders. Some common inherited disorders for which genetic tests are available include cystic fibrosis, sickle cell anemia, hemophilia A, Duchenne muscular dystrophy, Huntington's disease, fragile X syndrome, and many others. People who are concerned whether they or other family members carry a defective gene should consult with a genetic counseling professional.

Two examples serve to illustrate the complex issues surrounding genetic testing. Symptoms of Huntington's disease do not appear until midlife or later. Folksinger Woody Guthrie died of Huntington's disease, and his son, Arlo Guthrie, did not know whether he had inherited the abnormal gene from his father. (Arlo had a 50–50 chance of having inherited the gene. The genetic test for Huntington's disease had not yet been developed.) Arlo took the chance and had his children before he reached the age when symptoms appear. Luckily, Arlo did not inherit the gene from his father, so his children would not get Huntington's disease either.

If a parent has died of Huntington's disease, the children of that parent can be tested for the presence or absence of the gene. Suppose a child finds out at age 15 that the Huntington gene has been passed on and that symptoms likely will begin to appear in midlife followed by disability and premature death. For a child or young adult to cope with that knowledge may well be too much of a psychological burden. Some people whose families have a history of members with Huntington's disease choose not to know or to be tested; others want to know their status. Either choice is difficult and may result in serious psychological stress whether the result is positive or negative. (A negative result may produce overwhelming feelings of guilt if a sibling's result is positive.)

Another dilemma arises with breast cancer susceptibility genes. The risk of developing breast cancer in women is strongly influenced by inheriting one or both cancer susceptibility genes called *BRCA1* and *BRCA2*. Inheriting both susceptibility genes means a woman has an 80% to 90% probability of developing breast cancer at some time in her life, usually while quite young. In families whose female members have a high incidence of breast cancer, young women can be tested for the presence of these susceptibility genes. If both genes are found to be present, a young woman is faced with two demoralizing choices. She can worry and wait for signs of breast cancer. Or she can elect to have prophylactic mastectomy in which both breasts are surgically removed while she is young to avoid the development of breast cancer later in life.

In Great Britain, women who carry breast cancer susceptibility genes can choose to have a child using *in vitro* fertilization. A single cell from the embryo can be tested to make sure it does not carry *BRCA1* or *BRCA2* genes before it is implanted. In this way, parents can be sure the harmful genes will not be passed on to their child.

Genetic tests for serious diseases are a great medical advance but also create serious psychological and ethical problems. Any person thinking about getting a genetic test should consult a genetic counselor before proceeding with such tests. Knowing what your disease risks are can change your life forever. And if others obtain the results of your genetic tests, it could lead to insurance or employment problems.

Prenatal Testing

Prospective parents can be tested for the presence of genetic abnormalities that might be passed on to their child(ren). Also, it is possible to test if a fetus *in utero* is affected by a genetic abnormality. One such procedure is **amniocentesis** (**Figure 15.4**). In this procedure, fetal cells are obtained by removing a sample of amniotic fluid from the womb around the 15th week of pregnancy. Although amniocentesis is very safe, there is still a small risk of harming the fetus or inducing a miscarriage. The physician should discuss the risks and benefits of the procedure as part of the genetic counseling. Amniocentesis is performed so that prospective parents can decide whether to continue the pregnancy or abort the fetus. The decision is generally made after discussion with their physician and a counselor.

The fetal cells obtained by amniocentesis are grown in the laboratory and tested for biochemical and genetic abnormalities. Examination of the chromosomes in the karyotype analysis also identifies the sex of the fetus, but this information is provided only if the pregnant woman specifically requests it. (Although most people in American society are joyful at the birth of either a boy or a girl, in other countries, male children are still considered more desirable. In fact, determination of a female fetus by amniocentesis and karyotype analysis is the most common cause of elective abortion in many countries.)

Another prenatal procedure called **chorionic villus sampling (CVS)** can be performed as early as 8 weeks after conception. This earlier test provides information regarding the health of the fetus, allowing the parent(s) to make an earlier decision with respect to terminating the pregnancy.

A noninvasive form of prenatal testing is **ultrasound scanning**, which is used to visualize the developing fetus

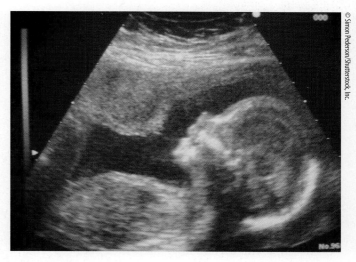

■ **Figure 15.5**

Ultrasound Scanning
Image of a fetus obtained by ultrasound scanning. Such ultrasound scans reveal the position of the fetus and may also indicate certain physical abnormalities.

(**Figure 15.5**). Ultrasound scans use high-frequency sound waves that bounce back from the various tissues in the fetus with different intensities. The sound waves reflected from the fetus are displayed on a screen, and the image is interpreted by a physician trained in the use of this technique.

TERMS

amniocentesis: a procedure in which amniotic fluid is removed from the uterus and tested to determine whether genetic or anatomical defects exist in the fetus

chorionic villus sampling (CVS): a prenatal procedure used to determine whether genetic or anatomical defects exist in a fetus; an alternative to amniocentesis

ultrasound scanning: use of sound waves to visualize the fetus in the womb

---

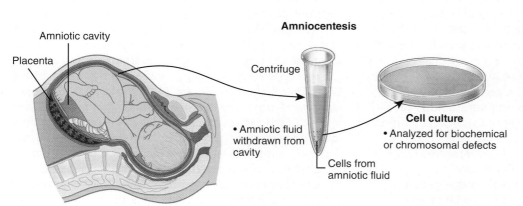

Amniocentesis

Amniotic cavity

Placenta

Centrifuge

• Amniotic fluid withdrawn from cavity

Cells from amniotic fluid

Cell culture
• Analyzed for biochemical or chromosomal defects

■ **Figure 15.4**

Amniocentesis
In the diagnostic procedure called amniocentesis, a sample of the fluid that surrounds the developing fetus is collected. Both the fluid and the fetal cells it contains are then analyzed for biochemical or chromosomal defects.

Ultrasound scans are used to detect multiple fetuses and to determine the location of the placenta, which is important if amniocentesis is to be performed. The scans can gauge the fetus's head size, thereby providing determination of the age of the fetus. Abnormal brain development and neural tube defects also can be diagnosed with an ultrasound scan.

Genetic Discrimination

One of the potential harmful consequences of genetic testing is the possibility of discrimination against a person because he or she carries a particular gene that predisposes the person to a disease. We all understand what discrimination based on sex or race means, and laws have been passed to prevent racial or sexual discrimination in employment, housing, the armed services, and in other public settings. Although rarely described in genetic terms, racial and sexual discrimination are actually a form of genetic discrimination because sex and skin color are determined by the genes that were inherited from parents.

Employers and insurance companies are the organizations most interested in knowing what defective genes a person may have inherited. Companies would obviously prefer not to hire someone who is likely to have a serious health problem after working a few years. Such a person is costly to a company because of wasted training, lost work, and costs of health benefits. A company's health insurance plan might even be canceled if the benefits paid become too high.

> In nature there is no blemish but the mind. None can be called deformed but the unkind.
>
> *William Shakespeare,* Twelfth Night

Health insurance and life insurance companies also would like to have information about a person's genetic profile so that they could select members who are "good" risks and reject those who are "poor" risks. Insurance companies are profit driven, like all companies, and usually can obtain information about genetic tests from a person's medical record. Thus, everyone needs to be very cautious in allowing others to have access to their medical records.

After more than 10 years of intense effort to deal with the problems of genetic discrimination, the Genetic Information Nondiscrimination Act (GINA) was finally passed by Congress and signed into law in 2008. The law forbids:

- An employer from firing or not hiring a person based on information obtained from genetic testing
- Insurance companies from denying health or life insurance to persons based on information obtained from genetic tests
- Companies from charging higher premiums for persons with disease susceptibility genes

It is hoped that the federal law will make people feel safer if they choose to undergo the increasing number of genetic tests that are available and not fear reprisal from employers or insurers.

Gene Therapy Cures Sickle Cell Disease

Sickle cell disease occurs when an individual inherits from each parent abnormal copies of the hemoglobin gene. The abnormal genes produce abnormal hemoglobin proteins, large molecules in the blood responsible for carrying oxygen to all cells in the body. The abnormal hemoglobin proteins tend to stack, causing the red blood cells that carry them to become crescent or sickle shaped (hence the name of the disease) instead of biconcave discs characteristic of normal red blood cells. The crescent-shaped red blood cells clog small blood vessels, producing many symptoms of oxygen deprivation, including pain.

Sickle cell disease first arose in tropical, malarial regions of the world. In a quirk of evolution and natural selection, the presence of one abnormal hemoglobin gene helps protect individuals against infection by the parasite that causes malaria. Those who inherit one copy of the abnormal hemoglobin gene are said to have *sickle cell trait*; they have no symptoms of sickle cell disease because their other normal hemoglobin gene makes sufficient normal hemoglobin to keep them well. Also, they are less likely to die from malaria compared those who carry two abnormal copies of the hemoglobin gene.

Drugs and transfusions have been mainstay treatments for sickle cell disease for many years. In March 2017, a team of French physicians and scientists inserted a normal hemoglobin gene into the bone marrow of a teenage boy with sickle cell disease; after 2 years he was producing sufficient normal hemoglobin to stay well (Ribiel, 2017). It is hoped that this gene therapy treatment will prove sufficiently successful such that it can become a standardized cure. This would represent an enormous success for gene therapy in curing a serious inherited disease. In the United States alone, approximately 900,000 persons have sickle cell disease, mostly Americans of African descent whose ancestors acquired the mutated form of the gene in Africa. Worldwide, as many as 275,000 babies are born annually with sickle cell disease.

Treating Hereditary Diseases

Very few of the thousands of known hereditary diseases can be treated effectively. Phenylketonuria (PKU) is an exception; it can be managed if the affected newborn is diagnosed at birth. Because PKU is treatable and because the test is accurate and inexpensive, all newborns in the United States are tested for PKU. The amino acid phenylalanine is present in any normal diet and, if it is eaten by a child with PKU, it accumulates in the blood, affecting brain development and causing intellectual disabilities. A person with PKU lacks an enzyme that is essential for the chemical breakdown of the phenylalanine present in most proteins, including proteins in milk. Thus, any baby with PKU is immediately put on a phenylalanine-free diet, which must be maintained at least until, and often beyond, puberty.

Mandatory testing for inherited metabolic (chemical) disorders in newborns varies from state to state. With modern technology, a single drop of blood taken from the heel of a newborn can be tested for at least 40 different inherited metabolic disorders. One problem with the tests is that for every infant who actually has an inherited disorder, up to 60 false positives also result. These false-positive results must be ruled out by further tests, during which time parents will continue to worry. Each metabolic disorder creates its own set of medical problems, some of which may be treatable and others not.

Gene Therapy

Thousands of human disorders are caused by inheriting an abnormal gene. Because genes contain the information for making proteins, inheriting an abnormal gene results in a malfunctioning protein that often is manifested as a disease. People with sickle cell anemia inherit abnormal genes for hemoglobin synthesis. In cystic fibrosis, the defective protein is in cell membranes that determine how chemicals enter and exit many cells. And in muscular dystrophy, proteins that are used to build muscle are defective. The problem for medical science is how to cure these inherited diseases.

Occasionally, the defective protein can be manufactured and injected into patients to replace the missing one, as in the treatment for hemophilia. In other cases, drugs are used to lessen the severity of symptoms, as in cystic fibrosis and sickle cell anemia. However, because a fundamental gene is defective in all of the cells in a person's body, these kinds of treatments do not permanently cure the patient. That is the goal of **gene therapy**, an experimental method that uses genes to treat or prevent disease. Researchers are testing several approaches to gene therapy, including (1) replacing a mutated/defective gene that causes disease with a healthy copy of the gene; (2) inactivating, silencing, or "knocking out" a gene that is functioning improperly; and (3) introducing a new, different gene into the body to help fight a disease.

Since elucidation of the complete chemistry of the human genome in 2001 (U.S. National Human Genome Research Institute, 2016), scientific understanding of how genes work, and hence ways to alter malfunctions, has deepened. More and more genes have been identified and obtained to be used in gene therapy trials involving replacing or silencing malfunctioning genes by a variety of techniques. The hope is that the normal gene will function once it is in the cells, and that the protein will be produced in sufficient quantity to cure the inherited disease permanently.

The logic of gene therapy is sound; however, in practice it has proved exceptionally difficult to overcome the technical and biological obstacles. In 2000, it appeared that gene therapy had its first major success. Several children in France suffering from a severe inherited immune system disease were given healthy genes, and their immune systems began functioning normally. The normal genes were transferred to their cells using what was thought to be a harmless virus as a vector to carry the genes into cells. Scientists hailed the results. By the end of 2002, however, two of the children had contracted leukemia, presumably from the virus that had been used in the gene therapy experiment. The use of this method of gene therapy was suspended, and scientists are searching for other means of transferring genes to cells.

After decades of setbacks for gene therapy techniques to cure inherited diseases, there are now some significant successes (Lewis, 2014). A few patients with hemophilia, a serious inherited blood disorder, have been helped through insertion of normal genes into their cells. Gene therapies for inherited immune diseases, blindness, and lung disease are in development or have been approved for use. Researchers are looking to develop therapies for Alzheimer disease, diabetes, heart failure, and cancer.

Although gene therapy is a promising treatment option for a number of diseases (including inherited disorders, some types of cancer, and certain viral infections), the technique remains risky and is still under study to make sure that it will be safe and effective. Gene therapy is currently being tested only for diseases that have no other cures.

Embryonic Stem Cells

A generation ago there was great consternation and public debate over the ethical and social issues associated with *in vitro* fertilization (IVF). Today, the benefits and risks of IVF are widely accepted, and millions of children, many of whom have reached reproductive age themselves, have been conceived using assisted reproductive technologies. However, the ability to create human embryos in the laboratory has led to research with unused laboratory-derived embryos to generate **embryonic stem cells**. Such cells hold great promise for treating presently incurable diseases such as Parkinson's disease, amyotrophic lateral sclerosis (ALS), spinal injuries, and type 1 diabetes.

TERMS

embryonic stem cells: cells derived from human fertilized eggs and grown in laboratory dishes; stem cells have the capacity to differentiate into many different tissues and organs

gene therapy: a technique for replacing defective genes with normal ones in certain tissues of a person affected with a hereditary disease

A human being begins with a fertilized egg that develops over a span of nine months in the uterus into a fully developed infant. When a human embryo develops to the point where it contains several hundred cells, it is called a blastocyst (**Figure 15.6**). The internal cells in the blastocyst are embryonic stem cells because they possess the capability of developing into specific tissues such as lung, heart, liver, brain, and so forth when they are exposed to specific environmental factors that cause them to differentiate (become specialized). In the laboratory, cells can be removed from early-stage embryos and grown in large numbers in laboratory dishes, where some develop into stable embryonic stem cell lines that can be stored or grown under special conditions during which they develop into specialized cells and tissues. Stem cell lines retain the potential for developing into specific tissues almost indefinitely. When injected into organs in the body, stem cells can replace tissues that may have been damaged or destroyed by disease.

For example, mouse embryonic stem cells have been injected into the pancreas of diabetic mice where the cells developed into pancreatic cells capable of producing insulin. The research with mice suggests that some forms of human diabetes (type 1) might be helped by the use of human embryonic stem cells.

A major goal of stem cell research is to develop lines of stem cells that contain an individual's own genetic information (Phimister, 2005). This can be accomplished as follows. Cells are removed from a patient with a serious disease. Several nuclei are removed and injected into human eggs from which the nuclei have been carefully removed (enucleated eggs). Each egg with the patient's cell's nuclei will develop into a blastocyst in a laboratory dish. Then single cells are removed and grown into stable embryonic stem cell lines. If this is successful, the individualized stem cells can be used to treat the patient's disease without concern about rejection because the genetic information in the stem cells is the same as in the patient's own cells.

Embryonic stem cell research is exceptionally controversial in the United States. Supporters of such research point to its enormous potential for relieving human suffering and treating incurable diseases. Opponents believe that every human embryo, regardless of how it was created, is a potential "person" and that the "soul" enters when fertilization takes place or when an embryo exists. Despite ethical concerns and scientific setbacks, it seems likely that stem cell therapies will eventually be developed and used successfully to treat serious diseases.

Genome Editing

The genome is the entirety of all the DNA in an organism's cells. The composition of a human's genome is established at conception and remains unchanged for life, although small parts of a genome can change depending on interactions with the environment. For example, sunlight (ultraviolet radiation) acting on skin cells can alter their DNA, causing some of them to become redder or darker, or even cancerous.

In 2015, scientists discovered a way to change precisely, easily, and inexpensively the composition of a person's DNA using a method of **genome editing**, also referred to as *gene editing* or *gene splicing*, called *CRISPR/Cas-9*. This method allows segments of DNA to be changed, added, removed, or distributed to different locations within cells. For example, if ultraviolet radiation in sunlight has damaged some part of the DNA in a person's skin cells, genome editing could be employed to snip out the affected DNA and replace it with an undamaged copy of the original or a piece customized in some other way. Genome editing using CRISPR/Cas-9 is being explored in research on a wide variety of diseases, including single-gene disorders such as cystic fibrosis, hemophilia, and sickle cell disease. The method may also be

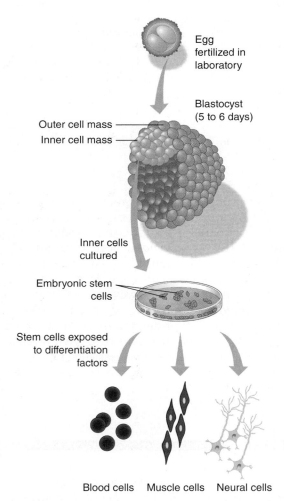

Egg fertilized in laboratory

Blastocyst (5 to 6 days)

Outer cell mass
Inner cell mass

Inner cells cultured

Embryonic stem cells

Stem cells exposed to differentiation factors

Blood cells   Muscle cells   Neural cells

■ **Figure 15.6**

Isolation of Embryonic Stem Cells
A fertilized egg is allowed to develop in the laboratory until it contains several hundred cells. Some of these cells are spread on laboratory dishes where they grow into colonies of embryonic stem cells. These cells can be grown almost indefinitely; when they are exposed to certain environments, they differentiate into cells characteristic of specific tissues and organs.

instrumental in treating and preventing more complex conditions such as some types of heart disease, mental illness, and infections.

Ethical concerns arise when genome editing is used to alter the genomes in eggs and sperm or the DNA of embryos. Such changes would be passed from one generation to the next. This would be beneficial to any potential parent who carried a harmful gene, such as Huntington's disease or hemophilia. However, the technology could be used to enhance normal human traits such as height, musical ability, or intelligence. This is the reason sperm/egg and embryo genome editing are currently illegal in many countries.

TERMS

genome editing: a method to precisely add, change, or remove segements of DNA

Critical Thinking About Health

1. A friend who is about 25 years old has just learned that she is pregnant. The woman smokes cigarettes and likes to party on weekends. Based on what you have learned about the causes of congenital defects in this chapter, make a list of all the behavioral, dietary, and lifestyle changes you would recommend to your friend to help ensure that she gives birth to a healthy child. Discuss the rationale for each of your recommendations.

2. Abortion is one of the most controversial issues in American society. At one end of the spectrum of views are people who think that all abortions should be prohibited for any reason whatsoever, even if the life of the pregnant woman is in jeopardy. At the other extreme are people who believe that each pregnant woman should have complete freedom to do whatsoever she chooses with respect to her pregnancy because it is her body. Evaluate these two views of abortion and present your own views in as much detail as possible. Substantiate each of your views.

3. Are scientists obliged to inform nonscientists of results of their research that might bear on suscepti- bility to a serious disease? Here is an example.

   A scientist is studying the DNA from patients who have died from cancer of the pancreas. She is trying to discover any genes that may be involved in the development of the disease. She finds that the DNA of many patients with pancreatic cancer carry mutations that are known to cause other cancers. One such mutation is *BRCA2*, which is a well-established risk factor for breast and ovarian cancer in women. Should the scientist inform relatives of pancreatic cancer patients of her discovery so they can be tested

   for *BRCA2*? Even though most cancer susceptibility genes increase risk, they do not make cancer inev- itable. If you agree they should be informed, how should relatives be notified and what support should be offered? On the other hand, should relatives not be told since there is no certainty they will develop pancreatic cancer and there is no established rule or law that says relatives should be informed of harm- ful mutations found in a relative's DNA?

4. A few years ago, the U.S. military ordered all service personnel to have a blood sample taken so that the DNA of each individual's cells could be analyzed and the pattern placed on file, much as the FBI keeps files of fingerprints of criminals and others. The reason the military wants each person's DNA analyzed is so that remains can be positively identified in case that person dies in a future conflict. One soldier refused to give a blood sample in violation of a direct order and was ordered to stand before a court martial. The soldier argued that he had no assurance that his DNA information would be kept private and would not be used for purposes of discrimination or to his detri- ment in other ways.

   a. Do you think the military is justified in wanting each person's DNA on file?

   b. In what ways might the DNA information be used to the detriment of the soldier either in the military or after his release from military service?

   c. Discuss the pros and cons of having the DNA profile of every person in the United States on file in a federal agency so that any person could be positively identified by law enforcement authorities, government agencies, or other orga- nizations, should the need arise.

Chapter Summary and Highlights

Chapter Summary

The hereditary information in every human being is con- tained in long, chainlike molecules of DNA. The mole- cules of DNA, in turn, are packaged into 46 chromosomes, 23 of which come from each parent. All of the information needed to construct a human being is contained in about 3 billion pairs of four different chemical letters: A, G, C, and T. Every human trait, from skin color to the propen- sity for athletic and intellectual ability, is contained in this massive "Book of Life." In the 1990s, scientists decided to decipher the exact sequence of the 3 billion elements in one person's DNA. The U.S. government funded the idea and established the Human Genome Project. The goal of sequencing a complete human genome was reached in

2003, when the entire sequence was published online. The cost of this project was $2.7 billion. In the years following this amazing accomplishment, the complete DNA sequences of some viruses, bacteria, yeast, plants, and animals were obtained. This became possible because the cost of sequencing DNA dropped dramatically as the process became automated and computerized. Today, the cost of sequencing all of the DNA in a person is only a few thousand dollars.

Because of these advances in sequencing DNA, a rev- olution has occurred in our understanding of inherited (genetic) diseases. A defect in a single gene can cause a genetic disease such as sickle cell anemia, muscular dystrophy, cystic fibrosis, hemophilia, and thousands of others. Genetic defects can be identified in prospective parents, and new genetic and reproductive technologies help prevent the defective genes from being passed on to children. Diseases such as cancer, heart disease, diabetes, and other chronic conditions are caused not by a single gene but by many genes that together increase a person's risk. Companies can sequence your DNA and inform you of your risk for hundreds of diseases … if you want to know. Scientists can now reconstruct human history and population migrations by analyzing the DNA of modern people. You might be interested to know that everyone carries a few genes from our Neanderthal ancestors. Personalized medicine is a new medical specialty based on analyzing patients' DNA and tailoring treatments to their specific genes. Cancer patients receive drugs that are most likely to destroy their particular tumors. Personalized medicine means that most treatments in the future will be customized to the patient's particular set of genes. The genetic revolution is likely to generate even more spectacular results than the Internet and communication revolution of the recent past.

Highlights

- Every newborn inherits 23 chromosomes and about 20,000 genes from each parent. Inheriting abnormal chromosomes or abnormal genes can result in an inherited disease.
- Genetic information is carried in DNA.
- Congenital birth defects are observed at birth in about 1 of 50 newborn babies in the United States. Abnormal development of the fetus during pregnancy can be caused by environmental factors, abnormal genes that were passed on from one or both parents, or a combination of both.
- Ultrasound, amniocentesis, and chorionic villus sampling are prenatal diagnostic procedures that can determine whether fetal development is normal or whether there is a physical or biological defect.
- Taking prescription or illegal drugs, drinking alcohol, or becoming infected by viruses during pregnancy also can harm the fetus. If drugs or alcohol are used by a pregnant woman, especially in early pregnancy, the fetus may abort spontaneously or the newborn may suffer growth deficiencies, intellectual disabilities, or other problems.
- Couples who are at higher-than-average risk for having a child with a genetic abnormality should undergo genetic counseling before and after pregnancy is established.
- Modern genetic diagnostic tests can detect genes responsible for hundreds of hereditary diseases; however, only a few can be treated successfully.
- Genetic discrimination may occur when people find out that they or others carry genes that predispose them to diseases and disorders. A federal law prohibits genetic discrimination.
- Gene therapy is a promising new method of treating genetic diseases.
- Embryonic stem cells are derived from early-stage embryos produced in the laboratory. Such cells have the potential to differentiate into any desired tissues. Such cells may help cure serious diseases.
- Genome editing, also referred to as *gene editing* or *gene splicing*, allows segments of DNA to be changed, added, removed, or distributed to different locations within cells.

For Your Health

Inheritance can have a major effect on health and disease. Do "My Family Medical History" (Exercise 15.1 in the Workbook) for your medical records.

References

Enattah, N. S., et al. (2002). Identification of a variant associated with adult-type hypolactasia. *Nature Genetics, 30,* 233–237.

Gibbons, A. (2006). There's more than one way to have your milk and drink it, too. *Science, 314,* 1672.

Hagerman, R. J., & Hagerman, P. J. (2008). Testing for fragile X gene mutations throughout the life span. *Journal of the American Medical Association, 300,* 2419–2421.

Hook, E. B. (1984). Chromosomal abnormality rates at amniocentesis and in live-born infants. *Journal of the American Medical Association, 249,* 2034–2038.

Itan, Y., et al. (2010). A worldwide correlation of lactase persistence phenotype and genotypes. *BMC Evolutionary Biology, 10,* 36. Retrieved from http://www.biomedcentral.com/1471–2148/10/36

Kaiser, J. (2012). New cystic fibrosis drug offers hope, at a price. *Science, 335,* 645.

Lewis, R. (2014, March). Gene therapy's second act. *Scientific American*, 53–57.

Phimister, E. G. (2005). A tetraploid twist on the embryonic stem cell. *New England Journal of Medicine, 353*, 1046–1054.

Ribeil, J.-A. (2017). Gene therapy in a patient with sickle cell disease. *New England Journal of Medicine, 376*, 848–866.

U.S. National Human Genome Research Institute. (2016). An overview of the Human Genome Project. Retrieved from https://www.genome.gov/12011238/an-overview-of-the-human-genome-project/

Suggested Readings

Brownlee, C. (2005, April 9). Code of many colors. *Science News*, 232–234. Evaluates the never-ending controversy about biology and race.

Couzin-Frankel, J. (2011). What would you do? *Science, 331*, 662–665. This article presents several real-life problems resulting from genetic testing and asks "What would you do?" Read this article to discover the serious consequences of genetic testing that uncovers unanticipated or unwanted truths.

Epstein, D. (2013). *The sports gene—inside the science of exceptional athletic performance.* New York: Current. A sports writer and former track-and-field athlete writes about the contribution of specific genes to athletic ability. All sports now banish the use of drugs to improve performance. But genes may be far more important, especially for sprinters and long-distance runners. We can't ban specific genes in athletes; or can we?

Gawande, A. (2004, December 6). The bell curve. *The New Yorker*, 82–91. A doctor describes the complexities of getting treatment for a common inherited disease, cystic fibrosis.

Hall, M., & Olopode, O. I. (2005). Confronting genetic testing disparities. *Journal of the American Medical Association, 293*, 1783–1785. Explains the many problems associated with genetic testing.

Nuzzo, R. (2008, June 2). Nabbing suspicious SNPs. *Science News*, 20–24. An excellent short article describing how the hundreds of disease susceptibility genes are being discovered.

Omenn, G. S. (2009, Summer). From human genome research to personalized health care. *Issues in Science and Technology*, 51–56. A thoughtful examination of what the new discoveries in genetics will mean to individuals' health and medical care.

Saey, T. H. (2009, April 25). Shared differences. *Science News*, 16–20. A lucid, easy-to-understand article that explains how mistakes in genes encoded in DNA result in susceptibility to physical and mental disorders.

Venter, C. (2007). *A life decoded: My genome, my life.* New York: Viking. The personal story of the man who beat everyone in the race to sequence the human genome.

Young, S. (2014). Genetic surgery. *MIT Technology Review, 117*, 55–59. New techniques for rapidly and accurately changing bits of information in human DNA may soon make it possible to correct serious genetic flaws, restore normal gene function, and cure serious diseases. Scientific reality is poised to catch up with science fiction.

Recommended Websites

GeneWatch

The Council for Responsible Genetics (CRG) publishes a monthly magazine called *GeneWatch*. CRG is an activist organization that focuses public attention on the moral and ethical issues of the genetic advances in medicine, food, and technology.

The Human Genome Project

Information on the scientific, medical, ethical, legal, and social aspects of medical genetics.

U.S. National Center for Birth Defects and Developmental Disabilities

Information on causes and prevention of birth defects.

PART FIVE

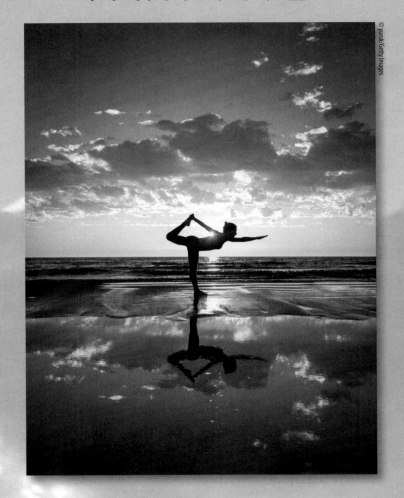

© yurok/Getty Images

Explaining Drug Use and Abuse

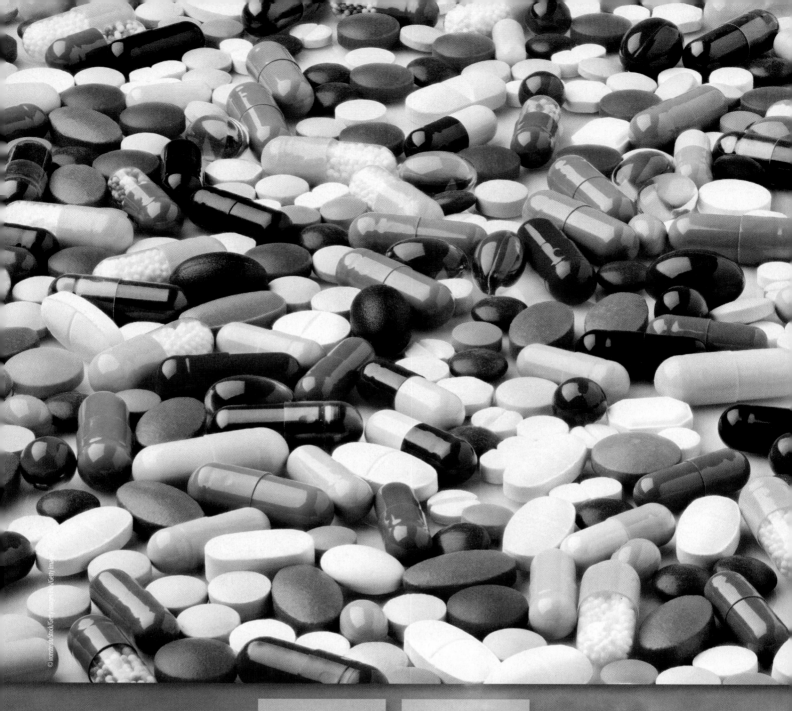

Health
Tips

Don't Overdose on Over-the-Counter Pain Killers

Screen Addiction to Video Games, the Internet, TV Binge Watching, and Smartphones

Wellness
Guide

Risk Factors for Addiction

What to Do with Expired or Unused Medicines

CHAPTER 16

Using Drugs and Medications Responsibly

Learning Objectives

1. Explain the difference between a drug and a medicine.

2. Explain the concept of a drug receptor and its relation to drug side effects.

3. Describe the logic of a double-blind drug effectiveness study.

4. Give examples of the overuse of legal drugs in American society and the influences of drug advertising on drug use.

5. Explain the FDA's drug approval process.

6. Define *addiction, physical dependence, habituation, tolerance,* and *withdrawal.*

7. Describe the different effects of the major classes of psychoactive drugs: stimulants, depressants, marijuana, hallucinogens, PCP, and inhalants.

8. Describe the health hazards of using anabolic steroids.

For thousands of years, people have been ingesting substances to heal themselves, change consciousness, produce sleep, drive out evil spirits, and promote tribal and family harmony. For most of that time, such substances were obtained by chewing the leaves of a particular plant, brewing a tea from a plant's bark or roots, or mixing a potion made up of plant and animal materials, as the three witches in Shakespeare's *Macbeth* did when they concocted "eye of newt and toe of frog, wool of bat and tongue of dog." Today, some substances used for healing or nonmedicinal purposes are still obtained from plant and animal tissues or extracts, whereas others are substances manufactured by modern chemical and biological technologies.

No matter how they are obtained, many substances are of enormous value in relieving pain, preventing disease, and facilitating healing. However, indiscriminate or inappropriate use and overuse of substances also are major problems in our society. For example, overuse of antibiotics has led to the creation of antibiotic-resistant bacteria, against which many antibiotic drugs are no longer effective. Recently, opium-like substances (*opioids*), intended for medicinal use as pain relievers, have become widely abused, often to the point of serious illness and death. Tobacco and alcohol are responsible for many millions deaths annually (**Figure 16.1**). Millions of people become sick and thousands die from unforeseen adverse reactions to prescription medications (U.S. Department of Health and Human Services, 2017). And everyone has

> Too much of a good thing is wonderful.
>
> *Mae West*

heard of the $40 billion per year "war on drugs," which is concerned with the social and legal problems associated with the use of amphetamines, cocaine, heroin, and other illegal substances.

The use of drugs in our society has become so commonplace and accepted that many people automatically turn to drugs to solve their physical, mental, and emotional problems, failing to appreciate the values of nondrug alternatives and to understand the associated dangers and health hazards of drug use of any need. When someone is stressed, anxious, depressed, or tired, or if they have a headache or stomach upset or chronic pain, they believe that taking drugs is the *only* source of relief. Although many medicines are extremely valuable, reliance on drugs to solve life's problems is much more likely to mask rather than to solve them, and may also open the way for chemical dependency.

What Is a Drug?

A **drug** is a single chemical substance that alters the structure or function of one or more of the body's biological processes. The alteration can start, stop, speed up, or slow down a process, depending on the specific drug and its effect. A **medicine** is a drug (or combination of drugs) that is intended to (1) prevent illness, as vaccines do; (2) cure disease, as antibiotics do; (3) aid healing, as heartburn medications do; or (4) suppress symptoms, as pain relievers do. Not all drugs—for example, alcohol and nicotine—are medicines.

Drugs are usually classified according to the particular biological process they affect rather than by their chemical properties. For example, all substances that increase urine production, regardless of their chemical structure, are called *diuretics*, those that reduce pain are *analgesics*, and those that produce nervous system excitation are *stimulants*.

Drug Laws

American society regulates chemicals that change physiology (the definition of a drug) by placing them into one of five groups:

1. Chemicals that are presumably so potent that only a doctor can permit their use so as to limit any harm that might arise from their use (so-called prescription drugs)
2. Chemicals that are not so potent or dangerous that consumers can obtain them directly from stores or other sellers (so-called nonprescription or over-the-counter drugs)
3. Chemicals, plant extracts, and vitamins that consumers can obtain directly from stores or other sellers, which are called *dietary supplements* rather than drugs, even though biologically they act as drugs
4. Tobacco and alcohol, which are addictive drugs with no therapeutic value and are used by choice for a variety of reasons

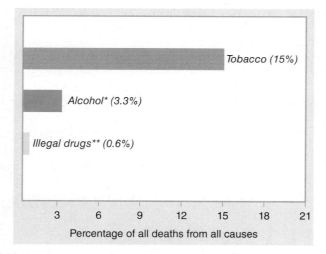

■ Figure 16.1

Percentage of All-Cause Annual Deaths from Drug Use, United States

*Includes deaths from alcohol-related car crashes.
**Deaths associated with suicide, homicide, motor vehicle injury, HIV infection, pneumonia, violence, mental illness, and hepatitis.
Adapted from Trinidad, J. T., et al. (2016). Using literal text from the death certificate to enhance mortality statistics: Characterizing drug involvement in deaths. Centers for Disease Control and Prevention, National Center for Health Statistics, *National Vital Statistics Reports, 65*(9). Retrieved from https://www.cdc.gov/nchs/data/nvsr65/nvsr65_09.pdf

5. Chemicals that are considered so dangerous to users and society that they are outlawed (so-called illegal or illicit drugs)

It is important to realize that regardless of its legal category, no drug is entirely safe. Any substance that can alter physiology has the potential to be harmful. The federal government screens only prescription drugs for potential harm. For chemicals in the other four categories in the preceding list, consumers are responsible for learning the risks and benefits.

The United States spends billions of dollars each year on the "war on drugs." It is important to see that this expenditure is about enforcement of laws and not necessarily about protecting health. This is not to say that there should not be laws regarding drug use. For health reasons, however, it is wise not to think of legal drugs as safe and good and of illegal drugs as harmful and bad. The situation is much more complex than that. This is why the healthiest course of action is to be a cautious, knowledgeable consumer of drugs of any kind.

How Drugs Work

Many drugs act by binding to **receptors** on the surface of, or within, specific cells in the body. A drug–receptor interaction is akin to a key (the drug) fitting into a lock (the receptor) (**Figure 16.2**). When a drug binds to a cell's receptor, it alters one or more biological processes of the cell. Frequently, a drug may chemically resemble a natural body component, such as a hormone or a neurotransmitter, which interacts with the receptor as part of normal functioning. The drug binds to the receptor in place of the natural substance and thereby alters physiology.

For example, the receptors for many antibiotics are on structures within bacteria that are responsible for manufacturing vital bacterial proteins. When an antibiotic binds to its receptor in a bacterium, it blocks the manufacture of bacterial proteins, the bacteria die, and the infection stops. The receptors for many antidepressant drugs are located in the brain on cells that utilize the neurotransmitter serotonin. When an antidepressant binds to its receptor, serotonin transport into those cells is blocked, and depression is relieved.

Pharmacogenetics

A major assumption in the prescribing of drugs is that everyone's body uses a drug in the same way. This is the reason that drugs have "standard" dosages and expected side effects and that adverse reactions occur in only a small number of people. However, doctors and scientists know that individuals respond to drugs differently, sometimes quite dramatically. The degree to which a person responds to a drug can depend on that person's genetic makeup. The primary products of genes, proteins, facilitate nearly all the body's chemical reactions. Just as variations in genes produce different eye color pigments, genetic variations determine how the body responds to a particular drug and how it is eliminated from the body. This is why one person may tolerate and respond positively to a particular dose of a drug while another person may respond weakly, have an adverse reaction, or even die. In some instances, scientists can now determine which of a person's genes may affect her or his response to a particular drug. This is the science of **pharmacogenetics**.

For example, the drug *warfarin* is used to prevent the formation of potentially fatal blood clots. To be effective and safe, the amount of warfarin in a person's blood must be maintained within narrow limits; too little may allow a clot to form, and too much may cause internal bleeding. It's been determined that individuals differ genetically with regard to how they utilize and excrete warfarin. Genetic tests are now available so doctors can match the appropriate dose of warfarin with a patient's corresponding genetic profile. The goal of pharmacogenetics is to identify many of the genes that affect drug responses and adverse effects. The hope is that one day drugs can be tailored to a patient's specific biology to produce optimum benefit with minimal risk.

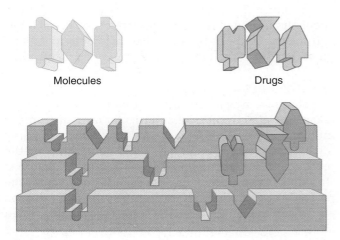

Molecules   Drugs

■ Figure 16.2

Bindings of Drugs to Cellular Receptor Sites
The molecular structures of many drugs are similar to molecules normally produced in the body. The drugs attach to receptor sites on cells and alter the physiological functioning of organs and tissues.

TERMS

drug: a single chemical substance that alters one or more of the body's biological functions

medicine: drugs used to prevent, treat, or cure illness; aid healing; or suppress symptoms

pharmacogenetics: tailoring drugs to a particular individual to match her or his biology

receptor: protein on the surface or inside of a cell to which a drug or natural substance can bind and thereby affect cell function

■ **Figure 16.3**

Common Side Effects of Drugs of Abuse
The functions of almost every organ or system in the body can be unintentionally altered by the effects of a drug.

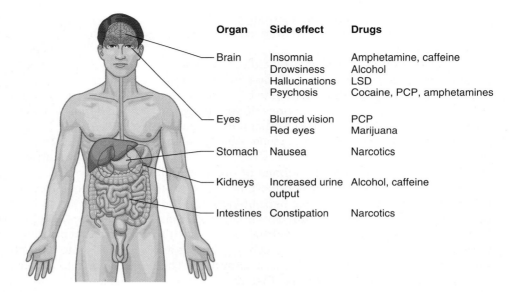

Organ	Side effect	Drugs
Brain	Insomnia	Amphetamine, caffeine
	Drowsiness	Alcohol
	Hallucinations	LSD
	Psychosis	Cocaine, PCP, amphetamines
Eyes	Blurred vision	PCP
	Red eyes	Marijuana
Stomach	Nausea	Narcotics
Kidneys	Increased urine output	Alcohol, caffeine
Intestines	Constipation	Narcotics

Unintended Harmful Effects of Drugs and Medicines

Even though a medicine may be intended to have a single effect, it often has more than one because it binds to a variety of receptors in or on different cells, causing **side effects** (**Figure 16.3**), which may be minor or severe. Some side effects include allergic reactions (**drug hypersensitivity**); harm to developing embryos and fetuses (**teratogen**); or physical dependence.

A drug also may be harmful if the drug taker has a condition that is aggravated by that drug. A medical reason for not taking a drug is called a **contraindication**. For example, a history of blood vessel disease is a contraindication for taking birth control pills. The need to screen for contraindications is one reason that many medicines are available only by prescription.

Side effects are examples of **adverse drug reactions (ADRs)**. These are unintended, unpleasant, and/or harmful reactions to a medicinal product resulting from errors in prescribing and administering a medicine; misuse or abuse by a patient; use of a medicine for a medically unapproved reason; unwanted effects associated with cumulative drug exposure; withdrawal reactions; and susceptibility factors such as genetic, pathological, and other biological differences (Colemen & Pontefract, 2017). Between 5% and 10% of patients experience ADRs; they can occur in both in-hospital and outpatient settings. Higher rates are found in elderly patients who are likely to be taking multiple medications for several long-term illnesses (*polypharmacy*).

An adverse reaction to a drug that gets little attention is the **rebound effect**. This is the reemergence of symptoms for which a drug is administered after the drug is suddenly stopped or the dose lessened. Often the symptoms that emerge after stopping the drug are more severe than the original symptoms. Rebound effects have been described for a variety of medications, including antihistamines to control symptoms of hay fever (allergic rhinitis), eczema (atopic dermatitis), insomnia, anxiety, high blood pressure, and certain pain medications. When symptoms from the rebound effect occur, physicians and patients are lured into restarting the drug at a higher, more effective dose. This, however, leads to further rebounds when the drug is discontinued. An alternative is to taper reduction of the drug to allow the body to adjust to lower doses. A severe rebound effect may prompt a patient and physician to explore nonpharmacological alternatives.

Medical practitioners should be knowledgeable about the side effects and contraindications of drugs, but sometimes these are overlooked. About one-third of hospital stays are extended because inappropriate medications are administered or medications are managed improperly by medical staff. Consumers of medications are wise to remember that all drugs and medicines have the potential for harm. They should learn as much as they can about the intended use and side effects of their drugs, and they should ask their medical providers to explain the rationale for the medications prescribed (**Table 16.1**).

Effectiveness of Drugs

The dose of a drug is the amount that is administered or taken. The effectiveness of a particular dose of a drug is influenced by a person's body size, how rapidly the drug breaks down and is eliminated, and sometimes by the presence of other drugs and foods recently consumed (**Table 16.2**). A drug's effectiveness also depends on the person's expectations of the drug's efficacy (placebo effect) and the person's mental state. For example, when stressed or anxious, many people require higher doses of analgesics to relieve pain than when they are relaxed. Most drugs have a narrow range of effectiveness; that is, doses that produce intended results. In excess, many drugs are toxic and some are lethal. If the dose is too low, insufficient therapeutic effect may result.

Table 16.1

Latin Terms Commonly Used in Prescriptions

Latin	Abbreviation	Meaning
ante cibum	ac	before meals
bis in die	bid	twice a day
gutta	gt	drop
hora somni	hs	at bedtime
oculus dexter	od	right eye
oculus sinister	os	left eye
per os	po	by mouth
post cibum	pc	after meals
pro re nata	prn	as needed
quaque 3 hora	q 3 h	every 3 hours
quaque die	qd	every day
quater in die	qid	four times a day
ter in die	tid	three times a day
†, ††, or †††		1, 2, or 3 (of the dosage form, such as tablets)

market, manufacturers of ibuprofen advertised heavily in medical journals to get physicians to recommend or prescribe the new drug. One advertisement showed that after 4 hours, Nuprin, the trade name for one ibuprofen drug, relieved headaches about 8% more effectively than acetaminophen (**Figure 16.4**). From a holistic health perspective, however, the more significant result is that almost 40% of headache sufferers got the same relief with a placebo. Thus, 4 of 10 headache sufferers found relief simply by believing that they had taken a pain-relief medicine.

An even more remarkable placebo effect is shown by the ability of balding men to stimulate hair growth simply by believing that they are using a hair-stimulating drug called Rogaine. Pfizer, the manufacturer of Rogaine, advertises extensively, emphasizing the effectiveness of

The effects of a drug or medicine are often determined scientifically by performing a **double-blind-placebo controlled trial**, which involves administering the drug and a look-and-taste-alike placebo to matched groups of patients. Neither the people administering the drug nor the patients know who is receiving the drug and who is receiving the placebo. Only after the trial is over is the code revealed that tells which patients received the drug and which the placebo. What is most remarkable about many of these drug trials is not that drugs show a therapeutic effect but that placebos often are almost as effective as the drugs.

In 1984, ibuprofen was introduced into the over-the-counter market. Because aspirin and acetaminophen compounds commanded over 90% of the pain-reliever

TERMS

adverse drug reactions (ADRs): unintended, unpleasant, and/or harmful reactions to a medicinal product

contraindication: any medical reason for not taking a particular drug

double-blind-placebo controlled trial: when neither the person receiving the drug nor the person administering the drug knows whether patients receive a placebo or the drug

drug hypersensitivity: an allergic reaction to a drug

rebound effect: the reemergence of symptoms for which a drug is administered after the drug is suddenly stopped or the dose lessened

side effects: unintended and often harmful actions of a drug

teratogen: any environmental agent or drug that alters development of a fetus

Table 16.2

Drug and Food Interactions That Should Be Avoided

If you take	Avoid	Because
Erythromycin or penicillin-type antibiotics	Acidic foods: pickles, tomatoes, vinegar, colas	These antibiotics are destroyed by stomach acids.
Tetracycline-type antibiotics	Calcium-rich foods: milk, cheese, yogurt, pizza, almonds	Calcium blocks the action of tetracycline.
Antihypertensives (to lower blood pressure)	Natural licorice (artificial is OK)	A chemical in natural licorice causes salt and water retention.
Anticoagulants (to thin blood)	Vitamin K: green leafy vegetables, beef liver, vegetable oils	Vitamin K promotes blood clotting.
Antidepressants (monoamine oxidase inhibitors)	Tyramine-rich foods: colas, chocolate, cheese, coffee, wine, avocados	Tyramine elevates blood pressure.
Diuretics	Monosodium glutamate (MSG)	MSG and diuretics both increase water elimination.
Thyroid drugs	Cabbage, brussels sprouts, soybeans, cauliflower	Chemicals in these vegetables depress thyroid hormone production.

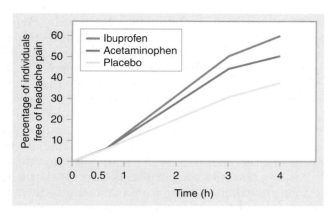

■ **Figure 16.4**

A Study of the Effectiveness of Ibuprofen Versus Acetaminophen in Relieving Headaches
Note that almost 40% of headache sufferers get relief from a placebo and no medicine.

Adapted from Schachtel, B. P., et al. (1996). Nonprescription ibuprofen and acetaminophen in the treatment of tension-type headache. *Journal of Clinical Pharmacology, 36*, 1120–5.

Rogaine compared with a placebo solution applied to the scalp. Rogaine produces minimal to moderate growth of new hair in 33% of patients receiving the drug. However, a placebo containing no active ingredient produces minimal to moderate hair growth in 20% of patients. Although this fact is ignored by the advertising, it means that one in five men who have pattern baldness (an inherited trait) can stimulate new hair growth simply because they believe they are using a drug. How the mind changes physiology to accomplish this is unknown. The point, however, is never to underestimate the power of your mind to act like a drug and help you to heal an injury or cure an illness.

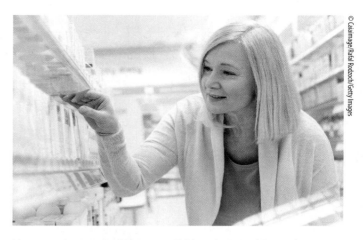

More over-the-counter drugs are available in the United States than anywhere else in the world.

The Medicating of Americans

Americans consume an enormous quantity of drugs. In the United States, about 4.5 billion drug prescriptions are filled each year at an annual cost of nearly $385 billion. About 60% of American adults use a prescription medicine each month; 15% use five or more prescription drugs per month (**Table 16.3**). In addition, there are about 100,000 different kinds of nonprescription drugs, or **over-the-counter (OTC) drugs**, purchased, for which Americans pay nearly $34 billion a year. Millions of people use herbal extracts and teas as medicines, and millions more take vitamins, not as nutritional supplements but to prevent or cure diseases. Indeed, when Americans are sick, four out of five times they self-treat with OTC drugs and alternative medicines.

Many drugs sold in the United States are **psychoactive**; that is, they alter thoughts, feelings, and sensations.

Don't Overdose on Over-the-Counter Pain Killers

People take pain-relieving drugs for headaches, backaches, arthritis, joint pain, and many other conditions. Because pain-relieving drugs such as acetaminophen (Tylenol) and ibuprofen (Advil, Motrin) are sold over the counter (OTC), most people assume they are safe and that you can take as much as you need until you get relief. Those assumptions are incorrect. Acetaminophen, ibuprofen, and many other OTC drugs can be as dangerous as their prescription counterparts if not taken as directed on the package and with caution.

Acetaminophen is the most commonly reported cause of poisoning in the United States. Taking more than 4,000 milligrams a day can cause liver failure. Indeed, acetaminophen poisoning is the most frequent reason for liver transplantation in the United States. Because of the dangers of acetaminophen overdose, the U.S. Food and Drug Administration (FDA) asks manufacturers to limit the amount of the drug to 325 milligrams per tablet. Although beneficial to consumers, this request ignores the fact that acetaminophen is sold not only as tablets but also as liquids, suppositories, and chewables and that it also is a component of cold remedies, allergy medicine, and opioid pain medications. If a person takes several acetaminophen-containing medications, overdose is quite possible.

Many people take both acetaminophen and ibuprofen to relieve pain or they take more than the recommend dose. Taking both of these drugs simultaneously increases the risk of an overdose.

People should read carefully all of the ingredients in OTC medications before taking them. Consult a healthcare professional to determine what dose and combination of drugs are safe. If you think you have symptoms of an acetaminophen overdose such as sweating, nausea, vomiting, diarrhea, or jaundice, you need help immediately. Often the fastest way to get help for any drug overdose or poisoning is to call 911 or get to a hospital emergency room.

Table 16.3

Percentage Prevalence of Prescription Drug Use in the United States

Category	Percentage (%) of Adults
Men (any prescription)	52
Women (any prescription)	65
Age > 65 years (any prescription)	90
Condition	
High blood pressure	27.0
High blood lipids	18.0
Depression	13.0
Pain	11.0
Diabetes	8.2
Acid stomach	7.8
Thyroid disease	6.4
Anxiety	6.1
Seizures	5.5
Asthma	5.2
Antibiotics	4.2
Coagulation	4.0
Irregular heartbeat	2.7
Muscle pain/stiffness	2.5
Nasal congestion	2.5

Data from Kantor, E. D., et al. (2015). Trends in prescription drug use among adults in the United States from 1999–2012. *Journal of the American Medical Association, 314*, 1818–1831.

Psychoactive drugs include tranquilizers, sleeping pills, and mood modifiers. About 52 million Americans use alcohol regularly, another 20 million smoke cigarettes or chew tobacco for the stimulant effects of nicotine, and more than one-third of adult Americans ingest caffeine daily for its stimulatory effects. In addition, about 24 million Americans regularly use illegal drugs.[1]

As a group, older persons tend to take the most drugs, usually because they have several chronic medical conditions. It is not uncommon for some older people to take 10 or more different medications daily, which may have been prescribed by different physicians at different times. Occasionally, these drugs interact with each other to cause additional problems. That's why it is important for older people and their families and caregivers to keep a list of all medications and their doses and to inquire of health providers about possible harmful drug interactions.

In American society, the belief that drugs are legitimate and desirable solutions to life problems is pervasive. About half of all doctor visits are for nonmedical or mental health issues that manifest as fatigue, lethargy, gastrointestinal upset, aches and pains, and sleeplessness. Often patients expect healthcare providers to prescribe a medicine, and just as often, healthcare providers feel obligated to offer some remedy, even if medicines are not the solution.

Being healthy means, among other things, being responsible for the drugs you use. You do not have to resort to "chemical coping" for emotional problems. You can resist being pushed into pill popping by drug company advertising. Seeking alternatives to prescription or OTC drug use may be the most healthful action you can take.

Drug Company Advertising

The American pharmaceutical industry is among the most profitable of all industries. Because the largest share of pharmaceutical company profits comes from the sale of prescription medications, pharmaceutical companies invest considerable resources in educating and persuading physicians to prescribe their products. Besides physicians and other healthcare professionals, consumers also are targets of drug company product promotion in the form of **direct-to-consumer advertising (DTCA)**, especially in magazines and on television and the Internet.

In 1997, the Food and Drug Administration (FDA) relaxed its regulations regarding the advertising of prescription drugs directly to consumers (the United States and New Zealand are the only industrialized nations that permit this), and pharmaceutical companies quickly found that direct-to-consumer advertising (DTCA) is very profitable.

Direct-to-consumer advertising is designed to encourage consumers to demand advertised drugs from their doctors in the belief that the drugs they see advertised are superior, whereas unadvertised, lesser known drugs are inferior. This creates pressure on doctors to prescribe advertised drugs even if other, equally effective (and sometimes less costly) medications are available.

Since the inception of DTCA, the FDA and medical organizations have frequently chastised pharmaceutical companies for making misleading claims in their advertising. In general, DTCA overstates or overemphasizes the benefits of a drug. The FDA requires drug companies to include all of a drug's risk information. In print ads, this is usually in a section called the "Brief Summary," which lists the side effects of the drug and which can be quite long. Broadcast ads are allowed to include only the most important risk information as long as the ads tell viewers or listeners how to get the full FDA-approved prescribing information.

TERMS

direct-to-consumer advertising (DTCA): the marketing of prescription drugs to consumers to stimulate demand for a drug

over-the-counter (OTC) drugs: drugs that do not require a prescription

psychoactive: any substance that primarily alters mood, perception, and other brain functions

---

[1] These data pertain to Americans over the age of 18.

The FDA and You

In 1906, the U.S. Congress passed the Federal Food and Drugs Act, which ultimately gave rise to the Food and Drug Administration, to ensure the safety of products sold as foods or medicines. The original 1906 law was revised and strengthened in 1938 as the Federal Food, Drug, and Cosmetic (FDC) Act. Prior to passage of the law, anyone could put anything in a package or bottle and sell it as a food or medicine. The FDA regulates the safety of nearly all foods (the U.S. Department of Agriculture [USDA] oversees meat and poultry), all prescription and over-the-counter drugs (but not dietary supplements) and medical devices, cosmetics, and animal feed.

A major function of the FDA is the approval of new prescription drugs, a process that usually proceeds in the following way:

Step 1: Someone discovers or invents a chemical that in laboratory animals shows promise as a medicine. Often this is a scientist at a research university or a medical school. Financial support for the research comes from tax dollars in the form of grants administered by the U.S. government's National Institutes of Health or the National Science Foundation. Occasionally, the initial research is carried out by drug-company researchers or academic scientists who receive financial support from a drug company to carry out specific research.

Step 2: Based on laboratory studies, a drug company decides that a chemical has promise as a human medicine and applies for FDA approval to conduct tests on people. These tests cost many millions of dollars, for which the drug company pays. There are three kinds of tests, or trials, each carried out on a different group of people:

Phase 1 trial: The test drug is given to 50 to 100 healthy volunteers to determine its safety by giving different doses of the drug.

Phase 2 trial: The test drug is given to several hundred people with the disease or condition to test its effectiveness.

Phase 3 trial: The test drug is given to as many as 3,000 to 5,000 people with the disease or condition to determine the drug's overall efficacy.

Step 3: If the test drug passes all three trials, the pharmaceutical company can apply to the FDA for approval to manufacture and market the drug. A public meeting is convened in Washington, D.C., at which interested parties testify before a panel of scientists on whether the new drug meets criteria for approval, that is, safety, effectiveness, and need. At the end of a day or two of testimony, the scientific panel sends its recommendation to the FDA. It is up to the FDA to accept or reject the panel's recommendations.

Step 4: After a drug is approved and made available to consumers, its safety and efficacy are monitored (so-called postmarket evaluation). That's because unknown problems with a drug can arise once it's in widespread use. Preapproval testing by a drug company takes place on only a few thousand people. That's enough to uncover obvious problems with a new drug. However, some drugs cause problems only in a small percentage of people, and these problems are not evident until many thousands or millions of people take the drug. If postapproval experience shows that a drug is dangerous, the FDA can require that the drug carry a warning label or revoke approval and the drug can no longer be sold.

The standard procedure for testing a new drug can take 2 years or more. However, if, while in testing, a new drug for a life-threatening condition shows promise and there are no alternative drugs, the FDA can grant a drug company accelerated, conditional approval ("fast-track approval") to market the drug. To obtain fast-track approval the drug company must promise that it will continue testing the drug in the postapproval period and be prepared to withdraw the drug from distribution if unknown problems are uncovered. Fast-track drugs can be sold without warnings or special restrictions, and patients may not be aware that a drug is still under study. After fast-track came into being in 1997, dozens of drugs have been withdrawn because they caused serious complications and, in some cases, death.

In 2004, a very popular anti-inflammatory drug called Vioxx (rofecoxib) was withdrawn from the market for increasing the risk of heart disease and stroke. Prior to approval, the drug had been tested for its ability to reduce arthritis symptoms while causing less stomach irritation and damage than other pain medicines. During the initial testing phases, the increased risk of heart attack and stroke from taking Vioxx was suspected from clinical observations and on biological grounds. Nevertheless, neither the pharmaceutical company (Merck) nor the FDA warned doctors and consumers of the potential life-threatening risks. Congress and the FDA are now requiring that all tests be reported to the approval committee, not just the ones chosen by the sponsoring drug companies. Because serious health problems caused by a new drug may not appear until the drug has been prescribed for millions of people, Public Citizen's Health Research Group suggests that all consumers adopt this rule: *Do not use any new drug that has been on the market for less than 5 years if any older, effective drug is available.*

For most medical conditions, safe, effective drugs that have been on the market for decades are the ones to use. Follow the 5-year rule unless you have a serious medical problem that can only be treated with a newer drug.

In 2007, the U.S. Congress passed a law giving the FDA more authority over postmarketing surveillance and approval of new drugs.

Screen Addiction to Video Games, the Internet, TV Binge Watching, and Smartphones

Do . . .

- you often stay on-screen longer than you intended to ("just a few more minutes")?
- your academics suffer because you spend too much time on-screen?
- you check your social media and email before starting something you must do, including sleep?
- others complain about the amount of time you spend on-screen?
- you feel depressed, moody, or nervous when off-screen, which goes away once you are back on-screen?
- you sometimes try to limit the amount of time you spend online and fail?

If you answered "yes" to any of the above, then you may be on the road to screen addiction.

The word *addiction* is almost always applied to drug use. However, because of recent advances in brain science, addiction can refer to a set of reward, motivation, and memory processes in the brain that underlie addiction to a variety of behaviors, including drug use, uncontrolled overeating, sexual activity, compulsive gambling, compulsive video game play, TV binge watching, and extensive use of the Internet and smartphones.

Although no scientific evidence suggests that excessive screen time carries the same health risks as tobacco smoking and alcohol or opioid abuse, some research suggests that overuse of screen devices is associated with increased risk of anxiety, depression, stress, overweight, lack of sleep, social isolation, and the masking of underlying mental health problems such as depression or anxiety (Substance Abuse and Mental Health Services Administration, 2017).

As of yet, scientists have not determined the daily amount of screen time that could be deemed to be unsafe. However, you can get a sense of how screen time may be affecting your life by keeping a diary/journal of your on-screen activities for 1 week. Count your daily texts, tweets, and the number of times you check Instagram, Facebook, and Snapchat. Keep a log of time spent playing video games, using the Internet, and TV binge watching. Notice and record when you find yourself anticipating or fantasizing about going on-screen again, or if you snap, yell, or act annoyed if someone bothers you while you are on-screen. If you think you are developing an addiction to on-screen activities, consult your campus health center for recommendations and referrals.

Drug Misuse, Abuse, and Addiction

Each year, a large number of Americans regularly use drugs that are not intended as medicines (U.S. Substance Abuse and Mental Health Services Administration, 2016):

- 138 million Americans, or 51% of the population, drink alcohol.
- 52 million Americans, or 18% of the population, use tobacco products, principally cigarettes.
- 27 million Americans, or 9% of the population, use an illegal drug (principally marijuana) or abuse a psychotherapeutic medication[2] for nonmedical reasons.

The human body is capable of tolerating and eliminating small quantities of virtually any substance or drug with no permanent harmful effects. However, it may be harmful to ingest large doses or to use a drug often even in small quantities. Each year, abuse or misuse of prescription drugs is responsible for more than 1.2 million visits to hospital emergency rooms. Generally, using any drug to the point where health is adversely affected or the ability to function in society is impaired can be defined as **drug abuse**. Characteristics of drug abuse include the following:

- Failure to fulfill major obligations at work, school, or home (e.g., repeated absences or poor work performance; absences, suspensions, or expulsions from school; neglect of children or household)
- Recurrent substance use in situations in which it is physically hazardous (e.g., driving an automobile or operating a machine)
- Recurrent substance-related legal problems (e.g., DUIs, arrests for substance-related disorderly conduct)
- Continued substance use despite having persistent or recurrent social or interpersonal problems caused or exacerbated by the effects of the substance (e.g., arguments with spouse, physical fights)

Drug abuse refers not to the type or amount of a drug taken but to whether or not the person taking the drug is personally or socially impaired. If a drug is used to mask anxiety or facilitate undesirable behaviors, it is being abused. If a drug is used continually to combat the effects of stress, it is being abused. If pleasure is experienced only when a drug is taken, the drug is being abused. If someone cannot control their personal use of a drug, it is being abused.

Most of the commonly abused drugs are psychoactive substances that affect thoughts, perceptions, feelings, and moods; in other words, they change consciousness (**Table 16.4**). Consciousness is the state

TERMS

drug abuse: persistent or excessive use of a drug without medical or health reasons

---

[2] These data pertain to Americans over the age of 12.

Table 16.4

Classifications of Drugs That Affect the Central Nervous System

Drug classification	Common or trade name	Medical uses	Effects of average dose	Physical dependence	Tolerance develops
Opiates	Codeine Darvon Demerol Fentanyl Heroin Methadone Morphine Opium Oxycontin Percodan Vicodin Dextromethorphan	Analgesic (pain relief) Cough suppressant	Blocks or eases pain; may cause drowsiness and euphoria; some users experience nausea or itching sensations	Marked	Yes
Sedatives	Amytal Nembutal Phenobarbital Seconal Doriden Quaalude Halcion	Sedation, tension relief	Relaxation, sleep; decreases alertness and muscle coordination	Marked	Yes
Minor tranquilizers	Dalmane Equanil/Miltown Librium Valium Xanax	Anxiety relief, muscle tension relief	Mild sedation; increased sense of well-being; may cause drowsiness and dizziness	Marked	No
Major tranquilizers (phenothiazines)	Mellaril Thorazine Prolixin	Psychosis control	Heavy sedation, anxiety relief; may cause confusion, muscle rigidity, convulsions	None	No
Alcohol	Beer Wine Distilled liquor	None	Relaxation; loss of inhibition; mood swings; decreased alertness and coordination	Marked	Yes
Inhalants	Amyl nitrite Butyl nitrite Nitrous oxide	Muscle relaxant, anesthetic	Relaxation, euphoria; causes dizziness, headache, drowsiness	None	?
Stimulants	Benzedrine Biphetamine Desoxyn Dexedrine Methedrine Preludin Ritalin	Weight control; relief from narcolepsy, fatigue, and hyperactivity in children	Increased alertness and mood elevation; less fatigue and increased concentration; may cause insomnia, anxiety, headache, chills, and rise in blood pressure; organic brain damage after prolonged use	Mild to none	Yes
Cocaine	Cocaine hydrochloride	Local anesthetic, pain relief	Effects similar to stimulants	Marked	No
Cannabis	Marijuana Hashish	Relief of glaucoma, asthma, nausea accompanying chemotherapy	Relaxation, euphoria, altered perception; may cause confusion, panic, hallucinations	Mild to none	No
Hallucinogens	LSD PCP Mescaline Peyote Psilocybin	None	Altered perceptions, visual and sensory distortion; mood swings	None	Yes
Nicotine	(In tobacco)	None	Altered heart rate; tremors; excitation	Yes	Yes

of being aware of one's mental processes. Each of us has a "normal" state of consciousness, although many people would have difficulty describing what they mean by "normal." However, everyone knows when his or her state of consciousness deviates from normal—for example, when drunk, extremely angry, sad, or depressed. A high fever can alter consciousness even to the point of hallucinations.

There are numerous activities not generally regarded as consciousness-altering that produce changes in consciousness comparable in many respects to those produced by psychoactive drugs. Long-distance runners may experience a change of consciousness that is described as a "runners' high"; dancing can produce psychic "highs" and even ecstatic states of consciousness, which is the goal of the whirling dervishes who practice particular forms of Sufi dancing. Fasting can produce profound changes in consciousness, which is why prolonged fasts are often part of religious training. Many "thrill" activities, such as riding on roller coasters, shooting the rapids on river rafts, or bungee-jumping, change consciousness and presumably are enjoyed for that reason. Put into this perspective, ingesting psychoactive drugs is only one of many ways people change their consciousness.

> Freedom's just another word for nothing left to lose.
>
> *Janis Joplin*

Taking psychoactive drugs to alter consciousness is particularly dangerous because the cognitive, emotional, and behavioral processes that the drugs alter are required for harmonious adaptation to one's environment. Drugs that induce pleasant emotions can give a false sense of benefit. Drugs that block uncomfortable emotions (e.g., sadness, fear, pain) can impair useful defenses. Furthermore, regular use of psychoactive drugs can alter the biology of the brain to the point that drug using becomes a goal in itself, irrespective of any desire to alter thoughts and emotions (**Figure 16.5**).

Addiction

One of the many dangers of drug abuse is **addiction**, which is a progressive, chronic condition that is characterized by the following:

- *Compulsion:* An overwhelming preoccupation, desire, or drive to use a drug, which can include obsessive thinking about a drug and drug-seeking and drug-hoarding behavior
- *Loss of control:* The inability to control use of a drug or loss of control over one's behavior because of taking a drug (e.g., impulsive actions, verbal or physical violence, impulsive sexual behavior)
- *Continued drug use despite adverse consequences:* The tendency not to stop drug use in the face of arrest, job loss, family breakdown, and health problems
- *Distortions in normal thinking:* Not admitting that problems are the result of drug taking (denial)

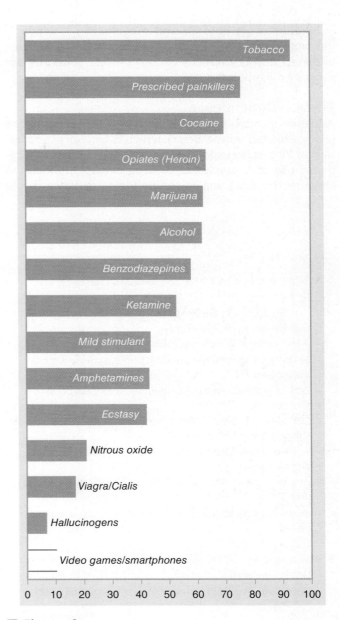

■ Figure 16.5

Addiction Potential

More than 5,700 individuals over age 18 from more than 40 countries reported their experience of commonly used drugs. The data show respondents' assessment of the addiction potential of various drugs. Note that both legal and illegal drugs can be highly addictive.

Data from Morgan, C. J. A., et al. (2013). Harms and benefits associated with psychoactive drugs: findings of an international study of active drug users. *Journal of Psychopharmacology, 27*, 497–506.

Many people who are addicted to drugs have coexistent mental health issues, such as depression, bipolar disorder, panic disorder, generalized anxiety disorder, and antisocial and dependent personality.

TERMS

addiction: physical and psychological dependence on a drug, substance, or behavior

Addiction is chronic and progressive: It tends to get worse over time. Family members who wait for an addicted family member to "get better" generally are severely disappointed.

Physical Dependence

Addiction is often associated with **physical dependence** (also called *tissue dependence*), which is biological adaptation to long-term exposure to a drug. First-time or infrequent use of a psychoactive drug causes intoxication because the drug upsets the biological balance in the brain. With continued use of a psychoactive drug, actual physical changes take place in brain tissues to adapt to the continual presence of the drug.

Both legal and illegal drugs can cause physical dependence. The legality of a drug is more a function of social, political, and economic considerations than the drug's toxicity or pharmacology. From a personal and community health standpoint, alcohol causes far more harm than all other drugs combined, yet it is legal.

The legal status of drugs changes with social customs and people's beliefs. In the 1920s and 1930s, alcohol was

---

Risk Factors for Addiction

Biologically Based Risk Factors (e.g., genetic, neurological, biochemical)	**Leading to This Effect**
• A less subjective feeling of intoxication	• More use to achieve intoxication (warning signs of abuse absent)
• Easier development of tolerance; liver enzymes adapt to increased use	• Easier to reach the addictive level
• Lack of resilience or fragility of higher (cerebral) brain functions	• Easy deterioration of cerebral functioning, impaired judgment, and social deterioration
• Difficulty in screening out unwanted or bothersome outside stimuli (low stimulus barrier)	• Feeling overwhelmed or stressed
• Tendency to amplify outside or internal stimuli (stimulus augmentation)	• Feeling attacked or panicked; need to avoid emotion
• Attention deficit hyperactivity disorder and other learning disabilities	• Failure, low self-esteem, or isolation
• Biologically based mood disorders (depression and bipolar disorders)	• Need to self-medicate against loss of control or the pain of depression; inability to calm down when manic or to sleep when agitated

Psychosocial and Developmental "Personality" Factors	
• Low self-esteem	• Need to blot out pain, gravitate to outsider groups
• Depression rooted in learned helplessness and passivity	• Need to blot out pain; use of a stimulant as an antidepressant
• Conflicts	• Anxiety and guilt
• Repressed and unresolved grief and rage	• Chronic depression, anxiety, or pain
• Posttraumatic stress disorder (as in veterans and abuse victims)	• Nightmares or panic attacks

Social and Cultural Environment	
• Availability of drugs	• Easy, frequent use
• Chemical-abusing parental model	• Sanction; no conflict over use
• Abusive, neglectful parents; other dysfunctional family patterns	• Pervasive sense of abandonment, distrust, and pain; difficulty in maintaining attachments
• Group norms favoring heavy use and abuse	• Reinforced, hidden abusive behavior that can progress without interference
• Misperception of peer norms	• Belief that most people use or favor use or think it's "cool" to use
• Severe or chronic stressors, as from noise, poverty, racism, or occupational stress	• Need to alleviate or escape from stress via chemical means
• "Alienation" factors: isolation, emptiness	• Painful sense of aloneness, normlessness, rootlessness, boredom, monotony, or hopelessness
• Difficult migration or acculturation with social disorganization, gender or generation gaps, or loss of role	• Stress without buffering support system

illegal in the United States, but marijuana was legal. During the early twentieth century, opium, morphine, and cocaine were openly advertised and sold in the form of tonics and cough syrups. Coca-Cola, concocted by a Georgia pharmacist in 1886, was sold as both a remedy and an enjoyable drink. "Coke" contained cocaine until 1906, when the cocaine was replaced by caffeine.

Tolerance

Tolerance is an adaptation of the body to a drug so that larger doses are needed to produce the same effect. Thus, the longer one uses a drug, the more of that drug one must consume to produce the desired effect. Because not all parts of the body become tolerant to a drug to the same degree, these higher doses may be dangerous. For example, a heroin or barbiturate user can become tolerant to the psychological effects of the drug, but the user's respiratory center in the brain, which controls breathing, does not. If the person takes a high dose of heroin or barbiturate to overcome tolerance to the drug's psychological effects, the brain's respiratory center may cease to function as a result of the overdose, and the person may stop breathing.

Withdrawal

A consequence of physical dependence is the experience of withdrawal (or abstinence syndrome), which occurs when the body adapts to the absence of a drug on which it has become physically dependent. Withdrawal is often uncomfortable, and it may be fatal. For example, someone physically dependent on heroin may experience anxiety, pain, sweating, muscle cramps, frightening hallucinations, and fatal seizures when deprived of the drug. Indeed, for those who have experienced withdrawal, the fear of experiencing it again may become a greater motivator to continue drug use than the effects of the drug itself.

With many drugs, **withdrawal symptoms** are the opposite of the drug's primary effects. In general, withdrawal from central nervous system depressants, such as alcohol, opiates, tranquilizers, and sedatives, leads to symptoms such as hyperexcitedness, anxiousness, irritability, and susceptibility to seizures. Withdrawal from stimulants, such as cocaine, amphetamines, and caffeine, on the other hand, can produce sleepiness, depression, and loss of consciousness.

Psychological Dependence

Besides physical dependence, drugs can create **habituation** or **psychological dependence**, which is manifested as an intense craving for the drug. Habituation becomes injurious when a person becomes so consumed by the need for the desired drugged state that all of that person's energy is siphoned into compulsive drug-seeking behavior. Physically addicting drugs such as heroin, alcohol, and nicotine often produce habituation. As a consequence of compulsive drug-seeking behavior, relationships, jobs, and families may be destroyed.

Stimulants

Stimulants are substances that increase the activity of the central nervous system. These drugs include cocaine, amphetamine, amphetamine-like drugs, and caffeine. Their main effects are an increase in mental arousal and physical energy and production of a state of euphoria, which is why they are referred to as "uppers." Stimulants also can cause restlessness, talkativeness, and difficulty sleeping. Long-term use of stimulants tends to produce physical and psychological dependence.

Cocaine

Cocaine is obtained from the leaves of the coca shrub, *Erythroxylum coca*, a plant indigenous to the Andes. For thousands of years, inhabitants of Peru, Bolivia, and Colombia have chewed coca leaves to obtain a moderate stimulant effect intended to overcome fatigue. After the Spanish conquest of the Inca empire in the sixteenth century, coca leaves were introduced to Europe and later to North America. In the late nineteenth century, Angelo Mariani, a Corsican, received a medal from the pope for manufacturing an extract of coca leaves that "freed the body of fatigue, lifted the spirits, and induced a sense of well-being." In the United States in the 1880s, Atlanta pharmacist J. C. Pemberton mixed extracts of coca leaves and kola nuts to produce Coca-Cola, claimed at the time to be not only refreshing but also "exhilarating, invigorating, and a cure for all nervous afflictions." Today, of course, Coke no longer contains cocaine, although cocaine-free extracts of coca leaves are still used for flavoring. Sigmund Freud extolled the use of cocaine as a mood elevator, a possible antidote to depression, and a treatment for morphine addiction. However, witnessing a friend's severe

---

TERMS

cocaine: a stimulant drug, obtained from the leaves of the coca shrub, that causes feelings of exhilaration, euphoria, and physical vigor

habituation: psychological dependence arising from repeated use of a drug

physical dependence: a physiological state that depends on the continuous presence of a drug; absence of the drug may cause discomfort, nervousness, headaches, and sweating (withdrawal symptoms) and sometimes death

psychological dependence: dependence that results because a drug produces pleasant mental effects

stimulants: substances that increase the activity of the central nervous system

tolerance: a condition in which increased amounts of a drug or increased exposure to an addictive behavior is required to produce desired effects

withdrawal symptoms: uncomfortable and sometimes dangerous reactions that occur after a person stops taking a physically addicting drug

and terrifying psychotic reaction to cocaine tempered Freud's enthusiasm for the drug.

As an illegal recreational drug, cocaine is most commonly taken into the body by sniffing ("snorting") it as a white powder, injecting it directly into the bloodstream (an obvious risk factor for AIDS), or smoking "free base" or "crack" cocaine. Each of these methods rapidly produces euphoria, a sense of power and clarity of thought, and increased physical vigor. The drug's effects last from minutes to an hour, depending on the dose and the route of administration into the body. After the initial high, users tend to experience a letdown ("crash") and an intense craving for more of the drug.

Cocaine increases heart rate and blood pressure. Continued use of the drug can result in appetite and weight loss, malnutrition, sleep disturbance, and altered thought and mood patterns. Frequent cocaine sniffing can inflame the nasal passages and cause permanent damage to the nasal septum. An overdose can cause seizures or death. Pregnant women who ingest cocaine risk giving birth to cocaine-addicted babies, who may be permanently disabled or even die in infancy.

Cocaine produces tolerance, physical dependence, and withdrawal. The potential for psychological dependence is great, probably the greatest among all psychoactive drugs. Some people develop such a strong craving for the drug that their lives are consumed by their cocaine habit.

Amphetamines

Amphetamines are manufactured chemicals that stimulate the central nervous system. The most common amphetamine substances are dextroamphetamine, methamphetamine, dextromethamphetamine, and amphetamine itself. Amphetamines are usually taken orally, but they can also be injected ("mainlined") and smoked. The effects of an oral dose usually last several hours. Slang terms for amphetamines include "dexies," "footballs," "orange," "bennies," "peaches," "meth," "crystal," "speed," and "ice."

Although amphetamines may be used medically to treat narcolepsy and attention deficit hyperactivity disorder (ADHD), they are principally used (illegally) to produce feelings of euphoria, increased energy, and greater self-confidence; an increased ability to concentrate; increased motor and speech activity; a perception of improved physical performance; and appetite suppression. Besides being used by those wishing to experience an amphetamine high, these drugs are frequently abused by people who fight sleep, such as students cramming for exams, entertainers, and truck drivers.

Excessive amphetamine use can cause headaches, irritability, dizziness, insomnia, panic, confusion, and delirium. The user often experiences a "crash," which occurs when the stimulants wear off, during which he or she usually is very depressed and tired and sleeps for long periods.

Prolonged use of amphetamines can lead to tolerance, especially for the euphoric effects and for appetite suppression. Amphetamines can cause mild physical dependence and create a psychological dependence and a particular pattern of use called the "yo-yo," which is a cycle of amphetamine use for the stimulatory effect followed by use of a depressant to sleep, followed by more amphetamines the next day to get going. Chronic use can cause an amphetamine psychosis, consisting of auditory and visual hallucinations, delusions, and mood swings.

A particularly dangerous form of amphetamine is "ice"—a smoked form of pure methamphetamine hydrochloride. The inhaled drug reaches the brain almost immediately, producing a high that can last for several hours. Because the drug can be so easily inhaled, the potential for compulsive use, tolerance, and abuse is also very great. This amphetamine is manufactured at clandestine laboratories; the purity of the drug varies considerably from one laboratory to another, which adds to the risks of abusing it.

Amphetamines used illegally by some college students to promote alertness when studying, preparing assignments, or taking tests are the prescription medications Adderall and Ritalin. Adderall is a combination of amphetamine and dextroamphetamine; Ritalin is an amphetamine derivative, methylphenadate. These drugs are medically indicated for the treatment of ADHD. Several million prescriptions for them are written for children and young adults diagnosed with ADHD, so these drugs are widely available. Patients or their siblings sell ADHD medicine to other students, who tend to use it periodically rather than chronically. That they are medicines may lead users to believe incorrectly that they are harmless. These drugs are potent stimulants with unpleasant side effects, and in high doses (such as when snorted), they can cause irregular heartbeat, stroke, and death.

Caffeine

Caffeine is a natural stimulant found in a variety of plants used in coffee, tea, chocolate, and soft drinks (**Table 16.5**). These beverages and foods are an integral part of American eating habits and may be enjoyed partly for their psychoactive properties.

The effects of caffeine are familiar to most people. They include decreased drowsiness and fatigue (especially when performing tedious or boring tasks), faster and clearer flow of thought, and increased capacity for sustained performance (for example, keyboarding faster with fewer errors). In higher doses, caffeine produces nervousness, restlessness, tremors, and insomnia and may have a negative effect on performance of complex tasks. In very high doses (10 grams, or about 100 cups of coffee), it can produce convulsions, which can be fatal.

In the past, caffeine was prescribed for a variety of complaints, but it is rarely used medically any more. However, it is still a key ingredient in more than a thousand over-the-counter drugs. For example, many "energizers" and "stay-awake" products are pure caffeine.

Table 16.5

Caffeine Content of Beverages and Chocolate

Item	Amount	Caffeine content (milligrams)
Coffee, generic brewed	8 oz	133 (range: 102–200)
Starbucks brewed coffee (grande)	16 oz	320
Starbucks vanilla latte (grande)	16 oz	150
Espresso, generic	1 oz	40 (range: 30–90)
Tea, brewed	8 oz	53 (range: 40–120)
Snapple fruit teas	16 oz	42
Arizona iced tea, green	16 oz	15
Mountain Dew	12 oz	54
Coca-Cola	12 oz	34
Diet Coke	12 oz	47
Dr. Pepper	12 oz	42
7-Up, regular or diet	12 oz	0
Fanta, all flavors	12 oz	0
5-Hour Energy Shot	2 oz	138
Rockstar Energy Shot	2.5 oz	200
Spike Shooter	8.4 oz	300
Rip It, all varieties	8 oz	100
SoBe No Fear	8 oz	83
Red Bull	8.3 oz	80
Jolt caffeinated gum	1 stick	45
Hershey's chocolate bar	1.55 oz	9
Hot cocoa	8 oz	9 (range: 3–13)
NoDoz (maximum strength)	1 tablet	200
Vivarin	1 tablet	200
Excedrin (extra strength)	2 tablets	130
Anacin (maximum strength)	2 tablets	64

Data from Caffeine Informer. (2015). Caffeine database. Retrieved from http://www.caffeineInformer.com-the-caffeine-database

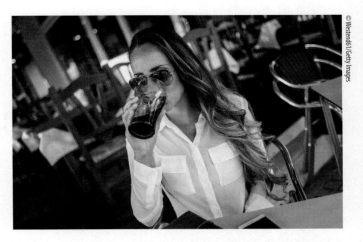

Most Americans consume more soft drinks than glasses of water. This can mean a significant daily intake of caffeine and calories.

entactogens), carry little or no risk for addiction, and, because they are ingested orally, no risk of contracting HIV/AIDS from injection. Despite these seeming benefits, club drugs can be dangerous, especially when taken together with alcohol or other drugs. Also, something sold as a club drug often is some other substance unknown—and possibly dangerous—to the user.

Ecstasy

Ecstasy is chemically 3-4 methylenedioxymethamphetamine, or MDMA. Some of its common nicknames are "Adam," "XTC," "Clarity," and "Essence." Ecstasy is a synthetic chemical; that is, it does not occur naturally in plants. The substance has a chemical structure similar to the stimulant methamphetamine and the hallucinogen mescaline, and it can produce both stimulant and psychedelic effects. Ecstasy is most often available in tablet form and is taken orally. It also is available as a powder; it is sometimes snorted and occasionally smoked, but rarely injected.

Ecstasy increases levels of the neurotransmitter serotonin in the brain, producing a high that lasts from several minutes to an hour. The drug's rewarding effects vary with the individual taking it and with the dose, purity, and the

Pain relievers, cough medicines, and cold remedies contain caffeine to counteract the drowsiness produced by other ingredients in these medications. Caffeine is also put into weight control and menstrual pain products because it increases urine output and water loss.

Psychological dependence may result from chronic use of caffeine, and tolerance to the stimulant effect may gradually develop. Mild withdrawal symptoms, such as headache, irritability, restlessness, and lethargy, may occur when caffeine use is stopped.

Club Drugs

Club drugs consist of several psychoactive chemicals that are used at parties, dances, festivals, and raves to enhance social experiences and increase sensory stimulation. These include Ecstasy, GHB, ketamine, and Rohypnol (flunitrazepam). Compared to marijuana, amphetamines, hallucinogens, and opiates, club drugs are believed to give a sense of emotional closeness and euphoria (so-called

TERMS

amphetamines: synthetic drugs that stimulate the central nervous system and sometimes produce hallucinogenic states

caffeine: a natural stimulant found in a variety of plants; commonly found in tea, coffee, chocolate, and soft drinks

club drugs: psychoactive chemicals used at parties, dances, festivals, and raves to enhance social experiences and increase sensory stimulation

Ecstasy (MDMA): a club drug with both stimulant and pleasurable effects

environment in which it is taken. Ecstasy can produce stimulant effects, such as an enhanced sense of pleasure and self-confidence and increased energy. Its psychedelic effects include feelings of peacefulness, acceptance, and empathy. Users claim they experience feelings of close-ness with others.

The risks associated with using Ecstasy are similar to those found with the use of amphetamines and cocaine:

- Confusion, depression, sleep problems, drug craving, severe anxiety, and paranoia during and sometimes weeks after taking the drug
- Muscle tension, involuntary teeth clenching, nausea, blurred vision, rapid eye movement, faintness, and chills or sweating
- Increases in heart rate and blood pressure
- Long-term damage to serotonin-producing nerve cells in the brain
- Liver damage with long-term use

Ecstasy-related fatalities have been reported. The stimu-lant effects of the drug, which enable the user to dance for extended periods, combined with the hot, crowded conditions usually found at raves, or parties, can lead to dehydration, hyperthermia, and heart or kidney failure.

GHB

GHB is chemically **gamma-hydroxybutyrate**. Its street names include "Georgia home boy," "liquid ecstasy," and "grievous bodily harm." GHB is ingested as a white powder or a clear, bitter-tasting liquid, which is often mixed with sweet alcoholic beverages to mask the bitter taste. This is often the way GHB is "slipped" into an unsuspecting person's drink. The drug's effects begin about 30 minutes after ingestion and can last several hours.

At low doses (–10 mg/kg body weight), GHB produces light sedation, increased sexual interest, relaxation, and short-term amnesia—the mental state sought in much of club drug use and that which increases the risk of sexual assault ("date rape"). At moderate doses (–20 mg/kg), users become lethargic. At large doses (–60 mg/kg), users can become comatose and stop breathing. More than half of the users of GHB at low doses experience unconscious-ness, vomiting, and profuse sweating.

After more than 60 deaths were reported from GHB use, the U.S. government classified the drug as a Sched-ule I controlled substance. Chemical precursors sold as dietary supplements (GBL, gamma-butyrolactone, and BD, 1-4-butane diol) are converted naturally to GHB in the body.

Ketamine

Ketamine is an anesthetic. Its street names include "K," "special K," "vitamin K," and "black hole." Mixing ketamine with MDMA (Ecstasy) is called "kitty flipping"; mixing it with MDMA and marijuana is called "EGK" (Ecstasy, ketamine, marijuana). "Trail mixes" are ketamine mixed with other drugs, such as methamphetamine, cocaine, Viagra, or heroin.

As a recreational drug, ketamine is generally ingested orally as a white powder or intranasally with an inhaler (called a "bumper"). It can also be administered by injec-tion. After oral ingestion, drug effects occur after about 30 minutes and last up to 3 hours. At very low doses, ket-amine can produce an out-of-body dissociative state and hallucinations (called "k-land"). At high doses, ketamine can produce muscular rigidity, bizarre behavior, psycho-sis, and social withdrawal.

Rohypnol

Rohypnol is a powerful tranquilizer. It reduces anxi-ety, inhibition, and muscular tension. At higher doses it can cause unconsciousness. Its effects are dangerously compounded when taken with alcohol or other sedating drugs. Chronic use can produce dependence and with-drawal symptoms.

Depressants

Depressants comprise a vast number of drugs whose com-mon effects include a reduced level of arousal, motor activity, and awareness of the environment and increased drowsiness and sedation. The depressants include alcohol and drugs that affect sleep: sedatives, hypnotics, and opi-ates. A number of other drugs, such as antihistamines and some medications used in the treatment of high blood pres-sure or heart disease, may also act as depressants. In low doses, depressants produce a mild state of euphoria, reduce inhibitions, or induce a feeling of relaxation. In high doses, they may impair mood, speech, and motor coordination.

Depressants are dangerous. All carry the potential for physical and psychological dependency, tolerance, unpleasant withdrawal symptoms, and toxicity from con-tinual use or overuse. Acute overdoses may produce coma, respiratory or cardiovascular collapse, and even death. Aggravating the potential for lethal overdose are the synergistic actions of depressants. That is, when taken together, two or more different depressants can produce a much stronger effect than the sum of both drugs. The most common synergistic effect occurs when people drink alcohol while taking depressant medications such as barbiturates or tranquilizers.

Sedative and Hypnotic Drugs

A **sedative** is a drug that promotes mental calmness and reduces anxiety. A **hypnotic** is a drug that promotes sleep or drowsiness. Because of their potential for induc-ing dependence, almost all sedatives and hypnotics are highly regulated and are available only by prescription. Nevertheless, sedative-hypnotics are among the most widely used drugs in the United States.

The most common sedative-hypnotics are drugs called benzodiazepines, more popularly known as **tranquilizers**. Medically, these drugs are used to relieve anxiety, promote relaxation, induce sleep, alleviate muscle spasm and lower back pain, treat convulsive disorders, and lessen the discomfort of alcohol and opiate withdrawal. Benzodiazepines are most helpful when used on a short-term basis (a few weeks) as an adjunct to psychotherapy or medical therapy. Long-term use (more than four months) increases the risk of both dependence and of not confronting and overcoming issues and symptoms for which the benzodiazepines were originally prescribed.

Barbiturates are sedative-hypnotic drugs that include barbituric acid and its derivatives: amobarbital (Amytal), pentobarbital (Nembutal), phenobarbital (Luminal), secobarbital (Seconal), and Tuinal (50% amobarbital plus 50% secobarbital). Because they are less safe than benzodiazepines, barbiturates tend not to be prescribed for medical conditions that call for sedative-hypnotic drug therapy.

Opiates

The **opiates** are a group of chemically related drugs that depress the central nervous system (e.g., morphine, heroin, codeine, Demerol [meperidine], Duragesic [fentanyl], Oxycontin [oxycodone], Percodan [aspirin and oxycodone], Vicodin [acetaminophen and hydrocodone]); cause physical dependence, habituation, and tolerance; and produce serious withdrawal symptoms. Opiates are derived from the opium poppy, *Papaver somniferum*, extracts of which have been used for thousands of years in a variety of cultures to produce euphoria, relieve pain, and treat various diseases.

Medically, opiates are used for pain relief, cough suppression, and treatment of diarrhea. They can be taken by mouth, injection, snorting, and smoking. Heroin is converted to morphine in the body, and the morphine is eventually excreted in urine, saliva, sweat, and the breast milk of lactating women (which means that nursing infants can become addicted). Because morphine crosses the placenta, a developing fetus may become addicted even before birth and may experience withdrawal symptoms after it is born.

Opiates are commonly abused substances, taken for their pain-relieving and psychoactive effects. The psychological sensations produced by opiates include feelings of warmth and belonging, relaxation, and mellowness. Regular use of opiates can produce tolerance to the psychological effects, constipation, loss of appetite, depression, loss of interest in sex, constriction of the pupil of the eye, disruption of the menstrual cycle, and drowsiness. Very large doses or prolonged use can be fatal because of respiratory failure.

About 7 million Americans are believed to use prescription opiates illegally for nonmedical reasons. The abuse of prescription opiates is responsible for thousands of emergency room visits and deaths from unintentional overdoses each year. Besides serious medical consequences, the demand for prescription opiates has created an epidemic of robberies at pharmacies.

The abuse of opiate painkillers is driven by their wide availability. Millions of Americans are afflicted with chronic pain and receive these drugs from their physicians, many of whom do not have sufficient training in pain management to forestall abuse. Also, pharmaceutical companies aggressively market these drugs. Furthermore, opiates are easily obtained illegally. Anyone who needs opiates to deal with legitimate medical conditions should discuss with their physician the risks and benefits of this course of treatment.

Marijuana

Marijuana is another name for the plant *Cannabis sativa*, which grows in temperate climates all over the world. Species of this plant have been cultivated for thousands of years as a source of hemp fiber used to make clothing and rope or for a substance that, when ingested, produces euphoria, a sense of relaxation, mood elevation, altered perceptions of space and time, and heightened sensory awareness. Marijuana ingestion also produces increased hunger (the "munchies") and dry mouth.

The principal psychoactive ingredient in marijuana is a chemical called delta-9-tetrahydrocannabinol (THC). This substance is found in the plant's leaves, buds, seeds, and resins. THC can be ingested by smoking the dried and crushed flowers and leaves or by eating food that has been prepared with marijuana as an ingredient. THC is chemically similar to natural substances in the brain, called *endocannabinoids*, that modulate appetite, pain sensation, mood, memory, and other processes by binding to specific receptors in brain tissue. THC binds to the same cannabinoid receptors.

Hashish (a resin generally smoked in a special pipe) is a highly potent derivative of marijuana obtained from the sticky resin found on the flowers and leaves of marijuana plants. *Ganja*, another derivative of marijuana,

---

TERMS

gamma-hydroxybutyrate (GHB): a dangerous club drug with unpleasant side effects

hashish: the sticky resin of the *Cannabis* plant

hypnotics: central nervous system depressants used to induce drowsiness and encourage sleep

ketamine: an anesthetic used as a club drug

marijuana: a psychoactive substance present in the dried leaves, stems, flowers, and seeds of plants of the genus *Cannabis*

opiates: central nervous system depressants derived from the opium poppy

Rohypnol: a powerful tranquilizer used as a club drug

sedatives: central nervous system depressants used to relieve anxiety, fear, and apprehension

tranquilizers: central nervous system depressants that relax the body and calm anxiety

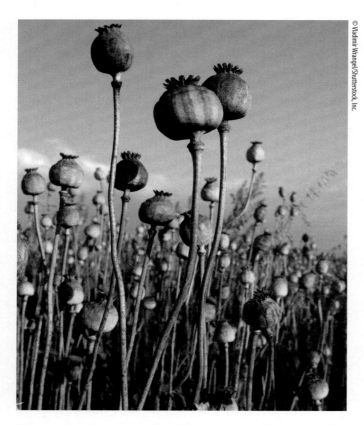

Opium poppies (*Papaver somniferum*), from which morphine is obtained.

are removed from the plot to prevent seed formation and to allow more of the female plant's energy to be directed into the growth and formation of psychoactive compounds.

Besides its intended psychoactive effects, marijuana ingestion may evoke confusion, anxiety, panic, hallucinations, and paranoia. Speech and short-term memory may be impaired, which may be interpreted as humorous changes in one's normal mental state. However, because perception, motor coordination, and reaction time are also impaired, driving a car or operating other machines while intoxicated with THC is unsafe. Marijuana use may also aggravate an existing mental health problem.

Some of the possible health dangers of long-term marijuana use include the risk of bronchitis caused by marijuana smoke, increased heart rate and blood pressure, and possibly a slight depression of immune system functions. Marijuana smoke, like tobacco smoke, contains carcinogens.

Brain imaging studies support a body of psychological research showing an association between heavy marijuana use and impairment in short-term memory and attention, loss of internal control, and reduced learning while a person is intoxicated, but not beyond the time of marijuana use. Heavy, extended marijuana use is associated with lower performance in school and at work, lower educational attainment, and other illicit drug use.

Marijuana use or possession is illegal in many countries (exceptions include Canada, Czech Republic, Portugal, Spain, The Netherlands, Uruguay, and Portugal). As of 2017, several states in the United States permit marijuana for recreational use, more than half of states permit marijuana for treatment and relief of medical conditions, and

consists of the dried tops of female plants. *Bhang* (called "ditch weed") is made from parts of the plant that contain lesser amounts of THC. *Sinsemilla* (from the Spanish word "without seeds") is a potent form of marijuana derived exclusively from female plants. All male plants

---

What to Do with Expired or Unused Medicines

Can you use expired drugs?

Many solid drugs in their original unopened containers can retain 90% of their potency for about 5 years after the expiration date on the label. Exposure to heat, humidity, and water can shorten a drug's useful lifetime. Drugs-in-solution are generally less stable. There are no reports of toxicity from degradation products in currently available drugs.

Disposing of prescription and over-the-counter drugs and inhalers

Check the product label or instructions. Contact local law enforcement or your household trash and recycling service for guidance. You can search online for "Controlled Substance Public Disposal Locations."

Although certain drugs can be flushed down the sink or toilet, the FDA and EPA prefer more environmentally friendly disposal efforts. If a disposal program is not available in your area:

- Remove the prescription or over-the-counter drug from its original container and mix it with an undesirable substance, such as used coffee grounds, dirt, or kitty litter, to make the contents less appealing to children and pets and unrecognizable to people who may intentionally go through the trash seeking drugs.

- Place the mixture in a sealable bag or other container to prevent leaking.

- Scratch out all identifying information on the prescription label to make it unreadable.

- Do not give your medicine to friends. Something that works for you could be dangerous for someone else.

Data from The Medical Letter on Drugs and Therapeutics, 57, 164–165. Reprinted in *Journal of the American Medical Association*, 57, 164–165. U.S. Food and Drug Administration (2016). How to Dispose of Unused Medicines. Retrieved from https://www.fda.gov/ForConsumers/ConsumerUpdates/ucm101653.htm

a few permit growing psychoactive-free marijuana for production of hemp used in manufacturing. Despite the fact some states permit growing and using it, marijuana is nevertheless considered by the federal government as a Schedule I Controlled Substance, putting it in the most dangerous category of drugs.

Hallucinogens

The **hallucinogens** comprise a variety of chemical substances derived from as many as 100 kinds of plants as well as by chemical synthesis in the laboratory (**Table 16.6**). Despite their chemical differences, hallucinogens share the ability to alter perception, thought, mood, sensation, and experience. The similarity of their effects to psychotic hallucinatory experience is one reason they are called hallucinogens, but in many respects the psychedelic drug experience is not the same as a psychotic hallucination. Psychotic hallucinations are generally auditory and frightening, and the hallucinator believes them to be real. Drug-induced hallucinations tend to be visual, usually are enjoyable, and the individual is aware that the experience is unusual and is not part of his or her normal state of consciousness.

Hallucinogens are most often ingested orally, either by eating the plant itself or by ingesting powder containing the active chemical. Normally, a hallucinogenic drug begins to take effect in 45 to 60 minutes. The first effects are physical: sweating, nausea, increased body temperature, and pupil dilation. These symptoms eventually subside, and the psychological effects become manifest within an hour or two of ingestion. Depending on the particular substance and the amount ingested, the "trip" lasts anywhere from 1 to 24 hours. Perhaps the most commonly used hallucinogen is **LSD** (D-lysergic acid diethylamide), commonly called "acid."

A common feature of the hallucinogenic experience is the suspension of the normal psychic mechanisms that integrate the self with the environment. The distortion of self–environment interactions makes the user extremely open to conditions in the surroundings. For this reason, experience in any particular drug episode is highly influenced, for better or worse, by the environmental setting in which the trip takes place and by the "psychic set"—the expectations and attitudes—of the user.

Phencyclidine (PCP)

Phencyclidine, or **PCP**, also known as "angel dust," "hog," "crystal," and "killer weed," was developed originally for medical use as an animal anesthetic. But because of the drug's many adverse effects, it was removed from legal sale and became an illegal recreational drug. In the 1960s, phencyclidine was called the "PeaCePill"—a serious misnomer in view of the drug's effects.

The effects of PCP are variable: Depending on the dose and the route of administration, it can be a stimulant, a depressant, or a hallucinogen. Some of the intended effects are heightened sensitivity to external stimuli, mood elevation, relaxation, and a sense of omnipotence. Some of the common unintended effects are paranoia, confusion, restlessness, disorientation, feelings of depersonalization, and violent or bizarre behavior. In high doses, the drug can cause coma, interruption of breathing, and psychosis.

> Insanity is doing the same thing over and over again and expecting a different outcome.
>
> *Albert Einstein*

Many admissions to psychiatric emergency rooms are for PCP intoxication. The drug impairs perception and muscular control, and users are prone to accidents such as falling from heights, drowning, walking in front of moving vehicles, and collisions while driving under the influence of the drug. PCP does not induce tolerance or physical dependence, but because it is eliminated slowly from the body, chronic users may experience the drug's effects for an extended period.

Table 16.6

Substances Considered to Be Hallucinogenic or Psychedelic

Substance or active ingredient	Common name
D-lysergic acid diethylamide	LSD
Trimethoxyphenylethylamine	Mescaline (peyote)
2,5-dimethoxy-4-methylamphetamine	STP
Dimethyltryptamine	DMT
Diethyltryptamine	DET
Tetrahydrocannabinol	Marijuana (cannabis)
Phencyclidine	PCP
Psilocybin	Mushrooms

TERMS

hallucinogens: psychoactive substances that alter sensory processing in the brain, producing visual or auditory sensations that are not real (i.e., that are hallucinatory)

LSD: a powerful hallucinogenic chemical; ingestion alters brain chemistry and produces a variety of hallucinogenic and behavioral effects

phencyclidine (PCP): drug that, depending on the route of administration and dose, can be a stimulant, depressant, or hallucinogen; originally developed as an animal anesthetic

The effects of PCP are unpredictable and frequently unpleasant, if not terrifying and life-threatening. PCP produces more unwanted and dangerous symptoms of drug intoxication than any other psychoactive substance. Drug dealers often surreptitiously mix PCP with marijuana or cocaine or sell PCP while claiming it to be LSD, DMT, or some other drug. Because PCP is relatively easy to manufacture, it is one of the more readily available and dangerous of the illegal recreational drugs.

Inhalants

Inhalants are a wide variety of chemical substances that vaporize readily and when inhaled produce various kinds of depressant effects similar to those of alcohol. Like alcohol, inhalants are depressants of the central nervous system. Generally, their intended effect is loss of inhibition and a sense of euphoria and excitement. Unintended effects include dizziness, amnesia, inability to concentrate, confusion, impaired judgment, hallucinations, and acute psychosis.

Inhalants commonly used for recreational purposes include the following:

Commercial chemicals, such as model airplane glue, nail polish remover, shoe polish, paint thinner, and gasoline, and substances such as acetone, toluene, naphtha, hexane, and cyclohexane

Aerosols—found in aerosol spray products

Anesthetics, such as amyl nitrite, nitrous oxide ("laughing gas"), diethyl ether, and chloroform

Because they are vaporous, these substances enter the body rapidly. The fumes are usually inhaled from plastic bags. The intoxicant effects are often felt within minutes, and the high lasts less than an hour. Regular users tend to be preteens and others without the money to buy other drugs. Some adults use amyl nitrite ("poppers") during sexual relations, believing that the drug enhances the sexual experience. Some medical personnel are frequent users of nitrous oxide, or "laughing gas," because it is easily available.

The inhalant chemicals do not produce tolerance or withdrawal, nor do they induce physical dependence. However, they are dangerous. In addition to any harm resulting from uncontrolled behavior (such as driving while intoxicated), these chemicals damage the kidneys, liver, and lungs and can upset normal heartbeat.

About 2 million adolescents between the ages of 12 and 17 use inhalants, some beginning as young as age 7. Signs of inhalant use that adults can watch for include paint stains on clothing, red and runny eyes, chemical breath odor, sores around the mouth, and a drunken demeanor.

Anabolic Steroids

Anabolic steroids are synthetic derivatives of the male hormone testosterone. These derivatives of testosterone promote the growth of skeletal muscle and increase lean body mass. Anabolic steroids were first abused by elite athletes seeking to improve performance. Today, athletes and nonathletes use steroids to enhance performance and also to change physical appearance.

Anabolic steroids are taken orally or injected, typically in cycles of weeks or months rather than continuously. Users frequently combine several different types of steroids to maximize their effectiveness while minimizing negative side effects, a process known as stacking. Anabolic steroids produce increased lean muscle mass, strength, and ability to train longer and harder. Side effects of anabolic steroid use include liver tumors, jaundice, fluid retention, high blood pressure, severe acne, and trembling. Shrinking of the testicles, reduced sperm count, infertility, baldness, and development of breasts have been observed in males. In females, growth of facial hair, changes or cessation of menstrual cycle, enlargement of the clitoris, and deepened voice are among the side effects.

Reducing Drug Use

Almost everyone takes drugs of one kind or another at one time or another. People take drugs to relieve headaches, heartburn, tension, cramps, fatigue, and anxiety. Drugs are used to get to sleep and to stay awake. They are used for body problems and emotional problems. When used appropriately, prescription drugs can play a vital role in the treatment and prevention of disease.

However, as a society we are overmedicated and overly dependent on drugs. The healthiest approach is to be as free of drugs as possible. Wellness is not achieved by taking drugs. No drug should ever be taken casually,

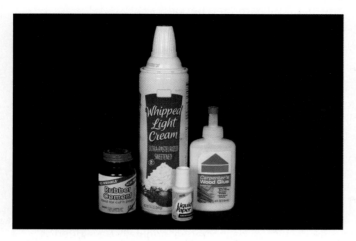

Inhalants are dangerous but unfortunately often readily available to kids looking for a "rush."

whether prescribed, over the counter, or offered in a social setting. Each person should learn when drugs are necessary to maintain or restore health and when the benefits of the drug outweigh the risks.

All drugs are dangerous, and illegal recreational drugs are especially so because you cannot be sure of either the quality or the strength. The use of most recreational drugs is illegal, and if caught, users and sellers are prosecuted as criminals. Still, many people in American society, especially young people, experiment with one or more illegal drugs. Experimenting with drugs is just that: You are taking a chance of getting caught, or getting high and causing an accident, or getting the wrong dose and dying.

■TERMS■

inhalants: vaporous substances that, when inhaled, produce alcohol-like intoxication

Critical Thinking About Health

1. The accompanying graph shows the results of a test of a new drug. Four groups of patients were involved. Group 1 received a placebo; group 2, 20 mg of the drug; group 3, 40 mg; and group 4, 80 mg.
   a. Do the data support the hypothesis that the drug is effective? Why or why not?
   b. What percentage of people get well without the drug? What's a likely explanation?
   c. What's the maximum percentage of people that can be expected to get well from taking the drug?
   d. If 80 mg produces the desired effect in the largest number of people, why didn't the experimenters report the effects of 100 mg?

2. Bob Kozlo came home from work early one day. Upon hearing his dad's car pull up in the driveway, Jamie, Bob's 16-year-old son, quickly disposed of the joint he and his friend Max were sharing. Mr. Kozlo, who as a teenager also had experimented with marijuana, smelled the telltale odor and knew immediately what Jamie and Max had been up to.
   a. Should Mr. Kozlo ignore this situation or take some kind of action, and if so, what should he do?
   b. Should he tell Max's parents?

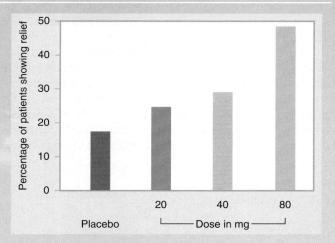

c. What is your opinion of teenagers experimenting with marijuana or any other drugs, including alcohol and tobacco?

3. Why are some drugs illegal? What characteristics distinguish a legal drug from an illegal one? If you had unlimited power and resources, what would you do to solve the illegal drug problem in the United States?

4. In what ways has substance use and abuse touched your life?

Chapter Summary and Highlights

Chapter Summary

Before recorded human history, our ancestors accidentally left containers of ripe fruit or wet grains out in the open where microorganisms began the process of fermentation. When they drank the liquid, their thoughts and behaviors changed. They liked it. They had discovered alcohol. So began a systematic search for leaves, roots, flowers, or mushrooms that could alter thoughts, feelings, and sensations or cure various ailments. Human history and drugs became forever entwined. The shamans, witch doctors, and healers became powerful forces for new knowledge.

A drug is a chemical substance that can produce a change in human (and animal) physiology. The change can be beneficial or harmful, fast or slow acting, long lasting or temporary, addicting or nonaddicting. Many of the most effective drugs used today to treat physical and mental ailments are derived from substances originally discovered in nature. Alcohol, nicotine, opium derivatives, marijuana, and cocaine are still the most widely used drugs. Whether a drug is legal or illegal today has nothing to do with the drug's effectiveness, usefulness, or safety. Consumption of alcohol (and smoking tobacco) causes far more disease and death than all illegal drugs

combined. Prescription drugs do great good as well as great harm. To preserve your health, think carefully about what drugs you ingest or inhale.

Drug abuse is a major problem in today's societies. Drug abuse really means overuse of a drug to the point where a person cannot function and has lost control of his or her life. Addiction or dependence on alcohol, heroin, cocaine, prescription pain killers, tranquilizers, or "uppers and downers" is an example of drug abuse. A person also can become physically or mentally tolerant to a drug, which means that larger doses are needed to achieve the desired effect. All drugs, legal and illegal, have secondary effects that may be dangerous or undesirable. When using any drug, be aware of undesirable side effects or adverse reactions. There are many ways to cope with life's problems without immediately seeking a drug-related solution.

Highlights

- People have been ingesting drugs throughout recorded history for a variety of reasons, including altering thoughts and feelings, curing illness, and facilitating social interaction.

- A drug is a chemical substance capable of producing a change in physiology. Most drugs react by binding to receptor sites in or on cells, which alters biological activity.
- Legal or illegal, medical or nonmedical, drug use in the United States is widespread. Drug use is encouraged by extensive advertising by the pharmaceutical industry.
- The Food and Drug Administration requires the testing of new drugs for safety and efficacy before they are approved for sale.
- Drug abuse is the overuse of a drug, often to the point of loss of control. Many drugs of abuse are psychoactive, meaning that they alter thoughts, feelings, and perceptions. Many psychoactive drugs cause physical dependence; some cause psychological dependence.
- Tolerance is the adaptation of the body to repeated drug use so that ever-increasing doses of the drug are required to produce an effect.
- The most commonly used psychoactive drugs in the United States include stimulants (cocaine, amphetamine, caffeine), depressants (sedatives, tranquilizers, hypnotics), opiates, marijuana, hallucinogens, cocaine, and Ecstasy.
- The medical use of marijuana has been legalized in several states but is illegal by federal law.

For Your Health

That consumption of prescription and over-the-counter medicines, dietary supplements, alcohol, tobacco, and other nonmedicinal chemicals is commonplace does not mean that these substances are harmless. Do Exercise 16.1 in the Workbook, "Being Knowledgeable About Drugs," to learn more about the substances you ingest. Further enhance your knowledge about drugs and medicines by doing the other exercises for Chapter 16 in the Workbook.

References

Caffeine Informer. (2015). Caffeine database. Retrieved from http://www.caffeineinformer.com/the-caffeine-database

Colemen, J. J., & Pontefract, S. K. (2017). Adverse drug reactions. *Clinical Medicine*, 16, 481–485.

Hanson, G. R., Venturelli, P. J., & Fleckenstein, A. (2001). *Drugs and society* (6th ed.). Sudbury, MA: Jones and Bartlett Publishers, p. 95.

Hanson, G. R., Venturelli, P. J., & Fleckenstein, A. (2012). *Drugs and society* (11th ed.). Burlington, MA: Jones & Bartlett Learning.

Murphy, S. L. (2012). Deaths: Preliminary data for 2010. *National Vital Statistics Report*, 60(4). Retrieved from http://www.cdc.gov/nchs/data/nvsr/nvsr60/nvsr60_04.pdf

Schachtel, B. P., et al. (1996). Nonprescription ibuprofen and acetaminophen in the treatment of tension-type headache. *Journal of Clinical Pharmacology*, 36, 1120–1125.

U.S. Department of Health and Human Services. (2017). Adverse drug events. Retrieved from https://health.gov/hcq/ade.asp

U.S. Substance Abuse and Mental Services Administration. (2016). *Key substance use and mental health indicators in the United States: Results from the 2015 National Survey on Drug Use and Health*. HHS Publication No. SMA 16-4984, NSDUH Series H-51. Retrieved from https://www.samhsa.gov/data/sites/default/files/NSDUH-FFR1-2015/NSDUH-FFR1-2015/NSDUH-FFR1-2015.pdf

Suggested Readings

Alter, A. (2017). *The rise of addiction technology and the business of keeping us hooked*. New York: Barnes and Noble. Explains how it is possible to become addicted to electronic technologies such as video games and smartphones in the same ways people become addicted to drugs and gambling, and how technology companies take advantage of screen addiction to make money.

Aviv, R. (2014, May 5). Prescription for disaster. *The New Yorker*, 50–59. A cautionary tale of the dire social and personal consequences associated with the overuse and over prescribing of pain-relief drugs.

Avorn, J. (2005). *Powerful medicines: The benefits, risks, and costs of prescription drugs*. New York: Vintage. Suggests policy reforms to improve the current system of drug development.

Bower, B. (2014, March (22). The addiction paradox. *Science News*, 16–20. Many people take antianxiety drugs in order to function and accomplish daily tasks. If someone taking these has an accident that requires prescription pain medications, they can die from a potent interaction of the drug combination. And, if you are addicted to narcotics, you should tell your physician before taking any antianxiety drug.

Gaidos, S. (2016, July 9). Addiction protection. *Science News,* 22–25. Discusses the possibility of developing a vaccine to prevent opioid abuse. A renowned advocate of alternative medicines explains how we can protect ourselves from taking unnecessary medications and avoid damaging our health by overusing drugs.

Hanson, G., Venturelli, P. J., & Fleckenstein, A. (2014). *Drugs and society* (12th ed.). Burlington, MA: Jones & Bartlett Learning. A useful text.

Koob, G. F., et al. (2014). *Drugs, addiction, and the brain.* San Diego: Academic Press. The director of the National Institute on Alcohol Abuse and Alcoholism and renowned neurobiologist explores the molecular, cellular, and neurocircuitry systems in the brain that are responsible for drug addiction.

Lee, M. A. (2013). *Smoke signals: A social history of marijuana—medical, recreational, and scientific.* A clearheaded survey that stretches from 2700 B.C. to the Obama administration.

Weil, A. (2017). *Mind over meds: Know when drugs are necessary, when alternatives are better, and when to let your body heal on its own.* New York: Little Brown.

Recommended Websites

National Council on Alcoholism and Drug Dependence, Inc.
NCADD's Alcohol & Drug Information discusses addiction and how it can be treated.

Public Citizen Health Research Group
A nonprofit organization that publishes a monthly magazine, *Worst Pills—Best Pills*, which warns of dangerous prescription drugs. The organization also reports on FDA actions and the drug industry.

U.S. National Institute of Drug Abuse
A division of the National Institutes of Health dedicated to improving drug abuse and addiction prevention, treatment, and policy.

Health Tips

Smoking: Playing the Odds

Smoking and Periodontal Disease

Benefits of Quitting Smoking

Global Wellness

Make Every Day World No Tobacco Day

Wellness Guide

Smoking: Not Much Fun Facts

Stages of the Quitting Process

Women and Cigarette Advertising

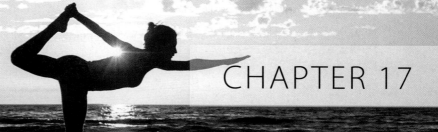

CHAPTER 17

Eliminating Tobacco Use

Learning Objectives

1. Describe the hazards of cigarette smoking.

2. Identify and explain the physiological effects of tobacco.

3. Describe the hazards of using e-cigarettes, hookahs, bidis, clove cigarettes, and smokeless tobacco.

4. Discuss the effects of smoke on nonsmokers, including children.

5. Explain why some people smoke.

6. Identify ways to quit smoking.

7. Describe the various ways to limit tobacco's damage to society.

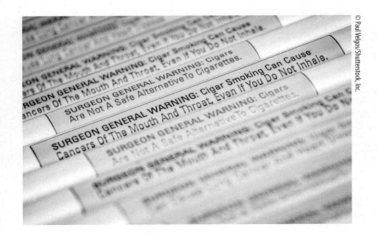

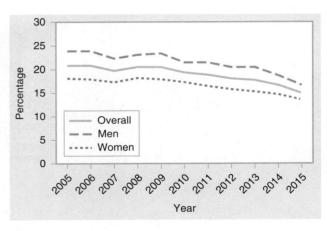

■ **Figure 17.1**

Percentage of Americans Who Smoke Cigarettes, by Age Group, 2005–2015

Data from Jamal, A., et al. (2016, November 11). Current Cigarette Smoking Among Adults – United States, 2005–2015. Morbidity and Mortality Weekly Report, 65; 1205–1211. https://www.cdc.gov/mmwr/volumes/65/wr/mm6544a2.htm

By now, this message and other warnings about the dangers of smoking have reached just about everyone and the number of American cigarette smokers is at an all-time low (**Figure 17.1**). Despite the warnings, however, about 36 million Americans aged 18 and older are cigarette smokers, making nicotine the most used addictive drug in the United States.

Smoking kills more people than AIDS, car accidents, alcohol use, homicides, illegal drugs, suicides, and fires combined. It contributes substantially to deaths from cancer (especially cancers of the lung, esophagus, oral cavity, pancreas, kidney, and bladder), cardiovascular disease (i.e., coronary disease, stroke, and high blood pressure), lung disease (i.e., chronic obstructive pulmonary disease and pneumonia), burns, and problems in infancy caused by low birth weight. Each year about 440,000 Americans die as a result of smoking (**Figure 17.2**); this accounts for one in five deaths in the United States annually. Included in this total are approximately 1,300 children who die from in-home fires caused by cigarettes. Worldwide, about 6 million people die from smoking each year. On average, smokers die about 10 years earlier than nonsmokers. Tobacco use is the single most preventable cause of death in the United States.

The economic costs of smoking are staggering. Cigarette smoking costs the United States more than $300 billion in healthcare costs and lost productivity annually. Only 17% of those costs are covered by smokers themselves in the form of cigarette taxes, direct costs, and health insurance. The remaining smoking-related costs are borne by nonsmokers. On average, each pack of

> Cigarettes are the only legal product that, when used as intended, cause death.
>
> *Louis W. Sullivan,* former secretary of U.S. Department of Health and Human Services

Smoking: Not Much Fun Facts

Erectile dysfunction (ED). Many studies confirm that smoking increases the risk of men not being able to get and/or maintain an erection (Biebel et al., 2016). The risk is related to the number of cigarettes a man has smoked in his life. Recovery of erectile function is possible only if a man stops smoking and has not been a smoker for a long time. Smoking contributes to ED by altering the function of pelvic blood vessels.

Tooth decay. Tobacco smoking increases the risk of tooth decay (dental caries) in adults (Benedetti et al., 2013).

"Light" cigarettes. Cigarettes labeled "low-tar," "mild," "light," or "ultralight" are not less harmful to health than regular cigarettes. That's because smokers of these kinds of cigarettes inhale more deeply or smoke more cigarettes in order to maintain a constant dose of nicotine. This perpetuates exposure to the many harmful chemicals in burning tobacco leaf.

Money pit. Assuming a pack of cigarettes costs $8, a pack-a-day smoker's habit would cost $2,920 a year. If, instead of buying cigarettes, a beginning freshman smoker stopped smoking and invested the money spent on cigarettes at 3.5% per year return, on graduation day nearly 4 years later the student would have $11,268.05. Congratulations! Buy a nice graduation present.

Genetic changes in immune cells. Smoking alters the activity of a gene in blood cells that is instrumental in immune system function. This may be one explanation of the observation that smoking compromises immune function (Stampfli & Anderson, 2009).

Impaired brain function. Compared to children who breathe smoke-free air, children chronically exposed to environmental tobacco smoke (secondhand smoke) score lower on math, reading, and problem-solving tests (Park et al., 2014).

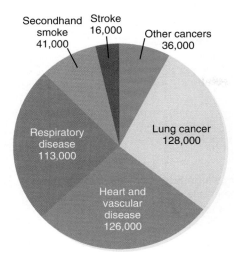

■ **Figure 17.2**

Annual Deaths Attributable to Cigarette Smoking in the United States

Data from Centers for Disease Control and Prevention. (2016). Tobacco-related mortality. Available at http://www.cdc.gov/tobacco/data_statistics/fact_sheets/health_effects/tobacco_related_mortality/.

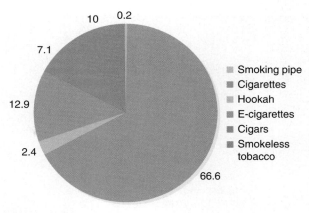

■ **Figure 17.3**

Tobacco Product Used "Every Day" or "on Some Days" by American Adults Age 18 and Older

Data from Hu, S. S., et al. (2016, July 15). Tobacco product use among adults— United States, 2013–2014. *Morbidity Mortality Weekly Report, 65,* 685–691.

cigarettes sold costs American society about four dollars in smoking-related health expenses.

Tobacco Use in the United States

About 16.7 million American men and 13.6 million American women smoke cigarettes. The prevalence of smoking among adult Americans has declined in recent years as the social views of cigarette smoking have become more negative, taxes on cigarettes have increased, laws have been passed to prohibit smoking in public buildings and

work sites, and the federal government has increased its efforts to enhance public health by restricting tobacco marketing to youth. Unfortunately, about 30% of the decline in cigarette smoking in recent years has been offset by increased use of other tobacco products, such as moist snuff, waterpipes, small cigars, and e-cigarettes (**Figure 17.3**).

According to the National Student Health Surveys, conducted by the American College Health Association (2016a, 2016b), a large majority of American and Canadian college students refrain from using nicotine-delivery products (**Table 17.1**). Smoking among Americans younger than age 18 increased during the 1990s but has declined since then (**Figure 17.4**). Smoking among youth is particularly troublesome because adolescence

Table 17.1

Percentage of American and Canadian College Students Using Nicotine-Delivery Products

	Cigarettes				Cigars or Little Cigars				Hookah				Smokeless Tobacco				E-Cigarettes				Marijuana			
	U.S.		Canada		U.S.		Canada		U.S.		Canada		U.S.		Canada		U.S.		Canada		U.S.		Canada	
	M	F	M	F	M	F	M	F	M	F	M	F	M	F	M	F	M	F	M	F	M	F	M	F
Never	71	80	69	75	71	81	72	86	73	79	78	84	85	96	90	97	77	87	82	88	57	61	57	59
Not in last 30 days	16	13	17	15	22	10	21	13	21	18	18	18	10	3	8	3	15	20	13	9	20	21	22	24
1–2 days in last 30 days	5	3	4	3	5	1	4	1	3	2	2	2	2	0	1	0	3	1	3	2	7	7	7	7
3–29 days in last 30 days	2	1	2	1	0	0	0	0	0	0	0	0	0	0	0	0	1	0	1	0	3	2	3	2
Daily	3	2	4	3	0	0	0	0	0	0	0	0	2	0	0	0	2	0	0	0	4	2	4	2

Data from American College Health Association. (2016). *American College Health Association—National College Health Assessment II, Canadian Reference Group Data Report, Spring 2016.* Hanover, MD: American College Health Association; American College Health Association. (2016). *American College Health Association—National College Health Assessment II, Undergraduate Student Reference Group Data Report Spring 2016.* Hanover, MD: American College Health Association.

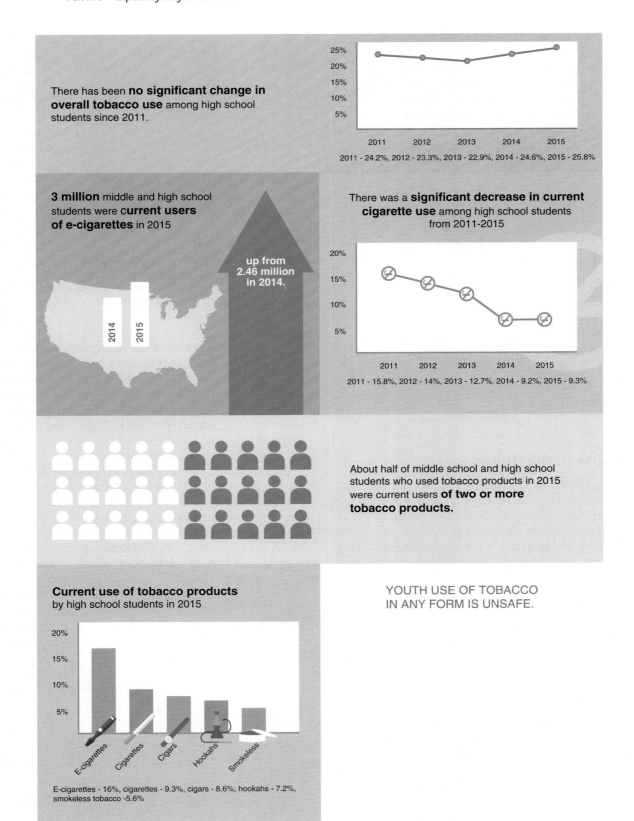

There has been **no significant change in overall tobacco use** among high school students since 2011.

2011 - 24.2%, 2012 - 23.3%, 2013 - 22.9%, 2014 - 24.6%, 2015 - 25.8%

3 million middle and high school students were **current users of e-cigarettes** in 2015

up from 2.46 million in 2014.

2014   2015

There was a **significant decrease in current cigarette use** among high school students from 2011-2015

2011 - 15.8%, 2012 - 14%, 2013 - 12.7%, 2014 - 9.2%, 2015 - 9.3%

About half of middle school and high school students who used tobacco products in 2015 were current users **of two or more tobacco products.**

Current use of tobacco products
by high school students in 2015

E-cigarettes   Cigarettes   Cigars   Hookahs   Smokeless

E-cigarettes - 16%, cigarettes - 9.3%, cigars - 8.6%, hookahs - 7.2%, smokeless tobacco -5.6%

YOUTH USE OF TOBACCO IN ANY FORM IS UNSAFE.

■ **Figure 17.4**

Tobacco Use Among Middle and High School Students—United States, 2011–2015
Reproduced from U.S. Centers for Disease Control and Prevention, Office on Smoking and Health, National Center for Chronic Disease Prevention and Health Promotion

is when regular use and dependence on tobacco begin. According to the Centers for Disease Control and Prevention (2016), among adults who smoke daily, 90% had done so by age 18. Every day nearly 2,100 young people under age 18 try their first cigarette and 1,000 of them become daily smokers. In 2009, the U.S. Congress passed a law to protect the health of young people by prohibiting the sale of cigarettes or smokeless tobacco to people under age 18, cigarette packages with fewer than 20 cigarettes, cigarettes and smokeless tobacco in vending machines and other impersonal modes of sale, and free samples of cigarettes and smokeless tobacco products. The law also prohibits tobacco brand name sponsorship of any athletic, musical, or other social or cultural event, or any team or entry in those events, and the sale or distribution of items, such as hats and T-shirts, with tobacco brands or logos.

What Is Tobacco?

Tobacco used for smoking, chewing, or snuff is the processed product of the leaves of the plant *Nicotiana tabacum*. This plant is indigenous to the Western Hemisphere, where it grows best in semitropical climates.

Tobacco was introduced to European societies in the sixteenth century by the Spanish returning from voyages to the Americas. The Spanish had learned about smoking from Native Americans, who used tobacco much as it is used today. In fact, the word "tobacco" is an Indian word referring to the pipe used to smoke the minced or rolled leaf of the tobacco plant.

The smoking habit spread quickly in Europe, fueled by tobacco imports from Spain's colonies. By the nineteenth century, changing social customs had caused tobacco smoking to be replaced largely by tobacco chewing; even more popular was the habit of sniffing tobacco in the form of snuff. Not until the 1880s, when the cigarette-making machine was invented in

the United States, did cigarette smoking become the predominant form of tobacco use worldwide. Camel cigarettes, introduced in 1913, ushered in the modern era of smoking in the United States. By coincidence, the American Cancer Society was established in the same year.

Processing tobacco for consumption involves harvesting the tobacco leaves and curing them by any one of several drying methods. The cured tobacco leaves are shredded, and various types of leaves are blended into commercially desirable mixtures. Often flavorings and colorings are added, as well as chemicals that facilitate even burning. Finally, the mixture is used to manufacture cigarettes, pipe tobacco, and chewing tobacco or is wrapped in specially cured tobacco leaves to make cigars.

The most familiar chemical constituent of tobacco is **nicotine**, but when tobacco is burned, approximately 4,000 other chemical substances are released and carried in the smoke. These chemicals include acetone, acrolein, carbon monoxide, methanol, ammonia, nitrous dioxide, hydrogen sulfide, traces of various mineral elements, traces of radioactive elements, acids, insecticides, and other substances. Besides these chemical compounds, tobacco smoke also contains countless microscopic particles that contribute to the yellowish brown residue of tobacco smoke known as **tar**, a documented cause of lung cancer. Nicotine is responsible for tobacco addiction. Forty-three of the other chemicals in tobacco are known to cause cancer (**carcinogens**).

Physiological Effects of Tobacco

Most of the physiological effects of tobacco smoking are attributable to the pharmacological effects of nicotine. The most prominent effects include increased heart rate, increased release of adrenaline, and a direct stimulatory effect on the brain, which combine to produce the mild "rush" cigarette smokers may experience when they light up. It also lowers skin temperature and reduces blood flow in the legs and feet. Nicotine is also responsible for the nausea and vomiting experienced by most beginning

Smoking: Playing the Odds

If you like to gamble, here are the odds of dying from lung cancer for smokers as compared to nonsmokers.

Cigarettes per day	Increased risk	
	Men	Women
1 to 4	3-fold	5-fold
5 to 9	11-fold	12-fold
10 to 14	17-fold	18-fold
15 to 19	10-fold	20-fold

Overall, 90% of lung cancers are caused by cigarette smoking.

TERMS

carcinogens: substances that can cause cancer in people and other animals

nicotine: an addicting chemical in tobacco that produces rapid pulse, increased alertness, and a variety of other physiological effects

tar: the yellowish brown residue of tobacco smoke

Make Every Day World No Tobacco Day

May 31 of each year is World No Tobacco Day, sponsored by the World Health Organization (WHO) to remind everyone about the health risks and social costs of tobacco use and to encourage the world to reduce and eventually end tobacco consumption. In 2016, about 22% of the world's population (1.2 billion people) smoked tobacco (about 6 trillion cigarettes); about 6 million people died of smoking-related causes, 80% of them in low- and middle-income countries. By 2025, WHO and its partner organizations aim to reduce the prevalence of smoking worldwide to about 18%.

In 2005, almost all of the countries of the world signed a treaty called the Framework Convention on Tobacco Control (FCTC) to combat worldwide tobacco use. The treaty states, "Every person should be informed of the health consequences, addictive nature, and mortal threat posed by tobacco consumption and exposure." The treaty calls for all countries to take action to protect people from tobacco smoke and children and nonsmokers from exposure to secondhand smoke. Some actions taken by countries to rein in tobacco consumption included comprehensive bans on tobacco advertising, promotion, and sponsorship, as well as other tobacco packaging and labeling measures, such a health warnings.

Some countries totally ban smoking advertising and promotion, especially to children. The United States opposes this position on the ground that it violates the constitutional right to free speech.

Some countries require that one-third to one-half of a cigarette packet carry health warnings and images showing the consequences of smoking. Some also ban the use of the words *light*, *low tar*, and *mild* in cigarette ads because these words deceive consumers into thinking that products labeled as such are not dangerous.

In observance of World No Tobacco Day 2016, WHO introduced suggestions for standardizing the packaging of tobacco products as part of a comprehensive approach to reducing smoking. The suggested packaging is without much graphics or color ("plain packaging") in order to reduce attractiveness, eliminate tobacco packaging as a form of advertising and promotion, prohibit design techniques that suggest that tobacco products are not harmful, and increase the visibility of health warnings. In 2012, Australia became the first country to use plain packaging for tobacco products. Follow-up research has indicated that plain packaging can reduce positive perceptions of smoking and dissuade tobacco use. The research supports governments deciding to implement plain cigarette packaging measures as part of comprehensive smoking prevention efforts (Smith et al., 2015).

Besides controlling advertising and promotion and insisting on health warnings on packets, countries reduce tobacco use by taxing tobacco products. A 10% price increase reduces consumption by about 4% in high-income countries and by 8% in low-income countries. Some countries also try to limit the importation of cigarettes.

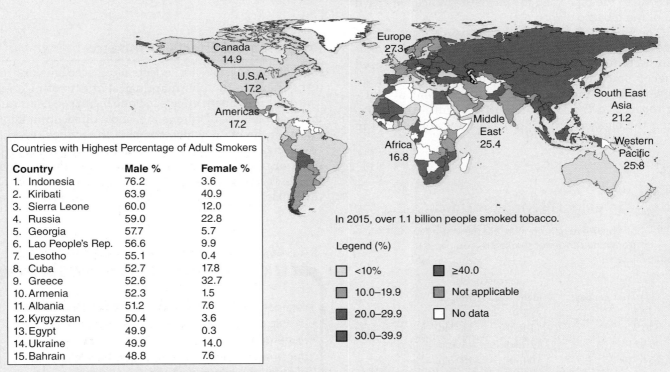

Percentage of Adult Male Smokers in Regions of the World

Canada 14.9 · U.S.A. 17.2 · Americas 17.2 · Europe 27.3 · Middle East 25.4 · Africa 16.8 · South East Asia 21.2 · Western Pacific 25.8

In 2015, over 1.1 billion people smoked tobacco.

Countries with Highest Percentage of Adult Smokers		
Country	**Male %**	**Female %**
1. Indonesia	76.2	3.6
2. Kiribati	63.9	40.9
3. Sierra Leone	60.0	12.0
4. Russia	59.0	22.8
5. Georgia	57.7	5.7
6. Lao People's Rep.	56.6	9.9
7. Lesotho	55.1	0.4
8. Cuba	52.7	17.8
9. Greece	52.6	32.7
10. Armenia	52.3	1.5
11. Albania	51.2	7.6
12. Kyrgyzstan	50.4	3.6
13. Egypt	49.9	0.3
14. Ukraine	49.9	14.0
15. Bahrain	48.8	7.6

Legend (%)

☐ <10%	■ ≥40.0
■ 10.0–19.9	■ Not applicable
■ 20.0–29.9	☐ No data
■ 30.0–39.9	

Data from World Health Organization, Global Health Observatory data, Prevalence of Tobacco Smoking. Retrieved from: http://www.who.int/gho/tobacco/use/en

smokers. Addiction to nicotine is largely responsible for perpetuating a smoker's habit.

Some harmful cardiovascular effects of cigarette smoking probably result from nicotine and carbon monoxide, which are believed to contribute to the development of heart and blood vessel disease. A host of other harmful chemicals in tobacco contributes to the development of cancer and diseases of the respiratory tract. Among these chemicals are benzo-a-pyrene, aza-arenes, N-nitrosamines, and radioactive polonium. Polonium is a product of the breakdown of radioactive lead, a natural constituent of soil. Radioactive particles in the soil become deposited on sticky tobacco leaf hairs and eventually become part of tobacco smoke. Radon, a radioactive gas, is also present in tobacco smoke inhaled both by the smoker and nonsmoker via secondhand smoke. These radioactive substances can become trapped in tiny air sacs in the lungs, where they induce cancerous changes in lung tissue.

Nicotine Delivery Systems

Cigars

Because cigar smokers generally do not inhale cigar smoke, it is often mistakenly assumed that cigar smoking is not harmful. However, compared with nonsmokers, cigar smokers who do not inhale have 3 times the risk of dying of lung cancer, and cigar smokers who inhale have 11 times the risk of death from lung cancer. Cigar smokers, whether they inhale or not, have a greater risk of death from cancer of the lip, tongue, mouth, throat, esophagus, larynx, pancreas, and bladder. Because cigars have more tobacco than cigarettes, and because they often burn for much longer, they give off greater amounts of secondhand smoke. In general, secondhand smoke from cigars contains many of the same poisons (toxins) and cancer-causing agents (carcinogens) as cigarette smoke but in higher concentrations. It was not until the year 2000 that health warnings became required on cigar packages.

Hookahs

Hookahs are water pipes used to smoke flavored tobacco (e.g., apple, mint, cherry, chocolate, coconut, licorice, cappuccino, and watermelon). Hookahs are also known as *narghile, argileh, shisha, hubble-bubble,* and *goza.* Hookah smoking is generally a group activity with the pipe mouthpiece passed from person to person over the course of an hour or more. Hookahs originated about 800 years ago in Persia (now Iran) and India. Today, hookah smoking is popular around the world.

Many believe that hookah smoking is safer than smoking, chewing, or sniffing tobacco. However, hookah smokers inhale large amounts of nicotine, many of the same chemicals that are in cigarette smoke, tar, metals, and various chemicals arising from the combustion of the flavorings and other additives. A typical 1-hour-long hookah smoking session involves 200 puffs, while an average cigarette is 20 puffs. The volume of smoke inhaled during a typical hookah session is about 90,000 milliliters, compared with 500 to 600 milliliters inhaled when smoking a cigarette. Just as with secondhand cigarette and cigar smoke, nonsmokers in the vicinity of hookah consumption also inhale the chemical-laden smoke.

The presence of nicotine and many hundreds of different chemicals from burned tobacco and the flavorings in hookah smoke are cause for concern. Nicotine is highly addictive and also contributes directly to heart and blood vessel disease. Nicotine addiction can foster ever-increasing hookah use and hence increased exposure to the toxic agents in hookah smoke. Also, nicotine addiction from hookah smoking can facilitate transition to smoking cigarettes or chewing tobacco with their associated negative health outcomes. The harmful chemicals in hookah smoke are the same as in cigarette smoke that are associated with lung cancer, respiratory illness, heart disease, low birth weight, and periodontal disease. Sharing a hookah may increase the risk of transmission of tuberculosis, viruses such as herpes or hepatitis, and other illnesses.

Bidis and Kreteks

Bidis are small, thin, hand-rolled cigarettes imported to the United States, primarily from India and other Southeast Asian countries. They comprise tobacco wrapped in a *tendu* or *temburni* leaf (plants native to Asia) and may be secured with a colorful string at one or both ends. Bidis can be flavored (e.g., chocolate, cherry, mango) or unflavored. **Kreteks**, also referred to as **clove cigarettes**, are imported from Indonesia and typically contain a mixture of tobacco, cloves, and other additives. Bidis and kreteks are falsely believed to be less harmful than commercial American cigarettes. Bidi smoke contains three to five times the amount of nicotine as a regular cigarette and places users at risk for nicotine

---

TERMS

bidis: small, thin hand-rolled cigarettes

hookahs: water pipes used to smoke flavored tobacco

kreteks (clove cigarettes): cigarettes with cloves and other additives

nicotine: an addicting chemical in tobacco that produces rapid pulse, increased alertness, and a variety of other physiological effects

addiction. Bidi smoking increases the risk of oral cancer, lung cancer, stomach cancer, esophageal cancer, coronary heart disease and heart attack, emphysema, and chronic bronchitis. Kretek smoking increases the risk of lung damage that can lead to abnormal lung function (Duong, 2017).

E-Cigarettes

E-cigarettes ("E" for electronic) are devices that deliver to the body nicotine, flavorings (e.g., fruit, mint, and chocolate), and other chemicals via an inhaled vapor, which is the reason using e-cigarettes is called "vaping." Typically, e-cigarettes are composed of a rechargeable, battery-operated heating element, a replaceable cartridge that contains nicotine or other chemicals, an atomizer that, when heated, converts the contents of the cartridge into an inhalable vapor, and the chemical propylene glycol that helps the vapor stay moist. Propylene glycol is widely used in foods and medicines to keep products moist. Whereas this chemical is harmless when eaten, its effect on the lungs when inhaled is unknown. E-cigarettes are often made to resemble cigarettes, cigars, and pipes and, for those who wish to camouflage their use, nontobacco items such as pens and USB memory sticks.

The prototype of e-cigarettes was invented by a Chinese pharmacist in 2003; e-cigarettes entered the U.S. market around 2007. Since then, their use and popularity have increased dramatically. Seeing a market opportunity and a way to control a competing product, the giant tobacco companies are now marketing e-cigarettes.

Purveyors of e-cigarettes maintain that the devices are a preferred form of nicotine ingestion since they do not deliver the hazardous chemicals released in burning tobacco. Although some e-cigarettes have been marketed as smoking cessation aids, much as FDA-approved nicotine-containing gum, patches, and inhalers are, there is no conclusive scientific evidence that e-cigarettes promote successful long-term quitting. Even if smokers quit tobacco successfully by using e-cigarettes, they are still addicted to nicotine, which could increase the possibility they would resume smoking. Also, there are concerns that the millions of young people who start using e-cigarettes will become addicted to nicotine and eventually become tobacco smokers. Furthermore, the vapor in e-cigarettes may eventually damage lung tissue. Tests have shown that the vapor contains tiny amounts of heavy metals (known to be carcinogenic) that are released from the solder in the metal coil.

As long as the manufacturers do not claim that e-cigarettes have any therapeutic value, they are unregulated by the Food and Drug Administration (FDA). In many states, there are no restrictions on the sale of e-cigarettes to minors. Should studies indicate that e-cigarettes pose a danger, the FDA has announced that it is prepared to issue regulations concerning the manufacture and sale of e-cigarettes, just as it does for tobacco products.

That e-cigarette use is increasing among U.S. adolescents and adults is cause for concern. One concern is the potential of e-cigarettes to cause acute nicotine toxicity, characterized by vomiting, rapid or pounding heart rate, abdominal cramps, agitation, muscle twitching, confusion, convulsions, rapid or difficulty breathing, coma, fainting, and headache. Long-term effects of nicotine exposure include accelerated coronary and peripheral vascular disease and stroke, high blood pressure, slow wound healing, pregnancy problems, ulcers, and esophageal reflux.

Smokeless Tobacco

Smokeless tobacco is available in two main forms: **chewing tobacco** and **snuff**. Chewing tobacco is processed into three different forms: loose leaf, firm/moist plug, and twist/rope chewing tobacco. A portion of chewing tobacco is either chewed or placed in the mouth and held in place between the lower lip and gum. Snuff is made from powdered or finely cut tobacco leaves and is available in two forms, dry and moist. In many European countries, dry snuff is inhaled through the nose. However, in the United States a pinch of snuff is placed in the mouth and held in place between the cheek and gum, referred to as "snuff dipping." Dipping snuff is highly addictive and exposes the body to levels of nicotine equal to those of cigarettes. **Moist snuff** is made from air- and fire-cured tobacco leaves that are processed into fine particles, flavored, and packaged in moist form in round, flat containers. Moist snuff is considered the most hazardous form of smokeless tobacco because of the methods used in processing it.

Tobacco for chewing and sniffing has been used for many centuries. Smokeless tobacco use by both men and women flourished until the end of the nineteenth century. At this time, scientists discovered that bacteria and viruses could survive in saliva and be spread by air. Spitting into spittoons and onto barroom floors became unacceptable and even unlawful in many public places. Cigarettes replaced chew and snuff.

Chewing tobacco became fashionable again in the 1970s when the dangers of cigarette smoking became clear. Cigarettes were publicized as carcinogenic, and advertisers promoted smokeless tobacco as being a healthy alternative to cigarette smoking, which it is not. Smokeless tobacco creates dependence on nicotine just as cigarette smoking does. It leads to cancer of the mouth, lip, and gum.

It also causes other diseases of the mouth, such as hard white patches on the gums (leukoplakia) and inflammatory lesions of the gum (gingivitis). The majority of these lesions are benign, but about 2% to 6% of cases develop into cancer. Some users show a marked increase in blood pressure, which is a major factor in heart disease.

Smokeless tobacco has also been linked to other health problems. Taste-enhancing sugars and sweeteners found in loose chewing tobacco may lead to tooth decay. Abrasive ingredients found in tobacco cause receding gums in areas where the tobacco is held for long periods between the teeth and lower lip or the teeth and the cheek. Tobacco users often experience halitosis (bad breath) or a loss of taste and smell.

Social consequences of using smokeless tobacco include yellow and brown stains on the teeth, clothing, and automobile; the tobacco may cling to teeth, lips, tongue, and clothing. Spitting tobacco juice disgusts others.

The health risks of smokeless tobacco have become increasingly apparent, and various steps have been taken to alert the public to this problem. In 1986, the Comprehensive Smokeless Tobacco Health Education Act was passed. This bill banned all smokeless tobacco ads on television and radio, and mandated that health hazard warnings be placed on all tobacco packages. However, advertisements in print media and at car races and rodeos have increased the use of smokeless tobacco among young people. Male athletes are particularly at risk because of intensive marketing targeted to adolescent males, distribution of free smokeless tobacco to college athletes, promotions by professional athletes, and the convenience of using smokeless tobacco during games.

Smoking and Disease

Almost from the beginning of tobacco use in Europe and America, people have been concerned about the possible harmful effects of smoking. Medical reports of the eighteenth and nineteenth centuries cited tobacco smoking as a cause of cancer of the lip, tongue, and lung. Years of research since then has established smoking to be a risk factor in the development of coronary artery disease; lung cancer; bronchitis; emphysema; cancer of the larynx, lip, and oral cavity; cancer of the bladder and stomach; duodenal ulcer; and allergies (**Figure 17.5**).

Furthermore, the death rate from cancer, heart disease, and respiratory diseases is higher among cigarette smokers than among nonsmokers. In fact, smoking decreases a person's life expectancy by an average of 10 years. Smokers between the ages of 35 and 70 have death rates several times higher than those who have never smoked.

Lung Cancer

Lung cancer is responsible for more deaths among men and women than any other type of cancer. Each year approximately 225,000 persons receive a diagnosis of lung cancer and about 160,000 people die of this disease. Smoking is responsible for almost 90% of lung cancers among men and more than 70% among women. In recent years, among American men, lung cancer incidence and death rates have declined, reflecting several decades of decline in active smoking and exposure to environmental tobacco smoke that together cause about 90% of lung cancer. In contrast, among American women, lung cancer incidence and death rates have increased, although the rate of increase has slowed in recent years. It is hoped that female lung cancer incidence and death rates will soon begin to decline as they have for men.

The increase in lung cancer deaths is the principal reason that the overall cancer death rate continues to rise. If lung cancer death rates are excluded from the statistics, the death rate from cancer would have been falling steadily for many years, principally because of preventive efforts and improved diagnosis and treatment. This situation is ironic as well as tragic, for lung cancer is one of the most preventable of all diseases. People simply need to stop (or never start) smoking cigarettes.

Heart Disease

Smoking cigarettes increases the risk of heart disease. Smoking can increase tension in the heart muscle walls, speed up the rate of muscular contraction, and increase the heart rate. As the heart's workload increases, so does the need for oxygen and other nutrients. Smoking also reduces the amount of high-density lipoprotein (HDL) cholesterol (i.e., the "good" cholesterol), there by facilitating plaque formation and abnormal blood clotting.

Bronchitis and Emphysema

Bronchitis and **emphysema** are respiratory diseases sometimes classified with asthma as **chronic obstructive pulmonary diseases (COPD)**. Each of these diseases is

---

▌TERMS▐

bronchitis: inflammation of the bronchi of the lungs as a result of irritation; often accompanied by a chronic cough

chewing tobacco: a form of shredded smokeless tobacco; chewed or placed in the mouth between the lower lip and gum

chronic obstructive pulmonary diseases (COPD): diseases that restrict the ability of the body to obtain oxygen through the respiratory structures (bronchi and lungs); include asthma, bronchitis, and emphysema

e-cigarettes: electronic devices that deliver via inhaled vapor nicotine, flavorings, and other chemicals; called "vaping"

emphysema: a progressive degeneration of the lung alveoli, causing breathing and oxygen assimilation to become more and more difficult

moist snuff: a form of snuff made from air- and fire-cured tobacco leaves; most hazardous form of smokeless tobacco

snuff: a form of smokeless tobacco; made from powdered or finely cut leaves

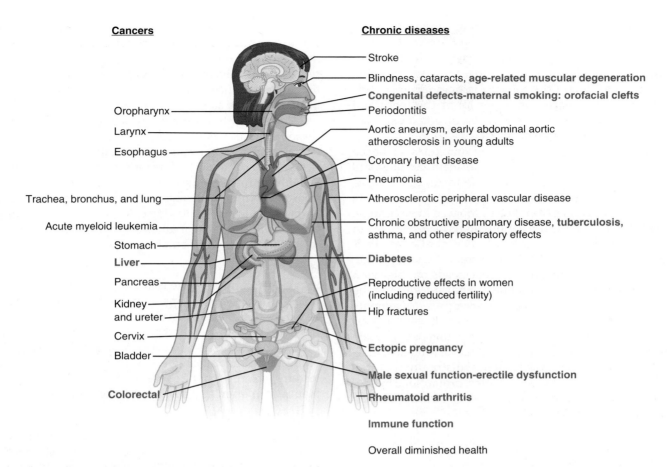

Figure 17.5

Health Effects of Tobacco Use

Reproduced from U.S. Department of Health and Human Services. (2014). The Health Consequences of Smoking 50 Years of Progress. A Report of the Surgeon General, Executive Summary, 2014. Atlanta, GA: U.S. Department of Health and Human Services, Centers for Disease Control and Prevention, National Center for Chronic Disease Prevention and Health Promotion, Office on Smoking and Health.

associated with breathing difficulty caused by obstruction or destruction of some part of the respiratory system. Often persons suffer from more than one of these conditions at the same time.

Bronchitis is an inflammatory condition of the upper part of the respiratory tract, principally the **trachea**, the main airway. Bronchitis is characterized by excessive production of mucus by cells that line the airways, which causes the major symptoms of bronchitis, such as a continual cough (smoker's cough) and the production of large amounts of sputum. Some affected people also experience shortness of breath, particularly during exertion.

Apparently, excessive production of mucus by the glands of the bronchi is a reaction to irritation caused by cigarette smoke. Fortunately, the pathology that produces the symptoms of bronchitis can be almost completely reversed by quitting smoking, reducing exposure to polluted air, or both. However, many people "live with" their persistent cough for many years and are not concerned

with the message their body is giving them. If the disease is left to run its course, sufferers increase their vulnerability to other respiratory illnesses, and the airways may become irreversibly damaged.

Smoking is the primary cause of emphysema, which results from the destruction of the tiny air sacs deep in the lungs called **alveoli** (**Figure 17.6**). Each lung contains millions of alveoli; across their thin membranes the function of breathing is accomplished—the exchange of the respiratory gases, oxygen and carbon dioxide.

Emphysema is a disabling condition in which the walls of the air sacs in the lungs lose their elasticity and are gradually destroyed. The lungs' ability to obtain oxygen and remove carbon dioxide is impaired, requiring the heart to work harder, which results in the heart becoming enlarged. Emphysema involves a slow, irreversible process of alveolar destruction; as the disease progresses, affected people have greater and greater trouble breathing.

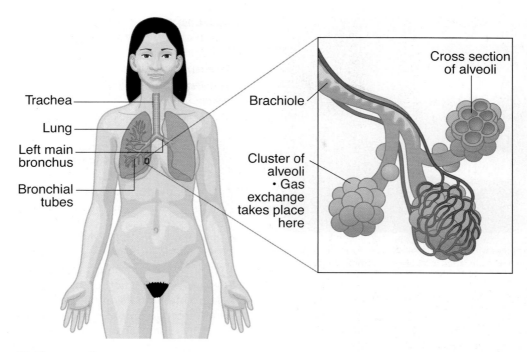

■ **Figure 17.6**

Respiratory System
Provides oxygen and removes carbon dioxide. Oxygen enters and carbon dioxide leaves via tiny air sacs in the lungs called alveoli. The rest of the respiratory system facilitates gas exchange in the alveoli.

Tobacco Smoke's Effects on Nonsmokers

Nonsmokers who are exposed to tobacco smoke run a significant health risk. People who work or live in environments heavily laden with tobacco smoke inhale the same smokeborne substances as do smokers. In fact, about two-thirds of the smoke from a burning cigarette enters the environment.

Environmental tobacco smoke (ETS), also called secondhand smoke, contains the same 4,000 chemicals that inhaled tobacco smoke does, but the concentration is greater because ETS is unfiltered. Annually, about 7,000 nonsmoking American adults die of lung cancer and about 30,000 die from heart disease as a result of exposure to ETS. Also, breathing ETS increases the severity of asthma in children and is responsible for thousands of cases of bronchitis and pneumonia in children younger than 18 months.

A nonsmoker in a smoke-filled room can inhale in one hour the equivalent of a cigarette's worth of nicotine, carbon monoxide, and carcinogenic substances. Also, many people are allergic to tobacco smoke, which can produce eye irritation, headache, cough, nasal congestion, and asthma. Nonsmokers forced to inhale tobacco smoke for long periods, such as workers in enclosed smoke-filled workplaces, can suffer impaired lung function equivalent to that of smokers who smoke 10 cigarettes a day.

Smoking and Periodontal Disease

Periodontal disease (unhealthy gums and teeth) leads to loosening of teeth; receding, swollen, or bleeding gums; and, eventually, tooth loss. About 4% of the U.S. population suffers from periodontal disease. Until recently, periodontal disease was thought to be due to plaque buildup resulting from poor dental hygiene and to inflammation of the gums caused by bacteria (*gingivitis*). However, new studies suggest that as much as 50% of periodontal disease may be due to the effects of smoking tobacco or marijuana (Shariff et al., 2017). Smoking cigarettes and marijuana reduces oxygen supply to the gums, leading to inflammation and destruction of gum tissue. If you have been looking for a really good reason to stop smoking, the possibility of destructive periodontal disease, loss of teeth, and thousands of dollars in dental bills should do the trick.

TERMS

alveoli: tiny air sacs in the lungs that exchange oxygen and carbon dioxide

trachea: upper part of respiratory tract

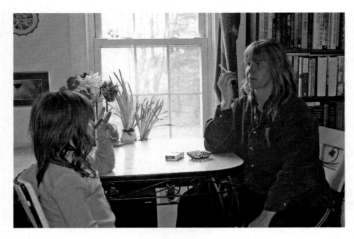

Children who live in homes where adults smoke have more respiratory problems than children who are raised in smoke-free environments.

Effects of Parental Smoking on Children

Parental smoking harms children, beginning in pregnancy and continuing throughout a child's life. Smoking is a risk factor for spontaneous abortion, newborn death, and sudden infant death syndrome (SIDS). A pregnant woman exposed to environmental tobacco smoke (ETS) risks giving birth to a low-birth-weight infant. Compared to children raised in a nonsmoking environment, children exposed to ETS have a higher risk of bronchitis, pneumonia, and other respiratory tract infections. They also are at higher risk for asthma and ear infections.

Why People Smoke

Most smokers begin their habit in their teen years, emulating friends, parents, celebrities, film stars, or cigarette ad models. Teenagers also smoke to attain acceptance in their peer group. About half of those who experiment with smoking continue the habit into adulthood. Despite the unpleasant taste, the initial adverse physiological reactions to smoke and nicotine, and the knowledge that tobacco smoke causes cancer and other life-threatening diseases, some continue to smoke because of an unusually high susceptibility to nicotine addiction (DiFranza, 2008). Other factors that contribute to the development and maintenance of regular smoking include the following:

- *Stimulation.* Some people experience a psychological lift from smoking. They say that smoking helps them to wake up in the morning and organize their energies. They often report that smoking increases their intellectual capacities.
- *Handling.* Some people enjoy the mere handling of cigarettes and smoking paraphernalia, such as lighters.
- *Pleasurable relaxation.* Some smokers say they smoke simply because they like it. Smoking brings them pleasure and relaxation and is often practiced to enhance other pleasurable sensations, such as the taste of food and alcoholic beverages. However, smoking actually dulls the taste buds.

- *Reducing negative feelings (crutch).* Approximately 40% of smokers say they smoke because it temporarily helps them deal with stress, anger, fear, anxiety, or pressure (**Figure 17.7**). Although many smokers attribute smoking to relieving psychological distress, studies indicate that the opposite is often the case: smoking contributes to psychological distress because of the biological effects of nicotine on the brain (Taylor et al., 2014). People with chronic mental illness or substance-use disorders are at highest risk for smoking.
- *Craving.* Some people crave cigarettes and have no other explanation for their habit except that they have a frequent need to smoke, regardless of the tension-relieving effects that smoking might bring.
- *Habit.* Some smokers light up only because of habit. They no longer receive much physical or psychological gratification from smoking; often they smoke without being aware of whether they really want the cigarette.

Some individuals smoke occasionally, claiming not to be addicted to smoking and able to stop at any time. Often they smoke for social reasons, that is, to share this activity with smoker-friends in social situations. The health risk of occasional social smoking, although probably less than regular, pack-a-day smoking, is not negligible. Compared to never smokers, current smokers who consistently smoke 10 or fewer cigarettes per day over their lifetime are over twice as likely to develop smoking-related cancer, especially lung cancer

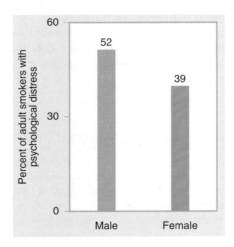

■ Figure 17.7

Smoking and Psychological Distress
Does smoking relieve psychological distress, as many smokers attest? It doesn't appear to be that way. Researchers measured psychological distress among nearly 38,000 American adults who smoked at least 100 cigarettes during their lifetime and, at the time of measurement, reported smoking every day or on some days. Measurements were made with the Kessler psychological distress scale, which produces scores for feelings of sadness, nervousness, restlessness, worthlessness, and feeling like everything is an effort in the past 30 days. The results showed that about half of male smokers and one-third of female smokers, have considerable psychological distress.

Data from Jamal, A., et. al. (2016) Current Cigarette Smoking Among Adults—United States, 2005–2015. *Morbidity and Mortality Weekly Report, 65,* 1205–1211.

(Inoue-Choi et al., 2018). Among lifelong smokers of 10 or fewer cigarettes per day who quit smoking, the risks of smoking-related cancer diminish as the duration of cessation increases. Thus, even low-level smokers need to quit now to protect their long-term health. Any exposure to cigarette smoke carries some risk. Furthermore, social smokers are probably more likely to increase smoking in certain circumstances, such as a stressful life situation, and become regular smokers.

Quitting Smoking

Mark Twain once quipped, "Giving up smoking is easy. I've done it a hundred times."

Whereas that little joke is intended to show how difficult stopping smoking can be, it also confirms research that shows stopping smoking is a process, not an event. Often, people think about stopping for a period of time before they even consider trying, and sometimes people go through one or more cycles of stopping and starting up again before they quit permanently. These tries and retries are part of the stopping process.

The smoking habit is part biological (addiction to nicotine), part psychological (smoking alters mood and provides pleasure), and part social (smokers smoke with other smokers). Because smoking involves several parts of a smoker's life, quitting successfully generally requires examining how smoking is integrated into one's life, and then planning and adopting alternative experiences that meet the biological, psychological, and social needs that smoking satisfies.

Successful smoking cessation plans center on a predetermined **quit date**—the day that the smoker stops smoking completely. Prior to the quit date, the smoker can prepare for stopping by

- Cutting back on the number of cigarettes smoked each day.
- Identifying which cigarettes will be the hardest to give up (e.g., first of the day; after a meal) and planning alternative activities for after the quit date.

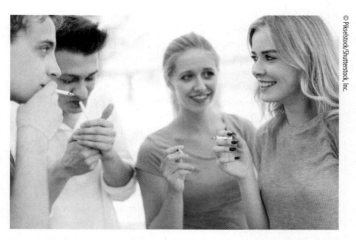

Smoking begins at an early age when peer acceptance is highly sought after.

Benefits of Quitting Smoking

The immediate health benefits of quitting smoking are substantial:

- Heart rate and blood pressure, which are abnormally high while smoking, begin to return to normal.
- Within a few hours, the level of carbon monoxide in the blood begins to decline. (Carbon monoxide reduces the blood's ability to carry oxygen.)
- Within a few weeks, people who quit smoking have improved circulation, produce less phlegm, and don't cough or wheeze as often.
- Within several months of quitting, people can expect substantial improvements in lung function.
- Within a few years of quitting, people will have lower risks of cancer, heart disease, and other chronic diseases than if they had continued to smoke.
- In addition, people who quit smoking will have an improved sense of smell, and food will taste better.

Data from National Cancer Institute. (2014). Harms of Cigarette Smoking and Health Benefits of Quitting. Retrieved from http://www.cancer.gov/about-cancer/causes-prevention/risk/tobacco/cessation-fact-sheet#q7

- Identifying and preparing to do without the benefits of smoking and finding alternative activities to meet the needs that smoking provides (e.g., stress management).
- Asking friends and family to offer support while quitting.
- Seeking professional smoking cessation counseling and support from smoking cessation groups. Nationwide telephone counseling is available at 1-800-QUIT NOW.
- During the first few weeks of the quitting process, planning to stay away from smoking stimuli (e.g., not going to bars, not hanging out with friends who smoke, not smoking at breaks with coworkers, not smoking in the car).
- Considering using **nicotine replacement therapy** (nicotine patch, gum, or nasal spray) in conjunction with smoker cessation counseling (Appolino & Glantz, 2017) to lessen the effects of nicotine withdrawal and prescription drugs, such as Wellbutrin (bupropion) and Chantix (varenicline), which lessen the urge to smoke.

TERMS

nicotine replacement therapy: using nicotine-containing gum, skin patches, nasal sprays, or inhalers to temper the symptoms of nicotine withdrawal when quitting smoking

quit date: the day a smoker designates as the one on which she or he will stop smoking completely

People stop smoking for a variety of reasons: to reduce the risk of early death from heart or lung disease; to enjoy, once again, the unpolluted taste of food; to please non-smoking loved ones; to eliminate the ever-present ashes and smell of cigarette smoke from their homes and cars; and to fulfill a simple, yet important, commitment to be healthy. Frequently, a positive change in other aspects of life leads to cessation of smoking. For example, many people who take up meditation, t'ai chi ch'uan, jogging, or other physical activity lose the desire to smoke and stop smoking. Free information for people who want to learn more about smoking and help with quitting smoking is available from the Centers for Disease Control and Prevention (1-800-QUIT-NOW and http://www.cdc.gov/Tobacco/).

Reducing Tobacco's Damage to Society

Tobacco is the only legal consumer product that causes disability and death when used as intended. To replace the thousands of adult tobacco users who die each day, tobacco companies must recruit new users, generally from youth.

Since the first Surgeon General report in 1964 on the health hazards of smoking, there has been an ongoing battle between doctors and health organizations and the tobacco industry. At stake is influencing the behavior of millions of smokers and prospective smokers, especially teens. The health groups try to persuade people not to smoke or to quit smoking; the tobacco industry encourages them to smoke.

> A good plan executed right now is better than a perfect plan executed next week.
>
> *General George S. Patton*

Made public in the 1990s, tobacco industry secret documents revealed that for more than 40 years, tobacco companies misled and lied to the public about the harmful, addictive effects of tobacco. Moreover, it was revealed that tobacco companies targeted and manipulated young people into starting smoking. The tobacco industry knows that today's teenager is tomorrow's potential regular customer. As the Campaign for Tobacco-Free Kids points out, the tobacco industry is addicted to advertising to children.

In 2009, the U.S. Congress passed the Family Smoking Prevention and Tobacco Control Act. Following are the provisions of this law:

- Tobacco-product manufacturers must list the ingredients and additives they put into tobacco products so consumers can know what they are being exposed to. Any harmful chemicals and additives are liable to regulation.
- Cigarettes with fruit, spice, and other flavorings that appeal to youth are banned. One exception is menthol, an ingredient in 25% of all cigarettes sold and 75% of all cigarettes sold to African Americans. Menthol could be banned if found to be harmful.
- The FDA has the authority to regulate the use of words such as *light*, *mild*, and *low* in promotional materials and on packages, because they incorrectly imply that such products are less harmful than regular tobacco products.
- Warning labels about the dangers of tobacco are larger and more prominently displayed on promotional materials and on packages.

Stages of the Quitting Process

Quitting smoking is a process involving five stages. The more one knows about the quitting process, the more likely one is to stop smoking and to have the confidence to remain tobacco free. The five stages of the quitting process are as follows.

Precontemplation Stage
Smokers in the precontemplation stage spend little time thinking about their smoking and may not see it as a problem. They see more negatives about quitting than positives, resulting in low motivation for stopping, even though they know that smoking carries serious health risks.

Contemplation Stage
Smokers in the contemplation stage are aware of the benefits of stopping and think about their smoking—and even about quitting—but they feel ambivalent about actually stopping. They may think about the negative aspects of smoking and the positive aspects associated with quitting, yet doubt that the long-term benefits associated with quitting will outweigh the short-term costs. Such ambivalence is a normal part of the quitting process and may last several months or even years.

Preparation
Smokers in the preparation stage have made the decision to quit and are taking steps to get ready to stop smoking. They see the cons of smoking as outweighing the pros and say things like "I've got to do something about this—this is serious," or "Something has to change. What can I do?"

Action Stage
Smokers in the action stage are actively trying to stop smoking. They may try several different techniques, believe they have inner strength to quit, and tend to seek help and support. They develop plans to deal with both personal and external pressures that may lead to slips (i.e., smoking a cigarette), and they use short-term rewards to sustain their motivation.

Maintenance Stage
Smokers in the maintenance stage have learned to anticipate and handle temptations to smoke. They remain aware that what they are striving for is personally worthwhile and meaningful and are patient with themselves, recognizing that it often takes a while to let go of old behavior patterns and adopt new ones. They see "slipping" not as failure but as a learning experience and remind themselves of how much progress they have made.

Each year in the United States, the tobacco industry spends billions of dollars to promote its products and to recruit new smokers. Cigarette advertising relies heavily on imagery portraying smoking as enjoyable and smokers as attractive, sexy, slim, and of high social status. Tobacco advertising in magazines for women and African Americans has increased in recent years, as has advertising of smokeless tobacco, with the erroneous implication that this form of tobacco consumption is safe. Besides print advertising, tobacco companies promote their products by sponsoring rock concerts, sporting events, and travel excursions. Some tobacco companies even support health research and smoking cessation programs, not only for the public relations benefits but also to obtain scientific information that can appease regulators and consumers without harming sales.

Another tactic is offering price discounts to retailers, which reduces the price of tobacco products and thus makes them more available to youth. Because increasing the cost of tobacco products decreases their use, many states have increased taxes on tobacco products. Every 10% increase in the price of cigarettes reduces consumption by 4%. Another youth-recruiting tactic is the marketing of candy- and fruit-flavored cigarettes and smokeless tobacco.

> We must always follow somebody looking for the truth, and we must always run away from anyone who finds it.
>
> *Andre Gide*

To reduce tobacco's damage to society, in 1998, 46 states and 7 large tobacco companies settled the states' lawsuits to recover their tobacco-related healthcare costs. The settlement, called the Master Settlement Agreement (MSA), totaled $206 billion, to be paid to the states over 25 years.

In addition to the MSA payments, the cigarette companies agreed to pay $5.15 billion over 12 years into a trust fund to compensate tobacco farmers and others for anticipated financial losses resulting from the implementation of the MSA. The states also signed a separate agreement with the leading smokeless tobacco company, United States Tobacco, that contains many of the same public health provisions as the MSA.

The MSA provided numerous restrictions and prohibitions on the tobacco industry, including bans on the following:

- The use of cartoons in tobacco advertisements
- The targeting of youth in advertising, promotions, or marketing, including free sampling
- The use of most outdoor advertisements, including billboards and signs and placards in arenas, stadiums, shopping malls, and video game arcades
- The distribution of apparel and merchandise with brand-name logos
- Payments to promote tobacco products in films, TV, and theater productions
- Distributing free samples of cigarettes any place where underage persons may be present

- Tobacco company lobbying against any proposed laws that limit youth access to tobacco
- Tobacco industry attempts to limit or suppress research on the health effects of smoking

Other ways to reduce tobacco's damage to society include the following:

- Raise taxes on cigarettes and other tobacco products.
- Create more smoke-free public places, including work sites, restaurants, and bars. Twenty-seven states and hundreds of local municipalities have banned smoking in essentially all public places.
- Provide comprehensive smoking cessation programs for all smokers who want to quit (about 70% of current smokers).

To continue the effort to reduce tobacco's damage to society and to counter the $1 million an hour the tobacco industry spends on cigarette advertising and promotion, the Centers for Disease Control and Prevention (CDC) produces its own antismoking ads called "Tips from Former Smokers" (TIPS). TIPS encourage people to quit smoking by showing the toll that smoking-related illnesses takes on smokers and their loved ones. Many of the people in TIPS ads started smoking in their early teens, and some were diagnosed with life-changing diseases before they were age 40. Some are nonsmokers who developed serious illnesses from exposure to secondhand smoke.

TIPS ads are placed in or on television, radio, print (magazines), out-of-home (billboards, bus shelters), theater, and online through digital video, display, search, and mobile channels, Facebook, Twitter, and YouTube. The TIPS campaign includes paid ads and public service announcements in English and Spanish, and it focuses on reaching low socioeconomic groups, which have high smoking rates.

Since its launch in 2012, TIPS has proved to be very successful (Neff et al., 2016). Evaluation of the 9-week long second TIPS ad campaign in 2016 showed that it was

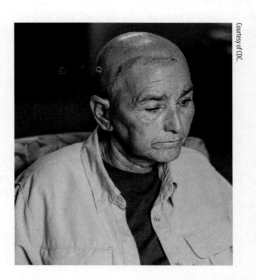

Rose, 59, Texas; diagnosed with lung cancer that spread to her brain.

Women and Cigarette Advertising

For more than 80 years, advertising by American tobacco companies has enticed women to smoke by associating cigarettes with sexiness, slimness, elegance, fun, independence, social and economic success, and even health! Tobacco advertising targeting women began in the 1920s, with messages such as "reach for a Lucky instead of a sweet" to establish an association between smoking and slimness. In the first year of this ad campaign, sales of Lucky Strike cigarettes increased 300%, mirroring the general rise in smoking among American women. In 1923, women consumed 5% of all cigarettes sold. By 1929, the number had grown to 12%, and by 1933, it was 18%. Currently, about 15% of American women smoke.

Between 1965 and 1977, the percentage of women who smoked peaked at 34%, in no small part due to the advertising cunning of the Virginia Slims ad campaigns. Not only did the name of the product and the body shapes of the models promoting it associate smoking with slimness but also the product's advertising slogan, "You've come a long way, Baby," co-opted women's desires for social and economic equality, emancipation from rigid gender role stereotyping, and empowerment. These same themes are common today. To counter women's concerns about the health risks of smoking, cigarette advertising uses images of models engaged in exercise or pictures of white-capped mountains against a background of clear blue skies.

Besides advertising, the tobacco industry has targeted women by offering the following:
- Cigarette brand clothing and other accessories
- A yearly engagement calendar and a catalog featuring clothing, jewelry, and accessories coordinated with the themes and colors of a product's print advertisement and product packaging
- Gifts, including mugs and caps, bearing a product's label in colors coordinated with the advertisement and packaging
- Discounts on turkeys, milk, soft drinks, and laundry detergent with the purchase of tobacco products
- Color-coordinated items in multiple-pack containers
- Free tickets to films and concerts

About 175,000 American women die from cigarette-caused diseases each year. Lung cancer has surpassed breast cancer as the leading cause of cancer deaths among women. And if that's not enough, the beauty editor of *Harper's* points out that "smokers' skin wrinkles up to 10 years sooner than that of nonsmokers."

Check out these online museum exhibits on women and cigarette advertising.
- *Selling Smoke*, Yale University Library: http://exhibits.library.yale.edu/exhibits/show/sellingsmoke
- Stanford University, Clayman Institute for Gender Research: http://gender.stanford.edu/news/2012/stanford -researchers%E2%80%99-cigarette-ad-collection-reveals -how-big-tobacco-targets-women-and

responsible for an estimated 1.83 million additional quit attempts, 1.73 million smokers intending to quit within 6 months after the end of the campaign, and 104,000 6-month sustained quits. These results were similar to those of the first 12-week 2012 TIPS campaign. As of 2017, TIPS' total cost was about $48 million: $480 per smoker who quit, $2,819 per premature death prevented, $393 per year of life saved, and $268 per year of healthy life gained. The bottom line is that TIPS works.

To complement TIPS, in 2014, the U.S. Food and Drug Administration (FDA) launched Real Costs, an educational program for youth aged 12 to 17 years that is distributed on TV, radio, the Internet, and in magazines and movie theaters. Real Cost's themes include the harmful effects of smoking on skin, the many toxic chemicals in tobacco smoke, and that tobacco addiction is about losing control of your life to a drug habit rather than a statement of independence. Evaluation of Real Cost showed that those who saw the ads were 30% less likely to start smoking than those who didn't, resulting in about 350,000 fewer youths aged 11 to 18 not starting to smoke between February 2015 and March 2016 (Farrelly et al., 2017). The TIPS website is http://www.cdc .gov/tobacco/campaign/tips/.

Critical Thinking About Health

1. Smoking takes a toll on everyone—those who smoke and those who do not. Government officials estimate that cigarette smoking costs the nation about $100 billion a year in healthcare costs and lost productivity. These costs are borne equally by nonsmokers and smokers.
   a. Should nonsmokers pay for the healthcare expenses of people who smoke? Why or why not?
   b. Should cigarettes be taxed by the government to cover their full cost to society, which could lessen tobacco consumption, put tobacco growers out of business, and drastically reduce tobacco companies' profits?

2. Purchase a popular magazine and count the number of cigarette ads in that issue. Review each ad and respond to the following questions:
   a. Who is the ad targeting? (e.g., women, men, young, old)
   b. How is the ad appealing to its target audience? (e.g., sex, friends)
   c. Besides the warning label (which is required by law), does the ad mention any other negative effects of smoking?
   d. What does the ad imply will happen if you smoke that brand of cigarette?

3. Over the last three decades, cigarettes have been shown to be hazardous to one's health. Smokeless tobacco was once thought to be a substitute for cigarette smoking, and its popularity increased during the 1970s and 1980s. You have been asked to return to your high school to discuss the negative consequences of tobacco.
   a. Identify two primary reasons for a young person not to begin using tobacco products.
   b. Respond to the following young athlete's question: "I don't smoke cigarettes because they are nasty. I use chew instead—my grandpa told me it wasn't bad. What can happen to me? I'm not inhaling tobacco."

4. More than half of U.S. states and all Canadian provinces and territories either entirely or in certain instances prohibit smoking in the workplace, public buildings, restaurants, and bars. The intention of these rules is to protect people from nonconsensual exposure to harmful toxins in tobacco smoke.
   a. What is your opinion about laws prohibiting smoking in public areas?
   b. Do you think that laws prohibiting smoking of tobacco products in certain public places should extend to smoking systems that do not rely on burning tobacco, such as e-cigarettes and possibly marijuana?

Chapter Summary and Highlights

Chapter Summary

The only products legally sold around the world that have no medicinal value and that are known to cause disease and death are cigarettes and other tobacco products. A major reason countries permit this is that political leaders benefit financially. Some countries are financial partners of tobacco companies and actively promote cigarettes to their citizens. In the United States, corporations have been granted the same constitutional rights as individuals. They have freedom of speech and the right to donate as much money as they want to issues that affect their business and to political candidates. When the U.S. government wanted to put stronger health warnings on cigarette packages, tobacco corporations went to court to block the stronger warnings, arguing that doing so infringed on their right to free speech. Despite decades of research showing that smoking cigarettes or being exposed to secondhand smoke can cause heart disease and cancer, tobacco companies are free to advertise and promote their products. Smoke at your own health risk.

Each year in the United States about 440,000 deaths (about one in every five deaths) are caused by smoking cigarettes or being exposed to cigarette smoke in the environment. For comparison, about 30,000 persons die in car crashes in the United States each year. Many American smokers would like to quit smoking; millions already have. Quitting smoking is not easy because nicotine, the psychoactive ingredient in tobacco, is one of most addictive drugs known to science. Tobacco smoke contains more than 4,000 different chemicals, some of which are known to cause cancer. Tobacco's harmful effects on the body accrue over many years before symptoms of disease appear. The most important health decision you can make is to not smoke. If you do smoke … STOP.

Highlights

- No public health message is disseminated as widely as the warning on every package of cigarettes and in every cigarette advertisement that cigarette smoking is dangerous to your health.
- Despite the overwhelming evidence that cigarette smoking is associated with higher death rates from cancer, heart disease, and respiratory diseases, approximately 36 million American adults smoke. Smoking also is associated with a higher risk of emphysema and bronchitis.

- Cigarette smoking is responsible for 440,000 American deaths per year, far more than AIDS, auto accidents, and drug use combined. Smoking increases the risk for heart disease, lung cancer, respiratory diseases, and cancers of all kinds.
- Smoking tobacco comes from the processed leaves of the plant *Nicotiana tabacum*. Tobacco smoke contains more than 4,000 chemicals, including nicotine—which is responsible for many of tobacco's drug effects, including physical dependence—and 43 others that are known to cause cancer.
- Smokeless tobacco is not a healthy alternative to smoking tobacco; it causes cancers of the lip and mouth. Cigar smoking also is harmful.
- Children are harmed by breathing parents' tobacco smoke. Pregnant women who smoke risk the health of their babies.

- Environmental tobacco smoke contains the same 4,000 chemicals and 43 carcinogens that inhaled tobacco smoke does, thus affecting the health of nonsmokers.
- People smoke cigarettes because of physical dependence on nicotine and a variety of psychological and social rewards that come from smoking.
- Smokers can stop smoking either on their own or with the help of a stop-smoking program.
- The advertising of cigarettes largely is aimed at young people and contributes to recruiting them to the smoking habit.
- In 2009, the U.S. Congress passed the Family Smoking Prevention and Control Act to give the Food and Drug Administration authority to regulate the promotion and sale of tobacco products.
- In 2012, the CDC established a successful antismoking advertising campaign called TIPS.

For Your Health

Smoking is the worst thing one can do to one's health. If you smoke or know someone who does, take the first step to quitting by doing the "Why Do I Smoke?" questionnaire (Exercise 17-1 in the Workbook). Carry on with the quit process by doing the other exercises for this chapter in the Workbook.

References

American College Health Association. (2016a). *American College Health Association—National College Health Assessment II, Canadian Reference Group Data Report, Spring 2016.* Hanover, MD: American College Health Association.

American College Health Association. (2016b). *American College Health Association—National College Health Assessment II, Undergraduate Student Reference Group Data Report Spring 2016.* Hanover, MD: American College Health Association.

Appolino, D., & Glantz, S. (2017, August 17). Tobacco industry research on nicotine replacement therapy: "If anyone is going to take away our business it should be us." *American Journal of Public Health, 107,* 1636–1642. doi: 10.2105/AJPH.2017.303935

Biebel, M. G., et al. (2016). Male sexual function and smoking. *Sexual Medicine Reviews, 4,* 366–375.

Benedetti, G., et al. (2013). Tobacco and dental caries: A systematic review. *Acta Odontologica Scandinavica, 71,* 363–371.

Centers for Disease Control and Prevention. (2016). Youth and tobacco use. Retrieved from https://www.cdc.gov/tobacco/data_statistics/fact_sheets/youth_data/tobacco_use/

DiFranza, J. R. (2008, May). Hooked from the first cigarette. *Scientific American, 298,* 82–87.

Duong, M., et al. (2017). Effects of bidi smoking on all-cause mortality and cardiorespiratory outcomes in men from south Asia: An observational community-based substudy of the Prospective Urban Rural Epidemiology Study (PURE). *Lancet Global Health, 5,* e168–e176.

Farrelly, M. C., et al. (2017). Association between the Real Cost media campaign and smoking initiation among youths—United States, 2014–2016. *Morbidity Mortality Weekly Report, 66,* 47–50.

Inoue-Choi M., et al. (2018). Association between long-term low-intensity cigarette smoking and incidence of smoking-related cancer in the national institutes of health-AARP cohort. *International Journal of Cancer, 142,* 271–280.

Jamal, A., et al. (2016). Current cigarette smoking among adults—United States, 2005–2015. *Morbidity Mortality Weekly Report, 65,* 1205–1211. Retrieved from https://www.cdc.gov/mmwr/volumes/65/wr/mm6544a2.htm?s_cid=mm6544a2_w

Neff, L. J., et al. (2017). Evaluation of the National Tips from Former Smokers Campaign: The 2014 longitudinal cohort. *Preventing Chronic Disease, 13,* E42. Retrieved from https://www.ncbi.nlm.nih.gov/pmc/articles/PMC4807436/

Park, S., et al. (2014). Environmental tobacco smoke exposure and children's intelligence at 8–11 years of age. *Environmental Health Perspectives, 122,* 1123–1128. Retrieved from https://ehp.niehs.nih.gov/1307088/

Shariff, J. A., et al. (2017). Relationship between frequent recreational cannabis (marijuana and hashish) use and periodontitis in adults in the United States: National Health and Nutrition Examination Survey 2011 to 2012. *Journal of Periodontology, 88,* 273–280.

Smith, C. N., et al. (2015). Plain packaging of cigarettes: Do we have sufficient evidence? *Risk Management and Healthcare Policy, 8,* 21–30. Retrieved from https://www.ncbi.nlm.nih.gov/pmc/articles/PMC4396458/

Stampfli, M. R., & Anderson, G. P. (2009). How cigarette smoke skews immune responses to promote infection, lung disease, and cancer. *Nature Reviews Immunology,* 9, 377–384.

Taylor, G., et al. (2014). Change in mental health status after smoking cessation: A systematic review and meta-analysis. *British Medical Journal, 348,* g1151. (http://www.bmj.com/content/348/bmj.g1151)

Suggested Readings

Appolino, D., & Glantz, S. (2017, August 17). Tobacco industry research on nicotine replacement therapy: "If anyone is going to take away our business it should be us." *American Journal of Public Health,* 107, 1636–1642. doi: 10.2105/AJPH.2017.303935. Researchers cite internal tobacco industry documents to show how tobacco companies developed and marketed nonsmoked nicotine replacements (NRTs) for cigarettes after finding that many smokers used NRTs to supplement smoking rather than to quit.

Benowitz, N. L. (2010). Nicotine addiction. *New England Journal of Medicine,* 362, 2295–2303. A thorough description of how nicotine affects the brain to cause tobacco addiction.

Bill & Melinda Gates Foundation. (2017). Tobacco control. Retrieved from http://www.gatesfoundation.org/What-We-Do/Global-Policy/Tobacco-Control. This international health foundation lays out its strategic framework to reduce tobacco-related death and disease in developing countries by preventing the initiation of new smokers, decreasing overall tobacco use, and reducing exposure to secondhand smoke.

Brandt, A. M. (2009). *The cigarette century.* New York: Basic Books. A thorough history of changing attitudes toward smoking in the United States and the scientific discoveries that exposed the dangers of smoking and the litigations against tobacco companies that followed.

Jacobs, M. (1997). *From the first to the last ash: The history, economics, and hazards of tobacco.* Cambridge: Community Learning Center. Retrieved from http://healthliteracy.worlded.org/docs/tobacco/index.html. A brief, comprehensive history of tobacco use in the Americas.

Kessler, D. (2001). *A question of intent: A great American battle with a deadly industry.* New York: Public Affairs. The former director of the FDA describes the agency's battle to regulate the tobacco industry and to document the deadly consequences of smoking.

U.S. Department of Health and Human Services. (2014). *The health consequences of smoking—50 years of progress: A report of the Surgeon General.* Atlanta: U.S. Department of Health and Human Services, Centers for Disease Control and Prevention, National Center for Chronic Disease Prevention and Health Promotion, Office on Smoking and Health.

World Health Organization. (2015). *WHO report on the global tobacco epidemic 2015.* Retrieved from http://www.who.int/tobacco/global_report/2015/en/. Addresses the global tobacco epidemic and the steps that can be taken to reduce tobacco use and save lives.

Recommended Websites

Be Tobacco Free
(http://betobaccofree.gov)

Centers for Disease Control and Prevention Tobacco Information and Prevention Source (TIPS)
Everything you ever wanted to know about smoking and tobacco use.

Clearing the Air
Smoking cessation guide from the National Cancer Institute.

Quit Smoking Program
From the Canadian Lung Association.

The Quit Net
A quit-smoking website produced by the Boston University School of Public Health.

You Can Quit Smoking
A guide from the U.S. National Institutes of Health.

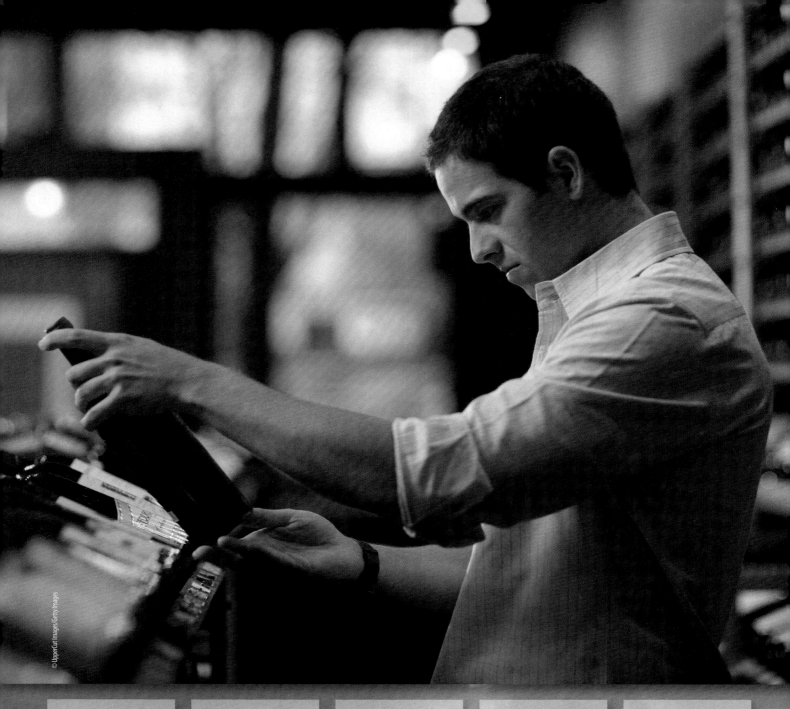

© UpperCut Images/Getty Images

Health Tips

Signs of Alcohol Overdose/Poisoning

Are You a Problem Drinker?

Dollars & Health Sense

Marketing Alcohol to Youth

Global Wellness

Alcohol Abuse Is a Worldwide Problem

Managing Stress

Breaking Addictive Behaviors

Wellness Guide

One Student's DUI Experience

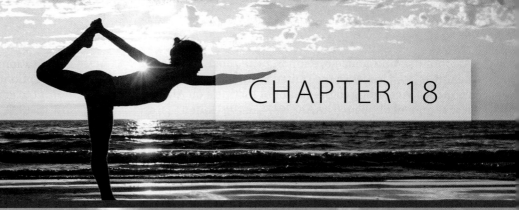

CHAPTER 18

Using Alcohol Responsibly

Learning Objectives

1. Discuss the prevalence of drinking, types of drinking, reasons for drinking, and attitudes toward drinking among college students.

2. Describe the effects of alcohol on the body.

3. Describe how alcohol is absorbed into the body and how this absorption relates to blood alcohol concentration.

4. Discuss the effects of alcohol on behavior, including sexual behavior.

5. Describe the long-term effects of alcohol overconsumption.

6. Describe alcohol use disorder.

7. Explain the stages of alcoholism.

8. Describe how alcohol affects one's significant others and the help that is available for both the family and the alcoholic.

Alcohol use and abuse are among the most significant health-related issues in the United States and many other countries. According to the National Institute on Alcohol Abuse and Alcoholism (NIAAA, 2017), in the United States, misuse of alcohol is responsible for nearly 90,000 deaths a year, shortening the lives of those who died by an average of 30 years, and for 10% of deaths among working-age adults aged 20 to 64 years. Each year, worldwide, alcohol is responsible for 3.3 million deaths, accounting for about 6% of total global deaths (World Health Organization, 2015). Although they receive much more attention from governments and the news media, drugs other than alcohol cause far fewer health problems than alcohol does (**Figure 18.1**).

It is likely that humans have been drinking alcohol since someone noticed the psychological effects of drinking some berry juice that had been left too long in an earthen jar. Through the ages, drinking fermented grains (beer); fermented berries, grapes, and fruits (wine); and the distilled products of natural fermentation ("hard" liquors) has been commonplace in many human societies. Alcohol is used in some religious ceremonies; is taken as medicine; is used to seal contracts, agreements, and treaties; and is offered to display hospitality. Alcohol consumption has been an integral part of American life since the landing of the *Mayflower* at Plymouth Rock. Even so, many people regard drinking as a social evil and drunkenness as a sin. The U.S. government tried to legislate alcohol use out of American lives in 1919 with the Volstead Act, a constitutional amendment that prohibited the sale and consumption of alcoholic beverages ("Prohibition"). This attempt to control alcohol consumption failed, however, and in 1933, Prohibition was repealed by another amendment to the Constitution.

Today, alcoholic beverages are available in many varieties, not only beer, wine, and traditional distilled liquors, but also a variety of premixed cocktails, often sweetened with sugar and containing various flavors, and malt liquors, inexpensive, high volume (24–40 ounces per bottle), sweetened, flavored products with the alcohol equivalent of five standard beers.

Approximately 70% of U.S. adults have at least one drink per year; 56% have at least one drink per month, and about 20% of Americans are lifetime abstainers from drinking alcohol (SAMSHA, 2015). A significant percentage of young Americans between the ages of 12 and 17 years consume alcohol regularly (**Table 18.1**). Approximately 9% of the U.S. population drinks excessively, putting them at risk for alcohol-related health and social problems. Excessive alcohol use is associated with thousands of divorces, as many as 80% of the incidents of family

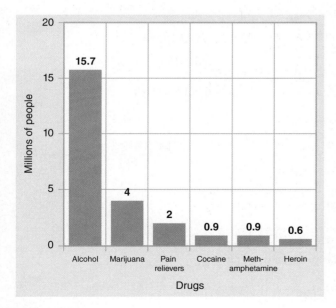

■ **Figure 18.1**

Number of Americans Older than 12 with Substance Abuse Disorders

Data from Center for Behavioral Health Statistics and Quality. (2016). Key substance use and mental health indicators in the United States: Results from the 2015 National Survey on Drug Use and Health (HHS Publication No. SMA 16-4984, NSDUH Series H-51). Retrieved from http://www.samhsa.gov/data/. Data are for civilian, noninstitutionalized Americans over age 12. Values may include people who have use disorders for more than one substance.

Signs of Alcohol Overdose/Poisoning

No one expects to die from partying, but it can happen. Alcohol is a potent central nervous system depressant, and too much of it can inhibit the brain's respiratory center, leading to death or irreversible brain damage. Also, alcohol is toxic, so when too much has been consumed, the body vomits it out. However, alcohol can inhibit the gag reflex, so instead of going out of the body, vomit gets sucked into the lungs and causes death from asphyxiation. Even if someone has passed out from ingesting too much alcohol, alcohol in the intestines continues to be absorbed into the body, increasing the risk of death. Don't assume an intoxicated person will be fine by sleeping it off. Know the signs of alcohol poisoning:

- Confusion, stupor, coma, or the person cannot be roused
- Vomiting
- Seizures
- Slow breathing (fewer than eight breaths per minute)
- Irregular breathing (10 seconds or more between breaths)
- Low body temperature, bluish skin color, paleness

If you suspect alcohol poisoning, don't try to sober the person up with black coffee, a cold bath or shower, or walking it off. Those methods don't work. Call 911 right away. You don't want to feel responsible for an alcohol-related tragedy. And don't worry that your friend may become angry or embarrassed afterward. Remember, you cared and did the right thing.

Modified from National Institute on Alcohol Abuse and Alcoholism. (2017). College Drinking—Changing the Culture. Facts about alcohol poisoning. Retrieved from http://www.collegedrinkingprevention.gov/parentsandstudents /students/factsheets/factsaboutalcoholpoisoning.aspx

Table 18.1

Alcohol Consumption by American Youth Aged 12 to 17 Years

	8th Graders (%)	10th Graders (%)	12th Graders (%)
Had 1 drink in prior 30 days	9.7	21.5	35.3
Ever been drunk	10.9	28.6	46.7
Drunk in last year	7.7	23.4	37.3
Drunk in past 30 days	3.1	10.3	20.6

Center for Behavioral Health Statistics and Quality. (2016). Key substance use and mental health indicators in the United States: Results from the 2015 National Survey on Drug Use and Health. HHS Publication No. SMA 16-4984, NSDUH Series H-51. Retrieved from http://www.samhsa.gov/data/

$2.00 per drink. In addition, alcohol abuse is linked to a long list of medical problems (Molina et al., 2014) **(Figure 18.2)**.

Alcohol use has long been a part of social events, such as parties, dinners, weddings, ball games, and picnics. The liquor industry encourages alcohol use by advertising in newspapers and magazines and on radio and television. No direct link between advertising alcoholic products and alcohol abuse has been established. However, public health, medical, and legal professionals are concerned that advertising associating drinking with athletic prowess, material wealth, social prestige, and sex encourages irresponsible drinking behavior.

Drinking on Campus

Each year several college students die from alcohol poisoning as a consequence of ingesting massive quantities of alcohol (See the Health Tips box.). In its coverage of these tragic occurrences, the national media remind Americans that drinking is as much a part of going to college as is going to class. Indeed, American college students spend more money on alcoholic beverages each year than they do on textbooks and soft drinks combined.

About 80% of North American college students drink alcohol at least once in a while **(Table 18.2)**. Much

violence, 40% of crimes, and millions of hours of school and job absenteeism. Yearly, about 120 million Americans admit to alcohol-impaired driving, about 1 million are arrested for driving while intoxicated, and nearly 11,000 die from alcohol-related traffic collisions, accounting for 31% of all driving fatalities (Centers for Disease Control and Prevention, 2017). Excessive alcohol consumption costs the U.S. economy about $280 billion per year, or

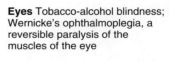

■ **Figure 18.2**

Medical Problems Associated with Alcohol Abuse

Brain Impaired memory and other cognitive functions, most notably alcohol-related dementia. Impaired vitamin B_1 (thiamin) absorption, causing Wernicke-Korsakoff syndrome, characterized by impairment of memory and learning ability, apathy, and degeneration of the white brain matter

Esophagus Esophageal varices, an irreversible condition in which the person can die by drowning in his own blood when the varices open

Liver An acute enlargement of the liver, which is reversible, as well as irreversible cirrhosis of the liver

Muscles Alcoholic myopathy, a condition resulting in painful muscle contractions

Blood and bone marrow Coagulation defects and anemia

Eyes Tobacco-alcohol blindness; Wernicke's ophthalmoplegia, a reversible paralysis of the muscles of the eye

Pharynx Cancer of the pharynx is increased 10-fold for drinkers who smoke

Heart Alcoholic cardiomyopathy, a heart condition

Lungs Lowered resistance is thought to lead to greater incidences of tuberculosis, pneumonia, and emphysema

Spleen Hypersplenism

Stomach Gastritis and ulcers

Pancreas Acute and chronic pancreatitis

Rectum Hemorrhoids

Testes Atrophy of the testes

Nerves Polyneuritis, a condition characterized by loss of sensation

Table 18.2

Alcohol Consumption Among North American College Students

	Males (%)		Females (%)	
	U.S.	Canada	U.S.	Canada
Consumption in prior 30 days				
Never	22.7	17.2	20.1	14.4
Prior to but not in past 30 days	15.2	14.2	17.3	15.4
1–9 days	45.9	52.0	50.3	57.4
10–29 days	15.0	14.5	11.7	12.2
All 30 days	1.3	1.6	0.6	0.6
Number of drinks when last "partied"				
4 or fewer	45.1	45.2	66.2	55.3
5	11.2	10.6	12.6	12.9
6	9.6	8.2	9.6	10.4
7 or more	34.1	34.7	13.0	21.4
Number of times in last 2 weeks having 5 drinks or more				
N/A (don't drink)	25.8	24.0	21.5	18.1
None	34.0	39.7	46.6	48.4
1–2	24.5	27.4	20.7	25.7
3–5	12.1	9.0	6.9	6.0
6 or more	3.6	2.5	1.8	1.8
Marijuana use in the prior 30 days[a]				
N/A (never)	57.0	56.7	60.9	59.3
Any	22.8	20.9	18.4	16.5
Consequences of drinking				
Did something I later regretted	35.0	36.0	34.6	38.9
Forgot where I was/ what I did	32.2	28.7	29.3	29.4
Had unprotected sex	22.5	23.8	20.4	24.3
Physically injured myself	14.9	17.7	13.0	18.6
Other[b]				
Most/all the time when partying or socializing in the prior 12 months				
Used a designated driver	81.7	75.6	89.5	86.7
Stayed with same friends	79.5	89.9	90.4	89.9
Ate before/during drinking	77.2	78.2	82.7	82.8
Kept track of how many drinks	60.1	60.6	70.7	63.2
Other[c]				

[a] Marijuana use for comparison.

[b] <5%: Trouble with police; sex without consent; injured another; suicidal ideation.

[c] <30%: alternate types of drinks; avoid drinking games; don't drink at all; set a number of drinks prior to drinking; have a friend tell when reached limit; pace drinks to one or two per hour.

American College Health Association. (2016a). American College Health Association—National College Health Assessment II: Canadian Reference Group Data Report Spring 2016. Hanover, MD: American College Health Association; American College Health Association. (2016b). American College Health Association—National College Health Assessment II: Undergraduate Student Reference Group Data Report Spring. Hanover, MD: American College Health Association.

college student drinking takes place when "partying"—social events at which one is expected to "let loose," drink alcohol to excess (becoming "hammered" or "wasted"), and behave atypically (e.g., doing something "outrageous"; having sex with a stranger). When partying, about 50% of male college students and 35% of female college students consume five or more drinks (American College Health Association, 2016a, 2016b).

> O God, that men should put an enemy into their mouths to steal away their brains! That we should with joy, pleasure, revel, and applause, transform ourselves into beasts.
>
> *Shakespeare,* Twelfth Night

Participants view partying as a way to reduce the tensions of academic stress, meet new people, prove their social competence, and just have fun. However, often, nonparticipants view partying, especially the emphasis on excessive alcohol consumption, as foolishly dangerous (**Figure 18.3**). They point out that excessive alcohol consumption impairs one's judgment, thus increasing the risks for being involved in a motor vehicle crash, of an unintended pregnancy, acquiring a sexual infection, and being either a perpetrator or victim of sexual assault.

College students who regularly drink to excess are more likely

- To miss class
- To get behind in schoolwork
- To do something they regret
- Not to use protection when engaging in sex
- To engage in unplanned sexual activity
- To get into trouble with campus police
- To damage property
- To get injured

1,825 deaths from alcohol-related unintentional injuries, including motor vehicle crashes

600,000 unintentional injuries

696,000 assaults by another student who has been drinking

97,000 victims of sexual assault or date rape

400,000 students have unprotected sex and more than 100,000 are too intoxicated to know if they consented to having sex

150,000 students develop an alcohol-related health problem

3,360,000 drove under the influence of alcohol

110,000 arrested for an alcohol-related violation such as public drunkenness or driving under the influence

■ **Figure 18.3**

Some Consequences of High-Risk College Drinking

Modified from National Institute of Alcohol Abuse and Alcoholism. (2017). Alcohol facts and statistics. Retrieved from https://www.niaaa.nih.gov/alcohol-health /overview-alcohol-consumption/alcohol-facts-and-statistics

- To engage in dangerous driving behaviors
- To disturb, insult, quarrel with, or assault others
- To require care from others while being sick from drunkenness

College athletes are much more likely than nonathletes to engage in both heavy and binge drinking. A study of over 16,000 college students found that, compared to nonathletes, intramural and club athletes were more likely to have three or more drinks per occasion and intercollegiate athletes were more likely to have five or six drinks per occasion (Marzell et al., 2015). Intramural/club athletes tended to drink more at fraternity and sorority parties, at on-campus parties, off-campus, at bars, and outdoors, whereas, perhaps because of stricter schedules, intercollegiate athletes drank more at Greek and on-campus parties. Because athletes tend to be visible on campus, their drinking behaviors contribute to the overall campus atmosphere regarding drinking and students' perceptions and expectations of campus norms concerning alcohol use.

The behaviors of excessive drinkers can affect non–binge drinkers and alcohol abstainers. So-called **secondhand binge effects** include the following:

- Being interrupted while studying
- Being awakened at night
- Having to take care of a drunken fellow student
- Being insulted or humiliated by a drunken student
- Being pushed, hit, or assaulted by a drunken student
- Being the victim of sexual assault

Although the majority of college students either do not drink or limit their drinking behavior to partying, about 25% abuse alcohol to a degree that it adversely affects their academic progress, personal relationships, and health. About 20% of college students meet criteria for alcohol abuse and dependence (National Institute on Alcohol Abuse and Alcoholism, 2017).

In general, the cultural attitude of the campus regarding alcohol use has a tremendous influence on student drinking behavior. A campus culture that encourages legal and responsible alcohol use and discourages underage drinking, binge drinking, and alcohol-induced antisocial behavior promotes responsible behavior among the students (Wechsler & Nelson, 2008). The opposite is true for a campus that has few or no student alcohol-use policies and at which students perceive that just about anything goes with regard to alcohol use. College students who drink heavily tend to view campus attitudes toward drinking as liberal. Students with the most enthusiastic attitudes toward drinking are typically the heaviest drinkers.

Breweries and liquor distributors are especially active on college campuses, spending millions of dollars each year on advertising in campus newspapers and promoting their products by sponsoring "pub nights," giving away items with product logos, and underwriting some of the costs of college athletic events.

To reduce the degree of excessive drinking among students, college campuses work to change the campus culture regarding alcohol use. Irresponsible drinking is not viewed as a rite of membership in campus organizations (e.g., clubs, athletic teams, fraternities, sororities), as an acceptable way to lessen social anxiety in party or other social situations, as the definition of partying, as an acceptable means to deal with academic stress, or as a rite of passage to adulthood and independence from parental control.

How Alcohol Affects the Body

Composition of Alcoholic Beverages
The alcohol in beverages is a chemical called **ethyl alcohol (ethanol)**. There are many other kinds of alcohol, such as methyl alcohol and isopropyl alcohol. Most alcohols are poisonous if ingested in small amounts. In large amounts, even ethanol is toxic, but the body has ways to detoxify and eliminate it, given enough time.

The amount of ethanol in a commercial alcoholic product usually is listed on the product label (beer is the exception). The amount of alcohol in beer and wine is usually given as the percentage of the total volume. Beer, for example, is generally about 4% alcohol, although some beers contain more or less (so-called light beers have nearly the same alcohol content as regular beers). Wine is about 12% alcohol. The amount of alcohol in distilled or "hard" liquors (e.g., scotch, vodka, bourbon, tequila, rum) is given in terms of **proof**, a number that represents twice the percentage of alcohol in the product. Thus, an 80-proof whiskey is 40% alcohol; 100-proof vodka is 50% alcohol.

Most standard portions of alcoholic drinks contain about the same amount of alcohol (**Figure 18.4**). For example, a 12-ounce beer that is 5% alcohol contains 0.6 ounces of alcohol. The same amount of alcohol is in a 5-ounce glass of wine. The alcohol content of a mixed drink made of 1.5 ounces of 80-proof spirits (40% alcohol) contains 0.6 ounces of alcohol. So, a can of beer, a malt liquor, a glass of wine, and a mixed drink contain approximately the same amount of alcohol. Thus, the perception that a beer is less alcoholic than a glass of wine or a mixed drink is wrong. Note that some malt liquors and ales are 6% to 8% alcohol; fortified wines, such as sherry and port, are 18% alcohol; and some distilled liquors are 100 proof (50% alcohol).

TERMS

ethyl alcohol (ethanol): the consumable type of alcohol that is the psychoactive ingredient in alcoholic beverages; often called grain alcohol

proof: a number assigned to an alcoholic product that is twice the percentage of alcohol in that product

secondhand binge effects: negative experiences caused by another's binge drinking

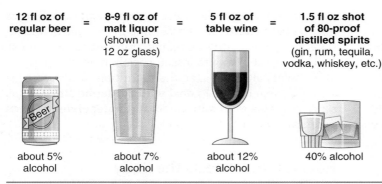

about 5%
alcohol   about 7%
alcohol   about 12%
alcohol   40% alcohol

The percent of "pure" alcohol, expressed here as alcohol by volume (alc/vol), varies by beverage.

■ **Figure 18.4**

A 12-ounce serving of regular beer, a 9-ounce serving of a regular malt liquor, a glass of wine, and a mixed drink have about the same amount of alcohol. So don't be fooled by the type of drink.

Reproduced from National Institute of Alcohol Abuse and Alcoholism, "What is a Standard Drink?". Retrieved from https://www.niaaa.nih.gov/alcohol-health/overview-alcohol-consumption/what-standard-drink

How Alcohol Is Absorbed, Excreted, and Metabolized

After alcohol is ingested, it is readily absorbed into the body through the gastrointestinal tract. About 20% of ingested alcohol is absorbed by the stomach and the rest by the small intestine. The alcohol is then carried through the bloodstream to all the body's tissues and organs. Although not strictly a food (it contains no protein, vitamins, or minerals), alcohol does contain calories—in fact, 7 calories per gram (almost twice as many calories per gram as sugar). A regular serving of beer, wine, or a mixed drink has between 100 and 150 calories.

Several factors affect the rate at which alcohol is absorbed into body tissues. For example, food in the stomach—especially fatty foods or proteins—slows the absorption of alcohol. Nonalcoholic substances in beer, wine, and cocktails can also slow absorption of alcohol. The presence of carbon dioxide in beverages, such as champagne, sparkling wines, beer, and carbonated mixed drinks, increases the rate of alcohol absorption. That is why people feel intoxicated more quickly when drinking champagne or beer, especially on an empty stomach. The higher the alcohol content in a drink, the faster it is absorbed.

The concentration of alcohol in the blood is called the **blood alcohol content (BAC)**, which is measured in grams of alcohol per deciliter of blood. A simple way to estimate BAC is to assume that ingesting one standard drink per hour (one beer, one glass of wine, one mixed drink), which contains approximately one-half ounce of ethyl alcohol, produces a BAC of 0.02 in a 150-pound male. Thus, the BAC of an average-sized man who drinks five beers during the first hour at a party will be 0.10; this level of alcohol in the blood violates the drinking-and-driving laws of most states. This shorthand method of approximating BAC changes depending on a person's body size, body composition (e.g., muscle, fat), and sex. All other things being equal, after ingesting the same amount of alcohol, the BAC of a large person is less than that of a smaller person because the alcohol is diluted more in the large person's tissues. Women tend to have a higher BAC from the same number of drinks as men because they generally weigh less than men, have proportionately more body fat (which does not absorb alcohol as readily as muscle and other tissues), have sex hormones that tend to increase alcohol absorption and decrease its elimination, and tend to absorb more alcohol from the stomach.

Alcohol is eliminated from the body in two ways. About 10% is excreted unchanged through sweat, urine, or

---

Marketing Alcohol to Youth

Alcohol use is a major health issue among youth. Several thousand middle and high school students report getting drunk every day. Between 20% and 25% of high schoolers report consuming five drinks in a row during the prior 2 weeks. Alcohol use is responsible for more than 5,000 deaths per year among persons younger than 21 years. Americans spend about $280 billion on alcohol each year; underage drinking accounts for about $40 billion of alcohol sales.

To help curtail alcohol use by youth, the Institute of Medicine, a division of the National Academy of Sciences, and Congress's Sober Truth on Preventing Underage Drinking Act (STOP ACT) want to reduce exposure of youth to alcoholic beverages and alcohol advertising and marketing directed at them.

Each year, youth (ages 12–20) are exposed to billions of alcohol advertisements on TV, radio, the Internet, and in magazines; brand naming in popular music; and product placements in films for youth audiences (Center for Alcohol Marketing and Youth, 2015). About 40% of TV ads are placed on cable TV shows with a large youth audience. The U.S. Surgeon General and a variety of youth health advocates want alcohol companies not to advertise in programming in which youth represent more than 15% of the audience.

Although the alcohol industry has voluntarily agreed not to advertise its products when 12- to 20-year-olds make up more than 28.4% of the audience, research shows that about 11% of alcohol advertising is placed when the audience is greater than 30% youth (Ross et al., 2016). Beverage companies that claim they are not contributing to the underage drinking problem and helping to develop a new generation of alcoholics are doing just what the cigarette companies did for decades—deny everything as long as the product is legal and profitable.

breath (hence the use of breath analyzers to test for drinking). The portion of alcohol that is not excreted (about 90%) is broken down primarily by the liver (metabolized), ultimately winding up as carbon dioxide and water. The liver detoxifies alcohol at a rate of about one-half ounce per hour; there is no way to speed up the process. Sobering-up remedies, such as drinking a lot of coffee, taking a cold shower, or engaging in vigorous exercise, do not accelerate the rate at which the liver removes alcohol from the body.

The Hangover

An occasional consequence of drinking too much alcohol is a **hangover**, which may involve stomach upset, headache, fatigue, weakness, shakiness, irritability, and sometimes vomiting. The frequency and severity of hangovers vary. The particular factors in alcohol that cause a hangover are unknown, but several causes have been suggested:

- When alcohol is present in the body, normal liver functions may slow to break down the alcohol. This slowdown may reduce the amount of sugar the liver releases into the blood, resulting in temporary hypoglycemia and its resultant fatigue, irritability, and headache.
- Alcohol may inhibit REM sleep, resulting in fatigue, irritability, and trouble concentrating.
- **Congeners**, which are chemical substances in an alcoholic beverage, or the breakdown products produced in the liver may cause a hangover.
- **Acetaldehyde**, a toxic substance produced when the liver breaks down alcohol, may be responsible for hangover symptoms.

The best way to deal with a hangover is to sleep, to drink juice to replace lost body fluid and blood sugar (alcohol increases urine output), and perhaps to take an analgesic for a headache. Ingesting more alcohol will only prolong the hangover symptoms.

The Effects of Alcohol on Behavior

Pharmacologically, alcohol acts as a central nervous system depressant, which means that it slows certain functions in some parts of the brain. In moderate amounts, alcohol may affect the parts of the brain that control judgment and inhibitions, which is why many people have a drink or two at a party to help "loosen up" or to become less shy and more able to interact freely with others. While some people may talk or laugh more than usual, others may become boisterous, argumentative, irritable, or depressed.

The behavioral effects of alcohol depend on the BAC (**Table 18.3**). At a BAC of 0.02, the "loosening-up" effects of alcohol manifest. At a BAC of 0.10, the depressant effects of the drug become pronounced, the person may become sleepy, and motor coordination is affected. Speech may become slurred and postural instability may become noticeable.

TERMS

blood alcohol content (BAC): the amount of alcohol in the blood

hangover: unpleasant physical sensations resulting from excessive alcohol consumption

congeners: flavorings, colorings, and other chemicals present in alcoholic beverages

acetaldehyde: a toxic substance produced when the liver breaks down alcohol

---

Table 18.3

Behavioral Effects of Alcohol in a 150-Pound Male

Number of drinks	Ounces of alcohol	BAC* (g/dl)	Approximate time for removal	Effects
1 beer, glass of wine, or mixed drink	½	0.02	1 hour	Feeling relaxed or "loosened up"
2½ beers, glasses of wine, or mixed drinks	1¼	0.05	2½ hours	Feeling "high"; decrease in inhibitions; increase in confidence; judgment impaired
5 beers, glasses of wine, or mixed drinks	2½	0.10	5 hours	Memory impaired; muscular coordination reduced; slurred speech; euphoric or sad feelings
10 beers, glasses of wine, or mixed drinks	5	0.20	10 hours	Slowed reflexes; erratic changes in feelings
15 beers, glasses of wine, or mixed drinks	7½	0.30	15–16 hours	Stuporous, complete loss of coordination; little sensation
20 beers, glasses of wine, or mixed drinks	10	0.40	20 hours	May become comatose; breathing may cease
25–30 beers, glasses of wine, or mixed drinks	15–20	0.50	26 hours	Fatal amount for most people

*BAC, blood alcohol content.

Alcohol's effects on motor skills, judgment, and reaction times make driving after drinking extremely dangerous. Even after just one or two drinks, although an individual may not be legally drunk, reaction time, perception, and judgment are impaired. Approximately 32% of the nearly 34,000 highway fatalities each year involve people who are intoxicated. Highway accidents are among the leading causes of death in the United States. The American College Health Association reports that about 10% of American and Canadian college students drive after ingesting alcohol (American College Health Association, 2016a).

Each year there are more than 120 million self-reported episodes of alcohol-impaired driving in the United States. Men in the 21 to 24 age group have the highest frequency of alcohol-impaired driving; men in the 25 to 34 age group have the second-highest frequency.

By contrast, the rate of alcohol-impaired driving among women in the same age groups is one-fourth that of their male peers. The frequency of alcohol-impaired driving declines in late middle-age.

Besides impaired driving, alcohol consumption contributes to arguments, fights, jeopardized relationships, employee absenteeism, school failure, and lost jobs. Alcohol is linked to anger and violence in several ways. Alcohol blunts self-control and other brain functions, thus enabling impulsive outbursts of anger and violence towards others and oneself and inattention to potentially violent social situations. Neurobiological dependence on alcohol can lead to failing to fulfill commitments and responsibilities to sustain oneself and one's family. Most homicides, assaults, robberies, sexual offenses, and incidents of domestic violence are alcohol-related (NCADD, 2015).

One Student's DUI Experience

Early in the morning last summer, I was arrested for driving under the influence of alcohol (DUI).

It's not easy to recall what actually happened—I see it through a fog, as if I am watching someone else.

The actual arrest is the blurriest. I was running for those few moments on pure adrenalin and fear. For a while, I don't even think I was breathing.

It's hard to explain the exact emotions.

It's hard to explain what it feels like to want more than anything to be sober.

It's hard to explain losing complete control of your life for even a short time.

It is hard to explain the feeling of handcuffs.

It's hard to explain what it feels like to sit in a holding cell and bite your lip in the hope of not going to sleep.

One thing for sure is that when those flashing lights appeared in my rearview mirror, all the rationalizations that got me into that car vanished. "It's just around the corner," "I need to get a friend home," or "No one is on the road at this hour"—none of them mean a thing—zero.

At the jail, it took what seemed like days to be fingerprinted and photographed and to fill out the required forms. Each step was just a little more humiliating than the last.

I am still overwhelmed at how a single, incredibly poor judgment could affect so many parts of my life.

The ramifications will be with me in various ways for the next 3 years—which is as far ahead as I have ever cared to plan.

These shock waves include probation for 3 years, an exorbitant increase in the cost of my car insurance, a restricted driver's license for 90 days (which was agreed upon in lieu of 2 days in jail), and a $600 fine, to name a few.

Many of the ramifications cannot be quantified. There was the call home, a couple of days of generally feeling lousy, and the unshakable sense that I had proven myself a fool.

Through all of it, however, I have some things to be thankful for.

On the top of that very short list is the fact that I didn't kill anyone.

Having struggled to come to terms with the arrest, it is impossible to imagine...for that there is no atonement.

Also on that list is the discovery of some very supportive people in my life, all of whom said not that what happened was okay, but that I was going to be okay. I turned to my parents and friends for help, and no one turned away—I am thankful.

Whether this column will keep anyone from driving drunk is doubtful. If I had read this column before my arrest, I would have thought of a hundred reasons why it would never have applied to me—but I would have been wrong.

Weight	Drinks (2-hour period) 1½ oz liquor or 12 oz beer											
100	1	2	3	4	5	6	7	8	9	10	11	12
120	1	2	3	4	5	6	7	8	9	10	11	12
140	1	2	3	4	5	6	7	8	9	10	11	12
160	1	2	3	4	5	6	7	8	9	10	11	12
180	1	2	3	4	5	6	7	8	9	10	11	12
200	1	2	3	4	5	6	7	8	9	10	11	12
220	1	2	3	4	5	6	7	8	9	10	11	12
240	1	2	3	4	5	6	7	8	9	10	11	12

Effects of drinking on driving

Be careful driving
BAC = up to 0.05%

Driving will be impaired
BAC = 0.05%–0.08%

Do not drive
BAC = 0.08–0.10%

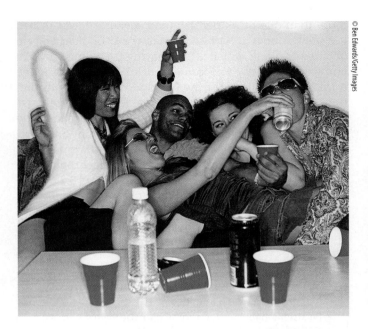

Drunkenness at parties can lead to actions and feelings that one regrets the next day—and sometimes for much longer.

Sexual Behavior

The effects of alcohol on sexual desire and performance vary from person to person, and depend on the BAC. In some individuals, small amounts of alcohol may dispel uncomfortable feelings about sex and may facilitate sexual arousal. Higher amounts of alcohol (a BAC of 0.10 or more) may cause problems for males, such as difficulty getting and maintaining an erection or ejaculating, and for females, such as inadequate vaginal lubrication and difficulty reaching orgasm. Even at moderate BACs, some individuals are too intoxicated to give and receive sexual pleasure.

Alcohol consumption may contribute to a variety of undesired consequences of sexual behavior. While intoxicated, people can forget to use birth control correctly or simply ignore the practice altogether and thus become unintentionally pregnant. Not using condoms or having sex with a stranger increases the risk of transmission of sexually transmitted diseases (STDs) and AIDS. Alcohol can blur one's judgment and can lead to unintended sexual experiences.

Although estimates vary, as many as 40% of sexual assaults reported by college students occur when the perpetrator, the victim, or both have been drinking alcohol (Abbey et al., 2014).

Other Effects of Alcohol

Alcohol can impair the functioning of body organs other than the brain. Alcohol can irritate the organs of the gastrointestinal (GI) tract—the esophagus, stomach, intestine, pancreas, and liver—causing upset or irritation, nausea, vomiting, or diarrhea. Alcohol can also dilate arteries and cause bloodshot eyes. Dilation of arteries in the arms, legs, and skin can cause a drop in blood pressure and decrease body heat, explaining why people occasionally feel flushed when they drink. Giving alcohol to people to "warm them up" actually produces the opposite physiological effect.

Alcohol should not be ingested simultaneously with other central nervous system depressants such as tranquilizers, sedatives, and antihistamines, which are found in cold medicines. In many instances, the depressant effects of alcohol and the other drug interact so that the combined effects of the two drugs are greater than the simple additive effects of either drug taken separately. Seemingly reasonable amounts of alcohol taken with another depressant drug can dangerously suppress brain function and respiration (Table 18.4).

Long-Term Effects

Long-term heavy drinking can affect immune, endocrine, and reproductive functions and can cause neurological problems, including dementia, blackouts, seizures, hallucinations, and peripheral neuropathy. Various cancers associated with heavy drinking include cancers of the lip, oral cavity, pharynx, larynx, esophagus, stomach, colon, rectum, tongue, lung, pancreas, and liver. Long-term

---

Table 18.4

Alcohol and Drugs That Don't Mix

Alcohol should not be consumed when taking drugs such as these.

Drug	Dangerous interaction
Allergy/cold/flu/cough medicine containing loratadine (Claritin), diphenhydramine (Benadryl), chlorpheniramine (Tylenol Allergy Plus), or dextromethorphan (Robitussin)	Drowsiness, possible overdose
Anxiety/epilepsy medicine containing lorazepam (Ativan), alprazolam (Xanax), paroxetine (Paxil), phenytoin (Dilantin), clonazepam (Klonopin), or phenobarbital	Drowsiness, breathing problems, overdose
Pain/arthritis pain medicine containing ibuprofen (Advil, Motrin), aspirin, acetaminophen (Tylenol), oxycodone (Percocet), or hydrocodone (Vicodin)	Ulcers, stomach bleeding, liver damage
Medicine for sleep problems such as zolpidem (Ambien), eszopiclone (Lunesta), or diphenhydramine (Sominex)	Drowsiness, impaired breathing, overdose

For more information, see National Institute on Alcohol Abuse and Alcoholism. (2014). Harmful interactions. Retrieved from http://pubs.niaaa.nih.gov/publications/medicine/medicine.htm.

heavy drinking can also increase the risk of chronic gastritis, hepatitis, hypertension, cirrhosis of the liver, and coronary heart disease.

Chronic alcoholic men may become "feminized," with breast enlargement and female body hair patterns. Chronic alcoholic women may experience menstrual disturbances, loss of secondary sex characteristics, and infertility. Women who drink heavily experience more gynecological problems and have surgery more often than women who do not.

Fetal Alcohol Syndrome

Alcohol can harm the health of anyone, man or woman, young or old. Even a fetus can be damaged by alcohol. Numerous kinds of birth defects and intellectual disabilities may result from ingestion of alcohol by pregnant women—a condition known as **fetal alcohol syndrome**. Fetal alcohol syndrome is estimated to be the third leading cause of birth defects and intellectual disabilities among newborns. Because the harmful effects on the fetus are believed to occur during the first few weeks of prenatal development, a time during which much of the nervous system is being formed, women should refrain from drinking alcohol if they are trying to become pregnant or if they suspect they are pregnant. The level of alcohol in the fetus's blood may be several times greater than the BAC of the mother. This explains why even a couple of drinks early in pregnancy can endanger normal fetal development.

Health Benefits of Alcohol

Many studies have shown an association between consuming a small amount of alcohol (about a drink per day) and a lower risk of heart disease and stroke (Nutrition Source, 2017). The benefits of alcohol consumption were first reported among people in France, where it was noted that despite a diet high in fat, the rate of heart disease is low. This anomaly became known as the "French paradox." At first, the French paradox was explained by the fact that red wine is widely consumed in France, and that substances in red wine, called flavonoids, produced the heart-healthy effects. However, several studies have shown that the healthful effects of drinking are not specific to the type of drink, and hence such effects are caused by ethanol. Moderate alcohol consumption is heart-healthy because it increases blood levels of high-density lipoproteins (HDL, so-called good cholesterol). Alcohol consumption also may reduce the risk of blood clots, gallstones, and type 2 diabetes. No benefit is associated with heavy drinking (four or more drinks per day). While not discounting possible healthful biological effects of moderate alcohol consumption, researchers also note that a drink with the evening meal can dampen the stress of a busy day, and that social interaction with friends—drink or not—can contribute to health.

Alcohol Use Disorder (AUD)

Most people who consume alcohol engage in moderate drinking, which is men having two or fewer drinks per day (and 14 or fewer drinks per week) and women having not more than one drink per day (and seven or fewer drinks per week). About 27% of Americans age 18 or older engage in binge drinking, which is men having five or more drinks and women having four or more drinks in 2 hours. Binge drinking typically raises the blood alcohol concentration (BAC) to 0.08 or higher, which is the legal limit for driving in most states. About 7% of Americans engage in heavy alcohol use, which is men having more than four drinks on any day or more than 14 drinks per week and women having more than three drinks on any day or more than seven drinks per week. About 6% (9.8 million men and 5.3 million women) of Americans aged 18 and older have an **alcohol use disorder (AUD)**, a pattern of uncontrollable alcohol use that is socially and personally harmful (**Figure 18.5**).

Lack of Control
- More alcohol is consumed in larger amounts or over a longer period than is intended.
- Persistent inability to control alcohol use even if personally desired.
- Considerable interest and effort in obtaining, using, and recovering from the effects of alcohol.
- Craving or otherwise strongly wanting to consume alcohol.

Social Impairment
- Failure to fulfill obligations at work, school, or home due to alcohol use.
- Continued alcohol use despite social or interpersonal problems resulting from doing so.
- Disengagement from important social, occupational, or recreational activities due to alcohol use.

Risky Use
- Persistent alcohol use in personally hazardous situations.
- Continued alcohol use despite knowledge it is causing significant personal problems.

Biological Changes
- Tolerance, as defined as needing increasingly more alcohol to become intoxicated and/or becoming less intoxicated using the same amount of alcohol.
- Withdrawal symptoms, which are unpleasant biological reactions due to abstaining from drinking.

■ **Figure 18.5**

Manifestations of Alcohol Use Disorder (AUD)
The extent of AUD is determined by the number of symptoms over a period of time. *Mild AUD* is two to three symptoms in the prior 12 months. *Moderate AUD* is four to five symptoms in the prior 12 months. *Severe AUD* is six or more symptoms in the prior 12 months.

Data from NIAAA. (2016). Alcohol Use Disorder: A Comparison Between DSM–IV and DSM–5. Retrieved from https://pubs.niaaa.nih.gov/publications/dsmfactsheet/dsmfact.pdf

TERMS

alcohol use disorder: alcohol consumption that causes distress or harm; also known as alcoholism or alcohol abuse

fetal alcohol syndrome: birth defects and mental disabilities caused by ingestion of alcohol by the mother during pregnancy

Alcohol Abuse Is a Worldwide Problem

The World Health Organization (WHO) estimates that nearly 62% of the world's teen and adult population (about 4 billion people) never or very rarely consume alcohol (World Health Organization, 2015). The remaining 38% consume beer, wine, distilled spirits, or homemade beverages, ingesting an average of 6.2 liters per person of pure ethyl alcohol a year. This is the volume equivalent of alcohol in 220 standard drinks in North America. The amount of alcohol consumed varies considerably by country (Table 18.5). In general, populations in high-income countries consume more alcohol per person than those in low-income countries. Worldwide about 16% of drinkers aged 15 years or older engage in heavy episodic drinking.

Alcohol misuse is responsible for 3.3 million annual deaths worldwide (5.9% of total deaths), more than HIV/AIDS, tuberculosis, sanitation problems, and high cholesterol. Alcohol problems include intoxication (drunkenness), neurobiological dependence (alcoholism), and causation of dozens of types of injuries and chronic diseases, including esophageal cancer, liver cancer, cirrhosis of the liver, homicide, epileptic seizures, motor vehicle accidents, assault, domestic violence, homicide, and suicide (Table 18.6). About 5% of all disease worldwide is alcohol related. Alcohol consumption has been identified as a component cause for more than 200 health conditions.

Recognizing that alcohol-related problems are the result of a complex interplay between individual use of alcoholic beverages and cultural, economic, physical environment, political, and social forces, in 2010, 193 countries reached consensus on a World Health Organization Global Strategy to produce national rules and recommendations to reduce harmful use of alcohol (WHO, 2016). These strategies include measures to control supply and/or affect the demand for alcoholic beverages, altering hazardous drinking patterns, and implementing health services to treat problem drinkers. For example, countries have limited alcohol use by instituting high alcohol taxes, restricting alcohol advertising, and limiting availability by outright prohibition, rationing, and state monopolies; promoted beverages with low or no alcohol content, and regulated, the density of alcohol outlets, hours, days of sale, drinking locations, and minimum drinking age; and

instituted health promotion campaigns and school-based education. Also, countries have established strict drinking-and-driving laws to reduce alcohol-related car crashes, injuries, and deaths. For example, in most European countries, the legal limit for alcohol in the blood (blood alcohol content, or BAC) is 0.05%; in some countries it is near zero. (In the United States it is 0.08%.) In some countries, failing a test for blood alcohol content results in immediate suspension of one's driver's license.

Table 18.6

Alcohol-Related Illness, Worldwide

Illness	Percent (%) of all alcohol-related illness	
	Male	Female
Neuropsychiatric	26.1	18.8
Cardiovascular diseases	10.6	33.6
Gastrointestinal diseases	12.5	17.6
Intentional injuries	12.1	3.2
Cancers	8.2	10.2
Infectious diseases	6.7	7.2
Neonatal diseases	0.2	0.5

About 5% of all illness in the world is alcohol related. This table shows the degree to which certain medical conditions and illnesses contribute to all alcohol-related illness. Note that a person can have more than one type of disease or injury due to alcohol consumption. Neuropsychiatric conditions include alcohol use disorders, epilepsy, withdrawal-induced seizures, depression, and anxiety disorders. Cardiovascular diseases (CVD) include heart disease, stroke, high blood pressure, and atrial fibrillation. (The beneficial effects on the heart of alcohol consumption are nullified by heavy drinking.) Gastrointestinal diseases include liver cirrhosis and acute and chronic pancreatitis. Intentional injuries include suicide and violence (risk is proportional to alcohol intake). Cancers include those of the mouth, nasopharynx, other pharynx and oropharynx, larynx, esophagus, colon and rectum, liver, pancreas, and female breast. Risk is proportional to alcohol consumption, although consumption as low as one drink per day increases the risk for female breast and other types of cancer. Infectious diseases include pneumonia and tuberculosis due to weakening of the immune system. Neonatal diseases include fetal alcohol syndrome (FAS) and preterm birth complications. World Health Organization. (2014). Global status report on alcohol and health, 2014. Retrieved from http://www.who.int/substance_abuse /publications/global_alcohol_report/en/

Table 18.5

Alcohol Consumption Patterns in Selected Countries

Country	% Current drinkers		Alcohol consumption (liters/year)		% Types of beverages			% Alcohol use disorder	
	Male	Female	Male	Female	B*	W*	S*	Male	Female
Argentina	70	48.3	19.5	10.9	41	48	5	9.0	2.5
Belarus	91	71	30.9	12.8	17	5	47	29.8	5.5
Canada	80.3	74.9	18.8	7.4	51	22	27	10.2	3.6
France	94.5	93.3	18.4	7.7	19	56	23	8.8	2.5
Iran and Kuwait				Almost zero					
Kenya	43.9	16.3	14.6	10.1	20	15	22	1.8	1.4
Japan	76.4	61.9	13.7	6.7	19	4	52	4.6	1.0
New Zealand	84.8	74.5	18.6	8.5	83	34	15	4.5	1.9
South Africa	56.3	26.3	32.8	16.0	48	18	17	10.0	4.2
Sweden	75.1	63.3	17.1	8.8	37	47	15	12.6	5.3
Thailand	45.4	14.9	30.3	5.2	27	0	13	9.1	3.4
United States	75.2	63	18.1	7.8	50	17	33	10.7	4.2

Adapted from: World Health Organization. (2014). Global status report on alcohol and health, country profiles. Retrieved from https://www.who.int/substance_abuse /publications/global_alcohol_report/profiles/en/

* B = Beer; W = Wine; S = Spirits

Alcohol Use Disorder (AUD) is characterized by alcohol-related impairment or distress and/or neurobiological dependence (addiction) on alcohol, otherwise referred to as **alcoholism**. AUD can be mild, moderate, or severe depending on the degree of impairment and neurobiological dependence.

Alcoholism, the most severe form of AUD, is characterized by an intense craving for alcohol, compulsive drinking behavior, an inability to control one's drinking, and physical dependence on alcohol. Withdrawal symptoms, including anxiety and stress, and **delirium tremens (DTs)**, characterized by hallucinations and uncontrollable shaking, may occur when a person affected by alcoholism is deprived of alcohol.

> I don't even know what street Canada is on.
> *Al Capone*

AUD can cause numerous negative consequences. Job and school performance can be impaired, family relationships and friendships can be destroyed, and drunk driving may cause financial problems, injuries, legal problems, and fatalities. Because alcohol supplies calories, excessive drinkers are rarely hungry. They may have vitamin deficiency syndromes, which result in mental confusion and loss of muscular coordination.

The cause or causes of problem drinking, AUD, and alcoholism are complex and the subject of considerable scientific research. Before the advent of modern psychology and medicine, alcohol abuse was thought to be a manifestation of immorality and irreligiousness. Some people still hold that view, but many healthcare professionals interpret alcohol abuse as a biologically based behavioral disorder or a medical disease involving the alteration of genes and physiological systems. For example, some people may be more susceptible to abusing alcohol because of variations in the ways their bodies break down or excrete alcohol or because of variations in the ways their brains respond to alcohol. Some experts resist considering alcohol abuse a disease because doing so may remove the sense of personal and social responsibility for problem drinking. Others argue that calling alcohol abuse a "disease" fosters successful treatment because it removes the stigma, lessens guilt, and offers a supervised and presumably scientifically based plan for treatment.

The Stages of Alcoholism

A large body of research suggests that alcoholism develops in four stages. Stage 1 is psychological attachment to alcohol. Most people consume alcohol to accompany other experiences, like having wine to enhance a meal or a beer at a ball game. Because alcohol can lessen anxiety and facilitate "feeling good," some people become very attracted to creating this alcohol-induced state of mind, and over time increase their intake of alcohol, not as an adjunct to other experiences, but to create the alcohol-induced drug experience itself. With regular ingestion of alcohol, the brain adjusts to the frequent, if not continual, presence of alcohol such that increasing amounts are needed to produce the expected, desired effects. This is **tolerance**. If drinking continues, eventually the original mental rewards of drinking become overshadowed by the unpleasant experience of not drinking, even for a short period of time. This unpleasant mental and bodily state is called **withdrawal**. The process eventually culminates in intense craving for alcohol and a lifestyle devoted to satisfying it.

In the second stage of alcoholism, tolerance for alcohol increases and individuals become more preoccupied with drinking. For example, when invited to a party they may ask what alcoholic beverages will be served rather than who is going to be there. In this stage, problem drinkers may sneak drinks often and may deny that they are drinking too much. **Blackouts** may also occur. Blackouts are periods in which others observe the drinker as behaving normally or abnormally, but the drinker has no recall of events that happened while drinking.

The third stage of alcoholism is characterized by loss of control over how much alcohol is consumed. The person may not drink every day but cannot control the amount of alcohol consumed once drinking has begun. In this stage, the problem drinker may rationalize drinking behavior and actually believe that there are good reasons for heavy drinking. The person may still carry out responsibilities (e.g., housework, job, schoolwork) for some time and may employ a series of strategies to prevent family rejection, including promises to stop drinking. Often alcoholics' extravagant measures to prove they do not have a drinking problem appear successful, but eventually they begin drinking heavily again. At this point the problem with alcohol is sometimes blamed on the kind of drinks preferred or on the usual place of drinking; as a result, problem drinkers may change to a different form of alcoholic beverage or to a different place in which to drink.

In the fourth stage, the alcoholic is dependent on the drug, and drinking behavior consumes nearly all aspects

Are You a Problem Drinker?

The CAGE questionnaire is a diagnostic tool for alcohol problems.

C = Concern by the person that there is a problem
A = Apparent to others that there is a problem
G = Grave consequences
E = Evidence of dependence or tolerance

Answer these questions:
1. Have you ever felt that you should **C**ut down on your drinking?
2. Have you ever become **A**nnoyed by criticism of your drinking?
3. Have you ever felt **G**uilty about your drinking?
4. Have you ever had a morning **E**ye opener to get rid of a hangover?

One "yes" response indicates possible alcohol abuse.

of life. Friends and family have resigned themselves to the problem and may be angry or ignore the alcoholic. At this stage of alcoholism the person may miss work or school occasionally. The health consequences of alcohol abuse may intensify and the person may need medical attention and even hospitalization. When physical addiction to alcohol occurs, continual drinking is needed to prevent withdrawal symptoms. Drinking for days at a time (a **bender**) may take place. The great majority of alcoholics do not wind up on "skid row" but instead struggle with their problem within their families and communities.

Alcohol Use Disorder and the Family

Alcohol Use Disorder (AUD) can severely stress a family, causing nondrinking family members mental and emotional suffering and sometimes financial hardship. Seventy-six million Americans, about 43% of the population, have been exposed to severe AUD in their family, including 11 million children under the age of 18.

Close relatives of a problem drinker can experience a variety of emotions, ranging from joy and relief when the problem drinker stops drinking for a time to depression and feelings of failure when the problem drinker begins drinking again. Family members can feel anger, shame, guilt, pity, and constant anxiety. Some try to cope by assuming responsibility for the problem; others may be designated scapegoats and blamed for the drinker's problem with alcohol. Some may withdraw in silence, whereas others try to maintain their sense of humor. These behaviors are all defenses against the family's psychological distress.

Like the problem drinker, family members may deny the problem, try to rationalize it, and isolate themselves from friends and relatives, and, in some cases, actually feel responsible for the drinker's problem. This **enabling**, or protection process, keeps the problem drinker from feeling responsible for his or her drinking—which is part of the paradox experienced by families of alcoholics. In their attempts to protect the alcoholic, family members may unwittingly contribute to the drinking problem; they may try to protect the alcoholic from serious social consequences of excessive drinking, for instance, making excuses for absenteeism from work or school.

Al-Anon is an organization that helps spouses, families, and friends of alcoholics. Alateen is a similar organization that helps children of alcoholics. Al-Anon and Alateen help family members understand how alcoholism has affected their lives and help them to explore the family relationships that contribute to the alcohol problem. Family therapy (with or without the problem drinker's participation) may help a family find ways to cope with the problem and regain harmony in their family life.

Children of Alcoholics

Children growing up in families in which one or both parents have a drinking problem may experience neglect, emotional deprivation, abuse, an unstable family environment, and sometimes violence. As a result, they may have developed thought, emotion, and behavior patterns that impair their personal lives and relationships in adulthood. Children of alcoholics, often referred to as COAs, are at a high risk of becoming alcoholics themselves.

Many COAs learn as children to block from their awareness the truth of their situation—both the fact of a parent's alcoholism and also the emotional distress resulting from it. This tendency is referred to as **denial**. The consequences of denial can go beyond issues of parental alcoholism to become a generalized way of approaching life. As adults, many COAs are constricted in their capacities to see the world as it really is and to experience emotional fulfillment.

Breaking Addictive Behaviors

It's a little known fact, but it was psychologist Carl Jung who inspired the Alcoholics Anonymous program. Frustrated with a client unable to change his alcoholism, Jung suggested that his only hope for recovery was to purposefully have a spiritual experience to rid himself of this addictive habit. So, Roland H. did just that. After conquering his addiction, he went on to share this experience with Edwin T., then Bill W., who then went on to co-found Alcoholics Anonymous.

In response to a letter from Bill W., Jung wrote, "His craving for alcohol was the equivalent, on a low level, of the spiritual thirst of our being for wholeness, expressed in medieval language: the union with God. You see alcohol in Latin is *spiritus*, and we use the same words for the highest religious experience as well as for the most depraving poison. The helpful formula therefore is: *Spiritus contra spiritum*." (Spiritual crises require spiritual cures.)

TERMS

alcoholism: loss of control over drinking alcohol

bender: several days of continued drinking

blackout: failure to recall normal or abnormal behavior or events that occurred while drinking

delirium tremens (DTs): hallucinations and uncontrollable shaking caused by withdrawal of alcohol in alcohol-dependent individuals

denial: refusal to admit you (or someone else) have a drinking problem

enabling: denial of, abetting, or excusing another's addictive behaviors

tolerance: biological adaptation to alcohol use such that increasing amounts of alcohol are needed to produce the expected, desired effects

withdrawal: unpleasant physiological and psychological symptoms in alcohol-dependent individuals when refraining from drinking

Many COAs have a negative self-image and a tendency to be hypercritical of themselves. As children, they believe themselves to be the cause of their parents' erratic, and sometimes violent behavior. Indeed, sometimes the parents reinforce this assumption by blaming their children for their own alcohol-related problems. The children not only come to believe themselves to be "bad" but also tend to believe they are responsible for everyone else's emotions. They can become so other-focused that they have no lives of their own, a characteristic called **codependency**.

Another consequence of growing up in an alcoholic family is the tendency to try to control situations and other people. Because family life was unstable and painful, many COAs come to believe that their interpersonal environment is likely at any moment to become emotionally painful, violent, or disruptive. Thus, COAs tend to be constantly anxious and hypervigilant for signs of danger. To minimize the threat (experienced as criticism, abandonment, or abuse), COAs tend to be compliant and agreeable and actively try to please others. Believing that others cannot be trusted and that the world must be made safe, COAs also try to be totally self-reliant and in control of their lives.

Denial, a negative self-image, the tendency to take responsibility for others, the need to control oneself and the environment, and other characteristics help a COA survive childhood in an alcoholic family. Unfortunately, in adulthood these same "survival" strategies limit the opportunity to grow and develop unique individual qualities and to experience healthy interpersonal relationships. Fortunately, these self-limiting beliefs and behaviors can be changed through awareness and professional help.

Treatment Options for AUD

The situation of problem drinkers and alcoholics is serious but not hopeless. Recovery is possible if the person is strongly motivated to stop drinking and to address motivations for alcohol use.

Sometimes the motivation to stop drinking comes in the form of a threat—a drinking-related legal problem or illness, severe disruption of family life, the loss of a job. The motivation to stop drinking can also come from the person's own resolve to stop his or her self-destructive behavior and to stop feeling helpless, hopeless, and confused.

Alcoholics Anonymous (AA), the worldwide nonprofit self-help organization, has assisted many people to get on the road back to wellness and enjoyment of life. AA bases its program on total sobriety, anonymity, and a step-by-step program of recovery. The environment at AA meetings is relaxing, caring, and open. Members share their experiences, strengths, and hopes with each other, with the goal of helping new and old members identify and learn more about their own problems with alcohol. Practical tips on how to remain sober are shared, and telephone numbers are exchanged so that a member can contact another member if stressful situations arise that previously led to drinking.

Alcoholics Anonymous emphasizes that sobriety is a state of mind, which means that recovering from a drinking problem involves changing values, attitudes, and lifestyles. The AA program helps problem drinkers honestly examine their feelings, recognize their limitations, and accept responsibility for past wrongs. For problem drinkers, remaining sober is an ongoing process, which involves finding new ways to satisfy emotional, spiritual, and social needs.

Besides AA, problem drinkers can receive help from individual and group psychotherapy. Many therapists are trained specifically to help problem drinkers and their families recover. Also, certain medicines may help. Disulfuram (Antabuse) causes uncomfortable physical and mental feelings when alcohol is ingested. Naltrexone can help reduce the craving for alcohol. Acamprosate reduces withdrawal symptoms.

Responsible Drinking

Each person has the option of drinking or abstaining from alcohol. Each of you has the responsibility for determining the occasions for drinking and the amounts of alcohol that you consume. If you drink, here are some guidelines to remember:

- Make sure that alcohol use improves your social interactions and does not harm or destroy them.
- Drink slowly and avoid mixing alcohol with other drugs.
- Be sure that using alcohol enhances your general sense of well-being and does not make either you or other persons feel disgusted with your actions.
- If you plan to drink, decide beforehand that you will not drive and designate someone who will not drink to be the driver.

In addition to being responsible for your own drinking habits, you can also help others to drink responsibly. Respect the wishes of the person who chooses to abstain from drinking and don't push drinks on people at parties. If you are giving a party, be sure to provide alternatives to alcohol. You may also offer places to sleep for those who have been drinking and should not drive home. Remember to eat when you drink and to provide food at your parties.

There is no evidence to indicate that total abstinence from alcohol is necessary for health and wellness. On the other hand, there is a great deal of evidence showing that excessive alcohol use can destroy personal health and family relationships, can cause traffic deaths and suicides, and can produce birth defects in newborns. We believe that you can significantly improve your health and happiness by developing responsible drinking habits while you are young and maintaining moderate drinking habits throughout life.

TERMS

codependency: a relationship pattern in which the nonaddicted family members identify with the alcoholic

Critical Thinking About Health

1. After about a month it was clear that inviting Chris to be their roommate had been a brilliant move. With a 3.9-plus GPA, Chris was a fountain of help with every subject from history to chemistry. Getting into law school was a foregone conclusion. The real question was how to get Chris on "Jeopardy!"

    When midterm exams rolled around, the roommates noticed that Chris was coming home every day with a 12-pack of beer—six cans would disappear before dinner and the rest disappeared as the night's studying progressed. Although Chris showed no signs of impairment from ingesting this quantity of alcohol, the roommates were concerned.
    a. What concerns might the roommates have? If you were Chris's roommate, would you be concerned?
    b. Given Chris's obvious success in school and the fact that Chris shows no outward sign of impairment, would you agree or disagree that Chris has a problem with alcohol?
    c. Do you think Chris's roommates should try to change Chris's drinking behavior, or is it none of their business?

2. "I don't like alcohol all that much. And it's never fun to wake up and find that you vomited all over yourself and don't remember doing it. There have been times I don't know how I got home, and I only hope that whoever drove the car wasn't as wasted as I was. Still, you need it. There's no better way to destress after a hard week of school. And you need to drink so you can be loose at a party. No one wants to dance with a loser, much less have sex with them."

    What is your opinion of this person's attitude? Do you disagree with this student's philosophy? Explain your reasons.

3. Every summer, State U. invites the parents of incoming students to "Parents' Day," a chance to visit the campus and talk to faculty, students, and administrators. Last summer, Dr. Meredith, one of the university's newest faculty members, gladly volunteered to give a "sample lecture" on paleontology to the parents and to chat with them at the luncheon in the Faculty Dining Room.

    A father of an incoming female student engaged Dr. Meredith in conversation about his daughter's likely experiences living in the college dormitory and swimming on the swim team.

    "My daughter's never been away from home before," said the father. "I want to be sure she'll be OK."

    Dr. Meredith silently gulped hard, for he knew that the dormitories had the reputation for massive illegal drinking during the first month or two of the school year, and that the swim coach would drink beer with the team members after swim meets.
    a. Does the father have anything to be concerned about?
    b. Should Dr. Meredith tell the father about alcohol use at the college?
    c. To avoid having to encounter another parent with similar concerns, Dr. Meredith vowed never again to help out at Parents' Day. What else could Dr. Meredith do to avoid such unpleasant experiences? Remember that Dr. Meredith is new at the university and without tenure.
    d. What is the campus climate toward tolerating alcohol use among students on your campus?

4. A college needs an electronic scoreboard for its football stadium, and a beer company is willing to buy it in exchange for exclusive advertising rights on the scoreboard and in the football game programs. The college president is against this deal, arguing that it promotes drinking on campus. However, the athletic director and the president of the alumni association favor it, arguing that it's vital to have the new scoreboard and, besides, "beer and college always have gone together and always will, and there's nothing wrong with it."
    a. Do you favor or object to the scoreboard deal?
    b. Do you agree or disagree with the college president about the fact that advertising promotes drinking?
    c. Do you agree or disagree with the athletic director and alumni president that beer and college always have and always will go together?

Chapter Summary and Highlights

Chapter Summary

Offering someone an alcoholic drink is a sign of hospitality and friendship in many cultures and countries around the world. Small amounts of alcohol can reduce the tensions of personal interactions and help calm anxieties and uncertainties pertaining to proper behavior in unfamiliar social encounters. Taking a small amount of wine is an important part of Christian religious services. Celebrating weddings, births, anniversaries, and other festive occasions with champagne is commonplace. Taken in large quantities, alcohol can lead to garrulity, boisterous, aggressive behavior, and eventually to drunkenness and unconsciousness. Many drinkers do not have the ability to control their consumption of alcohol, and develop an alcohol use disorder, a major health problem wherever alcoholic beverages are readily available.

The destructiveness of alcohol misuse is evidenced by high rates of domestic violence, date rape among college students, child abuse and neglect, and violence of many kinds. Drinking and driving is a hazard to oneself, other drivers, and pedestrians. One-third of all traffic fatalities involve drinking and drunkenness. Even a small amount of alcohol in the body affects judgment and driving skills. For a variety of reasons, many people choose not to drink. If you choose to drink, set limits for yourself. When drinking, do not engage in activities that may harm yourself or others. "One for the road" is the most dangerous invitation you will ever receive.

Highlights

- Alcohol abuse is a major drug problem in the United States. Consumption of alcohol is responsible for one-third of all highway fatalities and for numerous social, family, and health problems.
- Alcoholic beverages contain ethyl alcohol, which is produced by the action of yeast on sugar (fermentation) in grains and the juices of berries and fruits. Beer and wine are direct products of fermentation; "hard" liquor, such as whiskey, vodka, rum, and brandy, is made from distilled fermented liquids. Most standard portions of alcoholic beverages contain a one-half ounce of ethyl alcohol.
- Social and normative influences on drinking behavior are evident in specific drinking patterns among college students. Drinking on campus increases the risk of academic problems, unintended pregnancy, and violence, including sexual assault.
- Alcohol enters the bloodstream within minutes after ingestion. The physical and behavioral effects of alcohol depend on the blood alcohol content (BAC). A BAC of 0.02 produces a "loosening-up" effect. A BAC of 0.08 seriously impairs motor coordination and judgment; in most states it is illegal to drive with a BAC of 0.08.
- Frequent and constant use of alcohol can lead to an alcohol use disorder, consisting of neurobiological dependence and tolerance for the drug (alcoholism). Alcohol use disorder develops in stages, starting with the inability to control drinking and advancing to complete neurobiological dependence.
- Alcoholics may encounter severe health problems, and their personal lives, family relationships, and friendships may be disrupted. Millions of children who grew up in families where one or both parents were alcoholics experience personal problems as adults that stem from their childhoods.
- Organizations such as Alcoholics Anonymous and individual or group psychotherapy can help people recover from problem drinking and alcoholism. Alcohol abuse can be prevented by taking responsibility for one's drinking behavior.

For Your Health

It's common for users of alcohol not to be aware that their level of alcohol use is unhealthful and perhaps even dangerous to themselves and to others. You can find out if your drinking behavior is unhealthful by doing the CRAFFT or AUDIT questionnaires in Exercise 18.1 in the Workbook. And, if it is, do Exercise 18.2 in the Workbook, "Cutting Down on Drinking."

References

Abbey, A., et al. (2014). Review of survey and experimental research that examines the relationship between alcohol consumption and men's sexual aggression perpetration. *Trauma Violence Abuse, 15,* 265–282.

American College Health Association. (2016a). *American College Health Association—National College Health Assessment II: Canadian Reference Group Data Report, Spring 2016.* Hanover, MD: American College Health Association.

American College Health Association. (2016b). *American College Health Association—National College Health Assessment II: Undergraduate Student Reference Group Data Report, Spring 2016.* Hanover, MD: American College Health Association.

Center for Alcohol Marketing and Youth. (2015). Reducing youth exposure to alcohol advertising on cable TV. Retrieved from http://www.camy.org/resources /reports/alcohol-advertising-monitoring/alcohol -advertising-compliance/index.html.

Centers for Disease Control and Prevention. (2017). Impaired driving: Get the facts. Retrieved from https://www.cdc.gov/motorvehiclesafety/impaired _driving/impaired-drv_factsheet.html

Marzell, M., et al. (2015). Examining drinking patterns and high-risk drinking environments among college athletes at different competition levels. *Journal of Drug Education, 45,* 5–16.

Molina, P. E., et al. (2014). Alcohol abuse: Critical pathophysiological processes and contribution to disease burden. *Physiology (Bethesda), 29,* 203–215.

National Council on Alcohol and Drug Dependence (NCADD). (2015). Alcohol, drugs, and crime. Retrieved from https://www.ncadd.org/about-addiction /addiction-update/alcohol-drugs-and-crime

National Institute of Alcohol Abuse and Alcoholism (NIAAA). (2017). Alcohol facts and statistics. Retrieved from https://www.niaaa.nih.gov

/alcohol-health/overview-alcohol-consumption/alcohol-facts-and-statistics

National Institute on Alcohol Abuse and Alcoholism. (2017). A snapshot of annual high-risk college drinking consequences. Retrieved from http://www.collegedrinkingprevention.gov/statsSummaries/snapshot.aspx

National Institute on Alcohol Abuse and Alcoholism. (2017). *College drinking*. Retrieved from http://pubs.niaaa.nih.gov/publications/CollegeFactSheet/CollegeFactSheet.pdf

Nutrition Source. (2017). Alcohol: Balancing risks and benefits. Retrieved from https://www.hsph.harvard.edu/nutritionsource/alcohol-full-story/#possible_health_benefits

Ross, C. S., et al. (2016). Alcohol advertising compliance on cable television, October–December (Q4)2015. Center on Alcohol Marketing to Youth. Retrieved from http://www.camy.org/_docs /resources/reports/alcohol-advertising-monitoring/CAMY_CableTV_2015_Q4.pdf

Substance Abuse and Mental Health Services Administration (SAMSHA). (2015). National Survey on Drug Use and Health (NSDUH). Retrieved from https://www.samhsa.gov/data/sites/default/files/NSDUH-DetTabs-2015/NSDUH-DetTabs-2015/NSDUH-DetTabs-2015.htm#tab2-41b

Wechsler, H., & Nelson, T. F. (2008, July). What we have learned from the Harvard School of Public Health College Alcohol Study. *Journal of Studies on Alcohol and Drugs, 69,* 481–490.

World Health Organization. (2014). *Global status report on alcohol and health, 2014.* Retrieved from http://www.who.int/substance_abuse/publications/global_alcohol_report/msbgsruprofiles.pdf?ua=1

World Health Organization. (2015). Fact sheet on alcohol. Retrieved from http://www.who.int/mediacentre/factsheets/fs349/en/

Suggested Readings

Brown, S., & Lewis, V. (2002). *The alcoholic family in recovery: A developmental model.* New York: Guilford. Explains how families deal with abstinence and establish a more stable, yet flexible, family system.

Centers for Disease Control and Prevention. (2017). Alcohol and public health 2017. Retrieved from http://www.cdc.gov/alcohol/faqs.htm. Answers a variety of common questions about alcohol use and abuse.

Grant, B. F., et al. (2015). Epidemiology of DSM-5 Alcohol Use Disorder: Results from the National Epidemiologic Survey on Alcohol and Related Conditions III. JAMA *Psychiatry, 72,* 757–766.

Hart, A. B., & Kranzler, H. R. (2015). Alcohol dependence genetics: Lessons learned from genome-wide association studies (GWAS) and post-GWAS analyses. *Alcoholism, Clinical and Experimental Research, 39,* 1312–1327.

Harvard University Nutrition Source. (2017). Moderate drinking can be healthy—but not for everyone. You must weigh the benefits and risks. Retrieved from https://www.hsph.harvard.edu/nutritionsource/alcohol/

Koob, G. F. (2013). Theoretical frameworks and mechanistic aspects of alcohol addiction: Alcohol addiction as a reward deficit disorder. *Current Topics in Behavioral Neuroscience, 13,* 3–30. An eminent neuroscientist discusses the biology of alcohol addiction.

Loyola Marymount University, Los Angeles. (n.d.). History of alcohol use. Retrieved from http://academics.lmu.edu/headsup/forstudents/historyofalcoholuse. Discusses patterns of alcohol use, abuse, and dependence; the developmental course of alcohol problems within a community or population; and factors that are associated with an increased risk or susceptibility in a population for developing alcohol-related problems, alcohol abuse, or dependence.

Mayo Clinic. (2017). Alcohol use disorder. http://www.mayoclinic.org/diseases-conditions/alcohol-use-disorder/basics/definition/con-20020866

National Institute on Alcohol Abuse and Alcoholism. (2015). *Women and alcohol.* Retrieved from http://pubs.niaaa.nih.gov/publications/womensfact/womensFact.htm. Explains the particular risks and realities of drinking among women.

Nelson, T. F., et al. (2013). Efficacy and the strength of evidence of U.S. alcohol control policies. *American Journal of Preventive Medicine, 45,* 19–28. Ten U.S. alcohol policy experts identified and rated the efficacy of alcohol control policies for reducing binge drinking and alcohol-impaired driving among both the general population and youth and the strength of evidence informing the efficacy of each policy.

Porter, W. (2015). *Alcohol explained.* Santa Cruz, CA: Create Space. Explains how alcohol affects human beings on a chemical, physiological, and psychological level, from those first drinks right up to chronic alcoholism.

Vallee, B. L. (1998, June). Alcohol in the Western world. *Scientific American,* 80–85. A distinguished scientist examines the history of the role of alcohol in Western civilization.

Recommended Websites

Alcohol Problems and Solutions
Information compiled by Professor David Hanson, SUNY Potsdam.

Alcohol and Public Health
The Centers for Disease Control and Prevention's online resource for information on alcohol use and abuse.

College Drinking: Changing the Culture
Research-based information on the nature and extent of dangerous drinking among students.

Getting Help
Links to Alcoholics Anonymous, Al-Anon, Alateen, and other alcohol-problem resources.

National Institute on Alcohol Abuse and Alcoholism
A reliable source of information on treatments for alcoholism and ongoing research on alcohol abuse.

PART SIX

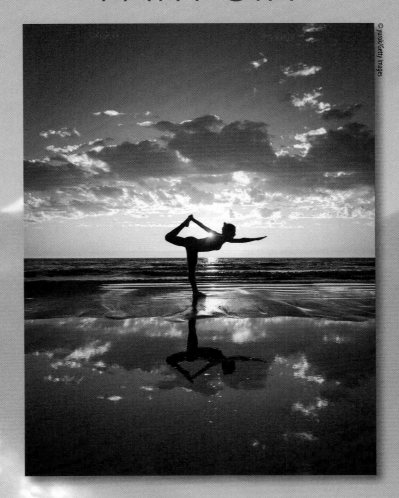

© yuruk/Getty Images

Making Healthy Choices

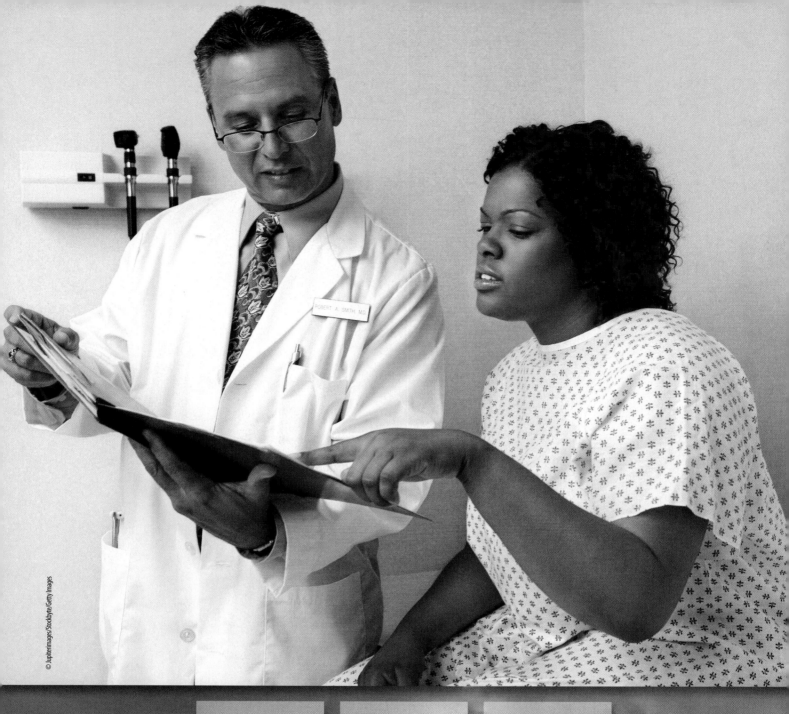

© Jupiterimages/Stockbyte/Getty Images

Dollars & Health Sense

Unhealthy Lifestyles Raise Healthcare Costs

Managing Stress

Healthcare Professionalism Versus Religious Belief

Wellness Guide

Interacting with Your Physician

How Does Your Hospital Rate?

Hope Helps Healing and Recovery

CHAPTER 19

Making Decisions About Health Care

Learning Objectives

1. Describe what you need to know to be an intelligent healthcare consumer.

2. Discuss the roles of several kinds of healthcare providers.

3. Compare the four main kinds of private health insurance available in the United States.

4. Explain which populations are served by Medicare and Medicaid.

5. Discuss several reasons why healthcare costs are high in the United States.

6. Compare health care and health insurance in Canada and the United States.

7. Discuss some of the problems with the quality of U.S. health care and frequency of medical errors.

8. Discuss the disparities of medical care based on patients' sex, race, and ethnicity.

9. Compare the pros and cons of organ transplants for donors and recipients.

10. List five kinds of cosmetic surgeries that are commonly performed.

Everyone needs health care at some time—for vaccinations, physical exams and diagnostic tests, and treatment when sick. Occasionally, people need to be hospitalized for serious illness, injury, or surgery.

Modern medicine is highly technological. The consumer of healthcare services must be able to evaluate the risks and benefits of diagnostic tests, treatments, recommended drugs, or surgery to influence and make decisions that affect her or his health. Understanding your rights as a patient and knowing how to communicate your concerns and needs to health professionals will help you stay healthy and help in the healing process when you become sick.

Modern medical care, especially hospitalization and pharmaceuticals, can be very expensive—too expensive for most people to pay for on their own. Most countries in the world have systems to help people pay for medical services; for example, in Canada, the UK, Japan, and other industrialized countries, the central government, through the collection of taxes, is the single payer of nearly all medical costs. In the United States, about 39% of medical care costs are federal and state government funded with tax dollars (Kaiser Family Foundation, 2017). The rest is paid by people themselves and through employer-funded insurance for employees. Prior to 2010, about 40 million Americans could not afford medical care and did not have access to government or private funding. In that year, however, the U.S. Congress passed the Affordable Care Act with the goal of ensuring that all Americans receive quality medical care.

Quality health care and the cost of medical services are among people's most important concerns. Both state and federal governments have been trying to ensure that all citizens have some form of health insurance and can receive health care when needed, but millions of Americans do not have health insurance.

> God heals and the doctor takes the fee.
>
> *Ben Franklin*

Being a Wise Healthcare Consumer

Making wise decisions about your health is part of self-care and self-responsibility. As healthcare consumers, we need to make important decisions about the health products we purchase, the health services we select, and the information we receive.

Behaviors that can help protect you from health fraud and unnecessary medical procedures include the following:

- Being well informed and knowing how to make healthy decisions
- Seeking reliable sources of information
- Being skeptical about health claims appearing in news media or advertising
- Avoiding unlicensed practitioners
- Selecting practitioners with great care and asking questions about fees, diagnoses, treatments, and alternative treatments and obtaining second opinions

- Reporting healthcare fraud and wrongdoing to government regulating agencies

Being a wise healthcare consumer starts with three basic principles: (1) working in partnership with your healthcare provider, (2) sharing in healthcare decisions, and (3) becoming skilled at obtaining health care.

Communication is extremely important in a physician–patient relationship. It is the policy of the American Medical Association that "the patient has the right to receive information from physicians and to discuss the benefits, risks, and costs of appropriate treatment alternatives." Many physicians want to fully inform patients of their medical situation and options, although some do not. A physician may feel that her or his religious beliefs or moral values justify not being fully open with patients regarding their options (Combs et al., 2011). Alternatively, physicians also may recommend unnecessary tests and procedures to boost profits for themselves or their employers or to avoid being sued for medical malpractice. For all of these reasons, you should choose a healthcare provider in whom you have complete confidence and trust.

As a partner in your own health care, you are best served by managing minor health problems. At the first sign of a health problem for which you seek professional help, you should observe and record symptoms so that you and your healthcare provider can better manage problems. When visiting your healthcare provider, be prepared; you only have a limited time with him or her. Prepare a checklist of questions you want to ask, as well as a list of your symptoms and any medications or other treatments for your symptoms. During your visit, state your concerns, describe the symptoms, and ask questions regarding prescribed drugs, the diagnosis, and treatment recommendations. Be open and honest when asked about sexual activity, smoking and drinking behavior, use of prescription or illegal drugs, or other questions you might feel too embarrassed to answer. Being truthful with healthcare providers is essential if you want your health restored.

The second principle in being a wise healthcare consumer is shared decision making. In partnership with your healthcare provider, you should participate actively in every medical decision. You have this right except in the emergency room, where informed consent is not necessary. There are numerous ways to share in healthcare decisions: (1) Let your doctor know what you want, (2) do your own research, (3) ask why a test or treatment is recommended, (4) ask about alternatives, (5) consider watchful waiting as an alternative to immediate treatment, (6) state your healthcare preferences, and (7) accept responsibility for the course of treatments.

Being skilled at obtaining health care is the third principle. By communicating and partnering with your healthcare provider, you can become skilled in purchasing healthcare services. There are many ways to cut the cost of health care without affecting the quality: (1) Exercise self-care and self-responsibility, (2) seek health care from a primary healthcare provider, (3) reduce unnecessary

Healthcare Professionalism Versus Religious Belief

A physician has a professional obligation to provide all patients nondiscriminatory access to medical services. A pharmacist has a professional obligation to fill all prescriptions for patients without discrimination. These tenets may seem obvious, but they are not practiced all of the time. Claiming violations of their "conscience," some physicians refuse to perform an abortion or refer a patient to another physician who will perform it. Some pharmacists refuse to fill a prescription for emergency contraception sought by a rape victim and even refuse to return the prescription so that she can take it to another pharmacy.

At least 45 states now have "laws of conscience" that allow healthcare professionals to refuse any service that violates their conscience. Besides not performing an abortion, the list of healthcare services that could be denied includes:

- Refusing to counsel a patient about the availability of emergency contraceptive pills or even to write a prescription for such pills, even for a rape victim
- Refusing to counsel infertile couples as to their options using new reproductive technologies

- Refusing patients' requests that the use of painful or futile treatments be withheld or stopped
- Refusing to vaccinate a child for chicken pox (or even to tell parents about its availability) because the vaccine was developed with the use of tissue from aborted fetuses
- Refusal by a pharmacist to fill any prescription for birth control pills
- Refusal to counsel patients as to their end-of-life options or to follow their health directives

There was a time when healthcare professionalism meant doing the utmost in every situation to relieve suffering and to help others in distress. Are we entering a period when personal autonomy is more important than relieving suffering, and when "conscience" overrides professional ethics? The author C. S. Lewis wrote: "Of all tyrannies, a tyranny sincerely exercised for the good of its victims may be the most oppressive. It would be better to live under robber barons than under omnipotent moral busybodies. The robber baron's cruelty may sometimes sleep, his cupidity may at some point be satiated; but those who torment us for our own good will torment us without end for they do so with the approval of their own conscience" (Charo, 2005).

medical tests, (4) reduce drug use, (5) use specialists only when necessary, (6) use emergency services only for actual emergencies, and (7) use hospitals only when recommended by a physician.

Choosing a Healthcare Provider

Today's healthcare system is extraordinarily complex. For most people "going to the doctor" is the most obvious choice. But the doctor is one component of a medical system that includes nurses, physician assistants, physical therapists, paramedics, and a broad range of technical specialists—people who take blood and x-rays, perform invasive diagnostic tests, change dressings, make casts for broken bones, assist in rehabilitation, and many other functions. Besides doctors and other medical specialists, there are other healthcare providers who use alternative medicines, sometimes in conjunction with conventional, Western medicine. These include chiropractors, naturopaths, massage therapists, acupuncturists, herbalists, and many others. Deciding what kind of healthcare provider you need for your particular problem is the first step in being a wise healthcare consumer.

All physicians are trained in and practice modern (Western) medicine that is based on modern scientific principles, experimentation, and clinical trials that determine the efficacy of treatments or medicines. Traditional medicines (mostly Eastern) are based on thousands of years of observation and theories of the universe and of human biology that differ from modern science. Traditional medicine practiced in China, India, Tibet, and other Asian countries is based on herbal remedies and

the balancing of human physiology with the elements of nature. Most Asian countries now use a combination of Western and traditional medicines. In the United States, some physicians now incorporate elements of alternative medicines into their practices. People choose healthcare providers for many different reasons—past experience, knowledge, cultural preferences, affordability, and personal convictions.

Healthcare Providers

The delivery of health care to the U.S. population is carried out by an enormous number of people trained in many different specialties (see **Table 19.1**). Physicians, of course, are the primary source of medical advice and care, but their tasks would be impossible to carry out without the help of others. A description of some important healthcare providers is presented here.

Physician Assistants

Physician assistants (PAs) are trained in many aspects of patient care. They work independently and with the supervision of a physician. PAs supervise other members of the physician's health team and perform complex diagnostic and therapeutic procedures. In busy offices, most patients spend more time interacting with the office PA than with the doctor. The PA can spend more time with the patient than the physician does and usually can answer most of the patient's questions regarding medications or operations.

Nurses

Registered nurses (RNs) are trained to promote health, advise patients on how to prevent disease, and assist

Table 19.1

Selected Medical Specialties

After receiving their M.D. degree, physicians can specialize. This involves several additional years of training. Medical specialty boards certify physicians in a specialty by examination. Some medical specialties are described below.

Specialty	Specific focus
Allergy and immunology	Prevention, diagnosis, and treatment of allergic disease
Anesthesiology	Administration of drugs to prevent pain or to induce unconsciousness during surgical operations or diagnostic procedures
Cardiology	Diagnosis and treatment of diseases of the heart and blood vessels, including such problems as heart attacks, hypertension, and stroke
Dermatology	Diagnosis and treatment of skin diseases
Endocrinology	Care of medical problems that result from abnormalities in the endocrine (hormone) system in the body
Family practice	General medical services for patients and their families
Geriatrics/gerontology	Concerned with problems of the elderly
Hospitalist	A physician who cares only for patients admitted to a hospital
Internal medicine	Diagnosis and nonsurgical treatment of internal organs of the body
Neurology	Diagnosis and nonsurgical treatment of diseases of the brain, spinal cord, and nerves
Obstetrics and gynecology	Care of pregnant women and treatment of disorders of the female reproductive system
Oncology	Diagnosis and treatment of all forms of cancer
Ophthalmology	Medical and surgical care of the eye, including prescription eyeglasses
Orthopedics	Diagnosis and treatment of abnormalities in bone and muscle, especially injuries resulting from sports activities
Pathology	Examination and diagnosis of organs, tissues, body fluids, and excrement
Pediatrics	Medical care of children, usually up to teenage years
Preventive medicine	Prevention of disease through immunization, good health care, and concern with environmental factors
Psychiatry	Treatment of mental and emotional problems
Public health	Subspecialty of preventive medicine that deals with promoting the general health of the community
Radiology	Use of radiation for the diagnosis and treatment of disease
Urology	Treatment of male reproductive system and urinary tract and treatment of female urinary tract

in the care of patients. Hospital RNs are in frequent contact with sick patients and monitor their progress, administer medications, and record progress and problems. RNs assist physicians during treatments, surgeries, and examinations. Nurses may specialize in such areas as surgical, cancer, maternity, or emergency room care. Other areas of specialization include home health nurses, occupational health nurses, and public health nurses.

Nurse practitioners are RNs with additional training and skills that enable them to provide many primary care services. They take medical histories and perform physical exams. They also counsel patients and make preliminary diagnoses before referring patients to a physician.

Emergency Medical Technicians

Emergency medical care is delivered at home and accident sites by emergency medical technicians (EMTs) and paramedics. EMTs work in hospitals and with police and fire departments. Paramedics have more advanced training that enables them to perform a variety of emergency procedures for sick or injured people needing immediate attention. A trained paramedic will recognize a heart attack victim and begin cardiopulmonary resuscitation (CPR). EMTs and paramedics are trained in ways to safely move seriously injured people and can communicate with hospital physicians to determine the best course of emergency treatment.

Physical and Occupational Therapists

Physical therapists (PTs) are trained to restore function, improve mobility, and relieve pain of patients suffering from an injury or disease. They try to maintain, restore, and promote overall fitness. Physical therapists usually work in hospitals or medical clinics and work with patients who are referred by a physician for physical therapy. PTs help patients regain mobility and strength and train them in exercises that can further hasten their recovery.

Occupational therapists (OTs) help people in the workplace perform their daily tasks even if they have some disability or injury. They can help workers who spend long hours at a computer or checkout counter to avoid physical and mental stress and avoid a repetitive motion injury. They are trained counselors and often work with PTs to help workers recover from illness or injury.

Sports Medicine

Sports medicine involves the coordinated efforts of many different kinds of healthcare providers and specialists. Because sports or exercise injuries can derive from physiological, psychological, or environmental causes, a variety of specialists is needed for prevention, treatment, and rehabilitation of injuries sustained in physical activities. Surgeons, trainers, coaches, physical therapists, psychologists, and other healthcare providers are all involved.

Sports medicine originated in ancient Greece and Rome where athletic training and contests were a part of everyday life. Modern sports medicine dates from 1928

Interacting with Your Physician

- You should choose a physician you trust and in whose medical skills you have complete confidence. Take the time to find a primary care physician who can satisfy your medical needs. He or she should be someone to whom you can openly express your health concerns.

- Clear and open communication between you and your physician is essential. You should understand the nature of your medical problems and the reasons for any tests that are ordered. You should feel free to ask about different treatment options. You are entitled to all the information pertaining to your condition in language you can understand.

- You should feel confident enough to share with your physician any emotional problems you may have or any stress in your life. This information may be important in arriving at an accurate diagnosis and treatment recommendation. If you are upset in your interaction with a physician, the art of healing is not being practiced.

- Before going to a physician's office, try to relax your mind and body by practicing a meditation or image visualization exercise. This will help calm you when you are discussing your problems with the physician.

- Always remember how suggestible your mind is during a medical consultation. What the physician says about your condition can be as important in the healing process as the treatment. If the physician is positive and encouraging, the likelihood of a cure is increased.

- The most difficult but essential discussions you need to have with your healthcare provider are the ones that make you feel embarrassed or ashamed; for example, those surrounding substance abuse problems; sexual and relationship problems and abuse; uncontrolled eating; and excessive stress, anxiety, depression, and other mental health issues. Remember that disclosures with your healthcare provider are confidential, and that not withholding important information is your part of the bargain in being a good patient. Even if your primary care physician is not able to treat your condition, you are likely to be referred to a competent health professional who can. It is crucial that you follow up on recommendations to obtain help. The sooner a problem is addressed, the more likely you are to have a positive outcome and to feel better.

when an Olympic Committee organized the first congress of sports medicine. Today's sports medicine specialties include cardiology, orthopedic surgery, biomechanics, and traumatology, as well as nutrition, drug, and psychological counselors.

Most sports injuries such as abrasions, blisters, and localized tenderness usually are minor and heal without medical attention. However, if they do not heal or if you experience any of the following symptoms, you may need to consult a sports medicine specialist:

- *Comparative weakness:* When one side of the body feels weaker than the other does.
- *Muscle cramps:* A sudden, intense pain caused by a muscle locked in spasm.
- *Numbness:* Loss of sensation in some part of the body; may also be recognized by a tingling or prickling sensation.
- *Reduced range of motion:* Inability to move some part of your body through its normal range of motion.
- *Sprains:* These vary in severity but involve pain, swelling, and torn muscles or ligaments.

Seeing the Doctor

The majority of people who go to a doctor have minor complaints, have come for a routine checkup or follow-up of some chronic problem, or may simply need some kind of reassurance. In general, patients fall into three categories: (1) those who think they are sick and are, (2) those who think they are well but are actually sick, and (3) the "worried well" who are not sick but seek reassurance that they are not sick. This last group may account for as many as half of all patients who are seen by family practice physicians.

Although some physicians encourage annual checkups, most studies show that frequent medical exams for people who are basically healthy are unnecessary. How often you see a physician depends on your personal needs, but many people go to a physician for minor complaints and illnesses that may not require medical attention (**Table 19.2**). Often people are asking more from their doctors than just medicine.

Patient satisfaction with health care usually depends on what occurs in the physician's office. The quality of health care depends to a great degree on the interaction between the physician and the patient. Anxiety about what may be wrong, long waits to see the physician, and a seemingly endless number of tests can contribute to patients' stress. You can increase the chance of a successful encounter with your healthcare provider if you have a clear understanding of what you want to accomplish during your office visit.

Diagnosis is separate and distinct from treatment. In any illness, there are two important choices: first, admitting that you are sick and finding out what is wrong, which is the process of the **diagnosis**; and second, deciding what is the best course of treatment, based on the diagnosis.

TERMS

diagnosis: the cause of a disease or illness as determined by a physician

Table 19.2

The 20 Most Common Reasons for Doctor Visits

One in eight people goes to the doctor without any complaint or symptom.

Rank	Reason	Rank	Reason
1.	Progress visit, not otherwise specified	11.	Knee symptoms
2.	General medical examination	12.	Back symptoms
3.	Postoperative visit	13.	Stomach and abdominal pain, cramps, and spasms
4.	Cough	14.	Gynecological examination
5.	Medication, other and unspecified kinds	15.	Well-baby examination
6.	Hypertension	16.	Shoulder symptoms
7.	Prenatal examination, routine	17.	Low back symptoms
8.	For other and unspecified test results	18.	Types of surgery
9.	Counseling, not otherwise specified	19.	Symptoms referable to throat
10.	Diabetes mellitus	20.	All other reasons

Adapted from Centers for Disease Control and Prevention. (2013). *National ambulatory medical care survey: 2013 summary tables.* Retrieved from http://www.cdc.gov/nchs/data/ahcd/namcs_summary/2013_namcs_web_tables.pdf

For example, suppose you have had a slight pain in your chest and the diagnostic tests indicate that you have partial blockage of a coronary artery. One physician might recommend dietary changes, exercises, and a drug to control the pain. Another physician might insist on immediate surgery to correct the condition. Only by obtaining as much information as possible can you make a decision that feels right to you.

Hospitals

At some time in your life you will likely need to use a healthcare facility, whether a hospital for planned surgery, a birthing center, an emergency room, or, as you, your parents, or friends become older, nursing home facilities. To make wise decisions concerning healthcare facilities, it is important to understand the types of facilities available and whether they meet your needs.

Most Americans will be admitted to a hospital at some time during their lives. For many people the hospital experience is confusing and frightening. To cope with this unpleasant reality, one should understand a hospital patient's rights.

On admission to a hospital, a patient is required to sign a consent form delegating all decisions regarding his or her care to the hospital and physicians. In most instances, physicians obtain informed consent for any invasive procedure, either diagnostic or therapeutic, before

How Does Your Hospital Rate?

Use this list of organizations to find ratings of hospitals on a number of criteria.

Organization	Website
Consumer Reports magazine	http://www.consumerreports.org/health/hospitals/ratings
Medicare	http://www.medicare.gov/hospitalcompare
Hospital Inspections	http://www.hospitalinspections.org
The Joint Commission	http://www.qualitycheck.org/
The Leapfrog Group	http://www.hospitalsafetygrade.org
U.S. News and World Report	http://www.health.usnews.com/besthospitals/rankings

proceeding. But the amount of information that is given to the patient and how well a patient understands the proposed treatment usually depend on many factors that affect communication between the patient and the physician. The American Hospital Association publishes *The Patient Care Partnership* to describe the situations and questions most often encountered by hospital patients (https://www.aha.org/advocacy-issues/communicatingpts/pt-care-partnership.shtml). Ask for this when in a hospital.

The most frustrating and anxiety-producing situations for a patient are not understanding what is going to happen and, even worse, not knowing what is happening while being subjected to unfamiliar and uncomfortable procedures. Except in the case of a life-threatening emergency that demands immediate action, you have the right to be fully informed of all medical procedures and the reasons for them. As a patient, you have the responsibility for deciding what you want done. Once you have made that decision, you should understand how to cooperate fully with the healthcare team to gain the most benefit.

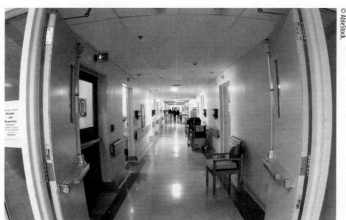

For many people, the hospital is an impersonal and confusing place. Developing good communication with healthcare providers and knowing your rights as a consumer can help combat those feelings.

Hospital Emergency Room (ER)

If you or someone with you thinks you are experiencing a medical emergency, such as a heart attack, stroke, or severe asthma attack, emergency services should be accessed immediately (call 911) for advice or to dispatch emergency medical first responders (emergency medical technicians, or EMTs) in an ambulance or other emergency vehicle. If transport to a hospital emergency room (ER) is required, that facility is bound by law to accept you and to diagnose the problem and initiate treatment, if required, regardless of your ability to pay. If you do not have health insurance, you may be transferred to a public hospital for further care.

Health Insurance

Health insurance is a system intended to pay some or all of the costs of a person's medical, surgical, and hospital care. The basic principle of health insurance is that individuals contribute money regularly (usually monthly) to a fund from which contributors can withdraw money to pay for their medical expenses. In some countries, such as Canada and Mexico, all health insurance is provided by a government-run system paid for by taxes. This is called *single-payer*, *universal*, or *public health insurance*. An alternative to a single-payer system is having each person obtain medical insurance from a private insurance company, similar to buying car insurance. Often private health insurance is obtained through one's employer with the employer bearing the cost. The medical insurance system in the United States and some other countries is a combination of public (Veterans, Medicare, Medicaid) and private (employer, self) funding (**Figure 19.1**).

Many kinds of health insurance are available in the United States depending on a person's age, employment status, medical history, and financial resources. Large

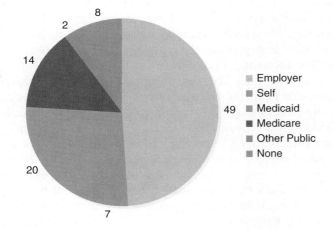

■ **Figure 19.1**

Adult Health Insurance Coverage in U.S., by Percent

Data from Kaiser Family Foundation (2017). Health Insurance Coverage of the Total Population. http://www.kff.org/other/state-indicator/total-population/

employers generally pay for health insurance for their employees and dependents. The U.S. government provides health insurance for federal employees, members of the armed services, and veterans and their dependents. Federal, state, and local governments provide health insurance for the elderly and the disabled. However, the U.S. government does not provide universal health insurance for all citizens as is the case in most other industrialized nations.

Types of Private Health Insurance

Private health insurance plans fall into two broad categories: (1) fee-for-service plans (also called indemnity plans), and (2) some form of **managed care** plan, which includes health maintenance organizations (HMOs), preferred provider organizations (PPOs), and point-of-service (POS) plans. About 90% of all Americans who have health insurance are enrolled in some kind of managed care plan. One of the primary goals of all managed care plans is to control costs of health care. Important features of each health insurance plan are outlined in the following subsections.

Fee-for-Service Plans

Fee-for-service (indemnity) health insurance plans allow a person complete freedom in choosing a physician or a hospital. For a fixed monthly fee, these plans will pay some fraction of the patient's medical costs, usually 80%.

Although most indemnity plans give a person great flexibility in choosing healthcare providers, many restrict the kinds of services they will pay for. Most will not pay for routine physical exams, immunizations, drug abuse programs, and mental health services. Subscribers to these plans must understand what healthcare services are covered and what are not and be sure they fit their needs. Also, paying 20% of the costs may be no hardship for minor healthcare needs. However, if a major illness requires surgery and hospitalization, costs can run into hundreds of thousands of dollars; 20% of such a large sum may be more than most people can afford.

Health Maintenance Organizations

Health maintenance organizations (HMOs) are prepaid health insurance plans that are an alternative to private insurance. HMOs are characterized by four principles

---

TERMS

health insurance: a system intended to pay some or all of the costs of a person's medical, surgical, and hospital care

health maintenance organization (HMO): an organization (either nonprofit or for-profit) of physicians, hospitals, and support staff that provides medical services to members

managed care: systems of health care in which the primary goal is to reduce costs

defined by Congress in the Health Maintenance Organization Assistance Act of 1973: (1) an organized system of health care that accepts the responsibility to provide health care, (2) an agreed-upon set of comprehensive health maintenance and treatment services, (3) a voluntarily enrolled group of people in a specific geographic region, and (4) reimbursement through a prenegotiated and fixed payment schedule on behalf of the enrollee. An example of a large, successful HMO is the Kaiser-Permanente Medical Care Program, in which physicians emphasize early detection of illness and disease prevention.

Some HMOs have experienced criticism. In contracts between physicians and HMOs, physicians may be prohibited from recommending certain expensive procedures that are not covered by the HMO; they also may receive bonuses for not recommending referrals or for other services. Physicians may also be prohibited from disclosing the conditions of their contracts; this so-called gag rule has been severely criticized and has generated a backlash against some HMOs. Although managed health care is well established, some health-care analysts believe that eventually health care will have to evolve into some form of more equitable, universal coverage for all Americans.

Choosing the best HMO for your needs is difficult, especially if choices are limited by your place of employment or financial resources. However, some guidelines may help. Some independent organizations attempt to rate the quality of HMOs. Check carefully what each HMO offers, especially for emergency care or for chronic conditions. If you are enrolled in an HMO, find a physician that you trust and with whom you can communicate freely. If you are not satisfied with a diagnosis or treatment, consult another doctor or ask for a second opinion.

Preferred Provider Organizations

Preferred provider organizations (PPOs) are a combination of the traditional fee-for-service healthcare plan and an HMO. Employers or insurance companies negotiate low fee-for-service rates with selected hospitals and healthcare providers in a specific geographic region. Participants in PPOs must use one of the "preferred" providers if they want their medical bills paid. If a participant opts for care from a nonprovider, he or she will be charged a substantial fee. Group health insurance costs are reduced for both an HMO and PPO in exchange for a guaranteed pool of patients.

Point-of-Service Plans

This is a twist that some HMOs offer. Usually a primary care physician in an HMO is required to refer you to a specialist who is also a member of the same HMO. However, in a point-of-service (POS) plan, you can be referred to a physician who is not a member and still receive coverage. However, if you choose to go to an outside physician without a referral, then you will have to pay all or part of the costs.

Choosing a health insurance plan requires time and thought. Take into account your particular health needs.

Don't be afraid to ask questions. Any plan that includes drug coverage will be considerably more expensive than one that does not include such coverage.

Public, Government-Provided Health Insurance

The U.S. government provides health insurance for about 37% of Americans through three programs: the Veterans Administration, Medicare, and Medicaid, and their various subsidiary programs (Kaiser Family Foundation, 2017). The U.S. government has been involved in supplying health insurance to veterans, but not other citizens, since the birth of the Republic. Today, the U.S. Department of Veterans Affairs, also called the Veterans Administration, or VA, serves 9 million veterans in more than 1,000 clinics and hospitals.

In 1965, the U.S. Congress created Medicare, which provides health insurance for people over age 65, for people under age 65 who are disabled, and for persons with permanent kidney failure. All eligible Medicare beneficiaries, on reaching age 65, automatically are enrolled in Medicare, Part A, which covers hospital costs, rehabilitation in a skilled nursing facility, and hospice care for the terminally ill. Enrollment in Medicare, Part B, is voluntary, but most beneficiaries choose to enroll. Part B pays for 80% (after a $100 deductible) of physicians' services, emergency room visits, laboratory fees, diagnostic tests, and other medical expenses.

In 1966, during its first year, Medicare had 19 million enrollees; by 2015 the number had increased to about 55 million and is expected to jump to 80 million by 2030 (Centers for Medicare and Medicaid Services, 2014). Medicare now insures one in every seven Americans; that ratio will increase to one in every five by 2030. Because of the projected rising costs of Medicare, the federal government is seeking ways to reduce costs. Possibly some benefits will be curtailed or eliminated and the payments to doctors and hospitals may be lowered. Also, given that the average life span has increased dramatically in the past 50 years, it is possible that the eligible age for Medicare will be increased from 65 to 68 or 70.

Also in 1965, Congress established Medicaid, which provides health insurance for people who are economically disadvantaged and cannot pay for medical care. Medicaid provides health insurance for certain poor people in the United States. To be eligible for Medicaid benefits, an individual must be on welfare, have dependent children, or receive supplementary Social Security income for persons who are aged, blind, or disabled. In addition, Medicaid covers nursing home care for many elderly Americans.

Medicaid is a joint federal and state program that, together with the Children's Health Insurance Program, provides health coverage to 75 million, mostly low-income Americans. Medicaid is the single largest source of health insurance coverage in the United States. The federal

Unhealthy Lifestyles Raise Healthcare Costs

Although many factors contribute to high healthcare costs in the United States, some contribute much more than others. If you were asked to make a list, you would probably include physicians' salaries, hospital costs, drug prices, overuse of diagnostic tests, billing fraud, and many others. But you should also include diseases resulting from unhealthy

lifestyles. The Centers for Disease Control and Prevention (CDC) has found that 75% of U.S. healthcare spending goes to treating "preventable" chronic diseases, such as type 2 diabetes and obesity.

Annually, through their tax dollars, U.S. citizens are spending $190 billion treating obesity, $245 billion treating diabetes, and hundreds of billions more on cardiovascular diseases and cancers that were caused by unhealthy lifestyles and behaviors.

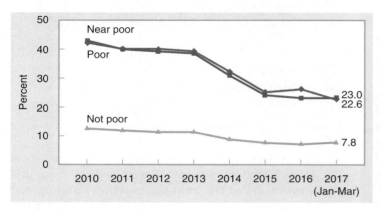

■ Figure 19.2

Percentage of Uninsured Adults by Socioeconomic Status, 2010-2017
The percentage of uninsured adults aged 18-64 declined from 2010 to 2017 because of the Affordable Care Act. The decline is greatest among those categorized as poor and near poor, designated according to the U.S. Census Bureau's determination of the Federal Poverty Level, FPL. Poor = 0-100% of the FPL; near poor = between 100% and 200% of the FPL; not poor = greater than 200% of the FPL. In 2017, the FPL for individuals = $12,060; family of 2, $16,240; family of 4 = $24,600 (complete data at https://www.healthcare.gov/glossary/federal-poverty-level-FPL/).

Data from Cohen R.A. et al. (2017). Health insurance coverage: Early release of estimates from the National Health Interview Survey, January–March 2017. National Center for Health Statistics (www.cdc.gov/nchs/nhis/releases.htm).

government sets minimum standards for eligibility for Medicaid, and all 50 states participate in the Medicaid program to at least that level. However, eligibility for Medicaid benefits varies widely among the states, and each state can determine to what extent it will provide insurance beyond the minimum federal guidelines.

In 2010, Congress passed the Affordable Care Act (ACA) to address a number of weaknesses in the provision of health and medical care in the United States, especially the fact that at the time over 40 million Americans had no medical insurance of any kind. To remedy this, the ACA mandated that every person in the country have health insurance, either through a public plan, employer coverage, or a self-financed individual insurance plan, with the federal government subsidizing the cost for those who could not afford it. Moreover, the ACA extended to the states the option to provide Medicaid coverage to all individuals with incomes less than 138% of the federal poverty level. This is called the Medicaid

Expansion. As of 2017, the ACA was responsible for providing health insurance for over 28.1 million people, many of whom were of low income (Cohen et al., 2017) (**Figure 19.2**).

Healthcare Costs

Why Healthcare Costs Continue to Rise

Anyone who has been to a physician, filled a prescription, paid a health insurance premium, or been admitted to a hospital realizes how expensive medical care is. Many factors contribute to the high cost of health care in the United States: physician salaries and fees, cost of prescription drugs, malpractice insurance, cost of hospital rooms and emergency services, and cost of health insurance. Another significant factor is the aggressive marketing of medical technologies, new drugs, and tests to physicians and also directly to patients. The overzealous use of diagnostic technologies distinguishes U.S. medical care from that in other major industrialized countries. The United States leads the world in organ and bone marrow transplants, coronary artery bypass surgeries, and **magnetic resonance imaging (MRI)** use. Although MRI is an important diagnostic tool for many medical problems, ownership of an expensive MRI machine by a hospital demands frequent use to pay for it, even if not warranted. Also, to stay competitive, almost every hospital must have one.

Another reason for high healthcare costs is waste in a variety of forms (Gawande, 2015). The Institute of Medicine (2013) estimates that 31% of healthcare dollars (about $765 billion) is wasted (**Figure 19.3**). About half of the wasted money is lost to inflated charges,

■TERMS■

magnetic resonance imaging (MRI): use of a strong magnetic field to produce images of internal parts of the body; especially useful for soft tissues

preferred provider organization (PPO): physicians who belong to the organization provide medical care at reduced costs that are negotiated by the organization

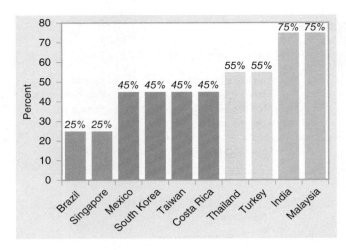

■ Figure 19.3

Sources of Financial Waste in U.S. Health Care (Billions of Dollars Per year)
Data from Institute of Medicine (IOM). 2013. Best Care at Lower Cost. Washington, DC: National Academies Press.

■ Figure 19.4

Average Cost of Medical Procedures of Most-Traveled Destinations Compared to the United States
Data from Patients Beyond Borders. (2017). *Medical tourism statistics and facts.* Retrieved from http://www.patientsbeyondborders.com/medical-tourismstatistics -facts

administrative costs, and fraud. The greatest waste comes from unnecessary healthcare services, with people being unnecessarily treated and prescribed drugs they do not need. Although the extent and sources of healthcare financial waste have been identified, no solution has yet been adopted.

Other factors contributing to rising healthcare costs are unhealthy lifestyles and an aging population. The epidemic of obesity contributes to a bevy of chronic diseases, the most notable being type 2 diabetes. Diseases caused by smoking or alcohol are costly and preventable in principle. And, as the population ages, older Americans acquire chronic ailments that require more medical attention, including costly drugs and surgery.

Medical Tourism

Because of the extraordinarily high cost of medical and dental procedures in the United States, 1.4 million *medical tourists* now seek treatment in other countries, combining travel, vacation, and health care in one trip. Thailand, India, Argentina, Costa Rica, Mexico, Israel, South Korea, and other countries are frequent destinations for medical tourists. A comparison of prices for some common surgeries in the United States and in four other countries shows why medical tourism has become so popular (**Figure 19.4**).

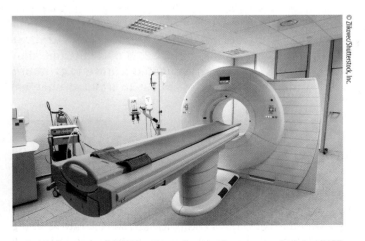

Computed tomographic (CT) scans and magnetic resonance imaging (MRI) help physicians make the correct diagnosis of an injury or disease.

Many hospitals overseas are accredited by a U.S. organization called the Joint Commission International (www.jointcommissioninternational.com). This nonprofit agency checks hospitals every 3 years and uses the same standards used to accredit American hospitals. Also, many surgeons working overseas have been *board certified*, which means that their qualifications are the same as surgeons working in U.S. hospitals. The American Board of Medical Specialties (www.abms.org) lists thousands of surgeons working in other countries who are board certified.

All medical procedures entail risks, whether done in the United States or other countries. Patients should do as much research as possible by checking sites on the Internet, such as the Centers for Disease Control (https://cdc.gov/features/medicaltourism /index.htm), and talking with patients who have undergone procedures overseas. It is important to ask questions about follow-up care. Communicate with the overseas surgeon if possible. Sometimes it is wise to work with an overseas travel company that can make all of the medical arrangements.

Healthcare Costs in Other Countries

Other industrialized nations, such as Canada, Great Britain, France, Germany, and Japan, spend about half as much as the United States on healthcare costs and still manage to provide health insurance for all of their citizens (**Table 19.3**). Some claim that the United States has the best health care in the world, which justifies the high cost. This may be true if you are a kidney dialysis patient or need a heart transplant. But the United States also has a lower life expectancy and a higher infant mortality rate than do many other industrialized countries.

Table 19.3

Per Capita Medical Care Spending in Developed Countries

Country	Per capita spending in U.S. dollars
United States	9,892
Switzerland	7,919
Norway	6,647
Germany	5,550
Sweden	5,487
Australia	4,708
Canada	4,643
France	4,600
Japan	4,519
United Kingdom	4,192
Italy	3,391
Israel	2,775
Mexico	1,080

Data from Organisation for Economic Co-operation and Development (OECD). (2016). Total expenditure on health per capita in 2016. Retrieved from https://data.oecd.org/healthres/health-spending.htm

Table 19.4

Health Status Rank of the United States Among 11 Developed Countries

Health factor		U.S. rank
Effective care	Treatment and prevention	3
Safe care	Harmful medical errors	7
Coordinated care	Providers work as a team	6
Patient-centered care	Heeding patient's needs and preferences	4
Cost-related access problems	Cost impedes access to care	11
Timeliness of care	Wait time for care	5
Efficiency	Administrative and legal costs	11
Equity	Gender, ethnicity, geographic location, SES*	11
Healthy lives	Infant mortality; healthy life expectancy	11
Overall		11

*SES, socioeconomic status.

Data from Davis, K., et al. (2014). *Mirror, mirror on the wall, 2014 update: How the U.S. health care system compares internationally.* Retrieved from http://www.commonwealthfund.org/publications/fund-reports/2014/jun/mirror-mirror

Some critics of U.S. health care advocate adopting Canada's model to provide universal health care for all citizens. There are arguments for and against this position. The most compelling reason is to provide everyone with basic health care. However, under the Canadian system, people must wait for some diagnostic tests and many kinds of elective surgery. People with conditions that are not immediately life threatening, such as colon cancer, usually wait a month or more for recommended treatment and surgery.

Many Canadian doctors opt to practice in the United States because they can earn more money; this creates a shortage of surgeons and other medical specialists in Canada. Also, Canada is experiencing a severe physician shortage partly because physicians are not allowed to have a private practice outside of the National Health Care system.

Canada saves considerable money because its healthcare administration costs are much less than administration costs in the United States. On average, the United States spends $752 more annually per citizen in administrative costs for health care than is spent in Canada.

Researchers from Johns Hopkins University compared the health systems of 11 developed countries (Davis et al., 2014). Comparative factors included healthcare quality, access, efficiency, equity, health status, and infant mortality. Their principal findings were that the United Kingdom ranked first among the 11 countries in providing quality heathcare outcomes. And despite the fact that it spends much more money per capita on health care than any of the 11 countries, the United States ranked last overall (**Table 19.4**).

Ranking U.S. health care seventh in safety, the data indicate that efforts to improve patient safety, implemented by Congress in 2005, can be strengthened. Each year, between 250,000 Americans die from medical errors in hospitals (Makary & Daniel, 2016). Approximately half of these deaths are preventable. Hospital-based medical errors are the third leading cause of death in the United States.

The data indicate that access to health care in the United States can be problematic for certain social groups and income levels. The United States is the only country of the 11 that does not provide a single-payer system of universal health care. Opponents of universal health care often argue that government-run systems engender long wait times for care. The data from the study show that wait times in the United States for primary care tend to be the same as in other countries. However, wait times for specialist care, which may or may not be immediately necessary, tend to be short compared to in other countries.

Almost all medical experts agree that the quality of U.S. health care needs to be improved. It makes no sense that receiving health care carries the same risk of death that bungee jumping and mountain climbing do (about 100 deaths per 100,000 encounters). The U.S. Centers for Medicare and Medicaid Services provides information on how well hospitals care for patients with certain medical conditions or surgical procedures as well as results from a survey of patients about the quality of care they received during recent hospital stays. Information on the quality of care hospitals provide is available at https://medicare.gov/hospitalcompare/search.htm.

Healthcare Disparities

Most Americans want for themselves and their families affordable, efficient, and high-quality medical care. One major factor in achieving these desires is taking personal responsibility for one's own health and the health of family members. Another major factor is reducing as much as possible health disparities among social groups. *Health disparity* generally refers to a higher burden of illness, injury, disability, or mortality experienced by one population group relative to another group. *Healthcare disparity* typically refers to differences between groups in health coverage, access to care, and quality of care.

Ample research has shown that health disparities adversely affect groups of people who have systematically experienced greater obstacles to health based on their race or ethnicity; religion; socioeconomic status; education, gender; age; mental health; cognitive, sensory, or physical disability; sexual orientation or gender identity; geographic location; or other characteristics historically linked to discrimination or exclusion. Other determinants of health disparities include availability and access to a high-quality education, nutritious food, decent and safe housing, affordable and reliable public transportation, culturally sensitive healthcare providers, clean water and nonpolluted air, and access to affordable quality health care.

The effects of race and sex on how long someone lives is an example of a health disparity. In 2016, average life expectancy at birth in the United States was 79.8 years. Among white females, life expectancy at birth was 82 years, for African American females, 78.8 years; for white males, 77.5 years; and for African American males, 72.5 years (**Figure 19.5**). There also are health disparities related to infectious diseases and diseases of the immune system. Approximately 2 million Hispanics/Latinos in the United States have asthma, and Puerto Rican Americans have almost three times the asthma rate of the overall Hispanic population. African Americans are diagnosed with asthma at a 28% higher rate than whites. Systemic lupus erythematosus is two to three times more common among African American women than among white women. African Americans are at greater risk than whites for diabetes, chronic kidney disease, and cardiovascular disease. About 80% of all tuberculosis cases in the United States occur in racial and ethnic minorities, particularly Hispanics, Asians, and African Americans.

> At one time I had ambitions, but I had them removed by a doctor in Buffalo.
>
> *Tom Waits*

Organ Transplants

Most major human organs now can be transplanted, including kidney, liver, heart, lung, and pancreas, as well as eye and skin tissues. Organs can be transplanted from cadavers (people who have died suddenly, usually in accidents) and from living donors as well. About 34,000 Americans receive organ transplants each year; however, about 125,000 individuals seek them.

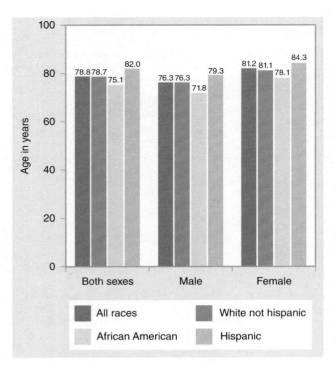

■ **Figure 19.5**

Racial Differences in Life Expectancy at Birth in the United States in 2015

Data from Centers for Disease Control and Prevention, 2016 *Health, United States,* Table 15. Retrieved from https://cdc.gov/nchs/hus/contents2016.htm#015

More than 71,000 people in the United States have donated an organ to another person, often a family member. Kidney donations are the most frequent because everyone has two kidneys, and one kidney can be donated without seriously affecting the donor—providing the remaining kidney continues to function normally. So, there is always an unknown element of risk. If the kidney donor is a young person, in his or her 20s or 30s, for example, the donor may lose the remaining kidney to infection or injury later in life and have to go on a waiting list for a kidney transplant. Because of this possibility, some hospital transplant centers prefer to transplant organs from older persons, but this also means the donor is at additional risk from the transplantation procedure, especially if she or he is not in the best of health.

No federal guidelines or state laws regulate who can donate and who can receive an organ. Each hospital or organ transplant center makes its own rules. Critics of live organ transplants argue that, because of the lack of official guidelines or standards, a person really cannot give informed consent. For example, no data are kept on the subsequent health or medical problems of living donors. Some hospital records indicate that 15% to 67% of live liver donors experience infections or other complications following the transplantation. But there are no laws requiring that records be kept on the fate of live donors. Some live donors feel that they were inadequately informed before the donation and received insufficient medical care afterward.

Because there are not nearly enough cadaver donors available to meet the burgeoning demand from people with failing organs, live donors will continue to play an important role. A parent at age 70 may be quite comfortable donating a kidney to save a child. But a young person considering donating an organ to save a much older person should carefully contemplate the risks and benefits to both parties. Each potential live donor presents a unique situation that can be resolved only by discussions among everyone involved, including doctors, spouses, family members, and others who may be affected by the decision.

Medicalization of Human Behaviors and Traits

Medicalization refers to medical consideration of conditions, behaviors, or traits that generally were not regarded as illnesses or medical problems. Once medicalized, these conditions are deemed to require treatment of some kind, such as psychotherapy, medication, or surgery. Once a condition has been medicalized, payment to doctors by health insurers is permissible.

The first significant human behavior to be medicalized was homosexuality (Conrad, 2007). For years homosexuality was stigmatized in the United States and other countries as a "disease" that required treatment with drugs, psychotherapy, and other methods. Homosexuality was officially demedicalized in the United States in the 1970s and is now viewed as a normal variation in a human trait, just as variation exists in intelligence and athletic ability. But medicalization of other human behaviors, conditions, and traits has increased markedly in recent years.

For centuries, people considered personal choice to be the reason for smoking tobacco and drinking alcohol, even to the point of undesirable health and personal consequences. Although many still hold this view, in recent decades both smoking and the overuse of alcohol have been medicalized; smokers and heavy drinkers now are encouraged to seek treatments for these unhealthy behaviors.

Drug companies have been quick to see the potential profit in medicalizing human conditions and traits. For years human growth hormone (hGH) was in short supply, but now it is available in unlimited amounts thanks to modern biotechnology. Children who are at the low end of the average distribution in height are now diagnosed with "idiopathic short stature" and are eligible to be treated with injections of hGH for years, provided that their parents can afford the expense of such injections. Children who are completely normal thus become stigmatized by the medicalization of their shortness. The psychological harm that is done to these children may far outweigh the maximum of 2 inches in height that they may gain from the treatments.

Drug companies have made enormous profits from the medicalization of "male aging problems" such as erection problems and baldness. These conditions and their drug solutions are presented daily to TV viewers as permitted by direct-to-consumer advertising. The advertising of prescription drugs directly to consumers is banned in all countries except for the United States.

Hope Helps Healing and Recovery

When faced with a serious health problem such as cancer or diabetes, signs of dementia, or disability from an accident, individuals tend to react with anger, despair, depression, or even thoughts of suicide. Confronting a serious health issue requires courage as well as competent intervention by physicians and other healthcare professionals. Improving the chances of recovery and restoring health requires active participation in all aspects of the care. To effectively assist in recovery requires dealing with one's personal mental state to become positive and hopeful about recovery.

Any form of treatment is substantially helped by a patient's hope for success (Harris & DeAngelis, 2008). We all know someone who has fully recovered from cancer or who returned to full activity after a serious accident. Athletes who are strongly motivated to recover from what appears initially to be a career-ending injury often recover to compete again. The body and mind are capable of remarkable feats of healing when aided by hope and a positive attitude. At first, hope may have an element of pretense, but as one small improvement follows another, the hope becomes real and so does the healing. Those who do not give up usually get up.

Active, inattentive children in classrooms are often diagnosed with attention deficit hyperactivity disorder (ADHD) and are treated with stimulant drugs that help many of them to quiet down. Parents and teachers benefit from the calmer home and classroom environments. The diagnosis of ADHD has been extended to older populations who are said to suffer from "adult ADHD," which expands the potential for drug therapy.

Obesity is a serious health problem for a large segment of the American population. Most often, obesity results from overeating and a lack of physical activity. The causes of obesity are rooted in individual lifestyle choices, social forces that promote sedentary living, and the mega-industrialization of the food supply that provides products for consumption that increase the risk of overweight and obesity. Because changing lifestyle, social, and economic forces is difficult, obesity has been medicalized. Pharmaceutical researchers are competing to find drugs that can stop weight gain or promote weight loss. Increasingly, the recommended medical treatment for obesity is bariatric surgery, which removes a portion of the stomach to prevent a person from overeating.

Individuals are still free to take responsibility for their health. They do not have to accept being medicalized for

TERMS

medicalization: medical treatment of conditions, behaviors, or traits that generally were not regarded as illnesses or medical problems

some behavior or condition that requires them to be treated. We urge all of our readers to accept responsibility for their health and to adopt behaviors and attitudes that foster health and well-being.

Precision Medicine

Much of current medical care is based on the premise that every patient with a particular set of symptoms or diagnosis should get the same treatment; that is, one that has been shown in rigorous testing to be effective in a large number of people. **Precision medicine** (also called *personalized medicine*) is different. Precision medicine is based on the premise that an individual's health and disease can be managed based on that person's unique characteristics, including, and especially, his or her genetic makeup. Precision medicine has become especially helpful in treating certain cancers. Precision medicine is possible because thousands of specific mutations (changes in genes) have been identified that are causally involved with specific diseases. Thus, a patient's DNA can be examined for disease-causing changes and medicine can be offered for that specific situation, particularly cancers. For example, a drug is now available that can control the symptoms of a very specific type of cystic fibrosis, a serious inherited condition that reduces lung function. However, only about 4% of cystic fibrosis patients have the specific type that responds to the drug; the other 96% do not benefit. Precision medicine means that each cystic fibrosis patient must be tested to determine if she or he carries the specific genetic mutation whose deleterious effects can be reversed by the drug.

In 1988, a drug called *herceptin* was approved for treating breast cancer. However, it was found to be effective in less than one third of women with breast cancer. Ultimately it was determined that herceptin was effective only in cases in which the cancer was caused by a particular gene, called *HER2*. Physicians treating breast cancer patients can use the techniques of precision medicine to determine if tumors in a breast cancer patient carry the *HER2* gene and will respond positively to herceptin.

Colorectal cancer is caused by many different mutations. A drug called *Vectibix* (panitumumab) can be effective in treating seven types of colorectal cancer; different drugs must be used for other colorectal cancer patients. The anticancer drug Keytruda (pembrolizumab) is intended for people who carry a specific genetic abnormality that prevents cells from repairing damage to DNA (Garber, 2017). When cancer in just about any tissue arises, this genetic abnormality, which is present in about 1% of people, can be identified by genetic testing and the antitumor drug pembrolizumab can be prescribed.

Cosmetic Surgery

For people who can afford it, **cosmetic surgery** is used to alter physical appearance. In 2015, about 12 million cosmetic surgical and nonsurgical procedures were performed in the United States (**Table 19.5**). In addition to

Table 19.5	
Most Frequent Cosmetic Surgeries in the United States, 2012	
Procedure	Number
Minimally Invasive	
Botulinum toxin type A	6.7 million
Soft tissue fillers	2.4 million
Chemical peel	1.3 million
Laser hair removal	1.1 million
Microdermabrasion	800,000
Cosmetic Surgical	
Breast augmentation	280,000
Nose reshaping	218,000
Eyelid surgery	203,000
Liposuction	222,000
Tummy tuck	128,000

Data from American Society of Plastic Surgeons. (2016). 2015 Plastic surgery statistics report. Retrieved from http://www.plasticsurgery.org/news/press-releases/new-statistics-reflect-the-changing-face-of-plastic-surgery.

cosmetic surgeries, about 5.2 million reconstructive plastic surgical procedures were performed. Women received 91% of all cosmetic surgeries, and men the remainder. Botox injections to remove wrinkles and age lines on the face are the most popular nonsurgical procedures among both men and women.

Large HMOs such as Kaiser and other health insurance organizations are now offering cosmetic surgery to their members for a fee, usually discounted from fees charged by private physicians. Cosmetic surgery is seen as a way to make money that can finance other medical services. Dermatologists and plastic surgeons perform the majority of the cosmetic surgeries, but many physicians now offer botox and collagen injections to their patients. As the population continues to age, it is anticipated that the boom in cosmetic surgeries will also grow.

Most cosmetic surgeries are safe, especially if performed by a board-certified physician. However, complications such as infections, scarring, and undesirable outcomes also occur. Liposuction is one of the more popular procedures. It is used to remove subcutaneous fat from various parts of the body to sculpt it into a more attractive shape. A variety of complications can result from liposuction, some of which can be serious or fatal, so it is not a procedure to undergo lightly and without considerable investigation of possible undesirable outcomes.

TERMS

cosmetic surgery: surgery performed not for any medical condition but solely to enhance appearance or correct visible effects of aging

precision (personalized) medicine: tailoring treatments to the genetic makeup of individual patients

Critical Thinking About Health

1. Congressman John Sockittoim from Arkansas has been working on a bill to solve the Medicare financial crisis. In trying to generate more funds for Medicare and Medicaid, he has proposed a 10% tax on all cosmetic surgeries that are not done out of medical necessity (such as breast reconstruction after mastectomy) but solely for enhancing physical appearance. He argues that people who can afford cosmetic surgery can also afford to support the basic medical needs of people less fortunate. Decide whether you approve or disapprove of this tax and discuss your reasons.

2. Have you ever been hospitalized for an illness or injury? Describe the condition that caused you to be hospitalized, and discuss the care and tests that you experienced in the hospital. What things were the most positive and healing in the hospital? What things were the most distressing and unhealthy about your hospital experience? Suggest ways (based on your experience) that hospitals might improve the care they provide to patients.

3. The Medicare program, like the Social Security program, will face a fiscal crisis in the near future. The money that is collected by these two federal programs will not cover their costs unless they are restructured. Congress has proposed a new Medicare system for retired persons in which each worker would be required to put away a percentage of earnings during working years to pay for medical needs after retirement. This means that workers would now have to contribute additional money for future health care. Discuss whether you think this is the proper solution to solve Medicare's financial problems. Can you propose any other alternatives to provide the Medicare program with the money that is needed and that you think would be fair? Or do you think the federal government should not be involved in providing health care for retired persons at all?

4. Joe Windam is in the hospital with liver failure. Joe is only 32 years old but has been a heavy drinker most of his life, just like his father. He also contracted a hepatitis C infection several years ago that has contributed to his liver disease. Joe has been out of work for over a year and does not have any health insurance. The only hope that Joe has is a liver transplant; without a new liver, Joe will probably die in a few months. Do you think Joe should be given a high priority for a liver transplant because of his young age? Who should pay the several hundred thousand dollars in hospital and doctor bills? How should the priority for liver transplants be assigned, since there are not enough livers available for all the patients who need them?

Chapter Summary and Highlights

Chapter Summary

The Affordable Care Act (ACA) was designed to help the more than 40 million uninsured Americans pay for health care through insurance. ACA has been popular with millions of uninsured Americans, especially those with preexisting conditions, who previously could not obtain health insurance. Under ACA, many low- and moderate-income Americans receive subsidies from the federal government to help pay for their health insurance. However, for a variety of reasons, many political and having more to do with dislike of President Obama than health care, ACA has also been unpopular with some Americans. Nearly all lawmakers agree that the original version of the ACA will be altered to fix problems and make programs run smoother. Those who dislike the ACA periodically challenge parts or all of the law with the goal of overturning it. Should any of these challenges be successful, it is possible that millions of Americans will, once again, be unable to afford health insurance.

The United States spends twice as much money on health care per citizen compared to any other industrialized country in the world. Most other countries guarantee comprehensive health care for all of their citizens. The only option a person without health insurance has in the United States is to go to a hospital emergency room (ER), where doctors are required by law to diagnose and treat any person regardless of ability to pay. However, once a person is discharged from the ER, he or she does not have access to follow-up care and may have to return repeatedly to the ER. America still has a long way to go to provide affordable, comprehensive health care to all citizens and also to a large noncitizen population.

Everyone requires medical care at some time in their lives. Be prepared with questions when you go to see a doctor and make sure you understand what you need to do to recover. Also, remember that a diagnosis is just one aspect of the patient–physician interaction and treatment options are distinct from the diagnosis. The doctor may recommend surgery for a torn ligament, but you may opt for physical therapy and time to heal. Be wary of unnecessary tests and procedures. Imaging machines are very costly, so hospitals and physicians need to use them often to pay for them. Always remember that *prevention* is often the best medicine. Immunizations prevent many infections; accidents can be prevented by not taking unwarranted risks and paying attention to what you are doing; overweight and obesity can be prevented by not eating processed foods and sugar-laden sweets and sodas and increasing activity level. Daily vigorous movement helps prevent many chronic illnesses.

Highlights

- Everyone needs medical care at some time in his or her life. Knowing what to ask and what to expect from your physician and the healthcare system is essential.
- The physician's responsibility is to find the cause and oversee treatment of illness. The patient's responsibility is working in partnership with the healthcare provider, sharing in healthcare decision making, and becoming skilled at obtaining health care.
- Besides physicians, there are a variety of healthcare specialists, some of whom work in conjunction with a person's primary care physician and some of whom work independently, often through physician referral.
- Admission to a hospital is often an unsettling experience. Patients should be aware of their rights and ask questions that will ease their concerns and reduce errors.
- Health care is increasingly provided by large organizations of physicians and hospitals, called preferred provider organizations or health maintenance organizations.
- The costs of medical care in the United States have grown so rapidly that some form of healthcare reform is needed. Forty-six million Americans lack health insurance and access to health care.

- The Affordable Care Act (ACA), passed by Congress in 2010, is intended to provide all U.S. citizens with health insurance.
- Drug, hospital, and medical errors account for thousands of deaths in the United States each year. Medical errors are the eighth leading cause of death.
- Healthcare providers include physicians, nurses, physical therapists, occupational therapists, physician assistants, and specialists in sports-related injuries.
- Disparities in health care exist depending on a patient's sex, race, ethnic origin, or geographical location in the country.
- Organ transplants from live donors are becoming more frequent and pose problems for donors and recipients.
- Medicalization of human behaviors such as smoking, drinking, and overeating has transferred responsibility for the resulting health problems from individuals to physicians. The normal human trait of short stature also has been medicalized.
- Millions of Americans spend billions of dollars each year on various kinds of surgical and nonsurgical cosmetic procedures to improve appearance.

For Your Health

For your personal health records and to share with your healthcare providers, complete the "My Medical History" questionnaire in the Workbook. Use the other exercises for this chapter in the Workbook to sharpen your skills as a healthcare consumer.

References

Blumberg, A., & Davidson, A. (2009). Accidents of history created the U.S. health system. National Public Radio. Retrieved from https://www.npr.org/templates/story/story.php?storyId=114045132

Centers for Disease Control and Prevention. (2013). *National ambulatory medical care survey: 2013 summary tables.* Retrieved from http://www.cdc.gov/nchs/data/ahcd/names_summary/2013_names_web_tables.pdf

Centers for Medicare and Medicaid Services. (2014). *2014 Annual Report of the Federal Hospital Insurance and Federal Supplementary Insurance Trust Funds.* Retrieved from http://www.cms.gov/Research-Statistics-Data-and-Systems/Statistics-Trends-and-Reports/ReportsTrustFunds/downloads/tr2014.pdf

Charo, R. A. (2005). The celestial fire of conscience—refusing to deliver medical care. *New England Journal of Medicine, 352,* 2471–2472.

Cohen R. A., et al. (2017). Health insurance coverage: Early release of estimates from the National Health Interview Survey, January–March 2017. National Center for Health Statistics. Retrieved from https://www.cdc.gov/nchs/nhis/releases.htm

Combs, M. P., et al. (2011). Conscientious refusals to refer: Findings from a national physician survey. *Journal of Medical Ethics, 37,* 397–401.

Conrad, P. (2007). *The medicalization of society: On the transformation of human conditions into treatable disorders.* Baltimore: Johns Hopkins University Press.

Davis, K., et al. (2014). *Mirror, mirror on the wall, 2014 update: How the U.S. healthcare system compares internationally.* Retrieved from http://www.commonwealthfund.org/publications/fund-reports/2014/jun/mirror-mirror

Garber, K. (2017). In a major shift, cancer drugs go "tissue-agonistic." *Science, 356,* 1111–1112.

Gawande, A. (2015, May 11). Overkill. *The New Yorker,* 42–53.

Harris, J. C., & DeAngelis, C. D. (2008). The power of hope. *Journal of the American Medical Association, 300,* 2919–2920.

Institute of Medicine. (2013). *Best care at lower cost.* Washington, DC: National Academies Press.

Kaiser Family Foundation. (2017). Health insurance coverage of the total population. Retrieved from http://www.kff.org/other/state-indicator/total-population/

Makary, M. A., & Daniel, M. (2016). Medical error—the third leading cause of death in the U.S. *BMJ, 353.* doi: https://doi.org/10.1136/bmj.i2139

Merck Manual, Consumer Version. (2017). Retrieved from http://www.merckmanuals.com/en-ca/home

Patients Beyond Borders. (2017). *Medical tourism statistics and facts.* Retrieved from http://www.patientsbeyondborders.com/medical-tourism-statistics-facts

Suggested Readings

Annas, G. J. (2004). *The rights of patients: The authoritative ACLU guide to the rights of patients.* Carbondale: Southern Illinois University Press. The country's foremost expert on medical ethics describes tragic cases and the need for patients to exercise their rights as patients.

Begley, S. (2011, July). The *best* medicine. *Scientific American*, 50–55. With so many drugs available, some cheap and some costly, how do doctors know what to prescribe? This article explains how research can determine what is the *best* medicine.

Begley, S. (2011, August 22 & 29). The one word that can save your life. *Newsweek*, 30–35. Discusses why many widely used diagnostic tests and procedures are not only unnecessary in most cases, but also dangerous.

Callahan, D. (2009). *Taming the beloved beast? How medical technology costs are destroying our healthcare system.* Princeton, NJ: Princeton University Press. More and more medical technology will lead to unsustainable cost increases and destroy the healthcare system.

Gawande, A. (2017). *Being mortal.* New York: Picador. A surgeon and professor at Harvard Medical School examines the frequently deleterious and inhumane consequences of reliance on a medical approach to end-of-life issues. Chosen "Best Book of the Year" by *The Washington Post, The New York Times Book Review,* NPR, and *Chicago Tribune*.

Gawande. A. (2017, January 23). Tell me where it hurts. *The New Yorker*, 36–45. Renowned physician and professor at Harvard Medical School and spokesperson for healthcare reform discusses how America's medical system and health insurance need to change.

Groopman, J. (2003, August 11). Sick with worry. *The New Yorker*, 28–34. An article that describes the large number of patients who have nothing wrong but who demand treatment.

Groopman, J. (2007, January 29). What's the trouble? *The New Yorker*, 36–41. An article describing how difficult it is sometimes for a doctor to arrive at the correct medical diagnosis.

Kaiser Family Foundation. (2012). *Focus on health care disparities.* Retrieved from http://kaiserfamilyfoundation.files .wordpress.com/2013/01/8396.pdf. Provides an introductory overview of health and healthcare disparities, including what disparities are and why they matter, the status of disparities today, and key efforts to address disparities, including provisions in the Affordable Care Act (ACA).

Merck Manual Consumer Edition (2018). A very helpful guide to understanding diseases and drugs. Retrieved from https://www.merckmanuals.com

Mukherjee, S. (2015). *The laws of medicine: Field notes from an uncertain science.* New York: TED Books. A physician and distinguished author of several highly acclaimed science books explains why the practice of medicine is still both an art and a science. Successfully treating many of today's health problems requires intuition as well as modern medical technology.

Sapolsky, R. (2005, December). Sick of poverty. *Scientific American*, 93–99. An article showing that poverty affects not only quality of life but length of life also.

Starr, P. (2011). *Remedy and reaction: The peculiar American struggle over healthcare reform.* New Haven, CT: Yale University Press. This book is a history of how and why ideological issues have affected the past century of rancorous debate on health insurance in the United States.

Recommended Websites

A Consumer Guide for Getting and Keeping Health Insurance
Guidelines for all states and the District of Columbia, from the Georgetown University Health Policy Institute.

Guide to Health Insurance
Discusses the basic forms of health coverage and includes a checklist to help compare plans.

Kaiser Family Foundation
Provides facts, analysis, and explanation on health policy issues to policymakers, the media, and the public.

Medicare
The U.S. government's health insurance program for seniors and persons with disabilities.

Organ Donors
Living Donors Online provides information for prospective organ donors.

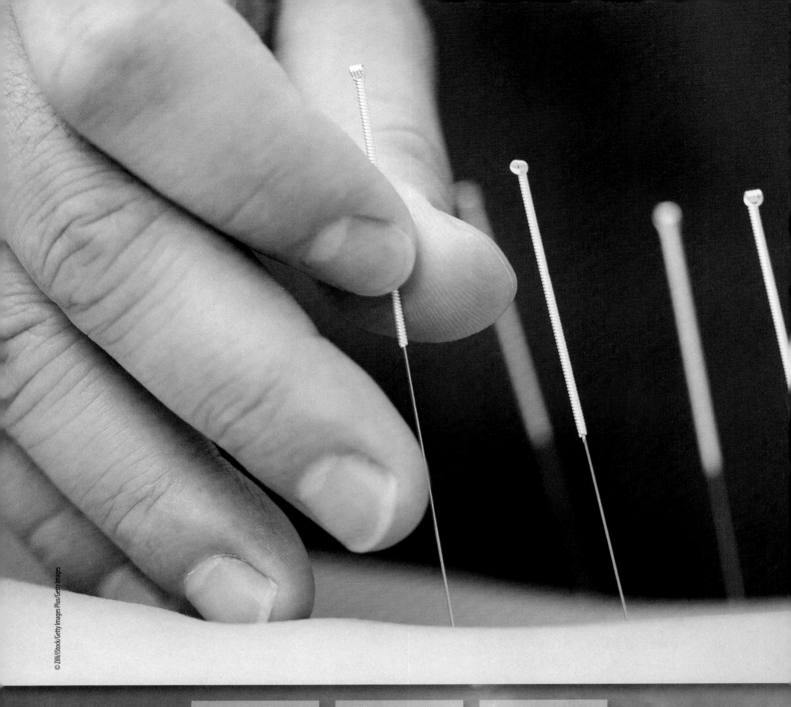

© Zilli/iStock/Getty Images Plus/Getty Images

Health Tips

Treating a Headache with Acupressure

Vitamin Supplements Are Not Always Safe

Dollars & Health Sense

Marketing "Miracle" Health Juices

Wellness Guide

Whole-Body Cryotherapy: No Cold, Hard Facts

CHAPTER 20

Exploring Alternative Medicines

Learning Objectives

1. Describe the main differences between modern medical care and alternative medicines.

2. Define the four categories of alternative medicines.

3. Discuss the philosophy and method of treatment in acupuncture, chiropractic, herbal medicine, and homeopathy.

4. Discuss the reasons why some people choose an alternative medicine in addition to, or instead of, modern medicine.

5. List reasons why herbal remedies may be dangerous.

6. Explain how biomagnetic therapy might help certain health problems.

7. Explain how you can protect yourself from being victimized by health fraud.

Although most people in the United States elect to visit a physician when they are sick, many seek alternatives to modern medicine for a variety of reasons. One important reason is cultural; persons raised in cultures that rely on herbal remedies and tribal healers to treat sickness often continue to use their own remedies even if they move to another country.

Some people who use **alternative medicine** do so because Western, scientific medicine has failed to relieve their suffering or cannot cure their disease. For example, people with terminal cancer for which no further treatments are available will often turn to some alternative medicine that offers hope, however faint, for prolonging life. People with chronic diseases such as arthritis, chronic fatigue syndrome, depression, or persistent allergies who do not respond satisfactorily to medical treatments often turn to alternative medicines for relief.

> You cannot teach a person anything. You can only help him to find it for himself.
>
> *Galileo*

Some surveys indicate that one-third to one-half of patients with serious medical problems use some form of alternative medicine in addition to conventional treatment. The alternative medicines that people use most frequently are herbal remedies, massage, megavitamin therapy, energy healing, and homeopathy. Some physicians in the United States have begun to address their patients' needs and preferences for alternative medicines. If an alternative medicine is used in conjunction with a conventional treatment, it is referred to as **complementary medicine** to indicate that both treatments complement one another. For example, a person with lower back pain might receive medications for pain and muscle relaxation as well as referral to a chiropractor or a massage therapist. A few doctors prescribe homeopathic remedies as well as prescription drugs for a variety of symptoms.

Sometimes the terms *complementary medicine* and *alternative medicine* are used interchangeably. Because many newly certified physicians incorporate some alternative medicines in their practices, these physicians are said to practice **integrative medicine**. Physicians practicing integrative medicine can offer patients advice on herbs, vitamins, homeopathic remedies, and many other alternative medicines. Today, many of the most prestigious medical schools in the United States have departments of integrative medicine that offer courses in complementary and alternative medicines.

Patients should always discuss with their physicians any alternative medicine that they are using because some herbs or treatments may interfere with any conventional therapy or prescribed drug that the patient is using. For example, some herbs are dangerous because they contain toxic substances; others interfere with the actions of prescribed drugs, thereby reducing the medicine's effectiveness. Also, many alternative medicines have not been scientifically tested in clinical trials or proven to be safe and effective. Finally, some practitioners of alternative medicines are not well trained and many practitioners are unlicensed. Anyone contemplating using an alternative medicine for a serious medical problem should obtain as much information as possible and discuss the problem with a qualified health practitioner.

In recognition of the growing use of alternative medicine, Congress established the Office of Alternative Medicine (OAM) in 1992. The task of OAM was to fund research that would test the validity and effectiveness of many alternative medicines, such as acupuncture, massage, hypnosis, biofeedback, yoga, macrobiotic diets, and others. In 1998, the National Institutes of Health turned the small OAM into a full-fledged research agency, today called the National Center for Complementary and Integrative Health (NCCIH). More than two-thirds of American medical schools now offer education and training in complementary and integrative health. A significant number of adult Americans use some form of alternative medicine (**Figure 20.1**).

The goal of NCCIH is to test nontraditional therapies that have a plausible scientific basis and that can help patients' unmet needs. To this end, NCCIH has funded large clinical trials of chondroitin sulfate and glucosamine in treatment of osteoarthritis, vitamin E and selenium in the prevention of prostate cancer, and the effect of *Ginkgo biloba* on slowing dementia and memory loss.

Even if scientific studies "prove" certain alternative therapies to be of no value, it is not certain that the public will heed the results. For example, the very principles of homeopathy (discussed later) preclude its being tested scientifically, and most of its medicines contain no active ingredients. Yet homeopathy is being used more and more

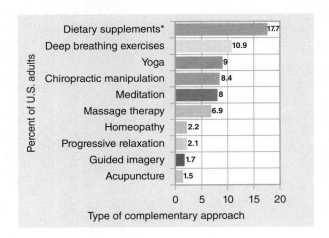

■ **Figure 20.1**

10 Most Used Types of Complementary Approaches to Health
Percent of U.S. adults who use different complementary approaches to health. Individuals can use more than one approach.
* indicates nonvitamin, nonmineral dietary supplement

Data from Clarke, T.C. et al. (2015, February 10). National Health Statistics Reports, 79. (www.ncbi.nlm.nih.gov/pmc/articles/PMC4573565/)

around the world, and millions of people attest to its therapeutic value in treating many diseases.

Defining Alternative Medicine

Alternative medicine can be divided into four broad categories based on the method of healing or intervention: (1) spiritual, psychic, or mental approaches, including prayer, meditation, hypnotherapy, and faith healing; (2) nutritional therapies, including change in diet, fasting, and the use of supplements; (3) therapies using herbs or other substances derived from natural sources, such as homeopathy, herbal medicine, or immune system boosters; and (4) physical therapies, such as chiropractic, acupuncture, massage, and yoga. **Table 20.1** presents a partial list of the hundreds of different alternative medicines.

Some alternative medicines, such as acupuncture and herbal remedies, have been used for thousands of years and would not have survived if people had not benefited. Other alternative medicines, such as homeopathy and chiropractic, are of recent origin and emerged partly as a response to the extraordinarily harsh practices of conventional medicine in the eighteenth and nineteenth centuries.

Before this century, irritants of all kinds were used to purge the body of unknown causes of illness. Bleedings, cuppings, leechings, enemas, and emetics (vomiting inducers) were all commonly used by doctors to treat diseases of which they had no real understanding. These treatments generally weakened the patient and often interfered with the natural processes of healing.

Today, patients with chronic diseases and pain still seek treatments that offer the promise of relief and that do little harm. The problem for the health consumer is knowing which alternative medicines might be of help and which ones are safe. To help you understand how to choose, some of the more widely used alternative medicines are described here.

Alternative Medicines

Ayurveda

Ayurveda refers to one of the world's oldest medical systems, which has been practiced in India for more than 4,000 years. Like other Asian medical practices, **Ayurvedic medicine** embodies a holistic approach to health; it teaches that health results from a balance of mind, body, and spirit, as well as a balance between people and the environment and their relationship to the cosmos. The word *Ayurveda* is from the Sanskrit and is a combination of two words: *ayur,* which means "life," and *veda,* which means "knowledge." Thus, health is knowledge of life. Ayurveda has been primarily practiced in the past by Buddhists or Hindus, but it is becoming increasingly popular in Western countries.

Ayurveda sees nature and people as being made of five elements or properties—earth, water, fire, air, and space; each element consists of both matter and energy. It is the interaction of these basic elements that gives rise to the universe and to human beings, who are viewed as being a microcosm or reflection of the macrocosm. Each element is associated with specific properties. For example, the earth element is dense and hard. Solid structures in the body, such as the skeleton, are derived from the earth element. The air element is cold and mobile. In the body, this element governs breathing and movement in the digestive tract. Thought, desire, and the will to do things also are under the control of the air element. The water element is fluid and soft and regulates the blood, secretions, and cerebrospinal fluid. The fire element is hot and light and regulates body temperature

Table 20.1

Partial List of Alternative Medicines and Healing Methods

Physical and nutritional	Mental and spiritual
Acupuncture	Ayurveda
Alexander technique	Biofeedback
Ayurveda	Christian Science
Feldenkrais technique	Co-counseling
Herbal medicine	Guided imagery
Kinesiology (touch for health)	Hypnosis
Macrobiotics	Meditation
Massage	Past lives therapy
No nightshade diet	Primal scream therapy
Qigong	Progressive relaxation
Reflexology	Psychic healing
Shiatsu	Magnetic therapy
T'ai chi ch'uan	Psychodrama
Yoga	Rebirthing

TERMS

alternative medicine: a therapy or healing procedure that is used *instead of* Western, scientific medical treatments

Ayurvedic medicine: a traditional form of preventive medicine and healing, involving mind, body, and spirit, practiced in India for thousands of years. Ayurveda is spreading to Western countries

complementary medicine: an alternative therapy that is used *along with* conventional medicine. Usually there is some scientific evidence for the effectiveness and safety of the complementary medicine

integrative medicine: combination of the practice of scientific, Western medicine with alternative medicines that are safe and effective for patients

and all aspects of digestion. Space plays a unique role in Ayurveda because it permits us to perceive sound and also regulates vibrations that affect the body. Harmony among these five elements in each individual (and in the world) produces health; disharmony in any of the elements produces disease.

The interaction of the body with the environment is further defined by the *doshas*, which mediate the functions of the body tissues and waste products. When the doshas are in balance, people experience health on all levels—physical, emotional, and spiritual. In holistic terms, these individuals are not just free of disease but experience optimal health. They have an abundance of energy and are intelligent and competent in all that they do. They enjoy good relations with other people and with the environment, and they are emotionally stable and happy. Spiritually, they are attuned with the cosmos. Imbalance in any of the doshas can produce mental, emotional, or physical illness. The goal of Ayurvedic medicine is to restore the balance of the doshas that is correct for each person.

An Ayurvedic physician diagnoses the patient's disease by a technique called pulse diagnosis, which is a highly developed skill in taking a pulse. Also, signs of illness are found by examination of the tongue, urine, and aspects of the body such as the condition of the nails, skin, and lips. Once the nature of the imbalance is determined, the physician provides various remedies. As with modern medicine, nutrition and exercise are among the primary recommendations. Ayurvedic medicine, however, does not define nutrition in terms of fats, proteins, vitamins, minerals, or food groups. Ayurveda recognizes six "tastes": salty, sweet, sour, pungent, bitter, and astringent. These tastes not only are sensations on the tongue but also effects on the body. Each taste is associated with a physiological function, such as elimination, condition of mucous membranes, amount of stress, and so on. The diet is adjusted to restore a balance of the tastes. Exercises such as yoga and t'ai chi are recommended; today, jogging may be included. Other techniques employed by Ayurvedic practitioners include massage, meditation, and herbal remedies. The success of Ayurvedic medicine is attested to by its long history and the increasing number of people who embrace its principles.

People who use Ayurvedic medicines need to use caution in making purchases. Most Ayurvedic medicines are made in Southeast Asia without regulation and sold in Asian grocery stores in the United States. About one in five products purchased in the Boston area was found to contain potentially harmful levels of heavy metals such as lead, mercury, and arsenic (Saper et al., 2008). At present, consumers have no way of knowing which products are safe and which ones contain heavy metals.

> Words are the most potent drug that mankind uses.
>
> *Rudyard Kipling*

Homeopathy

Of all the alternative medicines, **homeopathy** is the most widely used in America and around the world. Many physicians in the United States use some form of homeopathy in their practice of medicine. Homeopathy also is used by nurse practitioners, dentists, naturopathic doctors, chiropractors, acupuncturists, and veterinarians. Between 2 million and 3 million Americans take homeopathic remedies each year and spend upward of $200 million on homeopathic preparations. In European countries, homeopathy is widely used by physicians, and in India, there are more than 100,000 homeopathic practitioners.

Homeopathy is only about 200 years old and was founded by Samuel Hahnemann, a German pharmacologist and physician. The word *homeopathy* derives from two Greek words: *omoios*, meaning "similar," and *pathos*, meaning "feeling." Homeopathy is primarily a self-healing system that is assisted by very small doses of medicines or remedies. Hahnemann believed that tiny doses of a substance (a medicine) that evoked symptoms *similar* to the disease symptoms could, in some way, stimulate the body's natural defenses and promote healing. According to Hahnemann, homeopathy is based on four principles:

1. Substances that produce the same symptoms as the disease in an individual will cure that individual (Law of Similars).
2. Substances are tested by giving them to healthy subjects and observing symptoms (Law of Proving).
3. Smaller doses are more potent than undiluted solutions (Law of Potentiation or Law of Infinitesimals).
4. Vital forces must be released in the treated individual, which will result in reestablishing harmony (homeostasis) in the body.

For example, the substance *belladonna*, which is extracted from a poisonous plant, causes flushing and flulike symptoms when ingested by a healthy person. Thus, a homeopathic practitioner might use diluted doses of belladonna to treat the flu or high fever. The recommended dose of belladonna might be listed as 30x; this refers to the number of times that the original extract has been diluted. Practically, this means that one drop of the original extract is added to nine drops of water; then one drop of this solution is added to nine drops of water (or alcohol) and so on until 30 tenfold dilutions are reached. Statistically, the final solution is unlikely to have any molecules of belladonna in it. This is the primary reason that homeopathy is dismissed today as bogus by conventional medicine and Western science. Nonetheless, 200 years of experience and observation by patients and physicians show that it does help many patients suffering from many kinds of diseases.

Homeopathy began to be practiced extensively around 1830, a time when conventional medicine was particularly ineffective in treating epidemics of infectious diseases such as cholera, typhus, and scarlet fever. During this period, homeopathic doctors were significantly more successful in treating people than conventional doctors because the remedies worked, because people believed that they worked, or because of a combination of both. By 1890, at least 15% of conventional physicians used homeopathy and there were 22 homeopathic medical schools and more than 100 homeopathic hospitals operating in the United States.

In the 1800s, the American Medical Association (AMA) offered to include homeopaths in its organization. However, homeopaths chose to remain outside mainstream medicine, and the AMA began to harass and threaten physicians who practiced any form of homeopathy. In 1914, the AMA became the exclusive organization for licensing physicians to practice medicine; as a result, homeopathic medicine disappeared from the American scene for more than 50 years. In the 1970s, along with a general resurgence in alternative medicine, homeopathy again emerged as the choice of many sick people, either as a sole therapy or as an adjunct to conventional medical care.

Homeopathic practitioners use their remedies to evoke symptoms so that the body can recognize them and initiate a healing process from within. Homeopathy is used to treat both acute (infections, injuries) and chronic (arthritis, allergies, high blood pressure) conditions. It does not generally treat structural diseases or those stemming from long-term organic damage, such as cirrhosis, diabetes, chronic obstructive lung diseases, inherited diseases, neurological diseases, or cancer.

Homeopathic remedies are derived from plant, animal, microbial, and mineral sources. Examples of plant remedies include herbs, spices, foods, fragrances, and extracts from mushrooms and lichens. Mineral remedies include solutions of metals (copper, gold, tin, zinc), dilute solutions of acids, and substances derived from ores and rocks. Remedies derived from animal substances include venom from insects, spiders, and crustaceans, hormone extracts, and material taken from diseased tissues.

Chiropractic

Chiropractic was founded in the United States around 1900 by Daniel David Palmer, who had no scientific or medical training, but who believed throughout his life that he had a "calling" to heal people. At age 50, Palmer cured Harvey Lillard of deafness by manipulating his spine. Lillard had been deaf for 17 years after working stooped over in a mine. Palmer found a misaligned vertebra, which he manipulated; this allowed Harvey to straighten up for the first time in years and simultaneously restored his hearing. After several other cures by spinal manipulation, Palmer concluded that virtually all diseases are caused by *subluxed* (misaligned) vertebrae.

Palmer coined the name "chiropractic" (from the Greek *cheir,* meaning "hand," and *praktikos,* meaning "practical"; the two words are usually interpreted to mean "done by hand"). Two years later he opened the Palmer School for Chiropractic in Davenport, Iowa. In 1906, Palmer and his son, Bartlett Joshua (or B. J. Palmer), were arrested for practicing medicine without a license. Palmer was tried, convicted, and jailed. His son's case never came to trial.

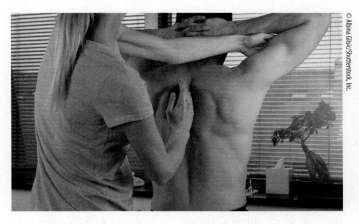

Chiropractic manipulations help many people who suffer from back pain and other musculoskeletal disorders.

B. J. Palmer took over the chiropractic practice and turned it into a multi-million-dollar business. B. J. was a genius at commercializing chiropractic, and he was the first to come up with the idea of mail-order diplomas. B. J.'s philosophy of chiropractic was summed up in his description of the spine: "The principal functions of the spine are to support the head, to support the ribs, and to support the chiropractor." Shortly after B. J. took over, chiropractic split into two distinct schools, which still exist today. One group, "the straights," adheres to the original idea that almost all diseases are caused by subluxion of the vertebrae. The other group was founded by John Howard, who believed that other factors also are involved in disease processes. This group became known as the "mixers," and practitioners of this philosophy include nutrition, relaxation, exercise, and other techniques, along with spinal manipulation, in their chiropractic practices.

Although chiropractors treat a wide range of diseases, 90% of patients seeking chiropractic help do so because of back pain, neck pain, or headaches. When the spine is in complete alignment, energy flows freely to all tissues and organs in the body and is the basis for health. **Subluxation** of vertebrae is the principal cause of disease according to chiropractic theory; subluxation can be caused by genetic disorders, falls, injuries, improper sleeping habits, poor posture, obesity, stress, or occupational hazards.

A number of research studies have demonstrated both short-term and long-term benefits of chiropractic

TERMS

chiropractic: an alternative medicine that uses manipulation of the spine and joints for healing

homeopathy: an alternative medicine that administers very dilute solutions of substances that mimic the patient's symptoms

subluxation: misalignment of a vertebra from its correct position

for chronic, disabling lower back pain. Other studies have concluded that chiropractic is cheaper and more effective in treatment of back pain and musculoskeletal disorders than conventional medicine. However, claims that chiropractic is effective in reducing blood pressure or relieving allergies or ulcers have not been substantiated by research.

Osteopathy

Osteopathy, like chiropractic, is basically treatment by manipulation of the spine and other structural parts of the body. Osteopathic physicians, called doctors of osteopathy (D.O.), undergo training that is as rigorous as the education of physicians, and generally osteopaths have the same medical privileges of prescribing drugs and performing surgery as do physicians. However, most practitioners of osteopathy rely primarily on physical manipulation and exercises for their patients' conditions.

Osteopathic medicine was founded in the United States by Andrew Taylor Still, who was born in Virginia in 1828. His father was a preacher–physician, and Andrew grew up observing his father treat patients. He eventually developed his own methods of healing, which depended heavily on manipulation. Today, there are hundreds of osteopathic hospitals in the United States and thousands of doctors of osteopathy.

Acupuncture

Acupuncture is an integral part of traditional Chinese medicine, and the use of acupuncture goes back at least 5,000 years. The accumulated knowledge of acupuncture was passed down over the centuries and recorded in a text called *The Yellow Emperor's Classic of Internal Medicine* written in the second or third century B.C. Although acupuncture has been used in China and other Asian countries for centuries, it became popular in the West only after President Nixon's visit to China in the 1970s. A *New York Times* reporter, James Reston, who was covering Nixon's trip, became ill and underwent an emergency appendectomy. He later wrote an article describing his acupuncture anesthesia, and American physicians began traveling to China to learn more about acupuncture.

The underlying principle of acupuncture is the existence of *qi* (pronounced *chi*)—the vital life force that circulates throughout the body and is carried by channels called **meridians**. There are 12 major meridians that connect all of the major organs, as well as a network of minor meridians. The meridians intersect with the surface of the body at many positions; these are the acupuncture points that are "needled" to restore balance to the qi to cure illness or relieve pain. According to Chinese medicine, an organ that is diseased or not functioning properly will manifest symptoms or signs on a corresponding meridian. These may include pain or ache, a change in temperature, sensitivity to touch, or a change in skin texture or color along the affected meridian. Thus, the acupuncturist must first diagnose the cause of the

Treating a Headache with Acupressure

Many people experience headaches caused by tension in the muscles of the neck and head. Often the tension alters blood supply to the brain, which causes a headache. Pressing acupressure points at two different locations may relieve the headache pain. The points are located just below the base of the skull, at the back of the head, just to the right and left of center.

Cup the back of your head with your fingers and use your two thumbs to press quite firmly just under the skull on either side of center. The thumbs should be an inch or so apart and away from the centerline of the skull. Press hard for up to a minute or until your thumbs become tired. Repeat the pressure two or three times. Breathe deeply while pressing. Notice if the pain has lessened or disappeared.

Two other acupressure points for headache relief are located on the back of each hand in the soft part between thumb and index finger. Using the thumb and index finger (or middle finger) of the opposite hand, press firmly on the acupressure point. This point may be sensitive, so press only as hard as is comfortable. Repeat on the opposite hand. Press these points for up to a minute and repeat several times. Notice if the headache pain has subsided.

illness by locating the affected meridians; then the correct acupuncture points can be treated.

In acupuncture treatment, very thin metal needles are inserted just under the skin at specific acupuncture points (**Figure 20.2**). Traditional Chinese medicine describes about 365 acupuncture points located along 14 meridians

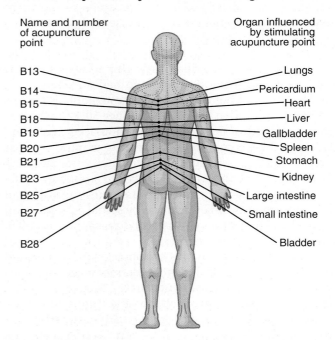

■ **Figure 20.2**

Acupuncture points supposedly influence the functions of internal organs.

in the body. Usually no more than a dozen or so needles are used. These remain in place for about a half hour, during which they may be twirled or connected to low-voltage generators to increase effectiveness in balancing qi. Sometimes heat is applied to the acupoint in a process called moxibustion. A small piece of an herb, *Artemisia vulgaris* (commonly known as mugwort), is either burned on the tip of the needle or placed on the acupoint.

In 2010, a scientific panel (Cochrane Review Groups) concluded that traditional acupuncture can be effective in relieving postoperative dental pain and in controlling nausea caused by surgery, chemotherapy, or pregnancy. Other conditions listed for which acupuncture may be effective include drug and smoking addiction, lower back pain, stroke rehabilitation, menstrual cramps, tennis elbow, headache, and carpal tunnel syndrome. Although there is no research to substantiate claims of effectiveness, acupuncture also is used to treat neurological disorders (Ménière's disease, trigeminal neuralgia), gastrointestinal disorders (ulcers, colitis, diarrhea), and respiratory disorders (asthma, rhinitis, sinusitis, bronchitis), as well as arthritic conditions. Acupuncture is effective in reducing the pain of osteoarthritis of the knee (Hinman et al., 2014). More than 20 million Americans suffer from this condition, which is caused by degenerating cartilage.

Acupuncture is also effective in the treatment of migraine and chronic tension headaches compared to routine care only, medical management, and sham acupuncture (Linde et al., 2016). However, many studies have shown that real acupuncture is no better than sham ("fake") acupuncture in reducing the frequency of migraine headaches. Acupuncture also exerts a powerful placebo effect. This highlights the problem of sorting out the scientific research on alternative medicines. Experimental designs are usually different, and conditions of the experiment vary from one research setting to another. Thus, the patient seeking relief for a condition usually acts on the recommendation of another person or on his or her own convictions about the effectiveness of an alternative medicine.

Herbal Medicine

Herbs have been used as medicines for centuries to treat every conceivable form of ailment. Ancient Chinese, Greek, and Roman societies compiled extensive *Pharmacopoeia* describing the uses and preparation of herbal remedies. One herbal compilation published by Nicholas Culpepper in the seventeenth century has gone through countless printings and lists more than 3,000 herbal remedies.

Herbal medicines consist of materials derived from plants and can be prepared as pills, teas, extracts, tinctures, salves, and other forms. In the 1780s, an English physician noted that one of his patients was cured of dropsy by drinking tea made from dried, powdered foxglove leaves. The physician, William Withering, made the connection between dropsy and heart disease. Subsequently, the chemical digitoxin in foxglove leaves was identified as the ingredient that helps heart functions.

Table 20.2

Herbs Used for Common Ailments

Herb	Use
Aloe	Burns, skin irritations
Black cohosh	Menstrual cramps, PMS, menopause
Chamomile	Digestion
Echinacea	Immune system stimulant
Feverfew	Reduces fever, helps migraine
Foxglove	Controls heart rhythm, angina
Garlic	Digestion, protects against high blood pressure
Ginger root	Motion sickness, cough
Ginkgo biloba	Dilates blood vessels, dementia
Ginseng	Reduces stress
Hawthorn	Lowers blood pressure, dilates blood vessels
Milk thistle	Protects damaged liver, prevents toxins from entering liver
Peppermint	Indigestion
St. John's wort	Depression
Saw palmetto	Enlarged prostate, improves urinary flow, anti-inflammatory agent
Senna	Strong laxative
Tea-tree oil	Skin and vaginal infections, acne
Valerian root	Mild sedative
Willow bark	Headache

Herbs and other plants have been the source for extracting and purifying modern drugs such as ephedrine, digitalis, atropine, reserpine, quinine, and most recently tamoxifen, used to treat breast cancer, and artemisinin, to treat malaria. Herbal medicines often contain a mixture of herbs, so it is difficult to know what component is involved in alleviating symptoms or in healing. Only with the advent of modern chemistry could plant materials be broken down into individual chemical components that can be tested for medicinal properties. Many herbal remedies are used for a variety of ailments and conditions (**Table 20.2**).

TERMS

acupuncture: an ancient Chinese alternative medicine that uses thin needles inserted into specific points on the body to produce healing energy

herbal medicines: materials derived from plants and other organisms that are made into teas, powders, and salves to treat diseases and injuries

meridians: the channels along the body where energy flows and where acupuncture points are located

osteopathy: an alternative medicine that uses manipulation and medicines for healing; osteopaths receive training comparable to that of physicians and can prescribe drugs

Herbal remedies can have the same potential for side effects and harm as prescription drugs. Some plants contain toxic chemicals along with the beneficial ones; the concentrations of both kinds of chemicals will vary from plant to plant and from one season to the next. Thus, one batch of herbs may be safe and effective, whereas another batch may be toxic, ineffective, or both. Without rigorous testing (which is required for prescription drugs), the safety and efficacy of herbal remedies cannot be ensured. Problems, side effects, and risks associated with some commonly used herbs are listed in **Table 20.3**.

Table 20.3

Risks and Side Effects Associated with Some Herbs

Echinacea
Allergic reactions, including rashes, increased asthma, and anaphylaxis (a life-threatening allergic reaction), especially if already allergic to related plants in the daisy family (ragweed, chrysanthemums, marigolds, and daisies)

Ephedra
Stroke, heart attack, and sudden death; worsening of cardiovascular disease, kidney disease, sleep disorders, and diabetes; nausea, anxiety, headache, psychosis, kidney stones, tremors, dry mouth, irregular heart rhythms, heart damage, high blood pressure, restlessness, sleep problems, irritation of the stomach, and increased urination

Garlic
Breath and body odor, heartburn, upset stomach, and allergic reactions; reduced ability of blood to clot (may be a problem during or after surgery and dental work)

Ginkgo biloba
Headache, nausea, gastrointestinal upset, diarrhea, dizziness, or allergic reactions; reduced ability of blood to clot (may be a problem during or after surgery and dental work)

Ginseng
Headaches, sleep, gastrointestinal problems, allergic reactions, lower levels of blood sugar (more likely to occur in people with diabetes)

Green tea
Contains caffeine, which can cause insomnia, anxiety, irritability, upset stomach, nausea, diarrhea, or frequent urination; contains small amounts of vitamin K, which can make anticoagulant drugs, such as warfarin, less effective

Kava
Drowsiness (avoid driving and operating heavy machinery), liver damage and (sometimes fatal) liver failure, abnormal muscle spasms or involuntary muscle movements; may interact with several drugs, including drugs used for Parkinson's disease

St. John's wort
Increased sensitivity to sunlight; anxiety, dry mouth, dizziness, gastrointestinal symptoms, fatigue, headache, and sexual problems; may increase or decrease the effects of other drugs, such as antidepressants, hormonal contraceptives, digoxin, warfarin, indinavir, and drugs used in organ transplantation

Valerian
Headaches, dizziness, upset stomach, and tiredness the morning after its use

Data from National Center for Complementary and Integrative Health. (2015). *Herbs at a glance*. Retrieved from http://nccih.nih.gov/herbs/herbsataglance.htm

An herb that helps reduce depression is *St. John's wort*. Clinical studies indicate that extracts of St. John's wort are as effective in treating moderate to severe depression as the prescription antidepressant drug *paroxetine* (Schmidt & Butterweek, 2015). However, a major problem with this herb is that it reduces the effectiveness of birth control drugs so that unanticipated pregnancies have occurred among depressed women taking St. John's wort. The herb also reduces the effectiveness of other prescription antidepressants, AIDS drugs, anticoagulants, and as many as 50% of all prescription drugs (Chen et al., 2012). Using this herb carries such sufficient risk that it should be used only on the advice of a physician who is familiar with its many effects.

Kava kava (or simply kava or awa) is an herbal drink used for thousands of years by people indigenous to islands of the Pacific such as Micronesia, Fiji, and Hawaii. Among these peoples, kava is imbibed mostly on ceremonial occasions, but kava beverages are also widely drunk in social settings as a relaxant and for stress reduction. In recent years, the use of kava in Europe, Canada, and the United States has blossomed into a major industry. Kava is sold as a drink, a tea, and as a powdered supplement in pill form. In 2002, a number of kava users, primarily in Europe, suffered severe liver damage and some died. Shortly thereafter, kava was banned in most European countries and Canada. It is still legal to sell and use kava in the United States, but the Food and Drug Administration (FDA) advises against its use. It is likely that the traditional preparation and use of kava, which is made by squeezing liquid from the bark on roots of the kava bush, is safe. However, in the West, extracts and pills are made from the bark as well as the roots of the plant. It appears that the bark contains toxic chemicals that are not present in the roots. In any event, drinking kava or taking kava supplements involves health risk and should be avoided.

Ephedra, also called *ma huang*, is a potent drug derived from the Chinese herb, *Ephedra sinica*. It is widely added

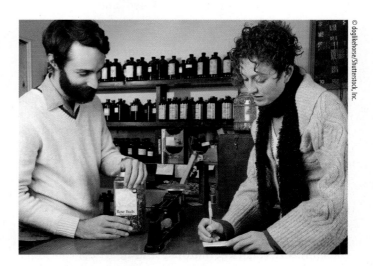

Herbal remedies are continuing to increase in popularity among Americans with a variety of ailments.

Vitamin Supplements Are Not Always Safe

Americans spend billions of dollars a year on vitamin, mineral, and other dietary supplements to ward off or cure every ailment known to science or to attain the fullest degree of health and wellness imaginable. Because the American dietary supplements industry is not regulated by the Food and Drug Administration, and only minimally by the Fair Trade Commission, it can sell just about anything to those who cannot resist the idea of improving health at no risk and at moderate cost. Unfortunately, consumers have no guarantee that a particular dietary supplement is safe, pure, or effective.

Vitamins have the reputation of being mandatory for good health, which they are. Inadequate intake of some vitamins can lead to deficiency diseases. Surveys of American eating patterns show that the diets of a large number of people are deficient in one or more vitamins (often vitamins A, D, folate, and some B vitamins), a situation for which they are encouraged to eat healthier foods. Although their intentions may be good, many people mistakenly believe that (1) vitamins out of a bottle are equivalent to vitamins in food and (2) if a little extra vitamins is good, then a lot of extra vitamins is better. They do not consider that without regulatory oversight something in a bottle may not even be what the manufacturer claims in its advertising or even on the product label. Also, large amounts of some vitamins are toxic (vitamins A, D, E, K, B_3, B_6). Claims that vitamin D can help alleviate depression, heart disease risk, fatigue, and muscle weakness have only the barest of scientific support. Yet, the mystique about this vitamin can lead people whose blood tests show their vitamin D levels to be normal to insist on taking vitamin D supplements. Too much vitamin D can cause nausea, vomiting, loss of appetite, and upset the balance of calcium and phosphorus needed for bone health. Vitamin supplements should only be taken when tests show evidence of a deficiency that is overcome with supplementation by a chemically pure product. No need to create health problems by taking unnecessary dietary supplements.

to dietary supplements as a stimulant to help people lose weight and is used by athletes to enhance performance. Ephedra contains the stimulant drug ephedrine, which is responsible for its desired effects and also unpleasant and dangerous side effects, including increased blood pressure and heart rate, psychiatric symptoms, and gastrointestinal problems. As a consequence of its effect on the heart, it can palpitations that may result in heart attacks and stroke in susceptible persons. Between 1997 and 2001, the U.S. armed forces documented 30 deaths among service personnel using ephedra products. In recent years, the deaths of several high-profile professional athletes were linked to ephedra supplements. In addition to deaths, thousands of people using ephedra products have reported adverse effects.

In April 2004, the FDA banned the sale of herbal and dietary supplements containing ephedrine. Ephedrine is banned only in weight loss supplements; it is used in various FDA-approved medications and in weight-loss products sold outside the United States. Many supplements marketed as ephedra remain legal by first removing the ephedrine.

The banning of ephedrine-containing supplements was the first time that the FDA banned a supplement under the procedures provided in the Dietary Supplement Health and Education Act (DSHEA) passed by Congress in 1994. This act gives the FDA the power to ban a supplement when there is compelling evidence of its potential health dangers. Vitamin and herbal supplements are a multi-billion-dollar industry in the United States, and suppliers of these products are opposed to any legislation that would dampen sales. For example, *ginkgo biloba* is one of the best-selling herbs; it is used as a memory booster and to help ward off senility in the elderly. However, taking *ginkgo biloba* can be quite dangerous if you are also taking a blood thinner medication for heart disease.

Scientific studies defining the risks and benefits of dietary and herbal supplements are not available for most supplements that people take. Manufacturers are not required to carry out tests that establish the safety and efficacy of a product before they sell it. Most vitamin and mineral supplements are safe if taken in reasonable amounts, and many Americans take them to supplement a diet that may be deficient in essential nutrients. However, herbal medicines pose a significant risk. Herbs contain chemicals that act as drugs, but the actual amounts of the active chemicals in most herbal medicines are not known or may be misrepresented on the label. Anyone planning on using an herbal medicine should consult a knowledgeable healthcare provider about its risks and benefits. Any adverse reactions to an herbal medicine should be reported to health authorities.

Many herbs are now being added to foods to increase marketability and sales. Herbs are added to sodas, fruit drinks, cereals, and many other kinds of foods. Remember that food is for eating enjoyment and maintaining health. Herbs are for treating ailments or diseases. Do not confuse the functions of food and herbs, and do not consume any herb in food "just because it might help me feel better."

Naturopathy

Naturopathy is a uniquely American approach to health that arose in the late nineteenth century. The term was introduced by Dr. John Sheel in 1895; the principles of naturopathy as a system of healing and way of living

TERMS

naturopathy: an alternative medicine that uses nutrition, herbs, massage, and other techniques to promote healing

Whole-Body Cryotherapy: No Cold, Hard Facts

Athletes! Listen up! Is freezing your body a good way to relieve soreness from competition, practice, and individual workouts? Cryotherapy—sitting in a tub or cabin and having your body blasted with air made frigid (−180°F, or −118°C) by treating it with liquid nitrogen—is all the rage. Thought to have originated in Japan in the 1970s to treat severe joint pain in people with multiple sclerosis and rheumatoid arthritis, whole-body supercooling is also used to treat dementia. However, no scientific studies have substantiated any therapeutic benefit from cryotherapy for any symptom (Costello et al., 2015). In 2016, the FDA issued a warning that whole-body cryotherapy had no legitimate medical use and could cause harm from frostbite, burns, and eye damage (not to mention feeling unpleasant).

Treating an injury or soreness with ice or a cold pack is a time-honored and helpful practice to limit tissue damage and aid healing. Unlike a cryotherapy tank, a cold pack lowers the skin temperature by about 45°F (7°C), enough to slow blood flow to injured tissue and biological reactions that cause inflammation and pain. That some sports stars have acknowledged using cryotherapy is insufficient medical justification for using it, despite what advertisers and purveyors of cryotherapy (which can cost $300 a session) claim.

---

were formulated by Benedict Lust in 1902. In the early 1900s, more than 20 naturopathic schools of medicine trained naturopathic doctors (N.D.), but with the rise of conventional medicine, naturopathy all but disappeared from the American health scene. However, it experienced a revival in the 1970s, along with other alternative medicines.

Naturopathy's approach to health emphasizes the prevention of disease and the individual's responsibility for a healthy lifestyle. Naturopathy draws on all available alternative medicines, as well as aspects of conventional medicine. However, it does reject the use of surgery and drugs. If there is a single unifying concept to naturopathy, it is that the body possesses the "energy" or "intelligence" to heal itself. In that sense it is similar in philosophy to Ayurvedic and Chinese medicine.

The eight basic principles of naturopathy are as follows:

1. The human body possesses an innate ability to heal itself.
2. It is the duty of the naturopathic practitioner to find and treat the underlying cause of illness, not simply the symptoms.
3. The naturopathic practitioner is first and foremost a teacher who must educate the patient on how to prevent illness and restore health.
4. The naturopathic practitioner must employ therapies that "do no harm." Surgery and drugs are not recommended.
5. The focus is mainly on prevention of illness. The patient's lifestyle is examined in detail, and recommendations are made to reduce health risks and to foster health.
6. Good nutrition is an essential goal of naturopathy. Without a healthy diet, the body invites illness.
7. The treatment must involve the whole person, not just an organ or part of the body. A person's physical, mental, emotional, and spiritual states must be evaluated and altered as necessary to promote health.
8. The ultimate goal of naturopathy is optimal health, not just the absence of disease.

These principles of naturopathy are essentially those of modern holistic medicine. The emphasis of the medicine of the future should be to prevent disease by educating patients in the health benefits of good nutrition and in helping them reduce destructive health behaviors such as smoking, drinking, or using recreational drugs. Also, people must find ways to reduce stress, anxiety, and emotional turmoil if they are to enjoy optimal health. In the modern world, these are difficult tasks even for a motivated individual.

Naturopathic doctors receive training that is as complete as a medical school that awards the M.D. degree. A naturopathic doctor who has graduated from one of the half dozen schools offering degrees in naturopathy is well equipped to diagnose and treat a wide range of diseases. It is the approach to healing that distinguishes the N.D. from the M.D., although many physicians with an M.D. practice naturopathic medicine even though they also can prescribe drugs and recommend surgery. Because naturopathy eschews the use of surgery and drugs, naturopathic doctors do not treat acute illness or conditions that require emergency care. People usually consult a naturopathic doctor to construct a lifestyle that will prevent illness and promote overall optimal health.

Therapeutic Massage

Therapeutic massage is a hands-on therapy in which touch is used to heal. Cave paintings dating back approximately 15,000 years depict injured people being treated with what looks like massage. The use of massage to heal is described in ancient Chinese, Greek, and Roman texts. Seemingly miraculous cures have been reported over the centuries by the "laying on of hands" by people believed to have divine powers, such as priests, shamans, and holy persons. Despite its effectiveness as an alternative medicine, some people still regard massage as a guise for sexual stimulation. However, therapeutic massage administered by a trained and licensed professional is a highly effective form of therapy for many conditions.

Human touch is essential to normal development of infants and children and to health in general. Americans tend to touch one another much less than people in other cultures. Psychologists who observe the number of times people touch one another in cafes or other public places report that, on average, Americans touch one another less frequently than almost any other culture in the world. In similar situations, Parisians touch one another more than 100 times per hour and Puerto Ricans almost 200 times per hour! Cultural anthropologists report that cultures that are more physically affectionate toward infants and children have lower rates of adult violence such as domestic and sexual abuse.

The most immediate effect of therapeutic massage is improved blood circulation. As the skin is stretched and the muscles are kneaded, the amount of blood returning to the heart is increased, and toxins released into the blood can be excreted more readily. Enhanced circulation also supplies more oxygen to tissues and to the brain. Massage benefits digestion and elimination, and it hastens wound healing. Massage also eases muscle pain caused by strain or injury; it may stimulate the release of endorphins and enkephalins, pain-relieving chemicals synthesized in the body.

There are certain conditions and diseases in which therapeutic massage should *not* be used because of the possibility of causing further damage to tissues or organs. These are as follows:

- Recent bone fractures or severe sprains
- Herniated disk in the spine
- Excessive blood pressure
- Areas of the body in which hemorrhage has occurred
- Any acute inflammation of the skin or joints
- Blood conditions such as phlebitis and thrombosis
- Severe varicose veins
- Certain kinds of cancer

Therapeutic massage involves five basic kinds of manipulation of a person's skin and muscles. The first is an extended gliding stroke with the whole hand or thumb. This warms the skin and relaxes muscle tension. The next is a kneading motion in which muscles are grabbed and lifted. This relieves soreness and improves circulation. Friction manipulation is used around joints and thick muscles. Repeated circular movement of the hands can help break up adhesions. The hands also can be used in a chopping or tapping motion to stimulate the skin and muscles; this chopping is used when muscles are spastic or cramped. Finally, the fingers or flattened hands are pressed into muscles and "vibrated" for a few seconds. This vibration stimulates nerves and circulation in the area.

Massage therapists are required to pass a licensing exam in most states. Many people claim to be massage therapists who are not licensed or who have limited training. Making sure a therapist is licensed and talking to people who have benefited from that therapist are good ways to ensure that your experience will be helpful. Even if you do not have a specific medical condition that needs massage therapy, getting a massage is relaxing and refreshing.

Some specific forms of massage are these:

Swedish massage: uses long strokes, kneading of muscles, and friction techniques on the outer layers of the body. Also uses active and passive movement of joints.

Shiatsu and acupressure massage: both techniques use pressure on specific points of the body to treat pain and improve body functions. In Shiatsu, pressure may be applied with fingers, elbows, or feet. In acupressure, fingers are used.

Lomi lomi massage: an ancient Hawaiian healing art that is a form of spiritual massage used to restore mind–body harmony.

Rolfing: developed by Ida Rolf to realign the body by deep (and often painful) massage of underlying myofascial tissues. Rolfing is also called structural integration.

Rosen massage: uses gentle touch and verbal communication to relieve suppressed emotions locked into musculature from past traumatic incidents.

Trigger point massage: uses finger pressure on "trigger points" in painful or inflamed areas of muscle to break the cycles of spasm and pain.

Aromatherapy

Aromatherapy is a centuries-old alternative medicine in which the essential oils of plants (many of which are fragrant) are administered so that chemicals contained in the oils are absorbed into the body and act as drugs. In that sense, aromatherapy is similar to herbal medicine or to conventional drug therapy. Since the 1980s, aromatherapy has increased in popularity among Americans seeking alternative medicines and now is a more than $300 million annual business.

Priests and healers in the ancient world used oils and perfumes to treat illnesses and as a prevention against disease. In the Egyptian Ebers Papyrus, which dates to about 1500 b.c., there are descriptions of more than 800 plant and herbal remedies, many of which are fragrant oil extracts. The modern medicinal use of plant oils and fragrances, as well as the term *aromatherapy*, derives from a French chemist who began to study the healing power of plant oils in the 1930s. He became interested after burning his hand in his family's perfume factory. He plunged his burned hand into a vat of lavender oil for relief and discovered that the burn healed rapidly and without scarring.

TERMS

aromatherapy: use of fragrant extracts of plants to promote healing

therapeutic massage: promotes relaxation and healing by massage of the skin and muscles

Marketing "Miracle" Health Juices

In recent years, a multi-billion-dollar business has developed—primarily on the Internet—in marketing exotic juices that proponents claim can cure almost any disease as well as boost longevity and energy. The juices are primarily derived from such fruits as pomegranate, mangosteen, goji, and noni. Pomegranates are probably familiar to most people, but the other plants are of Asian origin and are rarely seen in U.S. markets. The fruits of these plants contain antioxidants (as do many fruits and vegetables), which are advertised as cures for cancer, diabetes, heart disease, macular degeneration, Alzheimer's, and other serious diseases.

The current health fad in exotic fruit juices began in 2003, with the mass marketing of POM, a mixture of pomegranate and grape juice that sold for $5 for a 16-ounce bottle. Pomegranates contain phytochemicals that act as antioxidants; cranberries, blueberries, and strawberries also contain significant amounts of phytochemicals. Marketers recommended that people drink at least 8 ounces of pomegranate juice a day, which would mean spending $75 a month or more for this juice.

For centuries, people in Asia have been using the fruit and bark of the *mangosteen* to treat stomach and skin problems. In the United States, shrewd marketers set up a pyramid scheme of salespersons and multiple websites to hype the benefits of mangosteen juice. (It is usually mixed with nine other juices.) Health claims for mangosteen juice include boosting the immune system, enhancing physical performance, improving the respiratory system, and supporting the health of bone and cartilage. (Such claims do not violate any laws because they do not refer to specific diseases.)

Another popular tropical fruit product is *noni,* which grows in the wild on most Pacific islands, including Hawaii. When ripe, noni fruits soften rapidly and exude a foul-smelling and equally foul-tasting liquid. Proponents of noni claim that it will cure almost anything. A 32-ounce bottle costs between $40 and $50, and it is recommended that people drink 1 to 3 ounces a day for whatever ails them. Scientific studies to date do not support any of the health claims posted on noni websites.

The most recent addition to the booming business in functional health juices is *goji* juice, which is derived from small berries that grow in mountainous regions of China and Tibet. For centuries extracts of goji berries have been used in Chinese herbal remedies for a variety of conditions, including poor vision and cough. In contrast to noni's unpleasant taste and smell, goji juice is delicious, with a delightful blend of sweet and sour flavors. It is as easy to drink as a glass of lemonade. But at $40 to $50 a bottle for wild-berry juice, it's a rich person's drink. And, with the current craze for goji juice, the Himalayan plants are rapidly becoming extinct. The best thing that can be said for all these "antioxidant" juices is that they probably do no harm to health. These fruit juices do not cure cancers or extend life, as many of their proponents claim, but they are making some companies and salespeople very rich.

Some of the most popular aromatherapy oil extracts are derived from the following:

- The leaves of eucalyptus and peppermint
- The fruits and blossoms of oranges and lemons
- The flowers of lavender and roses
- Woods such as camphor and sandalwood
- Cinnamon bark, lemongrass, fennel, and rosemary
- Dried spices such as clove and fresh garlic bulbs

Essential oils made from plant extracts are very concentrated and contain hundreds of chemicals that can act as drugs. Thus, only minute amounts of oils are used, and a person practicing aromatherapy needs to be knowledgeable about the kinds of chemicals present in different extracts and their effects on the body. Aromatherapists treat people by prescribing oils that can be inhaled directly, applied to the skin as part of a massage, or added to a hot bath, in which case the oils are both absorbed and inhaled. Aromatherapy is used to treat infections, pain, arthritis, skin disorders, headaches, digestive disorders, and other conditions.

Although aromatherapy has been used for thousands of years, there is no scientific evidence that it cures any disease. It is critical that patients using aromatherapy (or other alternative medicine) inform their physicians as to what oils, herbs, or supplements they are using to avoid serious complications from drug–drug or drug–herb interactions.

Biomagnetic Therapy

Biomagnetic therapy (also called magnetic therapy) involves the use of static magnetic fields or pulsed magnetic fields created by electrical currents to treat a wide variety of ailments, especially pain. Biomagnetic therapies have been used for thousands of years, primarily in non-Western countries, to treat pain, inflammation, stress, fractures, and other health problems. The ancient Greeks discovered lodestone, a naturally magnetized substance, and thought that it had healing properties.

The earth has a magnetic field, and because all life developed in the earth's magnetic field, it is argued that the functions of damaged cells can be improved with biomagnetic therapies. Most of the evidence for the effectiveness of biomagnetic therapies comes from testimonials, which do not constitute scientific proof. In general, it is difficult to design randomized, placebo-controlled studies using magnets to treat specific conditions. However, a few positive studies have been carried out. The use of high-energy, pulsed magnetic fields to treat severe depression has met with some success. Also, bone healing has been accelerated with the use of electrical currents and magnetic fields, and some people claim to have experienced pain relief using small electrical generators.

However, despite numerous claims, use of static field magnets to treat a wide variety of health concerns has not been substantiated by scientific studies. Magnets are put under beds to reduce pain and stress or to cure other conditions. Magnets placed in shoes are used to treat pain. Magnetic bracelets are worn for many health reasons. And magnetized water is a booming business. Americans spend more than $300 million each year on various forms of biomagnetic therapies. Yet scientific studies showing that biomagnetic therapies are effective are rare and usually negative, including treatment of plantar heel pain by inserting magnets into shoes, or using magnets to reduce muscle strain or pain after exercise (Pittler et al., 2007).

The use of magnets may produce benefits by virtue of the placebo effect. Anything that a person believes in strongly can produce a healing effect through the mind's capacity to alter chemistry and physiology in distant parts of the body. Biomagnetic therapies, especially ones using static magnetic fields, do no harm. People spend money on many kinds of health aids to find relief from pain and other problems. Whether money spent on biomagnetic therapies is well spent is a matter of personal choice.

Quackery

Quackery is a term that refers to the sale of useless potions, devices, or other substances that promise to heal or cure the buyer of whatever ails him or her. People (quacks) who sell bogus medical products may actually believe in the products' worth and, consequently, are not committing fraud, which involves knowledge of the worthlessness of the products. Legally, it is difficult to separate quackery and fraud.

Quackery has a long history, and during the eighteenth and nineteenth centuries, traveling entertainers sold all sorts of nostrums and potions in towns all over America. Some of these potions actually contained "feel good" substances such as opium and cocaine. Quackery in the United States was dealt a serious blow with the passage of the Pure Food and Drug Act in 1906, which made the sale of worthless medicines illegal. But over the years, sales of useless health products have grown continuously. Ten years ago, the FDA estimated that 38 million Americans purchased a fraudulent health product in the previous year. The most prevalent fraudulent products listed by the FDA are the following:

- Fraudulent arthritis products
- Fake cancer clinics
- Bogus AIDS cures

- Penis enlargement pills and devices
- Instant weight-loss schemes
- Fraudulent sexual aids
- Useless baldness remedies
- False nutritional schemes
- Useless muscle stimulators
- Candidiasis hypersensitivity cures

Why do people buy useless and/or dangerous health products? Why are people easily fooled by quackery? Perhaps because they believe more in magic than in science (Offit, 2014). If you want to safeguard your health and your pocketbook, you should check on any product or treatment that is not provided by a licensed healthcare provider. A reliable source of information about fraudulent products can be found at www.quackwatch.com.

Choosing an Alternative Medicine

Many people are satisfied with the care they receive from modern medicine and the physicians who treat them. However, many Americans also seek alternative medicines to complement conventional treatments. And some persons choose to rely on alternative medicines exclusively. For many kinds of chronic sickness, alternative medicines may provide relief and healing.

> There is no medicine that cures stupidity.
>
> *Japanese proverb*

It often is wise to begin with the least invasive form of treatment before undergoing surgery or taking drugs that can also do harm. Our society is gradually coming to the view that healing can be accomplished by both conventional and alternative medicine. And, as we have pointed out repeatedly, the belief of the patient in a particular treatment, physician, acupuncturist, or chiropractor may be what heals.

TERMS

biomagnetic therapy: use of magnetic fields to treat pain, ailments, and diseases

quackery: promotion and sale of unapproved and worthless products, especially for medical problems and health enhancement

Critical Thinking About Health

1. Suppose that you have been in an auto accident and have a whiplash injury to your neck. It is some months since the accident and your doctor says that your neck has healed and that she cannot find anything wrong. However, you still have pain and difficulty moving your head. What alternative medicines would you now consider to relieve your symptoms? Discuss the rationale behind your choice of alternative medicine(s). If you have actually experienced such an accident, describe the healing process that you went through.

2. Describe any herbal remedy that you are now taking and the condition for which it is being used. Answer each of the following questions and discuss your reasons for taking this remedy and how you think it has helped you (if it has).

   a. Have you investigated whether this herbal remedy has been studied in clinical trials and found to be effective?

   b. Have you investigated whether there are any dangers associated with taking this herb?

   c. Have you discussed taking this herbal remedy with a physician?

3. Therapeutic touch (TT) is a technique widely used by nurses to alleviate suffering and promote healing in patients with a wide variety of ailments, including cancer. TT claims that nurses achieve healing and relief by sensing and manipulating a "human energy field" that is felt above the patient's body. A recent scientific study of TT found that, under controlled laboratory conditions in which nurses had to sense the presence of the experimenter's hand over one of their own without being able to see the person on the other side of a screen, nurses were unable to score significantly above chance (i.e., they had a 50% chance of being correct). The scientists concluded that nurses who practice TT are unable to detect a human energy field, that TT is bogus, and that further professional use of TT is unjustified.

   a. Do you agree with the scientists' conclusions?

   b. Think of reasons why the experiment might not be a valid test of TT and explain your criticisms in detail.

   c. Can you devise an experiment that you think would be better in proving or disproving that TT had beneficial effects on patients?

4. Studies of acupuncture have consistently shown that it is more effective when used on Chinese patients in China than when it is used on patients in the United States. In addition to being more effective on individual patients, more diseases respond to acupuncture treatments in China than when the same diseases are treated with acupuncture in the United States.

   a. Make a list of as many reasons that you can think of that would explain these observations (e.g., American acupuncturists are not as proficient as Chinese acupuncturists).

   b. Discuss each of the items on your list and describe how it would explain the observed difference.

   c. Pick one of the items that you have identified and design a scientific experiment that would prove whether your hypothesis is true or not.

Chapter Summary and Highlights

Chapter Summary

The medical care model familiar to most Americans is a science-based Western medicine that seeks to uncover the biochemical, microbial, physiological, neurological, or behavioral cause for disease and illness. Once a diagnosis is made, a cure is sought using surgery, pharmaceuticals, and psychological and behavioral changes. However, alternative medicines are also widely used around the world as well as in the United States. Hundreds of alternative medicines fall into a few categories: spiritual and mental interventions, nutritional therapies, herbal remedies, and physical and movement therapies. Some of the more widely used alternatives to Western medicine are massage, acupuncture, Ayurveda, and herbal remedies that have been used for thousands of years throughout Asia and Latin America. Some of these alternative medicines have been tested by scientific methods and have proved to be effective for some conditions.

Americans spend billions of dollars every year on vitamin and herbal supplements, energy elixirs, and substances to enhance physical appearance or to increase sexual experience. Many of the alternative health products Americans buy produce little or no benefit despite a manufacturer's claims. Some products, especially ones manufactured outside North America, may contain pesticides, heavy metals, or other toxic chemicals. Whereas prescription and over-the-counter drugs are regulated by a federal agency (FDA) in the

United States, vitamins, herbal supplements, and all products sold in nutritional supplement stores are not. Before you use any unconventional product or device to make yourself feel better, stronger, or happier, investigate carefully whether the product is safe and effective. Do not trust manufacturers' claims without independent verification. Every year, millions of Americans become victims of quackery.

Highlights

- Alternative medicine consists of hundreds of methods for dealing with sickness and disease in ways that are different from modern medical care performed by physicians.
- The broad categories of alternative medicine include spiritual and mental therapies, nutritional therapies, herbal remedies, and physical therapies.
- Homeopathy administers very dilute solutions of substances that are supposed to mimic the symptoms of sick persons and help the body cure itself of the disease.
- Chiropractic and osteopathy use manipulation of the spine and joints to treat musculoskeletal disorders and other diseases.

- Ayurveda and aromatherapy are ancient healing techniques.
- Acupuncture involves inserting very thin needles into specific points on the body to restore harmony to the functioning of tissues and organs.
- Herbal medicine uses mixtures of herbs in the form of pills, powders, teas, and tinctures to help the healing process. Some widely used herbs are ineffective.
- Some herbal remedies contain toxic chemicals, and some interact with prescription drugs to make them either more or less effective.
- There is little scientific evidence for the effectiveness of biomagnetic therapy in the treatment of disease, but many people use it for pain relief and for other health problems.
- Americans spend hundreds of millions of dollars each year on fraudulent health products and treatments; many are victims of quackery.
- Consumers of alternative medicine need to guard against fraudulent claims and unscrupulous persons who advertise therapies of unproved safety and of dubious value.

For Your Health

It's highly likely that if you're experiencing a health problem, someone you know can tell you of a nonstandard medical treatment that's sure to fix you right up. Does it?

Is it safe? Find out by consulting the scientific research on complementary and alternative medicine (Exercise 20.1, in the Workbook).

References

Chen, X. W., et al. (2012). Herb–drug interactions and mechanistic and clinical considerations. *Current Drug Metabolism*, 13, 640–651.

Cochrane Review Group (2010). *Acupuncture: Ancient tradition meets modern science. Cochrane Database of Systematic Reviews*. Retrieved from http://www.necommunityacupuncture.com/neca/acupuncture-ancient-tradition-meets-modern-sc

Costello, J. T., et al. (2015). Whole-body cryotherapy (extreme cold air exposure) for preventing and treating muscle soreness after exercise in adults. *Cochrane Database of Systematic Reviews*. doi: 10.1002/14651858. CD010789.pub2

Hinman, R. S., et al. (2014). Acupuncture for chronic knee pain: a randomized clinical trial. *Journal of the American Medical Association*, 312, 1313–1322.

Linde, K., et al. (2016, April 19). Acupuncture for the prevention of tension-type headache. *Cochrane Database Systematic Reviews*. doi: 10.1002/14651858.CD007587.pub2

Offit, P. A. (2014). *Do you believe in magic? The sense and nonsense of alternative medicine*. New York: Harper.

Pittler, M. A., et al. (2009). Static magnets for reducing pain: Systematic review and meta-analysis of randomized trials. *Canadian Medical Association Journal*, 177, 736–742.

Saper, R. B., et al. (2008). Lead, mercury, and arsenic in U.S. and Indian-manufactured Ayurvedic medicines sold via the Internet. *Journal of the American Medical Association*, 300, 915–923.

Schmidt, M., & Butterweck, V. (2015). The mechanisms of action of St. John's wort: An update. *Wiener Medizinische Wochenschrift*, 165, 229–235. doi: 10.1007/s10354-015-0372-7

Suggested Readings

American Cancer Society. (2014). *Complementary and alternative methods and cancer.* Retrieved from http://www.cancer.org/treatment/treatmentsandsideeffects/complementaryandalternativemedicine/complementaryandalternativemethodsandcancer/cam-and-cancer-toc. Provides reliable information about commonly available nontraditional therapies for people with cancer, including herbs, vitamins, minerals, mind/body/spirit, diet and nutrition, physical touch, and biological methods. Current research findings are explained in brief and understandable language.

Bausell, R. B. (2009). *Snake oil science: The truth about complementary and alternative medicine.* New York: Oxford University Press. The author gently debunks most alternative medicines but also believes that most of them *do* work because of the placebo effect.

Cochrane Review Group. (2010). *Acupuncture: Ancient tradition meets modern science. Cochrane Database of Systematic Reviews.* Retrieved from www.necommunityacupuncture.com/neca/acupuncture-ancient-tradition-meets-modern-ac. Leading scientists review the research on the therapeutic uses of acupuncture.

Kotsirilos, V., Vitetta, L., & Sali, A. (2011). *A guide to evidence-based integrative and complementary medicine.* London, U.K.: Churchill Livingstone. Discusses proven, research-based, nonpharmacologic treatments for common medical practice complaints including mind–body medicine, stress management techniques, dietary guidelines, exercise and sleep advice, acupuncture, nutritional medicine, and herbal medicine, and also includes advice for managing lifestyle and behavioral factors and complementary medicines that may impact the treatment of disease.

Mayo Clinic. (2014). *Complementary and alternative medicine.* Retrieved from http://www.mayoclinic.org/healthy-living/consumer-health/in-depth/alternative-medicine/art-20045267. Discusses the pros and cons of CAM.

Micozzi, M. (2010). *Fundamentals of complementary and alternative medicine.* Philadelphia: Saunders. Provides a complete overview of CAM, including homeopathy, massage and manual therapies, chiropractic, herbal medicine, aromatherapy, naturopathic medicine, and nutrition and hydration.

Recommended Websites

MedlinePlus on Alternative Medicine
This site is useful for checking on the validity or dangers of alternative medicines or therapies.

National Center for Complementary and Integrative Health
Education and resources from the U.S. National Institutes of Health.

Science Daily: Alternative Medicine News
Reports on current research.

Quackwatch.com
Good place to check for fraudulent products and treatments.

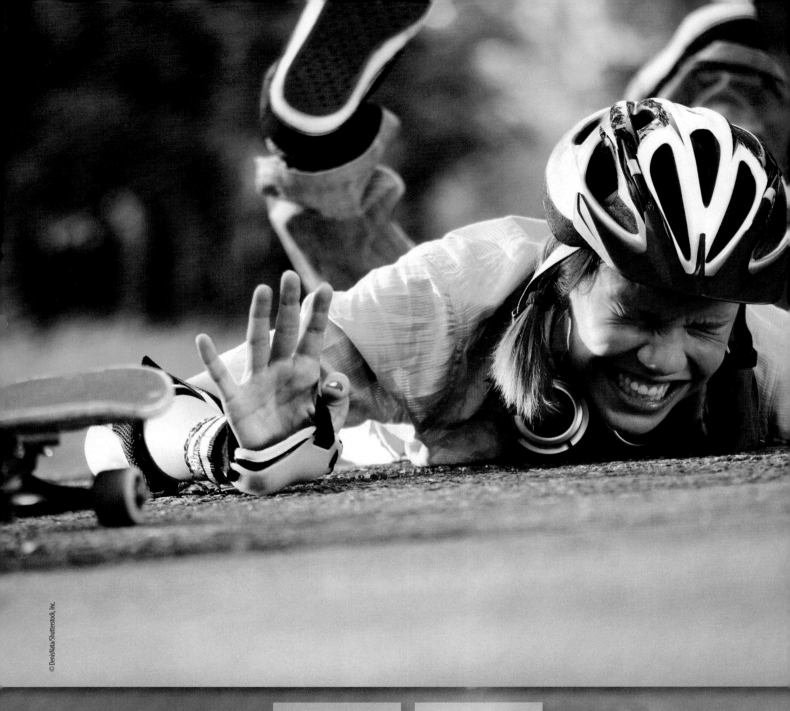
© Denislkata/Shutterstock, Inc.

Health Tips

Ways to Avoid Having a Motor Vehicle Accident

Driving Defensively

Avoid Falls at Christmas

Kids and Guns: Sometimes a Fatal Mix

Wellness Guide

Car Seat Recommendations for Children

Smoke Detectors Protect You from Fires

Prevent Computer-Related Injuries

College Athletes Opt for Health

CHAPTER 21

Accidents and Injuries

Learning Objectives

1. Define *safety, accidents,* and *unintentional injuries.*

2. Describe various strategies to prevent unintentional injuries.

3. Use the epidemiological triad to identify unintentional injury risk factors.

4. Describe the Haddon matrix and explain why it was developed.

5. Discuss various ways to prevent motor vehicle crashes, motorcycle accidents, bicycle accidents, and pedestrian accidents.

6. Describe various strategies to improve home and work safety.

7. Describe ways to prevent firearm injuries.

8. List the major sports with the highest risk of injury for boys and girls.

9. Describe the three grades of a concussion.

Injuries affect the health and well-being of millions of Americans every year. Unintentional injuries and accidents of various kinds are a far greater source of ill health and death than most people realize. Safety warnings and increased public awareness measures have reduced the number of unintentional injury deaths significantly since 1950 (**Figure 21.1**). In the United States, unintentional injuries are the leading cause of death among all persons aged 1 to 34 and the fourth leading cause of death among people of all ages.

> The best way to avoid something is to cause that which is to be avoided, to avoid you of its own accord.
>
> *Sufi proverb*

Many people believe accidents are chance occurrences over which people have no control. Whereas it is true that some accidents are the result of bad luck and chance events, a vast number of accidents and the injuries resulting from them are caused by social and economic conditions—unsafe roads and automobiles, unsafe homes and work sites—and personal factors, such as poor judgment, lapses in attention, recklessness, loss of emotional control, and mental states that are imbalanced by alcohol and drugs. Insofar as the environment can be made safer and individuals become more cautious, the number of unintentional injuries from accidents can be reduced.

Unintentional Injuries and Accidents

What is **safety**? The word *safety* is used in a wide context with various meanings for different individuals. Few experts or safety agencies can agree on a universal definition. "Is this a safe part of town to be in late at night?" "He is not a very safe motorcycle driver." "My daughter's safety has been a concern of mine since she obtained her driver's license." "Is that old ladder safe to use?" As you can see, the word *safe* or *safety* may be used in a variety of situations.

One way to tie all these different scenarios together is the word **accident**. As defined by the National Safety Council, an accident "is that occurrence in a sequence of events which produces unintended injury, death, or property damage. Accident refers to the event, not the result of the event."

Each year one in four Americans will sustain some type of serious injury that requires medical attention and that is a result of an accident. Injuries are a serious problem, but many individuals lack the necessary knowledge and skills to help themselves if a serious accident does occur. Injuries are the leading cause of disability in young people and cause more deaths in children than all the infectious diseases combined.

Unintentional injury refers to the *result* of an accident and its health consequences. Deaths from unintentional injuries result from motor vehicle accidents, home accidents (falls, fires, poisonings), workplace accidents, firearm accidents, and other causes (**Table 21.1**). The greatest number of deaths occur as a result of motor vehicle crashes, falls, and poisonings, including drug overdoses and toxicity. However, the age groups that are most likely to die in these kinds of accidents differ significantly.

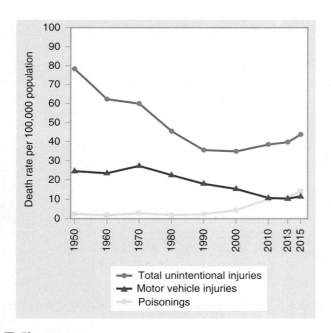

■ **Figure 21.1**

U.S. Death Rates per 100,000 Population Due to Unintentional Injuries, Motor Vehicle-related Accidents, and Drug Poisonings, 1950–2015

Death rates for unintentional injuries declined due to improved safety measures in homes, automobiles, and the workplace. Motor vehicle-related deaths declined due to improvements in automobile safety and reductions in driving after drinking alcohol. The increase in poisonings since 2000 is largely due to overdoses of heroin and prescription painkillers.

Data from National Center for Health Statistics. (2016). *Age-adjusted death rates for selected causes of death, by sex, race, and Hispanic origin: United States, selected years 1950–2015.* Retrieved from http://www.cdc.gov/nchs/data/hus/2016/017.pdf.

Table 21.1

Leading Causes of Unintentional Injury Deaths in the United States in 2014

Cause of death is ascribed to a single category even though many factors contribute to an accident.

Cause of death	Number of deaths
Poisonings	42,032
Motor Vehicle Accidents	33,736
Falls	31,959
Drownings	3,406
Exposure to smoke and flames	2,701
All others	22,094
Total unintentional injury deaths	**135,928**

U.S. National Center for Health Statistics. (2016). Deaths: Final Data for 2014. National Vital Statistics Reports, Volume 65, Number 4. Retrieved from http://www.cdc.gov/nchs/data/nvsr/nvsr65/nvsr65_04.pdf

10 Leading Causes of Injury Deaths by Age Group Highlighting Unintentional Injury Deaths, United States – 2016

Rank	<1	1-4	5-9	10-14	15-24	25-34	35-44	45-54	55-64	65+	Total
1	Unintentional Suffocation 1,023	Unintentional Drowning 425	Unintentional MV Traffic 384	Unintentional MV Traffic 455	Unintentional MV Traffic 7,037	Unintentional Poisoning 14,631	Unintentional Poisoning 13,278	Unintentional Poisoning 13,439	Unintentional Poisoning 9,438	Unintentional Fall 29,668	Unintentional Poisoning 58,335
2	Homicide Unspecified 132	Unintentional MV Traffic 334	Unintentional Drowning 147	Suicide Suffocation 247	Unintentional Poisoning 4,997	Unintentional MV Traffic 7,010	Unintentional MV Traffic 5,075	Unintentional MV Traffic 5,536	Unintentional MV Traffic 5,397	Unintentional MV Traffic 7,429	Unintentional MV Traffic 38,748
3	Unintentional MV Traffic 88	Unintentional Suffocation 118	Unintentional Fire/Burn 78	Suicide Firearm 160	Homicide Firearm 4,553	Homicide Firearm 4,510	Suicide Firearm 3,099	Suicide Firearm 3,873	Suicide Firearm 4,067	Suicide Firearm 5,756	Unintentional Fall 34,673
4	Homicide Other Spec., Classifiable 63	Homicide Unspecified 114	Homicide Firearm 68	Unintentional Drowning 103	Suicide Firearm 2,683	Suicide Firearm 3,298	Homicide Firearm 2,555	Suicide Suffocation 2,112	Unintentional Fall 2,679	Unintentional Unspecified 5,021	Suicide Firearm 22,938
5	Undetermined Suffocation 60	Unintentional Fire/Burn 107	Unintentional Suffocation 35	Homicide Firearm 95	Suicide Suffocation 2,100	Suicide Suffocation 2,643	Suicide Suffocation 2,199	Suicide Poisoning 1,736	Suicide Poisoning 1,538	Unintentional Suffocation 3,631	Homicide Firearm 14,415
6	Undetermined Unspecified 38	Unintentional Pedestrian, Other 82	Unintentional Other Land Transport 24	Unintentional Other Land Transport 64	Unintentional Drowning 530	Undetermined Poisoning 855	Suicide Poisoning 1,144	Homicide Firearm 1,420	Suicide Suffocation 1,474	Unintentional Poisoning 2,458	Suicide Suffocation 11,642
7	Unintentional Drowning 38	Homicide Firearm 64	Unintentional Pedestrian, Other 18	Unintentional Fire/Burn 52	Suicide Poisoning 426	Suicide Poisoning 767	Undetermined Poisoning 788	Unintentional Fall 1,238	Unintentional Suffocation 792	Adverse Effects 2,028	Suicide Poisoning 6,698
8	Homicide Suffocation 19	Homicide Other Spec., Classifiable 64	Unintentional Firearm 16	Unintentional Suffocation 39	Homicide Cut/Pierce 340	Unintentional Drowning 463	Unintentional Fall 515	Undetermined Poisoning 929	Homicide Firearm 738	Unintentional Fire/Burn 1,150	Unintentional Suffocation 6,610
9	Adverse Effects 18	Unintentional Firearm 34	Unintentional Struck by or Against 15	Unintentional Poisoning 28	Undetermined Poisoning 289	Homicide Cut/Pierce 420	Unintentional Drowning 396	Unintentional Drowning 478	Undetermined Poisoning 707	Suicide Poisoning 1,070	Unintentional Unspecified 6,507
10	Unintentional Natural/ Environment 18	Unintentional Poisoning 34	Unintentional Other Transport 14	Unintentional Firearm 23	Unintentional Fall 199	Unintentional Fall 326	Homicide Cut/Pierce 350	Unintentional Suffocation 419	Unintentional Unspecified 625	Suicide Suffocation 859	Undetermined Poisoning 3,827

Data Source: National Center for Health Statistics (NCHS), National Vital Statistics System.
Produced by: National Center for Injury Prevention and Control, CDC using WISQARS™.

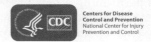

Centers for Disease Control and Prevention
National Center for Injury Prevention and Control

■ **Figure 21.2**

Ten Leading Causes of Unintentional Injury Deaths by Age Group, United States, 2016
Unintentional injuries are denoted by colored boxes.

Reproduced from U.S. Centers for Disease Control and Prevention. (2018). Retrieved from http://www.cdc.gov/injury/wisqars/leadingcauses.html

Teenagers and young adults are most likely to die in motor vehicle crashes, middle-aged persons by poisoning and drug overdose or toxicity, and the elderly by falls (**Figure 21.2**).

Unintentional injuries are the fourth leading cause of death among Americans exceeded only by heart disease, cancer, and chronic lower respiratory disease. The five leading causes of death from unintentional injury are motor vehicle accidents; falls; poisoning by solids, liquids, and drugs; fires and burns; and drowning. These risks have not changed since 1970. For most of the twentieth century, the rate of death from accidents steadily dropped because of increased safety and health efforts. However, in the last few years, there has been an increase in total deaths from unintentional injury, which should be a warning that greater attention to increased safety efforts is needed.

The causes of death from unintentional injury change with age. Poor diet, sedentary lifestyle, arthritis, decreased mobility, poverty, chronic diseases, or lack of access to primary medical care may contribute to injuries and accidental death as people get older. Persons older than age 75 are at highest risk of death compared to younger age groups from virtually all kinds of accidents—pedestrian and motor vehicle accidents, falls, choking, fires, and exposure to unusual natural heat or cold.

TERMS

accident: sequence of events that produces unintended injury, death, or property damage; refers to the event, not the result of the event

safety: an ever-changing condition in which one attempts to minimize the risk of injury, illness, or property damage from the hazards to which one may be exposed

unintentional injury: preferred term for accidental injury; result of an accident

Reducing Your Risk of Accidents

When considering accidents, their prevention, and their consequences, public health professionals focus on **accident mitigation**—methods to reduce damage caused by unplanned events—and **accident prevention**—ways to eliminate the occurrence of unintended injuries. Accident mitigation and prevention can be viewed in two contexts: (1) individual or personal and (2) environmental or community.

Many factors are involved in unintentional injury: knowledge, attitudes, beliefs, and behaviors; economic and social conditions; ability level of the performer of tasks; conditions of the environment; and alcohol and other drug use. Reducing these risk factors will lessen injuries, but more attention should be directed to prevention strategies. Their cost to society in direct medical care and lost productivity is many billions of dollars per year (Centers for Disease Control, 2017).

Attitudes and beliefs may be the most significant factor involved in unintentional injuries. Your individual attitude toward safety precautions greatly influences the likelihood of an injury. You may believe that safety precautions are a waste of time because you have no control over the situation (what will happen, will happen), or you may have a reckless attitude (you like to take risks).

Lack of knowledge and skills also plays a role in unintentional injury. In special circumstances, especially when performing a new procedure or task, lacking the proper knowledge or skills could result in unintentional injury (e.g., operating a new power tool before reading the instructions, operating a motorcycle the first time, or using a new kitchen appliance).

Socioeconomic factors also play a role in unintentional injuries. Some individuals may lack the necessary funds to replace unsafe or old equipment. Some may even lack the necessary funds to obtain proper training in safety-related matters. Safety training often is available through a local National Safety Council office on such topics as proper storage of household cleaning items, tool safety, and safety tips for the babysitter. Local health departments may also provide educational workshops on safety issues.

Attitudes and beliefs as well as the social setting can raise or lower the probability of an unintentional injury. For example, alcohol and drug use definitely affect the frequency of unintentional injuries. Prescribed medications, especially ones with a sedative effect, can increase the likelihood of an accident while operating a motor vehicle, motorcycle, or power tool.

The ability of the individual performing a task or activity may affect the probability of an unintentional injury. The person may be a child who is too young to perform a task competently. At the other end of the spectrum, an elderly individual may not be strong enough or steady enough to perform a simple task like sawing a piece of wood.

The environment can be the most unpredictable risk factor in unintentional injuries. Environmental risks include appropriate maintenance of streets, safe power transmission and sewage treatment, and laws that regulate the hazards of appliances and tools. Natural disasters such as floods, hurricanes, earthquakes, or tornadoes are also environmental risks. The devastation caused by natural disasters may affect us at some point in our lifetime. In 2011, thousands of people died in Japan from a tsunami that followed a stong earthquake. In 2005, the Gulf Coast of the United States was devastated by Hurricane Katrina, and the city of New Orleans was flooded. In 2008, a cyclone in Burma killed more than 10,000 people and an earthquake in China killed approximately 70,000 people, many of them children. Natural disasters can strike anyone, anywhere, and at any time.

Stress and fatigue contribute greatly to higher rates of unintentional injuries. Stress may interfere with your concentration when performing even a simple task or may distract you while you are engaged in an activity. Fatigue causes you to be less alert or have slower reaction times; fatigue affects your coordination, and, at worst, can cause you to fall asleep. It is not wise to attempt difficult tasks while you are fatigued or under stress.

> He who feels punctured must have been a bubble.
> He who feels unarmed must have carried arms.
> He who feels belittled must have been consequential.
> He who feels deprived must have had privilege.
>
> *Lao Tzu, The Way of Life*

Analysis of Unintentional Injury

Scientific studies of unintentional injury try to uncover why injuries occur, what factors play a role, and who or what age group is most at risk. Analysis of unintentional injury provides us with data that are necessary before effective educational, preventive, or enforcement strategies can be implemented.

Injury epidemiology, used to investigate risk factors that cause unintentional injuries, is analogous to the epidemiological model for disease. For injuries to result, three factors are involved: (1) the agent or source of energy exchange (i.e., mechanical, chemical, electrical, or thermal), (2) the vehicle for the transmission of mechanical energy (i.e., a car, truck, motorcycle, powerline, or poison), and (3) a host or object (i.e., a person, school building, or house) (**Figure 21.3**).

Most unintentional injuries involve many factors and interactions among risk factors. For example, cutting trees with a chain saw on a windy or rainy day may increase the risk of an accident, whereas choosing a dry, calm day might reduce the risk.

The Haddon matrix is one of the scientific models used in unintentional injury analysis. Developed by

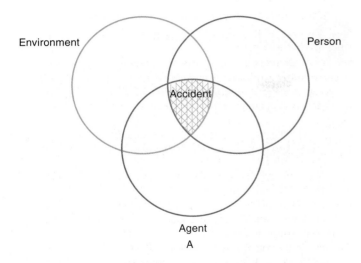

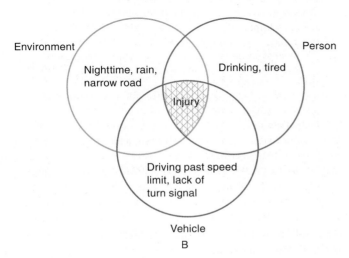

■ **Figure 21.3**

Epidemiologic Model for Unintentional Injuries
The model shows that (a) the environment, a person, and an agent
(car) interact to create conditions for an accident. Part (b) shows the
factors that increases the likelihood of an injury.

William Haddon Jr. in the 1960s, this model was used
originally to investigate motor vehicle risk factors and to
develop and implement programs to prevent or reduce
the occurrence of car accidents.

According to some estimates, "every two miles, the
average driver makes 400 observations, 40 decisions, and
one mistake. Once in every 500 miles, one of these mistakes
leads to a near collision, and once in every 61,000 miles,
one of these mistakes leads to a car crash" (Gladwell, 2001).
The Haddon matrix analyzes accidents in three phases:

- *Phase 1: Pre-event phase.* Includes factors that may
  determine whether an accident will happen; lack of
  knowledge or skills and alcohol use are the most significant factors.
- *Phase 2: Event phase.* Occurs when the host comes
  into contact with forces of energy. Many preventive measures, such as the use of helmets, seat belts, or
  protective goggles, are associated with this phase.

- *Phase 3: Postevent phase.* Includes emergency procedures provided after the injury has occurred. Preventive signaling devices, smoke and carbon monoxide
  detectors, or fire alarms will increase the speed with
  which help reaches an injured person. Emergency
  transportation and care of an injured or sick person
  occur in this phase.

All approaches to unintentional injury reduction include (1) educational and prevention strategies,
(2) stricter laws and regulations (e.g., mandates to enforce
seat belt and helmet compliance), and (3) better product
design and automatic protection devices (e.g., air bags,
child-proof car door locks, child-proof safety caps on
medicines).

Motor Vehicle Safety

Motor vehicle travel is a primary means of transportation
in North America and much of the world. Yet, for all its
advantages, injuries resulting from motor vehicle crashes
are a leading cause of death. Each year, approximately
33,000 Americans are killed in motor vehicle crashes, and
about 2.5 million suffer disabling injuries.

The National Highway Traffic Safety Administration
(NHTSA) estimates that alcohol was involved in 41% of
fatal crashes and 7% of all traffic accidents, fatal and
nonfatal. Approximately 3 in every 10 Americans will
be involved in an alcohol-related traffic accident some
time in their lives. Alcohol involvement in fatal crashes
during the day is 18% but rises to 61% at night. More
than 1 million drivers are arrested for driving under the
influence of alcohol or other drugs every year. Another
important statistic to be aware of is that in almost half of
pedestrian fatalities in which someone was hit by a car,
either the driver, the pedestrian, or both were intoxicated.
Heed the warning: *Do Not Drink and Drive.* Do not ride with
any driver who has been drinking. And do not go walking
on busy roads if you have been drinking.

Many accidents involving young persons occur
after dark, after parties, and after drinking. Alcohol in
the blood and brain impairs a driver's judgment, coordination, and reaction time. The effects of alcohol vary
considerably from one person to another, so even small
amounts of alcohol may impair driving skills and cause
an accident.

TERMS

accident mitigation: methods to reduce damage
caused by unplanned events

accident prevention: ways to eliminate the occurrence
of unintended injuries

injury epidemiology: the study of the occurrence,
causes, and prevention of injury

Ways to Avoid Having a Motor Vehicle Accident

Resolve to do the following each time you drive:

- Don't drive when sleep deprived.
- Wear the seat belt.
- Don't drive after consuming alcohol, marijuana, or other drugs.
- Don't interact with a cell phone or any screen device while driving.
- Don't speed or drive aggressively.

Remember: A motor vehicle accident injury occurs once every 13 seconds; a death occurs once every 12 minutes.

Driving Defensively

Driving defensively means not only taking responsibility for yourself and your actions but also keeping an eye on "the other guy." The National Safety Council offers the following guidelines to help reduce your risks on the road:

- Don't leave the driveway without securing each passenger in the car, including children and pets. Seat belts save thousands of lives each year!
- Remember that driving too fast or too slow can increase the likelihood of collisions.
- Don't kid yourself. If you plan to drink, designate a driver who won't drink. Alcohol is a factor in almost half of all fatal motor vehicle accidents.
- Be alert! If you notice that a car is straddling the center line, weaving, making wide turns, stopping abruptly, or responding slowly to traffic signals, the driver may be impaired.
- Avoid an impaired driver by slowing down, letting the driver pass, pulling onto the shoulder, or turning right at the nearest corner. If it appears that an oncoming car is crossing into your lane, pull over to the roadside, sound the horn, and flash your lights.
- Notify the police immediately after seeing a motorist who is driving suspiciously.
- Follow the rules of the road. Don't contest the "right of way" or try to race another car during a merge. Be respectful of other motorists.
- While driving, be cautious, aware, and responsible.

Teenagers between the ages of 16 and 17 have more car accidents than any other group, whether based on age or miles driven. For this reason, a majority of states have instituted a graduated driver licensing system (GDL) in an attempt to reduce the number of accidents among the youngest drivers. At least 43 states employ a three-stage GDL system for licensing teenage drivers. The system involves driver education classes, supervised driving lessons, restricted night driving, and prohibition on carrying teenage passengers. The results of GDL systems vary from state to state, and safety experts are still studying which aspects of the system are most effective in reducing accident risks among first-time drivers. New laws have been proposed that set a zero tolerance for blood alcohol for persons under age 21.

Many factors other than alcohol use contribute to motor vehicle fatalities and injuries; these include road conditions and speeding. The interaction between these two factors is particularly risky. In all severe accidents, rural and urban, exceeding the posted speed limit was the most common factor. Defects in a vehicle, such as faulty tires, brakes, headlights, or steering system, also contribute to the risk of motor vehicle accidents.

Driving can be difficult even when you are concentrating on the road and your surroundings. But driving while using a mobile phone can be distracting and a danger to the user and everyone on the road. At 55 miles per hour, a vehicle travels the length of a football field in 3.7 seconds, less time than it takes to read a text and respond with one tap on the keypad.

Using a mobile device while driving is much more distracting than having a conversation with someone in the car or listening to the radio. Doing business or having an argument with someone in a cell phone conversation increases the risk of an accident. Inattention to the task of driving is a contributing factor in about 80% of all motor vehicle accidents. The National Safety Council has recommended that "the best practice is to not use electronic devices, including cell phones, while driving. When on the road, drivers shall concentrate on safe and defensive driving and not on making or receiving phone calls, delivery of faxes, using computers, navigation systems, or other distracting influences."

Seat Belts

Lap/shoulder seat belts are the best protection against fatal injury in a crash. Seat belts are estimated to have reduced the risk of fatal injury to front seat occupants by almost 50% since 1980; it is estimated that hundreds of thousands of lives have been saved by seat belt use.

Seat belt use is at a record high. The national average for seat belt use in 2013 was 88%. Twelve states have averaged over 90%, the highest being Hawaii, with 97% of drivers using seat belts. Despite the increased use of seat belts, more than two-thirds of teenagers who died in crashes that occurred at night were not using seat belts. A national program called *Click It or Ticket* implemented in recent years has helped boost the use of seat belts across the nation. The value of consistent seat belt use by both drivers and passengers is incontrovertible; everyone should buckle up whenever riding in a car or truck.

Air bags provide additional protection but are not very effective by themselves except in a head-on collision; they should always be used in conjunction with a lap/shoulder seat belt. Government regulations, use of lap/shoulder seat belts and child safety seats, and installation of air bags

Car Seat Recommendations for Children

Motor vehicle crashes are the leading cause of death among children aged 3 to 14 years old. The use of safety seats by children riding in passenger cars reduces the risk of fatal injury by 71% among infants and by 54% among toddlers.

A car seat should be selected according to a child's age and size; it should fit in the vehicle and be used every time. Every car seat comes with the manufacturer's notification of height and weight limits and instructions for installing the car seat using the car's seat belt or latch system.

To maximize safety, children should ride in a car seat for as long as possible within the manufacturer's height and weight requirements. Every child should ride in the back seat at least through age 12.

Birth to 12 months
A child under age 1 should always ride in a rear-facing car seat. There are different types of rear-facing car seats. Infant-only seats can only be used rear-facing. Convertible and 3-in-1 car seats typically have higher height and weight limits for the rear-facing position, allowing you to keep your child rear-facing for a longer period of time.

1 to 3 years
A child should ride in a rear-facing car seat for as long as possible and until he or she reaches the maximum height or weight limit allowed by the car seat's manufacturer. Once a child

outgrows the rear-facing car seat, the child is ready to travel in a forward-facing car seat with a harness.

4 to 7 years
A child should ride in a forward-facing car seat with a harness until he or she reaches the top height or weight limit allowed by your car seat's manufacturer. Once a child outgrows the forward-facing car seat with a harness, it's time to travel in a booster seat, but still in the back seat.

8 to 12 years
Keep a child in a booster seat until he or she is big enough to fit in a seat belt properly. For a seat belt to fit properly the lap belt must lie snugly across the upper thighs, not the stomach. The shoulder belt should lie snug across the shoulder and chest and not cross the neck or face. To be safe, a preteen should still ride in the back seat.

A REAR-FACING CAR SEAT is the best seat for a young child. It has a harness and in a crash, it cradles and moves with a child to reduce the stress to the child's fragile neck and spinal cord.

A FORWARD-FACING CAR SEAT has a harness and tether that limits a child's forward movement during a crash.

A BOOSTER SEAT positions the seat belt so that it fits properly over the stronger parts of a child's body.

A SEAT BELT should lie across the upper thighs and be snug across the shoulder and chest to restrain the child safely in a crash. It should not rest on the stomach area or across the neck.

Reproduced from the U.S. National Highway Traffic Safety Administration (March, 2014). Retrieved from http://www.safercar.gov/parents/RightSeat.htm

have helped reduce the number of motor vehicle fatalities and injuries.

Americans are addicted to speed. Studies show that more and more Americans are driving faster than ever. Many Americans believe that speeding is a basic right, regardless of the posted speed limit. Automobile manufacturers build big, fast, heavy cars that can easily go over 100 mph, and many drivers get "high" by driving fast. Race car drivers are heroes to many Americans, and millions of people engage in the "sport" of racing modified cars. Speeding takes the lives of many young drivers as well as the lives of innocent passengers and drivers of other cars.

Along with drinking and speeding, *distracted driving* is a major contributor to automobile accidents. Among the many activities that distract drivers are eating a sandwich or hamburger (72%), kissing (29%), cell phone texting (28%), and taking off clothes (23%). Although it is not known how many of these activities contribute to accidents, it is well documented that talking on a cell phone while driving causes many accidents, injuries, and deaths. Each year in the United States about 28% of all car crashes (1.6 million) are directly attributable to talking or texting on a cell phone (Ship, 2010). With the enormous increase in cell phone use, distracted driving has become the focus of new laws across the country. So far,

31 states have passed legislation that restricts the use of a cell phone while driving.

Although hands-free devices are available, using a mobile device is nevertheless a powerful distraction from concentrating on driving. If the conversation is important or emotional, the distraction is even greater, and thus, so is the likelihood of an accident. Using a mobile device *safely* while driving requires first pulling off the road safely and stopping the car.

Motorcycle Safety

Motorcycles appeal to many individuals for various reasons: low cost to purchase, repair, and operate; the exciting feeling of open-air riding; and association with fellow motorcycle riders. However, higher risks include less crash protection than an automobile, and less visibility by other drivers. About 5,000 Americans die in motorcycle crashes each year. Motorcycle operators can ensure a safer ride by securing proper training in operational procedures and by using a helmet and proper protective clothing. Less than 10% of all motorcycle operators receive any formal training. Wearing a motorcycle helmet reduces the likelihood of fatal injuries in an accident by about 37%. Protective

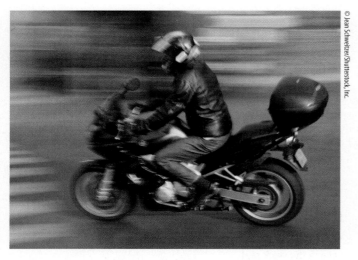

A helmet and protective clothing are essential to motorcycle safety.

clothing, such as long sleeves and pants, jackets, and boots, may lessen the chance for abrasions should an accident occur as well as protect from bad weather.

In 1966, Congress mandated that motorcycle riders and passengers in all states use helmets. If states did not enforce this mandate, they would lose federal highway funds. Although states were slow to enforce the federal motorcycle helmet mandate, by 1975, most had passed some form of helmet law for motorcycle riders (**Figure 21.4**); enforcement varies from strict to none. Only three states, Iowa, Illinois, and New Hampshire, do not have any kind of helmet laws.

Riding a motorcycle is significantly more dangerous than riding in a passenger vehicle. Although motorcycles represent only 3% of registered motor vehicles, motorcycles were involved in 13% of fatal accidents in 2009. Motorcycles are fun but, even with training, helmets, and protective clothing, are still a very risky activity.

All-Terrain Vehicles

Another popular vehicle, especially among the 16 and younger age group, is the all-terrain vehicle (ATV). These can be driven by anyone off road and almost anywhere they can be made to go. In addition to causing significant environmental damage to park lands, beaches, hiking trails, and pristine areas normally accessible only on foot, they also are responsible for many deaths and injuries. In 2014, over 100,000 injuries to young riders of ATVs were reported by hospital emergency rooms, about the same number as in previous years. However, only 324 deaths occurred among ATV riders, a significant reduction from previous years. Despite the reduced number of deaths among teenagers riding ATVs, more efforts are being made to reduce ATV accidents.

Some states have tried to legislate the use of ATVs but with little success. Kids can take their parents' vehicles with or without permission and can ride on public lands where roads are not policed.

Powered Two-Wheelers

Powered two-wheelers (PTWs) consist of a diverse group of vehicles, including powered scooters and mopeds. PTWs have small gasoline or electric engines and are manufactured not to exceed speeds of 30 mph, although they can be modified to attain speeds of 50 mph. PTWs are used on and off-road and for both basic transportation and recreation. PTWs are increasingly popular because of their low purchase price and maintenance costs, convenience, fun, ability to circumvent congested traffic, and relatively small carbon footprint.

Although lacking the size and power of conventional motorcycles, PTWs nevertheless carry a high injury risk. According to data from the French Institute of Science and Technology (Clabaux et al., 2017), PTW accidents are four to five times as likely to occur as conventional car crashes. It is estimated that PTWs account for about 15% of all traffic fatalities, or about 2,500 per year in

■ **Figure 21.4**

Motorcycle Safety
Nineteen states and the District of Columbia legally require all motorcycle riders to wear a helmet. Twenty-eight states have partial helmet laws, meaning that only some motorcycle riders must wear a helmet. Three states have no helmet laws.

Adapted from Insurance Institute for Highway Safety. (2017). *Motorcycle helmet use* (map). Retrieved from http://www.iihs.org/iihs/topics/laws/helmetuse/mapmotorcycle-helmets?topicName=motorcycles#map

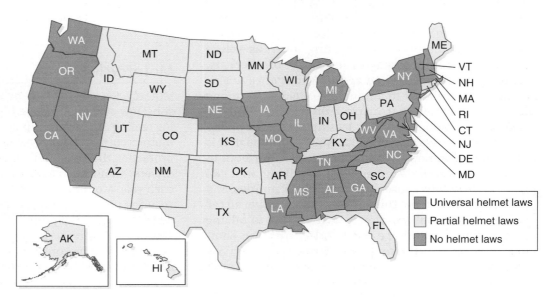

the United States. Half of fatally injured PTW users are younger than age 25.

Most serious and fatal PTW injuries result from collisions with a motor vehicle. PTWs are most vulnerable when a car is making a turn. Emergency braking can cause the rider to fall before the collision and possibly be thrown off the PTW after the collision. Wearing protective clothing can prevent some minor injuries. Wearing helmets can prevent severe head injuries. Safety experts agree that PTW helmet use should be mandatory. PTW drivers increase injury risk by speeding and lane splitting. Collision risks are minimized by using headlights during daytime, wearing fluorescent/retroflective clothing, and being mindful of dangerous road surface conditions and/ or small objects on the road.

PTW accidents are also caused by faulty vehicles— loose handlebars, wobbly wheels, failed brakes. Dangerous defects have resulted in recalls of thousands of PTWs. Since emergency braking a PTW can lead to loss of control, manufacturers are considering outfitting PTWs with antilock braking systems/combined braking systems (ABS/CBS) as found on motorcycles.

Many cities and countries have few laws regarding PTWs compared to laws for conventional motorcycles, including driving age, helmet use, traffic rules, use while intoxicated, and licensing of either driver or vehicle. Communities are increasingly recognizing that PTW safety requires more thorough licensing with higher age limits, more extensive driver training and testing, lower power-to-weight ratios, restricted top speed, and enforcement of quality manufacturing.

Pedestrian Safety

Each year in the United States, about 70,000 pedestrians are injured in motor vehicle accidents and about 4,500 are killed. About 80% of all pedestrian deaths and injuries involve children aged 5 to 9 who are either crossing or entering a street. Among young children, implementation of preventive strategies and educational efforts addressing safety procedures in traffic areas may reduce accidents. Many young children don't know what traffic signals or signs mean. Young children are also unable to judge the distance and speed of vehicles, which puts them in danger when trying to cross a busy intersection. Close supervision by adults helps prevent accidents; education of child-care workers is another preventive strategy.

The elderly are especially at risk for pedestrian injuries, as a result of failing eyesight, hearing, and mobility problems. Some pedestrian injuries occur when individuals dart into a busy street or are unable to see oncoming traffic because their view is blocked by a parked vehicle. Many pedestrian injuries involve joggers, runners, and walkers. Bright-colored clothes, especially reflective clothes, offer protection for pedestrians during both day and night. Also, just as alcohol impairs the judgment of motor vehicle operators, it impairs the judgment of pedestrians.

Whether an intersection is marked with a crosswalk does not seem to make a difference in pedestrian deaths among persons aged 65 and older. The important factor seems to be whether the intersection has a stop sign or signal. Pedestrians should always walk to a corner that has a stop sign or signal light; crossing in the middle of a block is dangerous even if there is a marked crosswalk.

Other preventive strategies can also help reduce the number of pedestrian injuries and deaths. Underpasses and overpasses in high-traffic areas, well-marked crosswalks, and pedestrian guardrails all offer protection for the pedestrian. Limiting traffic during peak hours of pedestrian traffic—for instance, before and after school or church—is also beneficial.

Bicycle Safety

Bicycle safety concerns have been increasing as more bicycles are used for exercise, recreation, and commuting to school or work. Few bicyclists wear a protective helmet every time they ride their bike, yet the single most

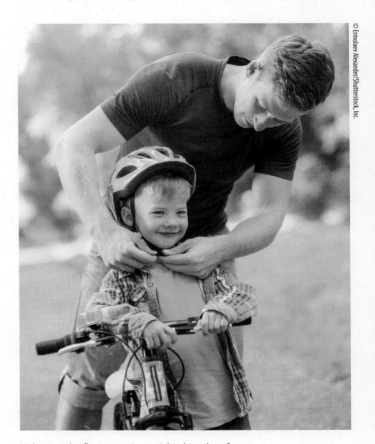

© Ermolaev Alexander/Shutterstock, Inc.

Helmet and reflector use is crucial to bicycle safety.

TERMS

Powered two-wheelers (PTWs): a diverse group of vehicles, including powered scooters and mopeds

important factor in reducing serious head injuries and bicycle deaths is the use of well-designed and effective helmets. The use of a helmet can reduce the chance of head and brain injuries by more than 60% should an accident occur. No state law requires adult bicyclists to wear helmets. Young riders are required to wear helmets in only 21 states and the District of Columbia. In 2015, almost half a million bicycle riders were injured seriously enough to require treatment; about 1,000 bicyclists died from injuries received in accidents.

Bicycle riders are required to follow the same rules of the road as automobile operators. But many bicycle riders lack knowledge of these rules, do not use proper hand signals, or ride on the wrong side of the street, contributing to bicycle injuries and fatalities. Also, lack of skill in handling a bicycle increases the risk of an accident. Individuals who purchase a new bicycle should be familiar with all its devices before riding it. Many young bicycle riders are unaware of the rules of the road or are too small to see over motor vehicles.

Bicycle riders need to wear bright, reflective clothing, and the bicycle itself should be properly equipped with reflectors and lights. A recent and dangerous phenomenon is wearing headphones while riding. Inability to hear the sounds of traffic, the honk of a horn, or a shout of warning may contribute to an accident. Construction of more bicycle paths, underpasses, overpasses, and guardrails along with defensive riding skills can reduce bicycle injuries and deaths.

Home and Community Safety

Accidental deaths in the home are gradually declining but are still a major source of injury and death. Accidents in the home take a special toll on both young and elderly persons. As the elderly population continues to grow, accidents in the home and community will increase. The main categories of home accidents include falls, poisonings, fires, suffocation, and drowning (**Figure 21.5**).

Disabling injuries occur more frequently in the home than in all automobile and workplace accidents combined. Disabling injuries of various kinds in the home number more than 30 million, and approximately 90,300 persons die from falls, poisonings, fires, and other accidents in homes. The annual cost of home and community injuries and deaths is more than $30 billion. Clearly, taking preventive measures to reduce accidents at home and in the community should be a high public health priority, especially in homes where very young and very elderly people live.

Falls

People of all ages fall, but most fatal injuries occur among elderly persons. Falls are the leading cause of deaths from unintentional injuries in the home and community. Children often fall because of their strenuous activities, but usually the injuries are minor and heal rapidly. However,

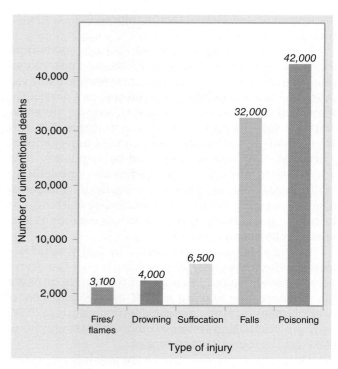

■ **Figure 21.5**

Approximate Number of Unintentional Injury Deaths at Home and in the Community, United States, 2014

Data from U.S. National Center for Health Statistics. (2017). Deaths: Final Data for 2017. National Vital Statistics Reports, Volume 65, Number 4. Retrieved from: http://www.cdc.gov/nchs/data/nvsr/nvsr65/nvsr65_04.pdf; U.S. Centers for Disease Control and Prevention (2015). Ten Leading Causes of Death and Injury. Retrieved from: http://www.cdc.gov/injury/wisqars/leadingcauses.html

children also fall down stairs, out of trees, from open windows, and from the backs of trucks. They fall while climbing, jumping, or running. People responsible for watching children at play must be alert to the danger of a fall.

Avoid Falls at Christmas

Every year, several thousand Americans suffer injuries from falls while decorating a Christmas tree. Be extra cautious during the holiday season and remember these tips when decorating a tree:
- Make sure any ladder you use is stable. If leaned against a wall, observe the 4 to 1 rule: If you climb 4 feet, the base of the ladder should be 1 foot from the wall; for 8 feet, the base should be 2 feet from the wall.
- Do not lean backward or sideways from the ladder. Keep feet in the center of each step.
- Do not overload the top of the tree with ornaments or lights.
- Do not place candles on or near the tree. A Christmas tree is a match waiting to be lit.
- Make sure Christmas tree lights are in good condition and will not spark or cause a wire to become hot. Test before stringing lights on trees.

Enjoy the holiday season and avoid accidents.

Falls are an especially serious problem for the elderly. Each year, 27% of Americans older than age 65 and 30% of Americans older than age 75 fall and suffer an injury (Bergen et al., 2016). Two-thirds of those who fall will suffer another fall within 6 months of the first fall. About 40% of all nursing home admissions result from injuries suffered in falls. It is no wonder that many older people have a fear of falling. When an elderly person falls, it can result in hospitalization and permanent loss of independent living.

The elderly need to take specific actions to avoid falls. Being physically active is important. Performing daily strength and flexibility exercises is helpful. Paying attention to balance and using canes or other walking aids may help avert a fall. Move slowly and carefully around the house and in the community. If an area is unfamiliar, an older person who is unsteady should ask someone to hold his or her arm for extra support.

Certain areas in the home are hazardous for falls. The kitchen, bathroom, and laundry room are dangerous because they often have wet floors. Stairs are also hazardous; a person may stumble while walking up or down, particularly if he or she is distracted or if the stairs are not well lit. Bumping into furniture or tripping over the legs of tables, chairs, or loose rugs are also common causes of falls. Many elderly persons fall over pets running free in the house.

Climbing ladders may be an invitation for a fall if a person is careless or the ladder is weak or unstable. When performing any activity in which a fall is possible, take extra safety measures, such as having someone hold the ladder that you are climbing.

Poisonings

A **poison** is any chemical substance that causes illness, injury, or death. Poisons enter the body by being ingested (medicines, drugs, mushrooms, shellfish, chemicals), inhaled (carbon monoxide, hydrogen sulfide), injected (bee sting, snake bite), or by contact with the skin (poison ivy, solutions that burn). Toxins arising from bacteria-contaminated foods are not considered poisons medically; illness and death resulting from them are considered diseases. Chemical poisons such as pesticides disturb essential biological reactions in the body and cause a variety of symptoms, even death. Some poisons cause only transitory symptoms; the body returns to normal once the poison is eliminated. However, some poisons cause permanent and irreversible damage.

Many cultivated and wild plants, trees, and bushes contain poisonous compounds. Eating the berries, seeds, roots, or leaves of unfamiliar plants can produce mild or severe symptoms of poisoning. Many common household plants are also poisonous, even the Christmas poinsettia. Collecting and eating wild mushrooms can be dangerous unless you are knowledgeable about what species are edible.

Young children, especially when they have just learned to crawl or walk, are particularly susceptible to poisoning accidents. Children are curious, active, and adventurous, and it is natural for young children to put things in their mouths, including nonfood items such as paint chips, dirt, marbles—almost any small object. When children are hungry, thirsty, or just curious, they are likely to ingest whatever is closest to hand—medicines, pills, household products, pesticides. Children between ages 1 and 5 years suffer the greatest number of accidental poisonings.

Precautions by manufacturers of drugs, solvents, paints, and other products have markedly reduced the number of accidental childhood poisonings. Child-resistant lids, tamper-proof caps, and internal seals help to prevent children from ingesting harmful substances. Precautions by parents and other child caregivers are essential to reduce the risk further. All household products and medicines should be kept out of reach of small children. Dangerous substances should be kept in locked cabinets. Small children should not be left unsupervised in areas like bathrooms, kitchens, and garages, where dangerous household products are stored.

There are several hundred poison control centers across the country (list at www.aapce.org). Should a poisoning accident occur, someone at a poison control center can give you immediate expert advice. Keep the number of a poison control center near the phone in case of emergency.

Illness or death from unintentional overdose of a prescription or nonprescription drug is considered poisoning. Such poisonings occur when a drug is taken accidentally, too much of a drug is taken accidentally, the wrong drug is given or taken in error, or an accident occurs in the use of a drug(s) in medical and surgical procedures. For example, acetaminophen (known as Tylenol in the United States and paracetamol in other countries) is one of the most widely used drugs for pain, headache, colds, and other symptoms. It also is a common cause of poisoning worldwide mostly from acute liver toxicity. Many people ingest excessive amounts of acetaminophen and develop toxic liver disease because they misunderstand dosing directions or fail to recognize that acetaminophen is found in more than one medication they are using.

Deaths in the United States from drug overdose have increased significantly in recent years (**Figure 21.6**). In great measure, the increase in drug overdose deaths is due to misuse of opioid prescription pain relievers such as hydrocodone (e.g., Vicodin), oxycodone (e.g., OxyContin, Percocet), oxymorphone (e.g., Opana), morphine, heroin, and synthetic opioids such as fentanyl. In 2017, over 2 million Americans were estimated to be addicted to opioids related to having received them medically for pain. Also,

TERMS

poison: any chemical substance that causes illness, injury, or death

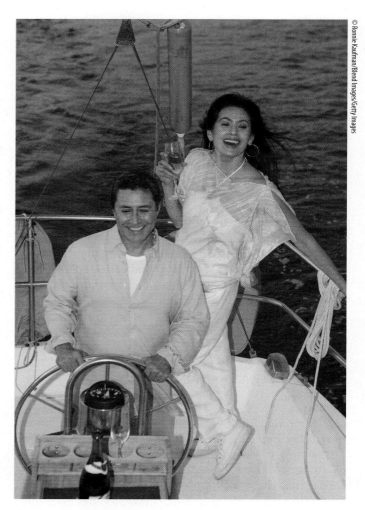

■ Figure 21.6

U.S. Deaths from Drug Overdose, 2010–2017

About 90% of drug overdose deaths are due to opioid misuse related to medically treated complaints of pain. Researchers have found that the increase in deaths due to opioid overdose occurs most frequently among middle-aged, non-hispanic white people with a high school diploma or less. This group's significant risk for opioid misuse is thought to be due to long-term, steady deterioration in economic and social wellbeing, which lead to increases in persons experiencing physical pain and poor health and mental health (Case, A. & Deaton, A., 2017).

Data from Hedegaard, H. et al. (2017, February). Drug overdose deaths in the United States, 1999–2015. National Center for Health Statistics Data Brief No. 273. Retrieved from https://www.cdc.gov/nchs/products/databriefs/db273.htm

Katz, J. (2017, June 5). Drug deaths in America are rising faster than ever. *New York Times*. Retrieved from https://www.nytimes.com/interactive/2017/06/05/upshot/opioid-epidemic-drug-overdose-deaths-are-rising-faster-than-ever.html?mcubz=0

Many boating accidents are associated with drinking alcohol while having fun on the water.

as many as 100,000 babies were born addicted to opioids and suffering consequent withdrawal (*neonatal abstinence syndrome*) because their mothers misused opioids during pregnancy. The annual cost of prescription opioid misuse in the United States to cover the costs of health care, lost productivity, addiction treatment, and criminal justice involvement is many billions of dollars annually.

Poisoning by gases and vapors is mainly caused by carbon monoxide. Carbon monoxide results from incomplete combustion in stationary motor vehicles, fireplaces, stoves, and appliances using natural or liquid propane gas. Engineering and manufacturing improvements to lower carbon monoxide emissions have contributed significantly to reducing the rates of unintentional carbon monoxide fatalities.

Drowning

About half of all drownings occur during June, July, and August, when many people are engaged in summer water activities. Recreation in large bodies of water, rivers, and streams provides the opportunities for accidental drowning.

When a person is under water and inhales water instead of air, an automatic muscular contraction of the larynx occurs that is called **laryngospasm**. This muscular reflex closes the body's main airway in an attempt to keep water from entering the lungs. The spasm continues as

long as the person is under water and within a few minutes can lead to death by suffocation. Once the laryngospasm relaxes, water enters the lungs. Only about 10% of people survive not breathing under water for as long as 6 minutes, and these victims will survive only if artificial respiration is applied immediately. Few people recover if breathing has stopped for as long as 10 minutes.

Scientific evidence does not support the widely held belief that swimming shortly after eating induces stomach cramps, thereby increasing the risk of drowning. However, it is true that after eating, blood is diverted to the stomach to assist digestion and consequently less oxygen may be available for muscles, which can lead to muscle spasms. This sequence poses no problem for a healthy person, but if a person is in poor health, is overweight, or has existing heart disease, the risk of drowning may be increased.

Knowing your swimming ability and avoiding swimming in dangerous waters are ways to reduce the risk of accidental drowning. Using a personal flotation device (commonly called a life jacket) while you engage in water sports can also reduce the risk of drowning.

Alcohol and other drugs may be the biggest predisposing factor in drowning for individuals aged

Smoke Detectors Protect You from Fires

Most deaths and injuries in fires result from inhalation of smoke and toxic gases that reach victims before the flames do. Survival depends on an early warning system that gives you time to vacate the premises at once. The best warning system available is a smoke detector, which cuts your risk of dying in a fire in half. The U.S. Consumer Product Safety Commission offers these suggestions about smoke detectors:

- Many localities require that you have a smoke detector in your home, so buy one—at least one. They're inexpensive and are available at most hardware stores and supermarkets. Check your local codes and regulations; they may require you to purchase a specific kind.
- Read the instructions that come with the detector for advice on where to install it. You should purchase at least one for every floor in your house. Preferably you should place one outside every bedroom.
- Manufacturers know what is best for their products and tell you how to care for them. Follow their instructions. Detectors can save lives, but only if you install and maintain them properly.
- Never disconnect a fire detector. If it goes off at wrong times because of heat from a stove or steam from a bathroom, move it to another location.
- Replace the battery annually (January 1 is an easy day to remember) or when you hear a "chirping" sound. And press the test button regularly to be sure the batteries work.
- Keep your detector clean. Dust, grease, or other materials can interfere with efficient operation. You may want to vacuum the grill work on the detector.

---

15 and older. Impairment of the individual's judgment may lead to the death of others as well, for example, operating a boat with passengers while intoxicated or drinking while supervising children who are in or near the water.

Choking and Suffocation

Choking to death as a result of an object lodged in the airway passage occurs more often than one might expect. Each year in the United States more than a thousand people die because a piece of food or a foreign object became stuck in their throats and caused them to stop breathing. Food that is swallowed without being chewed sufficiently is a common cause of choking and blockage of the air passage. Small bones from fish or chicken also can be swallowed inadvertently and become stuck in the airway. Sometimes dentures, fillings, or crowns become loose, are accidentally swallowed, and may cause the person to choke. Being intoxicated also increases the risk of swallowing improperly.

When the airway is completely blocked, a choking victim is unable to speak, breathe, or cough. A choking person often clutches his or her throat. If the object is not removed quickly, the victim may become unconscious and death may follow rapidly from lack of oxygen.

Elderly adults, especially those with Alzheimer's disease, Parkinson's disease, or pneumonia, are particularly susceptible to choking on food. A major reason for this difficulty in digesting foods is because of a lack of saliva, either because of aging or as a medication side effect. Foods such as hard candy or those requiring considerable chewing such as hot dogs, big pieces of meat, or large fruits like apples also pose a choking hazard. To reduce the risk of the elderly choking of food, the food industry in Japan has created easy-to-swallow foods that appear similar to regular foods but are processed to dissolve easily in the mouth.

Mechanical suffocation is another type of unintentional injury, occurring most frequently in young children up to four years old. A small child can get into tight spaces and become trapped or wedged, resulting in suffocation.

As infants become more mobile and inquisitive, the risk of entrapment and suffocation increases. Long cords dangling from appliances, draperies, or blinds should be placed well out of the way of a curious infant or toddler. Bulky bedding materials have been responsible for the suffocation of young children, especially fluffy comforters or infant bean bag cushions, and some household items, such as the bean bag cushion, have been recalled because of suffocation risks.

Anything stuck in the throat blocking the air passage can stop breathing and cause unconsciousness and death within minutes. Do not interfere with a choking person who can speak, cough, or breathe, but if a conscious person cannot speak, cough, or breathe, perform the following procedure immediately:

- Stand behind the person and wrap your arms around his or her middle just above the navel. Clasp your hands together in a double fist. Press in and up in vigorous thrusts. Repeat several times. This is called the *Heimlich maneuver*.

If the object is dislodged, take the person to a hospital immediately even if he or she seems all right. This is especially important if the swallowed object is a chicken or fish bone that may not have been completely dislodged. Also, if a bone has been swallowed, it can cause serious damage as it passes through the digestive system.

Fires

Two catastrophic fires in nightclubs in Chicago and Rhode Island in 2002 and 2003 focused the nation's attention on the deaths and injuries that can occur from fires. The fires in these two clubs spread rapidly, and exits were either

---

TERMS

laryngospasm: spasm of the larynx caused by inhaling water

locked or blocked. Hundreds of people were trapped in the buildings and died from burns or suffocation; hundreds more were seriously burned or injured.

About 360,000 residential fires occur in the United States each year. Those fires are responsible for about 13,000 injuries and 2,500 deaths and a loss of $7 billion. Fires in the home may be attributed to many factors: fireplaces, wood stoves, kerosene or space heaters, improper placement of appliances, faulty wiring of the house or appliances, grease fires in the kitchen (loose sleeves dangling over open flames), improper storage of combustible materials, or a careless smoker in the house.

Death rates from fires or burns have markedly decreased since the 1950s. Smoke detectors, portable ladders, and fire extinguishers have helped reduce fatalities. Also, many elementary school students are receiving annual training from local fire departments concerning fire safety. Prevention and education are, once again, the best strategies to eliminate unintentional injuries from fires and burns. Each household should have a planned escape route, smoke detectors placed at key locations throughout the home, and posted emergency phone numbers. Everyone should know how to operate a fire extinguisher and know exactly where it is kept, and in two-story houses, a portable ladder should be readily accessible.

Fire Retardants Fire retardants are chemicals added to clothing, drapes, furniture, bedding, and other fabrics to help prevent the spread of a fire should one start. Most fire retardant chemicals are toxic—they usually are carcinogenic when tested on laboratory animals, and they can pollute land and water and harm the environment. The amount of fire retardant chemicals added to fabrics and furniture is considerable—up to 5% of the fabric's weight. In the 1970s, two fire retardants (called *brominated tris* and *chlorinated tris*) that had been added to children's sleepwear for years were finally banned. These chemicals are carcinogenic and are absorbed into the body from pajamas and other bedding containing fire retardant chemicals. These substances are still added to the foam and fabrics used in furniture. The risk to health and to the environment far outweighs the risk of a fire in a home spreading from furniture. This is especially true now that most homes have smoke detectors. Also, all states, the District of Columbia, and Canada require that all cigarettes be fire-safe.

Firearms

Many Americans view ownership of guns as a constitutional right; others believe that it is a privilege and that ownership should be restricted and regulated. One aspect of firearms is incontrovertible—they cause thousands of deaths and injuries each year.

Firearm-related deaths fall into three categories: unintentional, intentional,

> The hour of departure has arrived and we go our separate ways—I to die and you to live. Which is better, God only knows.
>
> *Socrates*

Kids and Guns: Sometimes a Fatal Mix

Car accidents are the leading cause of unintentional death among children under age 18. The second leading cause of death in that age group is accidental or deliberate discharge of a firearm. Among all high-income countries in the world, 91% of firearm deaths of children younger than 14 years occur in the United States.

Every week about 50 American children die from a bullet wound (see table). Add nearly 5,800 nonfatal gun injuries in this age group annually, and it becomes clear that guns present a serious health risk to American children.

Gun-Related Deaths Among American Children by Age Group, 2012–2014

Age Group	Total	Homicide	Suicide	Unintentional
0–12 years	403	229	150	24
13–17 years	2,080	1,068	543	469

The vast majority of young children are killed in their homes, often unintentionally as a result playing with loaded guns or involvement in family violence and homicide among adults. Teens are just as likely to be killed by a firearm in a home or on the streets. Suicide by gun is almost always at home. The majority of children are killed with a handgun.

Protecting Kids from Firearm Death

Parents can take the following steps to help protect their children from death by firearm (University of Michigan Mott Children's Hospital, 2017):

- Parents who keep firearms at home should keep the guns locked and unloaded, with the ammunition locked in a separate location.
- Before a child goes to a friend's house, parents should ask the friend's parent whether the family has firearms in the house, and how they are stored. This can be part of all the usual things you would discuss before a visit, like allergies, snacks, sunscreen, etc.
- Parents of teenagers should store guns safely to lessen the risk of gun suicide attempt, even if their children have been educated about guns.

Fowler, K. A. (2017). Childhood firearm injuries in the United States. *Pediatrics, 140,* doi: 10.1542/peds.2017-2298

and undetermined. Studies show that having access to a firearm increases the risk of a firearm-related injury or death. If you keep one or more firearms in your home, you should be trained in their use and take all possible safeguards to prevent intentional or unintentional injury or death. All firearms should be locked away. Guns should never be stored loaded. Ammunition should be kept locked in a separate location.

Nonpowder guns such as pellet rifles (BB guns) and paintball guns are thought to be harmless. These guns, powered by compressed air, are often given to children

Prevent Computer-Related Injuries

Anyone who spends 30 to 40 hours a week in front of a computer screen risks some form of repetitive motion injury. Most injuries occur in the neck and shoulders; the elbow and wrist are the second most vulnerable areas. These injuries are due to the repetitive motions used to watch the screen and operate the keyboard.

People who spend many hours at a computer day after day should take precautions to reduce the risk of injury. Using an ergonomic chair and having the monitor and keyboard at comfortable positions and heights are important. Taking frequent breaks is also helpful. A recent study showed that forearm support boards can significantly reduce injuries to the neck and shoulders. Computer users should take all available measures to reduce the risk of musculoskeletal disorders.

Table 21.2

Repetitive Motion Disorders
These injuries affect muscles, tendons, and nerves.
Cervical radiculopathy:
People who look up to a computer screen or who balance a phone on their shoulder are at risk.
Pronator syndrome:
Mechanics, baseball pitchers, and barbers are at risk.
Carpal tunnel syndrome:
Typists, computer programmers, and potters are at risk.
Thoracic outlet syndrome:
Violinists and other musicians are at risk.
Cubital tunnel syndrome:
Truck drivers or other persons who keep their arms in fixed, flexed positions are at risk.
Distal ulnar neuropathy:
Meat packers, assembly line workers, and machine operators are at risk.

as gifts and are regarded as "toys." However, they are far from harmless. Each year, about 20,000 Americans are treated in hospital emergency rooms for nonpowder gun injuries; most of those injured are children between the ages of 5 and 14 years. The power of many of these guns can equal that of a 22-caliber rifle; when they are shot at someone at close range, they can kill, and several such deaths occur each year. Parents are advised not to let their children possess or use nonpowder rifles or pistols.

Work Safety

During the past century, unintentional injury deaths in the workplace were reduced by 90%. For 2015, the Bureau of Labor Statistics (2017) reported nearly 3 million workplace injuries requiring medical attention and about 4,800 deaths. Occupational injuries occur most often in manufacturing industries. Agriculture has the highest incidence of skin diseases and disorders, which may be attributed to agricultural workers' close contact with hazardous chemicals. Common occupational illnesses include skin disorders, respiratory conditions caused by inhalation of toxic substances, disorders associated with repeated trauma, poisonings, and dust-related diseases of the lungs. The incidence is suspected to be higher than reported because many workers do not seek medical attention for their illnesses or injuries.

Carpal tunnel syndrome is one of a group of injuries known as **repetitive motion disorders** (also called repeated trauma), caused by stress of a body part, resulting from repetitive motion for long periods (**Table 21.2**). Symptoms of carpal tunnel syndrome are burning, numbness, tingling, and stiffness of the hand, fingers, or wrist. Dentists, dental hygienists, supermar-

ket cashiers, seamstresses, musicians, factory workers, computer keyboard operators, and surgeons are at risk for carpal tunnel syndrome. Better product design, correct positioning of the operator and the tool, and limiting time spent at the same task are being investigated as possible solutions to the rising incidence of cumulative trauma disorders.

Sick building syndrome consists of a variety of symptoms reported by workers in modern office buildings. Recent investigations have found a correlation between pollutants in or near the building or a poor ventilation system and sick building syndrome. Much of the evidence of these symptoms is self-reported by the workers or documented by physicians. Symptoms include asthma, lung infections, dizziness, nausea, throat and eye irritations, fatigue, cough, and shortness of breath. Major causes of sick building syndrome include outdoor pollutants such as dust, airborne chemicals, auto emissions, and agricultural pesticides. Indoor causes include air conditioning contaminated by bacteria, molds, and other microorganisms and chemicals emitted from materials used in the construction of the building, such as formaldehyde in plywood. Buildings with little or no natural ventilation, such as skyscrapers, warehouses, and old factories, are particularly susceptible to sick building syndrome.

TERMS

repetitive motion disorders: disorders caused by repeated stress to a body part; carpal tunnel syndrome is a repetitive motion disorder

sick building syndrome: collection of symptoms reported by workers in some modern buildings

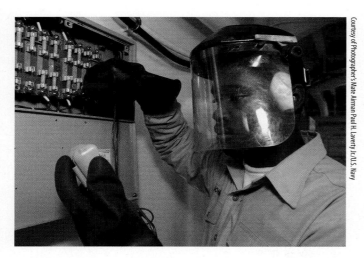

Workers should always wear the appropriate safety equipment while on the job.

Sports and Recreational Injuries

Millions of American youths engage in some kind of sport or physical activity, either with a school team, with organized leagues, in pick-up games, or just for fun. Playing sports is both fun and healthy. However, each year close to 4 million children, teenagers, and young adults wind up in hospital emergency rooms as a result of a sport or recreational injury. Approximately one-fourth of all emergency room admissions of persons aged 5 to 24 are due to a sports or recreational injury.

The most common sports injuries among boys result from playing basketball, football, or cycling. Among girls, basketball, soccer, and cycling cause the most injuries. The numbers do not indicate which sport is the most dangerous, because the number of people engaging in each sport is not known. Children between the ages of 5 and 14 are the most susceptible to injury; as children become older, the chance for injury declines. Boys are twice as likely as girls to visit an emergency room with a sports injury, but as more and more girls engage in sports, their number of visits is increasing. Coaches and parents have the obligation to see that protective gear is worn at all times and that recklessness is not a part of any game. It is useless (although all parents do it) to tell kids to be careful when they are playing sports or just having fun, but reasonable precautions should be taken by coaches, parents, and volunteers to prevent injuries, especially with young children.

In the past few years, activities called "extreme" sports have become very popular. Extreme sports include inline skating, snowboarding, mountain bicycling, rock climbing, kickboxing, skateboarding, and ultra-endurance racing. All of these activities, however fun and enjoyable, carry increased risk for injury. Everyone engaging in an extreme sport needs to weigh the risks against the enjoyment.

Traumatic Brain Injury and Concussion

Traumatic brain injury (TBI) is caused by a bump, blow, or jolt to the head (including shaking of babies) that results in impaired thinking or memory, altered movement or sensation (e.g., vision or hearing), personality changes, or emotional problems such as depression. Nearly 3 million TBIs occur in the United States every year.

Falls are the most common causes of TBI, accounting for nearly half of all TBI-related hospital visits. TBIs from falls occur frequently among the elderly, who may trip over objects in their homes or be unstable due to medication side effects that affect balance. Young people also are frequently affected by falls while playing or riding a bike. Being struck by or against an object is the second leading cause of TBI. TBIs can occur from collisions with others players in a game, being hit by a ball or bat, or bumping into a low beam in an old house. Motor vehicle crashes are the third leading cause of TBI-related injuries.

The severity of a TBI may range from "mild" (i.e., a brief change in mental status or consciousness) to "severe" (i.e., an extended period of unconsciousness or memory loss after the injury). About half of TBIs do not cause loss of consciousness or require medical intervention (DeKosky et al., 2010). About the same number of persons suffer a more serious TBI in which they do lose consciousness and suffer cognitive defects such as memory loss or changes in behavior. However, only a small number suffer from permanent brain damage that leaves them nonfunctional.

A **concussion** is a medically specific form of a traumatic brain injury, resulting from a bump, blow, or jolt to the head or body that causes the head and brain to move rapidly back and forth. This sudden movement can cause the brain to bounce around or twist in the skull, creating chemical changes in the brain and sometimes stretching and damaging brain cells. Concussions may cause

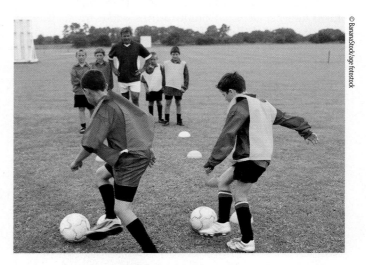

Soccer is a very popular children's sport. Teaching children proper techniques can prevent injuries.

College Athletes Opt for Health

Most college students (and their families) expect their college education to provide knowledge and skills that will facilitate attaining a satisfying job and a healthy future. Students do not expect to graduate from college with a brain injury that causes cognitive, emotional, and health deficits that might persist for life. Unfortunately, many college students who are active in intercollegiate athletics are at risk for traumatic brain injury (TBI) caused by a bump, blow, or jolt from a fall or a collision that causes the head and brain to move back and forth abruptly.

In 2014, athletes from major universities formed the National College Players Association (NCPA) to protect their health, academic progress, and well-being from brain and other injuries. Among the NCPA's goals are to minimize college athletes' risks for brain trauma and to prevent players from having to pay for their sports-related medical expenses. They also want to prohibit colleges from revoking an injured player's scholarship and establish and enforce uniform safety guidelines in all sports to prevent serious injuries and avoidable deaths (National College Players Association, 2017). Prompted by concern for athletes' long-term health, many colleges have developed rules to minimize head injuries. For example, before, during, and after football season limiting the number of weekly practices that involve live tackling to the ground and/or full-speed blocking. Also, to avoid pressure from coaches to return a player with a suspected brain injury to activity sooner than is medically responsible, medical personnel are hired and paid for by the student health service instead of the athletic department. Many schools make public their protocols for diagnosing and managing TBIs that conform to guidelines set by the American Academy of Neurology and the American College of Sports Medicine. Although originally focused on safety in football, the data on the prevalence of concussions and other head trauma among college athletes indicate that attention should be given to other concussion-prone sports (see the accompanying table).

Collegiate Athletes' Concussion Rates by Sport

Sport	Concussion rate per 1,000 athletic exposures
Men's wrestling	0.89
Women's ice hockey	0.78
Men's football	0.74
Women's soccer	0.54
Women's basketball	0.53
Women's lacrosse	0.45
Men's basketball	0.38
Women's volleyball	0.37
Men's lacrosse	0.30
Men's soccer	0.26
Women's softball	0.26
Men's baseball	0.09

Data from Hootman, J.M. et al. (2007). Epidemiology of collegiate injuries from 15 sports. *Journal of Athletic Training*, 42, 311–319.

problems with thinking, emotions, sensation, language, memory, communication, personality changes, depression, and the early onset of dementia. Many concussions are not life-threatening, however, the effects of a concussion can be serious. (**Table 21.3**).

Table 21.3

Signs and Symptoms of Concussion

- Can't recall events *prior to* or *after* a hit or fall.
- Appears dazed or stunned.
- Forgets an instruction, is confused about an assignment or position, or is unsure of the game, score, or opponent.
- Moves clumsily.
- Answers questions slowly.
- Loses consciousness *(even briefly)*.
- Shows mood, behavior, or personality changes.
- Headache or "pressure" in head.
- Nausea or vomiting.
- Balance problems or dizziness, or double or blurry vision.
- Bothered by light or noise.
- Feeling sluggish, hazy, foggy, or groggy.
- Confusion, or concentration or memory problems.
- Just not "feeling right," or "feeling down."

U.S. Centers for Disease Control and Prevention. (2015). Concussion Signs and Symptoms. Retrieved from https://www.cdc.gov/headsup/basics/concussion_symptoms.html

Concussions are among the most common kinds of injuries people experience, especially while engaging in strenuous physical activities. Sports and bicycle accidents account for the greatest number of concussions among children aged 5 to 14 years.

Chronic Traumatic Encephalopathy (CTE)

Repeated blows to the head such as occur in contact sports (football, soccer, hockey, boxing) can cause long-term damage to the brain even without concussions, referred to as **Chronic traumatic encephalopathy (CTE)**.

TERMS

chronic traumatic encephalopathy (CTE): destruction of nerve cells in the brain from repeated brain injury due to collisions and falls

concussion: a blow to the head that causes injury, temporary loss of consciousness, and possibly a period of amnesia upon awakening

traumatic brain injury (TBI): injury caused by a bump, blow, or jolt to the head that results in impaired thinking or memory, altered movement or sensation, personality changes, or emotional problems such as depression

CTE involves destruction of nerve cells in the brain causing declines in recent memory and thought processes, depression, impulsivity, aggressiveness, anger, irritability, suicidal behavior, and eventual progression to dementia. Initial signs and symptoms generally do not appear until many years after the brain trauma has occurred. Many retired professional football players have CTE. The National Football League (NFL) and other sports organizations now stress the need to reduce head injuries in sports. In 2010, the NFL placed a poster in every team's locker room warning players of the possible long-term effects of concussions. In 2013, the NFL agreed to set up a fund to pay for concussion-related health problems of approximately 18,000 retired NFL players.

Soccer players also experience concussions. These may occur from falls, head-to-head collisions, being hit by a kicked ball, or, more commonly, by repeated "headers" (using the head to intercept the ball in order to score or pass). Although an individual header may not cause any observable problem such as a concussion, brain damage from headers may accumulate over time. A professional soccer player may execute thousands of headers in practice and games over a career. Studies of professional soccer players show that some do exhibit signs of brain injury, loss of cognitive function, or both. Because of the growing concern over long-term brain damage from headers, it is recommended that children younger than age 14 who play soccer should not be allowed to use their heads to intercept a soccer ball at any time.

Well-designed protective helmets can reduce the chances of serious brain injuries in many sports. Although brain injuries among football and hockey players are the most publicized, they are much more common among skiers and snowboarders (Cuismano & Kwok, 2010). More than 100,000 winter sports enthusiasts suffer a TBI each year; many of the serious brain injuries and deaths could have been prevented if protective helmets had been worn.

A football helmet is now available that is equipped with sensors that measure the magnitude, location, and direction of each blow to a player's head. The data are wirelessly transmitted to a computer or mobile device on the sidelines that analyzes and evaluates the likelihood that the player may have suffered a concussion. The helmet is not cheap (about $1,000), but a number of NCAA colleges have ordered them for their players.

Taking Risks and Preventing Accidents

Risks cannot be avoided in life; accidents and unintentional injuries are a consequence of the risks we take. As soon as a child learns to crawl, he or she begins to take risks to explore and understand the environment. At each stage of life we take risks to learn and to expand our capabilities and experiences. We take a risk when we cross the street in traffic, run to catch a bus, or swing from the branch of a tree. When we go hiking or climbing or engage in sports, we are taking risks.

The important question YOU need to ask is: "What risks are necessary and acceptable for me to live the way I want to?" The answer will also, to some extent, determine your risk of unintentional injury. People differ enormously in their need for risk-taking behaviors. Some people thrive on high-risk endeavors, such as mountain climbing, racing cars, and skydiving. However, even people who live more sedate lives may be at risk for unintentional injuries because of destructive behaviors or unhealthy mental attitudes. Whatever your personal beliefs, a commitment to safe living can be made at any time.

Although unintentional injuries are usually not a laughing matter, one accident statistic does sound a humorous note. Saturday and Sunday are the two most dangerous days of the week for accidents and injuries.

Critical Thinking About Health

1. Briefly explain a recent injury that happened to you, a friend, or family member using the epidemiologic triad presented in Figure 21.3.
   a. What were the human factors involved in the injury?
   b. What were the environmental factors (physical as well as social) involved in the injury?
   c. What were the vehicle (or agent) factors involved in the injury?
      Which factor(s) could have been modified in such a way that may have prevented the injury from occurring?
2. Alcohol is a contributing factor in about half of motor vehicle fatalities. What are your campus and community doing to help prevent people, both young and old, from driving while intoxicated? Some questions to consider:
   a. Are there educational programs? If so, what are they and whom do they target?
   b. How would you design an educational program to keep your peers from drinking and driving?
   c. Are there seasonal programs that increase awareness about the dangers of drinking and driving (e.g., high school prom, Fourth of July)?
   d. What is the role of local law enforcement, both on and off campus, with regard to decreasing drinking and driving accidents and fatalities?
3. Federal, state, and local governments have written and passed laws and regulations that enforce certain safety behaviors that have an impact on the individual and/or community. Such laws regulate using a seat belt, restraining your child in a car seat, and wearing a helmet while riding a motorcycle or bicycle. Some people believe that the government (at any level) should not mandate laws regarding individual safety and injury prevention. Others believe that the government has a right to demand certain safe behaviors among its citizens for the public good. What's your opinion? Should the government be allowed to regulate individual safety behaviors? Explain why or why not.

Chapter Summary and Highlights

Chapter Summary

Many times during your life you will have an accident. Most accidents are minor: a cut, a burn, a bruise, a broken bone. Other accidents are more serious, resulting in significant injuries and often a long recovery. Some accidents are fatal. Children and old people are especially prone to accidents. Certain activities create opportunities that increase the likelihood of an accident. Driving a car is the most obvious example of an activity in which accidents frequently occur; riding a bicycle or motorcycle is another. Rodeo riders and professional football players engage in their activities knowing that they will be injured, if not this time, then very likely some time in the future. Because automobile, motorcycle, and bicycle accidents are frequent and the injuries suffered often serious, society devotes considerable effort and money to reducing accidents and mitigating injuries for these activities. Seat belts and air bags reduce injuries in a car crash; helmets and special clothing reduce injuries in bicycle and motorcycle accidents. A federal government agency monitors and enforces regulations that are designed to reduce workplace accidents. Workers may be required to wear special hats, masks, gloves, or clothing to reduce injuries from accidents. Companies are required to educate workers on safe practices and to provide a safe working environment. Sadly, safe practices are not always followed. In 2014, the owner of a coal mine was charged with murder for operating an unsafe mine in which more than a dozen miners died in a series of underground explosions. Overall, the coal industry owes the U.S. government more than $70 million in unpaid fines for violation of safety rules.

Just because accidents occur frequently does not mean that they are inevitable. You can increase or reduce your personal risk of an accident by your overall lifestyle and by how careful you are while performing hazardous tasks. For example, if you like to play sports, contact sports are more dangerous than noncontact sports. Ask yourself what kind of risks you are willing to take. Are you willing to jump off a cliff into a pool of water on a dare? When you go hiking or mountain climbing, do you take unnecessary risks. Even simple tasks like climbing a ladder, carrying groceries on an icy sidewalk, or using a table saw to cut some wood increase the risk of an accident. Taking a commercial airplane to get to a distant city is one of the safest things you can do; parachute jumping or sky diving for fun is not. You cannot and should not live your life in fear of accidents. Trying something new involves risk. You should decide, however, how much risk you are willing to take and engage in activities with which you are comfortable. When you are doing something for the first time or something that you know is dangerous, remind yourself to *Be Careful*.

Highlights

- Unintentional injuries and deaths cost Americans billions of dollars in medical costs as well as costs as a result of loss of work each year. Unintentional injuries and deaths are preventable!
- Many factors contribute to unintentional injuries: knowledge, attitudes, beliefs, and behaviors; economic and social factors; competence; environmental conditions; and use of alcohol and other drugs.

- The Haddon matrix was developed to assess motor vehicle risk factors and is used to develop prevention programs.
- A multidimensional approach to injury prevention includes education, prevention strategies, stricter laws and regulations, and better product design.
- One motor vehicle death occurs every 12 minutes.
- Alcohol is involved in more than half of all motor vehicle accidents.
- Motorcycle, all-terrain vehicles, and bicycle safety rules and equipment are keys to preventing accidents. Wear reflective clothing and obey safety rules.
- Safety in the home includes preventing falls, poisonings, drownings, choking, and fires.
- Work-related injuries have decreased steadily; however, they still cost employers and employees large amounts of time and money. Injuries to the back are most frequent, followed by legs, arms, and trunk. Proper work safety procedures can prevent the majority of work-related injuries.
- Millions of young people go to emergency rooms each year with a sport- or recreation-related injury. The highest percentage of injuries occur in basketball, cycling, football, and soccer.
- Concussions are serious injuries to the head that may or may not cause loss of consciousness. Protective head gear should be worn in all sports with a high risk of head injury.
- Accidents and injuries are a consequence of the many risks we take. Although most of what we do has some degree of risk, we can decrease that risk by increasing safety knowledge and taking safety precautions for physical activities we engage in.

For Your Health

What do you do to keep yourself safe from intentional injury? Do Exercise 21.1 in the Workbook "Preventing Intentional Injury" to assess your risks. Also do Exercise 21.2 "Preventing Unintentional Injury" to assess how you contribute to the risks for "accidents."

References

Bergen, G., et al. (2016). Falls and fall injuries among adults aged ≥ 65 years—United States, 2014. *Morbidity and Mortality Weekly Report, 65,* 994–998.

Bureau of Labor Statistics. (2017). Injuries, Illnesses, and Fatalities. Retrieved from: http://www.bls.gov/iif/

Case, A., & Deaton, A. (2017). Mortality and morbidity in the 21st century. Brookings Institution. Retrieved from https://www.brookings.edu/bpea-articles/mortality-and-morbidity-in-the-21st-century/

Centers for Disease Control and Prevention. (2017). *Injury prevention and control.* Retrieved from http://www.cdc.gov/injury/

Clabaux, N., et al (2017). Powered two-wheeler riders' risk of crashes associated with filtering on urban roads. *Traffic Injury Prevention, 18,* 182–287.

Cuismano, M. D., & Kwok, J. (2010). Skiers, snowboarders, and safety helmets. *Journal of the American Medical Association, 303,* 661–662.

Dekosky, S. T., Ikonomovic, M. D., & Gandy, S. (2010). Traumatic brain injury: Football, warfare, and long-term effects. *New England Journal of Medicine, 363,* 1293–1296.

Gladwell, M. (2001, June 11). Wrong turn. *The New Yorker,* 50–61.

Hootman, J. M., et al. (2007). Epidemiology of collegiate injuries from 15 sports. *Journal of Athletic Training, 42,* 311–319.

National Center for Health Statistics. (2015). *10 leading causes of injury deaths by age group, highlighted unintentional injury deaths, United States – 2012.* Retrieved from http://www.cdc.gov/injury/wisqars/pdf/leading_causes_of_injury_deaths_unintentional_injury_2015_1050w760h.gif

National Center for Health Statistics. (2016). *Age-adjusted death rates for selected causes of death, by sex, race, and Hispanic origin: United States, selected years 1950–2011.* Retrieved from http://www.cdc.gov/nchs/data/hus/2016/017.pdf

National College Players Association. (2017). *Mission and goals.* Retrieved from http://www.ncpanow.org/about/mission-goals

National Safety Council. (2017). *Injury facts 2017.* Itasca, IL: Author.

Ship, A. N. (2010). The most primary of care: Talking about driving and distraction. *New England Journal of Medicine, 362,* 2145–2147.

University of Michigan Mott Children's Hospital. (2017). Gun safety for children and youth. Retrieved from https://www.med.umich.edu/yourchild/topics/guns.htm

Suggested Readings

Dekosky, S. T., et al. (2010). Traumatic brain injury: Football, warfare, and long-term effects. *New England Journal of Medicine, 363*, 1293–1296. Describes in medical terms what happens to the brain following a blow to the head.

Gladwell, M. (2001, June 11). Wrong turn. The New Yorker, 50–61. An interesting look at why automobile safety measures may not be working as originally expected.

National Safety Council. (2017). Injury facts. Itasca, IL: Author. Presents the most current occupational, motor vehicle, home, community, state, and international injury statistics on deaths, nonfatal injuries, and their costs.

Levin, H., et al. (2014). *Understanding traumatic brain injury: Current research and future directions*. New York: Oxford. Medical experts explain the incidence and management of the neuropsychiatric aspects of traumatic brain injury.

Spellman, F. R., & Bieber, R. M. (2011). *Physical hazard control: Preventing injuries in the workplace*. Washington, DC: Government Institutes. Focuses on controlling physical hazards at work to prevent injury, illness, and death including layout and building design, safeguarding of machinery, confined space entry, noise, radiation, ergonomics, electricity, thermal stressors, hand tools, woodworking, welding, machining, mobile equipment, materials handling, and workplace violence.

Recommended Websites

Distracted Driving
The U.S. Department of Transportation's central clearinghouse for information, statistics, research, and commentary on distracted driving.

MedlinePlus on Accidents
Information on household, motor vehicle, childhood, and other safety issues.

National Center for Injury Prevention and Control
Statistics, fact sheets, and other information to help reduce morbidity, disability, mortality, and costs associated with injuries.

National Highway Traffic Safety Administration
Information about motor vehicle safety.

National Institute of Occupational Safety and Health
Dedicated to workplace safety and health.

National Safety Council
Information on preventing injuries and deaths at work, in homes and communities, and on the roads through leadership, research, education, and advocacy.

PART SEVEN

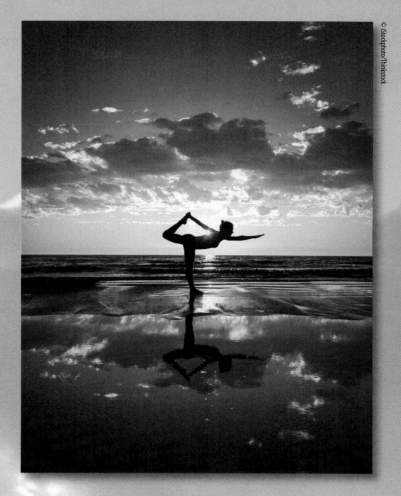

© iStockphoto/Thinkstock

Overcoming Obstacles

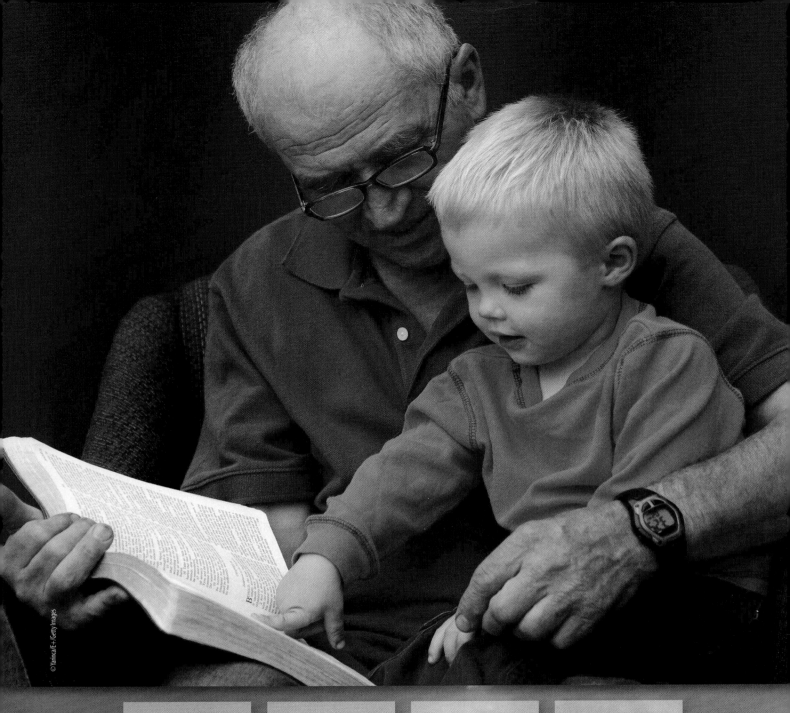

Health Tips

Steps You Can Take to Reduce the Risk of Dementia

The Surgeon General's Recommendations for Preventing Osteoporosis

Global Wellness

Japan's Aging Society

Can Beliefs Influence Life Span?

After Childhood and Adulthood There's Oldhood

Managing Stress

Giving Up Driving Is a Hard Decision

Wellness Guide

Spice Up Your Mind

Physical Exercise May Slow Aging

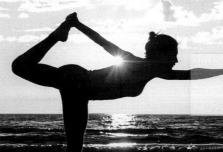

CHAPTER 22

Understanding Aging and Dying

Learning Objectives

1. Describe some of the biological changes that occur with aging.

2. Define *aging, maximum life span, average life span, life expectancy, ageism,* and *gerontology.*

3. Discuss some of the health and social issues that stem from the "graying" of the American population.

4. Briefly explain two major theories of aging processes.

5. Explain how undernutrition affects the aging process.

6. Describe some of the symptoms of Alzheimer's disease and Parkinson's disease.

7. Describe measures you can take while young to reduce the risk of dementia later in life.

8. Describe some of the causes of vision and hearing loss.

9. Describe several ways to reduce the risk of osteoporosis.

10. Discuss the stages of dying as explained by Kübler-Ross.

11. Explain the role of the two documents that constitute advance directives.

12. Briefly define the terms *physician-assisted suicide, hospice,* and *palliative care.*

13. Indicate steps you can take while young to help ensure a healthy old age.

Everything in the universe—plants, animals, mountains, planets, and stars—changes over time and eventually dies (plants and animals) or disintegrates and disappears (planets and stars). Our planet is aging in the sense that its resources are being used up and the environment is changing. The nuclear reactions that fuel the sun will eventually slow down, and the sun is expected to explode about 5 billion years from now.

> I don't want to achieve immortality through my work.
> I want to achieve immortality by not dying.
>
> *Woody Allen*

Many people associate aging with sickness, disability, loneliness, and increased inactivity. However, such negative views of aging are exaggerated; many older persons today are mentally, sexually, and physically active and continue to work well into their 80s or even 90s.

In America, negative views about aging are still prominent in movies, television, and, especially, advertising. The ideal American is portrayed as young, active, attractive, and wrinkle-free. Advertisements exhort people to retard the noticeable signs of aging by using face and body creams, dyes for graying hair, and special herbs or vitamins or by resorting to botox and other kinds of cosmetic surgery.

The normal processes of aging are not caused by disease, so aging cannot be cured. The noticeable effects of aging result from wear and tear on organs, bones, and tissues in the body that change and become less efficient over the years—muscles weaken, immune system functions decrease, and hormone-supported sex drive is reduced. Even the healthiest body wears out slowly. However, by developing healthy habits while young and by understanding aging processes, most people can remain vigorous and healthy until the very end of life.

Life expectancy in the United States is at an all-time high. In 2015, the average life expectancy for white men was 76.6 years, and for white women was 81.3 years. Life expectancy for African Americans was 72.2 years for men and 78.5 years for women. Between 1950 and 2009, the average life expectancy for Americans increased by about 10 years. However, to attain the average or better-than-average life expectancy, it is vital to adopt healthy behaviors and lifestyles while young.

America's Aging Population

Aging refers to the normal changes in body functions that occur after sexual maturity and continue until death. In an idealized situation, everyone would survive close to the maximum life span for the species; for human beings, **maximum life span** is about 120 years (**Figure 22.1**). The oldest person whose age has been reliably documented

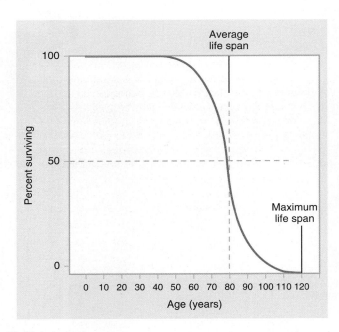

■ **Figure 22.1**

Survival as a Function of Years in an Idealized Aging Human Population

is Jeanne Calment, who died in Arles, France, on August 4, 1997. At the time of her death she was 122 years and 164 days old. She also had a brother who lived to 97 and other long-lived relatives, which suggests that her genetic makeup played a role in her longevity. The **average life span** is defined as the age at which half of the members of a population have died. Insurance companies use data based on actual populations to determine what insurance premiums are necessary to pay survivor benefits. **Life expectancy** is the average length of time that members of a population can expect to live. The average life expectancy at birth in the United States has increased by 30 years since 1900.

Genes are not the primary cause of aging. Although genes play a significant role in aging processes, studies show that the genes one inherits account for much less than half of the differences in life span among individuals. Evidence supporting this comes from the observation that identical twins who share identical genes generally die at quite different ages.

It seems counterintuitive but average life expectancy cannot be increased significantly by curing the major causes of death such as heart disease and cancer. Complete elimination of one or even both of these diseases would add only a few years to the average life expectancy after age 50 (**Figure 22.2**). Although curing major diseases is of inestimable benefit to those who die prematurely from them, their elimination has only a small effect on the average life expectancy of the entire U.S. population. However, slowing the aging processes can have a dramatic effect, allowing most people to live

Japan's Aging Society

The proportion of children in Japan's population has been declining for more than 30 years and reached an all-time low of 12.8% in 2014. By comparison, in the United States, the proportion of children in the total population is about 19.5%. Among 31 major industrialized nations, Japan has the fewest number of children younger than 14 years and the highest proportion of elderly. Currently, about 22% of Japan's population is 65 or older; by 2040, the number of elderly persons is expected to outnumber children by 4 to 1.

Today, Japan is one of the world's largest economies, but by 2050, the country is expected to lose 70% of its workforce.

A government report projects that Japan's population, now about 127 million, will shrink by one-third within 50 years and by two-thirds within a century. With a rapidly aging and shrinking population, Japan faces daunting economic and social problems in the coming years. To care for its elderly, the government is subsidizing the development of robotic caregivers.

Although Japan is at the forefront of countries with aging and shrinking populations, other major industrialized countries are expected to have similar problems to varying degrees. One solution is to increase immigration of young workers from underdeveloped countries, but this creates other social and economic problems.

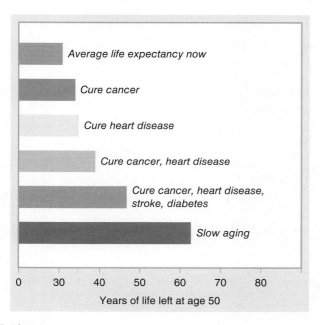

■ Figure 22.2

Increase in Average Life Expectancy After Age 50 Resulting from Curing Major Diseases or from Slowing Aging Processes
Eliminating cancer or heart disease as causes of death adds only a few years to the average life expectancy of the U.S population. However, if ways could be found to slow aging processes, as much as 60 years could be added to the average life expectancy after age 50.

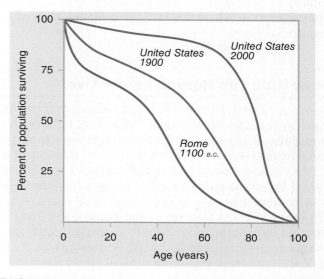

■ Figure 22.3

Approximate Survival Curves for Various Populations
The U.S population is beginning to approximate the idealized curve.

of every five Americans will be 65 years or older. This major demographic shift in population is expected to strain all areas of society—health care, Social Security, education, elder care, and voting patterns to name just a few.

almost 60 years beyond age 50. That is why scientists are studying the mechanisms of aging in the hope of finding ways to slow aging processes.

Because of disease, accidents, and other factors, actual populations do not survive according to the idealized situation but have followed various paths throughout history (**Figure 22.3**). The average U.S. life span has increased dramatically in the last century. Because of this, the number of older Americans also is rapidly increasing.

In 2015, the U.S. population was 320 million; in 2050, it is expected to increase to 438 million. By 2030, one out

TERMS

aging: normal changes in body functions that begin after sexual maturity and continue until death

average life span: the age at which half the members of a population have died

life expectancy: average number of years a person can expect to live

maximum life span: the theoretical maximum number of years that individuals of a species can live

The "graying" of America has caused social, medical, and economic problems. First and most important is the ability of the federal government to sustain Social Security payments in the future. At the present rate, the government has estimated that the Social Security system will run out of money within 30 to 40 years. To avoid this, Congress has begun to discuss ways to reform Social Security so that future retirees still will receive benefits. Although many older people are vigorous and healthy, a large number of people over age 65 have chronic illnesses and disabilities that require ongoing medical care, and some need expensive, long-term care. About 80% of older Americans have at least one serious chronic medical condition; about 20% have five or more chronic conditions. The costs of health care for the elderly are rising rapidly and will be a greater burden in the near future, which is why there is an urgent need for healthcare reform.

How Long Can Human Beings Live?

Some experts in **gerontology** (the science that studies the causes and mechanisms of aging) believe that populations in many countries are approaching the current maximum average life span, estimated at 85 to 90 years, although, as noted earlier, a few exceptional individuals live longer. One bit of evidence for a maximum average life span of 85 to 90 years comes from government estimates that show differences in the life expectancies of people in various countries (**Table 22.1**). Monaco tops the list. At the bottom of the list are countries in Africa where life expectancies are less than 40 years. The rapid decline in life expectancy in some African countries is primarily a result of deaths from AIDS, famine, and war.

The average life expectancy at birth for all Americans is about 78 years, but there are significant differences

---

Table 22.1

Average Life Expectancy at Birth in Various Countries

Countries at the top of the list have populations that are approaching the maximum average life expectancy for human beings. The countries at the bottom of the list (and others, primarily in Africa) have populations whose average life expectancies are 30 to 35 years less. This one statistic shows the tremendous inequality in health and opportunity that people experience from birth. Among the 224 countries for which data are available, the United States ranks 42nd in average life expectancy.

Country	Average Life Expectancy at Birth
Monaco	89.57
Japan	85.0
Singapore	85.0
Hong Kong	82.9
Israel	82.4
South Korea	82.4
Italy	82.2
Canada	81.9
France	81.8
United Kingdom	80.7
United States	79.8
Kuwait	78.0
Mexico	75.9
China	75.5
Iran	71.4
Russia	70.8
India	68.5
Kenya	64.0
South Africa	63.1
Afghanistan	51.3
Chad	50.2

Adapted from U.S. Central Intelligence Agency (2017). Country Comparisons: Life expectancy at birth. *World Fact Book*. Available at https://www.cia.gov/library/publications/the-world-factbook/rankorder/2102rank.html.

---

between the sexes and races that result from biology, socioeconomic factors, education, and access to health care. For example, white women outlive white men by about 5 years. The average difference in life expectancy between black Americans and white Americans is about 4 years. Studies suggest that socioeconomic factors are the strongest predictor. The lower a person is on a socioeconomic scale, the greater are his or her health problems and the lower the life expectancy.

> The older we get, the fewer things seem worth waiting in line for.
>
> *Will Rogers*

A slightly different picture of aging emerges from studies of people between the ages of 85 and 100—a group known as the "oldest old." Statistical studies of oldest old Scandinavians suggest that in the absence of disease,

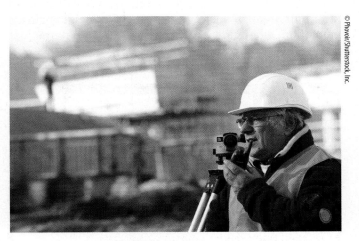

Many people continue to enjoy work long after the "normal" retirement age.

© Phovoir/Shutterstock, Inc.

senescent death (death from old age) could occur as late as 110 years. However, whether the maximum life expectancy for most people in the absence of disease is 85, 100, or 110 years, no human being is going to live to be as old as Methuselah, the biblical patriarch who is said to have lived for 967 years.

Theories of Aging

Biological Clocks Regulate Aging

Theories of aging fall into two broad categories. One ascribes aging to biological and genetic mechanisms that are specific for each species of animal and determine its maximum life span and rate of aging. The other theories focus on environmental factors that affect aging, such as nutrition, susceptibility to diseases, and exercise. Evidence for a "biological clock" that determines the maximum life span comes from measuring the amount of energy per gram of body weight consumed per day by mammals of different species. This energy consumption per day, called the **specific metabolic rate**, shows a striking correlation with the maximum life span of different species (**Figure 22.4**). Mammals that have the highest specific metabolic rate have the shortest life span; human beings have the slowest metabolic rate and the longest life span.

Longevity also has been associated with the number of heartbeats in individuals of different species. It is estimated that the total number of heartbeats for any mammal of any species is limited to about 1.5 billion beats before the heart wears out. In this model, longevity is determined by the rate of heartbeats. For example, shrews live only a few years and have hearts that beat thousands of times a minute. At the other extreme are elephants, whose hearts beat about once every 3 seconds and who live for more than 100 years. It is not clear whether a person's resting heart rate is a predictor of longevity, because many other environmental and lifestyle factors also must be taken into account.

Further evidence for a biological clock that governs aging comes from studying the growth of cells in the laboratory. Conditions have been established in which cells from various tissues of different animals can be grown under fixed laboratory conditions. The surprising result of these experiments is that cells grow and divide in a laboratory medium for a fixed number of generations and then die. The number of generations of growth is related to the maximum life span of the animal from which the cells were taken. Mouse cells only divide a few times, but human cells divide many times before dying. The inescapable conclusion from these experiments is that built into the cells of every animal is a genetically controlled clock that determines how many times cells can grow and divide before a signal tells them to stop.

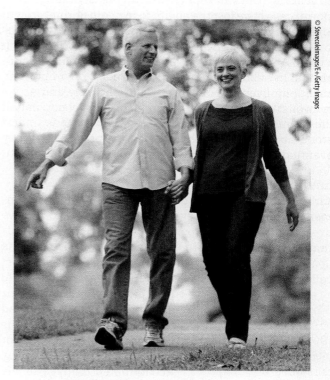

Shared activities are healthful at any age.

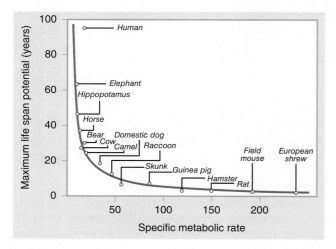

■ **Figure 22.4**

Correlation Between the Rate of Energy Consumed and Maximum Life Span Potential
Rate of energy consumption is calculated as energy per gram of body weight per day. Life span of various mammalian species is shown. The correlation suggests that the maximum human life span is a function of human biology and ultimately of human genes.

TERMS

gerontology: science that studies the causes and mechanisms of aging

specific metabolic rate: the amount of energy per gram of body weight consumed per day

Giving Up Driving Is a Hard Decision

One of the hardest choices older people have to make is deciding when to give up driving. Driving a car is a sign of independence; being able to come and go as one pleases often depends on driving. Having to stop driving means becoming more dependent on other people.

Even if a person is basically healthy, driving skills decline as we get older. The AARP lists these signs that it may be time to stop driving:

- Do I get nervous at intersections or when making left turns?
- Do I have trouble scanning far down the road to anticipate problems?

- Do I fail to notice red lights or traffic signs?
- Do cars suddenly seem to come out of nowhere?
- Do I generally feel nervous while driving?
- Do I have trouble looking over my shoulder when changing lanes?
- Do I have trouble seeing the sides of the road when looking straight ahead?
- Have I had a "close call" while driving in the past 6 months?

A distinguishing feature of cancer cells is that they are immortal when grown under the same laboratory conditions used for growing normal cells. Cancer cells grow and divide indefinitely as long as fresh nutrients are provided; cells taken from human tumors more than 50 years ago are still kept growing in the laboratory. Thus, cancer cells have lost the ability to regulate normal growth and aging both in people and in the laboratory.

Mutations discovered in specific genes in research animals such as worms and flies have produced individuals that live about twice as long as usual. More important, such long-lived worms and flies are healthy and active even as they pass the age at which the control population dies. Thus, it seems possible that when more is understood about how genes affect aging, people also may eventually live longer, healthier, and more active lives.

Environmental Factors Affect Aging

Although genetic factors contribute to aging, environmental factors play an even greater role. The longer we live, the more we are exposed to radiation and chemicals that can damage DNA in cells and, over time, cause the death of essential cells in the body. For example, most cells possess enzymes that repair damage to their DNA; loss of these cellular repair enzymes with age could lead to widespread cell death. This has been called the "error catastrophe" theory of aging. Accumulated damage to the chromosomes in cells may be responsible for development of cancer and also for aging.

> I don't believe in aging. I believe in forever altering one's aspect to the sun.
>
> *Virginia Woolf*

Another effect of exposure to radiation and chemicals is the production of very reactive molecules in cells, called free radicals. These substances are normally inactivated by cells, but as we age, our cells may be less able to cope with the damaging effects of free radicals. Free radicals also increase the damage to mitochondria, the complex structures in all cells that provide the energy for cellular growth and function. Without enough energy, cells become weak and possibly die; if too many cells die, organs function less efficiently and the person ages more rapidly. The mitochondrial error theory of aging is supported by animal studies. Mice have been genetically engineered so that the mitochondria in their cells accumulate mutations at a rapid rate. These mutations adversely affect essential mitochondrial functions. These mice age prematurely and die young.

Immune system functions also become less efficient with age, so that we become more susceptible to infections and diseases. Overall, aging is a complicated process brought on by a combination of genetic and environmental factors.

Alzheimer's Disease and Senile Dementia

In the absence of disease, normal mental functions can be maintained to age 100 or longer. However, many of the elderly have some loss of normal cognitive functions. The medical term for impairment or loss of cognitive functions in elderly persons is **senile dementia**.

The symptoms of senile dementia include the following:

- Loss of memory that increases over time
- Feeling confused
- Loss of problem-solving skills
- Suffering from delusions and agitated behavior
- Becoming lost in familiar settings
- Loss of interest in daily activities

Many medical conditions can cause dementia. A common cause is small strokes that gradually destroy cognitive functions in the brain. Neurodegenerative diseases such as Parkinson's disease, Huntington's disease, and Alzheimer's disease also cause dementia. In addition, viral and bacterial infections that cause HIV/AIDS, syphilis, tuberculosis, and meningitis also can give rise to symptoms of dementia.

The most common cause of dementia in the elderly is **Alzheimer's disease (AD)**, which accounts for more than half of all cases of dementia. AD is caused by damage to neurons in the brain, resulting in loss of cognitive functions, memory, mobility, and eventually death. Currently, more than 5 million Americans suffer from AD; worldwide there are an estimated 35 million cases. Late-onset AD usually is diagnosed after age 65, but the frequency of AD increases rapidly with age (**Figure 22.5**). By mid-century, it is estimated that 14 million Americans will have AD; worldwide the number is predicted to be in excess of 106 million people.

The disease is named for Alois Alzheimer, a German physician who, in 1907, described the abnormal brain structures he observed under the microscope in tissues obtained from patients who died from senile dementia. Alzheimer's findings at autopsy revealed what are still the diagnostic criteria for the disease: (1) the presence of bundles of tangled nerve fibrils called **tau tangles** in certain areas of the brain; and (2) the presence of plaques made of **amyloid protein**, which is localized in certain areas and blood vessels of the brain. How these changes affect the brain to produce loss of cognitive functions is still not understood.

Two forms of Alzheimer's disease are recognized, familial AD and sporadic AD. Familial AD, also known as early-onset AD, is a rare form of the disease that develops in individuals by age 50. This form has a strong genetic basis and often occurs in families in which many members suffer from AD at an early age.

A large, unique family in Colombia has been found in which dozens of family members develop Alzheimer's disease by age 50. A single abnormal dominant gene inherited from either parent is sufficient to cause early-onset AD among this group. By studying this gene, and other genes causing the familial form of AD, scientists hope to understand what causes late-onset (sporadic) AD, which is the form that occurs in almost 99% of cases. A gene called *APOE* is known to markedly increase the risk of AD in the average person. Inheriting one copy of

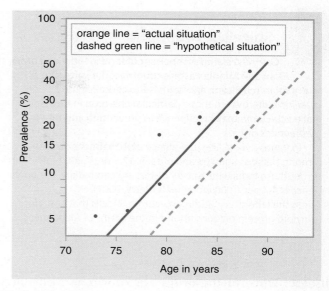

■ Figure 22.5

Benefits of Slowing Onset of Alzheimer's Disease (AD)
Alzheimer's disease (AD) increases linearly with age (orange line). The graph shows that if the onset of AD were delayed five years by a drug or other intervention, in this case from age 73 to 78, the prevalence of AD would decrease by half (dashed green line). This hypothetical reduction in the number of people with dementia would be an enormous benefit to families and society and would also substantially reduce health costs.

Courtesy Robert Katzman, University of California, San Diego.

this gene increases the risk of sporadic AD by a factor of 4; inheriting two copies of the gene, one from each parent, increases the risk 10-fold. A genetic test for this gene is available so individuals can find out if they are at higher-than-average risk of having AD in later life. However, finding out that you carry an *APOE* gene carries serious consequences, so anyone planning to take such a test must first undergo genetic counseling.

The sporadic form of AD may be caused by environmental factors that are undetermined as yet. The primary risk for sporadic AD is age. After diagnosis, AD can progress rapidly or slowly; the average time until death after diagnosis is 3 to 10 years.

Several drugs have been approved for treating the memory and cognitive losses that accompany Alzheimer's

Steps You Can Take to Reduce the Risk of Dementia

Generally speaking, actions that promote good health also reduce the risk of Alzheimer's disease and other forms of dementia later in life. Some research supports the following risk-reduction strategies:

Physical exercise: Moderate exercise such as walking several times a week.

Omega-3 fatty acids: Consuming more of these fatty acids that are found in fish.

Mental activity: Staying mentally active, even doing crossword puzzles or playing challenging games such as chess.

Healthy diet: Eating healthfully; maintaining normal weight.

Blood pressure: Strive to maintain normal blood pressure; 130/80 mm Hg.

▮TERMS▮

Alzheimer's disease (AD): a common cause of senile dementia and other symptoms, eventually leading to death

amyloid protein: an abnormal protein in the brain of patients with Alzheimer's disease

senile dementia: loss of cognitive functions in elderly people

tau tangles: aggregates of a brain protein called tau; a diagnostic indicator for Alzheimer's disease

Spice Up Your Mind

Curry is a staple component of food in India and other Asian and Middle Eastern countries. The spice that gives curry its aroma, flavor, and color is turmeric. Recently, scientists have discovered that a particular chemical in turmeric called *curcumin* may be effective in preventing and treating Alzheimer's disease.

In Pennsylvania, the prevalence of Alzheimer's disease among persons aged 65 and older is 17.5 per 1,000 individuals; in southern India where curry dishes are eaten daily, the prevalence is 4.7 per 1,000 individuals (Barry, 2007).

In the laboratory, adding curcumin to cells that contain amyloid protein plaques (found in the brains of Alzheimer's patients after death) rids the cells of the harmful protein. The evidence is thus building that curcumin really does have therapeutic potential for treating Alzheimer's disease. One problem with consuming curcumin in food or tablets is that the chemical does not easily enter the brain. Research shows that curcumin can be attached to nanoparticles to facilitate entry of the chemical into the brain. Mice with symptoms of memory loss and amyloid plaques in the brain show some improvement with this experimental treatment.

Taking curcumin as a supplement is not advised because dietary supplements are not regulated or tested for purity. Eating more curry dishes may be a good idea. Stick with yellow curry powder, which contains more turmeric than red curry powder.

---

disease. Three of the drugs are known as *cholinesterase inhibitors*: donepezil (Aricept), rivastigmine (Exelon), and galantamine (Razadyne). The other approved drug, memantine (Namenda), blocks the attachment of a specific neurotransmitter to cells. Clinical trials showed a very modest effect on symptoms of patients with moderate dementia, and only a minority of patients benefited at all. As one physician observed, "You can name 11 fruits in a minute instead of 10. Is that worth 120 bucks a month?" Still, many family members, caregivers, and physicians who are desperate to do something to slow the ravages of Alzheimer's disease are willing to pay the price. As AD progresses and behaviors become more agitated, antipsychotic drugs also are prescribed.

Until recently, AD could be confirmed only after death by examining the deceased person's brain for the presence of amyloid plaques. Now, a brain scan test (Amyvid test) is available that can confirm the amount of amyloid plaques in the brain of someone suspected of having AD. However, the test is only recommended for patients who already exhibit loss of memory and cognitive function. Since a diagnosis of AD has profound consequences for patients and their families, a well person should think long and hard before undergoing such a brain scan. Medicare does not yet pay for the Amyvid test. Despite this, hospitals in most large cities now offer the test.

Epidemiological studies show that people with more education (college graduates) are much less likely to develop Alzheimer's disease than are people with little or no education. A study of Catholic nuns who died between ages 76 and 100 has confirmed the importance of education. All of these Catholic nuns were college-educated and had a much lower prevalence of Alzheimer's disease than the general population. And among the few who did develop the disease, it could be shown by studying their brains after death that stroke was a primary trigger of the clinical symptoms of Alzheimer's disease.

It is not simply the level of education that helps to prevent the development of Alzheimer's disease. The key is to use the brain throughout life. Keep learning new things, explore new ventures—even doing crossword puzzles may help. It is now clear that brain cells continue to grow and establish new connections throughout life and that brain growth and health are dependent on mental stimulation. Just as exercise is necessary to maintain the body's fitness at all ages, exercising the brain is necessary to maintain mental functions (Marx, 2005).

Parkinson's Disease

Parkinson's disease (PD) is the second most common cause of neurodegenerative disease (after Alzheimer's disease) among older persons. About 1 million Americans suffer from PD, and about 60,000 new cases are diagnosed every year. Like other major neurological diseases such as Alzheimer's or Lou Gehrig's disease (ALS), Parkinson's disease is chronic and progressively worsens despite treatments that alleviate symptoms. PD was first described in 1817 by an English physician, James Parkinson, who described the symptoms as "the shaking palsy."

The four defining symptoms of PD are:

- *Tremor:* The tremor of a person suffering from PD involves a rhythmic back-and-forth motion of the thumb and forefinger that appears as if the patient is rolling a pill between the fingers. Although the tremor usually is observed in a hand, it can also arise in a foot or in the jaw.
- *Rigidity:* A basic principle of all movements of the body is that all muscles have opposing muscles. Movement occurs when one set of muscles contracts and the opposite set relaxes. The signals that tighten or relax muscles originate in the brain and are transmitted automatically to the muscles so that we make the movement that we desire. In PD patients, the signals from the brain are not coordinated, and the delicate balance between muscle tension and muscle relaxation is lost. In PD, the muscles stay constantly tensed and contracted, and the patient feels stiff and achy.

- *Bradykinesia:* This is probably the most distressing symptom of PD. Bradykinesia refers to the slowing down and loss of spontaneous movement. One moment, a person with PD is moving normally—crossing a street, for example—the next moment, the patient is frozen and cannot move, possibly in the middle of the crosswalk. Daily activities such as washing or putting on clothes may take hours because routine movements cannot be performed rapidly or continuously.
- *Postural instability:* Because PD patients have impaired balance and coordination of movements, they develop a tendency to lean forward or backward and to fall easily. As the disease progresses, walking becomes increasingly difficult; a patient may freeze in midstep and topple over if someone is not there for support.

The most effective drug used to treat PD is L-dopa (L-3,4-dihydroxyphenylalanine). Discovered in the 1960s, L-dopa delays the onset of the symptoms described and gives patients a period of time during which they can function more or less normally. Not all patients with PD are helped to the same degree by L-dopa, and not all symptoms of PD improve to the same degree. Today, L-dopa usually is taken with another drug, carbidopa (Lodosyn); this reduces the dose of L-dopa needed and increases its effectiveness. Although L-dopa therapy, in combination with other drugs, is effective for some time, eventually the drugs' effectiveness diminishes as the disease progresses. The hope for PD patients lies in new drugs that may be able to halt the loss of dopamine neurons in the brain or in direct replacement of neurons by transplantation of healthy tissues.

As with other neurodegenerative diseases, the causes of PD are both genetic and environmental. Several genes are linked to rare, inherited (familial) forms of PD, and numerous other genes are involved in the development of sporadic (not inherited) cases of PD. It is possible that the proteins produced by all of the genes associated with neurodegenerative diseases (AD, PD, ALS) change shape as people age, presumably as the result of time or exposure to environmental factors or both (Prusiner, 2012). As these altered proteins accumulate in the brain, they cause the normal proteins also to change. The altered proteins accumulate and form the plaques that are diagnostic of a neurodegenerative disease. These plaques can now be visualized using brain scan tests.

However, environmental factors such as exposure to pesticides and other chemicals that affect the functions of mitochondria, the energy-generating organelles in cells, also can result in PD. Studies with mice have shown that blocking mitochondrial functions with a specific chemical can cause the mice to develop symptoms that mimic those of PD. These preliminary results should further alert people to the potential serious, long-term dangers of pesticide exposure.

Parkinson's disease, Alzheimer's disease, and other forms of dementias affect millions of elderly people. These neurodegenerative diseases erode the quality of life for millions of elderly people, create enormous medical bills for families, and strain the resources and lives of caregivers. Medicines can provide some relief and perhaps slow the progression of the disease, but, ultimately, all neurodegenerative diseases are fatal.

Cognitive Impairment and the Right to Vote

Currently, in the United States there are approximately 3.3 million people age 65 and older with AD. That number is projected to increase to 13.5 million by 2050. Cognitive impairment occurs with other neurodegenerative diseases depending on their stage. Other conditions such as stroke, traumatic brain injury, and even obesity can cause cognitive impairment.

Physicians are required ro report diagnoses of cognitive impairment. A diagnosis of a neurocognitive disease can affect many aspects of life. One immediate and distressing consequence is revocation of the affected person's driver's license. Not being able to drive represents a serious loss of freedom and reduction in activities for most individuals with cognitive impairment.

Another consequence of the diagnosis of cognitive impairment is change in voting behavior. Many states now allow voting by mail weeks before actual voting day. Millions of Americans take advantage of this convenience. However, individuals who are cognitive impaired due to neurodegenerative disease may no longer be competent to make informed choices. Their ballot can be filled out by family members or caregivers who fill in their own choices and ask patients to sign the ballot or they may even sign for the individual. In such instances, there is no way to know who actually selected the candidates on mail-in ballots. Many elections are extremely close and may be decided by a few hundred or few thousand votes. To protect the legitimacy of elections it may be necessary to no longer allow those with neurogenerative diseases the right to vote, just as the right to drive is prohibited.

Osteoporosis

The skeleton provides a means of locomotion, protection of vital organs, and a readily available store of calcium and phosphorus. Only recently has it been recognized that the skeleton is a delicately balanced regenerating tissue, regulated as precisely as the destruction and synthesis of blood cells. The most common metabolic

---

TERMS

Parkinson's disease (PD): a neurodegenerative disease in which brain functions that control movements of the body are gradually lost

bone disease is **osteoporosis**, which results from many environmental factors such as poor diet, smoking, corticosteroid use, excess alcohol consumption, and lack of exercise. Genetic variation among individuals also may be an important factor in the development of osteoporosis in some individuals, but not others.

Osteoporosis occurs because the rate of bone breakdown exceeds the rate of bone renewal; many factors contribute to this. In older women, estrogen loss following menopause contributes to loss of bone material. In both older men and women, aging results in bone loss and increases the risk of fracture, depending on how much bone mass is reduced (**Figure 22.6**). Generally, the bone loss in women caused by low estrogen levels is significantly greater than the bone loss caused by normal aging processes.

The risk of osteoporosis in older women can be lessened by replacing the lost estrogen with **hormone replacement therapy (HRT)**. For many women, HRT has been beneficial because it reduces the risk of osteoporosis later in life. However, some studies showing that HRT increases slightly the risks of heart attack, stroke, and breast cancer have persuaded many postmenopausal women to forgo HRT therapy. On the other hand, other studies show that very low doses of estrogen may help prevent osteoporosis while avoiding the risks of standard HRT therapy. Estrogen supplementation in postmenopausal women also reduces the risk of Alzheimer's disease by about half. Thus, the use of HRT or low-dose estrogen may benefit some postmenopausal women. Making an informed decision is difficult, but discussing all options with one's health provider is important.

The best way to avoid osteoporosis is to build up as much bone mass as possible while young through a healthy diet with sufficient calcium, vitamin D, and exercise. Only 10% of American children get enough calcium or vitamin D or exercise enough to prevent osteoporosis later in life. Even children can be diagnosed with low bone mass that will only worsen as time goes on. After

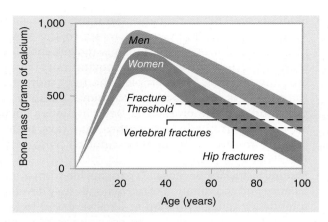

■ Figure 22.6

Changes in Bone Mass in Aging Men and Women
The risk of bone fracture from osteoporosis occurs when bone mass falls below a theoretical threshold and even a slight strain can cause a fracture.

maturity, calcium and vitamin D still are needed to maintain bone mass. Consuming at least a gram of calcium daily is recommended, but nutritional surveys indicate that half of all Americans do not consume that amount. Vitamin D is essential because it assists in the absorption of calcium and in bone formation. Milk is advocated as the best bone-building food. It contains large amounts of calcium and is fortified with vitamin D to facilitate calcium absorption.

Osteoporosis can be treated in two different ways. Either the breakdown of bone can be slowed or the synthesis of new bone can be accelerated. In principle, both of these mechanisms can be treated with drugs,

The Surgeon General's Recommendations for Preventing Osteoporosis

- Be sure you are getting the recommended daily amounts of calcium and vitamin D. High levels of calcium are found in milk, leafy green vegetables, soybean products, and cheese. Vitamin D is synthesized in the skin by sunlight exposure. People getting insufficient amounts of these substances should take supplements.
- The average adult younger than age 50 needs about 1 gram of calcium per day and 200 International Units (IU) of vitamin D. One cup of fortified milk provides 302 milligrams of calcium and 50 IU of vitamin D.
- Adults should maintain a healthy weight and exercise at least 30 minutes daily. Weight-bearing and balance exercises also are recommended.
- Do not smoke.
- Take steps to reduce the risk of falls at home, at play, and at work.

   Information on bone health and osteoporosis can be obtained by calling toll-free 860-642-2663.

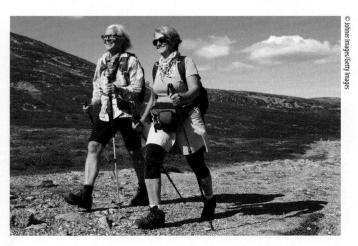

Regular exercise is important for reducing the risk of osteoporosis.

but in practice only one or the other is effective, not both. The class of drugs that reduces bone breakdown (also called remodeling or bone resorption) is bisphosphonates. These drugs have proved effective and result in an increase in bone mass in postmenopausal women by about 1% per year. The drug that stimulates new bone formation is a fragment of the parathyroid hormone. This drug can increase bone mass by as much as 10% in a year, but it has some drawbacks. It must be taken daily, there are risks of side effects, and the regained bone mass is lost when the therapy is stopped. The first bisphosphonate to treat osteoporosis, alendronate (Fosamax), was introduced in 1995. Since then, three other bisphosphonate drugs have been approved to treat osteoporosis. Generally, these drugs have been proven safe and effective, and millions of women have used them to prevent and treat osteoporosis. However, they can cause a rare kind of fracture of the thigh bone without any stress or injury. Because of this risk, women are advised to be more cautious in using bisphosphonates. Some physicians recommend discontinuing use of bisphosphonate if a postmenopausal woman has been taking the drug for many years, depending on the patient's particular risk for osteoporosis (Shane, 2010).

In 2004, the Surgeon General issued a report documenting the impending public health crisis of osteoporosis. Currently, 10 million Americans older than age 50 are suffering from osteoporosis and millions more are at risk. The report estimates that by the year 2020, just a few years from now, *half* of all Americans older than age 50 will be at risk of life-threatening fractures caused by osteoporosis. At present, osteoporosis is the cause of more than 1 million fractures every year in people older than age 50. The most frequent kinds of fractures are:

- Hip fractures—300,000
- Vertebrae fractures—250,000
- Wrist fractures—250,000
- Other bone fractures—300,000

About 20% of senior citizens who have a hip fracture die from complications of the fracture; another 20% wind up in a nursing home.

It is difficult for young, active people to think about building up their bone mass while young. However, a healthy diet consisting of green leafy vegetables and milk (not soda) and lots of exercise will go a long way toward keeping your body strong and active later in life. The Surgeon General issued this report to alert the nation to adjust their lifestyles in ways that will ensure adequate bone mass throughout life.

Age-Related Vision Loss

Another major health problem for the elderly is loss of vision as a result of **age-related macular degeneration (AMD)**. The central portion of the retina consists of a structure called the macula, which contains

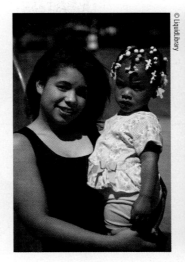
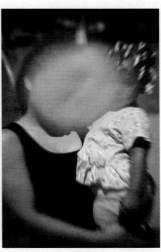

Loss of vision (right) caused by macular degeneration.

specialized cells that give the eye the capacity to see fine detail. (See **Figure 22.7**.) For reasons that are still undefined, these cells begin to die in some people as they age. AMD progresses slowly over years and eventually means that people can no longer drive, read normal print, watch television, recognize faces at a distance, or perform tasks involving small objects. Macular degeneration does not affect peripheral vision, so complete blindness does not occur and affected individuals can still be active in many ways.

About 2 million Americans over age 50 have vision loss caused by AMD. About 2% of people between the ages of 65 and 74 and about 14% of people older than age 75 are affected. Because the U.S. population is expected to age rapidly in coming years, the number of older people with macular degeneration is expected to increase markedly by the year 2020.

Macular degeneration occurs in two forms: age-related dry macular degeneration is the most common, occurring in about 90% of patients. The other form is caused by proliferation of blood vessels in the macula; this form is called age-related wet macular degeneration.

TERMS

age-related macular degeneration (AMD): loss of vision as a result of death of cells in a region of the eye called the macula; loss of vision progresses slowly over several years

hormone replacement therapy (HRT): administration of estrogen to menopausal and postmenopausal women to help prevent symptoms of menopause, osteoporosis, and heart disease

osteoporosis: a condition in older people, particularly women, in which bones lose density and become porous and brittle

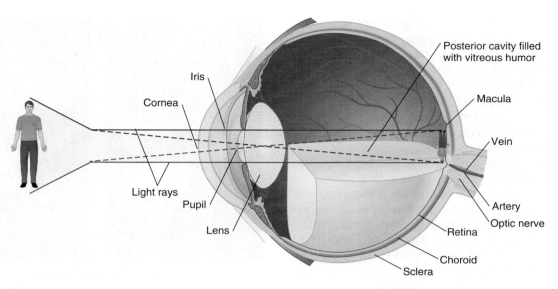

■ Figure 22.7

Diagram of the Human Eye Showing Key Structures
As people age, changes may occur in the pupil and macula that affect vision. The lens may become cloudy (cataract formation) due to changes in the proteins making up the lens. Normal vision can be restored by replacing the cloudy lens with a plastic lens in what is known as cataract surgery. If cells in the macula begin to die, a more serious condition called macular degeneration (AMD) results. Once AMD starts, it gradually worsens over time. There is no treatment or way to prevent AMD; some older people are affected while others are not. Although people with AMD have more and more difficulty seeing things, they usually do not become completely blind.

This is the most serious form because loss of vision progresses rapidly; occasionally the dry form may convert to the wet form. The wet form can be treated with laser surgery, which may be able to slow the progression of the damage. A drug, ranibizumab (Lucentis), also has been approved for treating the wet form of macular degeneration. However, the drug must be injected monthly, and each dose costs about $2,000. The injections must be continued indefinitely.

There are no approved treatments for the dry form of macular degeneration. However, in many people the loss of vision proceeds rather slowly so that many years pass after the initial diagnosis before legal blindness occurs. The progression of the dry form of macular degeneration can be slowed by daily antioxidant supplements consisting of vitamin C, vitamin E, beta-carotene, zinc oxide, and copper oxide (van Leeuwen et al., 2005). Taking these antioxidants when damage to the macula was minimal substantially slowed the progression of the disease and preserved functional vision for a longer period of time than vision was preserved in a control group of patients who did not take daily antioxidants.

Age-Related Hearing Loss

Age-related hearing loss refers to hearing loss experienced by people as they get older that interferes with understanding normal conversation. Hearing loss is the third most common chronic health condition among older Americans after high blood pressure and arthritis. About 4 million Americans older than 65 have hearing loss and difficulty understanding normal conversations. Some age-related hearing loss is inevitable as sensitive cells of the inner ear die or become less functional. However, much hearing loss is caused by exposure to noise and is referred to as noise-induced hearing loss. Even a single exposure to an extremely loud noise such as an explosion or a blast of sound from a loudspeaker can produce some permanent hearing loss. Lifetime exposure to loud noises such as driving in urban traffic, using power tools, listening to loud music, and working in noisy factories may also result in a gradual but permanent hearing loss.

Protecting your hearing while young is essential to preserving as much hearing as possible when you become old. Avoid explosions from firecrackers and guns or take precautions to protect your hearing. Always wear ear plugs or ear muffs designed to reduce environmental noise when operating any kind of noisy equipment. Even vacuum cleaners and hair dryers may exceed safe noise levels. Your hearing is precious; protect it at all times.

Stress, Telomeres, and Aging

Telomeres are short segments of DNA at the ends of chromosomes in every cell of the body. Their purpose is to retain the functional integrity of the DNA during cell division by protecting the ends of chromosomes. In early life the telomeres are long. Over time and cycles of cell

Physical Exercise May Slow Aging

Physical exercise has long been recommended for older people to help them remain physically fit, to prevent weight gain, and enhance balance to prevent falls. In addition to maintaining physical vigor, exercise may actually have a beneficial effect on the structural integrity of chromosomes. Structures at the ends of chromosomes (called *telomeres*) are responsible for preventing the loss of genes near the ends each time a chromosome duplicates.

Telomeres wear away little by little as we age; if telomeres become too short, cells die. If too many cells die, organs fail and we may die. Scientists have examined the length of telomeres in cells taken from older people who exercised and from people who were sedentary. The most active people had telomeres that were considerably longer than ones from people who did not exercise at all (Ludlow et al., 2013). The conclusion of the study was that exercise may slow aging by preventing chromosome destruction and consequent death of cells in the body.

Can Beliefs Influence Life Span?

Just how powerful are thoughts and feelings in influencing health? Can beliefs affect the duration of a person's life? A survey of the causes and ages of death among Chinese Americans shows that strongly held beliefs can affect the cause of death and how long a person lives (Phillips, Ruth, & Wagner, 1993).

In Chinese astrology, a particular phase—metal, water, wood, fire, or earth—is associated with the year of a person's birth. Also associated with each phase is susceptibility to particular diseases (see table). According to Chinese astrology and medicine, being born in a particular year makes a person more likely than usual to succumb to diseases associated with the phase of their birth year. An analysis of almost 30,000 death certificates of Chinese Americans showed that people with the predicted combination of birth year and disease susceptibility died two to five years before white Americans with the same diseases and phases.

The more traditional the Chinese lifestyle of the person, the shorter their life was once they contracted the disease associated with their birth year. The most plausible explanation of the findings is that Chinese Americans who believe in the predictions of Chinese astrology are the most likely to succumb to the disease that they expect will kill them. It appears that beliefs not only affect health through the onset of disease but also affect life span.

Birth year ends in	Phase	Susceptibility to
0 or 1	Metal	Pulmonary diseases
2 or 3	Water	Kidney disease
4 or 5	Wood	Cirrhosis of liver
6 or 7	Fire	Heart attack
8 or 9	Earth	Cancer, diabetes, ulcers

division, the telomeres progressively shorten until they cannot protect chromosomes very well or at all, and cells malfunction (become *senescent*) or die. Thus, telomeres may play a vital role in the aging process. Indeed, some inherited conditions involving premature aging are associated with malfunctions in telomere biology.

Far more significant for the average person's health are research findings showing the deleterious effects of compromised mental health on the length of telomeres and presumed acceleration of brain and bodily illness. For example, prolonged stress (Revesz et al., 2016) and depression (Verhoeven et al., 2017) are associated with telomere shortening. From these results we can see that an unhealthy state of mind can accelerate aging and accompanying illness. Telomere length can be measured by clinical tests.

Thinking About Aging

When you are young, thinking about aging usually is the last thing on your mind. You look at your parents and grandparents and cannot really imagine what it feels like to be 60 or 80 years old. Aging is something that happens to everyone irrespective of how successful they have been in living a "healthy" life. Of course, efforts that are implemented while you are young to care for your physical, emotional, mental, and spiritual health will help to maintain well-being when you are old. But there is no guarantee. Things happen. Life is a journey. Nothing in

life is predictable. The main thing is to have the resiliency, understanding, and spiritual strength to cope with changes.

Acceptance of change is crucial to "successful" aging. When you get older, physical strength may diminish, but hopefully you no longer need to lift heavy objects. You walk more instead of being "on the run." Having time to cook at home and being able to enjoy fresh foods are daily pleasures. You have time to read, think, and meditate. You

TERMS

age-related hearing loss: loss of hearing with advancing age; some loss of hearing may be caused by exposure to loud noise earlier in life

telomeres: DNA at the ends of chromosomes that protect the integrity of genetic information during cellular replication

have more time for art, gardening, reading, exercise, and socializing. Small things like watching a full moon rise from the ocean are special events. You are more aware of the spiritual side of nature and people.

Health and aging are lifelong processes, not goals that can be set and achieved with concentrated effort. At any age, you can take steps to improve your health now and later in life.

End-of-Life Decisions

With few exceptions, the media portray aging as a time of life beset with sickness, inactivity, and deterioration of physical, sexual, and mental functions. These negative views of aging are used to sell products and do not truthfully portray the experiences of most older Americans.

> I don't mind dying…
> I just don't want to be there when it happens.
> *Woody Allen*

Of all human fears, for most people, none is greater than the fear of death. When we are young, thoughts of death and dying are rare. Instead we are occupied with living, learning, and daily activities. We can't imagine that someday we will die. As we grow older and see parents, relatives, and friends die, we become more aware of our own mortality. We may begin to ponder our own eventual death.

Fear of aging and death may lead to anxiety and stress that may hasten aging processes. A few of the many fears that people associate with aging are cancer, poverty, being victimized, becoming disabled, memory loss, and sexual inadequacy. Most of these fears are unfounded, but they diminish quality of life. Chronological age often does not correlate with biological age. Some people feel and act young even if old.

Death can strike without warning in the form of an accident or an unexpected heart attack. However, for most people, thoughts of death do not occupy their daily lives until very old age. People in their 70s and 80s realize the inevitability of death and may modify their lives and affairs accordingly.

Steve Jobs, CEO of Apple computer and Pixar Animation Studios, was diagnosed with terminal pancreatic cancer in 2004 and died in 2011 at age 56. In an eloquent address to the Stanford University graduation class, Jobs described what this experience did for him.

> Remembering that I'll be dead soon is the most important tool I've ever encountered to help me make the big choices in life. Because almost everything—all external expectations, all pride, all fear of embarrassment or failure—these things just fall away in the face of death, leaving only what is truly important. Remembering that you are going to die is the best way I know to avoid the trap of thinking you have something to lose. (Jobs, 2005)

Most people would prefer to die peacefully in their sleep after living a full, satisfying life. Some may be fortunate to die like this, but others may have to endure considerable pain and suffering for years. In addition to wondering how they are going to die, people usually wonder what will happen to them after death. Christianity provides a heaven where one's "soul" can exist in the grace of God for all eternity. Buddhism embraces a belief in reincarnation; after a series of deaths and rebirths a person can attain "Buddhahood," a perpetual state of enlightenment.

In our society, death is not discussed openly, although this is beginning to change. Dying people are often isolated in hospitals and their care is left to physicians who may perform unwanted or unnecessary treatments. Sterile, impersonal death in a hospital or nursing home has increased many people's fears of death and the process of dying.

Stages of Dying

People have different attitudes toward death and dying. In conversations with many persons who were facing death, Elisabeth Kübler-Ross (1975) identified five distinct stages in the process of dying. Not all persons experienced all stages, but most experienced some of them. These stages of dying are (1) denial and isolation, (2) anger, (3) bargaining, (4) depression, and (5) acceptance.

The work of Kübler-Ross has found widespread acceptance, especially among counselors and those who help dying patients, but it has also received criticism. The main objection is that the studies were not conducted scientifically but were based on personal observation and interpretation. Another criticism is that because the stages of dying that Kübler-Ross proposed have been widely accepted and publicized, some dying patients may feel obliged to follow the stages she described.

More and more it is recognized that dying, like living, is an individual, personal matter. People can do as poet Dylan Thomas recommended and "Rage, rage against the dying of the light." Or they can embrace the idea that "with a better understanding of aging, it will become easier to accept the fact that life ends" (Campion, 1998).

Advance Directives

In 2005, the widely publicized case of Terri Schiavo created a national controversy. On February 25, 1990, Terri Schiavo suffered a heart attack that was triggered by complications of an eating disorder. The heart attack interrupted the flow of blood to her brain. Although medical intervention kept her alive, she suffered extensive, permanent brain damage and survived in what is medically described as a "persistent vegetative state," a condition in which no detectable cognitive brain function remains.

Terri Schiavo was kept alive for 15 years by means of a feeding tube that supplied nutrition and water. Her husband, Michael Schiavo, insisted that his wife would not have wanted to be kept alive in this way and wanted the feeding tube removed. Terri Schiavo's parents were adamantly opposed to this action and insisted that their daughter be kept alive by any and all means. The battle over Terri Schiavo ultimately involved the governor and legislature of the state of Florida, the U.S. Congress, the Supreme Court, and President George W. Bush (Bloche, 2005). In the end, the courts allowed the feeding tube to be removed and Terri Schiavo died on March 31, 2005 (Annas, 2005).

The Terri Schiavo case made millions of Americans realize the importance of executing **advance directives** so that family and health providers know exactly what their wishes were regarding medical care should they become unable to function on their own behalf. Advance directives are particularly important for the elderly but should be executed by young people as well. Terri Schiavo was only 26 when she suffered her heart attack.

Advance directives typically consist of two distinct documents. A **living will** explicitly states your desires for or rejection of specific treatments should you become unable to communicate. A living will should indicate your wishes with respect to artificial ventilation, CPR (cardiopulmonary resuscitation), tube feeding, and do-not-resuscitate (DNR) orders as well as other treatments. A living will is signed and witnessed, and copies are given to your personal physician as well as to family members and others whom you trust.

A living will should be as detailed as possible but may not cover all circumstances in a medical emergency. If you suffer a heart attack and someone calls 911, paramedics are required by law to administer CPR irrespective of what is stated in a living will. Only after you reach a hospital can the provisions in a living will be respected by physicians and hospital staff.

Another important document is a **healthcare power of attorney** in which you designate a spouse, family member, or close friend as the person responsible for health decisions in the event you are unable to make such decisions. The person you designate must be 18 years or older and cannot be one of your healthcare providers. Together, a living will and healthcare power of attorney make up your advance directive.

States differ considerably in the forms and terminology of advance directives. Help in understanding and completing advance directive forms can be obtained at a number of websites. Forms and instructions for each state can be obtained at www.compassionandchoices.org.

Everyone should execute advance directives to avoid a tragedy like Terri Schiavo's. Filing advance directives with your physician and family does not mean that you give up the right to make your own health decisions. Advance directives are used only if you become incapacitated and are unable to communicate.

Medical Aid in Dying

Medical aid in dying is an end-of-life medical practice in which a mentally capable, terminally ill adult with less than 6 months to live may request medication from her or his doctor for self-administration to bring about a peaceful death if her or his suffering becomes unbearable.

In 1997, Oregon passed the Death with Dignity Act, which legalized medical aid in dying in that state. In the first year after the bill passed, 23 persons received prescriptions for lethal medications, and 15 actually took the medicine and died. In 1999, physicians prescribed lethal medications to another 33 patients, but some died before they could take the drugs. In Oregon in 2016, 204 medical-aid-in-dying prescriptions were written by about 200 different physicians; 133 people actually took the medication and died. Over the 20 years that Oregon's Death with Dignity Act has been in effect, fewer than 1,000 individuals have requested a lethal prescription, and even among those many elected to die from their disease. It is clear from these numbers that, so far, there has not been a rush among terminally ill patients in Oregon to end their lives.

In the practice of medical aid in dying, a terminally ill patient who is mentally competent must express a desire to die on a number of occasions. Then a second physician is be consulted. If both physicians agree that the patient is mentally competent (not clinically depressed) and has an incurable, painful disease, one physician supplies the patient with the drugs for ending life.

Despite growing public support for medical aid in dying in the United States, there is still great resistance to its use, including among physicians, and clergy. As of 2014, Oregon, Washington, Vermont, California, and Montana are the only states that permit medical aid in dying. Thirty-four other states still have laws that explicitly criminalize any form of assisted suicide.

There is general agreement that end-of-life care needs to be improved substantially. Studies show that of the more than 2 million people that die each year in the United States, almost half of hospitalized patients suffer serious pain in the days preceding death. And

---

▌TERMS▐

advance directive: legal documents that express your desires regarding treatments should you be unable to communicate. A living will and a healthcare power of attorney constitute an advance directive

healthcare power of attorney: designates someone to make healthcare decisions for you if you are unable to communicate

living will: a legal document that expresses your wishes regarding treatment if you become unable to make your own medical decisions

medical aid in dying: a physician assistance to help a patient who no longer desires to live because of pain or an incurable illness to die

only about one-third of patients in nursing homes receive adequate pain relief. Two national health-care organizations have proposed that every physician attending to a dying patient should make the following six promises:

1. You will have the best of medical treatment, aiming to prevent exacerbation, improve function and survival, and ensure comfort.
2. Your care will be continuous, comprehensive, and coordinated.
3. You and your family will be prepared for everything that is likely to happen in the course of your illness.
4. Your wishes will be sought and respected, and they will be followed whenever possible.
5. We will help you consider your personal and financial resources and we will respect your choices about their use.
6. We will do all we can to see that you and your family will have the opportunity to make the best of every day.

The public discussion over end-of-life treatments and legal options and problems has been active in the United States for more than a quarter of a century and is still far from being resolved. In 1990, the U.S. Supreme Court did rule that withholding or withdrawal of life support from dying patients who can no longer be helped medically is legal.

Palliative Care

Palliative care is a newly recognized branch of medicine that focuses on noncurative treatments for the dying. The World Health Organization (WHO) defines palliative care as follows:

- Affirms life and regards dying as a normal process
- Neither hastens nor postpones death
- Provides relief from pain and other distressing symptoms
- Integrates the psychological and spiritual aspects of patient care
- Offers a support system to help patients live as actively as possible until death
- Offers a support system to help families cope with the patient's illness and death

When a person elects palliative care, the emphasis of treatment shifts from prolonging life to enhancing the quality of life that remains, preserving a person's dignity, and relieving suffering. Usually, a team of health professionals, in consultation with the patient and family, will decide if palliative care is appropriate.

Many opponents of medical aid in dying embrace the concept of palliative care and believe that it is more in accord with the ethics of medical practice. Now that palliative care is seen as a reimbursable form of therapy by many health insurance programs, eventually all terminally ill patients may have access to such care and no longer have to fear prolonged pain and suffering.

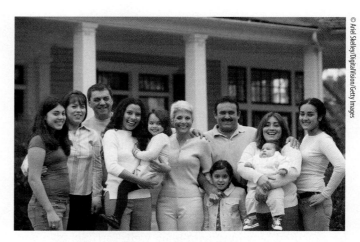

Strong family ties are healthy for young and old alike.

The Hospice

The term **hospice** originally applied to medieval Christian hospitals caring for the poor, the aged, and the sick. Hospices also provided refuge for people on religious pilgrimages. Providing physical necessities, medical care, and spiritual comfort was the primary purpose of the early religious hospices. In the United States there are more than 6,000 hospices offering comprehensive care for terminally ill patients. The goal of a hospice is to meet the total health needs—physical, psychological, and spiritual—of patients who have weeks or months to live. Medications are given to ease pain, but heroic treatments are not attempted. Family and friends are free to visit with the patient in a comfortable setting, whether it is in a patient's home or a hospice facility.

The hospice philosophy is that dying is part of living and should not be resisted with every weapon in the modern medical arsenal. Hospice care is designed to control pain and make patients comfortable, but staff also are trained to discuss emotional and spiritual issues relevant to death. Counseling and social services are available in hospices, and close family members are encouraged to participate in daily activities.

In 1982, Congress passed the Medicare Hospice Benefit Act. This law ensures that Medicare will pay hospice costs for any terminally ill patient whose projected life expectancy is 6 months or less. In 2008, most hospices were enrolled in the Medicare plan. Overall, about one in three Americans now dies under hospice care either at home or in a hospice facility.

Healthy Aging Depends on a Healthy Lifestyle

With the dramatic upward shift in average life expectancy in the United States and other countries, finding ways to improve health in elderly people has become a major

After Childhood and Adulthood There's Oldhood

We're all familiar with the periods of childhood and adulthood. But you don't hear much about "oldhood." Childhood is the time of considerable physical, emotional, and social development, for which there are expectations, guidelines, rules, teachers, mentors, and laws. Most cultures have a marker for when childhood ends and adulthood begins, such as turning 18 or getting married. Unlike childhood, adulthood is given over to meeting the demands of work/career, marriage, parenthood, and other responsibilities, and their attendant stresses and strains. Oldhood, which also has markers, such as turning 65 or retiring from an occupation, is often seen as a time of diminishing capacity and opportunity. However, as with any other time in the life span, if one has one's health and financial and social support, oldhood can present an enormous diversity of opportunities for new experiences, work, creativity, and joy. There are fewer responsibilities and stress, and more time for exercise, sleep, and indulging one's intellect, and even engaging in a long-put-off passion. Oldhood may be the final epoch of life, but it does not have to be the least rewarding.

Persons surviving to age 55 today can expect to live, on average, another 25 years; those surviving to age 75 can expect to live another 10 to 12 years. Many of these older people are relatively healthy and the length of time that they will be disabled before death is short. In general, people who live to the oldest ages without disabilities are those who have practiced good nutrition, were physically and mentally active, and did not use tobacco or drink alcohol excessively.

More and more attention is being paid to the role of nutrition in healthy aging. Increased consumption of fresh fruits and vegetables is thought to slow the aging processes; those containing antioxidant chemicals are regarded as particularly potent antiaging foods. These include avocado, berries, broccoli, cabbage, carrots, citrus, grapes, onions, tomatoes, and spinach. Coffee and tea also contain significant amounts of antioxidants. But according to believers in the antioxidant theory of aging, supplements still are needed to ensure that you are getting sufficient amounts of antioxidant vitamins and minerals.

Every age of life provides opportunities for growth and satisfaction. Even though we have no way of knowing when serious illness or death will confront us, we do have control of how we live each day and the satisfactions we find in life. The way we choose to live when we are young will greatly affect our health later. For example, smoking while young increases the likelihood of developing cancer and heart disease later. Drinking alcohol to excess and taking unnecessary chances invite accidents that can cause death or permanent disability. Although each person's life span is partly determined by genes, environmental factors, such as nutrition, exercise, and lifestyle, are also important in determining not only how long we live but how well we live.

challenge. Generally, increasing age is associated with increasing disability and functional impairments, such as loss of mobility, sight, or hearing. One goal of gerontology is to find ways to minimize or postpone the disabilities that accompany aging so that quality of life extends to, or close to, the end of life.

The scientific evidence is now quite overwhelming that most of the disability and long-term medical care in elderly persons results from major chronic diseases that were already present in midlife. The most significant predictors of a healthy old age are low blood pressure and low serum glucose levels, not being obese, and not smoking cigarettes while young. These factors are also important in predicting such diseases as cardiovascular disease, cancer, and diabetes. Thus, the evidence points to the importance of developing healthy habits while young if the "golden years" are going to be enjoyed with one's physical and mental abilities intact.

TERMS

hospice: a place for terminally ill patients to spend the time before death in an environment that attends to their physical, emotional, and spiritual needs but does not administer any further treatments; hospice care also can be given in a patient's home

Critical Thinking About Health

1. In 2017, researchers Angus Deaton and Anne Case at Princeton University reported that the mortality rate among male and female Caucasian Americans aged 50-54 had been increasing 0.5% a year between 1997 and 2014. This is contrary to the overall U.S. mortality rate, which had been steadily declining for more than 100 years, and also contrary to the trends in mortality rate in many other industrialized countries, which are relatively stable or declining. Deaton and Case determined that the increase in mortality rate was related to more suicides, prescription drug overdoses, and deaths from alcohol abuse. Imagine that you are part of the Angus/Dean research team and you've been tasked to determine the reason(s) underlying these causes of death. What lifestyle, social, and environmental factors would you consider? Check out the Dean/Case study at https://www.brookings.edu/bpea-articles/mortality-and-morbidity-in-the-21st-century/

2. Imagine that you have just learned that your mother is suffering from terminal cancer that cannot be treated. The physician estimates that death can occur at any time within a few months and that your mother's pain will be considerable. Although drugs can alleviate some of the pain, the doctor honestly does not know how effective the pain relief will be. Your mother is 75 years old and is aware of her condition. When you and she discuss her condition, she expresses a strong desire not to suffer to survive a few weeks or months. She asks you to help her obtain drugs that she can use to end her life peacefully whenever she chooses.

   Describe how you would feel in such a situation and what actions you would take. Would you discuss the problem with her physician, with a religious counselor, or with someone else? Would you be concerned about legal problems if you did obtain the lethal drugs and give them to your mother? Would you tell your mother that you want to keep her alive at all costs and you will do all that you can to reduce her suffering? Make a list of all the steps you would take in this situation, and explain your reasons for each action.

3. Make a list of all the health-related factors in your life that you think might play a role in how healthy you will be at age 70 (e.g., you smoke cigarettes, you are significantly overweight). After thinking about the list you have made, ask yourself if some behaviors or lifestyle factors are worth changing to help ensure that you will enjoy a healthy old age. Or perhaps you feel that it is not worth worrying about old age now and that the important thing is to enjoy life at the present time. Discuss these different views and try to develop a personal philosophy of aging that is right for you.

4. Because both of your grandmothers have Alzheimer's disease, the other members of your family are very concerned over their own future mental health, even though both of your parents are only in their 50s. Having read that a particular gene contributes to the risk of Alzheimer's disease and that doctors can test for the presence of this gene, your mother and father have been discussing the advisability of getting the test. They also have asked if you would like to be tested for the Alzheimer's gene. What advice would you give them? Would you want to be tested for the Alzheimer's susceptibility gene? Discuss in detail the reasons for your advice to them and the decision you would make for yourself.

Chapter Summary and Highlights

Chapter Summary

When we are young, we rarely think about growing old or dying. When we are old, we often think about what we could have done when we were young to make us healthier now that we are old. But every stage of life has its different perceptions, needs, worries, and goals. At 17, your primary goal was probably getting the attention from someone you admire; at 77, your goal may be getting through the day without pain. Many young people today will live into their 80s, 90s, or older. How well, active, and mentally alert you will be depends, in large measure, on how much attention you pay to your health and lifestyle while young. Living a long, healthy life depends on the genes you inherited and the lifestyle you lead. For the same reasons you put money into a retirement account to ensure financial security in your later years, you should think about banking some healthy habits when you are young. Maintaining a healthy weight and diet, not smoking, and getting regular exercise are some ways to invest in a healthy old age. It's even worth visualizing playing several sets of tennis, playing 18 holes of golf, or possibly running a marathon when you are 80 years old. As the great Yankee catcher Yogi Berra once quipped, "It is very hard to make predictions...especially about the future." Dying is like that. We never know how many days and years we are allotted. So, rather than fearing death, we should engage in and enjoy life day by day. Life can be envisioned as a voyage. Some days are slow, calm, and without incident; others are turbulent, frenzied, and stormy; still others are beautiful and rewarding. Accept each day and what it offers. One thing is certain; all things change with time, including your loves, despairs, failures, and successes. It is difficult to make light of death, but Woody Allen came close when he remarked, "I don't mind dying; I just don't want to be there when it happens."

Highlights

- Aging and dying are natural stages of life. People should strive to remain physically, emotionally, mentally, and spiritually active at all stages of life regardless of chronological age.
- The maximum human life span is approximately 115 years; the average life span in many countries is 80+ years, which means that half of the people in those countries will live to be 80 years of age or older.
- The average age of the population in the United States is rising rapidly, increasing healthcare costs and causing problems for the Social Security system.
- Aging is partly determined by genes and partly by environmental factors that cause cellular damage. Caloric restriction slows aging in laboratory animals but is impractical in people.
- Loss of cognitive abilities in the elderly is called senile dementia; the major cause of mental deterioration is Alzheimer's disease.

- Parkinson's disease is a neurodegenerative disease that affects movement.
- Bone loss in the elderly causes osteoporosis.
- The major cause of vision loss in the elderly is macular degeneration.
- Advance directives consist of executing a living will and a healthcare power of attorney.
- Palliative care is treatment that does not cure but that relieves pain and suffering of dying patients and deals with the distress of family members.
- Hospice care provides terminally ill patients with medical, emotional, and spiritual support during the final weeks or months of their lives.
- Successful aging depends on maintaining a healthy weight; eating a nutritious, balanced diet; getting lots of exercise; and keeping mentally active.

For Your Health

Even if scientists one day find ways to extend the human life span, individuals won't be able to make much use of those discoveries if they are not otherwise healthy. Do the "Heathy Aging" questionnaire (Exercise 22.1 in the Workbook) to see how well you are doing to make your later years healthy.

References

Annas, G. J. (2005). "Culture of life" politics at the bedside—the case of Terri Schiavo. *New England Journal of Medicine, 352,* 1710–1715.

Barry, P. (2007, September 15). Curry powder. *Science News,* 167–168.

Bloche, M. G. (2005). Managing conflict at the end of life. *New England Journal of Medicine, 352,* 2371–2373.

Campion, E. W. (1998). Aging better. *New England Journal of Medicine, 338,* 1064–1066.

Jobs, S. (2005). Graduation address at Stanford University, June 12.

Kübler-Ross, E. (1975). *Death: The final stage of growth.* Englewood Cliffs, NJ: Prentice Hall.

Ludlow, A. T., et al. (2013). Do telomeres adapt to physiological stress? Exploring the effect of exercise on telomere length and telomere-related proteins. *Biomed Research International, 2013*(2013), 601368. doi:10.1155/2013/601368

Marx, J. (2005). Preventing Alzheimer's: A lifelong commitment? *Science, 309,* 864–867.

Phillips, D. P., Ruth, T. E., & Wagner, L. M. (1993, November 6). Psychology and survival. *Lancet, 342,* 142–145.

Prusiner, S. B. (2012). A unifying role for prions in neurodegenerative diseases. *Science, 336,* 1511–1512.

Revesz, D., et al. (2016). Baseline biopsychosocial determinants of telomere length and 6-year attrition rate. *Psychoneuroendocrinology, 67,* 153–162.

van Leeuwen, R., et al. (2005). Dietary intake of antioxidants and risk of age-related macular degeneration. *Journal of the American Medical Association, 294,* 3101–3107.

Verhoeven, J. E., et al. (2015). The association of early and recent psychosocial life stress with leukocyte telomere length. *Psychosomatic Medicine, 77,* 882–891.

Suggested Readings

Critser, G. (2010). *Eternity soup: Inside the quest to end aging.* New York: Harmony Books. If you are one of those people who wonders what it might be like to live forever (or at least longer than you can imagine), this book can give you some idea of what scientists are pursuing.

Fins, J. J. (2006). *A palliative ethic of care: Clinical wisdom at life's end.* Sudbury, MA: Jones and Bartlett. An excellent discussion of palliative care and end-of-life decisions.

Gawande, A. (2007, April 30). The way we age now. *The New Yorker,* 48–57. An intimate portrait of how one elderly person copes with aging.

Kinsley, M. (2014, April 26). Have you lost your mind? *The New Yorker*, 24–31. Between 1946 and 1964, about 79 million babies were born in the United States. This group is known as the baby boomers. In 2015, the first of this group will turn 70 and the ranks of the elderly will swell rapidly in subsequent years. Many of the baby boomers will develop Alzheimer's disease or other forms of dementia. How will society cope with their care?

Kirkwood, T. (2010, September). Why we can't live forever. *Scientific American*, 42–49. Understanding the aging processes may help us live longer and healthier lives, but not dying is not going to happen.

Nuland, S. B. (2007). *The art of aging: A doctor's prescription for well-being.* New York: Random House. A famous physician, now in his 70s, offers advice on how to age successfully.

Sanders, L. (2011, March 12). Memories can't wait. *Science News*, 24–28. A good discussion of the causes of Alzheimer's and approaches being taken to detect changes early in the disease and to treat patients before dementia becomes noticeable.

Stix, G. (2010, June). Alzheimer's: Forestalling the darkness. *Scientific American,* 51–57. As populations age and the prevalence of Alzheimer's increases, scientists are looking for ways to forestall or prevent dementia. This article explains how the research is being conducted.

Recommended Websites

Compassion and Choices
Offers help and advice on end-of-life decisions. Provides advance directives tool kit. Helped design Oregon's Death with Dignity Act.

HospiceNet
Information and education about hospice and other death and dying issues, including bereavement and end-of-life caretaking.

My Health Directive.com
This site also provides information and help with advance directives.

National Right to Life
The National Right to Life Committee supplies living wills that instruct physicians to use all techniques available to preserve life.

NIH Senior Health
Health information for older Americans from the U.S. National Library of Medicine.

U.S. Administration on Aging
General information on aging.

U.S. National Institute on Aging
Information on research on aging problems.

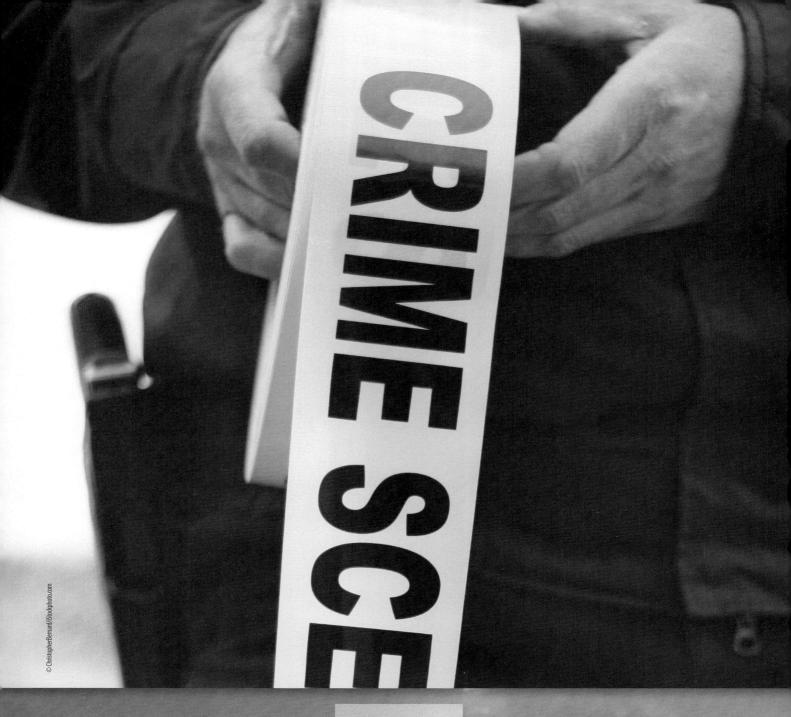

Health Tips

Hotline for Domestic Violence Help

How to Prevent Date Rape

Preventing Sexual Assault

CHAPTER 23

Violence in Our Society

Learning Objectives

1. Describe the different kinds of interpersonal violence.

2. Explain ways that violence affects health.

3. List the kinds of violence and abuse that can lead to posttraumatic stress disorder.

4. Describe the different forms of child abuse.

5. Define *sexual assault, forcible rape*, and *acquaintance rape*.

6. Discuss the reasons that underlie forcible rape and acquaintance rape.

7. Define *elder abuse* and the factors that contribute to it.

8. List and describe the different kinds of hate crimes.

9. Discuss some of the ways that firearms increase the risk of homicide and suicide among young people.

10. Discuss how media violence contributes to aggression and violence among children.

Anger, aggression, hostility, and violence are inherent to all animals, including humans. Their major biological roles are to aid in the acquisition of food, mates, territory, and other resources and to ward off danger to self and offspring and, in some species, family and community as well. As intelligent as humans are, they seem unable to control biologically rooted rage and violent behavior. Compared to other animals, modern humans have sophisticated weapons and ways to assault, vanquish, and kill, sometimes out of need, but most often out of greed. In addition, we kill others and ourselves, not for self-defense or the acquisition of material wealth, but because of ideas, beliefs, prejudices, insults, and a host of hurts that are conjured up in our minds. The goal of modern societies—as yet unrealized—is to develop ways to prevent and control human aggression and violence.

> In war, truth is the first casualty.
>
> Aeschylus (525–456 B.C.)

Violence is a physical or verbal behavior in which the intent is to harm, injure, or destroy someone or something. Human beings are unique in understanding the future possibility of injury and death and so will fight for many reasons, including being threatened by loss of personal freedom. People also have many intangible things to fear—fear of being hungry, fear of being poor, fear of being attacked, and fear of being unwanted or unloved are examples. All of these fears can provoke violent behavior.

Some people use violence as a means of gaining power over others. In its simplest form, power is the ability to satisfy one's needs and desires. Power and its accompanying violence manifest in society in a variety of ways—as rape, domestic violence, child abuse, elder abuse, homicide, suicide, terrorist attacks, gang fights, and wars between nations.

About 17,000 persons die in the United States every year from homicide, and more than 2 million persons are injured in violent attacks. Homicide is the second leading cause of death among persons aged 15 to 24, and suicide is the third in the same age group. The consequences of violence in society are broken families, battered women, abused children, and countless unnecessary injuries and deaths.

To treat the effects of violence on the minds and bodies of people is expensive, difficult, and often unsuccessful. The *only* solution to violent human behavior, as with other serious diseases, is prevention. Although some people believe that violence in human societies is inevitable, many others do not and choose to live nonviolent lives and work to end violent behaviors.

Intimate Partner Violence

Intimate partner violence (IPV) refers to physical, sexual, or psychological harm by a current or former intimate partner or spouse. Women are the most likely victims of IPV, but both heterosexual and homosexual men also are affected. Until recently, the public generally viewed intimate partner violence as rare. However, IPV and other forms of domestic violence are now recognized as major public health problems. IPV is regarded as one of the most serious, preventable public health problems, affecting more than 32 million Americans at one time or another in their lives.

Several categories of IPV are recognized by health experts:

- *Physical violence:* the intentional use of physical force on another person that has the potential for causing injury, disability, or death. Physical violence may include scratching, pushing, kicking, punching, grabbing, biting, choking, and use of weapons.
- *Sexual violence:* (1) use of physical force to compel another person to engage in a sexual act against his or her will; (2) any sexual act against a person who is unable to understand the act or to indicate unwillingness to engage in a sexual act, for example, a person might be too drunk or intimidated to prevent the act; and (3) abusive sexual contact.
- *Threats of physical or sexual violence:* use of words, gestures, or weapons to communicate the intent to cause physical injury or death.
- *Psychological or emotional violence:* use of acts, threats of acts, or coercive measures that cause the victim to feel humiliated, embarrassed, diminished, or frightened; denying a victim access to friends, money, or food.
- **Stalking:** behavior that causes victims to feel a high level of fear of physical or sexual violence.

Studying IPV is difficult because it often is not discussed openly by family members or even by abused individuals. It is estimated that fewer than half of all cases of family violence are reported to authorities, but the extent of physical and sexual attacks on women in the United States is alarming (**Table 23.1**). More women are treated in hospital emergency rooms for IPV injuries each year than for muggings, rape, and traffic accidents combined. And battering during pregnancy is the leading cause of birth defects and infant mortality.

In trying to reduce the epidemic of intimate partner violence, the federal government has declared each October as National Domestic Violence month. Extra efforts are made during this period to increase public awareness of domestic violence and to educate people on how to prevent it.

People who experience battering or rape by a partner or acquaintance not only have medical problems but also may suffer from anxiety, depression, chronic pelvic pain, gastrointestinal upset, substance abuse, obesity, or headaches. Assaulted individuals may also develop symptoms of *posttraumatic stress disorder (PTSD)* and its variants,

Table 23.1

Estimated Number of U.S. Women Who Have Experienced Intimate Partner Violence

Violent acts	Number
Rape	44.8 million
Sexual coercion	17.3 million
Unwanted sexual contact	34.2 million
Unwanted noncontact sexual experiences*	37.1 million
Physical violence	57.6 million
Psychological aggression by intimate partner	65.1 million

*Includes exposing sexual body parts, being made to look at or participate in sexual photos or movies, and/or being harassed in a public place in a way that felt unsafe.

Data from Smith, S., et al. (2017). *The National Intimate Partner and Sexual Violence Survey: 2010–2012 Summary Report*. Atlanta, GA: National Center for Injury Prevention and Control, Centers for Disease Control and Prevention. Retrieved from http://www.cdc.gov/ViolencePrevention/pdf/NISVS-StateReportBook.pdf

Hotline for Domestic Violence Help

If you or someone you know is subject to domestic or interpersonal violence of any kind, professional help should be obtained as quickly as possible. Advice and assistance can be obtained by calling the following hotline: U.S. Government's National Domestic Violence Hotline: 800-799-SAFE (7233).

battered person syndrome or rape trauma syndrome. Symptoms of PTSD include the following:

- Reexperiencing the traumatic event(s) through recurrent intrusive images, thoughts, dreams of the trauma, and "flashbacks"—having a sense of reliving the trauma, including reexperiencing the disturbing emotions.
- Intense reactions to things that symbolize the traumatic experience. For example, in recovering from a rape, victims may intensely fear being in locales that resemble the scene of the assault.
- Some people may experience nausea when thinking of the rape, and some may have difficulties with sexual relations.
- Being unable to recall the trauma (denial), or being able to "make the mind go somewhere else" to avoid the pain associated with the memory of the trauma (dissociation). Victims may feel detached or estranged.
- Manipulation of others and the environment as a way to keep things calm and under control. Victims may become compliant as a way to avoid real or imagined abuse.
- Persistent arousal symptoms, such as difficulty falling or staying asleep, being edgy, jumpy, irritable, and sometimes irrationally angry. Victims may have difficulty concentrating, be hypervigilant to their surroundings, and have an exaggerated startle response.

Many long-term health consequences are associated with battering, rape, and sexual abuse. For example, traumatized individuals tend to be more susceptible to arousal by stimuli that makes it difficult for them to differentiate normal aches, pains, and sensations from signals of disease, leading to increased incidence of seeking help from health professionals. Also, emotional upset and guardedness can produce painful muscle tension and skeletal misalignment. Chronic anxiety can lead to gastrointestinal

upsets. Alcohol, nicotine, and other drugs may be used to block out memories of abuse and to alleviate uncomfortable emotions and physical sensations that accompany memories of the assault or abuse.

Recovering from the trauma of relationship violence requires patience and support. Victims are encouraged to seek psychological counseling from professionals who specialize in helping victims of relationship violence and to join support groups of other assaulted individuals. Support can hasten healing and recovery and help restore the trust that is shattered by assault. Support groups can also provide a place to stay if the victim needs to escape the abuser, or the group can offer companionship if the victim is afraid to be alone.

Causes of Domestic Violence

There is no single cause of domestic violence, but contributing factors include the following:

- A high level of conflict and stress in the family
- Male dominance and the view that women and children are men's property
- Cultural norms that permit family violence
- Displays of violence on TV and in other media
- Being raised in a violent family
- Alcohol and drug abuse
- Victim-blaming ("people get what they deserve")
- Denying the existence of physical violence or sexual abuse

Women who are at the greatest risk for serious injury from domestic violence include those with male partners who abuse alcohol or drugs, are unemployed or intermittently employed, have less than a high school

TERMS

intimate partner violence (IPV): physical, sexual, or psychological harm by a current or former intimate partner or spouse

stalking: behavior that causes victims to feel a high level of fear of physical or sexual violence

violence: a physical or verbal behavior in which the intent is to harm, injure, or destroy someone or something

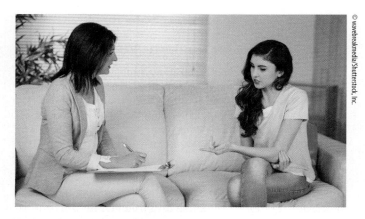

Being able to tell an understanding person what happened helps.

education, and are former husbands or boyfriends of the women.

Ways to prevent domestic violence include providing shelters, safe houses, and other protective environments for abused women; reducing contributing social and economic factors (unemployment, poverty, and racism); holding the abusers accountable for their actions; training law enforcement and healthcare professionals to recognize and intervene in cases of domestic violence; training everyone in nonviolent conflict resolution; and reducing the amount of violent imagery on TV, in films, and in popular music. Physicians also are receiving more training in recognizing, treating, and helping victims of domestic violence, most of whom are women, find shelter and support.

Domestic violence does not only affect adults who are in an abusive relationship; children who share the abusive environment also suffer (**Table 23.2**). Resolution of conflicts between parents or partners is essential to the long-term health of children. And children who grow up in physically or sexually abusive environments are much more likely to find themselves in abusive relationships as adults.

Table 23.2

Symptoms of Parental Violence in Children

Children who are exposed to parental violence are subject to a variety of symptoms.

Behavioral symptoms

Aggression	Tantrums	Immaturity	Delinquency

Emotional symptoms

Anxiety and depression	Low self-esteem	Anger	Withdrawal

Cognitive symptoms

Poor performance in school	Poor language skills

Physical symptoms

Eating disorders	Poor motor skills	Sleep problems	Retarded growth
Psychosomatic disorders			

Maltreatment of Children

Child abuse is physical, mental, or sexual maltreatment or neglect of a child. In recent years, child abuse has gained widespread public attention when numerous clergy were found to have sexually abused and molested youths in their care and who were involved in church activities. Hundreds of sexually abused victims broke years of silence to describe how they were sexually maltreated by clergy when they were young. Many described how seriously their lives had been damaged by their traumatic childhood experiences. In addition, some day care operators have been charged with child abuse, but, in some cases, the charges turned out to be unfounded. Young children have vivid imaginations and can easily be led by an investigator into agreeing with things that the investigator describes. However, confirmed cases of child abuse indicate that the problem of maltreatment of children is as serious a problem as intimate partner violence.

Each year in the United States, over 3 million documented cases of child abuse occur. (Many more cases occur but are not reported.) Among these cases, about 17% are physical abuse, 8% are sexual abuse, and 75% are neglect. About five children die each day in the United States from neglect and physical abuse. The Centers for Disease Control and Prevention (CDC) reports that about 2% of infants in the United States younger than the age of 1 suffer from neglect or abuse, often in the first few weeks of life. A large number of these cases are related to drug abuse by one or both parents.

Child abuse affects children physically (e.g., broken bones, burns, or even death) and emotionally (e.g., they may become abusive themselves, suicidal, or withdrawn). Effects are both short and long term and invariably devastating to all victims. As the abused child reaches age 10 and older and becomes more independent, he or she may feel in a hopeless situation and may run away from home. The consequences for many runaways are dismal: teenage prostitution, illicit drug and alcohol use, higher rates of juvenile crimes, and higher school dropout rates. Child abuse is costly to society and directly or indirectly affects everyone.

A particularly disturbing form of child abuse is **shaken-baby syndrome (SBS)** in which infants are violently shaken by adults either to punish them or to stop them from crying. SBS affects as many as 1,400 infants each year. Shaken infants can be identified by physicians and trained personnel by a collection of symptoms that result from the violent shaking. Any kind of violent shaking of an infant is a crime.

Child abuse involves several forms of maltreatment, all of which invariably lead to serious harm.

Physical Abuse When intentional force of any kind that results in injury is used on a child, the child has suffered physical abuse. Physical force that is used to discipline or control a child or adolescent that causes serious physical and psychological injury is child abuse. Often a parent is venting anger over some other issue that is irrelevant to the child's behavior; the child is the unwitting victim of the anger and knows that the punishment is unjust. The younger the child, the more likely a serious injury will result from the use of physical force. Shaking a baby repeatedly to get it to stop crying, or for any other reason, can cause death.

Emotional Abuse Psychological abuse can cause severe emotional distress and can produce illness and violent behavior that may lead to suicide or homicide. Being screamed at repeatedly and told that one is worthless, stupid, or defective can permanently damage psychological and social development.

Sexual Abuse Sexual contact between adults and children is forbidden both by cultural taboos and by criminal law. Although it is difficult to determine with accuracy the prevalence of child sexual abuse in the United States, some surveys have found that in the United States as many as 15% of women and 6% of men have experienced sexual abuse as children. Because this subject is not one that most people are willing to discuss, the prevalence of child sexual abuse may be higher than reported. Sexual abuse of children may result in depression, anxiety, and general dysfunction later in their lives.

Neglect This is probably the most common form of maltreatment of children. Neglect includes failure to provide a child with adequate nourishment, proper clothing, and prescribed medications or to oversee a child's hygiene. Neglected children are left to their own devices for long periods without adult supervision, and many neglected children engage in self-destructive behaviors.

Social Aspects of Child Maltreatment

Because many cases of child abuse go unreported, reliable data are difficult to obtain; also, abusers and the abused usually do not offer information freely. As a result, much information on child abuse has been incorrect or misleading.

Males tend to abuse children at a higher rate than females. However, no unique factors have been found that distinguish male abusers of children from female abusers. Male children are abused more frequently and seen by parents as more deserving of harsh treatment than female children. Male children even blame themselves more than female children do for their own maltreatment.

Two-thirds of all abused children are between the ages of 5 and 17. Preteen children are more vulnerable to abuse because they lack both physical strength to resist child abuse and knowledge about what is normal and abnormal behavior. Infants are abused less frequently than older children, but are at greater risk of death than older children, especially when shaken. As children pass the age of 15, they are more likely to be abused by peers than by family members.

Children with physical or mental disabilities such as blindness, deafness, intellectual disability, or cerebral palsy are at a greater risk for child abuse than others. Being vulnerable because of the physical disability or the stress created by caring for a disabled child can provoke abuse. Children who are temperamental, impulsive, aggressive, depressed, or hyperactive are also at a higher risk for being abused. These behaviors create parental stress that may contribute to child abuse.

Lack of knowledge and skills about child care may predispose parents to child maltreatment, possibly because of frustration and stress created by the needs of a child and its apparent lack of cooperation. Males who are primary caregivers usually have received little or no training regarding child care.

The same holds true for adolescent mothers and mothers with low levels of education, for example, high school dropouts. They, too, lack the knowledge and skills necessary for adequate child care. This lack places them in a stressful situation in which abuse is more likely to occur. These mothers feel they have no one to turn to for help, and they may not even know where to obtain help. In frustration, they abuse their children.

If the family lives in an unsafe neighborhood, family members may feel afraid to venture out to seek help for their problems. This fear results in even more isolation and may exacerbate family conflicts and abuse. Other reasons for child abuse are social isolation, lack of friends, dangerous neighborhoods, or lack of access to transportation.

Child Maltreatment Prevention

Child abuse prevention programs can help parents reduce the stress that is a risk factor in child abuse. These programs emphasize educating parents on how to care for their children and how to avoid abuse. Different stress reduction programs have been developed for adolescent mothers, young parents, fathers who have never been in charge of child care before, working mothers, single parents, step parents, and siblings who are in charge of child care. Stress management programs are particularly important in communities where unemployment rates are high.

Conflict resolution programs can also help prevent child abuse. If people are able to manage conflict without using physical force, the risk of child abuse is lower. Both anger mediation programs and conflict resolution

---

TERMS

child abuse: physical or mental injury, sexual abuse or exploitation, maltreatment, or neglect of a child by a person who is responsible for the child's welfare

shaken-baby syndrome (SBS): a form of child abuse in which an infant is violently shaken by an adult

programs have been shown to help lower rates of child abuse. Training in life and social skills for all individuals involved with child abuse is recommended. Training in parenting skills for both males and females of all ages is also strongly suggested. This training also helps to educate about resources for assistance.

Sexual Violence

Sexual violence is any sexual act that is perpetrated against a person's will. Sexual violence includes a completed, nonconsensual sex act (i.e., rape), an attempted nonconsensual sex act, abusive sexual contact (i.e., unwanted touching), and noncontact sexual abuse (e.g., threatened sexual violence, exhibitionism, verbal sexual harassment). All types involve victims who do not consent, who are unable to consent, or who are unable to refuse to allow the act.

Rape and Sexual Assault

The word *rape* comes from the Latin *rapere*, which means to seize or take by force. Originally, the word meant the looting and destruction of an enemy's village, town, or city and the capture of its citizens to be used as slaves. The idea that to be raped is to be vanquished persists today, as when referring to the inhumane destruction of a town or city (e.g., the "rape" of the city of Nanking in 1937) or being defeated in an endeavor ("I was raped on that exam").

More commonly, the word **rape** refers to nonconsensual sexual behavior, generally penile penetration of a bodily orifice. In the conduct of a rape, a victim also may be beaten, have her or his life threatened, or be killed. The combination of forced sexual penetration and nonsexual violence is **sexual assault**. Sexual assault is committed not for sexual gratification but for the desire to control, harm, humiliate, and dehumanize the victim.

In North America, rape and sexual assault are crimes. Although varying by jurisdiction, rape is generally defined as nonconsensual penetration by force or threat of force of a bodily orifice, including the mouth, rectum, or vagina. Penetration generally means by penis, although it also may include objects or other body parts such as fingers. *Nonconsensual* means the victim is incapable of giving legal consent because of mental development, physical disability, being intoxicated (e.g., with alcohol or drugs), or being unconscious. Types of rape include the following:

- *Date or acquaintance rape:* The victim and perpetrator know each other.
- *Marital rape:* The victim and perpetrator are married.
- *Stranger-rape:* Forced sexual contact by a stranger.
- *Gang-rape:* Rape by two or more perpetrators.
- *Statutory rape:* Sexual activity with a legally underage person.

According to the U.S. Department of Justice (Planty et al., 2016), approximately 300,000 adult American women and 90,000 adult American men report being raped each year. And because rape is largely an underreported crime, these data are thought to represent only about 40% of actual rape incidents. More than half of all rapes of women (54%) occur before age 18; 22% of these rapes occur before age 14. Among men, 75% of all rapes occur before age 18 and 48% of these occur before age 14.

Because the vast majority of perpetrators of sexual assault are men, it is theorized that gender role attitudes and expectations facilitate the occurrence of many rapes. For example, the belief that to be masculine is to be aggressive encourages some men to use sexual violence to gain control over others. This leads to expressions such as "women like a powerful man" and "women like being raped." Also, some men believe that a sexual conquest proves masculinity. Believing that the male role is to be dominant, some men try to take what they want regardless of how their behavior may harm others. Moreover, some men receive support from male peers for sexually abusive behavior. The expectation that the male takes the lead in sex fosters misunderstandings and frustration. A woman's "no" to a sexual advance can be misinterpreted as a signal to continue until finally the woman stops or pulls away, which frustrates the male and leads to anger-induced aggression. This gives rise to expressions such as "I didn't believe her when she said no."

Men who sexually assault women can be characterized either as anger motivated or power motivated. Anger-motivated assaults (about 20% of rapes) are generally motivated by an intense hatred of women. They tend to be committed by a stranger who threatens the victim with a knife or other weapon. Indeed, for victims, dying is a major fear during the attack. Perpetrators of power-motivated sexual assault (about 80% of rapes) are someone the victim knows who wants to control the victim rather than harm or injure her or him. The following are some common myths about sexual violence.

- Sexual violence is most often an attempt to control, harm, or overpower a victim; it is not motivated by sexual attraction, passion, or sexual deprivation.
- Most incidents of sexual violence are not reported to friends, family, or the authorities.
- Most incidents of sexual violence occur in the victim's immediate environment and are premeditated and planned.
- In most incidents of sexual violence the perpetrator knows the victim.
- Sexual violence is perpetrated by people from all socioeconomic, educational levels, and ethnic backgrounds.
- Victims do not secretly want to be sexually violated.

Acquaintance Rape

Acquaintance rape, or date rape, occurs when a person known to the victim uses verbal or physical force to coerce the victim into having sex. About 80% of rapes in

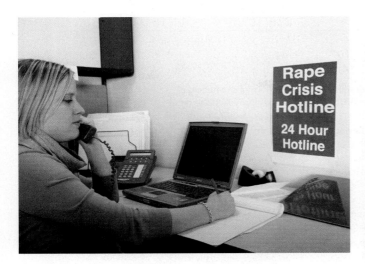

Many communities have crisis centers for rape victims.

the United States are committed by someone the victim knows. About half of all rapes occur on dates, at parties, or in other social situations. About 10% of American women are victims of rape or attempted rape in their lifetimes. Among men who are raped, more than half know their attacker. Acquaintance rape carries the same legal penalties as sexual assault committed by a stranger.

Women of high school and college age are the most vulnerable to acquaintance rape. Every year, more than 100,000 forcible rapes are reported in the United States. This number is probably low because many rapes are not reported by the victim.

Cultural views on sexual relationships between men and women play a significant role in acquaintance rape. Many young women who are victims of attacks that meet the legal definition of rape do not know that what happened to them was sexual assault. Victims may believe that a sexual assault can be committed only by a stranger

or they may blame themselves for the act. A rapist may not realize that the victim's refusal really means NO. Aggressive males mistakenly believe that when women say no, men should insist. A significant proportion of men whose actions meet the legal definition of sexual assault believe they have not committed sexual assault.

Consequences of Acquaintance Rape

Victims of acquaintance rape often suffer serious, long-term psychological effects. Compared with victims of stranger rapes, acquaintance rape victims tend to blame themselves for what happened. They often have difficulty trusting people in later relationships. It may take acquaintance rape victims longer to recover, particularly if the rape involved physical violence. Acquaintance rape victims are less likely than other rape victims to seek crisis services, tell someone, report the incident to the police, or seek counseling. Family and friends may not provide the same support for acquaintance rape victims as they might offer victims of stranger rape. If victims tell friends or family, the severity of the attack may be minimized or the victim may be blamed for the sexual assault.

If a woman has had too much to drink or has been drugged and is unconscious, she cannot consent to any sexual act. Having sex with a woman who is unconscious or semiconscious is defined as an act of rape. Certain substances are known as "date rape drugs." Rohypnol (also called "Roofies," "rope," "activesex") is an odorless, tasteless compound that can be added to a person's drink that will render the person unconscious. People who commit rape on drugged victims are sentenced to long terms in prison if convicted.

Consequences of Sexual Assault

Sexual assault can have many harmful and lasting consequences for victims, families, and communities. For example, being raped exposes victims to pregnancy and acquiring a sexually transmitted disease, including HIV/AIDS. Another common consequence is a sense of having been personally violated. Also, an assault victim may experience for months or years chronic pelvic pain,

How to Prevent Date Rape

Be wary of a relationship that is operating along classic stereotypes of dominant male and submissive, passive female. The dominance in ordinary activities may extend to the sexual arena.

Be wary when a date tries to control behavior or pressure you in any way.

Be explicit with communication. Don't say "no" in a way that could be interpreted in any way as a "maybe" or "yes."

Avoid ambiguous messages with both verbal and nonverbal behavior. Saying "no" and permitting heavy petting creates confusion or ambiguity.

First dates with an unknown companion may be safer in a group.

Avoid remote or isolated places where help is not available.

Avoid becoming intoxicated while on a date.

TERMS

acquaintance rape: (also known as "date rape") sexual assault occurring when the victim and the rapist are known to each other and may have previously interacted in some socially appropriate manner

rape: nonconsensual sexual behavior, generally penile penetration of a bodily orifice

sexual assault: the combination of nonconsensual sexual penetration (rape) and nonsexual violence, such as battery, the threat of harm, or homicide

sexual violence: violent actions that include rape, incest, attempted rape, and unwanted sexual touching

Table 23.3

Feelings Reported by Sexual Assault Victims

Fear	Embarrassment	Shame	Guilt	Anxiety
• Fear of death • Fear of rapist	• Embarrassed to discuss details • Embarrassed about their bodies	• Destruction of self-esteem, self-worth, self-respect • Ashamed at having the medical exam • Ashamed at having to perform a sexual act to stay alive	• Feelings of shame and of having provoked the rape • Feeling of blame for the assault	• Shaking • Nightmares • Difficulty sleeping or sleeping all the time • Constantly reminds self what "should or shouldn't have" been done
Stupidity	**Vulnerability**	**Concern**	**Anger**	**Loss of control**
• Feels stupid for engaging in risk-taking behavior(s) • Feels stupid for being too trusting	• General fear of people • Paranoid feelings • Intensely heightened awareness of environment	• Will the rapist get psychiatric help? • What will happen to offender if rape is reported?	• Toward assailant • Toward self • Toward men and women in general, especially if they resemble assailant	• Small decisions seem monumental • Unsure about self or actions

gastrointestinal disorders, migraines and other frequent headaches, back pain, and facial pain. Victims may also be susceptible to alcohol and other drug abuse, principally to block out memories and anxieties associated with the attack. Common feelings reported by sexual assault victims are listed in **Table 23.3**.

Victims of sexual assault face both immediate and long-term psychological consequences, referred to as **rape trauma syndrome**. Immediately following an assault and continuing for days to several weeks, victims may display one of the three possible responses: (1) frequent crying and appearing agitated, hysterical, and anxious; (2) appearing calm and emotionally in control, as if nothing happened; and (3) shock and disbelief, being disoriented, confused, and unable to carry out normal tasks.

Recovering from sexual assault requires patience and support. Sexual assault survivors are encouraged to seek psychological counseling from rape-recovery or trauma professionals. Also, joining a support group of other assaulted individuals can be helpful in releasing the shame and horror associated with the assault. Support and understanding from family, friends, intimate partners, and the community are also valuable.

Sexual Violence at American Colleges and Universities

According to the American College Health Association (2016), each year about 3% of American college women and 1% of American college men experience attempted or completed sexual assault against their will. Approximately 90% of sexual assaults on college campuses are committed by someone the victim knows. Most acquaintance rapes occur when people involved are at a party or studying together in a dorm room. College students are the most vulnerable to acquaintance rape during the first few weeks of the freshman and sophomore years. Actual "date rape" tends to occur at the beginning of a dating relationship.

Acquaintance rape among college students is sometimes interpreted as a result of miscommunication between those involved. This theory holds that men are socialized to believe that women initially resist sexual advances to preserve their reputation as "moral," and because of this, they prefer to be overcome sexually. If a woman says no, a man is to proceed as if she said yes. In addition, some men believe that if a woman is labeled or perceived as a "tease" or "loose," she is asking for sex. Men view certain cues as evidence that a woman is interested in having sex; wearing revealing clothing, agreeing to go to his room, or complimenting the man during the date.

Alcohol use among offenders, victims, or both is associated with most rapes among college students. Alcohol can reduce the capacity to verbally or physically resist a rapist.

College acquaintance rape victims suffer the same psychological harms as other rape victims. In addition, college acquaintance rape victims may leave school for fear of facing their attacker on campus.

Many victims, perpetrators, and others in the campus community often do not interpret forced sex by a victim's dating partners or intimate partner as criminal sexual assault. They believe the myth that rape is only committed by strangers. Thus, forced sex by an acquaintance is something other than rape.

What to Do After a Sexual Assault

A person who has been sexually assaulted is advised to do the following:

- Contact a rape-crisis hotline.
- DO NOT shower, bathe, douche, change or destroy clothing, or straighten up the area where the sexual assault occurred (if indoors) because these actions would destroy important evidence.
- Go to the nearest hospital emergency room.
- Notify the police.
- Seek professional counseling.

Preventing Sexual Assault

- When you go out, always take your cell phone and $20–$30 for emergency transportation. Tell someone where you are going.
- Trust your feelings. If you feel you are in danger, get yourself to safety immediately. If you are confronted, blow a whistle or yell "FIRE." Do not yell "help" or "rape" as people are more likely to respond to a general emergency than an assault.
- Be aware of your surroundings. Know where you are going.
- Stay in well-lit areas. Use a shuttle service after dark. Never walk alone at night and avoid taking roads or paths where there are few people.
- After entering your car, do not dawdle. Drive away immediately.
- Do not leave a party, concert, game, or other social occasion with someone you just met or do not know very well.
- Always travel in groups.
- Check out a first date or a blind date with friends. Insist on going to a public place such as a movie, sporting event, or restaurant and meet the person there.

- Avoid targeting yourself by not allowing your photo and personal information to be published for distribution to the campus community.
- Think about how close you want to get to the person with whom you have a relationship, and clearly state your limits.
- If someone is coming on to you forcefully, say "NO" firmly and with force. Don't try to protect that person's feelings; don't smile; use the word *rape* to show what is really going on. Get away or scream if you assess it is safe to do so. Lie if you must. Say you have herpes, gonorrhea, or some other transmissible disease.
- Avoid date rape drugs, such as Rohypnol, GHB, and ketamine. Pour and prepare all drinks you consume (alcoholic and nonalcoholic).
  - Do not leave your drink alone on the table or bar.
  - Keep your hand over the bottle or top of your glass.
  - Do not drink out of large, open containers, such as punch bowls.
  - Do not trade or switch drinks with others.
  - Do not drink something if it looks or tastes "different."
  - Watch for signs of drug effects in friends and help them.

Each person's reaction to being sexually assaulted is different, and it is natural that each victim's pain and needs are unique. All victims of sexual assault should seek counseling from someone they trust.

Elder Abuse

Elder abuse is defined as the physical, sexual, or emotional maltreatment or financial exploitation of an adult aged 60 or older. The abuse or neglect may be by a spouse, child, relative, professional caregiver, or friend. More than 1 million elderly persons are victims of abuse each year in the United States.

A variety of abusive methods are used by caregivers in the domestic setting to control the elder persons under their care. These include screaming and yelling (the most frequent form of abuse), physical restraint, forced feeding or medicating, blows and slaps, and threats to send the person to a nursing home.

However, the abuse is not all one way. Elder persons who are disabled or immobilized also use abusive methods to control their caregivers. Elder persons scream and yell, pout and withdraw, refuse food and medication, cry or become emotional, throw objects, and threaten to call the police. As with other forms of abuse, the reasons for the abusive behaviors by both persons in the relationship are many. Alcohol plays a role in many situations, and emotional illness contributes, as does mental impairment on the part of one or both parties.

Despite increased public attention to the problems of elder abuse, much maltreatment of elders still remains hidden to a large extent. The reason much elder abuse

remains hidden or undocumented is that many elderly people are concerned about the family's privacy and fear public exposure and embarrassment. The victim also may feel shame at having raised a child who has now become abusive. If the child is stealing money, the elderly parent may fear that the child will be sent to jail if the abuse is reported. And, despite the abusive treatment, the elder person may feel that the situation is preferable to being sent to a nursing home. Elder abuse is likely to become an even greater problem in the future, as more and more people live to be age 80 or older and as the number of people with dementia increases.

Firearm Violence

Firearm violence is nonmilitary violence committed with the use of a gun with or without criminal intent. Criminal gun violence includes intentional homicide (except if ruled justifiable), and assault with a deadly weapon. Noncriminal

TERMS

rape trauma syndrome: Immediate and long-term psychological difficulties, including PTSD, from having been raped
elder abuse: physical, sexual, or emotional maltreatment or financial exploitation of an adult aged 60 or older
firearm violence: nonmilitary violence committed with the use of a gun with or without criminal intent

Table 23.4

Rates of Firearm Violence Among Several Developed Countries

Country	Guns per 100 people	Homicides per 100,000
United States	88.8	10.2
Switzerland	45.7	3.84
Finland	45.3	3.64
Canada	30.8	2.44
Austria	30.4	2.94
Norway	31.3	1.78
Germany	30.3	1.10
New Zealand	22.6	2.66
Italy	11.9	1.28
Ireland	8.6	1.03
United Kingdom	6.2	0.25
Netherlands	3.9	0.46
Japan	0.6	0.06

Modified from Bangalore, S. & Messerli, F.H. (2013). Gun ownership and firearm-related deaths. *The American Journal of Medicine*, 126, 873–876, with permission from Elsevier.

gun violence includes accidental or unintentional injury or death. The United States has the highest rate of firearm violence among peer nations (**Table 23.4**). Compared to other high-income countries (e.g., Canada, Switzerland, the UK, and Japan), in the United States, deaths from firearms are 10 times higher, from firearm homicides 25 times higher, from firearm suicides 8 times higher, and from unintentional firearm deaths 6 times higher (Grinshteyn & Hemenway, 2016). Each year about 35,000 Americans die from gunshot wounds; slightly more than half of the deaths are from suicide.

> Every gun that is made, every warship launched, every rocket fired signifies, in the final sense, a theft from those who hunger and are not fed, those who are cold and are not clothed.
>
> *President Dwight D. Eisenhower (1953)*

In response to mass killings in recent years at schools, movie theaters, nightclubs, and concerts, many Americans—gun owners and nongun owners alike—believe that gun violence is a very big problem in the United States, and many support strengthening gun control laws (Igielnik & Brown, 2017). For example, nearly 90% of gun owners and nongun owners favor preventing mentally ill persons from purchasing a gun; 80% favor barring those on no-fly lists from purchasing a gun; and more than 50% favor the creation of a federal database for tracking gun sales. Furthermore, many agree that a major cause of gun violence is the ease with which people can obtain guns. Research on firearm use suggests that more scrutiny of prospective gun buyers and more safety features on guns (such as fingerprint recognition) would reduce firearm violence.

Gun violence in the United States costs about $2 billion in medical costs and an estimated $100 billion in other costs. Living in a house where there are guns increases the risk of homicide by about 170% and the risk of suicide by about 460% (Wintemute, 2008). States with the least strict gun ownership laws also have the highest rates of firearm-related deaths; states with stringent gun control laws have the lowest rates of firearm-related deaths (Fleeger et al., 2013).

Firearms are the second leading cause of death among young people between the ages of 10 and 24. A national survey found that 1 student in 12 admitted to carrying a firearm within the past month, either for defense or assault. People living in homes in which guns are kept have a risk of suicide that is five times greater than for people living in homes without guns. Surveys also show that the vast majority of teenage suicides are accomplished with guns.

Hate Crimes

A **hate crime** is an unlawful act committed against a person, group, or place that is motivated by hate or bias. Bombing a church, synagogue, or mosque because it represents places of worship of particular faiths is a hate crime. Attacking a gay person because of his or her sexual orientation is a hate crime. Attacking a person because of his or her gender or nationality is a hate crime. In general, any act of violence that is motivated in whole or in part by the victim's race, religion, ethnicity, gender, sexual orientation, disability, or age is a hate crime.

> War is but a spectacular expression of our daily conduct.
>
> *Krishnamurti*

In 1990, the U.S. Congress recognized the increasing frequency and seriousness of such crimes and required the FBI to keep statistics on the number and kinds of hate crimes in the country. Hate crimes are prosecuted first as a particular crime and, in addition, as a hate crime. Additional penalties are added if the person is convicted of a hate crime. Shooting someone is homicide; shooting the person because he or she is African American, Jewish, or Latino is both a homicide and a hate crime.

There is a difference between freedom of speech and a hate crime. Freedom of speech, no matter how offensive, is protected under the U.S. Constitution. Biased views and verbal attacks cannot be prosecuted as hate crimes.

However, if someone because of hate or prejudice advocates the committing of a crime, such as incitement to riot, to destroy property, or to actually hurt someone, then the person has committed a crime. Hate crimes, unfortunately, are a worldwide phenomenon. Nazi war crimes were hate crimes. Genocide in Rwanda was a hate crime. Killing of Muslims of one sect by Muslims of another sect is a hate crime. Hate in any guise is destructive both to the people who are hated and to those who hate.

Bullying

Bullying is unwanted, aggressive behavior among school-aged children that involves a real or perceived power imbalance. The behavior is repeated, or has the potential to be repeated, over time. Bullying includes making threats, spreading rumors, attacking someone physically or verbally, and excluding someone from a group on purpose. There are three main types of bullying: verbal, social, and physical. Cyberbullying is verbal or social aggression carried out through technology. Some types of bullying are illegal, such as harassment, hazing, and assault. The Centers for Disease Control and Prevention (2014) reports that 28% of U.S. students in grades 6–12 experienced bullying, 20% of U.S. students in grades 9–12 experienced bullying, and approximately 30% of young people admit to bullying others in surveys.

Many students who are subjected to daily taunts, harassment, or bullying suffer from mental and physical problems, and many may be forced to leave school. Recognizing that harassment and bullying of certain students may lead to violent behavior, including suicide and murder, many school districts have instituted "no bullying" policies at school and on school buses. The rules encourage students to report to teachers and parents instances of bullying involving any kind of verbal or physical abuse. However, most bullying occurs outside of the school's jurisdiction; for example, most bullying is now done by texting a victim's mobile phone or by putting derogatory comments on social networking websites.

Bullying on the Internet is known as *cyberbullying*. Posting derogatory remarks about someone on a social media site can be viewed by many others who are connected to the site. Cyberbullying of a victim by many postings can produce enormous stress and emotional harm to the person being harassed online. Some instances of cyberbullying have led students to commit suicide rather than endure further humiliation. In 2011, a study at the University of Hawaii concluded that as many as 1 in 10 students at the university had been exposed to cyberbullying.

Tyler Clementi was an 18-year-old violinist enrolled at Rutgers University in New Jersey in 2011. Unbeknownst to him, his roommate had hidden a video camera in the dorm room they shared in order to record a sexual encounter between Clementi and another male student. After recording the sexual encounter in the dorm room, the roommate posted the video on YouTube. Shortly thereafter, Clementi jumped from the George Washington bridge and died. Cyberbullying is not just a harmless form of student hazing; it can be as deadly as being shot with a gun. Following widely publicized suicides resulting from bullying, Massachusetts and New Jersey enacted laws to protect students from bullying of any kind.

Although laws may help reduce bullying, they are unlikely to stop it, just as gun laws do not eliminate homicides and suicides. Each one of us needs to ask ourselves how we would feel if tormented and harassed by bullying. As individuals and as a society, we need to stop bullying wherever we encounter it. We need to become as outraged by bullying as we are by the sexual abuse of a child.

Violence in America

By almost any measure or statistic, the United States is a violent country. The United States has a larger percentage of homicides, suicides, rapes, and other forms of interpersonal violence and more people in prisons than any other industrialized country. From its beginning, America has had a history of violence. Immigrants from Europe established colonies in the New World and eventually killed or subjugated all of the Native Peoples in North America. The country engaged in a horrific Civil War over slavery and other issues. Americans own more guns than citizens of other industrialized countries.

Since 1970, the number of persons in U.S. prisons has increased sixfold (Bureau of Justice Statistics, 2012). This means that approximately 1 out of every 100 U.S. citizens is behind bars. The United States has about 5% of the world's population, yet 25% of the entire world's prison population is in the United States. A disproportionate number of people in U.S. prisons are black, poor, or both; overall about 10 million Americans are sent to prison each year.

This dismal picture of crime and violence in the United States is further darkened by the number of prison inmates who are innocent, especially those convicted of violent crimes such as rape and murder. Advances in forensic DNA technologies have made it possible to revisit hundreds of convictions and demonstrate that an innocent person was sent to prison, sometimes to death row. As of 2017, the Innocence Project, a New York–based legal organization, has secured the release of about 350 prisoners. The Innocence Project was established in 1992 to investigate wrongful convictions. As of July 2017, 351 prisoners had been released, 20 of whom had been on death row. The majority of wrongful convictions were of minority males. The convictions were overturned largely based on analysis of DNA evidence recovered from the crime scene and preserved along

TERMS

bullying: unwanted, aggressive behavior among school-aged children that involves a real or perceived power imbalance

hate crime: any unlawful act committed against a person, group, or place that is motivated by hate or bias

with other evidence. Some of the released prisoners had been on death row for 20 years. Others had served more than 30 years before their cases were reexamined and reversed. More than half of the innocent prisoners were black Americans. Astonishingly, almost 40% of those convicted had confessed to their crimes although they knew they were innocent; many confessed to avoid a death sentence. Although hundreds of prisoners have had their convictions reversed in the past 20 years, thousands more will remain in prison because in many cases the evidence, especially DNA, has been lost or destroyed. In America, justice for all is still a work in progress.

Being arrested, convicted of a crime, and sent to prison is obviously not a healthy situation for individuals, their families, or society. Every year, the U.S. prison system puts thousands of inmates into solitary confinement for the safety of other prisoners or for not following prison rules. Some prisoners may spend years in solitary confinement with virtually no contact with other people. Is this humane? Experiments with primates raised in captivity show that infant monkeys separated from their mothers shortly after birth become withdrawn and mentally ill. Prisoners of war or hostages who have endured long years of isolation exhibit brain abnormalities when they are examined after being released. One physician notes that "Without sustained social interaction, the human brain may become as impaired as one that has received a traumatic injury" (Gawande, 2009).

Violence and its consequences are profoundly unhealthy to individuals and to society. British and European nations have long recognized the mentally destructive consequences of solitary confinement and have devised other ways to control violent behavior among prison inmates. Violent words can be as mentally destructive as violent actions. Committing yourself to a life of nonviolence might be the most healthy action you can take to facilitate lifelong health.

Critical Thinking About Health

1. Imagine that you are in a debate in school over this question: "Should all Americans over 21 years of age be allowed to own (a) a handgun, (b) a rifle, (c) a semi-automatic weapon, or (d) an automatic weapon?"

   Take a position on this issue with respect to owning or not owning guns in general. If you favor the ownership of guns, give your reasons for owning or not owning each of the four categories of guns. If you do not favor the ownership of guns, explain your reasons. Whatever side of the issue you are on, discuss whether you believe that ownership and availability of guns contribute to violence and crime in America.

2. You and Jennifer have been close friends for more than 15 years (since you both were in high school). Jennifer has recently divorced and has a 5-year-old son, Timmy, who is a "handful" in your view. You and Jennifer have shared many thoughts and feelings over the years. One day after work you stop by to see how Jennifer is doing. You notice that Timmy is limping and has several bruises on his legs. When you comment on Timmy's limp, Jennifer looks at the boy sharply and says, "You fell out of a tree. Isn't that right, Timmy?" The boy mumbles, "Yes" and limps from the room. Jennifer seems tense and doesn't want to talk. You soon leave, but not before you smell alcohol on her breath.

   Do you think that this might be a case of child abuse? If so, what do you think your actions should be? In your discussion, indicate whether you are a male or female. Do you think a male or female friend of Jennifer's would act differently in this situation?

3. Volunteer to help at a retirement or nursing home in your community. Ask the older persons what they enjoy and dislike most about being elderly. Observe how many of the persons living there are mentally incompetent in your judgment and to what degree. Make a report of your findings and observations. Describe how your views of the elderly have changed as the result of your volunteer work.

4. By all statistical measures, the United States is the most violent society among all industrialized countries in the world by a large margin. The United States has more forcible rapes, more battered women, more homicides, and more suicides than any other industrialized nation on a per capita basis. Discuss why you think our society is so violent and what could be done to change its violent nature.

Chapter Summary and Highlights

Chapter Summary

There is no sugarcoating the facts. By any measure or standard, American society is by far the most violent of any developed country in the world. Per capita, the United States reports more rapes, homicides, and suicides than other developed countries with large populations. We also have a larger percentage of our population in prison than any other country. Sickening news reports of child molestation and rape are frequent occurrences. Domestic violence has come under greater public scrutiny because several prominent athletes were formally charged with that crime. Date rape has become so pervasive that most colleges and schools have instituted programs and policies to stem rapes on and around their campuses. Random shootings of fellow students and by teenagers in schools are frequently reported. Disgruntled partners and spouses use spyware to follow every move and conversation of ones they presume to love. Police resort to excess violence time after time in city after city in the guise of "keeping the peace." What is so terribly wrong with American society that it accepts and tolerates so much violence?

Everybody must find an answer to this question for themselves. What would cause someone to become violent enough to beat, rape, or shoot another person? Ask yourself if you have a problem with anger, drugs, alcohol, or any condition that might cause you to commit a violent act. Violence is reduced one person at a time, one day at a time, one incident at a time. The human species has a long history of violence. It may have contributed to the survival of those who lived in an environment of "kill or be killed." But uncontrolled violence only poisons a modern society. Live a life in which you do not have to resort to violence. If a majority of people in America became advocates of nonviolence, society would change. It might mean the end of war as a way to resolve differences. Is that so bad?

Highlights

- Domestic violence includes relationship abuse and child abuse. Violence refers to use of force and power.
- Child maltreatment encompasses physical abuse, emotional abuse, sexual abuse, and neglect.
- People who have been assaulted may experience anxiety, depression, substance abuse, headaches, and other medical problems. These are symptoms of posttraumatic stress disorder (PTSD). Many long-term consequences of sexual abuse are associated with PTSD.
- Acquaintance rape, or date rape, occurs when a person known to the victim uses force or power to coerce the victim into having sex. Women of high school and college age are most vulnerable to acquaintance rape.

- Child maltreatment is a form of domestic violence that reaches across all social, economic, racial, ethnic, geographic, and educational barriers.
- Education is the key to all forms of violence prevention, including firearm violence, relationship abuse, acquaintance rape, and child abuse.
- The United States exceeds all other developed nations in the per capita rate of rapes, homicides, and suicides and in the percentage of its population in prisons.
- Violence and the presence of handguns in schools mirror our communities and generate fear.
- Violence is not an essential part of human behavior, and many societies in the world are nonviolent.

For Your Health

How well are you protecting yourself from crime? Do Exercise 23.1 in the Workbook to find out.

References

American College Health Association. (2016). *National College Health Assessment Spring 2016 Reference Group Data Report.* Retrieved from http://www.acha-ncha.org/docs/ACHA-NCHA-II_ReferenceGroup_ExecutiveSummary_Spring2016.pdf

Bangalore, M. D., & Messerli, F. H. (2013). Gun ownership and firearm-related deaths. *American Journal of Medicine, 126,* 873–876.

Black, M. C., et al. (2011). *The National Intimate Partner and Sexual Violence Survey (NISVS): 2010 summary report.* Atlanta, GA: National Center for Injury Prevention and Control, Centers for Disease Control and Prevention. Retrieved from http://www.cdc.gov/violenceprevention/pdf/NISVS_Report2010-a.pdf

Bureau of Justice Statistics. (2012). *Jail inmates at midyear 2011.* Retrieved from http://www.bjs.gov/index.cfm?ty=pbdetail&iid=4235

Centers for Disease Control and Prevention. (2014). *Facts about bullying.* Retrieved from http://www.stopbullying.gov/news/media/facts/#listing

Fleegler, E. W., et al. (2013). Firearm legislation and firearm-related fatalities in the United States. *JAMA Internal Medicine, 173,* 732–740.

Gawande, A. (2009, March 30). Hellhole. *The New Yorker,* 36–45.

Grinshteyn, E., & Hemenway, D. (2016). Violent death rates: The U.S. compared with other high-income OECD countries, 2010. *American Journal of Medicine, 129,* 266–273.

Igielnik, R., & Brown, A. (2017). Key takeaways on Americans' view of guns and gun ownership. Pew Research Center Report. Retrieved from www.pewresearch.org/fact-tank/2017/06/22/key-takeaways-on-americans-views-of-guns-and-gun-ownership/

Planty, M., et al. (2016). *Female victims of sexual violence, 1994–2010.* Bureau of Justice Statistics. Retrieved from http://www.bjs.gov/content/pub/pdf/fvsv9410.pdf

Wintemute, G. J. (2008). Guns, fear, the Constitution, and public health. *New England Journal of Medicine, 358,* 1421–1424.

Suggested Readings

Finkelhor, D. (2014). *Childhood victimization: Violence, crime, and abuse in the lives of young people.* New York: Oxford University Press. A comprehensive analysis encompassing the prevention, treatment, and study of juvenile victims, unifying conventional subdivisions like child molestation, child abuse, bullying, and exposure to community violence.

Graffunder, C. M., et al. (2011). Through a public health lens: Preventing violence against women: An update from the Centers for Disease Control and Prevention. *Journal of Women's Health, 1,* 5–16. Explains how four core public health principles—emphasizing primary prevention, advancing the science of prevention, translating science into effective programs, and building on the efforts of others—can help prevent violence against women.

Kaye, D. H. (2010). *The double helix and the law of evidence.* Cambridge, MA: Harvard University Press. DNA testing has proved definitive in both convicting and exonerating persons accused of serious crimes. This book explains clearly how forensic DNA evidence is used and misused in criminal cases.

Maltz, W. (2012). *The sexual healing journey: A guide for survivors of sexual abuse* (3rd ed.). New York: Morrow. A comprehensive guide that helps survivors of sexual abuse heal from the past, improve relationships, and discover the joys of sexual intimacy.

Muscari, M. (2002). *Not my kid: 21 steps to raising a nonviolent child.* Scranton, PA: Ridge Row Press/University of Scranton. Discusses how media violence influences children and how parents can reduce their children's exposure to violent media.

Pinker, S. (2012). *The better angels of our nature: Why violence has declined*. New York: Penguin. Harvard psychology professor argues that despite the ceaseless news about war, crime, and terrorism, violence has actually been in decline over long stretches of history.

Rosen, M. (2016, May 14). Misfires in the gun control debate. A balanced discussion of why it has been impossible to regulate gun use and reduce gun violence in the United States. *Science News*.

U.S. Department of Health and Human Services. (2014). What is child abuse and neglect? Recognizing the signs and symptoms. Retrieved from https://www.childwelfare.gov/. Outlines the legal definition of child abuse and neglect, the different types of abuse and neglect, the signs and symptoms of abuse and neglect, and the impact of trauma.

Recommended Websites

Centers for Disease Control and Prevention
Resources on violence facts and prevention.

Initiatives Related to Domestic Violence
Legal and educational references for families, justice professionals, and mental health and social service professionals.

Minnesota Center Against Violence and Abuse
Research, education, and access to violence-related resources, from the University of Minnesota.

National Domestic Violence Hotline
Information and resources available from the telephone hotline (1-800-799-7233).

Partners Against Hate
Provides a training program that teaches ways to reduce hate and hate crimes.

Tolerance.org
Provides information and advice on how to reduce hate crimes, school violence, and other violence problems in society.

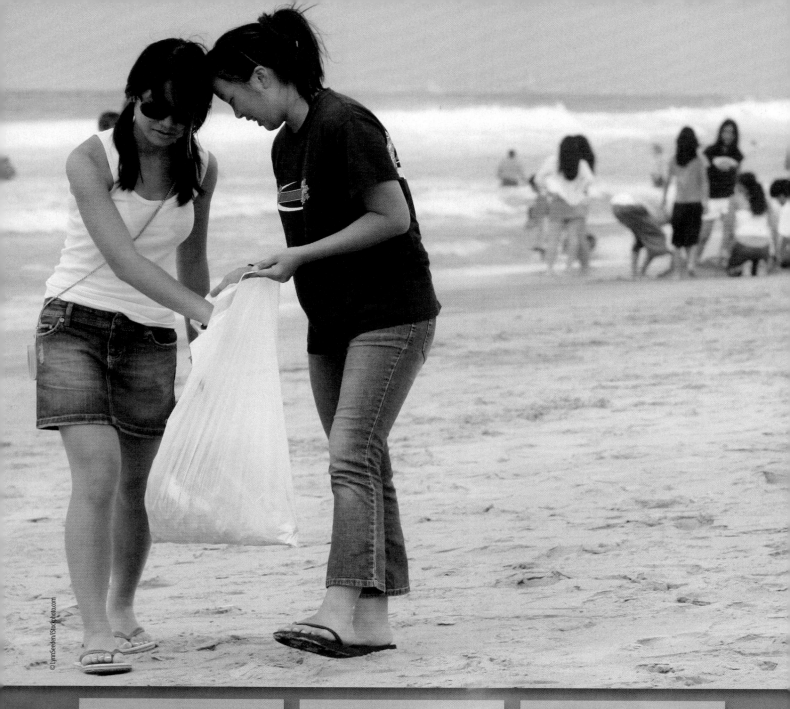

Health Tips

Where You Live Can Affect Your Health

Dispose of All Mercury Thermometers Safely

Compact Fluorescent Light Bulbs Contain Mercury

Good Riddance to the Plastic Bag

Recycle Anything—Safely

Precautions for Pesticide Use

Avoid Pesticide-Contaminated Fruits and Vegetables

Ways to Reduce Your Exposure to EMFs

Noise Pollution: Bad for Kids

Dollars & Health Sense

Bottled Water Battles

Plastic Microbeads and Microfibers Pollute Oceans and Seas

Global Wellness

Gaia: Can Earth Regulate Itself?

Wind-Based Electrical Power

Working Toward a Healthy Environment

Learning Objectives

1. Discuss the relationship between environment and health.

2. Describe the health effects of air pollution, including smog and the hole in the ozone layer.

3. Explain the greenhouse effect and the predicted consequences of global warming.

4. Describe the effects of lead on children's health and intelligence.

5. Describe substances that pollute water in the United States.

6. Discuss the impact of land pollution on food production and health.

7. Describe sources of pesticide contamination and their effects on health.

8. Explain the effects of endocrine disruptors.

9. Identify the potential health problems associated with noise pollution and EMFs.

10. Discuss how human population growth affects global health and environmental issues.

The term **environment** refers to all external physical factors that affect us. To survive, all animals, including human beings, require a certain amount of high-quality air, water, food, and shelter. If people are deprived of any essential environmental factors, or if the environment is polluted with toxic substances, health is adversely affected. Anyone who has experienced difficulty breathing smoggy, dusty, or smoke-filled air realizes the unhealthy effects of polluted air. Anyone who has become sick from consuming contaminated food or water knows the importance of sanitation and uncontaminated food in maintaining health.

To achieve optimal health, we must live in a high-quality environment. Unfortunately, the quality of many aspects of the environment is deteriorating from pollution, degradation, depletion of natural resources, and extinction of species. The effects of environmental pollution are long lasting and often irreversible. People and nations are beginning to appreciate the serious consequences of ongoing air, water, and land pollution that adversely affect health. Dramatic changes in personal lifestyles and industrial technology are likely to be required to reduce existing pollution and prevent future destruction of the environment.

Environmental problems are not restricted to the United States or even to industrialized countries; environmental problems are global. Worldwide problems include:

- Global warming from increased amounts of carbon dioxide and other pollutants in the atmosphere. Global warming will alter climate patterns, raise sea levels and flood coastlines, imperil the world's food supply, increase the frequency and distribution of infectious diseases, and create extremes in the weather.
- Land degradation caused by deforestation, desertification, and soil erosion. Land degradation undermines the ability of populations to grow food and protect fresh water supplies.
- Fresh water shortages caused by overpopulation, lack of modern sanitation in parts of the world, and outmoded irrigation practices.
- Air pollution from the burning of fossil fuels by industry and cars and trucks. Pollutants foul the air and cause respiratory disease, destruction of forests and lakes by acid rain, and destruction of atmospheric ozone, which increases the risk of cancer and other biological damage.
- Exposure to toxic industrial and agricultural chemicals, which cause cancer and disrupt normal biological functions in humans, animals, microorganisms, and plants.
- Extinction of species from global warming, destruction of tropical rain forests, overhunting and overfishing, habitat destruction from human activity, and the introduction of nonnative species into new environments.
- Nuclear, chemical, and biological problems due to industrial pollution and accidents.

Environmental health hazards stem from many different causes. Through the enactment and enforcement of environmental laws and regulations, the United States has made progress in reducing environmental pollution and its negative health consequences. The United Nations and the World Health Organization carry out research and sponsor programs to protect the environment and to improve health. However, governments and other organizations alone cannot solve environmental problems. Each individual must strive to reduce or eliminate air, water, and land pollution and to take steps to create a healthy environment. Human activities are at the root of almost *all* environmental pollution and consequent health problems.

Gaia: Can Earth Regulate Itself?

Life on Earth depends on a very precise range of climatic and chemical conditions. On a global scale, the temperature and the chemical composition of air, land, and water, as well as other natural processes we take for granted, must be relatively constant for life to survive. Since the dawn of the Industrial Revolution over 200 years ago, human activity has been altering the chemical balance of Earth, and it remains to be seen if Earth can tolerate these alterations.

In 1979, James E. Lovelock, an English chemist and engineer, published a book called *Gaia: A New Look at Life on Earth,* which proposed that a special, interdependent relationship exists between life (particularly human beings) and all the physical and chemical processes of the planet required to sustain biological life. Lovelock suggested that, in a sense, Earth was "alive" and chose the name of the Greek goddess of Earth, *Gaia,* to express the idea of a living planet. Lovelock described Gaia as "a complex entity involving the Earth's biosphere, atmosphere, oceans, and soil; the totality constituting a feedback or cybernetic system which seeks an optimal physical and chemical environment for life on this planet" (Lovelock, 1979).

The idea that Earth is a self-regulating system may be correct; however, there is little indication that people will alter their mistreatment of Earth any time soon. So, in a way, the Gaia hypothesis will be tested and all the world will see the results. Either Earth can adapt to the effects of human activity, or it cannot. And if it cannot, it is not unreasonable to predict that humans will become extinct. Extinction has been the fate of virtually all the species that ever existed on Earth; even the dinosaurs, who survived for about 150 million years, eventually became extinct.

Outdoor Air Pollution

Pure air is essential for healthy human life. Each of us breathes about 35 pounds of air per day—more than 6 tons over the course of a year. Fresh, clean air consists of about 21% oxygen, 78% nitrogen, and trace amounts of seven other gases. It is the oxygen in air that is essential for human life. If the oxygen content of the air drops below 16%, body and brain functions are impaired. If breathing stops for even a few minutes, a person becomes unconscious and will die unless breathing is quickly restored.

Since the beginning of the Industrial Revolution in the nineteenth century, the burning of fossil fuels (coal, oil, and natural gas) to power transportation and industry has progressively polluted the air with carbon dioxide, oxides of nitrogen and sulfur, soot, and small particles, some of which cause health problems. A variety of chemical substances used in modern societies pollute the air as well (e.g., chlorofluorocarbons, dioxin). Thus, technological advances over the past 200 years have created, as a by-product, pollution of the air we breathe and of Earth's atmosphere.

Smog

Everybody has heard of **smog**, a term first used in England to describe a hazardous combination of sulfurous chemicals emitted into the air from the burning of coal and the water vapor in fog. Smog causes breathing problems, coughs, bronchitis, and asthma and can even result in death among people with lung or heart diseases. In most U.S. cities, smog is not associated with fog but results from the action of sunlight on various chemicals and particles in the air that come from automobiles, oil refineries, electricity-generating plants, and other industrial sources. This is why it is called **photochemical smog**.

Photochemical smog consists of ground-level ozone, carbon monoxide, sulfur dioxide, nitrogen oxides, particulates, and volatile organic compounds (**Table 24.1**).

Ground-Level Ozone Ozone (O_3) consists of three atoms of oxygen, as compared with the oxygen we breathe, which consists of two atoms of oxygen (O_2). Whereas ozone in the upper atmosphere benefits life on Earth by shielding it from harmful ultraviolet radiation from the sun, high amounts of ozone at ground level are a major health hazard. Ground-level ozone is not emitted directly into the air from polluting vehicles or industries. Instead, it is formed when sunlight acts on two other pollutants, volatile organic compounds (VOCs) and oxides of nitrogen (nitrogen oxide and nitrogen dioxide).

Ozone can damage lung tissue, reduce lung function, and sensitize the lungs to other irritants. Exposure to even relatively low amounts of ozone for several hours can induce respiratory inflammation in healthy people during exercise. This decrease in lung function generally is accompanied by chest pain, coughing, sneezing, and pulmonary congestion. Ozone's effects on people with impaired respiratory systems, such as asthmatics, is usually more severe.

TERMS

environment: all external physical factors that affect us

photochemical smog: air pollution from the action of sunlight on emissions from motor vehicles and industrial sources

smog: air polluted by chemicals, smoke, particles, and dust

Table 24.1

Major Air Pollutants and Their Health Effects

These pollutants affect breathing, damage lungs, and cause a wide range of health problems. The primary sources of these air pollutants are industrial emissions, automobiles and trucks, and coal and oil burning in industry and homes.

Pollutant	Health effects and symptoms
Carbon monoxide gas	Low levels cause dizziness, headache, and fatigue. High levels lead to coma and death. Especially dangerous for persons with asthma and heart disease.
Carbon dioxide	A major contributor to global warming. Since 1970, yearly carbon dioxide emissions have increased 1% to 2% per year, reaching an all-time high in 2017.
Nitrogen oxide gas	Causes a smelly brown haze that irritates the eyes, nose, and lungs.
Sulfur dioxide gas	Sulfur dioxide gas is poisonous and irritates the eyes, nose, throat, and lungs. It kills plants and rusts metals.
Particulate matter (particles from dust and smoke that are less than 10 microns in diameter)	Causes throat irritation and permanent lung damage. Some industrial soot particulates may cause cancer.
Ozone (O_3)	In the stratosphere ozone protects us from UV light. Can be formed at ground level from nitrous oxides and organic compounds. Causes eye irritation, cough, and breathlessness.
Volatile organic compounds	Smog-forming chemicals, such as benzene, toluene, methylene chloride, and methyl chloroform. All VOCs can cause serious health problems.

Where You Live Can Affect Your Health

Living in a region with air polluted with industrial and automobile combustion waste is not only a nuisance but also a threat to life. Each year, 6.5 million people worldwide die prematurely from having to breathe air made toxic from industrial and auto pollution (Landrigan et al., 2017).

According to the American Lung Association's annual report *State of the Air 2017*, in the United States, about 39% of the population, around 125 million people, live in regions that have year-round unhealthful levels of either ozone or particulate pollution, or both. Most of these high-pollution regions are in the western states because of climate (high atmospheric pressure inversions), reliance on automobile transport, and exposure to smoke and soot from wildfires and wood-burning fireplaces. In the middle and eastern parts of the United States, high air pollution is due to industrial emissions from coal-fired power plants, refineries, and diesel-powered transportation. It should be noted that several regions of the country have extremely good quality air: Burlington-South Burlington, Vermont;

Cape Coral–Fort Myers–Naples, Florida; Elmira–Corning, New York; Honolulu, Hawaii; Palm Bay–Melbourne–Titusville, Florida; and Wilmington, North Carolina.

Since the passage of the Clean Air Act in 1970, air quality throughout the United State has improved tremendously. You can take measures to maintain that progress:

- Protect the Clean Air Act from changes that would weaken or dismantle key provisions that currently protect the lives and health of all Americans.
- Reduce carbon emissions from power plants to reduce ozone and particulate pollution and slow global warming.
- Retain state and federal clean vehicle emission standards to limit ozone and particulate pollution.
- Reduce emissions from new and working oil and gas production facilities to limit pollution from methane and volatile organic compounds.
- Improve the air pollution monitoring network to measure air quality in the 65% of communities that do not already do so.
- Drive less, use energy efficiently, and do not burn wood or trash.

Carbon Monoxide Carbon monoxide (CO) is a colorless, odorless, poisonous gas produced by incomplete burning of carbon-containing fuels. Three-fourths of CO emissions in the United States are from transportation sources, mostly motor vehicle exhaust. Other major CO sources are wood-burning stoves, incinerators, and industries.

When CO enters the bloodstream, it reduces the amount of oxygen that can be delivered to the body's organs and tissues. Exposure to high levels of CO can cause impairment of visual perception, manual dexterity, learning ability, and performance of complex tasks. If the air contains 80 parts per million (ppm) of CO, the oxygen supplied to the body is reduced by 15%. In heavy freeway traffic, the levels of carbon monoxide may reach 400 ppm. It is no surprise that many commuters in large cities who get stuck in traffic jams arrive home with headaches. Car mechanics and parking garage attendants, who are exposed to high levels of carbon monoxide for long periods, may develop health problems. Health threats from CO are most serious for those with heart disease.

Sulfur Dioxide Sulfur dioxide (SO_2) is produced when gasoline, diesel fuel, and coal or oil, all of which contain sulfur, are burned in cars, trucks, power plants, and industrial and home heating systems. Sulfur dioxide also is produced by active volcanoes. Sulfur dioxide can mix with water vapor to form sulfuric acid, a highly corrosive substance that can erode stone, pit metal, and damage living tissue. Exposure to SO_2 makes breathing difficult and aggravates existing respiratory and cardiovascular diseases. Sulfur dioxide in the air can combine with water to form acid rain (discussed later in this chapter), which damages aquatic ecosystems and forests in many parts of the world.

Nitrogen Oxides The major sources of nitrogen oxides are from transportation, electric power plants, and industrial

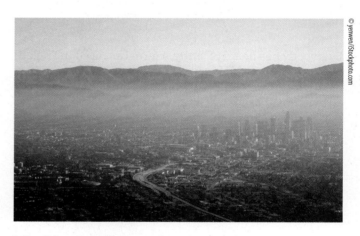
© yenwen/iStockphoto.com

Polluted, "smoggy" air over many large cities contributes to respiratory problems and other diseases.

boilers. Nitrogen oxides consist principally of nitrogen oxide (NO) and nitrogen dioxide (NO_2). In photochemical smog, nitrogen oxide is converted to NO_2, which is a brownish, highly reactive gas that can irritate the lungs, opening the way for bronchitis, pneumonia, and other respiratory infections. Nitrogen oxides also contribute to ground-level ozone and acid rain, and they may alter both terrestrial and aquatic ecosystems.

Particulate Matter Particulate matter (PM) is microscopic particles that arise principally from the burning of diesel fuel and coal. These particles are released into the air, causing the haze associated with photochemical smog and damaging soil and structures in the process. When inhaled, particulate matter damages the respiratory system and impairs breathing; the particles also aggravate existing respiratory and cardiovascular diseases.

Microscopic particles of many kinds and from many different sources are constantly being emitted into the air. It is now well documented that many of the fine particles that people breathe on a daily basis are harmful to health, impair lung function, and shorten life expectancy. The World Health Organization (WHO) estimates that 80% of city dwellers worldwide live in environments that do not meet WHO air quality standards. Breathing this highly polluted air, especially with its high levels of particulate matter, results in the premature deaths of over 3 million people annually. The Environmental Protection Agency monitors and measures two different sizes of particulate matter in the air, 2.5 micrometers (PM2.5) and 10 micrometers (PM10). These particles are extremely small; for comparison, a grain of fine beach sand has a diameter of about 90 micrometers.

The composition of PM2.5 particles includes emissions from gasoline and diesel engines, metals, and organic compounds, as well as from other sources. The composition of PM10 particles includes dust, pollen, mold, and other substances. Particle measurements are made in these two size ranges for convenience; in reality, however, air is polluted with particles of all sizes ranging from invisible nanoparticles to large particles originating in dust storms and from forest fires. Urban and industrialized areas have more air pollution from particulate matter than is found in rural areas.

The size of particulates is directly related to their potential for causing health problems. Particulates smaller than 10 micrometers in diameter pose the greatest problems because they can get deep into the lungs, and a percentage of those enter the bloodstream and travel to other parts of the body. Numerous scientific studies have linked exposure to particulate pollution to a variety of heath problems, particularly on days when air pollution is high. The health problems associated with particulate pollution include death in people with heart or lung disease, heart attacks, irregular heartbeat, asthma attacks, decreased lung function, and coughing or difficulty breathing. People with heart or lung diseases, children, and older adults are the most likely to be affected by particulate exposure. Air pollution is the 13th leading cause of mortality worldwide.

In considering healthy lifestyle changes, we usually think about giving up smoking and alcohol, or improving our diet and losing weight. But we rarely think about the quality of the air we breathe. When you think of moving away to go to school or to take a job, check into the quality of air in the area in which you choose to live. Although healthy young people can breathe polluted air for years without noticeable effects, eventually they may develop asthma, diminished lung capacity, heart disease, and other health problems.

Volatile Organic Compounds Volatile organic compounds (VOCs) are chemical substances that exist in the air as gases. About 50% of VOCs come from industrial and commercial processes such as oil refining, printing, painting, and dry cleaning. Another 40% of VOCs come from motor vehicle exhaust. Five percent come from power generation, and the rest from miscellaneous sources. In the presence of sunlight, some VOCs (called "ozone precursors") easily combine with other air pollutants to form ground-level ozone.

Besides contributing to photochemical smog, some VOCs are harmful to human health and are classified as hazardous air pollutants. VOCs cause eye, nose, and throat irritation; headaches, loss of coordination, nausea; damage to the liver, kidneys, and central nervous system; and some are suspected or known to cause cancer. The ability of VOCs to affect health depends on their innate toxicity and the degree and length of a person's exposure.

Children and Air Pollution Children who live in regions of high air pollution such as Los Angeles and Mexico City suffer a 10% to 15% decrease in lung function as compared with children who grow up where the air is less polluted. Early exposure to polluted air can damage the respiratory tract and can increase the risk of respiratory disease in adult life. Children are much more likely than adults to develop pollution-related lung damage because they inhale several times more air than adults, and they breathe faster, particularly during strenuous physical activity. In addition, they spend more time outdoors than any other segment of the population. The lungs in children and adolescents undergo steady development, with peak lung capacity reached between the ages of 20 and 25. Lung capacity remains stable for another 10 years and then gradually declines with age. Breathing polluted air while the lungs are still developing can decrease lung function later in life and contribute to the development of asthma, chronic obstructive lung disease, and cardiovascular disease.

Improving Air Quality

Prior to the 2008 summer Olympics in Beijing, the Chinese government took unprecedented steps to reduce the severe air pollution that covers the city almost constantly. In the years prior to the Olympics, the government planted millions of trees in and around the city. In the months leading up to the Olympics, the government ordered the shutdown of air-polluting industries for hundreds of miles around the city. Construction in Beijing was halted and traffic was sharply curtailed. Although not producing crystal clear air, these efforts did significantly improve air quality during the 2008 Olympics. This example shows that reducing air pollution is a matter of will and not a lack of scientific know-how.

Since the U.S. Congress passed the Clean Air Act and created the Environmental Protection Agency in 1970, Americans have supported a substantial reduction in air pollution. In 2016, about 78 million tons of air pollution were emitted into the atmosphere in the United States. These emissions mostly contribute to the formation of ozone and particulates, the deposition of acids, and visibility impairment. This degree of pollution represents a 67% reduction in total emissions of the major air pollutants (carbon monoxide, lead, nitrogen oxides, VOCs, PM10 and PM2.5, and sulfur dioxide) since 1980. This reduction in pollution occurred when U.S. gross domestic product increased 133%, vehicle miles traveled increased 92%, energy consumption increased 27%, and U.S. population grew by 38%. About 60% of air pollution is caused by emissions from cars, trucks, buses, aircraft, and ships. Today, there are about 1 billion privately owned cars in the world; by 2030, the number is expected to reach 2 billion. Car manufacturers will rejoice, but without substantial changes in transportation technology, the effects on air pollution are likely to be devastating.

A modern U.S. car with a catalytic converter to reduce emissions still produces about 20 pounds of carbon dioxide for every gallon of gas that is burned; this is a significant factor in global warming. Over an average 10-year life, each American car spews 50 tons of carbon dioxide into the atmosphere.

One major victory in the battle against air pollution was the elimination of lead in gasoline in the United States. The phaseout of leaded gasoline, which began in 1984, has markedly reduced the blood levels of lead in the U.S. population. The battle to eliminate lead in gasoline took more than 10 years to accomplish, which shows the amount of time and effort that goes into changing just one factor in air pollution. Efforts are ongoing to develop less-polluting fuels and vehicles.

When it passed the Clean Air Act and Clean Water Act in the 1970s, the U.S. Congress established the Environmental Protection Agency (EPA) to carry out the mandates of those and other environmental laws. When Congress and the presidential administration are pro-environment, the EPA tends to lock horns with industry, which resists changes in the design and manufacture of products intended to provide a clean environment on the grounds that the costs of doing so will weaken the U.S. economy. Often, industry tries to bolster its resistance by attempting to find flaws in scientific research.

The evidence that particulate matter in air is a health hazard is overwhelming, but industries argue that other air pollutants underlie the health problems and that particulates are not responsible. It required more than 10 years of heated debate and legal wrangling to prove that lead from gasoline was damaging the brains of young children. Many years of effort and research were devoted to showing that chlorofluorocarbons (CFCs) were destroying the ozone layer that protects Earth's surface from harmful UV irradiation. Eventually, both lead in gasoline and CFCs were banned. These two examples show that improving air quality can be accomplished with long-term effort.

A dramatic example of the air pollution caused by electricity-generating plants was provided by the August 2003 blackout that affected much of the Midwest and northeastern United States. Air samples collected over Pennsylvania a day after the shutdown of all plants in the region showed a 90% reduction in sulfur dioxide and a 50% reduction in ozone. Visibility increased by 25 miles.

Suddenly, the air was no longer hazy. Finding cleaner ways to generate electricity is another urgent problem that needs to be solved.

Carbon Dioxide, Global Warming, and Climate Change

Along with the gases oxygen (O_2) and nitrogen (N_2), carbon dioxide (CO_2) is a natural component of Earth's atmosphere. Plants use carbon dioxide to manufacture more plant material, and in the process, they give off oxygen that animals breathe. Carbon dioxide in air also is absorbed into oceans, where it forms carbonate-containing rocks for coral and other sea life.

Before humans began burning coal, oil, and wood in vast quantities to fuel the Industrial Revolution, the level of carbon dioxide in the atmosphere was fairly constant at about 290 parts per million (ppm). By 1920, the level of atmospheric CO_2 rose to about 300 ppm, and by 1950, it rose further to about 315 ppm. In early-2018, atmospheric CO_2 levels reached an all-time high of about 408 ppm. The rate of increase in CO_2 levels in the atmosphere is now about 2 ppm per year (U.S. National Oceanic and Atmospheric Administration, 2018).

In 1861, an English scientist pointed out that carbon dioxide is a good absorber of infrared (heat) radiation. When sunlight lands on Earth's surface, some of the energy in the light is radiated back toward space as infrared radiation or heat. Carbon dioxide absorbs the infrared radiation and thereby traps heat in the atmosphere. Because this process is analogous to how a garden greenhouse works, this phenomenon is called the **greenhouse effect** (**Figure 24.1**).

It became apparent in the 1990s that Earth's temperature is increasing (**Figure 24.2**) and that it is *not* due to natural fluctuations in the global climate; nearly all climate scientists now believe that the rise in global temperature is caused principally by increased levels of human-generated carbon dioxide (Intergovernmental Panel on Climate Change, 2017). The amount of methane gas in the atmosphere also is increasing. Methane is about 25 times more potent than CO_2 in causing global warming. However, because there is much less of it in the atmosphere as compared with CO_2, its contribution to global warming is still minimal. As the levels of these two gases in Earth's atmosphere continue to increase, so, too, will global warming. If humans continue to pump carbon dioxide, methane, and other greenhouse gases into the atmosphere even at reduced rates, it is predicted that sometime in this century the temperature of Earth will increase 5 to 10 degrees Fahrenheit. Five to 10 degrees may not seem like much, but in climatic terms it is a tremendous change. Some of the predicted effects of global warming include:

- A rise in sea level from the melting of ice masses in the Arctic, Antarctic, and on mountaintops sufficient to flood coastal and low-lying regions all over the world. A 3° increase in global temperature will raise sea level 1 to 3 feet. More than 600 million people live

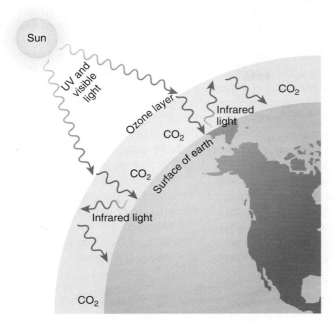

■ Figure 24.1

Greenhouse Effect

Carbon dioxide (CO_2) in Earth's atmosphere acts like the glass roof in a greenhouse. During the day, the sun's energy passes through Earth's atmosphere and warms the planet's surface. At night, heat energy is radiated back toward the atmosphere, but some is trapped by atmospheric carbon dioxide and other "greenhouse gases." Over time, the trapping of heat increases the temperature of the atmosphere causing global climate change.

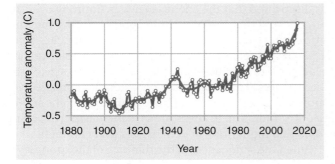

■ Figure 24.2

Global Temperature Changes (1880–2016)

Earth has warmed in the past 50 years. Since record keeping started in the 1880s, global temperatures have risen 0.85°C (1.53°F) due to rising carbon emissions stemming mostly from burning fossil fuels. This graph illustrates the annual (blue line) and 5-year (orange line) average change in global surface temperature relative to the composite average temperature of the time period 1951–1980, represented by the "zero degree" line. Note that mean average global temperatures began to rise about 1920. Sixteen of the 17 warmest years in the 136-year record have occurred since 2001, with the exception of 1998. The year 2016 ranks as the warmest on record.

Courtesy of NASA. Global Climate Change: Vital Signs of the Planet. Retrieved from https://climate.nasa.gov/vital-signs/global-temperature/

in coastal regions. Many would be forced to relocate, possibly resulting in massive refugee problems. During the past century, sea level rose 4 to 10 centimeters. The Arctic Ocean and tundra no longer are completely covered with ice during winter. Chunks of ice as large as Delaware have broken off the Antarctic ice shelf and have melted in the southern oceans.

> It ain't what we don't know that gives us trouble, it's what we know that ain't so that gives us trouble.
>
> *Will Rogers*

- A massive change in Earth's climate. Some tropical regions will become deserts while some temperate regions will become more tropical. In some parts of the world rainfall will increase, whereas in others it will decrease. Winters may become a bit more temperate with less snow, and summers may be hotter and more humid. Global climate change certainly will affect food production throughout the world in a variety of ways. Already, the natural habitats of many land- and water-living plants and animals have changed.

Wind-Based Electrical Power

The answer, my friend, is blowin' in the wind.

—*Bob Dylan*

The world uses about 20 trillion kilowatt hours of electricity every year. The bulk of this energy is supplied by coal- and oil-fired generating plants that emit enormous amounts of pollutants into the atmosphere. These plants also are a major contributor to global warming and create health problems for people who must breathe polluted air.

Researchers at Stanford University studied sustained wind speeds at 8,000 locations around the world. They concluded from their study that wind-based power generation is sufficient to meet the entire global demand for electrical power. It was estimated that the United States alone could use wind turbines to produce 14% of the world's total output of electrical energy.

The researchers point out that wind and other renewable energy could totally replace fossil fuels by 2030–2050 if societies were willing to undertake the challenge. Shifting to wind and other renewable energy sources would save about 3 million lives a year and also halt global warming and reduce air and water pollution.

TERMS

greenhouse effect: the ability of atmospheric carbon dioxide to reflect heat radiated from Earth back to Earth and to thereby raise Earth's temperature globally

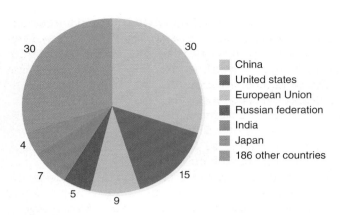

■ **Figure 24.3**

Carbon Emissions by Countries in Billions of Metric Tons
Total carbon emissions by various countries in billions of metric tons. These data include CO_2 emissions from fossil fuel combustion, as well as cement manufacturing and gas flaring.

- Many diseases, particularly insect-borne diseases, will spread to new regions. Dengue fever, previously unknown in South America, is now prevalent and has spread as far north as Texas. Malaria will spread widely to warmer areas, particularly those subject to large increases in rainfall from tropical storms, cyclones, and hurricanes. Increased weather variability has already contributed to the emergence of both hantavirus pulmonary syndrome and West Nile virus infections. Increased summer temperatures and humidity will threaten people who cannot take refuge in air-conditioned buildings.
- The number and intensity of violent storms—hurricanes, cyclones, drought, blizzards, and wildfires—will increase globally. Since 1992, record-setting storms have struck countries around the world and produced weather changes, including record rainfall, drought, hurricanes, and tornados in regions of the United States.

For decades, the United States was the world's largest emitter of carbon dioxide. However, in 2007, China's total carbon dioxide emissions surpassed those of the United States (**Figure 24.3**). As the economies of China, India, Brazil, and Russia grow, global warming and climate change are expected to continue to increase for the foreseeable future.

Reducing Your Carbon Footprint

Anxiety over global warming and its consequences for human health has prompted people to search for ways to reduce their individual contributions to CO_2 emissions. Your "carbon footprint" is a measure of how your lifestyle adds to CO_2 emissions and global warming. Some lifestyle changes that help curb further increases in global warming are obvious: Drive less and walk or ride a bicycle whenever possible. If you buy a new car, buy one with high fuel efficiency. Replace incandescent light bulbs with compact fluorescent and LED light bulbs, and reduce electrical power use wherever possible.

Other lifestyle changes are not as obvious. Changing your diet and where you buy food can lessen your carbon footprint. For example, about 15% of all CO_2 emissions due to human activities come from the transport of goods. Thus, the global economy is a major contributor to global warming. Buying goods, especially food, that are manufactured near where you live can reduce your carbon footprint. Changes in diet also have an impact. The food and agriculture industries account for about one-third of greenhouse gases. Eating meat and dairy products contributes considerably to global warming. The digestive systems of cattle emit tons of methane gas into the atmosphere. (Are you ready to eat fewer or no cheeseburgers to reduce your carbon footprint?) Reducing your carbon footprint may help in a small way to solve the problem of global warming. At the very least, reducing your carbon footprint may help you make dietary and lifestyle changes that make you healthier.

The Ozone Layer

The **ozone layer** consists of ozone molecules (i.e., three atoms of oxygen bonded together: O_3) that form a layer in the outermost region of the Earth's atmosphere. The ozone layer absorbs much of the dangerous ultraviolet (UV) light that is radiated from the sun and protects us from excessive exposure to UV radiation that can increase the risk of skin cancer and cataracts in the lens of the eye. The ozone in the ozone layer is the same chemical produced in photochemical smog. However, in the upper reaches of the atmosphere ozone protects life, whereas at ground level it is a toxic irritant.

A class of chemicals called **chlorofluorocarbons (CFCs)** has been widely used as refrigerant and propellant gases in cans during the twentieth century. These CFCs escape into the atmosphere and rise to the ozone layer, where they destroy ozone molecules. In the 1970s, it was discovered that the ozone layer was thinning over the Antarctic and that an **ozone hole** appears during the Antarctic spring (August to October). Ozone disappears completely in that region at that time. The ozone hole reached its largest size in 2006—about three times the size of the United States. The ozone hole occasionally spreads over populated areas of Asia and northern Europe. The intensity of UV radiation in these areas is increasing, exposing people to a higher risk of skin cancer and cataracts.

When the seriousness of the thinning of the ozone layer was realized, 31 industrialized countries agreed in 1987 to phase out the use of CFCs. Even though CFC use has now dropped significantly, the large amounts of these chemicals already in the atmosphere will persist for many decades.

Evaluating the Risks of Air Pollution

In evaluating the health hazards of toxic air pollutants, two important factors must be considered separately. **Emission** refers to the amount of a substance that is released into the atmosphere from an automobile or other source of air pollution. **Exposure** refers to the amount of the substance to which people are exposed. Frequently, emission can be high, while exposure is low. Alternatively, emission can be low, while exposure is high.

Table 24.2

Major Sources of Emission of a Pollutant Versus Major Sources of Exposure to It

Pollutant	Major emission sources*	Major exposure sources
Benzene	Industry; automobiles	Smoking
Tetrachloroethylene	Dry-cleaning shops	Dry-cleaned clothes
Chloroform	Sewage treatment plants	Showers
p-Dichlorobenzene	Chemical manufacturing	Air deodorizers
Particulates	Industry; automobiles; home heating	Smoker at home
Carbon monoxide	Automobiles	Driving; gas stoves
Nitrogen dioxide	Industry; automobiles	Gas stoves

*For many hazardous airborne pollutants, the health risk is not related significantly to the major source of emission (as shown in Figure 24.4).

For many air pollutants, such as carbon monoxide, benzene, and chloroform, the major sources of emissions are automobiles, industry, and sewage treatment plants, respectively. However, the major health risks from these substances are *not* from the sources of highest emission, but from gas stoves, cigarettes, and chloroform in shower water, respectively (**Table 24.2**).

To regulate all of the possible pollutants of the air is impossible, so it is important to identify both the sources of greatest emission and the sources of greatest exposure. For example, benzene is an important chemical used in many industrial processes; it also can cause leukemia in people who are exposed to it. Of all the benzene released into the air, 50% comes from automobiles. However, although cigarettes emit only a tiny amount of benzene compared with automobiles, at least half of the total population's exposure to benzene comes from smoking cigarettes (**Figure 24.4**). Even nonsmokers get most of their exposure to benzene from secondhand cigarette smoke as opposed to benzene from automobile exhausts. The most serious indoor air pollutant is cigarette smoke.

Indoor Air Pollution

Until recently in the United States and in other industrialized countries, indoor air pollution was primarily due to cigarette smoke that accumulated in enclosed spaces. People smoked in bars, restaurants, offices, airplanes, railroad cars—really, everywhere—and many indoor environments were hazardous to the health of nonsmokers as well as smokers (see **Table 24.3**). In the past several decades, smoking tobacco has been banned from bars, restaurants, offices, airplanes, railroad cars, hotel rooms, taxis, and many public gathering places. Protecting the quality of indoor air has been a major victory for health organizations and health authorities.

Elsewhere in the world, especially in impoverished countries, indoor air pollution still sickens and kills more than 2 million people every year. At least half of the world's more than 7 billion people live in extreme poverty. To cook food, they build fires that are fueled by organic matter—wood, charcoal, coal, dry vegetation, and dung—in cramped, enclosed living spaces. The smoke from fires used for cooking (and heating) causes extreme indoor air pollution that eventually sickens and kills the inhabitants. Children and women are at highest risk because they spend more time indoors.

The United Nations and member countries are trying to address this global health problem by developing simple stoves and nonpolluting fuels that can replace the toxic cooking fires used around the world. The goal is to develop and distribute 100 million safe cooking stoves to poor people in poor countries by the year 2020.

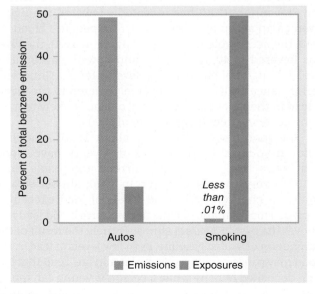

■ **Figure 24.4**

Benzene Emissions
Automobiles emit the greatest amount of benzene into the air—about 50% of the total. However, in terms of the amount of benzene that people inhale, most exposure comes from cigarette smoking.

TERMS

chlorofluorocarbons (CFCs): chemicals formerly used as coolants that are released into the atmosphere and that are responsible for destroying stratospheric ozone

emission: amount of substance that is released into the atmosphere

exposure: actual amount of the substance people are exposed to

ozone hole: an ozone-deficient portion of the atmosphere above Antarctica that has been steadily growing since the problem was first reported in 1985

ozone layer: a layer of ozone molecules located in the stratosphere in a diffuse band extending from 10 to 30 miles above Earth's surface

Table 24.3

Symptoms of Carbon Monoxide (CO) Poisoning

CO blood level (%)	Symptoms
0–2	No symptoms.
2–5	No symptoms in most people, but sensitive tests reveal slight impairment of arithmetic and other cognitive abilities. Levels of 2–5% are found in light or moderate smokers.
5–10	Slight breathlessness on severe exertion. Levels of 5–10% are found in smokers who inhale one or more packs of cigarettes per day.
10–20	Mild headache, breathlessness on moderate exertion. These levels are sometimes seen in smokers who are exposed to additional CO from other sources.
20–30	Throbbing headache, irritability, impaired judgment, defective memory, rapid fatigue.
30–40	Severe headache, weakness, nausea, dimness of vision, confusion.
40–50	Confusion, hallucinations, ataxia, hyperventilation, and collapse.
50–60	Deep coma with possible convulsions.
Above 60	Usually results in death.

Radon

Another form of indoor air pollution is **radon**, a radioactive gas that is invisible and odorless. Radon is naturally produced in the ground in areas that contain uranium ore. In New Jersey, for example, some homes built on top of rocks that contain uranium ore have over 100 times the safe level of radon in air inside the house. Homes also may be constructed from bricks or building materials that contain radioactive minerals, one of the decay products of which is radon gas. The radon is slowly released into the house over many years.

Long-term exposure to radon increases the risk of lung cancer. Uranium miners exposed to radon for years have a much higher risk of lung cancer than average. Cigarette smoking seems to act synergistically with radon; smokers who also are exposed to radon get lung cancer at rates much higher than individuals whose exposure is limited solely to cigarette smoke or solely to radon. The EPA estimates that radon exposure in homes is responsible for as many as 30,000 deaths a year from lung cancer. It is possible to test one's home for the presence of radon and to reduce the amount of radon if it is found.

Heavy Metal Pollution

Lead Lead is a heavy metal that is a serious threat to the health of millions of Americans, especially children. Lead contaminates air, land, water, and houses that still contain lead-based paints. Early symptoms of **plumbism** (lead poisoning) are loss of appetite, weakness, and anemia (**Table 24.4**). Lead poisoning also causes brain damage and is responsible for an enormous number of learning problems among children.

High lead levels in children not only cause learning and behavior problems but also are associated with criminal activity and arrest later in life (Wright et al., 2008). Studies involving children who had blood lead levels ranging from 4 to 37 micrograms per deciliter ($\mu g/dl$) showed that arrests and the violence of the crimes increased in proportion to the childhood blood lead level.

Table 24.4

Effects of Lead in People

Lead blood level ($\mu g/dl$)	Observable effects
10	Enzyme inhibition, learning disabilities
10–40	Red blood cells affected
40–50	Anemia, infertility (men)
50–60	Central nervous system effects, cognitive disabilities
60–100	Permanent brain damage, death

The crimes were committed when the subjects were aged 19 to 24 years. Any parent whose child is diagnosed with learning, behavior, or cognitive disabilities should have the lead level in the child's blood measured.

Over the past 50 years, the Centers for Disease Control and Prevention (CDC) has repeatedly lowered the figure given as an acceptable level of lead in people's blood. In 1960, the acceptable level was 60 $\mu g/dl$; in 1970, the level was lowered to 40, then to 20, and now the acceptable level is 10 $\mu g/dl$ of blood. Is that level safe? No. Children's performance on IQ tests is inversely related to the levels of lead in their blood and any level of lead is likely to have some adverse effect (Lanphear et al., 2005).

The good news is that only about 1% of American children younger than the age of 5 years have blood lead levels that exceed the current acceptable limit of 10 micrograms per deciliter. In 1980, almost 90% of American children had blood levels of lead exceeding 10 $\mu g/dl$. This dramatic decline in children's blood lead levels over the past 25 years is almost entirely the result of the elimination of leaded gasoline. Even low levels of lead in the blood may cause health problems later in life. Lead that has been deposited in bone while a person is young can return to the blood as a person ages and bone begins to break down. Recent studies suggest that the small amounts of lead released into the blood of older people may contribute to cardiovascular disease and heart attacks (Chen, 2013).

Poor children are at highest risk for having elevated blood lead levels because they live in old buildings that still contain lead-based paints. The paint flakes off walls and the lead becomes a component in house dust. Also, very young children like to eat paint flakes, which further elevates their blood lead levels.

Unfortunately, neurological damage from lead poisoning cannot be reversed by detoxification. The best way to prevent learning disabilities in children caused by lead pollution is to clean up the environment.

Lead is important to many industries, particularly the battery industry, so it is still an uphill battle to further reduce the amount of lead released into the environment and to clean up all sources of lead contamination. Despite the progress society has made in reducing lead contamination of the environment, the neurological development of millions of children is still at risk from lead toxicity.

Mercury In 1953, an epidemic of methylmercury poisoning occurred in several villages around Minamata Bay in Japan. Since that epidemic, mercury poisoning has become known as "Minamata disease." High levels of mercury in any form, but especially methylmercury, cause a variety of severe neurological symptoms, including blindness, deafness, coma, and death. Symptoms of low levels of mercury poisoning include hair loss and chronic fatigue. In 1970, high levels of methylmercury were found in Lake St. Clair in Canada, where a chemical plant had been discharging wastes. As a result, the U.S. Food and Drug Administration began testing lakes and rivers for mercury contamination. Based on these findings, sport fishing restrictions were implemented by many states because of high levels of methylmercury found in fish taken from contaminated streams and lakes.

Methylmercury is a worldwide environmental pollutant found in fresh water, land, and oceans. Methylmercury contamination of fish in both fresh water and oceans is now common. Because fetal development is especially sensitive to damage by mercury compounds, the EPA and Food and Drug Administration (FDA) jointly issued guidelines to limit fish consumption by pregnant

Compact Fluorescent Light Bulbs Contain Mercury

Compact fluorescent light bulbs (CFLs) use about one-fourth the amount of electricity as standard incandescent light bulbs and last 10 times longer.

CFLs contain mercury, a dangerous neurotoxin. Thus, they are a potential health hazard. Two billion CFLs contain 10 metric tons of mercury (Appell, 2007). If all the bulbs sold in the United States were CFLs, the mercury content would be 200 metric tons. Obviously, CFLs must not be disposed in the usual ways if a pollution disaster is to be avoided. Never throw a CFL into the trash! Many companies and stores have recycling programs.

If you break a CFL, open windows to help dissipate the mercury vapor. Use gloves and sticky tape to pick up glass fragments and powdery residue. Vacuum the area. Double-bag all the contents and dispose in a hazardous waste pickup if possible. For information on recycling CFLs, go to https://www.epa.gov/cfl/recycling-and-disposal-cfls.

women, women who plan to become pregnant, and nursing mothers:

- Do not eat shark, swordfish, king mackerel, tilefish, marlin, or bigeye tuna.
- Limit consumption of commercial fish to 12 ounces per week (about 2 meals).
- Fish with the lowest levels of mercury include shrimp, canned light tuna, salmon (wild), pollock, and catfish. (Albacore tuna has higher levels of mercury than light tuna.)

In the United States, coal-fired power plants are responsible for 40% of all mercury pollution. Mercury and other heavy metals are released into the air by the plant's smokestack and are carried around the world by air currents. Rain washes mercury from the air into lakes, rivers, and oceans, where it is transformed by bacteria into hazardous methylmercury. In 2011, the EPA ruled that, as a group, the nation's coal-fired power plants had to reduce their combined amount of mercury pollution by 90% by 2018. Although industry and Congressional opponents of the rule have delayed its full implementation, the energy industry is rapidly turning away from coal as a power source because cleaner fuels (natural gas and renewables) are less expensive, making upgrading old coal-fired plants and construction of new ones unwise. Until all coal-fired plants are taken out of commission, people living near them (especially children) are at risk for neurological damage.

Dispose of All Mercury Thermometers Safely

Many medicine cabinets in American homes still contain mercury thermometers. If one of these thermometers breaks and the mercury spills, dangerous levels of mercury may be inhaled as the mercury vaporizes, and the contaminated spot will release mercury for months or years.

If you have mercury thermometers, they must be disposed of at a hazardous waste site. Call local government officials to find out how to dispose of hazardous waste in your area. If mercury has spilled in your home, you should contact a hazardous waste expert to arrange a cleanup.

TERMS

plumbism: disease caused by lead poisoning

radon: a radioactive gas found in some homes that can increase the risk of cancer

Water Pollution

After air, water is the body's most essential requirement. We can survive without air for only a few minutes and without water perhaps for several days. The human body is composed of about 60% water, which is essential to every function carried out by organs in the body.

Agriculture, cities, and industry are enormous consumers of water. For example, producing 1 gallon of gasoline requires 5 gallons of water; brewing a barrel of beer consumes 1,000 gallons; a ton of newspaper takes about 50,000 gallons; a ton of steel requires 25,000 gallons; and irrigating an acre of orange trees requires almost 1 million gallons of water a year. A family of four uses about 400 gallons of water daily.

It was once believed that ethanol and other liquid fuels derived from food crops such as corn and soy would help reduce the use of petroleum fuels and all of its accompanying problems. What was initially overlooked in that assumption was the enormous amount of water required to grow corn and soy—several thousand gallons per acre. Thus, using food crops to produce fuels is unsustainable. Moreover, using food crops to produce fuel reduced the amount of available food, thus driving up the price of food and making it difficult for many people to afford to buy corn and soy products that are staples in many diets, especially in poor countries.

Water is continuously recycled in the environment by evaporation and rain. However, as more and more water becomes polluted from pesticides, chemicals, oil spills, and sewage, less and less water is suitable for human consumption and agricultural use. Of special concern is the chemical contamination of rivers, lakes, and underground water supplies, which provide most of our water needs. Around the world, safe, sufficient water supplies are stretched to the limit. Worldwide, it is estimated that about 1.2 billion people lack safe, unpolluted drinking water.

Waterborne diseases, such as cholera, typhoid fever, and dysentery, have been virtually eliminated in North America through sanitation and water treatment methods. In many communities, the water supplied to homes is purified by sedimentation, filtration, or chlorination. The addition of chlorine to water kills dangerous bacteria; however, it may create other health hazards. Interaction of chlorine with other chemicals in the water produces toxic substances, such as chloroform and chloramines, which are cancer-causing agents. The widespread use of detergents, herbicides, pesticides, fertilizers, and other chemicals also has contributed to increased water pollution.

Drinking Water

In the early 1970s, the Environmental Protection Agency found that the water supplies of many towns and cities were dangerously contaminated with pathogenic organisms and toxic chemicals. As a result, Congress passed the Safe Drinking Water Act of 1974, which covers 58,000 community water supply systems and another 160,000 private systems.

The act requires that these systems meet federal drinking water safety standards; but it is one thing to pass such a law and another thing to enforce it.

In 1996, Congress renewed the Safe Drinking Water Act of 1974. Under the new act, consumers must be notified whenever contaminants are found in drinking water and not merely when the water does not meet federal standards for contamination and safety. Community water systems in the United States must be tested for 80 contaminants. Each year, about 7% of community water systems report exceeding federal safety levels for at least one contaminant, which may be why so many people are buying and drinking bottled water.

The most dangerous and ubiquitous chemical found in drinking water is arsenic. This chemical, which occurs naturally in soils and water supplies around the world, is a well-known poison. In low doses, arsenic increases the risk of cancer; at higher doses that may occur in well water, arsenic causes skin eruptions, vomiting, diarrhea, pain, and death. Globally, at least 50 million people are at risk of arsenic poisoning from drinking arsenic-contaminated water.

Americans generally take for granted their (seemingly) endless supply of safe, clean water for daily needs (**Table 24.5**). Most of the people in the world, particularly in developing countries, are not so fortunate. More than a billion people in the world do not have access to safe, clean water. Those who do often must carry it in buckets from sources a long way from where they live. If rivers or wells run dry, they will die within days if they cannot find water.

Worldwide, including in the United States, water is becoming increasingly scarce. Vast underground water aquifers in the American West and South are being depleted. At least 36 states anticipate water shortages by 2020. The water table under Beijing, China, has sunk more than 200 feet since 1985.

The average American uses 100 or more gallons of water a day, more than people anywhere else in the world.

Table 24.5

Water Use

Average water use per person in the United States

Toilet	12 gallons/day
Shower	25 gallons/day
Bath	36 gallons/day
Personal faucet washing	3 gallons/day
Leaks	10 gallons/day
Garbage disposal	5 gallons/day
Washing machine	25 gallons/load
Dishwasher	10 gallons per load

Ways to conserve water

Check and fix leaks in faucets and toilets.

Install low-flush (1.6 gallon) toilets.

Install low-flow shower heads (2.5 gallons/minute).

Do not overwater lawn and gardens.

Do not leave hose running when washing car.

Bottled Water Battles

Annually, U.S. consumers buy about 8 billion gallons of bottled water. Bottled water is the fastest-growing segment of the beverage industry. The water bottled by the two largest distributors (Aquafina by Pepsi and Dasani by Coke) is usually reprocessed tap water. But tap water in the United States is the safest and purest in the world. Still, millions of Americans spend billions of dollars a year on bottled water.

There are many problems with bottled water. First, the bottled water may not be as pure or safe as people think. Some companies actually bottle tap water without any purification. About 50 billion plastic water bottles (1 billion pounds of plastic) are discarded each year, and only a few percent get recycled; the rest clutter streets and lots, pollute the oceans and waterways, or wind up in landfills. It takes an estimated 1.5 million barrels of oil to manufacture the plastic water bottles used each year, and then there is the energy used to transport the bottles to markets.

Maybe it's time to stop the bottled water craze. Buy a reusable bottle, fill it with tap water, and carry it with you. Enjoy.

It is estimated that, just to survive, a person needs about 10 to 15 gallons a day for drinking, cooking, and washing. In large cities such as New Delhi, India, about one-third of all the water is lost before it reaches consumers due to leaky, broken underground pipes. Many cities in the American West lose a comparable amount of water due to aging water pipes that leak. Water for drinking, agriculture, manufacturing, and other needs is going to become more difficult to obtain in the years ahead.

Land Pollution

Until relatively recently, little attention was paid to the disposal of garbage and solid wastes in landfills around the country. Now, however, communities are beginning to run out of space to dump what they want to get rid of. Each year in the United States, we junk about 8 million cars and trucks; 100 billion cans, bottles, and jars; and more than 200 million tons of garbage. The average American generates more than twice as much garbage as citizens of other industrialized countries.

Many old, abandoned solid waste disposal sites are dangerous to health because they contain hazardous materials that may be corrosive, flammable, or contain toxic chemicals (**Table 24.6**). In 1980, Congress passed the Superfund Act, which provides for the cleanup of the most dangerous

Good Riddance to the Plastic Bag

In 2007, the city of San Francisco became the first U.S. locale to ban the use of polyethylene (plastic) shopping bags. Since then, dozens of cities and states have followed San Francisco's lead. Nations that have banned or placed fees on the use of plastic bags include Bangladesh, Rwanda, and Italy. Cities in Australia, Mexico, England, Canada, Wales, China, and Thailand have also joined the ban.

More than a trillion plastic bags are used and discarded every year worldwide. The plastic bag is arguably the most environmentally destructive item ever invented. Plastic bags clog sewers and kill fish and seabirds of all kinds (seabirds pick up bits of plastic on the ocean surface to feed to chicks; when the chicks' stomachs are full of plastic, they die). Plastic bags and other debris destroy coral reefs. Discarded plastic bags collect water and provide a breeding ground for mosquitoes and diseases. In China, plastic bags are called "white pollution." Civilized societies may finally have had it with plastic bags as more cities and nations move to ban them. Many countries in Africa and Asia have banned single-use plastic bags entirely. In 2017, Kenya passed a law carrying a penalty of $40,000 and several years in prison for anyone using, selling, or manufacturing single-use plastic bags. Planet-saving alternatives to plastic bags include cotton, hemp, or sisal bags.

Table 24.6

Hazardous Wastes That Escape into the Environment Cause Many Health Problems

Millions of tons of these substances are discarded every year in the United States.

Substance	Source	Health effects
Mercury	Sludge from chloralkali plants; electrical equipment, fluorescent lights	Tremors, intellectual disabilities, loss of teeth, kidney damage, neurological damage
Arsenic	Arsenic trioxide from coal combustion and from metal smelters	Diarrhea, vomiting, paralysis, skin cancers
Cadmium	Waste from electroplating industry; paint containers, nickel-cadmium batteries	Lung diseases
Cyanide	Electroplating industry waste	Poisoning, interferes with cellular energy metabolism
Pesticides	Solid wastes and wastes in solutions	Multiple effects including rashes, respiratory and gastrointestinal symptoms, neurological disorders, hemorrhages

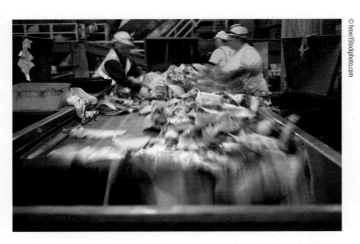

Reduce, reuse, recycle.

waste sites. By 2017, 394 Superfund sites had been cleaned up with 1342 remaining. Over 1,000 toxic waste sites await attention. It is estimated that 11 million Americans live within a mile of one of these Superfund sites, and their health is at some risk from exposure to toxic substances. You can find out where Superfund sites are located and whether you live near one of the listed sites. Go to http://www.epa.gov/superfund/search-superfund-sites-where-you-live to find out if you are living close to a Superfund site.

In 2014, China issued a shocking report documenting the extent of serious land pollution. The report concluded that 19.4% of all land used to grow food in China was seriously polluted. The most prevalent and serious contaminants included heavy metals (lead, cadmium, and mercury) along with high levels of pesticides. China uses more than twice the average amount of pesticides used on crops in other countries. Consumers of food grown in China are very concerned over possible adverse health consequences of consuming Chinese food products.

Americans are big consumers and big discarders. Every year millions of cars, tires, appliances, computers, TVs, paints and solvents, construction materials, and other objects, large and small, wind up in landfills or toxic waste disposal sites. To the extent that we continue to pollute the land we live on, the environment and our health will be adversely affected. Many items can be recycled with a little effort. Many communities have recycle programs for bottles, cans, plastic, and paper. Many organizations have recycle programs for old computers, cell phones, batteries, solvents used in printers, and other machines that contain toxic substances. Think of the environment when you consume and when you discard.

Pesticides

Soil, water, foods, and people have become increasingly contaminated with chemicals used to control weeds, insects, and plant diseases. Any chemical capable of killing an unwanted plant or animal is called a **pesticide**.

Specific kinds of chemicals that destroy specific organisms are **insecticides** (to kill insects), **fungicides** (to kill molds and fungi), **herbicides** (to kill weeds), and **rodenticides** (to kill rats and mice). Pesticides are important to the agriculture industry, which has claimed over the years that the abundance and quality of food grown in the United States depend on the use of chemicals to destroy crop pests. Although pesticides may contribute to agricultural productivity (this is contested by people who practice organic farming), widespread dissemination of pesticides in the environment has created health problems for people and animals.

Many pesticides have been found to be so dangerous that their use has been banned by the EPA, the federal agency that regulates pesticide use. One of the most widely used pesticides, DDT, was found to be carcinogenic and was banned by the EPA only after vast amounts had been released into the environment over decades of use.

Pesticides such as heptachlor, kepone, dieldrin, mirex, and toxophene also have been banned, and these chemicals have been off the market in the United States for a number of years. The quandary faced by the EPA is balancing the legitimate use of chemicals by agriculture and other industries while safeguarding public and environmental health.

Of particular concern is the agricultural pesticide *atrazine*. Each year about 76 million pounds of atrazine are used by farmers to control weeds. Most of the pesticide is used on corn, cotton, sugar cane, and sorghum crops. It also is used on some golf courses. Studies show that the pesticide is carried by runoff into lakes and streams and that fish and amphibians in atrazine-contaminated waters exhibit sexual deformities, sterility, and abnormal development of sexual organs. Large-scale studies show that birth defects across the United States increase about 10% during the months of April to June when most of the atrazine is released into the environment (Raloff, 2010).

Recycle Anything—Safely

Every day we throw out things that we know are toxic or hazardous to the environment or that we know should be recycled but we don't know where. We want to do the right thing and live responsibly, but it is just too time consuming to figure out where to get rid of the half-full paint cans, the old car battery, the obsolete cell phone, or the junk computer. So usually everything winds up in the garbage can and eventually in a landfill somewhere.

At the website http://www.earth911.com, you can find a nearby location where you can recycle almost anything. You simply type in the product that you want to dispose of and your zip code. You will see a list of locations in your area that accept that item for recycling or disposal. Help protect the environment that you live in and dispose of all hazardous materials safely.

Because of its widespread use, atrazine is now found in significant amounts in drinking water around the country.

Because of increasing concerns about the possible adverse effects of atrazine on human health and the environment, the pesticide has been banned in the European Union, though it is still widely used around the world. In 2014, atrazine was the second most widely used herbicide in the United States, Roundup being number one.

Most of the pesticides that accumulate in the bodies of young children come from the food that they eat. The good news is that switching the children's diet to organic foods lowers the concentration of agricultural pesticides in their bodies within a few days. Researchers measured the levels of various commonly used agricultural pesticides in children's urine samples. Within a few days of switching to organic fruits, vegetables, and grains, no pesticides could be detected in urine samples. Switching to foods grown without pesticides can substantially reduce the amount of potentially harmful chemicals absorbed into the body.

Generally, the health effects of pesticides on people and other animals are subtle. For the most part, pesticides do not cause sudden, severe sickness or death unless the amount of exposure is extremely high. The amount of

Avoid Pesticide-Contaminated Fruits and Vegetables

Listed below are fruits and vegetables that are most highly contaminated with pesticide residues and ones that are relatively free of pesticides.

Most contaminated	Least contaminated
Peaches	Onions
Apples	Avocados
Bell peppers	Sweet corn
Celery	Pineapples
Nectarines	Mangos
Strawberries	Asparagus
Cherries	Sweet peas
Pears	Kiwifruit
Imported grapes	Bananas
Spinach	Cabbage
Lettuce	Broccoli
Potatoes	Papaya

pesticide capable of causing death varies widely depending on the specific chemical as well as on individual susceptibility.

As a society, we are not ready to abandon the use of pesticides. However, as individuals we should restrict our use of pesticides as much as possible to protect ourselves and the environment. To achieve this goal, many people now grow their own vegetables without the use of pesticides. Others shop at stores that sell organic fruits and vegetables grown without the use of pesticides and herbicides.

Endocrine Disruptors

Endocrine disruptors are chemical substances, usually pesticides, in the environment that enter the body and interfere with the action of one or more hormones. Some endocrine disruptors mimic the effects of a hormone, causing overstimulation of a normally regulated biological process. Other endocrine disruptors block the actions of

Precautions for Pesticide Use

- Before you buy a pesticide product, read the instructions for use and any health and safety warnings. When mixing, do not increase the concentration of the pesticide above the label-recommended amount. Do not purchase the product if you can't use the pesticide properly (you may not have the right equipment). If you don't understand or feel completely comfortable with the health and safety information provided, get more information before you buy the product. Also, consider whether you have adequate storage space for the pesticide. A bigger bottle may be cheaper, but can you store it safely?
- Use the least toxic pesticide available for your pest control problem. Try to strike a balance between effective pest control and the safety of people, pets, and other nontarget organisms. Minimize skin and respiratory contact with pesticides. Wear rubber gloves. When you select gloves, consider both the solvent used in the pesticide formulation and the possibility that the pesticide itself can penetrate skin. You may want to use a respirator to guard against inhaling pesticide spray or dust.
- Use pesticides only for the uses for which they are intended. For instance, some wood preservatives are meant for outside use only, so don't use them inside the house!
- Don't leave seemingly empty pesticide containers where children can get them. Children have been poisoned by drinking from "empty" containers that actually contained leftover pesticide.
- Never smoke, eat, or drink while using pesticides.

TERMS

endocrine disruptors: chemical substances in the environment that interfere with the actions of one or more of the body's hormones

fungicide: a chemical that kills fungi and molds

herbicide: a chemical that kills weeds

insecticide: a chemical that kills insects

pesticide: a chemical that kills unwanted plants and animals

rodenticide: a chemical that kills mice and rats

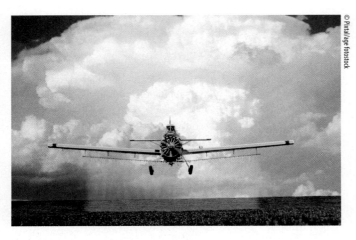

Large amounts of pesticides are routinely sprayed on major food crops.

normal hormones, thereby lessening or completely inhibiting a biological process. Because hormones are present in the body in very small amounts, only a small amount of an endocrine disruptor can affect hormone actions. Environmental endocrine disruptors include pesticides such as DDT, vinclozolin, endosulfan, toxaphene, dieldrin, and DBCP, and industrial chemicals and by-products such as polychlorinated biphenyls (PCBs), dioxins, and phenols, some of which are derived from soaps and detergents. Other potential endocrine disruptors include heavy metals, plastics, cosmetics, textiles, paints, lubricants, and sewage treatment effluent, which may contain a variety of natural and synthetic endocrine disruptors, including natural hormones from animal and human waste.

The Environmental Protection Agency carries out an Endocrine Disruptor Screening Program (http://www .epa.gov/endocrine-disruption) that focuses on possible effects of environmental chemicals on estrogen, androgen, and thyroid hormones. Estrogens, produced primarily by the ovaries and in small amounts by the adrenal glands, are responsible for female sexual development. Androgens, including testosterone, are responsible for male sex characteristics. Thyroid hormones control many biological processes such as growth, reproduction, development, and metabolism.

Hundreds of studies have shown high levels of endocrine-disrupting chemicals in the tissues of animals, including large mammals, birds, and fish. For example, the pesticide dicofol, chemically similar to DDT, is present in a lake in Florida as a result of dumping by a chemical company that used to operate on its shore. Dicofol mimics the action of estrogen and causes abnormalities in reproduction and in sexual development in alligators.

There is mounting evidence that endocrine disruption occurs in humans. For example, chronic exposure to the organophosphate pesticide *endosulfan* delays the onset of puberty in adolescent boys. This pesticide is widely used on squash, melons, strawberries, and other crops around the world. In the United States, more than a million pounds of endosulfan is used every year. Because it can pose unacceptable health risks to farm workers and wildlife and can persist in the environment, EPA is taking action to end the use of the pesticide endosulfan.

Before manufacturers can sell pesticides in the United States, the EPA must evaluate the pesticides thoroughly to ensure that they meet federal safety standards to protect human health and the environment. The EPA grants a "registration" or license that permits a pesticide's distribution, sale, and use only after the company meets the scientific and regulatory requirements.

In evaluating a pesticide registration application, the EPA assesses a wide variety of potential human health and environmental effects associated with use of the product. Potential registrants must generate scientific data necessary to address concerns pertaining to the identity, composition, potential adverse effects, and environmental fate of each pesticide.

Toxic Plastics

Plastic products are essential to virtually every aspect of modern-day life. Think of an object, and it is probably made of some type of plastic: eating utensils, tools, packaging, toys, bottles, shelving, plumbing pipes, and so on.

Plastics are derived from petroleum. Some plastics are made of one or several types of chemicals linked

Plastic Microbeads and Microfibers Pollute Oceans and Seas

Earth's seas and oceans are increasingly polluted with oil, chemicals, fertilizers, fishing lines, and garbage. But among the most hazardous pollutants are microscopic beads and fibers formed by the breakdown of millions of tons of discarded plastic objects of all kinds. These tiny particles are ingested by sea creatures and birds that mistake them as food. Tragically, adult birds pick up these bits of plastic and feed them to baby birds that subsequently die from lack of nutrients. These tiny plastic beads never degrade entirely.

Plastic microfibers from discarded fleece jackets, athletic clothing, yoga pants, and other apparel used to increase softness and sweat absorption are also a threat to sea creatures. With every wash, microfibers are released from the cloth and go down the drain and eventually into a river or the ocean. Fish and other sea life ingest the microfibers as they feed. Tests of water from the Great Lakes and New York Harbor show high concentrations of plastic. Testing of waters where oysters grow shows that they ingest microfibers. One possible solution to the plastic microfiber problem may be to require all washing machines to have filters engineered to capture the fibers on a screen before they can be released into the environment.

together in long arrays. In some circumstances, the end-product plastic is not harmful to health, but one or more of its individual components is. Thus, people involved in the manufacture of the plastic may be exposed to harmful effects of one or more of the component chemicals with which they work. Also, the plastic product may degrade and release its toxic chemical components into the environment. This is called leaching. Leach can occur when a plastic is heated, is exposed to microwave radiation, or comes into contact with liquids, fats, oils, and detergents. Types of plastics shown to leach toxic chemicals are polycarbonate, polyvinylchloride (PVC), and styrene. Other plastics may be harmful, but studies of their safety have yet to be carried out. In recent years, two chemicals used in the manufacture of plastics have been implicated in a number of developmental defects in animals and humans and in a variety of health problems.

Phthalates are used in the manufacture of plastic flooring, medical devices, cosmetics, and coatings on drugs. Phthalates are everywhere in the environment, and nearly 100% of humans have significant levels of phthalate in their bodies. Exposure to phthalates, particularly in fetuses and children, has been linked to a variety of developmental abnormalities (Mankidy et al., 2013). For example, phthalate exposure appears to increase the risk of allergy and asthma, abnormal breast development in pubertal boys, and early onset of puberty in girls. Phthalates in the body have an adverse effect on children's brain and sexual development. Phthalates impair sperm quality, reduce the level of reproductive hormones, affect thyroid functions, and alter the development of reproductive organs in boys.

Bisphenol-A (BPA) is a chemical used in the manufacture of polycarbonate plastic, a clear, hard plastic identified by the number 7 imprinted somewhere on the product. BPA is also found in the epoxy resins used as lacquers to coat metal products such as food cans, bottle tops, and water supply pipes. BPA has been linked to miscarriages, birth defects, and abnormal brain development in fetuses.

BPA was first synthesized in the 1930s in an effort to develop a synthetic estrogen but was abandoned in favor of diethylstilbestrol (DES), which proved to be a more effective estrogen. Subsequently, chemists discovered that BPA could be used to make polycarbonate plastic. Today, polycarbonate plastics are used in canned goods, water bottles, baby bottles, microwave cookware, and many other food-related products. As polycarbonate plastics age or when they are heated or exposed to strong detergents, BPA leaches out. Studies show that 92% of Americans have significant amounts of BPA in their bodies. BPA also leaches out of the resins used to coat food cans. One study showed that consuming one serving of canned soup daily for five consecutive days increased BPA in the body to extremely high levels (Carwile et al., 2011). Any health effects of such high transient increases in BPA are unknown.

Pregnant women and nursing mothers should avoid products made of polycarbonate plastic as much as possible. Do not use polycarbonate plastic water bottles or, if you do, do not wash them in hot water with detergent. Do not use baby bottles or baby gadgets that are made of polycarbonate plastic. Do not heat food in polycarbonate plastic containers. In general, try to avoid any food or beverage that is packaged in polycarbonate plastic.

Many studies suggest that BPA is a health hazard (Konieczna at al., 2015). In 2012, the FDA banned the sale of baby bottles and children's drinking cups made with BPA. The European Union and Canada have banned BPA use in baby bottles. However, the FDA has been reluctant to ban the use of polycarbonate plastics for food and beverage containers, claiming that studies do not suggest that the amounts of BPA found in all manner of packaging and in nearly everyone's body are harmful.

Monitoring Environmental Chemicals

To monitor the effects of potentially harmful environmental chemical pollution on human health, the Centers for Disease Control and Prevention (CDC) has been measuring the chemical load in a cross section of Americans every two years since the late 1990s. In its updated fourth National Report on Human Exposure to Environmental Chemicals, the CDC measured the levels of 148 chemicals in blood and urine samples taken from people of all ages (Centers for Disease Control and Prevention, 2017).

The measurement of environmental chemicals that are detectable in the body is called **biomonitoring**. Chemicals enter the body from air, water, food, dust, soil, or consumer products. Although the sensitivity of chemical tests has improved in recent years, the health effects of many environmental chemicals that accumulate in the body are unknown; more research must be done. The most recent report shows that levels of lead and *cotinine* (a chemical that measures exposure to secondhand cigarette smoke) have declined significantly, especially among children. However, the levels of organophosphate pesticides, phthalates, and other compounds known to cause health problems are increasing.

TERMS

biomonitoring: measurement of environmental chemicals present in the body that may harm health

bisphenol-A (BPA): chemical used to manufacture polycarbonate plastics; may cause abnormal brain development in fetuses and birth defects

phthalates: chemicals used in the manufacture of various plastics; may cause abnormal genital development in males and premature breast development in girls

Electromagnetic and Microwave Radiation

Electric power lines, appliances, motors, TV sets, microwave ovens, and power tools all emit very low-frequency **electromagnetic fields (EMFs)**. Except for Earth's electromagnetic field, all EMFs come from electricity that is generated by electrical devices of all kinds (**Table 24.7**). Only in the past few generations have people been exposed to the magnetic fields. Until recently, these EMFs were thought to be too weak to affect living organisms, so their impact on health was ignored.

Some epidemiological studies have found an association between the incidence of childhood leukemia and brain tumors and exposure to EMFs. Families that live close to high-voltage power lines or electrical distribution boxes tend to experience more sickness and more cancers. However, a very careful study of the risks of childhood leukemia and exposure to EMFs showed that the risk of cancer was not increased. On the other hand, studies suggest that exposure to EMFs among adult railway workers is associated with a higher risk for leukemia.

All of us are exposed to EMFs every day. An electric shaver or hair dryer puts out a strong EMF, although users are exposed for only a few minutes a day (**Figure 24.5**). If a person lives near a high-voltage transmission line, exposure to EMFs may be considerable depending on the distance between the house and the wires. And the exposure goes on day and night. Calculating EMF exposure, at best, yields crude approximations, one reason why the evidence regarding EMFs and harmful health effects is conflicting.

Cellular Phones

Digital cellular phones emit pulses of microwave radiation. Millions of Americans use cell phones, often for several hours a day. Any possible health consequences from long-term cell phone use by billions of people around the world are as yet unknown. Another uncertainty is the

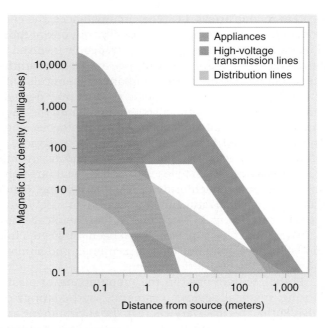

■ **Figure 24.5**

Strength of Magnetic Fields from Sources of Electromagnetic Fields (EMFs)

Small appliances produce strong fields, but the strength disappears within a few feet. High-voltage lines produce less dense magnetic fields, but they cover a large area.

Adapted from Florig, H. K. (2001). Alternative goals and policy mechanisms for radiation protection. *Health Physics, 80,* 397–400.

health consequences of working in modern offices that are filled with microwave radiation from a variety of electronic devices. People who use cell phones extensively should use a headset to keep the phone away from the head.

Some cancer researchers believe that long-term use of a cell phone might increase the risk of getting a brain tumor. Evidence that cell phone use is associated with brain tumors is suggestive, but not conclusive (Davis et al., 2013).

Table 24.7

Strength of Electromagnetic Fields from Household Sources

Many electrical appliances, especially ones with motors, produce very strong magnetic fields, but the strength of the field falls rapidly with increasing distance from the appliance.

	Intensity (milligauss) at distance from source	
Source	At 4 cm	At 20 cm
100-watt bulb	2.5	—
Refrigerator (back)	11	5
200-watt stereo	27	5
80-watt fluorescent bulb	34	18
Coffeemaker	90	7
Electric drill	600	6
Hair dryer	1,000	0.1

Ways to Reduce Your Exposure to EMFs

- Don't use an electric blanket or water bed heater unless it is a newer model with reduced EMFs.
- Use battery-operated shavers and hair dryers. Battery-operated appliances and toys do not put out EMFs.
- Don't sit too close to computers, TVs, fans, or light fixtures.
- If your work requires long exposure to EMFs, look for ways to reduce it. Do not sit too close to computer screens for long periods.
- If you rent or buy a house, choose one that is not near a high-voltage line or distribution transformer.

Based on current research, the risk to health from exposure to EMFs and cell phone radiation must be regarded as small compared with the risks of chemical pollutants in air, soil, water, and food. Moreover, our lives are so dependent on electricity and the gadgets that make life more comfortable that major changes in electrical use are not anticipated.

Noise Pollution

Have you ever been kept awake at night by a dripping faucet or a neighbor's party? Does the sound of sirens and horns put you on edge? Have you ever found yourself thinking, "If that noise doesn't stop, I'm going to scream"? Everyone is sensitive to noise, and excessive noise produces stress and can cause health problems. Noise interferes with sleep and over periods of time can cause fatigue, irritability, tension, and anxiety.

Sound activates the nervous system, thereby affecting functions of the endocrine, cardiovascular, and reproductive systems. Noise is a "stressor" and can increase blood pressure, alter hormone levels, constrict blood vessels, and cause intense pain at high levels.

Sound levels are measured in **decibels** (dB). The danger zone for hearing loss begins at about 85 dB, a level present on school buses crowded with kids or driving in freeway traffic with the window open (**Table 24.8**). Many daily activities expose us to sound levels that can permanently damage hearing. Millions of people in the United States are exposed to dangerous levels of sound every day that can cause hearing loss.

Noise Pollution: Bad for Kids

Most people have experienced difficulty carrying on a conversation in a noisy restaurant or bar or at a party. If it's too hard to get what's said, it's often easier to nod and just give up. Whereas adults may become annoyed when they are unable to understand what's being said because of distracting and interfering background noise, the same experience can be much more deleterious for toddlers and young children. Research confirms that children have increasingly poor sentence recognition when noise competes with meaningful talk because they have to expend more mental effort to identify meaningful stimuli correctly (Lewis et al., 2016). Background noise from music, television, interactive toys, computers, or people (adults or kids) yelling can result in permanent damage to normal speech development and comprehension. This is especially true for children with mild or serious hearing loss in one or both ears.

Some tips to help children learn and understand speech:

- Never let children use headphones. Not only can hearing be damaged by inadvertent loud sounds, but speech development also is can also be impaired.
- Speak slowly and clearly to children. Do not use "baby talk." Look at the child when speaking; do not shout from across the room.
- Repeat what you are trying to convey several times and enforce the information with an action. For example, "Let's put on your clothes," should accompany the act of dressing a child.
- Except for moments of danger or warning, shouting at a child who does not understand is counterproductive.
- Read to children often from their earliest days.

Table 24.8

Loud Noise Encountered Daily

A noise level above 85 dB can damage hearing and cause hearing loss over time.

Source of noise	Sound level (dB)
Firearms	140 to 170
Jet engines	140
Rock concerts	90 to 130
Amplified car stereos	140 (at full volume)
Portable stereos (e.g., iPods)	115 (at full volume)
Power mowers	105
Jackhammers	100
Subway trains	100
Video arcades	100
Freeway driving in a convertible	95
Power saws	95
Electric razors	85
Crowded school buses	85
School recesses or assemblies	85
Hair dryer	60 to 90
Normal conversation	40
Quiet room	10

Rock musicians and people who listen to loud rock music are particularly at risk for hearing loss. Members of many famous rock bands suffer from **tinnitus**, a persistent ringing in the ears, or have lost a significant amount of their hearing. Children are especially prone to turning up the volume and to listening to music with earphones

> We have met the enemy and he is us.
>
> Pogo
> *Walt Kelly*, cartoonist

at dangerously high sound levels. A nationwide study of hearing loss among American children and adolescents found that almost 15% had some degree of hearing loss at both the high and low end of audible frequencies

TERMS

decibel: a measure of noise level

electromagnetic fields (EMFs): a form of radiation produced by electrical power lines and appliances that may increase the risk of cancers

tinnitus: persistent ringing in the ears, often caused by repeated or sudden exposure to loud noises

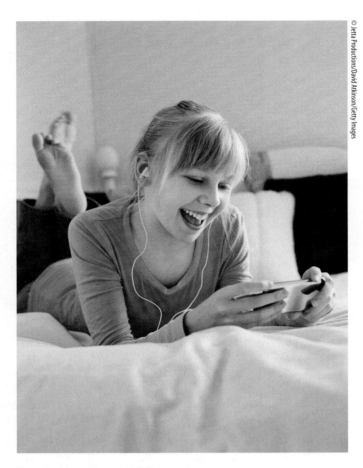

Keep the volume low to avoid hearing loss.

(Su & Chan, 2017). Some had hearing loss in only one ear; others had hearing loss in both ears.

Even a brief exposure to sustained loud noise can damage the sensitive structures of the inner ear. Hearing loss is caused not only by listening to loud music but also by noise in urban environments. The noise levels at sporting events, rallies, and other places where large numbers of people congregate can also contribute to hearing loss. Hearing loss is a major problem for the elderly. Protect your hearing while you are young; keep the volume down.

Many people live and work amid the din of urban life and have forgotten the rest and peacefulness that come with silence. If you have the good fortune to spend time at isolated spots in remote woods or mountains, you become aware of the beneficial effects of quiet. The human need for stillness was expressed eloquently in 1854 by Chief Seattle, after whom the modern city in Washington is named:

> There is no quiet place in the white man's cities. No place to hear the unfurling of leaves in spring or the rustle of insects' wings. But perhaps it is because I am a savage and do not understand. The clatter only seems to insult the ears. And what is there to life if a man cannot hear the lonely cry of the whippoorwill or the arguments of the frogs around a pond at night?

How Human Population Growth Affects Us

In 1960, the world's population was about 3 billion people. By 2013, the world's population more than doubled to 7.2 billion people. By 2050, the world's population is expected to reach 9.6 billion people, and by 2100, 11.3 billion (**Figure 24.6**). The fastest population growth today is occurring in Africa, which is expected to have 6 billion people by 2050, more than half the entire world population.

Young people aged 10 to 19 currently make up the largest age group in the world, accounting for about 20% of the world's total population. Virtually all of the population increase in the next 40 years is expected to take place in underdeveloped nations, especially in the world's poorest countries (**Table 24.9**). In contrast, the developed, industrialized nations are expected to be near zero population growth, except for the United States.

Of the 7.5 billion people living today, it is estimated that 1 billion have no access to clean water, 2 billion have inadequate sanitation, and 1.5 billion breathe polluted, unhealthy air. Human activities are resulting in the extinction of almost 10,000 plants and animal species a year. A few hundred years ago, the rate of extinction was about 10 species per year.

Deforestation; loss of native species of plants and animals; depletion of natural resources; and air, water, and land pollution are all related to too many people needing too many scarce resources. The demand for

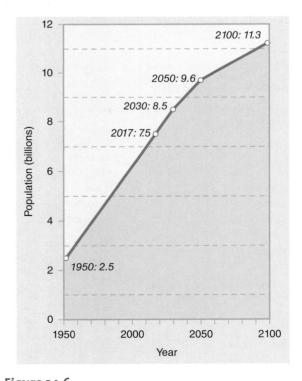

■ **Figure 24.6**

World Population from 1950 to 2050 (estimate)
Data from U.S. Census Bureau. (2011). World Population 1950–2050. Retrieved from http://www.census.gov/population/international/data/idb/worldpopgraph.php

Table 24.9

Countries Projected to Have the Largest Populations in 2050

By 2050, the world's population is predicted to increase to 9 or 10 billion people. Most of the population increase will occur in the poorest and least developed countries in Africa and Southeast Asia. The population of the United States is expected to increase by about 50%, while the populations of most European countries will decline. The estimates for 2050 do not take into account food scarcity, weather extremes, and social unrest and war caused by climate change.

	Population	
Country	2017	2050
India	1.3 billion	1.6 billion
China	1.4 billion	1.3 billion
United States	324 million	389 million
Nigeria	190 million	410 million
Indonesia	264 million	321 million
Pakistan	197 million	360 million
Bangladesh	164 million	201 million
Brazil	209 million	232 million
Ethiopia	104 million	190 million
Philippines	105 million	151 million

Data from U.S. Census Bureau (2014). International Data Base Country Rankings. Available at http://www.census.gov/population/international/data/idb/rank.php.

modern lifestyles and products adds to the destruction and pollution of the environment.

The actions, needs, and goals of people are at the root of all environmental problems and the ongoing destruction of nature. As the economies of nations become stronger and the aspirations of people around the globe increase, so does the rate of environmental destruction. Political and economic solutions to the population problem are acknowledged, but many nations are unable or unwilling to undertake the measures that might curb population growth. Some countries have family planning programs, but the success of these programs depends on educating people and in raising their standard of living so that they understand that large families are not in their best interest. Most of the world's population is opposed to any form of birth control, so the world's population is expected to continue to increase for at least the next 50 years.

The United States has made progress in slowing damage to the environment. Thanks to legislation, environmental lawsuits, and improved technology, air quality has improved, many waterways are cleaner than they were 20 years ago, and disposal of hazardous wastes into the environment has declined dramatically. While all this is good news, we have a long way to go in solving environmental and population problems. To most researchers who study human population dynamics, 11 billion people is certain to strain the carrying capacity of Earth, with the possible consequences of famine, pandemic disease, wars, catastrophic climate changes, and breakdowns in human societies.

The dinosaurs survived for about 150 million years and disappeared about 65 million years ago, presumably as a result of the earth being hit by a giant meteor that changed the climate drastically. According to anthropologists, the modern human species has been around for only about 3.5 million years. At the rate we are destroying habitat, using up Earth's resources, and polluting the environment, we may be hastening our own disappearance.

> In wilderness is the preservation of the world.
>
> *Henry David Thoreau*

What we call the beginning is often the end
And to make an end is to make a beginning.
The end is where we start from.

—*T. S. Eliot*
Four Quartets

Critical Thinking About Health

1. Check around your house or apartment, and make a list of all pesticides or herbicides that are stored anywhere. Decide which ones you really need to keep and which ones can be discarded. (Check with your local waste management authorities for proper disposal of pesticides and herbicides.) Make a list of how and when you use pesticides and what precautions you take when you use them. After doing this, write a report on how you can reduce your use and exposure to pesticides and herbicides.

2. If you, like many Americans, are committed to halting global warming by reducing your contributions to increasing levels of atmospheric carbon dioxide, consider these suggestions:

   a. Reduce your electricity use by 30%. What appliances use the most electrical energy and what changes can you make to reduce their use?

   b. Reduce the use of your automobile by 30% or more. What changes in your lifestyle can you make that will reduce your dependence on car transportation?

   c. Find out what industries release the most CO_2 in manufacturing their products. Are these products essential to your life, or would you be able to live without some of them?

3. The major global threats to the environment are (a) nuclear, chemical, and biological warfare; (b) pollution; (c) global warming; (d) land and ocean degradation; and (e) extinction of species of plants and animals. Indicate which of these global environmental problems is of the most concern to you personally. What can you personally do about the problem? What do you think governments should do about the problem? Discuss any effects that you think this problem will have on your life now and in the future.

4. If you had the option of living anywhere in the world, where would you choose to live? Is your choice largely determined by job opportunities, environmental concerns, access to a favorite sport (e.g., surfing), or by some other variable? Discuss your choice in detail, and explain the things that are most important to you in making your selection. Do you think your choice will be the same 10 years from now? Why might it change?

Chapter Summary and Highlights

Chapter Summary

Our planet was formed along with the rest of the solar system about 5 billion years ago. The first signs of life appeared perhaps 3 to 4 billion years ago. Over time, species of all kinds arose and became extinct as conditions on Earth changed. Just a few million years ago, the first human-like species appeared. Now there are about 7.2 billion of us living on Earth. To be in good health, a person needs unpolluted air, water, and food, as well as adequate shelter and a nutritious diet. Unfortunately, only a minority of people live in such conditions. Many of the world's peoples live in dire poverty, suffer many diseases, and die prematurely. Despite problems of disease, starvation, war, and genocide, the human population is predicted to reach 9.6 billion by the year 2050. Humans now occupy every ecological niche on the planet and have produced so much air pollutants that we have already altered Earth's climate with unpredictable future consequences for our survival. Like it or not, it is going to get hotter and hotter. Unpolluted air, water, and food will become scarce. With an additional 2 billion people on Earth by 2050, what will life be like?

You probably will be someone who will live to know the answer to this question. So, you have a vital interest in helping Earth survive and possibly recover from ongoing pollution and temperature rise. Think more about where to live than where to work when you finish college. Is the air relatively unpolluted most of the time? What is the source of the water where you plan to live? Are there farmers' markets or other nearby sources of fresh fruits and vegetables? These are questions that previous generations would have considered foolish. But Earth evolves. The dinosaurs lasted about 165 million years on Earth before becoming extinct in a matter of a few centuries. We have been around for a mere 5 million years or fewer. Extinction can happen to us in a very short time as well.

Highlights

- To maintain good health, people require adequate unpolluted air, water, food, and shelter.
- The air we breathe is often polluted with ozone, carbon monoxide, hydrocarbons, nitrogen and sulfur oxides, lead, cigarette smoke, and other contaminants.
- Global warming is expected to cause serious environmental disruptions in this century.
- The greenhouse effect and the ozone hole are examples of global environmental problems caused by human activities.
- Pollution of air, land, and water from heavy metals, such as lead, is particularly hazardous to health. Children with even small amounts of lead

or mercury in their bodies may suffer from learning deficits and growth retardation.

- Drinking water may be contaminated with chemicals or microorganisms that can cause disease.
- Pesticides, some of which are endocrine disruptors, can harm health, especially reproduction.

- Noise pollution can cause a wide range of health problems, including stress, tinnitus, and hearing loss.
- World population is expected to increase by 3 billion people in the next 50 years, severely taxing an already depleted environment and creating more health and environmental problems.

For Your Health

Personal health is affected by how much the physical and social environments support healthy attitudes and behaviors. Assess your personal contribution to the health of your environment by doing the "Environmental Aware-ness Questionnaire" (Exercise 24.1 in the Workbook). Do the other exercises for this chapter to learn more about clean air and water in your community.

References

American Lung Association. (2017). *State of the Air 2017*. Retrieved from http://www.lung.org/assets/documents/healthy-air/state-of-the-air/state-of-the-air-2017.pdf

Appell, D. (2007, October). Toxic bulbs. *Scientific American*, 30–31.

Carwile, J. L., et al. (2011). Canned soup consumption and urinary bisphenol A. *Journal of the American Medical Association, 306*, 2218–2219.

Centers for Disease Control and Prevention. (2017). *National report on human exposure to environmental chemicals*. Retrieved from http://www.cdc.gov/exposurereport

Chen, I. (2013, September). Lead's buried legacy. *Scientific American*, 28–29.

Davis, D. L., et al. (2013). Swedish review strengthens grounds for concluding that radiation from cellular and cordless phones is a probable human carcinogen. *Pathophysiology, 20*, 123–129.

Florig, H. K. (2001). Alternative goals and policy mechanisms for radiation protection. *Health Physics, 80*, 397–400.

Intergovernmental Panel on Climate Change. (2017). 46th *Annual report*. Retrieved from http://www.ipcc.ch/

Jurewicz, J., & Hanke, W. (2011). Exposure to phthalates: Reproductive outcome and children's health. A review of epidemiological studies. *International Journal of Occupational Medicine and Environmental Health, 24*, 115–141.

Konieczna, A., et al. (2015). Health risk of exposure to bisphenol A (BPA). *Roczniki Panstwowego Zakladu Higieny, 66*, 5–11.

Landrigan, P. J., et al. (2017). The *Lancet* Commission on pollution and health. *The Lancet. 391*, 462–512.

Lanphear, B. P., et al. (2005). Low-level environmental lead exposure and children's intellectual function: An international pooled analysis. *Environmental Health Perspectives, 113*, 894–899.

Lewis, D., et al. (2016). Effects of noise on speech recognition and listening effort in children with normal hearing and children with mild bilateral or unilateral hearing loss. *Journal of Speech, Language, and Hearing Research, 59*, 1218–1232.

Lovelock, J. E. (1979). *Gaia: A new look at life on Earth*. New York: Oxford University Press.

Mankidy, R., et al. (2013). Biological impact of phthalates. *Toxicology Letters, 217*, 50–58l.

National Oceanic and Atmospheric Administration. (2014). *Climate at a glance*. Retrieved from http://www.ncdc.noaa.gov/cag/time-series/global/globe/land_ocean/ytd/5/1880-2014

Raloff, J. (2010, February 27). Weed killer in the cross hairs. *Science News*, 18–20.

Su, B. M., & Chan, D. K. (2017). Prevalence of hearing loss in U.S. children and adolescents: Findings from NHANES 1988–2010. JAMA *Otolaryngology Head & Neck Surgery, 143*, 920–927.

U.S. Census Bureau. (2011). *World population 1950–2050*. Retrieved from http://www.census.gov/population/international/data/idb/worldpopgraph.php

U.S. Census Bureau. (2014). *International database country rankings*. Retrieved from http://www.census.gov/population/international/data/idb/rank.php

U.S. Energy Information Administration. (n.d.). *International energy statistics*. Retrieved from http://www.eia.gov/cfapps/ipdbproject/IEDIndex3.cfm?tid=90&pid=44&aid=8

Wright, J. P., et al. (2008). Association of prenatal and childhood blood lead concentrations with criminal arrests in early adulthood. *PLoS Medicine, 5*, e101.

Suggested Readings

Hoernschemeyer, D. L. (2014). *Healthy living in a contaminated world: How to prevent toxic chemicals from undermining your health*. North Charleston, SC: CreateSpace. Describes the health damages caused by specific chemicals and recommends actions that people can take to avoid exposure to them.

Holland, A. (2016, June). Preventing tomorrow's climate wars. *Scientific American*, 61–65. Future climate changes may increase international conflicts as countries face shortages of water and food, increased pollution, and encroachment of coastal lands by rising sea levels.

Kolbert, E. (2013). *The sixth extinction: An unnatural history*. New York: Henry Holt and Company. An award-winning science journalist examines the idea that we currently are involved in a human-produced mass extinction.

Lerner, S. (2012). *Sacrifice zones: The front lines of toxic chemical exposure in the United States*. Cambridge, MA: MIT Press. Case studies of 12 communities that confronted industrial and military pollution of their habitat.

Liberman, M. C. (2015, August). Hidden hearing loss. *Scientific American*, 49–53. Explains how excessively loud noise at sporting events, large concerts, restaurants, bars, and parties can gradually damage hearing in people of all ages.

Michael, A. J. (2017). *Climate change and the health of nations: Famine, fevers, and the fate of populations*. London: Oxford University Press. Nature does not care what people think. More than 99.9% of all species that have ever lived on Earth have become extinct. Humans are hastening our own demise. This book documents the bleak future due to climate change and its consequences to the planet.

National Oceanic and Atmospheric Administration. (2018). Trends in Atmospheric Carbon Dioxide. Retrieved from https://www.esrl.noaa.gov/gmd/ccgg/trends/

Pearce, F. (2006). *When the rivers run dry: Water—the defining crisis of the twenty-first century*. Boston: Beacon Press. The author believes the battle for water in the coming years will cause conflicts and create a global crisis.

Physicians for Social Responsibility. (2014). *The medical and public health impacts of global warming*. Retrieved from http://www.psr.org/resources/the-medical-and-public-health.html. Addresses the predicted effects of global warming on patterns of disease.

Recommended Websites

Center for Environmental Health
Information from the Centers for Disease Control and Prevention about environmental health topics.

Environmental Defense
Information and education about, and advocacy for, a clean environment.

Environmental Protection Agency
Information about air, water, land, and other types of pollution.

History of Lead Industry Advertising
The Cincinnati Children's Hospital depicts the lead industry's advertising campaign to counter the evidence implicating lead paint in children's deaths.

Intergovernmental Panel on Climate Change
Expert analysis from the World Meteorological Organization (WMO) and the United Nations Environment Programme (UNEP) on the scientific, technical, and socio-economic information relevant for the understanding of the risk of human-induced climate change.

National Report on Human Exposure to Environmental Chemicals
Presents the findings of the CDC's third report on the level of 148 potentially harmful chemicals that were measured in people's blood and urine.

National Safety Council
Fact sheets on the health effects of more than 80 toxic chemicals.

Office of Energy Efficiency & Renewable Energy
The official site of the U.S. Department of Energy Office of Efficiency & Renewable Energy.

Rocky Mountain Institute
The Rocky Mountain Institute provides independent analyses of energy policies.

Health Enhancement Methods

This appendix contains several methods for enhancing health and well-being. The techniques include mental imagery (Experiencing the Peacefulness of a Mountain Lake and Open Heart and Compassion Meditation), muscular stress reduction (Progressive Muscular Relaxation), and mind–body harmony exercises (Hatha Yoga Postures and T'ai Chi Movements). You may want to record the instructions on an audiotape so that you can listen to the instructions while focusing on the exercise.

Exercise 1
Experiencing the Peacefulness of a Mountain Lake

Imagine yourself walking alone in the early morning along a path leading to some nearby mountains. All around you are trees rustling in the breeze; the path is covered with soft leaves and pine needles. The air is cool but not cold; your body feels relaxed as you walk slowly through the woods. You become aware of the quietness of the surroundings, how different from the constant noise of city life. As you stroll along you hear the calls of different songbirds. You breathe in the cool air tinged with the fragrance of pine and eucalyptus. You walk through patches of sunlight and see the mountain peaks in the distance.

As you gradually walk higher, you notice the subtle sound of water cascading over rocks, and the sound mixes with the wind moving through the branches of the tall trees. Up ahead, a chipmunk is perched on an old stump of a tree, frozen in the moment as it decides which way to jump. Suddenly it is gone and you notice yellow, brown, and orange insects buzzing around the flowers on the bushes. The path begins to level off and the air turns slightly cooler. Now the path is more rocky, and as you come around a bend, a deep blue mountain lake comes

into view. You climb onto a boulder weathered smooth by water, wind, and time. You sit down on the boulder to see the entire lake.

Near the shore of the lake are tall green grasses, and spreading back from the shore are clusters of spruce, pine, aspen, and birch. You see a large bird perched on top of one tree in the distance. As you watch, the bird spreads its wings and swoops down over the lake, soars up again, and is gone. The peaks of the mountains surrounding the lake are mixtures of gray and white snow. As your eyes move from the lake to the peaks and back to the lake again, you become aware of the harmony of nature, how each part seems to be in balance with the other parts of the scene.

The sky is dotted with small puffs of white clouds that circle the peaks. The rock you are sitting on radiates the sun's warmth, and you feel your body relaxing, melting into the comfortable saddle of the rock. Your eyes return to the surface of the lake and now you notice the evenly spaced ripples moving across its surface.

As you become more aware of the wind-induced ripples on the otherwise still surface of the lake, you imagine that the ripples on the lake are the tensions in your body. You want your body to become as quiet and relaxed as the stillest part of the lake. As the cessation of the breeze causes the ripples to cease, so the cessation of thoughts in your mind causes the tension to disappear. As you watch the surface of the lake, all of your attention is focused on the ripples as they form, move toward the shore, and disappear.

Breathe slowly and deeply from your diaphragm and continue to focus on the stillness of the beautiful, clear mountain lake that you have created in your mind. Notice that you can make the surface of the lake as smooth as a mirror; as you do this, all of your tensions, thoughts, and worries also disappear, and your mind and body become fully relaxed. Hold onto this feeling of calm and relaxation for as long as you desire. Remind yourself that this is a place you can come back to in your mind time and time again whenever you feel tense, stressed, or angry. It's your personal safe haven that will always induce a feeling of calmness and relaxation.

Note: You can record this image-visualization exercise yourself or have a friend read it into a voice recorder so that you can simply listen to the instructions whenever you feel the need for some mental and physical relaxation. Also, the details of the image can be changed to suit your own experiences or imagination.

Exercise 2
Open Heart and Compassion Meditation

The heart is vital to life, and heart disease is still the number one cause of death in most industrialized countries. The heart is a pump; it circulates blood through the body. But symbolically, we think of the heart as the center of feeling; love flows from the heart. However, we also think of a *hardened heart*, one that may express mean, hateful, destructive, indifferent, and inconsiderate sentiments. What we feel in our heart symbolically can be manifested as stress and in physiological changes that may eventually produce illness. Fear, anger, or hate may contribute to heart disease as well as other ailments. A healthy goal is to rid the heart of acrimonious, destructive feelings and to develop feelings of love and compassion for others, even those who hurt us either deliberately or unwittingly. The following suggestions are designed to help you open your heart to feeling love and compassion for others.

- Sit quietly for a few minutes in a comfortable position on a chair or on the floor, and pay attention to your breathing. Feel the air come in through your nose and flow down into your lungs as the lungs expand and your diaphragm moves outward. Breathe in slowly and exhale slowly to a count of ten. Repeat this a number of times while noticing your body becoming more relaxed with each breath. It may help to repeat silently in your mind, "My body is calm and relaxed."
- After your breathing has become slow and even, focus your attention on the left side of your chest where your heart is located. Picture there a symbol you associate with love, such as a flower or some other object. If you visualize a flower, imagine it starting out as a bud and opening up into a full blossom.
- As you breathe in and out, see the flower or other object symbolic of your heart radiating love outward through your chest.
- Imagine some person to whom you want to send your love or deep feeling of compassion. Use your imagination to surround that person with the rays of your love and caring.
- Make the feeling of love or compassion as profound as you can. Feel the warmth of it in your chest.
- Realize that this love can be sent both to people whom you truly love as well as to people with whom you feel angry or frustrated. Use your imagination to beam your love and caring feelings to the person whose image you have in your mind. You may want to visualize the person at work or at home and see how the person responds to the feelings you are sending.
- Feeling and sharing love and compassion with others help to keep you emotionally and spiritually well.

Exercise 3
Progressive Muscular Relaxation

The following is a slight variation of a stress-reduction technique developed by a physician, Edmund Jacobson, in 1929, in Chicago. Our technique involves deliberately tensing various muscles in the body to varying degrees. For each area of the body listed in this exercise, tense the muscles for about five seconds (1) as hard as you can, (2) about half as hard as the first time, and (3) just the slightest tension. In so doing, you train your mind to recognize varying degrees of tension in different parts of the body and, more important, how to relax the tension. After performing these exercises for a while, your mind automatically recognizes tension building up in different parts of your body, and that awareness leads to relaxation of the tension.

In this exercise, we describe how to tense and relax various parts of the body that most commonly accumulate tension. After you have practiced progressive muscle relaxation exercises for a while, you can apply the same principles to any area of your body that needs to learn how to relax.

Jaws

Take a moment to feel the muscles of your jaws. Notice any tension, even the slightest amount. The jaw muscles can harbor a lot of undetected muscle tension. Now consciously tense the muscles of your jaws really tight, as tight as you can and hold it, even tighter, hold it. Now relax these muscles, exhale, and sense the tension disappear completely. You may even feel your mouth begin to open a little. Feel the difference between how these muscles feel now, compared with what you just experienced at 100% contraction. Feel the absence of tension. Now, contract these same muscles, but at half the full intensity, a 50% contraction. Hold the tension, keep holding, and now relax again. Feel how relaxed these muscles are. Compare this feeling of relaxation with what you felt before. By comparing the difference in tension levels, a greater sense of relaxation will surface. Once again, contract these same muscles, but with only a 5% contraction. A 5% contraction is a very slight twinge, with no motion whatsoever, just the acknowledgment that these muscles can contract. Now hold it, keep holding, and relax. Release any remaining tension so that these muscles are completely loose and relaxed. And sense just how relaxed these muscles are. To enhance this feeling of relaxation, take a comfortably slow, deep breath and sense how relaxed your jaw muscles have become.

Shoulders

Concentrate on the muscles of your shoulders and isolate these from the surrounding neck and upper arm muscles. Take a moment to sense these muscles. The shoulder muscles can hold a lot of undetected muscle tension resulting in stiffness. Symbolically, your shoulders carry the weight of all your thoughts, the weight of your worries and concerns. Now, consciously tense the muscles of your shoulder really tight, as tight as you can and hold it, even tighter, hold it. Now relax these muscles and sense the tension disappear completely. Sense the difference between how these muscles feel now compared with what you just experienced at 100% contraction. Once again, contract these same muscles, but this time only half as tight, a 50% contraction. Hold the tension, keep holding, and now completely relax these muscles. Sense how relaxed your shoulder muscles are. Compare this feeling of relaxation with what you felt before. By comparing the difference in tension levels, a greater sense of relaxation will surface. Finally, contract these same muscles at only 5%. A 5% contraction is a very slight twinge, with no motion whatsoever—just the acknowledgment that these muscles can contract, just a sense of the clothing touching the shoulder muscles. Now hold it, keep holding, and relax. Release any remaining tension so that these muscles are completely loose and relaxed. To enhance this feeling of relaxation, take a slow, deep breath and sense how relaxed your shoulder muscles have become.

Hands and Forearms

Concentrate on the muscles of your hands and forearms. Take a moment to feel these muscles, including your fingers, palms, wrists, and forearms. Notice the slightest bit of tension. Now consciously tense the muscles of each hand and forearm really tight by making a fist as tight as you can and hold it, as if you're going to punch something. Now release the fist and relax these muscles. Sense the tension disappear completely. Open the palm of each hand slowly, extend your fingers, and let them recoil just a bit. Sense the difference between how relaxed these muscles feel now compared with what you just experienced at 100% contraction. They should feel very relaxed. Now contract these same muscles at half the intensity, a 50% contraction. Hold the tension, keep holding, and now relax again. Sense how relaxed these muscles are. Compare this feeling of relaxation with what you felt before. By comparing the difference between tension

and relaxation, a more profound sense of relaxation will surface. Now, barely contract these same muscles. A slight contraction is like holding an empty, delicate eggshell in the palm of your hand. Try to imagine that. Now hold it, keep holding, and relax. Release any remaining tension so that hand and arm muscles are completely relaxed. To enhance this feeling of relaxation, take a slow, deep breath and sense how relaxed your forearm and hand muscles have become.

Abdominals

Really focus your attention on your abdominal muscles. Take a moment to sense any residual tension in either the muscles or organs of the abdomen. Now consciously tense your abdominal muscles really tight as if someone is about to punch you in the stomach and you want to block that punch. Contract as tight as you can and hold it, even tighter, hold it. Now relax these muscles and sense the tension disappear completely. Feel the complete absence of tension. Compare the difference between how these muscles feel now with what you just experienced at 100% contraction. Once again contract these same muscles, this time at half the full intensity. A 50% contraction is like preparing for a false stomach punch. You know they won't make contact, but just in case you want to be ready. Hold the tension, keep holding, and now relax again. Feel how relaxed these muscles are. Compare this feeling of relaxation with what you felt before. When you compare the difference between tension levels and this current state of relaxation, a greater sense of relaxation will follow. Finally, contract these same muscles so slightly you barely feel the clothing over your stomach area. Now hold it, keep holding, and relax. Release any remaining tension so that these muscles are completely relaxed. Sense just how relaxed these muscles have become. To enhance this feeling of relaxation, take a slow, deep breath and feel how relaxed your abdominal region has become.

Feet

Focus your attention on the muscles of your feet. Typically the muscles of the feet are not tense, but standing can produce a lot of tension. In addition, in the confinement of shoes, feet muscles become tense. Now consciously contract the muscles of your feet by scrunching your toes really tight, as tight as you can. Hold it, even tighter, hold it. Now relax these muscles and sense the tension disappear completely. You may even feel your feet become warm as they relax. Feel the difference between how these muscles feel now as compared with when they were tense. Once again contract these same muscles at half the tension. Hold the tension, keep holding, and now relax again. Compare this feeling of relaxation with the tension you felt at full tension. By comparing the difference in tension levels, a greater sense of relaxation will surface. Now, contract these same muscles only slightly. Now hold it, keep holding, and relax. Release any remaining tension so that these muscles are completely relaxed. Sense just how completely relaxed these muscles are. To enhance this feeling of relaxation, take a slow, deep breath and feel how relaxed your feet and whole body are now. Your whole body feels completely relaxed and calm.

Now lie still, and enjoy the complete feeling of relaxation.

Exercise 4
Hatha Yoga Postures *(Asanas)*

Yoga has been used for centuries as a way to relax the mind and body and to promote health and spiritual well-being. The following hatha yoga postures (or *asanas*) were chosen and arranged to reflect a typical yoga class. Each position should be done slowly and without pain. Go only as far into the posture as you can while maintaining full complete breaths. It is very important to breathe through each posture. Hold each posture for at least 30 seconds. If you feel any pain (especially in your knees or lower back), ease out of the pose until the pain subsides. Do not judge yourself. Yoga is not about reaching an ideal or being competitive; it is about moving your body, listening to your body, and increasing your flexibility over time.

If you find these postures enjoyable and helpful in reducing tension, you may want to enroll in a yoga class because it is very helpful to have an instructor. Also, DVDs are available that allow you to follow a course of instruction in your own home at your own convenience.

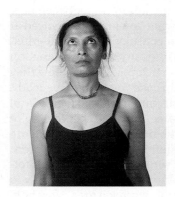
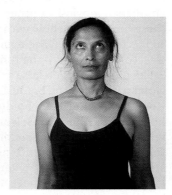

Eye Exercises Sitting comfortably on a chair or on the floor, lengthen the spine and relax the facial muscles. Be sure to breathe normally throughout the exercises. Without moving the head, move the eyes slowly and smoothly: (1) look up and keep looking up without blinking for a couple breaths and then look down and hold for a couple breaths; return to a neutral gaze; (2) look to the right and hold, and then to the left and hold; return to a neutral gaze; (3) slowly circle the eyes clockwise and then counterclockwise. Finish by rubbing the palms together quickly and vigorously to create heat and lightly cup the palms over closed eyes to soothe and relax them.

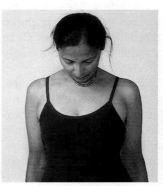
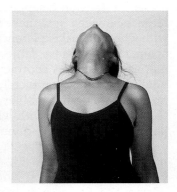
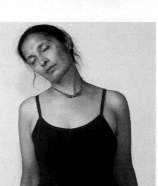
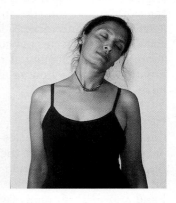

Neck Exercises (1) Keeping the torso upright, gently and slowly move the head forward, easing the back neck muscles long. Use the weight of the head to lengthen the muscles as you breathe easily in and out. Roll the head back up and tilt it on the top of the spine (which is at the level of the ears) as you gently ease the chin up toward the ceiling, allowing the head to tilt back only as far as is comfortable. Be careful not to crunch the neck; keep those muscles long. Roll back up and repeat forward and backward several times. (2) Tilt the head to the right, easing the right ear toward the right shoulder. Keep the shoulders level while you breathe through the stretch. Repeat to the left side.

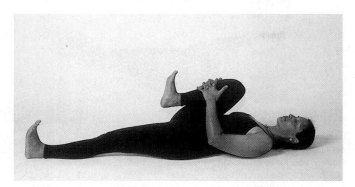

Wind Relieving Pose *(Pavanmuktasana)* Lie on your back, spreading your back along the floor. Bring the right knee toward the head and the right thigh toward the chest. Grasp the knee or behind the knee to pull the leg in closer, as you lengthen the left leg along the floor. Breathe easily in and out while you stay in this position. Bring the left knee up and in as you lengthen the right leg along the floor. Breathe easily in and out while you stay in this position.

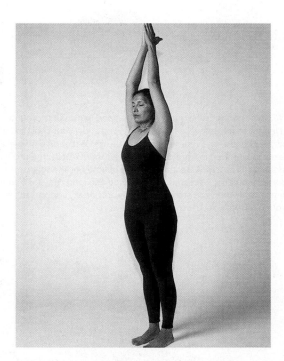

Mountain *(Tadasana)* Stand comfortably with your feet hip-width apart as you lengthen your head up off the top of the spine. Feel the weight of your arms dropping down and out to the sides of your body. Allow the arms to lengthen out wide to the sides as you float them up overhead, palms facing each other. (Be sure not to arch your back. If your back is arched, bring your hands out in front of you. Also, don't lock your knees.) Take a few easy sufficient breaths and gradually release the arms out and down to the sides.

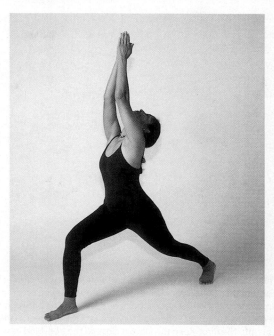

Warrior *(Virabhadrasana)* Come into Mountain pose and inhale an easy breath. Exhale on a "ha" sound as you step forward with your right leg into a lunge position. Check that your right knee is directly over your right foot (front to back and side to side). Straighten your left leg behind you as you ease the left heel toward the ground. Breathe easily a few times. If you feel comfortable, you can bring a slight arch in your back and look up at the ceiling. Lean forward over your right leg with your arms and trunk as you step your left foot forward to join your right and return to Mountain pose. Notice the sensations in your body as you allow the arms to float back down to your sides. Repeat with the left leg forward and the right leg behind.

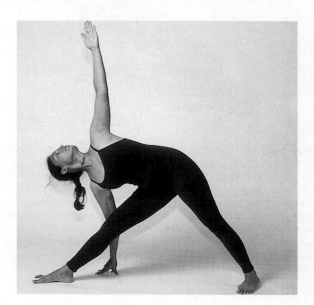

Triangle *(Trikonasana)* Come into Mountain pose. Step lightly to the right so your feet are about three feet apart and bring your arms out to the side at shoulder height, palms facing down. Rotate the right leg out from the hip joint to turn the knee and foot to the right. Inhale, and as you exhale, ease your hips to the left as you reach out with your right fingertips as far as you can. Find ease as you inhale. Exhale as you rotate the arms, the left up toward the ceiling and the right down toward your leg, palms facing forward. Turn the head to look up at your left hand. Continue to breathe. If you cannot breathe easily, bring your torso up a little. Return slowly to the upright position and repeat on the left side.

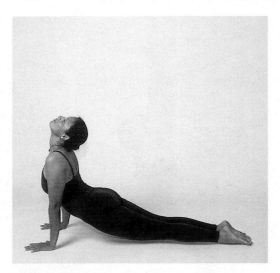

Cobra (Bhujangasana) Lie comfortably on the floor on your stomach, with your legs together. Soften your body into the ground as you breathe. Bring the palms to the floor under your shoulders, keeping wide between the shoulder blades. Lengthen your head forward and roll up, gently pressing the palms into the floor. Keep the elbows close to the body and ease the shoulders down, away from the ears. (Don't crunch the lower back. If you have any pain, be sure to come back down.) Breathe in and out a few times and ease down keeping the spine long.

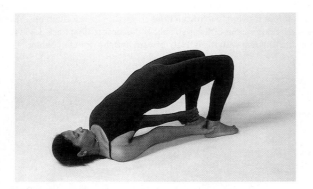

Bridge (Setu bandhasana) Lie on your back with your knees bent. Spread your shoulder blades wide and ease your lower back onto the floor. Slide your heels toward your buttocks, hip-width apart. Begin to lift your buttocks off the ground, sending your knees forward over your feet and gradually roll the back up off the ground toward the neck and shoulders. Clasp the hands underneath as you begin to straighten the elbows and ease the shoulder blades together behind you. Allow the breath to flow in and out with ease as you maintain this position. To come out of the pose, separate the hands, widen the shoulders and back, and slowly roll the back down onto the ground.

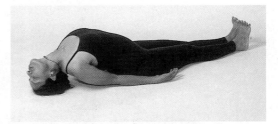

Fish (Matsyasana) Lie on your wide, long back with your legs together in front of you. Place your hands close together under your buttocks, palms down, arms straight, and elbows as close together as possible. Allowing the head to roll back, press your elbows into the ground as you expand your chest and torso forward and up, gently resting the crown of the head on the ground, and lengthening the front of your neck. Keep lengthening and expanding the torso as you breathe. Ease the heels of the feet forward and when you are ready, tuck the chin forward and slowly ease your back onto the ground. Release the arms out to the sides and rest, making note of the movement of your breath.

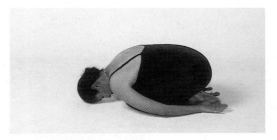

Child (Gharbasana) Come onto your knees and gently sit on your heels as you lengthen the spine. Lean forward as you allow your chest to come toward your knees. Rest your forehead on the ground or on a pillow. Allow your arms to lengthen in front of you, then let them rest on the ground. Soften the facial muscles, feel the massage of your organs against your thighs as you breathe. Spread your back wide and long. Stay for a couple of minutes, and when you are ready, gently and slowly support the torso with your hands as you return to kneeling.

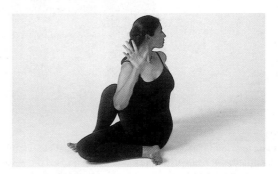

Spinal Twist (Matsyendrasana) Before you begin, sit with legs extended straight out in front of you. (If you can't sit comfortably, with your back straight, you may want to sit on the edge of a cushion or rolled up towel or blanket.) Then bend the left leg and put it to the right of your right knee. Bring the left knee as close to you as you can while keeping the foot on the floor. Grab the left knee in the crook of your right arm and pull on the arm to help bring your torso forward and up. Keep the right leg extended in front of you, opening the knee toward the floor, with the foot flexed. Inhale and bring the left arm out to the side at shoulder height and with palm down. As you exhale, take your arm, eyes, and head to the left, rotating slowly through the entire spine. Place the left arm down on the floor, close to your body, and support yourself into a more upright position. Follow the movement of your body as you breathe. Ease back out by unwinding the spinal rotation. Repeat on the other side, left leg down, right knee up, and twisting to the right.

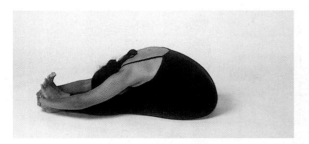

Stretch of the West *(Paschimottanasana)* Find comfort in sitting, with legs together and extended straight out in front of you. (If you can't sit comfortably, with your back straight, you may want to sit on the edge of a cushion or rolled up towel or blanket.) Put your fists on the floor next to your hips and press them into the ground as you lengthen your torso up. Keep the spine long and, without curving the back, ease your way forward by bending in your hip joints. Go only as far as you can with a straight back and be careful not to roll the shoulders forward. Open the backs of the knees into the floor, bring the toes toward you, and find ease in the body as you breathe. Notice where you feel sensation and slowly float the head and torso back up.

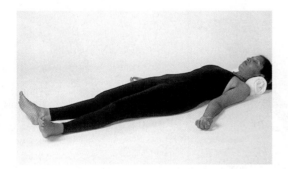

Corpse *(Savasana)* Slowly lower yourself onto your back. Resting on the floor, lengthen the neck muscles as you ease the head away from your feet. Wrap your arms around yourself and grasp your shoulder blades, easing them out to the sides. Lower the arms to the floor about 30 degrees out from the sides of the body, palms facing up. Gently press the lower back into the floor, then release it, allowing the natural curve of the spine to return. Lengthen the heels away from your torso, and let the heels roll out from the hips, feet opening out. Scan the body to find any areas of tension and let it go: in the face muscles, neck, shoulders, arms, torso, buttocks, abdomen and pelvis, legs, and feet. Rest here for at least 10 minutes as you follow the flow of your breath.

Exercise 5
T'ai Chi Movements

T'ai chi forms are sets of movements varying in length from five minutes to nearly one hour. The example illustrated here is an excerpt from a Yang style form. The orientation of the body is described in terms of north, south, east, and west directions. When starting, you should be facing north. Keep in mind that although the exercise is described as a series of steps, the movement is continuous.

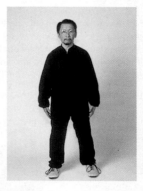

Starting Position Stand erect with feet shoulder-width apart, arms by your side, palms in toward the legs, chin up, and eyes looking directly ahead.

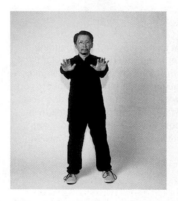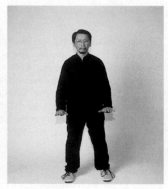

Beginning Position Leading with the wrists, raise your arms directly in front of the body to about shoulder level. Elbows should be slightly bent and shoulders relaxed. Leading with the elbows, slowly allow your arms and hands to return to starting position below waist level.

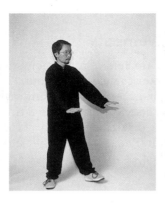
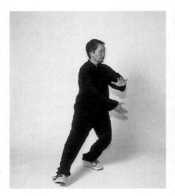
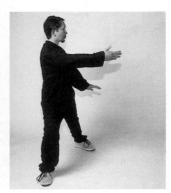

Right Hand Ward-Off   With your weight on your right foot, pivot your body left about 90 degrees. Keep your arms in front of you, palms down and at waist level. Once you've rotated your body, shift your weight to your left foot, bending at the knee. Bring your left hand up to mid-chest level, keeping the palm turned down. Keep your right hand at waist level but turn your palm up, keeping space between your hands. Step north with the right foot. Shifting your weight back to the right leg, extend your right arm and raise your right hand to shoulder level. Lower your left hand to waist level, keeping your palm down and your arm extended.

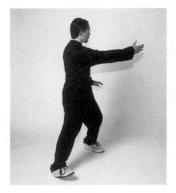
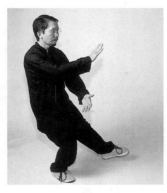
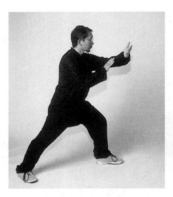
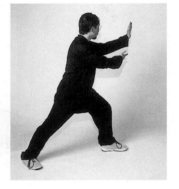

Left Hand Ward-Off   Shift your weight back to your left foot, bending at the knee. Pivoting on your right heel, bring your right foot in slightly toward your body. Move your right arm, bringing your arm and hand up to chin level and keeping your arm outstretched. Shift your weight to your right leg, bending at the knee. Set the left foot on its heel, pointing west. Turn the palm of your right hand outward and start pulling your arm in toward your chest, bending at the elbow. Pull your left arm across your body so that it is underneath your right arm, and turn the palm inward.

Grasp the Bird's Tail   Shift your weight forward to your left foot. While doing this movement, bring your left arm, still curved, across your body with the palm facing inward at chin level. Keep your right hand in front of you, palm facing outward. Turn the left hand out to face forward while pushing outward with both arms.

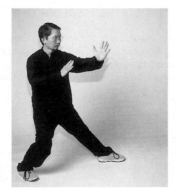
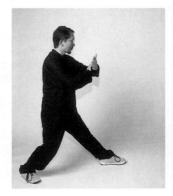
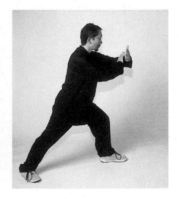

Rollback and Press   Shift your weight backward onto your right leg, bending at the knee, and rotate your body to the right. Pull your right arm back toward your chest, bending at the elbow and keeping your palm facing the same direction as your body and at shoulder height. Rotate your body to the left, keeping your right arm close to your chest. Pull your left arm across your body and bring your palm toward your right hand as if the two were touching. As you shift your weight forward onto your left leg, push through the movement by pushing both arms forward in front of your body as if the right arm were pushing the left arm out at the wrist.

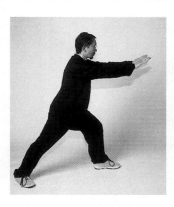 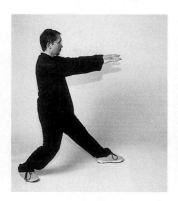 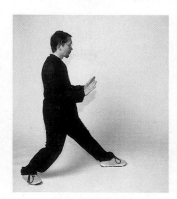 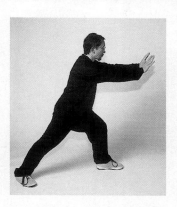

Push Continue to lean forward and extend your arms, turning both palms down with fingers pointing slightly upward. Release the wrists so the palms face down and pull back, shifting your weight to your right leg. Leading with your elbows, pull both arms down and toward your stomach. With your elbows bent, your forearms should be parallel to the floor with your palms facing forward. Shift your weight forward onto your left leg and extend your arms outward in front of you with palms continuing to face outward, as if you were pushing against a wall.

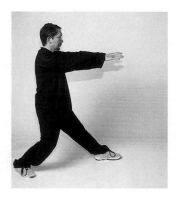 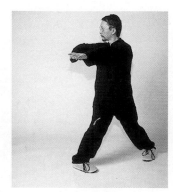

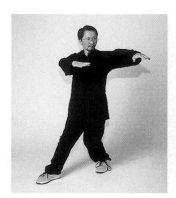 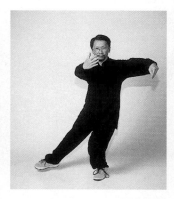 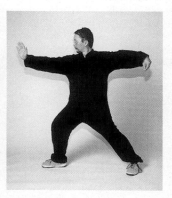

Holding a Single Whip With your arms still outstretched, release your wrists so your palms face the floor. Shift your weight back onto your right leg, bending at the knee. Keeping the right leg bent, pivot on your left heel, turning the foot in 90 degrees. Bend your right arm at the elbow and bring your right hand toward your chest, your palm continuing to face down. Keep your left arm extended out. Shift your weight to your left foot, bending at the knee, and pick up the right foot and step 45 degrees to the right. Keep your arms in the same position and rotate them around with your body. Your left hand points down toward the floor as you continue to shift your weight to your left foot, bringing the right foot off the floor and turning the leg outward (right foot points east). Turn the palm of your right hand to face toward you at chin level. Let the left wrist bend and the four fingers of the hand gather around the thumb to form a beak-hand. Shift your weight to the right onto your right leg and swing your right arm open so the palm faces outward. (The body and palm should now be facing east.) Keep your left arm out behind you.

Calendar of Events and Health Organizations

January

National Volunteer Blood Donor Month
American Association of Blood Banks
8101 Glenbrook Road
Bethesda, MD 20814
301-907-6977
www.aabb.org
Contact: Public Relations

February

American Heart Month
American Heart Association
7272 Greenville Avenue
Dallas, TX 75231
800-AHA-USA1
www.americanheart.org
Contact: Local chapters

National Children's Dental Health Month
American Dental Association
211 E. Chicago Avenue
Chicago, IL 60611
312-440-2593
www.ada.org
Contact: Public Information

National Child Passenger Safety Awareness Week
U.S. Department of Transportation
National Highway Traffic Safety Administration
400 Seventh Street, SW
Washington, DC 20590
202-366-0123
www.nhtsa.dot.gov

March

Hemophilia Month
National Hemophilia Foundation
116 West 32nd Street
11th Floor
New York, NY 10001
800-42-HANDI
www.hemophilia.org

National Kidney Month
National Kidney Foundation
30 E. 33rd Street, Suite 1100
New York, NY 10016
800-622-9010
www.kidney.org
Contact: Local chapters

National Chronic Fatigue Syndrome Awareness Month
**National Chronic Fatigue Immune Dysfunction
   Syndrome Foundation**
3521 Broadway
Suite 222
Kansas City, MO 64111
816-931-4777
www.ncf-net.org

National Nutrition Month
Academy of Nutrition and Dietetics
120 South Riverside Plaza
Suite 2000
Chicago, IL 60606-6995
800-877-1600
www.eatright.org

Red Cross Month
American Red Cross
National Headquarters
431 18th Street, NW
Washington, DC 20006
www.redcross.org
Contact: Public Inquiries

National Poison Prevention Week
Poison Prevention Week Council
4330 East West Highway
Bethesda, MD 20814
301-504-0580 x1184
www.poisonprevention.org
Third full week in March

April

National Alcohol Awareness Month
National Council on Alcoholism and Drug Dependence
20 Exchange Place, Suite 2902
New York, NY 10005
212-269-7797
www.ncadd.org

Cancer Control Month
American Cancer Society
1599 Clifton Road, NE
Atlanta, GA 30329-4251
800-ACS-2345
www.cancer.org
Contact: Local chapters

National Child Abuse Prevention Month
Prevent Child Abuse America
228 South Wabash Avenue, 10th Floor
Chicago, IL 60604
312-663-3520
www.preventchildabuse.org

Alcohol-Free Weekend
Rhode Island Council on Alcoholism and Drug Dependence
500 Prospect Street
Pawtucket, RI 02860
800-622-7422

World Health Day
American Association for World Health
1825 K Street, NW
Suite 1208
Washington, DC 20006
202-466-5883
www.thebody.com/aawh/aawhpage.html

National Minority Cancer Awareness Week
National Cancer Institute
NCI Public Inquiries Office
Suite 3036A
6116 Executive Boulevard, MSC8322
Bethesda, MD 20892-8322
800-4-CANCER (Cancer Information Service)
www.cancer.gov

May

Clean Air Month
American Lung Association
61 Broadway, 6th Floor
New York, NY 10006
212-315-8700
www.lungusa.org

Mental Health Month
Mental Health America
2001 N. Beauregard Street, 12th Floor
Alexandria, VA 22311
703-684-7722
www.nmha.org

National High Blood Pressure Month
National Heart, Lung, and Blood Institute
P.O. Box 30105
Bethesda, MD 20824-0105
301-592-8573
www.nhlbi.nih.gov

National Physical Fitness and Sport Month
President's Council on Fitness, Sports & Nutrition
200 Independence Avenue, SW
Humphrey Building, Room 738H
Washington, DC 20201
202-690-9000
www.fitness.gov

Older Americans Month
Administration on Aging
One Massachusetts Avenue
Suites 4100 & 5100
Washington, DC 20201
202-619-0724
www.aoa.gov

National Employee Health and Fitness Day
National Association for Health and Fitness
401 West Michigan Street
Suite 560
Indianapolis, IN 46202-3233
317-955-0957
www.physicalfitness.org
Third Wednesday in May

World No Tobacco Day
World Health Organization World No Tobacco Day
P.O. Box 3543
New York, NY 10163
212-601-8245
www.who.int/tobacco/wntd/en

June

Dairy Month
American Dairy Association
Interstate Place II
100 Elwood Davis Road
North Syracuse, NY 13212
315-472-9143
www.adadc.com

National Safety Week
American Society of Safety Engineers
1800 E. Oakton Street
Des Plaines, IL 60018-2187
847-699-2929
www.asse.org

July

National Therapeutic Recreation Week
National Therapeutic Recreation Society
22377 Belmont Ridge Road
Ashburn, VA 20148
703-858-0784
www.recreationtherapy.com

August

National Water Quality Month
Culligan International
One Culligan Parkway
Northbrook, IL 60062
847-205-6000
www.culligan.com

September

National Cholesterol Education Month
National Cholesterol Education Program
Program Information Center
P.O. Box 30105
Bethesda, MD 20824-0105
301-592-8573
www.ncbi.nlm.nih.gov
Contact: Information Center

National Sickle Cell Month
Sickle Cell Disease Association of America
200 Corporate Pointe
Suite 495
Culver City, CA 90230-8727
800-421-8453
www.sicklecelldisease.org

Treatment Works Month
**National Clearinghouse for Alcohol
   and Drug Information**
P.O. Box 2345
Rockville, MD 20852
800-729-6686
www.samhsa.gov

October

Domestic Violence Awareness Month
National Coalition Against Domestic Violence
1120 Lincoln Street
Denver, CO 80203
www.ncadv.org

Family Health Month
American Academy of Family Physicians
11400 Tomahawk Creek Parkway
Leawood, KS 66211-2672
800-274-2237
www.aafp.org

National Breast Cancer Awareness Month
Susan G. Komen Breast Cancer Foundation
5005 LBJ Freeway
Suite 250
Dallas, TX 75244
972-855-1600
www.komen.org

National Collegiate Alcohol Awareness Week
**Interassociation Task Force on Campus Alcohol and
   Other Substance Abuse Issues**
P.O. Box 100430
Denver, CO 80250
www.collegesubstanceabuseprevention.org
Starts the third Sunday in October

World Food Day
National Committee for World Food Day
2175 K Street, NW
Washington, DC 20437
202-653-2404
www.worldfooddayusa.org

American Heart Association's HeartFest
American Heart Association
7272 Greenville Avenue
Dallas, TX 75231
800-AHA-USA1
www.heart.org
Contact: Local chapters

National Adult Immunization Awareness Week
**National Coalition for Adult Immunization
   and National Foundation for Infectious Diseases**
4733 Bethesda Avenue
Suite 750
Bethesda, MD 20814-5278
301-656-0003
www.nfid.org
Last full week in October

November

National Alzheimer's Awareness Month
Alzheimer's Association
225 N. Michigan Avenue
Suite 1700
Chicago, IL 60601-7633
800-272-3900
www.alz.org

Great American Smokeout
American Cancer Society
1599 Clifton Road, NE
Atlanta, GA 30329-4251
800-ACS-2345
www.cancer.org
Contact: Local chapters

December

National Drunk and Drugged Driving Prevention Month
National Coalition Against Drunk Driving
8403 Colesville Road, Suite 370
Silver Spring, MD 20910
240-247-6004
www.ncadd.com

World AIDS Day
American Association for World Health
1825 K Street, NW
Suite 1208
Washington, DC 20006
202-466-5883
www.thebody.com/aawh/aawhpage.html

GLOSSARY

A

abortion: the expulsion or extraction of the products of conception from the uterus before the embryo or fetus is capable of independent life; abortions may be spontaneous or induced

accident: sequence of events that produces unintended injury, death, or property damage; refers to the event, not the result of the event

accident mitigation: methods to reduce damage caused by unplanned events

accident prevention: ways to eliminate the occurrence of unintended injuries

acetaldehyde: a toxic substance produced when the liver breaks down alcohol

acquaintance rape: (also known as "date rape") sexual assault occurring when the victim and the rapist are known to each other and may have previously interacted in some socially appropriate manner

acquired immune deficiency syndrome (AIDS): a syndrome of more than two dozen diseases caused by HIV

acupuncture: an ancient Chinese alternative medicine that uses thin needles inserted into specific points on the body to produce healing energy

addiction: physical and psychological dependence on a drug, substance, or behavior

adult attention deficit hyperactivity disorder (ADHD): difficulty focusing on activities, organizing and finishing tasks, managing one's time, following instructions, and/or being overly restless, "on the go," and perceived as not thinking before acting or speaking

advance directive: legal documents that express your desires regarding treatments should you be unable to communicate. A living will and a healthcare power of attorney constitute an advance directive

adverse drug reactions (ADRs): unintended, unpleasant, and/or harmful reactions to a medicinal product

aerobic: biological energy production using oxygen

aerobic training: exercise that increases the body's capacity to use oxygen

afterbirth: placenta and fetal membranes

age-related hearing loss: loss of hearing with advancing age; some loss of hearing may be caused by exposure to loud noise earlier in life

age-related macular degeneration (AMD): loss of vision as a result of death of cells in a region of the eye called the macula; loss of vision progresses slowly over several years

agency: the belief that one can influence the nature and quality of one's life, rather than believing that one's fate is determined by reacting to circumstances not in one's control

aging: normal changes in body functions that begin after sexual maturity and continue until death

alcoholism: loss of control over drinking alcohol

alcohol use disorder: alcohol consumption that causes distress or harm; also known as alcoholism or alcohol abuse

allergens: foreign substances that trigger an allergic response by the immune system

alternative medicine: a therapy or healing procedure that is used *instead* of Western, scientific medical treatments

alveoli: tiny air sacs in the lungs that exchange oxygen and carbon dioxide

Alzheimer's disease (AD): a common cause of senile dementia and other symptoms, eventually leading to death

amenorrhea: cessation of menstruation in a woman of reproductive age

amino acids: compounds containing nitrogen that are the building blocks of proteins and some neurotransmitters

amniocentesis: a procedure that involves aspiration of amniotic fluid from the uterus to detect certain abnormalities in the fetus

amnion: the inner membrane that forms a fluid-filled sac surrounding and protecting the embryo and fetus

amniotic fluid: fluid in the amniotic sac

amphetamines: synthetic drugs that stimulate the central nervous system and sometimes produce hallucinogenic states

amyloid protein: an abnormal protein in the brain of patients with Alzheimer's disease

anaerobic: biological energy production without using oxygen

anaphylactic shock: a severe allergic reaction involving the whole body that can cause death

androgenic anabolic steroids: synthetic male hormones used to increase muscle size and strength

aneurysm: a ballooning out of a vein or artery

angina pectoris: medical term for chest pain caused by coronary heart disease; a condition in which the heart muscle doesn't receive enough blood, resulting in chest pain

anogenital warts: hard growths caused by an infection with human papillomavirus (HPV) that appear on the skin of the genitals or anus

anorexia nervosa: disorder occurring most commonly in adolescent females, characterized by abnormal body image, fear of obesity, and prolonged refusal to eat, sometimes resulting in death

antibodies: proteins that recognize and inactivate viruses, bacteria, and other organisms and toxic substances that enter the body

antigens: foreign proteins on infectious organisms that stimulate an antibody response

antioxidants: substances that in small amounts inhibit the oxidation of other compounds

anxiety: the fear of an imaginary threat

aorta: the large artery that transports blood from the heart to the body

aromatherapy: use of fragrant extracts of plants to promote healing

arteries: any of a series of blood vessels that carry blood from the heart to all parts of the body

arteriosclerosis: hardening of the arteries

arthritis: a variety of chronic diseases involving inflammation, stiffness, and pain in joints of the body

artificial insemination: introduction of semen into the uterus or oviduct by other than natural means

asthma: a chronic disease involving inflammation and narrowing of the airways that makes it difficult to breathe

atherosclerosis: a disease process in which fatty deposits (plaques) build up in the arteries and block the flow of blood

atrial fibrillation ("a-fib"): rapid, erratic contraction of the upper chambers of the heart

autism spectrum disorder (ASD): a group of conditions characterized by degrees of impairment in interpersonal interaction

autogenic training: the use of autosuggestion to establish a balance between the mind and body through changes in the autonomic nervous system

autoimmune diseases: mistakes in the functioning of the immune system that cause it to attack tissues in the body

autonomic nervous system: the special group of nerves that control some of the body's organs and their functions

average life span: the age at which half the members of a population have died

Ayurvedic medicine: a traditional form of preventive medicine and healing involving mind, body, and spirit, practiced in India for thousands of years. Ayurveda is spreading to Western countries

B

B cells: cells of the immune system that produce antibodies

bacterial vaginosis (BV): infection of the vagina

bariatric surgery: weight loss surgery

basal body temperature (BBT) method: uses daily body temperature readings taken immediately after waking to identify the time of ovulation; approximately 24 hours after ovulation, the BBT increases

basal cell carcinoma: a form of skin cancer that usually can be removed surgically

basal metabolic rate (BMR): the amount of energy needed per day to keep the body functioning while at rest

basal metabolism: the minimum amount of energy needed to keep the body alive

bender: several days of continued drinking

benign tumor: a tumor whose cells do not spread to other parts of the body

bidis: small, thin, hand-rolled cigarettes

binge eating disorder: an uncontrolled consumption of large quantities of food in a short period of time, even if the person does not feel hungry

biofeedback: using an electronic device to "feed back" information about the body to alter a particular physiological function

biomagnetic therapy: use of magnetic fields to treat pain, ailments, and diseases

biomonitoring: measurement of environmental chemicals present in the body that may harm health

biopsy: removal of cells from a tumor for examination under a microscope

bipolar disorder: episodes of depression followed by episodes of mania

birth defect: an anatomical or functional abnormality present at birth that is inherited or caused by the effects of a chemical, such as alcohol

bisphenol-A (BPA): chemical used to manufacture polycarbonate plastics; may cause abnormal brain development in fetuses and birth defects

blackout: failure to recall normal or abnormal behavior or events that occurred while drinking

blood alcohol content (BAC): the amount of alcohol in the blood

blood pressure: measurement of the force with which the heart pushes blood through the circulatory system

body composition: the relative amounts of the body's major components

body dysmorphic disorder: a preoccupation with an imagined defect in one or more of one's body parts

body image: a person's mental image of his or her body

body mass index (BMI): a measure of body fatness, calculated by dividing body weight (in kilograms) by the square of height (in meters)

Braxton-Hicks contractions: normal uterine contractions that occur periodically throughout pregnancy

breasts: a network of milk glands and ducts in fatty tissue

bronchitis: inflammation of the bronchi of the lungs as a result of irritation; often accompanied by a chronic cough

bulimia: serious disorder, especially common in adolescents and young women, marked by excessive eating, often followed by self-induced vomiting, purging, or fasting

bullying: unwanted, aggressive behavior among school-aged children that involves a real or perceived power imbalance

burden of disease: the gap between the ideal of living to old age in good health and the current situation in which life is shortened by illness

C

C-reactive protein (CRP): a protein in blood that is a measure of chronic inflammation and risk of a heart attack

caffeine: a natural stimulant found in a variety of plants; commonly found in tea, coffee, chocolate, and soft drinks

calendar rhythm: estimation of fertile, or unsafe, days to have intercourse

calorie: the amount of energy required to raise 1 g of water from 14.5°C to 15.5°C

calorie dense: food items that contain considerable calories but are of little nutritional value

cancer: unregulated multiplication of cells in the body

cancer susceptibility gene: gene responsible for familial breast cancer and genes that cause susceptibility to colorectal cancer; increases the risk of a person developing cancer in his or her lifetime

capillaries: extremely small blood vessels that carry oxygenated blood to tissues

carbohydrates: the main source of biological energy; biological molecules consisting of one or more sugar molecules

carcinogens: substances that can cause cancer in people and other animals

cardiac catheterization: visualization of blocked coronary arteries by using a catheter and monitoring blood flow in coronary arteries; a dye is injected through the catheter

cardiologist: a physician who specializes in diseases of the heart

cardiopulmonary resuscitation (CPR): an emergency lifesaving procedure used to revive someone who has stopped breathing or suffered cardiac arrest

cardiorespiratory fitness: the degree to which the body can supply sufficient fuel and oxygen to produce sustained, effortful physical activity

cardiovascular disease (CVD): any disease that causes damage to the heart or the body's blood vessels

carotid endarterectomy: removal of fatty deposits in arteries in the neck to prevent a stroke

cell-mediated immunity: the response of T cells to infections

cellulose: a carbohydrate forming the skeleton of most plant structures and plant cells; the most abundant polysaccharide in nature and the source of dietary fiber

cervical cap: small latex cap that covers the cervix, used with spermicidal jelly or cream inside the cap

cervix: the lower, narrow end of the uterus

cesarean section (C-section): delivery of the fetus through a surgical opening in the abdomen and uterus

challenge situations: positive events that may involve major life transitions and may cause stress

chancre: the primary lesion of syphilis, which appears as a hard, painless sore or ulcer, often on the penis or vaginal tissue

chemical carcinogen: a chemical that damages cells and causes cancer

chemotherapy: use of toxic chemicals to kill cancer cells and treat some forms of cancer

chewing tobacco: a form of shredded smokeless tobacco; chewed or placed in the mouth between the lower lip and gum

chi: a Chinese term referring to the balance of energy in the body

child abuse: physical or mental injury, sexual abuse or exploitation, maltreatment, or neglect of a child by a person who is responsible for the child's welfare

chiropractic: an alternative medicine that uses manipulation of the spine and joints for healing

chlamydia: a sexually transmitted disease caused by the bacterium *Chlamydia trachomatis*

chlorofluorocarbons (CFCs): chemicals formerly used as coolants that are released into the atmosphere and that are responsible for destroying stratospheric ozone

cholesterol: a fatlike compound occurring in bile, blood, brain, nerve tissue, liver, and other parts of the body

chorionic villus sampling (CVS): a method to detect biochemical disorders and chromosomal abnormalities in the fetus

chromosomes: threadlike structures in the nuclei of cells that carry an individual's genetic information

chronic disease: a disease that persists for years or even a lifetime

chronic obstructive pulmonary diseases (COPD): diseases that restrict the ability of the body to obtain oxygen through the respiratory structures (bronchi and lungs); includes asthma, bronchitis, and emphysema

chronic traumatic encephalopathy: destruction of nerve cells in the brain from repeated brain injury due to collisions and falls

cilia: microscopic hairs in the lining of the bronchial tubes

circumcision: a surgical procedure to remove the foreskin from the penis

clitoris: erotically sensitive organ located above the vaginal opening

club drugs: psychoactive chemicals used at parties, dances, festivals, and raves to enhance social experiences and increase sensory stimulation

cocaine: a stimulant drug, obtained from the leaves of the coca shrub, that causes feelings of exhilaration, euphoria, and physical vigor

codependency: a relationship pattern in which the non-addicted family members identify with the alcoholic

cognition: the act or process of knowing

cognitive behavioral therapy (CBT): treatment of psychological distress by examining and changing thoughts that underlie it

cognitive reframing: choosing to see a situation from a different point of view

colostrum: yellowish liquid secreted from the breasts; contains antibodies and protein

combined hormonal contraceptives: pills, a skin patch, a vaginal insert, and injections that contain two kinds of synthetic hormones that are chemically similar to a woman's natural ovarian hormones, estrogen and progesterone

communicable disease: an infectious disease that is usually transmitted from person to person

complementary medicine: an alternative therapy that is used *along with* conventional medicine. Usually there is some scientific evidence for the effectiveness and safety of the complementary medicine

complex carbohydrates: a class of carbohydrates called polysaccharides; foods composed of starch and cellulose

concussion: a blow to the head that causes injury, temporary loss of consciousness, and possibly a period of amnesia upon awakening

condom: a latex or polyurethane sheath worn over the penis (male condom) or inside the vagina (female condom); can be both a barrier method of contraception and can act as a prophylactic against sexually transmitted diseases

congeners: flavorings, colorings, and other chemicals present in alcoholic beverages

congenital (birth) defect: any abnormality observed in a newborn that occurred during development

contact dermatitis: an allergic reaction of the skin to something that is touched

contraceptive sponge: a dome-shaped device coated with spermicide

contraindication: any medical reason for not taking a particular drug

coping: efforts to manage a stressful situation regardless of whether those efforts are successful

coping strategies: ways people devise to prevent, avoid, or control the emotional distress of unfulfilled needs

coronary arteries: two arteries arising from the aorta that supply blood to the heart muscle

coronary artery bypass graft (CABG): surgery to improve blood supply to the heart muscle by replacing the damaged portion of the artery with a graft

coronary heart disease (CHD): disease caused by fatty deposits in the heart's coronary arteries that impede or completely block the transport of oxygen and nutrients to the heart muscle cells

cosmetic surgery: surgery performed not for any medical condition but solely to enhance appearance or correct visible effects of aging

Cowper's glands: small glands secreting drops of alkalinizing fluid into the urethra

creatine: a natural substance in skeletal muscle tissue required for muscle contraction; which can also be purchased as a dietary supplement

cross-training: incorporating more than one activity into a regular activity plan

cystitis: inflammation of the bladder

cytokines: small molecules that coordinate the activities of B cells and T cells

D

date label: a manufacturer's or a store's assessment of when a food product is at peak quality; not related to when the product poses a potential health risk

decibel: a measure of noise level

defense mechanisms: mental strategies for avoiding unpleasant thoughts and emotions

defibrillator: an electrical device that can restart a heart that has stopped beating by delivering electrical shocks to it

delirium tremens (DTs): hallucinations and uncontrollable shaking caused by withdrawal of alcohol in alcohol-dependent individuals

denial: refusal to admit you (or someone else) have a drinking problem

deoxyribonucleic acid (DNA): a chemical substance that carries genetic information in all cells of all organisms

diagnosis: the cause of a disease or illness as determined by a physician

diaphragm: a soft, rubber, dome-shaped contraceptive device worn over the cervix and used with spermicidal jelly or cream

diastole: the pressure in the arteries when the heart relaxes (the lower number)

Dietary Reference Intakes (DRIs): recommended nutrient intakes intended to prevent chronic disease

dietary supplements: products that provide one or more of the 40 essential nutrients or nonessential vitamins, minerals, enzymes, amino acids, herbs, hormones, and nucleic acids

direct-to-consumer advertising (DTCA): the marketing of prescription drugs to consumers to stimulate demand for a drug

distress: stress resulting from unpleasant stressors

DNA (deoxyribonucleic acid): a chemical substance that carries genetic information in all cells of all organisms

double-blind-placebo controlled trail: when neither the person receiving the drug nor the person administering the drug knows whether patients receive a placebo or the drug

douching: rinsing the vaginal canal with a liquid; not an effective means of birth control or STD prevention

drug: a single chemical substance in a medicine that alters one or more of the body's biological functions

drug abuse: persistent or excessive use of a drug without medical or health reasons

drug hypersensitivity: an allergic reaction to a drug

dysmenorrhea: abdominal pain during menstruation ("menstrual cramps")

dysthymia: a long-lasting, mild form of depression

E

e-cigarettes: electronic devices that deliver via inhaled vapor nicotine, flavorings, and other chemicals; called "vaping"

Ecstasy (MDMA): a club drug with both stimulant and pleasurable effects

ectopic pregnancy: a pregnancy occurring outside the uterus, usually in a fallopian tube

elder abuse: physical, sexual, or emotional maltreatment or financial exploitation of an adult aged 60 or older

electrocardiogram (EKG): a test that shows the rate and rhythm of the heartbeat

electromagnetic fields (EMFs): a form of radiation produced by electrical power lines and appliances that may increase the risk of cancers

embryo: the developing infant during the first two months of conception

embryonic stem cells: cells derived from human fertilized eggs and grown in laboratory dishes; stem cells have the capacity to differentiate into many different tissues and organs

emerging infectious diseases: infections that newly appear, or re-emerge, within a vulnerable population of people or known infections that are suddenly spreading rapidly

emission: amount of substance that is released into the atmosphere

emotion-focused coping: appraising and accepting a stressful situation as not immediately changeable and adopting an attitude that lessens anxiety and brings comfort

emotional wellness: understanding emotions and knowing how to cope with problems that arise in everyday life and how to manage stress

emotions: patterns of brain activity that can arise spontaneously or in response to what is experienced, has been experienced, or believed to be experienced

emphysema: a progressive degeneration of the lung alveoli, causing breathing and oxygen assimilation to become more and more difficult

enabling: denial of, or excuses for, the excessive drinking by an alcoholic to whom one is close

endocrine disruptors: chemical substances in the environment that interfere with the actions of one or more of the body's hormones

endometrium: the inner lining of the uterus

endurance: the ability to move an object without becoming quickly fatigued

energy balance: when energy consumed as food equals the energy expended in living

environment: all external physical factors that affect us

ephedra: an herb that is a stimulant

epidemiology: a branch of science that studies the causes and frequencies of diseases in human populations

episiotomy: an incision in the perineum to facilitate passage of the baby's head during childbirth while minimizing injury to the woman

ergogenic aids: substances used to increase strength and endurance

erythropoetin: a hormone that increases the number of red blood cells, thus increasing the body's ability to carry oxygen to tissues

essential fat: necessary body fat required for normal physiological functioning

essential (primary) hypertension: high blood pressure that is not caused by any observable disease

essential nutrients: chemical substances obtained from food and needed by the body for growth, maintenance, or repair of tissues; not made by the body; must be obtained from food

ethyl alcohol (ethanol): the consumable type of alcohol that is the psychoactive ingredient in alcoholic beverages; often called grain alcohol

etiology: specific cause of disease

eustress: stress resulting from pleasant stressors

exposure: actual amount of the substance people are exposed to

F

failure rate: likelihood of becoming pregnant if using a birth control method for 1 year

fallopian tubes: the usual site of fertilization; a pair of tubelike structures that transport ova from the ovaries to the uterus

familial hyperlipidemia (FH): an inherited disease causing extremely high levels of cholesterol in the blood

fat-soluble vitamins: soluble in fat; there are four fat-soluble vitamins

fat substitutes: chemicals added to packaged foods to provide the taste and texture of fat but few or no calories

fatty acids: naturally occurring in fats, either saturated or unsaturated (monounsaturated or polyunsaturated)

fecal microbiota transplantation (FMT): transplanting fecal material from a healthy donor to the colon of an unwell person to create a healthful change in the patient's intestinal micrombiome

feedback: response of the receiver of a message to let the sender know the message was received

female athlete triad: combination of disordered eating, cessation of menstruation (amenorrhea), and weakened bones (osteoporosis)

fertility awareness methods: methods of birth control in which a couple charts the cyclic signs of the woman's fertility and ovulation, and/or uses basal body temperature, mucus changes, and other signs to determine fertile periods

fertility cycle: the near-monthly production of fertilizable eggs

fertilization: the fusion of a sperm cell and an ovum

fetal alcohol syndrome (FAS): birth defects and mental disabilities caused by ingestion of alcohol by the mother during pregnancy

fiber: a group of compounds that make up the framework of plants; fiber cannot be digested

firearm violence: nonmilitary violence committed with the use of a gun with or without criminal intent

flexibility: the degree to which one can rotate, bend, and twist a part of the body

flight-fight–freeze response: a defensive reaction that prepares the organism for conflict or escape by triggering hormonal, cardiovascular, metabolic, and other changes

first-stage labor: the beginning of labor during which there are regular contractions of the uterus

follicle-stimulating hormone: stimulates ovaries to develop mature follicles (with eggs); the follicle produces estrogen

food allergies: allergic responses to something that has been eaten

foreskin: a fold of skin over the end of the penis

Foundation Health Status: seven categories of health goals that represent the major public health concerns in the United States

fructose: a simple sugar found in fruits and honey

functional food: a food to which additional vitamins, minerals, herbs, or other substances are added to allow the manufacturer to make health claims

fungicide: a chemical that kills fungi and molds

G

gamma-hydroxybutyrate (GHB): a dangerous club drug with unpleasant side effects

gamma irradiation: nonchemical method of food preservation

gastric ulcers: open sores in the stomach from infection by the bacterium *H. pylori*

gender: social classification based on biological sex

gene therapy: a technique for replacing defective genes with normal ones in certain tissues of a person affected with a hereditary disease

general adaptation syndrome (GAS): a three-phase biological response to stress

generalized anxiety disorder: persistent and often non-specific worry and anxiety

genetic counseling: information to help prospective parents evaluate the risks of having or delivering a child with a genetic abnormality

genetic testing: medically supervised procedures that identify changes in chromosomes, genes, or proteins to confirm or rule out a suspected genetic condition or help determine a person's chance of developing or passing on to children a genetic disorder

genetically modified foods: agricultural plants and animals in which one or more genes from different organisms have been inserted also called *genetically modified organisms, or GMOs*

genome editing: a method to precisely add, change, or remove segments of DNA

gerontology: science that studies the causes and mechanisms of aging

glucose: the principal source of energy in all cells; also called *dextrose*

gluten: a mixture of proteins that occur naturally in wheat, rye, barley, and crossbreeds of these grains, which can damage the small intestine

glycogen: the form in which carbohydrate is stored in humans and animals

gonorrhea: sexually transmitted disease caused by gonococcal bacteria (*Neisseria gonorrhoeae*)

greenhouse effect: the ability of atmospheric carbon dioxide to reflect heat radiated from Earth back to Earth and to thereby raise Earth's temperature globally

guided imagery: using verbal suggestions to create one's own mental images that produce relaxation and feelings of harmony, and reduce stress

H

habituation: psychological dependence arising from repeated use of a drug

hallucinogens: psychoactive substances that alter sensory processing in the brain, producing visual or auditory sensations that are not real (i.e., that are hallucinatory)

hangover: unpleasant physical sensations resulting from excessive alcohol consumption

harm-and-loss situations: stressful events that include death, loss of property, injury, and illness

hashish: the sticky resin of the *Cannabis* plant

hate crime: an unlawful act committed against a person, group, or place that is motivated by hate or bias

health: state of sound physical, mental, and social well-being

healthcare power of attorney: designates someone to make healthcare decisions for you if you are unable to communicate

health insurance: a system intended to pay some or all of the costs of a person's medical, surgical, and hospital care

Health-related quality of life and well-being (HRQoL): a measure of health that includes non-medical factors

heart attack: death of, or damage to, part of the heart muscle caused by an insufficient blood supply

heart failure: when the heart is weakened to the degree it cannot pump blood throughout the body

hedonic eating system: motivation to eat by the psychological desire to experience a psychological reward, or pleasure from consuming food

hemicellulose: substances found in plant cell walls that are composed of various sugars chemically linked together

hemophilia: a hereditary disease (primarily in men) caused by lack of an essential blood clotting factor; results in excessive bleeding in response to any scratch or injury

hepatitis: serious disease of the liver caused by hepatitis virus A, B, C, or D; also caused by chemicals and alcohol

herbal medicines: materials derived from plants and other organisms that are made into teas, powders, and salves to treat diseases and injuries

herbicide: a chemical that kills weeds

hereditary (genetic) disease: any disease resulting from the inheritance of defective genes or chromosomes from one or both parents

herpes: a sexually transmitted disease caused by herpes simplex virus, HSV

high-density lipoprotein (HDL): the carrier of cholesterol from tissues to the liver for removal from the circulation; carrier of "good" cholesterol

histamine: a chemical released by cells in an allergic response; causes inflammation

histocompatibility: the degree to which the antigens on cells of different persons are similar

HIV antibody test: detects antibodies in blood that are produced in response to infection by HIV

homeopathy: an alternative medicine that administers very dilute solutions of substances that mimic the patient's symptoms

homeostatic eating system: integrated neurological and hormonal control of eating behavior based on the body's need for energy (calories)

hookahs: water pipes used to smoke flavored tobacco

hormone replacement therapy (HRT): administration of estrogen to menopausal and postmenopausal women to help prevent symptoms of menopause, osteoporosis, and heart disease

hormones: chemicals produced in the body that regulate body functions

hospice: a place for terminally ill patients to spend the time before death in an environment that attends to their physical, emotional, and spiritual needs but does not administer any further treatments; care also can be given in a patient's home

hostility: a personal trait characterized by an ongoing mistrust of others, cynicism, a personal emotional style of anger mixed with disgust and contempt, and a tendency to act out those feelings with overt aggression, snide comments, or criticism

human chorionic gonadotropin (HCG): a hormone produced during the first stages of pregnancy; it is used as a basis for pregnancy tests

human growth hormone: a naturally occurring pituitary hormone

human immunodeficiency virus (HIV): the virus that causes AIDS; it causes a defect in the body's immune system by invading and then multiplying within certain white blood cells

human leukocyte antigens (HLAs): antigens that are measured to determine the suitability of an organ for transplantation from donor to recipient

human microbiome: the total composition of bacteria, fungi, viruses, and other microorganisms that inhabit a human body

human papillomavirus (HPV): a genus of viruses including those causing papillomas (small nipplelike protrusions of the skin or mucous membrane) and warts

humoral immunity: the response of B cells to infections

hypertension: high blood pressure

hypnosis: a state of concentration and focused attention

hypnotherapy: the use of hypnosis to treat sickness

hypnotics: central nervous system depressants used to induce drowsiness and encourage sleep

hypothalamo-pituitary-adrenal (HPA) axis: a coordinated physiological response to stress involving the hypothalamus of the brain and the pituitary and adrenal glands

hysterectomy: surgical removal of the uterus

I

I-statements: statements beginning with "I"; positive communication skill

image visualization: use of mental images to promote healing and change behaviors

immune system: an interacting system of organs and cells that protect the body from infectious organisms and harmful substances

immunizations: vaccinations to prevent a variety of serious diseases caused by both bacteria and viruses

immunosuppressive drugs: drugs to suppress the functions of the immune system (e.g., after organ transplants)

immunotherapy: medically enhancing the body's immune system to fight cancer

incidence: the number of new cases of a particular disease

infertile: unable to become pregnant or to impregnate

ingredients label: label on a manufactured food that lists the ingredients in descending order by weight

inhalants: vaporous substances that, when inhaled, produce alcohol-like intoxication

injury epidemiology: the study of the occurrence, causes, and prevention of injury

insecticide: a chemical that kills insects

insoluble fiber: cannot be dissolved in water

insomnia: prolonged inability to obtain adequate sleep

integrative medicine: combination of the practice of scientific, Western medicine with alternative medicines that are safe and effective for patients

intellectual wellness: having a mind open to new ideas and concepts

intimate partner violence (IPV): physical, sexual, or psychological harm by a current or former intimate partner or spouse

intrauterine device (IUD): a flexible, usually plastic, device inserted into the uterus to prevent pregnancy

in vitro **fertilization (IVF):** a procedure in which an egg is removed from a ripe follicle and fertilized by a sperm cell outside the human body; the fertilized egg is allowed to divide in a protected environment for about 2 days and then is inserted into the uterus

ionizing radiation: radiation, such as x-rays, that can damage cells and cause cancer; also used to treat cancer

ischemia: an insufficient supply of blood to any part of the body; can cause fatal damage to the heart and brain

isometric training: a type of strength training

K

karyotype: visual display of all of a person's chromosomes that can detect chromosomal abnormalities characteristic of inherited diseases

ketamine: an anesthetic used as a club drug

kilocalorie: unit of energy; the amount of heat needed to raise 1 kilogram of water 1°C, equivalent to 1,000 calories

kreteks (clove cigarettes): cigarettes with cloves and other additives

L

labia majora: a pair of fleshy folds that cover the labia minora

labia minora: a pair of fleshy folds that cover the vagina

labor: the process of childbirth

lactase: enzyme secreted by glands in the small intestine that converts lactose (milk sugar) into simple sugars

lacto-ovo-vegetarian: one who excludes meat, poultry, and fish, but includes eggs and dairy products from diet

lacto-vegetarian: one who excludes meat, poultry, fish, and eggs, but includes dairy products from diet

lactose: a sugar formed by glucose and galactose chemically bonded together; found primarily in milk

laryngospasm: spasm of the larynx caused by inhaling water

Leading Health Indicators (LHIs): a set of high-priority Healthy People 2020 objectives and ways to achieve them

lecithin: an essential component of cell membranes

leukocytes: white blood cells that fight infections

life expectancy: average number of years a person can expect to live

lightening: the positioning of the fetus for birth by descent in the uterus

linoleic acid: an essential fat that must be obtained from food

lipids: fats such as cholesterol and triglycerides

lipoproteins: spherical particles that transport cholesterol and fat (TG) in the blood

liposuction: surgery used to remove fat under the skin to reshape parts of the body

literal message: a message that is conveyed by symbols

living will: a legal document that expresses your wishes regarding treatment if you become unable to make your own medical decisions

low-density lipoprotein (LDL): the carrier of "bad" cholesterol in blood

lowest observed failure rate: likelihood of becoming pregnant if using a birth control method consistently and as intended

LSD: a powerful hallucinogenic chemical; ingestion alters brain chemistry and produces a variety of hallucinogenic and behavioral effects

lupus erythematosus: an autoimmune disease that mostly affects women

luteinizing hormone: stimulates the release of the ovum (egg) by the follicle; the follicle produces progesterone

Lyme disease: a serious, difficult-to-diagnose infectious disease caused by bacteria deposited by ticks when they bite

lymph nodes: nodules spaced along the lymphatic vessels that trap infectious organisms or foreign particles

lymphatic system: a system of vessels in the body that trap foreign organisms and particles; the immune system is part of the lymphatic system

M

macrophages: specialized cells that destroy and eliminate foreign particles and microorganisms from the body

magnetic resonance imaging (MRI): use of a strong magnetic field to produce images of internal parts of the body; especially useful for soft tissues

major depression: a mental state characterized by feelings of hopelessness, helplessness, and self-recrimination

malaria: a disease of red blood cells that produces fever, anemia, and death

malignant tumor: a tumor whose cells spread throughout the body

mammogram: x-ray picture used to detect tumors in the breast

managed care: systems of health care in which the primary goal is to reduce costs

mandala: an artistic, religious design used as an object of meditation

mantra: a sound or phrase that is repeated in the mind to help produce a meditative state

marijuana: a psychoactive substance present in the dried leaves, stems, flowers, and seeds of plants of the genus *Cannabis*

masturbation: self-induced sexual stimulation

maximum life span: the theoretical maximum number of years that individuals of a species can live

medical aid in dying: a physician assistance to help a patient who no longer desires to live because of pain or an incurable illness to die

medical model: interprets health in terms of the absence of disease and disability

medication abortion: nonsurgical abortion using specific medications to stop pregnancy

medicalization: medical treatment of conditions, behaviors, or traits that generally were not regarded as illnesses or medical problems

medicine: drugs used to prevent, treat, or cure illness; aid healing; or suppress symptoms

meditation: focusing awareness on a self-produced inner sound ("mantra") or an external sound, or image, or one's breathing to lessen attentiveness to external stimuli

melanoma: a particularly dangerous form of skin cancer

menarche: the beginning of menstruation

menopause: the cessation of menstruation in midlife

menstrual cycle: the period of time from one menstruation to another

menstruation: the regular sloughing of the uterine lining via the vagina

mental health: a sense of optimism, vitality, and well-being, and intentional behaviors that lead to productive activities, fulfilling relationships with others, and the ability to adapt to change and cope with adversity

mental illness: alterations in thinking, emotions, and/or intentional behaviors that produce psychological distress and/or impaired functioning

meridians: the channels along the body where energy flows and where acupuncture points are located

mesothelioma: a form of lung cancer caused by asbestos

metabolic equivalents (METs): per-minute multiples of the amount of energy used while lying still

metabolic syndrome: a model embracing five risk factors that puts people who have at least three risk factors at risk for cardiovascular disease, diabetes, and premature death

metabolism: the process of obtaining energy and matter from the chemical breakdown of molecules obtained from food or from the body

metamessage: how the message is interpreted between sender and receiver

metastasis: the process by which cancer cells spread throughout the body

minerals: inorganic elements found in the body both in combination with organic compounds and alone

mini-pill: a progestin-only contraceptive pill

moist snuff: a form of snuff made from air- and fire-cured tobacco leaves; most hazardous form of smokeless tobacco

mononucleosis: an infectious disease caused by the Epstein-Barr virus, common among college-age adults

monounsaturated fatty acid: carries one less than all the hydrogen atoms it possibly could

morbidity: the number of persons in a population who are ill

mortality: death rate; number of deaths per unit of population (e.g., per 100, 10,000, or 1,000,000) in a specific region, age range, or other group

multiple sclerosis (MS): an autoimmune disease that affects the central nervous system

mutations: permanent changes in the genetic information in a cell; only mutations in sperm and eggs are inherited

myelin: a substance that sheaths and insulates nerve fibers in the brain and spinal cord

myocardium: muscular wall of the heart that contracts and relaxes

myotonia: muscle tension

MyPlate: a graphic to remind people of the composition of a healthy diet

N

narcolepsy: extreme tendency to fall asleep during the day

naturopathy: an alternative medicine that uses nutrition, herbs, massage, and other techniques to promote healing

nicotine: an addicting chemical in tobacco that produces rapid pulse, increased alertness, and a variety of other physiological effects

nicotine replacement therapy: using nicotine-containing gum, skin patches, nasal sprays, or inhalers to temper the symptoms of nicotine withdrawal when quitting smoking

nocebo effect: the opposite of the placebo effect; a harmless substance has harmful, undesirable, and adverse effects on health

nonessential amino acids: eleven amino acids required for protein synthesis that are synthesized by humans and are not specifically required in the diet

nutraceutical: a dietary supplement intended to prevent or treat an illness or disease

Nutrition Facts label: label on a manufactured food that lists the quantity of certain nutrients in the food and the percent daily value for those nutrients

nutritional calorie: unit of energy; often used interchangeably with the term *kilocalorie*

nutrient dense: food items that are high in nutrition in proportion to their calorie content

O

obesity: storage fat exceeding 30% of body weight

obsessive-compulsive disorder (OCD): persistent, unwelcome thoughts or images and the urgent need to engage in certain rituals

occupational wellness: enjoyment of what you are doing to earn a living and contribute to society

open-heart surgery: surgery performed on the opened heart while the blood supply is diverted through a heart–lung machine

opiates: central nervous system depressants derived from the opium poppy

opportunistic infection: any infectious disease in a patient with a weakened immune system; often occurs in AIDS patients

optimism: the thought process of imagining a high probability of attaining a goal

orgasm: the climax of sexual responses and the release of physiological and sexual tensions

osteopathy: an alternative medicine that uses manipulation and medicines for healing; osteopaths receive training comparable to that of physicians and can prescribe drugs

osteoporosis: a condition in older people, particularly women, in which bones lose density and become porous and brittle

ova: female eggs (singular, *ovum*)

ovaries: a pair of almond-shaped organs in the female abdomen that produce egg cells (ova) and female sex hormones

overload: the feeling that there are too many demands on one's time and energy from being confronted with too many challenges

over-the-counter (OTC) drugs: drugs that do not require a prescription

overuse injuries: injuries to muscles, tendons, ligaments, and joints resulting from too much exercise

ovo-vegetarian: one who excludes meats, poultry, fish, and dairy but eats eggs

ovulation: release of an egg (ovum) from the ovary

oxidation: the chemical term for the process of oxygen-present energy production

ozone hole: an ozone-deficient portion of the atmosphere above Antarctica that has been steadily growing since the problem was first reported in 1985

ozone layer: a layer of ozone molecules located in the stratosphere in a diffuse band extending from 10 to 30 miles above Earth's surface

P

pacemaker: an electrical device implanted in the chest to control irregular heartbeats

panic disorder: severe anxiety accompanied by physical symptoms

parasomnias: activities that interrupt restful sleep

Parkinson's disease (PD): a neurodegenerative disease in which brain functions that control movements of the body are gradually lost

pathogen: a disease-causing organism

pathologist: a physician who specializes in the causes of diseases

pedometer: a step counter

penicillin: an antibiotic produced by mold and capable of curing many bacterial infections

penis: the male's organ of copulation and urination

perceived social support: believing that support from one's social network is available if needed

percent daily value (PDV): percentage of the recommended daily amount of a particular nutrient found in a food

percutaneous transluminal coronary angioplasty (PTCA): a procedure to open blocked arteries

pessimism: the thought process of imagining a low probability of attaining a goal

pesticide: a chemical that kills unwanted plants and animals

pharmacogenetics: tailoring drugs to a particular individual to match his or her biology

phencyclidine (PCP): drug that, depending on the route of administration and dose, can be a stimulant, depressant, or hallucinogen; originally developed as an animal anesthetic

phobia: a powerful and irrational fear of something

photochemical smog: air pollution from the action of sunlight on emissions from motor vehicles and industrial sources

phthalates: chemicals used in the manufacture of various plastics; may cause abnormal genital development in males and premature breast development in girls

physical activity level (PAL): a measure of the amount of energy expended per day over and above that used for basal metabolism

physical dependence: a physiological state that depends on the continuous presence of a drug; absence of the drug may cause discomfort, nervousness, headaches, and sweating (withdrawal symptoms) and sometimes death

physical wellness: maintaining a healthy body by eating right, exercising regularly, avoiding harmful habits, and making informed, responsible decisions about your health

phytochemicals: chemicals produced by plants

Pilates: a system of stretching and strengthening exercises

placebo effect: healing that results from a person's belief in a treatment that has no medicinal value

placenta: the flat, circular vascular structure within the pregnant uterus that provides nourishment to and eliminates wastes from the developing embryo and fetus and is passed as afterbirth after the baby is born

plaque: deposit of fatty substances in the inner lining of arteries

plumbism: disease caused by lead poisoning

poison: any chemical substance that causes illness, injury, or death

polyunsaturated fatty acid: carries at least two fewer hydrogen atoms than it would if saturated

posttraumatic stress disorder (PTSD): physical and mental illnesses resulting from severe trauma

powered two-wheelers (PWTs): a diverse group of vehicles, including powered scooters and mopeds

precision personalized medicine: tailoring treatments to the genetic makeup of individual patients

preferred provider organization (PPO): physicians who belong to the organization provide medical care at reduced costs that are negotiated by the organization

premenstrual dysphoric disorder (PMDD): premenstrual symptoms severe enough to impair personal functioning

prevalence: the number of people within a population with a particular disease

problem-focused coping: appraising a stressful situation as changeable and making and attempting a plan for changing something to improve things

processed foods: industrial products derived from natural foods to which salt, sugar, oils and fats, and other chemicals are added to modify taste and consistency

progestin-only contraceptives: work by inhibiting ovulation and thickening of the cervical mucus; completely reversible

progestin-only implantation methods: inserting a 1.5-inch hormone-containing plastic rod under the skin, where it remains for 3 years

progestin-only injectable methods: injection of a 12-week supply of hormone, which is released at a steady rate

prolactin: a hormone produced by the anterior lobe of the pituitary gland that stimulates milk secretion

proof: a number assigned to an alcoholic product that is twice the percentage of alcohol in that product

prostate gland: gland at the base of the bladder providing seminal fluid

prostate-specific antigen (PSA) test: a blood test that detects a protein associated with abnormal growth of the prostate gland

protein: the foundation of every body cell; biological molecules composed of chains of amino acids

protein complementarity: combining sources of protein such that amino acid deficiencies in one are counterbalanced by abundances in another

psychoactive: any substance that primarily alters mood, perception, and other brain functions

psychological dependence: dependence that results because a drug produces pleasant mental effects

psychosomatic illnesses: physical illnesses brought on by negative mental states such as stress or emotional upset

pubic lice: small insects that live primarily in hair in the genital and rectal regions

puerperium: the 6 weeks after childbirth, also called postpartum period

Q

quackery: promotion and sale of unapproved and worthless products, especially for medical problems and health enhancement

quit date: the day a smoker designates as the one on which she or he will stop smoking completely

R

radiation therapy: use of high-energy radiation, such as x-rays, to kill cancer cells and treat some forms of cancer

radon: a radioactive gas found in some homes that can increase the risk of cancer

range of motion: the amount of rotating, bending, or twisting allowed by the anatomy of a joint

rape: nonconsensual sexual behavior, generally penile penetration of a bodily orifice

rape trauma syndrome: immediate and long-term psychological difficulties, including PTSD, from having been raped

rapid eye movement (REM) sleep: stage of sleep in which dreams occur

reactive hypoglycemia: occurring after the ingestion of carbohydrates, with consequent release of insulin

rebound effect: the reemergence of symptoms for which a drug is administered after the drug is suddenly stopped or the dose lessened

receptor: protein on the surface or inside of a cell to which a drug or natural substance can bind and thereby affect cell function

relative perceived exertion: awareness of one's relative response to exercise

relaxation response: the physiological changes in the body that result from mental relaxation techniques

repetitive motion disorders: disorders caused by repeated stress to a body part; carpal tunnel syndrome is a repetitive motion disorder

rheumatic heart disease: damage to the heart valves from bacterial infection

RICE: an acronym for rest, ice, compression, elevation; the first aid measures for sports injuries

rodenticide: a chemical that kills mice and rats

Rohypnol: a powerful tranquilizer used as a club drug

S

safety: an ever-changing condition in which one attempts to minimize the risk of injury, illness, or property damage from the hazards to which one may be exposed

saturated fat: generally solid at room temperature; comes from animal sources

scabies: infestation of the skin by microscopic mites (insects)

scrotum: the sac of skin that contains the testes

seasonal affective disorder (SAD): depressive symptoms that appear in autumn or winter and remit spontaneously in spring

second-stage labor: the stage during which the baby moves out through the vagina and is delivered

secondary hypertension: high blood pressure caused by a recognizable disease

secondary sex characteristics: anatomical features appearing at puberty that distinguish males from females

secondhand binge effects: negative experiences caused by another's binge drinking

sedatives: central nervous system depressants used to relieve anxiety, fear, and apprehension

sedentary behavior: a pattern of living that lacks sufficient physical activity for good health

self-disclosure: sharing personal experiences and feelings with someone

self-efficacy: the belief that one can carry out the actions required to accomplish a goal

self-esteem: the judgment one places on one's self-worth

semen: a whitish, creamy fluid containing sperm

seminal vesicles: glands that secrete a fluid that is a component of semen

seminiferous tubules: convoluted tubules in the testicles that produce sperm

senile dementia: loss of cognitive functions in elderly people

sexual assault: the combination of nonconsensual sexual penetration (rape) and nonsexual violence, such as battery, the threat of harm, or homicide

sexual orientation: the propensity to be sexually and romantically attracted to a particular sex

sexual response cycle: the four-phase physiological response to sexual arousal in both men and women

sexual violence: violent actions that include rape, incest, attempted rape, and unwanted sexual touching

sexually transmitted diseases (STDs): infections passed from person to person by sexual contact

shaken-baby syndrome (SBS): a form of child abuse in which an infant is violently shaken by an adult

sick building syndrome: collection of symptoms reported by workers in some modern buildings

side effects: unintended and often harmful actions of a drug

simple sugars: a class of carbohydrates called monosaccharides; all carbohydrates must be reduced to simple sugars to be digested

sinoatrial node: the region of the heart that produces an electrical signal that causes the heart to contract

smegma: a white, cheesy substance that accumulates under the foreskin of the penis

smog: air polluted by chemicals, smoke, particles, and dust

snuff: a form of smokeless tobacco; made from powdered or finely cut leaves

social anxiety disorder: fear of being observed and evaluated by others in social situations

social support: resources that one receives from others, particularly people in one's immediate social network with whom one has emotional bonds and/or social ties

social wellness: ability to perform social roles effectively, comfortably, and without harming others

socialization: the process by which social groups confer attitudes and expectations upon individuals

soluble fiber: nondigestible plant material that can dissolve in water

somatic symptom disorder: occurrence of physical symptoms without any bodily disease or injury being present

specific metabolic rate: the amount of energy per gram of body weight consumed per day

spectatoring: observing one's own sexual experience rather than fully taking part in it

spermicide: a chemical that kills sperm; particularly foams, creams, gels, and suppositories used for contraception

spiritual wellness: state of balance and harmony with yourself and others

squamous cell carcinoma: cancer of the top layer of skin; most are curable if removed early

stalking: behavior that causes victims to feel a high level of fear of physical or sexual violence

starch: complex chain of glucose molecules

statins: a class of drugs that block synthesis of cholesterol in the liver and reduce the amount of cholesterol in the blood

sterility: the state of permanent infertility

stimulants: substances that increase the activity of the central nervous system

storage fat: also called depot fat; energy stored as fat in various parts of the body

strength training: the use of resistance to increase one's ability to exert or resist force for the purpose of improving performance

stress: the sum of physical and emotional reactions to any stimulus that disturbs the harmony of body and mind

stressor: any physical or psychological situation that produces stress

stroke (brain attack): death of brain cells due to an insufficient supply of blood to the brain, resulting in loss of muscle function, loss of speech, or other symptoms

subluxation: misalignment of a vertebra from its correct position

sucrose: common refined table sugar; a molecule of glucose and a molecule of fructose chemically bonded together

sulfites: used as preservatives for salad, fresh fruits and vegetables, wine, beer, and dried fruit; in susceptible individuals, especially those with asthma, they can cause a severe reaction

surgical abortion: the most common abortion method, in which the uterus is emptied with the gentle suction of a manual syringe

syphilis: a sexually transmitted disease caused by spirochete bacteria (*Treponema pallidum*)

systole: the pressure in the arteries when the heart contracts (the higher number)

T

T cells: cells of the immune system that attack foreign organisms that infect the body

t'ai chi ch'uan: a Chinese martial arts system of movements that enhances freedom of movement and focus of mind

tar: the yellowish brown residue of tobacco smoke

target heart rate: the heart rate during strenuous exercise associated with inducing the training effect

tau tangles: aggregates of a brain protein called tau; a diagnostic indicator for Alzheimer's disease

telomeres: DNA at the ends of chromosomes that protect the integrity of genetic information during cellular replication

teratogen: any environmental agent that causes abnormal development of a fetus

testes: a pair of male reproductive organs that produce sperm cells and male sex hormones

therapeutic massage: promotes relaxation and healing by massage of the skin and muscles

third-stage labor: the stage during which the afterbirth is expelled

threat situations: events that cause stress because of a perception that harm or loss may occur

tinnitus: persistent ringing in the ears, often caused by repeated or sudden exposure to loud noises

tolerance: biological adaptation to alcohol use such that increasing amounts of alcohol are needed to produce the expected, desired effects

trachea: upper part of respiratory tract

training effect: beneficial physiological changes as a result of exercise

tranquilizers: central nervous system depressants that relax the body and calm anxiety

trans fatty acid: also trans fat, an artificial fat manufactured by chemically modifying monounsaturated and polyunsaturated fatty acids

traumatic brain injury (TBI): injury caused by a bump, blow, or jolt to the head that results in impaired thinking or memory, altered movement or sensation, personality changes, or emotional problems such as depression

triglyceride: dietary fat composed of fatty acids

tubal ligation: a surgical procedure in women in which the fallopian tubes are cut, tied, or cauterized to prevent pregnancy; a form of sterilization

tumor: a mass of abnormal cells

tumor viruses: viruses that infect cells, change their growth properties, and cause cancer

typical use failure rate: likelihood of becoming pregnant considering all the potential problems associated with a birth control method

U

ultrasound scanning: use of sound waves to visualize the fetus in the womb

unintentional injury: preferred term for accidental injury; result of an accident

universal donors: people whose blood is accepted by everyone during transfusion

universal recipients: people whose blood type is compatible with anyone else's blood

urethra: a tube that carries urine from the bladder to the outside

urethritis: an irritation or infection of the urethra caused by bacteria

urinary tract infection (UTI): inflammation and/or infection of the urethra and/or bladder, usually by bacteria

uterus: the female organ in which a fetus develops

V

vaccines: inactivated bacteria or viruses that are injected or taken orally; the body responds by producing antibodies and cells that provide lasting immunity

vagina: a woman's organ of copulation and the exit pathway for the fetus at birth

varicose veins: swelling of veins (usually in the legs) resulting from defective valves

vasectomy: a surgical procedure in men in which segments of the vasa deferentia are removed and the ends tied to prevent the passage of sperm

vasocongestion: the engorgement of blood in particular body regions in response to sexual arousal

vector: the carrier of infectious organisms from animals to people or from person to person

vegan: one who excludes all animal products from the diet, including milk, cheese, eggs, and other dairy products

vegetarian: one who consumes no meat, poultry, or fish

veins: blood vessels that return blood from tissues to the heart

ventricular fibrillation: a type of cardiac arrhythmia in which the ventricles (the lower chambers of the heart) quiver very rapidly and irregularly instead of contracting forcefully, resulting in the heart pumping little or no blood to the body

violence: a physical or verbal behavior, in which the intent is to harm, injure, or destroy someone or something

virtual reality therapy (VRT): use of computer programs to create virtual worlds that engage the mind in order to overcome pain and fear and to treat symptoms of posttraumatic stress disorder

vital statistics: numerical data relating to birth, death, disease, marriage, and health

vitamins: essential organic substances needed daily in small amounts to perform specific functions in the body

vulva: the female external genital structures

vulvovaginitis: inflammation of the vaginal region

W

water-soluble vitamins: soluble in water; there are nine water-soluble vitamins

wean: to discontinue breastfeeding, using other means to provide nutrients

well-being: qualities of life that include positive emotions (e.g.; happiness, contentment) and life satisfaction

wellness model: encompasses the physiological, mental, emotional, social, spiritual, and environmental aspects of health

Western blot: a test that measures the level of specific HIV proteins in blood

withdrawal: unpleasant physiological and psychological symptoms in alcohol-dependent individuals when refraining from drinking

withdrawal method: removing the penis from the vagina just prior to ejaculation; also called *coitus interruptus* or pulling out

withdrawal symptoms: uncomfortable and sometimes dangerous reactions that occur after a person stops taking a physically addicting drug

X

xenoestrogens: environmental chemicals that mimic the effects of natural estrogen; may cause cancer

Y

yoga: a system of exercises formulated in India thousands of years ago to unite one's mind and body

you-statements: statements beginning with "you"; negative communication skill

Z

zygote: the first cell of a new person, formed at fertilization

Health & Wellness

THIRTEENTH EDITION

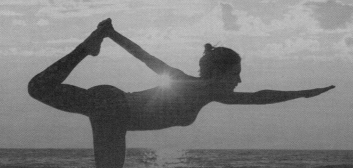

Gordon Edlin, PhD
Emeritus Professor of Genetics
University of California, Davis

Eric Golanty, PhD
Emeritus Professor of Health, Wellness, and Physical Education
Las Positas College

JONES & BARTLETT
LEARNING

1.1 My Health and Wellness Assessment

Directions

1. Complete the Health and Wellness Assessment on the following pages.

2. For each question, write the number (1 to 5) that corresponds to your response to each question in the Health and Wellness Assessment.

3. Calculate your scores for the six wellness categories (e.g., Emotional Health, Fitness and Body Care, etc.).

4. List two aspects of your personal health with which you are the most pleased and explain your reasoning.

   _____

   _____

   _____

5. List two aspects of your personal health with which you are the least pleased and explain your reasoning.

   _____

   _____

   _____

6. List three questions in the Health and Wellness Assessment that interested you and explain your reasons.

   _____

   _____

   _____

7. Indicate one or more aspects of your personal health that you would like to change and explain your reasons. Consider doing a Health Behavior Change project as a way to make a positive health change in your life.

   _____

   _____

   _____

   _____

   _____

8. Identify factors that prevent you from accomplishing your health goals.

   _____

   _____

   _____

   _____

   _____

Health and Wellness Assessment

Complete the following health and wellness inventory to gauge your present degree of wellness. For each question, write one of the following numbers:

5 if the statement is ALWAYS true

4 if the statement is FREQUENTLY true

3 if the statement is OCCASIONALLY true

2 if the statement is SELDOM true

1 if the statement is NEVER true

1. I am able to identify the situations and factors that overstress me. ___
2. I eat only when I am hungry. ___
3. I don't take tranquilizers or other drugs to relax. ___
4. I support efforts in my community to reduce environmental pollution. ___
5. I avoid sugar-sweetened beverages. ___
6. I rarely have problems concentrating on what I'm doing because of worrying about other things. ___
7. My employer (school) takes measures to ensure that my work (learning) environment is safe. ___
8. I carefully think about whether to use medications when I feel unwell. ___
9. I am able to identify certain bodily responses and illnesses as my reactions to stress. ___
10. I discuss with my healthcare practitioner the necessity of diagnostic x-rays and other scanning tests. ___
11. I try to change personal habits that are risk factors for heart disease, cancer, and other lifestyle diseases. ___
12. I avoid taking sleeping pills to help me sleep. ___
13. I try not to eat foods with refined sugar or high-fructose corn syrup as ingredients. ___
14. I accomplish goals I set for myself. ___
15. I stretch or bend for several minutes each day to keep my body flexible. ___
16. I support immunization of all children for common childhood diseases. ___
17. I try to prevent friends from driving after they drink alcohol. ___
18. I minimize my salt intake. ___
19. I don't mind when other people and situations make me wait or lose time. ___
20. I climb four or fewer flights of stairs rather than take the elevator. ___
21. I eat fresh fruits and vegetables several times a week (or daily). ___
22. I use sunscreen when I am exposed to sunlight for any length of time. ___
23. I read product labels to determine that the ingredients are not harmful to health. ___
24. I try to maintain a normal body weight. ___
25. I record my feelings and thoughts in a journal or diary. ___
26. I have no difficulty falling asleep. ___
27. I engage in some form of movement activity at least three times a week. ___
28. I take time each day to quiet my mind and relax. ___
29. I want to make and sustain close friendships and intimate relationships. ___
30. I obtain an adequate daily supply of vitamins from my food or vitamin supplements. ___
31. I rarely have tension or migraine headaches or pain in the neck or shoulders. ___
32. I wear a safety belt when driving or when I am a passenger in the front seat. ___
33. I am aware of the emotional and situational factors that lead me to overeat. ___
34. I avoid driving my car after drinking any alcohol. ___
35. I am aware of the side effects of the medicines I take. ___
36. I am able to accept feelings of sadness, depression, and anxiety, realizing that they are almost always transient. ___
37. I would seek several additional professional opinions if my doctor recommended surgery for me. ___

38. I agree that nonsmokers should not have to breathe the smoke from cigarettes in public places. ___
39. I think that pregnant women who smoke should stop in order to prevent harm to the developing fetus. ___
40. On most nights I get enough sleep to awaken feeling refreshed. ___
41. I ask my doctor why a certain medication is being prescribed and inquire about alternatives. ___
42. I am aware of the calories expended in my daily activities. ___
43. I am willing to give priority to my own needs for time and psychological space by saying "no" to others' requests of me. ___
44. I walk or bike instead of drive whenever feasible. ___
45. I eat a breakfast that contains about one-third of my daily need for calories, proteins, and vitamins. ___
46. I prohibit smoking in my home. ___
47. I try to forgive people who have been mean or unkind to me. ___
48. I seek medical attention only when I have symptoms or feel that some (potential) condition needs checking, rather than have routine yearly checkups. ___
49. I endeavor to make my home accident-free. ___
50. I ask my doctor to explain the diagnosis of my problem until I understand all that I care to. ___
51. I try to include fiber or roughage (whole grains, fresh fruits, vegetables, or bran) in my daily diet. ___
52. I can deal with my emotional problems without alcohol or other mood-altering drugs. ___
53. I check the calorie content of the packaged foods that I eat. ___
54. I require children riding in my car to be in infant seats or in child safety seats. ___
55. I try to associate with people who have a positive attitude about life. ___
56. I rarely eat snacks of candy, packaged pastries, or other junk food. ___
57. I know the signs of depression. ___
58. I am aware of the calorie content of the foods I eat. ___
59. I brush my teeth after meals. ___
60. (*for women only*) I regularly examine my breasts for any signs of cancer. (*for men only*) I am aware of the signs of testicular cancer. ___

How to Score

Write the numbers you've entered next to the question number in the columns below and total your score for each category. Then use the wellness status key to determine your degree of wellness for each category.

Emotional Health	Fitness and Body Care	Environmental Health	Stress	Nutrition	Medical Self-Responsibility
6 ___	15 ___	4 ___	1 ___	2 ___	8 ___
12 ___	20 ___	7 ___	3 ___	5 ___	10 ___
25 ___	22 ___	17 ___	9 ___	13 ___	11 ___
26 ___	24 ___	32 ___	14 ___	18 ___	16 ___
36 ___	27 ___	34 ___	19 ___	21 ___	35 ___
40 ___	33 ___	38 ___	28 ___	23 ___	37 ___
47 ___	42 ___	39 ___	29 ___	30 ___	41 ___
52 ___	44 ___	46 ___	31 ___	45 ___	48 ___
55 ___	58 ___	49 ___	43 ___	51 ___	50 ___
57 ___	59 ___	54 ___	53 ___	56 ___	60 ___
Total ___	Total ___	Total ___	Total ___	Total ___	Total ___

My Wellness Status

To access your status in each of the six categories, compare your total score in each column to the following key: **0–34**, need improvement; **35–44**, good; **45–50**, excellent.

How Is Your College or University Doing?

Have you received information from your college or university on the following topics?

	Yes	No
Alcohol use		
Anxiety		
Cold/flu/sore throat		
Depression		
Eating disorders		
Financial problems		
Grief and loss		
Healthy eating		
Helping others in distress		
Injury prevention		
Overuse Internet/video games/social media		
Overweight		
Physical activity		
Pregnancy prevention		
Prescription drug overuse		
Recreational drug use		
Relationship difficulties		
Self-harm		
Sexually transmitted diseases		
Sleep difficulties		
Suicide prevention		
Tobacco use		
Interpersonal violence		

1.2 Health Issues Affecting My Academic Performance

Directions

1. Use the chart below to indicate how much each health issue affects you.

Health Issue	Affects My Academic Performance		
	Rarely/Not at all	Sometimes	Frequently
Stress	_____	_____	_____
Cold/flu/sore throat	_____	_____	_____
Sleep difficulties	_____	_____	_____
Concern about family/friend	_____	_____	_____
Relationship difficulties	_____	_____	_____
Depression/anxiety	_____	_____	_____
Internet use/games	_____	_____	_____
Sinus infection	_____	_____	_____
Death of friend/family	_____	_____	_____
Alcohol use	_____	_____	_____

2. For any frequent health issue, describe how it affects your academic performance and offer strategies for lessening the frequency with which the issue occurs.

Student Workbook

1.3 My Definition of Health

Directions
Write a one-paragraph response to these questions:

- What is your personal definition of health?

_____

_____

_____

_____

_____

_____

_____

- How does your definition compare to the World Health Organization's definition of health (Chapter 1)?

_____

_____

_____

_____

_____

_____

_____

_____

1.4 My Health Behaviors

Health is a precious gift that you give yourself by living meaningfully and in harmony with your inner self and all that surrounds you. Researchers have found that the personal behaviors listed in the table below contribute to health.

Directions

1. List the behaviors in the table that are regular aspects of your life.

   _____

   _____

   _____

   _____

2. Identify one behavior that you would like to be part of your life right now and explain your reasoning. Consider doing a Health Behavior Change project (see workbook Exercise 1.6) to integrate one of these health behaviors into your life.

   _____

   _____

   _____

   _____

   _____

The Breslow Study	The Ornish Study
No smoking	No smoking
7–8 hours of sleep per night	No more than 10% of daily calories from fat
Body weight not less than 10% and not more than 30% of recommended for height and body frame	Daily meditation
Regular exercise	Daily exercise
Eating breakfast regularly	Vegetarian diet
Little between-meal snacking	Daily yoga
Little or no alcohol consumption (1–2 drinks per day)	Support group meetings twice a week

Data in column 1 are adapted from Breslow, L.,& Enstrom, J. E. (1980). Persistence of health habits and their relationship to mortality. *Preventive Medicine, 9*, 469–483; Camacho, T. C., & Wiley, J. A. (1983). Health practices, social networks, and change in physical health. In L. Berkman & L. Breslow, eds., *Health and ways of living: The Alameda County Study*. New York: Oxford University Press. Data in column 2 are adapted from Ornish, D., et al. (1998). Intensive lifestyle changes for reversal of coronary heart disease. *Journal of the American Medical Association, 280*, 2001–2007.

1.5 My Personal Vital Statistics

Enter the appropriate data about yourself. Date it and keep it for your personal records.

Height in inches (without shoes): _____

Weight in pounds (with clothes): _____

Highest adult weight: _____ pounds. At what age? _____

Lowest adult weight: _____ pounds. At what age? _____

Recommended weight for height (see text, Chapter 5): _____

Body mass index (see text, Chapter 5): _____

Resting heart rate (pulse): _____ beats per minute (see Chapter workbook Exercise 7.1)

Blood pressure: Systolic (top number): _____ Diastolic (bottom number): _____

Blood type: A _____ B _____ 0 _____ AB _____ Rh– _____ Rh+ _____

Total blood cholesterol: _____ LDL cholesterol: _____ HDL cholesterol: _____

1.6 Health Behavior Change Project

Design, carry out, and evaluate a project for changing a personal health behavior (e.g., stop smoking, learn a relaxation method, alter diet, begin an exercise plan).

The Health Behavior Change project has five steps:

Step 1. Project Declaration: You state what you want to do. Address the following:

1. The reasons for your choice
2. What you hope to learn or achieve and why
3. Any prior experiences that are similar
4. Your start and stop dates
5. The ways you will determine progress

Step 2. Research: You find four resources that provide information about your proposed Health Behavior Change project. Consult books, magazines, the Internet, or personal advisors to determine a way(s) to accomplish your goal(s). Because research in the health field is extensive, find resources that are no older than five years. For each of the four resources report the following:

- The title
- The author or writer
- The source: name of magazine, producer of video, affiliation of professional expert, Internet address
- Date of publication and pages on which the information appears

Step 3. Project Plan: You develop and describe a plan for carrying out your Health Behavior Change project. Describe what you plan to do for your Health Behavior Change project and the ways you will determine progress.

Step 4. Project Activity: You carry out your project for three weeks. Choose a start date. Keep a diary/journal of your activity. Note obstacles that get in the way of progress. At the end of each week, write a progress report that summarizes that week's experience, including obstacles you encounter.

Step 5. Assessment: You write an evaluation of your experience by:

- Summarizing your project plan and the health principles it represented
- Describing the experience of trying to accomplish your goal(s)
- Listing at least two things about your topic that you learned
- Describing what doing the project helped you learn about yourself
- Describing what you learned about how to change a health behavior
- Stating whether the project was worthwhile and why

2.1 Mindfulness Meditation

Follow the directions below to learn how to practice mindfulness meditation. Then, on each of six consecutive days, practice for 20 minutes. At the end of the six days, describe your experience. *Headspace* (https://www.headspace.com) is a free online mindfulness training program for computers and mobile devices.

Directions

Become comfortable: Find a quiet place where you can sit in a chair. Sit straight, uncross your legs, place your feet flat on the floor. Place your hands in your lap and take two easy, deep breaths. Then breathe easily and naturally. Bring your shoulders down from your ears.

Step 1. Focusing on the feet: Close your eyes for 10 seconds and focus your awareness on the sensation of the bottoms of your feet touching the insoles of your shoes. After you open your eyes, note what your mind was doing while your eyes were closed.

Step 2. Focusing on the back: Close your eyes for 10 seconds and focus your awareness on the sensation of your back touching the chair. After a couple of seconds with your eyes closed, open your eyes, take an easy breath, and note what your mind was doing while your eyes were closed.

Step 3. Focusing on the breath: Close your eyes for 10 seconds and notice your breathing. Don't change your breathing rhythm or pattern, just notice the breath going in and out of your body.

Now you know three basic meditation postures: feet on the floor, back against the chair, and focus on the breath. With a bit of practice, you will discover the posture that is best for you.

Step 4. Focusing for 30 seconds, and then 90 seconds: Become comfortable (see above). Choose one of the three meditation postures. Close your eyes, and focus your awareness on your feet, back, or breathing for 30 seconds. While you're meditating, if you notice your mind wandering, refocus your awareness on your feet, back, or breathing. When you think the 30 seconds has elapsed, open your eyes and take a breath.

What did you notice while you were meditating? Did you hear sounds? Did your mind wander? Did you think about your to-do list? Did you tell yourself this was silly? Did you feel sleepy? Did you relax? All of these reactions are common. Whenever you meditate, you can expect your mind to wander and to think. When you notice that it does, just notice, and refocus your awareness on your feet, back, or breathing. When you are ready, try meditating for 90 seconds.

Do the exercise again tomorrow for 5 minutes.

2.2 Autogenic Training

Autogenic training uses autosuggestion to balance and harmonize the mind and body. Autogenic training involves concentrating on one of six basic autogenic phrases for a few minutes each day for a week or more. After weeks or months of practice, you are able to attain a deep sense of relaxation, often within seconds. The six basic autosuggestions are as follows:

1. My arms and legs are heavy.
2. My arms and legs are warm.
3. My heartbeat is calm and regular.
4. My lungs breathe me.
5. My abdomen is warm.
6. My forehead is cool.

Directions

1. Place yourself in an environment in which you are comfortable and can relax. Turn off cell phones, pagers, computers, and music. Lock the door.
2. Sit or lie comfortably. Breathe comfortably.
3. Choose one of the autogenic phrases from the preceding list and silently (or aloud) repeat it seven times.
4. Open your eyes, stretch, and mentally note or "observe" the sensations in your body.
5. Repeat steps 3 and 4 five times, for a total of about 10 minutes.
6. After one week, carry out the exercise using a different autogenic phrase.

Note: The exact phrasing of any autogenic suggestion is not critical to its effectiveness. The words carry no particular power. Any suggestion can be rephrased so that it becomes comfortable, believable, and acceptable to you.

2.3 The Relaxation Response

Many students live fast-paced, hectic lives that are full of time pressures and stress. Trying to accommodate all of life's demands produces near continuous physiologic arousal, resulting in sleep disturbances, muscle tension, gastrointestinal symptoms, and an increased risk for cardio-vascular disease. The Relaxation Response is an automatic physiological pattern opposing nervous system arousal. Do it for 10 to 20 minutes each day to keep yourself centered and calm.

Directions

1. Place yourself in an environment in which you are comfortable and can relax. Turn off cell phones, pagers, computers, and music. Lock the door.
2. Sit or lie comfortably. Breathe comfortably.
3. Silently repeat the word *one*. If your mind wanders, as soon as you notice, refocus your attention on silently repeating the word one. Do not become angry or frustrated because you "aren't doing it right."
4. Do the exercise for as long as you are able. Try to work up to 20 minutes per day.

2.4 Image Visualization

Your mind has the power to promote your personal wellness and to help healing. By dwelling on negative thoughts and images, such as "I feel lousy," you increase the chance that you will feel that way. On the other hand, by thinking positive thoughts, such as "I feel great" or "Today is a good day," you can create positive feelings and positive behavioral outcomes. You can put healing suggestions into your mind, too. For example, you can suggest to yourself that a headache will go away in an hour or a cold will be mild.

Directions

Find a quiet, pleasant place where you can sit or lie down comfortably. Remove any uncomfortable clothing, eyeglasses, or contact lenses. Turn off the phone, TV, and computer. Give yourself permission to relax and decide what you are going to visualize. It's probably best to begin with something specific. You can visualize yourself being slimmer, giving up cigarettes, being successful in an upcoming job interview, or taking an exam while feeling confident and sure of the answers. You can visualize yourself becoming physically stronger or an area of your body becoming well.

Allow your eyes to close, and relax the muscles in the eyelids all the way—to the point where they are so relaxed and comfortable that you feel you are unable to pull your eyelids open. Then let your mind transfer that same comfortable, relaxed feeling to all the other parts of the body, one by one, from top to bottom—head, chest, arms, hands, back, stomach, legs, feet.

Imagine that you are floating on a white cloud bathed in warm sunlight. Everything is quiet and peaceful. You are warm and comfortable and serene. Allow your mind to visualize whatever scene or image it chooses that is related to what you want to improve or heal. Accept your mind's images. They are helping you to change, to feel better. Allow yourself to remain in this relaxed state while your mind continues to create pleasant, positive, beneficial images. Begin to notice how relaxed your body is and how good it feels.

Whenever your mind decides it wants to return to a fully awake state, you will automatically open your eyes and be fully aware of your surroundings. Notice how refreshed and relaxed you feel!

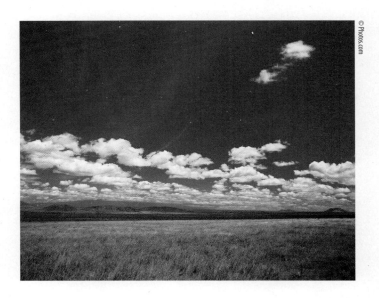

2.5 Progressive Muscle Relaxation

Developed by American physician Edmund Jacobson in 1938, Progressive Muscle Relaxation (PMR) involves tightening individual muscles or muscle groups for five seconds and slowly releasing to create a reflex relaxation.

Directions

On each of two consecutive days, practice PMR, following the directions below. You can start at your feet and progress toward your head or vice versa, whichever is most comfortable for you. Try voice-recording the directions so you don't have to refer to the printed page. Note: Some people experience muscle cramps while doing this exercise, especially in their feet. If a muscle cramps, either (1) straighten out the muscle, or (2) "breathe through" the muscle: Close your eyes and imagine that air is entering your body through the tight muscle instead of your lungs. If cramping or any other aspect of this exercise is uncomfortable, you may stop.

PMR Exercise (15–20 minutes)
Phase 1: Sinking into the floor
Put yourself in quiet, comfortable surroundings.
Shoes off, clothes loosened.
Lie on your back on a soft or padded surface.
Set feet slightly apart with palms facing upward.
Close your eyes; breathe naturally.
Observe thoughts without focusing on them.
As if it were a sponge, imagine the surface on which you are lying drawing tension from your body. As tension leaves your body, notice that it feels as though you are sinking into the floor.
Breathe naturally.
Lie quietly for at least two minutes.

Phase 2: Lower-body PMR
Focus your awareness on your feet. Breathe normally.
Keeping your heel on the floor, point the toes on your left foot away from you as far as you can. Hold five seconds and slowly release.
Repeat for right foot.
Rest, breathe naturally, and observe the sensation that follows.
Keeping your heel on the floor, point the toes on your left foot toward you as far as you can. Hold five seconds and slowly release.
Repeat for right foot.
Rest, breathe naturally, and observe the sensation that follows.
With leg outstretched, tighten the thigh muscles of your left leg. Hold five seconds and slowly release.
Repeat for right leg.
Rest, breathe naturally, and observe the sensation that follows.
Tense pelvic (butt) muscles. Hold five seconds and slowly release.
Rest, breathe naturally, and observe the sensation that follows.

Phase 3: Upper-body PMR
Tense stomach muscles. Hold five seconds and slowly release.
Rest, breathe naturally, and observe the sensation that follows.
With palms turned down and keeping your forearm on the floor, bend your left hand at the wrist and point the fingers back as far as they will go. Hold five seconds and slowly release.
Repeat for right hand.
Rest, breathe naturally, and observe the sensation that follows.
With palms turned up and keeping your forearm on the floor, bend your left hand at the wrist and point the fingers toward your face as far as they will go. Hold five seconds and slowly release.

Repeat for right hand.
Rest, breathe naturally, and observe the sensation that follows.
Tense muscles of the left upper arm. Hold five seconds and slowly release.
Repeat for right arm.
Rest, breathe naturally, and observe the sensation that follows.
Tense the muscles in your back. Hold five seconds and slowly release.
Rest, breathe naturally, and observe the sensation that follows.
Tense the muscles in your shoulders.
Hold five seconds and slowly release.
Rest, breathe naturally, and observe the sensation that follows.

Phase 4: Head and neck PMR

Tense the muscles in your neck. Hold five seconds and slowly release.
Rest, breathe naturally, and observe the sensation that follows.
Tense the muscles in your face. Hold five seconds and slowly release.
Rest, breathe naturally, and observe the sensation that follows.
Close your eyes and squeeze the lids tightly shut. Hold five seconds and slowly release.
Rest, breathe naturally, and observe the sensation that follows.

2.6 Quiet Time Exploration

For 3 weeks, experiment with different methods of relaxation to find one(s) that suits you and that you can practice indefinitely to enhance your health and well-being.

During Week 1

Experiment with three of the following relaxation techniques (or others of your choosing).

- Mantra meditation
- Breathing meditation
- Walking
- T'ai chi ch'uan
- Image visualization
- Progressive Muscle Relaxation
- Hatha yoga

During Week 2

Choose one technique and practice it for at least 3 days for 10 minutes each time.

During Week 3

Practice your chosen technique for at least 6 days for 20 minutes each day. For each day record the following information:

- The name of the relaxation activity you're doing
- The time you spent each day doing the activity
- What you experienced doing the activity
- Any obstacles that prevented you from carrying out a day's activity
- Strategies for overcoming any obstacles

2.7 The Power Write

You've probably heard of a power nap. How about a power write, a 5-minute exercise designed to focus your attention on something other than dealing with the stresses and hustle-and-bustle of daily life? When you realize that you're caught up in a whir of mental and physical activity that seems to separate you from yourself, power write about any of the following:

- A message from your body to you. What's going on right now?
- A conversation with someone you admire
- What is stressing you today
- What you find meaningful in life
- Some place you'd rather be right now and the reasons why

2.8 Massage

Everyone experiences tense muscles and soreness in parts of the body occasionally. Some parts of the body, such as the neck, shoulders, and back, are prime locations for accumulated tension. Mental and emotional distress can cause muscle tension and physical discomfort.

Massage is an excellent way to reduce physical tension and relax body muscles. In turn, a relaxed body facilitates a relaxed state of mind. All human beings need physical contact with other people. Babies and children are constantly seeking ways to be held, touched, and massaged by their caregivers. Mothers instinctively stroke and rub their infants. Unfortunately, as we grow older we tend to give and receive less physical contact.

Giving a Back Massage

Anyone can give a massage to another person. All that's required is the desire to make another person feel more comfortable and a willingness to be sensitive to another person's stiff muscles.

Learn by exchanging massages with friends and persons with whom you are comfortable and trust. The person being massaged can be sitting up or lying down. The area to be massaged should be free of clothing. Begin with the neck, using your thumbs to press the muscles on either side of the spine. Press firmly and smoothly away from the spine. Work down the back, always pressing down and away from the spine. Be sensitive to sore places or knots of tense muscles. Apply steady, gentle pressure to these areas until you feel the person relax or the muscles soften. As you become more experienced, you can use the heels of your hands or your knuckles to knead tense muscles. Always be sensitive to what the other person is feeling.

It helps to use a small amount of massage oil on your hands to reduce friction. You may want to play soft music or encourage the person to relax while you are massaging him or her.

Giving a Foot Massage

A foot massage is a relaxing, pleasant experience. The foot is a sensitive part of the body and often has places that are stiff or sore. Most people feel greatly relaxed after receiving a foot massage.

Begin by washing the person's feet with warm water. Rub the whole foot and ankle with a small amount of massage oil. Massage each toe and between each toe. Gently pull each toe to stretch the muscles and joints. You may hear the joint make a small cracking sound; this is normal. Massage the foot with your thumbs, fingers, or knuckles from top to bottom. Do one foot and then the other. It's easier if you cradle the foot in your lap. Be sensitive and gentle. Ask the person to tell you if any part hurts. Spend more time in places that are sore by gently pressing, rubbing, and massaging the area.

Always give a massage with your whole being—not just your hands. Be gentle, caring, and sensitive to what the other person is experiencing. A massage is an ideal way for two persons to become more in touch with their bodies and to release physical tension.

2.9 Leaving It at the River

Directions

1. Read the story of "Two Monks and the River."

Two Monks and the River

Two monks set out on their last day's journey to their monastery. At mid-morning they came upon a shallow river, and on the bank there stood a beautiful young maiden.

"May I help you cross?" asked the first monk.

"Why, yes, that would be most kind of you," replied the maiden.

So the first monk hoisted the maiden on his back and carried her across the river. They bowed and went their separate ways.

After an hour or two of walking, the second monk said to the first monk, "I can't believe you did that! I just can't believe it! We take vows of chastity, and you touched a woman. You even asked her! What are we going to tell the abbot when we get home? He's going to ask how our journey was, and we can't lie. What are we going to say?"

Another couple of hours passed and the second monk erupted again. "How could you do that? She didn't even ask. You offered! The abbot's going to be incredibly angry."

By late afternoon the two were nearing their home, and the second monk, now filled with anxiety, said, "I can't believe you did that! You touched a woman. You even carried her on your back. What are we going to tell the abbot?"

The first monk stopped, looked at the second monk, and said, "Listen, it's true that I carried that maiden across the river. But I left her at the river bank hours ago. You've been carrying her all day."

2. Which monk was the most stressed and why?

_____

_____

_____

3. Write a brief essay describing your interpretation of the story.

_____

_____

_____

_____

_____

_____

_____

_____

_____

_____

_____

4. When you are stressed or upset, what can you do to "leave it at the river"?

_____

_____

_____

_____

_____

_____

3.1 My Stressors

Directions

1. Use the chart below to indicate the degree to which each item is stressful for you.

Stressor	Stressful		
	Rarely/Not at all	Sometimes	Frequently
Academic			
Competition	_____	_____	_____
Schoolwork (difficult, low motivation)	_____	_____	_____
Exams and grades	_____	_____	_____
Poor resources (library, computers)	_____	_____	_____
Oral presentations/public speaking	_____	_____	_____
Professors/coaches (unfair, demanding, unavailable)	_____	_____	_____
Choosing and registering for classes	_____	_____	_____
Choosing a major/career	_____	_____	_____
Time			
Deadlines	_____	_____	_____
Procrastination	_____	_____	_____
Waiting for appointments and in lines	_____	_____	_____
No time to exercise	_____	_____	_____
Late for appointments or class	_____	_____	_____
Environment			
Others' behavior (rude, inconsiderate, sexist/racist)	_____	_____	_____
Injustice: seeing examples or being a victim of	_____	_____	_____
Crowds/large social groups	_____	_____	_____
Fears of violence/terrorism	_____	_____	_____
Weather (snow, heat/humidity, storms)	_____	_____	_____
Noise	_____	_____	_____
Lack of privacy	_____	_____	_____
Social			
Obligations, annoyances (family/friends/girl-/boyfriend)	_____	_____	_____
Not dating	_____	_____	_____
Roommate(s)/housemate(s) problems	_____	_____	_____
Concerns about STDs	_____	_____	_____
Self			
Behavior (habits, temper)	_____	_____	_____
Appearance (unattractive features, grooming)	_____	_____	_____
Ill health/physical symptoms	_____	_____	_____
Forgetting, misplacing, or losing things	_____	_____	_____
Weight/dietary management	_____	_____	_____
Self-confidence/self-esteem	_____	_____	_____
Boredom	_____	_____	_____

(continued)

Stressor	Stressful		
	Rarely/Not at all	Sometimes	Frequently
Money			
Not enough	_____	_____	_____
Bills/overspending	_____	_____	_____
Job: searching for or interviews	_____	_____	_____
Job/work issues (demanding; annoying)	_____	_____	_____
Tasks of Daily Living			
Tedious chores (shopping, cleaning)	_____	_____	_____
Traffic and parking problems	_____	_____	_____
Car problems (breakdowns, repairs)	_____	_____	_____
Housing (finding/getting or moving)	_____	_____	_____
Food (unappealing or unhealthful meals)	_____	_____	_____

2. For any frequent stressor, describe how it affects your life and offer strategies for lessening the frequency with which it occurs.

3.2 My Stress Reactions

Many people experience particular physical reactions to excessive stress. Here's a list of some common stress reactions. Check the rate at which you experience each reaction. Can you add some reactions that are not on the list?

Reaction	Once a day	Once every 2–3 days	Once a week	Once a month	Not in the last 2 months
Headaches	_____	_____	_____	_____	_____
Nervous tics and twitches	_____	_____	_____	_____	_____
Blurred vision	_____	_____	_____	_____	_____
Dizziness	_____	_____	_____	_____	_____
Fatigue	_____	_____	_____	_____	_____
Coughing	_____	_____	_____	_____	_____
Wheezing	_____	_____	_____	_____	_____
Backache	_____	_____	_____	_____	_____
Muscle spasms	_____	_____	_____	_____	_____
Itching	_____	_____	_____	_____	_____
Excessive sweating	_____	_____	_____	_____	_____
Palpitations	_____	_____	_____	_____	_____
Constipation	_____	_____	_____	_____	_____
Jaw tightening	_____	_____	_____	_____	_____
Rapid heart rate	_____	_____	_____	_____	_____
Impotence	_____	_____	_____	_____	_____
Pelvic pain	_____	_____	_____	_____	_____
Stomachache	_____	_____	_____	_____	_____
Diarrhea	_____	_____	_____	_____	_____
Frequent urination	_____	_____	_____	_____	_____
Dermatitis (rash)	_____	_____	_____	_____	_____
Hyperventilation	_____	_____	_____	_____	_____
Irregular heart rhythm	_____	_____	_____	_____	_____
High blood pressure	_____	_____	_____	_____	_____
Delayed menstruation	_____	_____	_____	_____	_____
Vaginal discharge	_____	_____	_____	_____	_____
Nail biting	_____	_____	_____	_____	_____
Heartburn	_____	_____	_____	_____	_____

3.3 How Susceptible Am I to Stress?

Some persons are more susceptible to the harmful effects of stress than others. The following inventory can give you an indication of your susceptibility. Score each item from 1 (almost always) to 5 (never) as it applies to you. A total score lower than 50 indicates you are not particularly vulnerable to stress. A score of 50 to 80 indicates moderate vulnerability, and a score of more than 80, high vulnerability—time to make some changes.

_____	1. I eat at least one hot, nutritious meal a day.
_____	2. I get 7 to 8 hours of sleep at least four nights a week.
_____	3. I am affectionate with others regularly.
_____	4. I have at least one relative within 50 miles on whom I can rely.
_____	5. I exercise to the point of sweating at least twice a week.
_____	6. I smoke fewer than 10 cigarettes a day.
_____	7. I drink fewer than five alcoholic drinks a week.
_____	8. I am about the proper weight for my height and age.
_____	9. I have enough money to meet basic expenses and needs.
_____	10. I feel strengthened by my religious beliefs.
_____	11. I attend club or social activities on a regular basis.
_____	12. I have several close friends and acquaintances.
_____	13. I have one or more friends to confide in about personal matters.
_____	14. I am basically in good health.
_____	15. I am able to speak openly about my feelings when angry or worried.
_____	16. I discuss problems about chores, money, and daily living issues with the people with whom I live.
_____	17. I do something just for fun at least once a week.
_____	18. I am able to organize my time and do not feel pressured.
_____	19. I drink fewer than three cups of coffee (or tea or cola drinks) a day.
_____	20. I allow myself quiet time at least once during each day.

TOTAL
SCORE _____

Adapted from Miller, L. H., and Smith, A. D. (1993). *The stress solution: An action plan to manage the stress in your life*. New York: Atria Books.

3.4 Warning Signs of Stress

Do you have any of these warning signs of stress?

	No	Yes
Trouble falling asleep	_____	_____
Difficulty staying asleep	_____	_____
Waking up tired and not well rested	_____	_____
Fatigue	_____	_____
Changes in eating patterns	_____	_____
Craving sweet/fatty/salty foods ("comfort foods")	_____	_____
More headaches than usual	_____	_____
Short temper/irritable	_____	_____
Recurring colds and minor illness	_____	_____
Muscle ache or tightness	_____	_____
Trouble concentrating, remembering, or staying organized	_____	_____
Depression	_____	_____

Student Workbook

3.5 My Life Changes and Stress

Directions

1. Mark any item in the Recent Life Changes Questionnaire (below) that has occurred in your life in the past month.
2. Total the number of life change units (LCUs) you have accumulated.
3. Refer to Chapter 3 of the text to determine if you are at risk for a health change.

Recent Life Changes Questionnaire

Life Event	Life Change Units		Life Event	Life Change Units	
	Women	Men		Women	Men
Death of son or daughter	135	103	Engagement to marry	47	42
Death of spouse	122	113	Moderate illness	47	39
Death of brother or sister	111	87	Loss or damage of personal property	47	35
Death of parent	105	90	Sexual difficulties	44	44
Divorce	102	85	Getting demoted at work	44	39
Death of family member	96	78	Major change in living conditions	44	37
Fired from work	85	69	Increase in income	43	30
Separation from spouse due to marital problems	79	70	Relationship problems	42	34
			Trouble with in-laws	41	33
Major injury or illness	79	64	Beginning or ending school or college	40	35
Being held in jail	78	71	Making a major purchase	40	33
Pregnancy	74	55	New, close personal relationship	39	34
Miscarriage or abortion	74	51	Outstanding personal achievement	38	33
Death of a close friend	73	64	Troubles with coworkers at work	37	32
Laid off from work	73	59	Change in school or college	37	31
Birth of a child	71	56	Change in your work hours or conditions	36	32
Adopting a child	71	54	Troubles with workers whom you supervise	35	34
Major business adjustment	67	47	Getting a transfer at work	33	31
Decrease in income	66	49	Getting a promotion at work	33	29
Parents' divorce	63	52	Change in religious beliefs	31	27
A relative moving in with you	62	53	Christmas	30	25
Foreclosure on a mortgage or a loan	62	51	Having more responsibilities at work	29	29
Investment and/or credit difficulties	62	46	Troubles with your boss at work	29	29
Marital reconciliation	61	48	Major change in usual type or amount of recreation	29	28
Major change in health or behavior of family member	58	50	General work troubles	29	27
Change in arguments with spouse	55	41	Change in social activities	29	24
Retirement	54	48	Major change in eating habits	29	23
Major decision regarding your immediate future	54	46	Major change in sleeping habits	28	23
			Change in family get-togethers	28	20
Separation from spouse due to work	53	54	Change in personal habits	27	24
An accident	53	38	Major dental work	27	23
Parental remarriage	52	45	Change of residence in same town or city	27	21
Change residence to a different town, city, or state	52	39	Change in political beliefs	26	21
			Vacation	26	20
Change to a new type of work	51	50	Having fewer responsibilities at work	22	21
"Falling out" of a close personal relationship	50	41	Making a moderate purchase	22	18
Marriage	50	50	Change in church activities	21	20
Spouse changes work	50	38	Minor violation of the law	20	19
Child leaving home	48	38	Correspondence course to help you in your work	19	16
Birth of grandchild	48	34			

Adapted from Miller, M. A. and Rahe, R. H. (1997). Life changes scaling for the 1990s. *Journal of Psychosomatic Research*, 43, 279–292, with permission from Elsevier Science.

3.6 Prioritizing Tasks: First Things First

Directions

1. Refer to your to-do list for today or create one for this exercise.

2. Sit or lie quietly for a few minutes to become mentally and physically relaxed (see note below).

3. Using a four-box chart, place each item on your to-do list in the appropriate box according to its urgency and importance (see example).

4. Carry out your tasks in this order: (1) urgent and important; (2) not urgent but important; (3) urgent but not important; and (4) not urgent and not important.

Note: Quieting yourself helps you distinguish the urgent/important tasks from the urgent/not important ones because urgency is a state of mind that makes tasks seem important even if they are not.

TO-DO

Call Jeremy
Poli sci quiz
Chem problem set
Mom b'day card
Send Monica email
Download music
Prof. Adams office hour
New shoes

		IMPORTANT	
		Yes	No
URGENT	Yes	Poli sci quiz Mom b'day card Prof Adams	Call Jeremy
	No	Send Monica email Chem problem set	Download music New shoes

3.7 Time Audit for Time Management

Directions

1. For three representative days in your life, keep a Time Diary (example below) in which you record your activities for every hour of the day. Make entries in your Time Diary two to three times a day. For example, at noon, record your activities since awakening; at 5:00 P.M. or so, record your activities since noon; at bedtime, record your activities since 5:00 P.M.

Time	Activity
6:00 A.M.	wake up
6:15 A.M.	shower/dress/eat
7:00 A.M.	go to school
8:00 A.M.	Chem lecture
9:30 A.M.	hang out in library/snack
10:30 A.M.	Psych lecture
12:00 noon	job
5:00 P.M.	go home

2. Calculate the average daily hours and percentage of a day's time spent in the following activities:

Time awake	_____hrs.	_____%
Time asleep	_____hrs.	_____%
Time traveling to and from work/school/activities	_____hrs.	_____%
Time spent at school	_____hrs.	_____%
Time spent studying/with schoolwork	_____hrs.	_____%
Time spent at job	_____hrs.	_____%
Time spent with family	_____hrs.	_____%
Time spent with friends	_____hrs.	_____%
Time spent with self	_____hrs.	_____%

3. Are you getting the recommended 7 to 8 hours of sleep per night? If not, what could you change to get more sleep?

_____

_____

_____

_____

4. Can you identify windows of time that you can devote to priority activities that now go neglected?

_____

_____

_____

_____

5. What did you learn from the Time Audit?

_____

_____

_____

_____

3.8 Are You a Procrastinator?

Do you label yourself a procrastinator? Are you haunted by undone tasks? People who label themselves as procrastinators would be wise to consider the ancient Chinese proverb, "The journey of a thousand miles begins with the first step." They tend to focus on the end result of their activities (the end of the "journey of a thousand miles") instead of steps required to get started. Doing this can make getting to the end so difficult that they become stymied and put off moving toward their goal. And the more they put it off, the more formidable it seems because time is closing in. The way out of this is to focus on the first step instead of the end result.

Directions

1. Identify ONE task or goal that you cannot seem to do or move toward. Write it down here: _____.

2. Ask yourself, "What simple thing can I do today to move me toward my goal?" For example, if you are procrastinating about doing an assignment, take your textbook or lecture notes out of your backpack and make them visible. Write down here what step you could take: _____.

3. Do the step you wrote down in step 2.

4. When you are ready, ask yourself, "What step can I take now to move me toward my goal?" For example, you may decide to open your textbook or flip through your notes. Write it down here: _____.

5. Do the step you wrote down in step 4.

6. Repeat steps 4 and 5 as many times as necessary to accomplish your goal. If all you can do is two steps, that's fine. At least you got started.

Note: Be alert for a voice in your head that tells you how lame you are for only doing a few steps or how lame this exercise is. This voice is trying to protect you from some harm it associates with accomplishing the goal. Sit quietly and "converse" with this voice (perhaps write out a dialogue) to lessen its effect on your behavior.

3.9 Minimizing In-Class Listening Errors

Ineffective learning skills are major contributors to academic stress. One group of ineffective learning skills consists of in-class listening errors, which are listed below. For each error on the list, indicate how likely you are to engage in that behavior using this scale:

1 = never, 2 = infrequently, 3 = sometimes, 4 = often, 5 = frequently

For behaviors marked with a 4 or 5, think of ways to limit their frequency.

In-Class Listening Errors

_____ 1. Calling the subject or speaker uninteresting or boring. Doing this allows you to "distance" yourself from the listening experience—to lose focus—and to daydream, chat, or sleep.
   The Efficient Listener says, "As long as I'm here, I'll focus on what's going on to gain as much as I can."

_____ 2. Criticizing the speaker's delivery. This allows you to distract yourself from the content of the message by focusing on the presentation.
   The Efficient Listener, while possibly noting that the speaker's delivery is sub par, nevertheless pays attention to the content and reserves judgment until the talk is over.

_____ 3. Getting worked-up with disagreements with the speaker's message. If you allow yourself to get caught up in challenging or contradicting the speaker (even silently in your mind), you are talking to yourself and no longer listening.
   The Efficient Listener pays attention to gather all the information before thinking about challenging what is said.

_____ 4. Listening only for facts. This risks focusing on retaining one fact and losing others.
   The Efficient Listener listens for main ideas and themes and notes facts that illustrate and support the main ideas. By having a structure, more facts are remembered.

_____ 5. Trying to outline the talk. This will work if the speaker's remarks are themselves organized. If not, the main ideas and themes can be lost while trying to find a pattern.
   The Efficient Listener notes main themes and ideas and organizes them later.

_____ 6. Faking attention. This is being present in body and not in mind.
   The Effective Listener accepts that attention will wander and learns to become aware of when attention is lost and to refocus the mind.

_____ 7. Tolerating or creating distractions. If someone is creating a distraction, tell the person that the behavior is distracting. If you cannot tell the person, raise your hand and ask the speaker to ask for order. If you lose your focus and create distractions, either take a deep breath to center yourself or excuse yourself from the talk so as not to distract others.

_____ 8. Evading or avoiding difficult material. This is a form of giving up. If you do not understand the material, rather than tune out, use your curiosity to try to learn something.

_____ 9. Letting emotion-laden words throw you off focus. Responding in your mind or verbally to emotionally charged ideas can distract you from the content. If you have a reaction to what is said, note it in your mind or jot down a word or two about it and then refocus your attention.

_____ 10. Letting your mind wander. People process what they hear in less time than it takes a speaker to talk. Don't let your mind wander in that brief period of time.
   The Effective Listener learns to "be still" by quieting the mind to keep focused during interims.

3.10 Image Visualization for Exam Anxiety

Because of school pressures and exam anxiety, students' health often suffers. Students suffer from tension and migraine headaches, stomach upsets, frequent infections, and a host of other mental and physical symptoms that are brought on or made worse by stress. Exam anxiety is learned behavior and it probably began quite early in your school life. (You may be able to recall the first time you experienced exam anxiety in school.) Like any learned behavior, exam anxiety can be unlearned or the response to it can be changed. There is absolutely nothing frightening or dangerous in exams themselves. Rather, the anxiety you experience is directly related to the importance you attach to your success on the exam. Obviously, if you feel that your whole life and future hinge on how well you score on an exam, you are constructing a situation that can cause severe anxiety and such physical symptoms as headaches and diarrhea.

Image visualization can be a powerful technique for reducing the panic and physical symptoms of exam anxiety. By using image visualization prior to an exam, you can teach your mind and body how to relax.

Directions

Step 1. Find a comfortable place in your house or apartment and a time when it is quiet. Pick an environment in which you feel secure and where there are no disturbing distractions. Sit in a comfortable chair or lie down on a couch, bed, or floor. The main thing is to get physically comfortable. If music helps you relax, you can play some of your favorite instrumental music, but it should not be so loud that it becomes intrusive.

Step 2. Close your eyes and ask your mind to recall a place where you felt content and happy. Let it be a place where you had the kind of positive feeling that you wish you had all the time. Use your imagination to reconstruct the scene or place where you felt comfortable and happy. It might be a vacation spot or a time when you were lying on a beach or hiking in the mountains. The main thing is to let your mind freely choose a place or memory that feels the most comfortable and to let yourself become totally involved in that scene. It's like having a daydream except that you are constructing your own dream. While your mind is engaged in this pleasurable memory, your body automatically relaxes.

Step 3. After your mind and body have become comfortable and relaxed, you can refocus your attention on an upcoming exam. You can visualize in your mind taking the exam while remaining relaxed and confident. Because your mind and body have already been relaxed and because you are secure and comfortable in your own environment, your mind will associate these positive feelings with the inner visualization of the exam. Use your imagination to project your mind into the future when you are taking the exam, being calm and confident as you write down the answers to the questions or write your essay.

Let your imagination construct all of the details of the exam situation. Visualize the exam room and where you are sitting; notice that you can read and understand the questions without any effort. Pay attention to how you feel as you take the exam and note the absence of anxiety and the absence of uncomfortable physical symptoms. Continue with the visualization until you feel comfortable with the experience and with the exam. Repeat this exercise for several days prior to the actual exam. When you take the exam you will be surprised at the absence of nervousness or anxiety; you will be even more surprised and pleased at the improvement in your grades.

CHAPTER 4

4.1 Keeping a Journal

Our emotions tell us how well we are fulfilling our life needs and how well we are achieving our life goals, but sometimes it is difficult to understand why we feel a certain way at a certain time. One way to clarify thoughts and feelings is to record them in a journal or notebook, which is something like a diary except that thoughts and feelings are recorded instead of specific events. Practice keeping a journal of your thoughts and feelings for a two-week period. Set aside a particular time each day, perhaps just before you go to sleep, to check in with your feelings by writing how you feel at that moment or how you felt that day and explaining why those feelings may have occurred.

- Use a special notebook for your journal.
- Write in a quiet place.
- Keep your journal private so you can be honest with yourself.
- Write continuously. Don't worry about grammar or spelling.
- Be expressive. Don't worry about making sense.

4.2 My Definition of Mental Health

Directions

List and describe five characteristics of a mentally healthy person.

1. _____
   _____

2. _____
   _____

3. _____
   _____

4. _____
   _____

5. _____
   _____

If you were (are) a parent, how would you ensure that your child(ren) manifests the five characteristics on your list?

_____
_____
_____
_____
_____
_____
_____
_____
_____
_____
_____

4.3 Saying No

Many people have a hard time saying no to the requests and demands made by others and an equally hard time saying yes to themselves for something they want. To be generous with time and energy is thought to be a virtue; to accommodate your own wishes, selfish. There are times, however, when saying no to others and yes to yourself is highly appropriate. Your emotions tell you those times. The time to say no is when saying yes makes you feel angry, stressed, resentful, or unwell. The time to say yes to yourself is when it increases physical, emotional, and spiritual well-being.

Think about some recent times when you said yes to others when you really wanted to say no. Write them down like this: I would have liked to have said no when _____ asked me to _____.

Prepare yourself to say no to the same or other requests the next time they occur. Imagine yourself saying no to another and firmly and politely dealing with the other person's response.

Learning to say no may take practice, so don't get discouraged if at first you find it difficult.

4.4 My Fears and Phobias

Many health behaviors are reflections of beliefs and attitudes that operate beneath the level of conscious awareness. Because these beliefs and attitudes in the mind are similar to programs in a computer, they can be changed. Your mind can create new, health-promoting programs to replace old, health-destroying ones.

Health problems often arise from destructive mental programs that have their origins in frightening life experiences, especially ones encountered early in life. If you can become aware of how such frightening experiences have programmed your mind and have thereby influenced your subsequent behavior, you can take steps to reprogram your mind and eliminate both the fear and the unwanted behavior.

Directions

Step 1. Identify your fears and phobias using the chart below.

Step 2. Sit or lie down in a quiet, comfortable place and allow your mind to recall experiences that may have caused one of your present fears—perhaps the one that bothers you the most. Allow yourself to relax your mind and body as much as possible, then let the images just freely enter your mind. When you encounter a frightening situation, imagine it taking place in a manner that is not frightening—in your mind, any scene can be changed so that you feel safe and comfortable. Let the situation resolve itself in a positive way. Remember, because everything is going on in your mind, you have complete control of all actions and events in your imagined scene.

Step 3. Practice this positive imagery until you feel that your fear is less intense.

Frightening situations or objects	No fear	Mild fear	Strong fear
Airplanes	_____	_____	_____
Birds	_____	_____	_____
Bats	_____	_____	_____
Blood	_____	_____	_____
Cemeteries	_____	_____	_____
Dead animals	_____	_____	_____
Insects	_____	_____	_____
Crowds of people	_____	_____	_____
Dark places	_____	_____	_____
Dentists or doctors	_____	_____	_____
Hospitals	_____	_____	_____
Dirt or germs	_____	_____	_____
Lakes or oceans	_____	_____	_____
Dogs or cats	_____	_____	_____
Other animals	_____	_____	_____
Guns	_____	_____	_____
Closets or elevators	_____	_____	_____
Heights	_____	_____	_____
Public presentations	_____	_____	_____
Loud noises	_____	_____	_____
Driving in a car	_____	_____	_____
Being shouted at	_____	_____	_____
Being rejected	_____	_____	_____
Walking alone at night	_____	_____	_____
Other fears	_____	_____	_____

4.5 My Sleep and Dream Record

Each morning for one week, assess your sleep behavior with the aid of a chart like the one below. Also record the details of your dreams in a journal or notebook. Hints for dream recording:

1. Keep a pen or a pencil and a pad of paper near your bed.
2. Remind yourself before going to sleep that you want to remember your dreams.
3. Write down your dreams immediately upon awakening.

	Sun	Mon	Tues	Wed	Thurs	Fri	Sat
Time to bed							
Time fell asleep (estimate on waking)							
Feelings before falling asleep							
Trouble falling asleep? (yes or no)							
Take sleeping aid? (e.g., milk or pills)							
Number of times awake in the night							
Time woke up							
Time got out of bed							
Feelings on awakening							
Dreams? (yes or no)							
Total sleep time							

4.6 How Can I Sleep Better?

College students are notoriously poor sleepers. Which of the healthy sleep habits listed below could you incorporate into your life? Explain your reasoning.

- *Establish a regular sleep time.* Give your own natural sleep cycle a chance to be in synchrony with the day–night cycle by going to bed at the same time each night (within an hour more or less) and arising *without being awakened by an alarm clock.* This will mean going to bed early enough to give yourself enough time to sleep. Try to maintain your regular sleep times on the weekend. Getting up early during the week and sleeping late on weekends may upset the rhythm of your sleep cycle.

- *Create a proper (for you) sleep environment.* Sleep occurs best when the sleeping environment is dark, quiet, free of distractions, and not too warm. If you use radio or TV to help you fall asleep, use an autotimer to shut off the noise after falling asleep.

- *Wind down before going to bed.* About 20 to 30 minutes before bedtime, stop any activities that cause mental or physical arousal, such as work or exercise, and take up a "quiet" activity that can create a transition to sleep. Transitional activities could include reading, watching "mindless" TV, taking a warm bath or shower, meditation, or making love.

- *Make the bedroom for sleeping only.* Make the bedroom your place for getting a good night's sleep. Try not to use it for work or for discussing problems with your partner.

- *Don't worry while in bed.* If you are unable to sleep after about 30 minutes in bed because of worry about the next day's activities, get up and do some limited activity such as reading a magazine article, doing the dishes, or meditating. Go back to bed when you feel drowsy. If you cannot sleep because of thinking about all that you have to do, write down what's on your mind and let the paper hold onto the thoughts while you sleep. You can retrieve them in the morning.

- *Avoid alcohol and caffeine.* Some people have a glass of beer or wine before bed to relax. Large amounts of alcohol, although sedating, block normal sleep and dreaming patterns. Because caffeine remains in the body for several hours, people sensitive to caffeine should not ingest any after noon.

- *Exercise regularly.* Exercising 20 to 30 minutes three or four times a week enhances the ability to sleep. You should not exercise vigorously within three hours of bedtime, however, because of the possibility of becoming too aroused to sleep.

4.7 How Do I Affect Others?

You can influence how others feel simply by your words and actions. When you sincerely say to someone, "You look terrific," you make that person feel good, thereby initiating a series of psycho-physiological processes that begin in the mind and affect hormonal and nervous regulation of the body in such a way that his or her wellness is enhanced. On the other hand, when you say to someone, "You look terrible," you can initiate physiological responses that are correspondingly negative.

Directions

Step 1. For one week keep a record of the remarks you make to others that may affect their health and well-being, either positively or negatively. For example:

To John: "I liked the way you handled your anger in that situation. How'd you do it?"

To Sue (who is overweight): "You sure do pack away the food. I don't see where you put it all."

Step 2. For one week try to avoid remarks that can hurt a person's feelings or make a person feel bad. Say positive things to the people you interact with. Tell others how well they look and how well they are doing things. Show them that you care how they feel. As people around you feel better, so will you.

4.8 Disarming Your Internal Critic

The Internal Critic is mental self-criticism. The Internal Critic says things like, "You can't do that!" or "Don't do it that way, you'll embarrass yourself." The Internal Critic can stop us from doing things for fear of shame and embarrassment, and it can make us feel generally incompetent and bad about ourselves.

You can learn to identify and disarm your Internal Critic by being alert for it. When the Internal Critic is activated, someone facing a challenge might say, "I can't" or "I'm confused." Sometimes a student verbalizes the Internal Critic's message, as in, "I'm too stupid to understand this."

Disarming the Internal Critic

1. *Name and Voice It.* Write or say what the Internal Critic says. Be sure to add the Internal Critic's emotional tone.

2. *Defend Yourself.* Say to the Internal Critic, "Don't talk to me like that!"

3. *Talk Back to It.* Write or say, "I hear you, but I'm going ahead anyway."

4. *Ignore It.* Acknowledge that the Internal Critic has been activated and say to yourself, "There's that Internal Critic again," and shift your mental focus to the task at hand.

5. *Try to Understand It.* Sometimes the Internal Critic is trying to protect you from an imagined hurt. Write an imaginary conversation with your Internal Critic in which you discuss its motive(s).

4.9 Constructing Your Personal House

Let the drawing of this house represent your personal life. Write a one-paragraph description for each of these parts of your house:

Foundation: Your life governing principles

Walls: Your means of physical and emotional support

Roof: Ways you protect yourself physically and psychologically

Chimney: Ways you relieve stress

Attic: Your fears

Chest: Highly personal things you are willing to share with another

Window: Things you are proud of

Door: Physical and psychological things you have borrowed from others

Mirror: How you see yourself (self-image, self-esteem, strengths, weaknesses)

Trash can: Things you want to get rid of

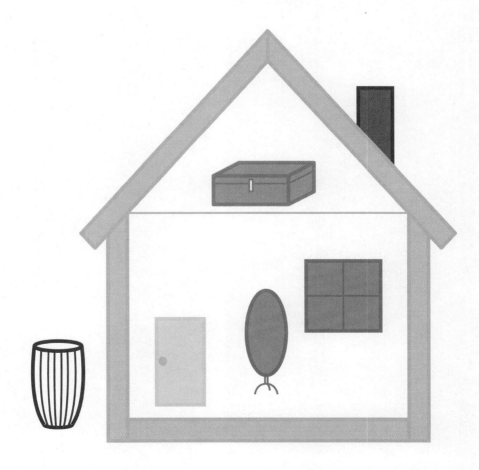

5.1 My Food Diary

Directions

For 2 days that are representative of your usual food consumption patterns, keep a list of everything you eat (see illustration below). Record:

- the name of each food item
- the quantity of each food item consumed
- the time of day each item was consumed
- whether consumption was part of a meal or as a snack
- whether you ate because of hunger or for other reasons
- your feelings at the time you ate
- the social circumstances surrounding eating (alone, with friends, with family, etc.)

Food	Quantity	Time of day	Meal or snack	Hungry? Other?	Feelings?	Social?
cereal	bowlful	6:30 AM	meal	hungry	sleepy	alone
banana	one					
milk, skim	cup					

Data Analysis

1. How close are you to the recommended Five-A-Day servings of fruits and vegetables?

   _____

   _____

   _____

   _____

2. Describe your snacking patterns.

   _____

   _____

   _____

   _____

3. Describe ways your feelings affect your food consumption.

   _____

5.2 My Estimated Daily Calorie Requirement

Estimate your daily calorie requirement using steps 1–4 below.

Step 1. I am _____ feet _____ inches tall.

Step 2. Calculate your total body mass units:

- Women: Allow 100 body mass units for the first 5 feet of height + 5 body mass units for each additional inch.
- Men: Allow 106 body mass units for the first 5 feet of height + 6 body mass units for each additional inch.

My total body mass units = _____.

Step 3. My activity factor is:

Sedentary = 13

Active = 15

Very active = 17

Step 4. Calculate your estimated daily calories by multiplying your body mass units by your activity factor:

(Body mass units) × (Activity factor) = _____ (my estimated calories)

5.3 My Dietary Analysis

Refer to your Food Diary and consult the U.S. Department of Agriculture's MyPlate website (http://www.choosemyplate.gov) to analyze the nutrient content of your diet and to obtain recommendations for improving the nutrient quality of your diet.

Directions

1. Log on to https://www.choosemyplate.gov/MyPlatePlan.

2. Click the Daily Food Plan link and enter the appropriate data for your age, sex, and level of physical activity to determine your nutritional recommendations. Print the response.

3. Go to the U.S.D.A. Food Composition Database (https://ndb.nal.usda.gov/ndb/) and enter the foods from your Food Diary for a day that is typical of your dietary pattern.

4. Add the values for calories (kcal) and grams of fiber, total fat, sugar, protein, iron, and sodium for each of the foods on your list.

_____ energy (calories/kcal)

_____ grams of fiber

_____ grams of total fat

_____ grams of sugar

_____ grams of protein

_____ milligrams of calcium

_____ milligrams of iron

_____ grams of sodium

5. How does your diet compare to the MyPlate recommendations? Do the same calculations as in Item 4 for the recommended diet you found in Item 2. A cup is 120 grams.

_____

_____

_____

_____

_____

_____

_____

_____

_____

_____

_____

_____

5.4 Can I Read a Food Label?

Go to the FDA's online food label (www.accessdata.fda.gov/scripts/InteractiveNutritionFactsLabel/#intro.whats-on-the-label) and respond to these questions:

1. Click on the Vitamin A link, then the Health Facts link. Which vitamin is considered "a nutrient of public health concern"?

2. How many added grams of sugar are in a serving of this product? A gram of sugar provides 4 calories of energy. How many calories from added sugar are contained in a serving of this product?

3. Click on the Sugars link, then the Health Facts link. How many calories from added sugar would be allowed for someone with a 2,000 calorie per day requirement? A soda contains about 120 calories of added sugar. What percentage of the daily allowable amount of added sugar would be obtained from consuming s snack consisting of one serving of this product and a soda?

4. How many more calories of added sugar would be consumed if a regular Milky Way candy bar were consumed for a sweet dessert? (Search "Milky Way food label.")

5. Click on the Ingredients Tab. How many sources of sugar are in this product? For a list of kinds of sugars that are added to foods, click on What's on the Label Tab, then the Sugars link on the label, then Action steps.

6. Click on the Resources Tab. Scroll down to and click on the National Nutrient Database link. What's the nutrient composition (grams protein, fat, carbohydrate, and fiber) of one slice of *DIGIORNO Pizza, pepperoni topping, cheese stuffed crust, frozen, baked?*

   Answers: 1: vitamin D. 2) 23; 23 x 4 = 92 calories per serving. 3) 10% x 2000 calories = 200 calories/day; 23 calories from the product + 120 calories from the soda = 143 calories consumed. Since 200 is the allowable amount, this snack provides 143/200 = 71.5% of allowable calories from added sugar. 4) a 52g Milky Way bar contains 31 grams of added sugar a 4 calories/gram = 124 calories. 5) corn syrup solids, apple juice concentrate, sugar, apples, orange juice concentrate, sugar.

5.5 Five-A-Day

Use your Food Diary (see Exercise 5.1) to determine the number of servings of fruits and vegetables you consume each day. For 3 weeks, try to increase by one (at most two) the number of servings a day of fruits and vegetables that you consume.

1. Keep a daily record of the number of servings of fruits and vegetables you consume.

2. Make a graph in which you record the number of servings of fruits and vegetables you consume each day over the 3-week activity period.

3. Identify any obstacles that prevented you from carrying out a day's activity.

4. Develop strategies for overcoming any obstacles that keep you from increasing the number of servings you consume.

5.6 My Fiber Consumption

1. Use your Food Diary (see Exercise 5.1) and this website (https://www.webmd.com/diet/healthtool -fiber-meter) to determine the number of grams of fiber you typically consume per day.

2. Make a list of foods that you will consume to bring your total number of grams of fiber consumed to 20–30 per day.

3. For 3 weeks, try to consume 20–30 grams of fiber per day. Keep a diary in which you:
   - Record the number of grams of fiber you consume and their sources.
   - Identify obstacles that prevented you from achieving your goal.
   - Identify and implement strategies for overcoming obstacles.

4. Record on a graph the number of grams of fiber you consume daily over the 3-week activity period.

5.7 Dietary Fat Consumption

Reduce fat consumption to 30% (or less) of daily calories.

1. Use your Food Diary and the U.S. Department of Agriculture's SuperTracker website (http://www.supertracker.usda.gov) to determine the percentage of total calories from saturated fat you typically consume each day.

2. Make a list of food exchanges that you will employ to lower your fat intake (e.g., piece of fruit for a candy bar, pasta for a hamburger, etc.).

3. For 3 weeks, alter your diet to lower your fat intake.

4. Keep a diary in which you record the following information:

   - The amount of fat grams and fat calories you consume each day

   - Any obstacles that prevented you from carrying out a day's activity

   - Strategies for overcoming any obstacles

5. Make a graph in which you record the percentage of total daily calories derived from fat during the 3-week action period.

5.8 My Soda Consumption

Soda is nutritionally inferior. Sodas with sugar contribute to weight gain. Try to limit or eliminate soda consumption using the following steps:

- For 1 week, keep a diary of your soda consumption; count how many sodas you consume each day.

- For the next 2 to 3 weeks, reduce soda consumption gradually by choosing alternative beverages, such as water, tea, or 100% juice (no sugary "juice drinks" or "energy drinks"). Note: Going "cold turkey" on sodas may produce caffeine withdrawal headaches for a couple of days. Cut back gradually.

- Continue to keep your soda consumption diary to record decreasing consumption. Record obstacles that get in the way of reducing soda consumption.

Student Workbook

6.1 Fast-Food Restaurant Research

Each day approximately 20% of the U.S. population eats at a fast-food restaurant. The reasons for patronizing such establishments are convenience (they are everywhere), perceived lack of time to shop and prepare meals at home, fast food's taste and texture, the need to mollify nagging children, and cost. Since fast food is so popular and prevalent, it is healthful to know the nutrient content of the fast food you consume. So...

Directions

1. Go to your favorite fast-food restaurant and ask the serviceperson for a copy of the brochure listing the nutritional content of that establishment's foods. (If you do not patronize such establishments, do the assignment for someone you know who does and share the information with her or him.)

2. Choose a fast-food meal that is typical for you. Refer to the restaurant's website or brochure, and for each of the meal's components list the following information:

   - Total calories
   - Grams of protein
   - Total grams of fat
   - Total grams of saturated fat
   - mg of cholesterol
   - mg of salt
   - Grams of fiber

3. Calculate the dollar cost of the energy content of the meal (divide total calories by the total cost). This tells you how much bang (energy) you are getting for your buck.

4. What percentage of your estimated daily calories is contributed by this meal?

   _____

   _____

5. Describe your experience obtaining the company's brochure at the restaurant.

   _____

   _____

6. List the reasons you patronize this establishment.

   _____

   _____

7. How frequently do you patronize fast-food restaurants?

   _____

   _____

8. What did you learn from this assignment?

   _____

   _____

Note: The U.S. Department of Agriculture's National Nutrient Dadatase provides ingredient information for fast foods (https://ndb.nal.usda.gov/ndb/) and lists the nutrient composition of fast foods. Most fast-food corporations list the nutrient composition of their products on the company website. Whereas it is possible to analyze the data for this assignment with that Web tool, it is more interesting and makes you a better health consumer if you go personally to the restaurant and ask for the data.

6.2 My Body Weight

My height in feet and inches (without shoes):_____.

My weight in pounds now (with clothes):_____.

My highest weight as an adult = _____ pounds, which I weighed when I was _____ years old.

My lowest weight as an adult = _____ pounds, which I weighed when I was _____ years old.

The recommended weight for my height and body frame is (see text Chapter 6): _____.

My body mass index* is _____.

(See the BMI chart in Chapter 6 or the online calculator at https://www.nhlbi.nih.gov/health/educational/lose_wt/BMI/bmicalc.htm.

The circumference of my body at my waist† is _____.

The circumference of my body at my hips is _____.

The ratio‡ of my waist/hip circumferences is _____.

---

*The body mass index (BMI) is the most common way doctors assess the relationship of body size and health. It is calculated by dividing a person's weight in kilograms by her or his height in meters squared: $BMI = wgt/(hgt)(hgt)$. A BMI between 18 and 24.9 is not associated with an increased risk of weight-related illness. (Note: The health risks for a BMI over 25 are less reliable for people who are muscular or have a large body frame.)

†A waist circumference of more than 40 inches in men and 35 inches in women indicates overweight.

‡A waist-to-hip ratio of 0.95 in men and 0.80 in women indicates overweight.

6.3 Managing My Weight

Develop a plan for weight loss/weight management.

1. Determine your healthy weight range by consulting the weight-for-height tables and BMI table in Chapter 6 of the text.

    My healthful body weight range is _____.

    My body mass index is _____.

2. If you wish to lose weight, make a plan that combines increased exercise and moderate calorie reduction to produce the loss of not more than one pound a week until body weight is reduced by 10%. List the types and duration of exercise you will do, foods that you will limit, and the length of time you will devote to a weight loss regime.

    Exercise I will increase:

    _____

    _____

    _____

    Foods I will limit:

    _____

    _____

    _____

    Time allotted to lose 10% of current body weight:

    _____

    _____

    _____

3. Increase exercise and limit certain foods (e.g., junk and fast foods, sodas).

4. Keep a daily record of exercise and dietary changes. For each day record the following information:
    *   The exercise changes you're doing
    *   The food changes you make
    *   What you experience
    *   Any obstacles that prevented you from carrying out a day's plan
    *   Strategies for overcoming any obstacles

5. Make a graph in which you record each day the number of minutes of exercise you do and the number of calories you don't consume.

6.4 My Body Image

Body image (more accurately, body esteem) is a self-appraisal of your body's size and shape.

Directions:

1. Do the Body Image questionnaire below.

    How do you feel about the appearances of these regions of your body?

	Quite satisfied	Somewhat satisfied	Somewhat dissatisfied	Very dissatisfied
Hair	❑	❑	❑	❑
Arms	❑	❑	❑	❑
Hands	❑	❑	❑	❑
Feet	❑	❑	❑	❑
Waist	❑	❑	❑	❑
Buttocks	❑	❑	❑	❑
Hips	❑	❑	❑	❑
Legs and ankles	❑	❑	❑	❑
Thighs	❑	❑	❑	❑
Chest or breasts	❑	❑	❑	❑
Posture	❑	❑	❑	❑
General attractiveness	❑	❑	❑	❑

2. Write an essay in which you respond to these questions:

    *   Which of your regular thoughts and actions are likely to enhance your body image?

    *   Which of your regular thoughts and actions are likely to be detrimental to your body image?

    *   How do social expectations of body size and shape affect your body image?

    *   How susceptible are you to media images of "ideal" body proportions for members of your sex?

    *   How could you become more satisfied with your body image?

CHAPTER 7

7.1 Putting Exercise Into My Life

1. Use your Time Audit (see Exercise 3.7 in Chapter 3) to identify four "windows" of time during the week to exercise.

2. Choose an activity that interests you and schedule it for your four "exercise windows."

3. Keep a diary of your exercise sessions. For each day record the following information:
   - The activity
   - The time you spent doing the activity
   - What you experienced while doing the activity
   - Any obstacles that prevented you from carrying out a day's activity
   - Strategies for overcoming any obstacles

4. Make a graph in which you record the number of sessions of exercise and their length each week.

7.2 Walking for Health

Everyone knows that physical activity is good for health. Those who are not active frequently say that they don't have time to go to the gym and/or that they hate to sweat. Aerobic activity (the kind in which you breathe hard and sweat) and strength training, while good for health if done in moderation so as to avoid injury, are not the only ways to be active. The easiest and cheapest form of physical activity is to walk.

The current minimum recommendation is to walk for a total of 150 minutes a week, which is about 20 minutes a day (1 mile). Forty minutes to an hour a day is best (3 miles). And you don't have to do the whole 20–60 minutes at once. You can break it up into segments.

If you like to count or like to challenge yourself, you can get a pedometer or mobile app that counts your steps. Try to walk 10,000 steps a day in any way you can. Keep a "walking log" in which you record the number of steps you take each day.

7.3 My Target Heart Rate Zone

Your target heart rate zone is the level of activity that leads to maximum conditioning. Activity below the target heart rate zone conditions little; activity above the target heart rate zone may be dangerous for some people.

The pattern of the preferred exercise session is shown in the following figure:

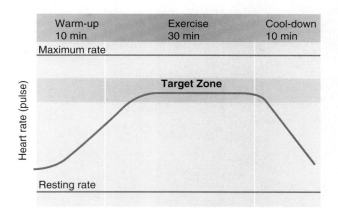

To compute your target heart rate zone:

1. Subtract your age from 220 (Example: For a 20-year-old person with resting heart rate of 80 beats/min: 220 − 20 = 200).
2. Subtract resting heart rate from number obtained in step 1 (200 − 80 = 120).
3. Multiply the result once by 0.65 and once again by 0.75 (120 × .65 = 78; 120 × .75 = 90).
4. Add resting heart rate to the results obtained in step 3 to give lower and upper heart rates of target zone (Lower limit: 78 + 80 = 158; upper limit: 90 + 80 = 170).

After your warm-up period and 10 minutes of activity, take your pulse and compare it to the heart rate for your target zone level of activity. If you are below your target zone heart rate, increase your activity. If above, slow down.

Measuring Heart Rate

Your heart rate, or pulse, is the number of times your heart beats per minute. When your heart beats, it pushes about a cup of blood into your circulatory system. At certain sites in the circulatory system you can feel when the blood from the most recent heartbeat arrives. These sites are where you measure your heart rate. The most commonly used are in the neck (carotid artery), the wrist below the thumb (radial artery), or the inner thigh (femoral artery). To measure your heart rate:

- Get a device that measures seconds.
- Place your first two fingers, not your thumb (it has a pulse and can confuse things), on one of the common measuring sites (neck, wrist, or inner thigh).
- Press a tiny bit to make solid contact with the tissue under the skin (including the artery).
- Move your fingers around until the sensation of the pulse is strongest.
- Look at your timing device and count the number of beats/pulsations in 15 seconds.
- Multiply the number of beats/pulsations in 15 seconds by 4 to get beats per minute.

7.4 My Fitness Index

The Harvard Step Test is a standardized measure of cardiorespiratory fitness. To carry out the Harvard Step Test, you need to be comfortably dressed (athletic clothes are best); you need a chair, stool, or bench 12–18 inches high, a stopwatch or clock with a second hand, a pencil and paper, and a metronome or some other method to produce a rhythmic 100–120 beats per minute, such as a recording of a march or some disco music. Once all this is assembled, you can begin.

1. Make a 15-second recording of your resting pulse and multiply by 4 to obtain your rate per minute.

2. Start the metronome or music; 120 beats per minute.

3. Step completely up on the bench with the left leg first, followed by your right leg, then step back down with the left leg first, followed by the right. The stepping should be done on a four-count: up-up-down-down; up-up-down-down....

4. Continue the exercise for 3 minutes unless you are more than 30 years old and have been rather inactive for more than six months. In that case, do the test for only a minute or two, whichever you think you can do. If you are sure you cannot do the test for even a few seconds, don't.

5. When the 3 minutes of exercise are through, immediately take your pulse. Record the number of heartbeats between 15 and 30 seconds after exercising. Make another heart rate measurement between 60 and 75 seconds; another between 120 and 135 seconds; another between 180 and 195 seconds; another between 240 and 255 seconds; and a final measurement between 300 and 315 seconds.

6. Multiply each of the 15-second heart rates by 4 to give the beats per minute. Record your data on the graph provided.

7. Compute your Fitness Index: Add the per-minute heart rates for the first 3 minutes after exercise. Then divide that number into 30,000.

Fitness index	Rating
Above 90	Excellent
80–89	Good
65–79	Average
55–64	Low Average
Below 55	Poor

Harvard Step Test Data Record

Time	Heartbeats per 15 Seconds	Heartbeats per Minute
At rest	_____ × 4 =	_____
15–30 sec.	_____ × 4 =	_____
60–75 sec.	_____ × 4 =	_____
120–135 sec.	_____ × 4 =	_____
180–195 sec.	_____ × 4 =	_____
240–255 sec.	_____ × 4 =	_____
300–315 sec.	_____ × 4 =	_____

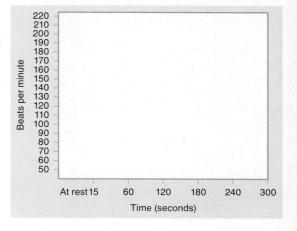

7.5 Increasing My Physical Fitness

1. Measure your level of fitness using the Harvard Step Test (see Exercise 7.4).

2. Measure your resting heart rate.

3. Determine your Target Zone heart rate (see Exercise 7.3).

4. Refer to your Time Audit to find at least four times per week when you can exercise for 30–60 minutes (see Exercise 3.7 in Chapter 3).

   My Fitness Index is _____.

   My resting heart rate is _____ beats per minute.

   My Target Zone heart rate is between _____ and _____ beats per minute.

5. Choose an aerobic activity that interests you and exercise at least four times a week for three weeks. Determine your heart rate at the end of each exercise session to see if you are exercising within your target zone.

6. Keep a diary of your activity. For each day record the following information:
   - The activity
   - The time you spent doing the activity
   - What you experienced doing the activity
   - Any obstacles that prevented you from carrying out a day's activity
   - Strategies for overcoming any obstacles

7. For each week record your resting heart rate and your Fitness Index.

8. Make a graph in which you record for the three-week period:
   - The number of sessions of exercise and their length
   - Your resting heart rate at the start and end of the project
   - Your Fitness Index at the start and end of the project

7.6 My Flexibility Index

Body flexibility is a fundamental aspect of feeling good and keeping your body healthy. Use this simple YMCA test to determine your degree of body flexibility, and continue to use it to determine your progress in becoming more limber.

1. Warm up with some stretching before the test.

2. Sit on the floor with your legs extended and feet a few inches apart.

3. With a piece of adhesive tape, mark the place where your heels touch the floor. Your heels should touch the near edge of the tape.

4. Place a yardstick on the floor between your legs and parallel to them. The beginning of the yardstick should be closest to you and the 15-inch mark should align with the near edge of the tape.

5. Slowly reach with both hands as far forward as possible. Touch your fingers to the yardstick to determine the distance reached. Do not jerk to increase your distance—this may cause damage to your leg muscles.

6. Repeat the exercise two or three times and record your best score.

Inches reached		Rating
Men	Women	
22–23	24–27	Excellent
20–21	21–23	Good
14–19	16–20	Average
12–13	13–15	Fair
0–11	0–12	Poor

7.7 Increasing My Flexibility

Increase your flexibility by undertaking a regular regime of stretching or yoga.

1. Measure your flexibility by using the flexibility test (see Exercise 7.6).
2. Refer to your Time Audit (see Exercise 3.7 in Chapter 3) to find at least four occasions per week when you can stretch for 10–20 minutes each time.
3. Choose a stretching regime (see text Chapter 7) that interests you and carry it out at least four times a week.
4. Keep a diary of your activity:
   - Record the number of stretching sessions you do each week.
   - Record the time spent in each session.
   - Record your physical and psychological experiences before and after each session.
   - Identify any obstacles that prevented you from carrying out a day's activity.
   - Develop strategies for overcoming any obstacles.
5. Make a graph in which you record the number of sessions of stretching each week. Determine your flexibility index (inches reached) at the end of each week.

7.8 The Sun Salute

The sun salute, a Hatha yoga exercise, is a series of 12 postures, or asanas, intended to be done in one flowing routine. Each of the 12 postures is held for 3 seconds. The entire routine should be done at least twice in succession, alternating the legs. The Sun Salute is an excellent way to stretch the body every morning or any time you may need to relax tense muscles and restore deep, regular breathing. Try it.

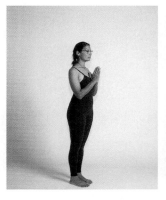

Position 1 Stand erect with your feet hip-width apart and palms together in front of your chest. Inhale and exhale slowly and calmly.

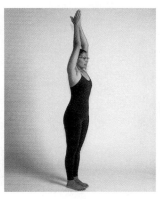

Position 2 Inhaling, raise your arms above your head, palms facing in. Lengthen through the spine, but do not arch your back.

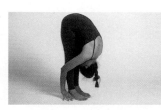

Position 3 Exhaling, bend forward from the hips, keeping your arms extended and your head hanging loosely between them. Keep your legs slightly bent and relax your neck and shoulders.

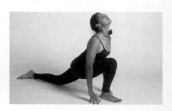

Position 4 Inhaling, bend both knees and place your palms flat on the floor by the outsides of your feet. Extend your left leg back. Stretch your chin toward the ceiling.

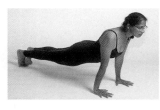

Position 5 Continue while holding the breath if you can—don't strain. Reach your forward leg back next to the other leg. Hold your body straight, supported by your hands and toes, with ankles, hips, and shoulders in a straight plane.

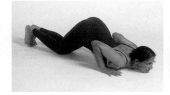

Position 6 Exhaling, lower your knees, chest, and chin or forehead to the floor, keeping your hips up and toes curled under.

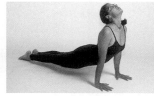

Position 7 Inhaling, bring the tops of your feet to the floor, straighten your legs, and come up to straight arms, opening the chest and stretching your chin toward the ceiling. Be careful not to overarch your lower back.

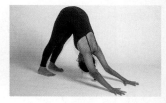

Position 8 Exhaling, curl your toes under and raise your hips into an inverted "V." Push back with your hands and lengthen your spine by reaching your hips upward. Keep your head hanging loosely.

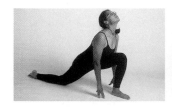

Position 9 Inhaling, lift your head and bring your left leg between your hands, keeping the right leg back. Raise your chin toward the ceiling.

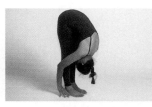

Position 10 Exhaling, bring your left foot forward so your feet are together. Bend forward from the hips, keeping your legs slightly bent and your upper body relaxed. If you can, touch your head to your knees and place your palms beside your feet.

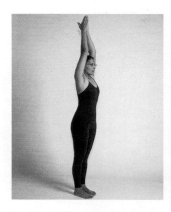

Position 11 Inhaling, slowly straighten up with your arms extended above your head. If you have any lower back pain, be sure to bend your knees.

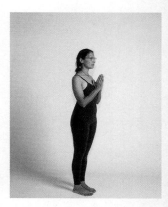

Position 12 Exhaling, bring your hands together in front of you. Close your eyes for a moment and feel the sensations in your body.

8.1 Listening Exercise

Directions

Ask someone to be the speaker for this exercise. Carry out steps 1–4 below. So that you can observe body language (very important for discerning the speaker's emotions), do the assignment in person, not on the phone or via email, IM, or text messaging.

Step 1. **Topic 1:** Ask the speaker to tell you something that's important to her or him. The first time you do this it's better that the topic not involve you personally or your relationship with the speaker. Let the speaker talk for up to 5 minutes.

Step 2. While the speaker is talking, just listen, and notice any urges you have to stop paying attention or to interrupt with suggestions or comments. Notice where your attention goes, for example, if your mind drifts to other topics or you daydream. Notice if you feel critical or if you have the urge to comment or advise.

Step 3. When the speaker has finished, tell her or him what you experienced. Share with the speaker if you were able to pay full attention to what was being said or if your mind was busy with something else. If you're new at this, you'll probably notice that it's difficult simply to listen.

Step 4. **Topic 2:** Do the exercise a second time. Ask the speaker to address a topic different from that addressed in step 1. Also, instead of telling the speaker your experience with listening, tell the speaker a paraphrase of what she or he said using

- an *emotion word* that describes the speaker's feelings (not yours!)
- a *because statement* that describes the reason for that emotion from the speaker's point of view (not yours!)

As a noun, the word *paraphrase* means a condensed rewording of a statement, given in simple language for clarity. As a verb, *paraphrase* means to render a paraphrase.

Example: The speaker talks about being worried that she has not found an occupation that seems interesting. The listener responds:

"You seem nervous because you haven't found a job you want to do in the future."
nervous = emotion word that describes the speaker's feelings
because you haven't found a job you want to do in the future = reason for the feelings

Do not offer the speaker

- your advice ("You should…")
- your opinion ("I think…")
- your judgments ("That's crazy/stupid/weird")
- your life history ("Here's what happened to me…")
- your predictions ("It/he/she will…")

At first, listening and paraphrasing may feel uncomfortable because it is not how we usually converse. But with a little practice you'll get good at it, and those with whom you communicate—family, friends, lovers, and coworkers—will appreciate you greatly for it.

Reaction Essay

Respond in writing to the following questions.

1. With whom did you carry out the Listening Exercise?

2. In step 1, what topic did the speaker address?

3. In step 1, what did you notice your mind doing while the speaker was talking?

4. In step 4, what was the topic of the speaker's remarks?

5. In step 4, write the paraphrase you offered the speaker, using the speaker's emotion word (not yours!) and the speaker's because statement (not yours!).

   Correct: "You're nervous because you cannot find a job you want to do."

   Incorrect: "The speaker was nervous about not finding a job."

   Incorrect: "I was bored because I've heard this complaint a million times."

6. What effect did this exercise have on your usual listening style?

8.2 My Sexual Attitudes

Write a one-paragraph response to the following questions. Your responses will be read only by the instructor and will be kept strictly confidential.

1. Describe how your current sexual attitudes and beliefs compare to those of your parents (give examples).

_____
_____
_____
_____

2. Describe the ways religious/spiritual values affect your sexuality and sexual behavior.

_____
_____
_____
_____

3. What is the importance of sex in human relationships?

_____
_____
_____
_____

4. By what criteria, if any, is sexual intercourse before marriage permissible? How would you advise your own child on having premarital sex?

_____
_____
_____
_____

5. Describe two social expectations of you as a member of your sex.

_____
_____
_____
_____

Complete the following statements based upon your experiences and thoughts.

6. When I was growing up, talking about sexual matters with my parents…

_____
_____
_____
_____

7. As a child and teenager I learned the most about sex from…

_____
_____
_____
_____

8. The way I reacted to how my body changed at puberty was…, especially…

_____

_____

_____

_____

9. My first significant sexual experience (not necessarily intercourse) taught me that…

_____

_____

_____

_____

10. From my parents' marriage I learned…

_____

_____

_____

_____

8.3 My Sexual Values

For each statement, indicate the response that most closely identifies your beliefs and attitudes. Use the following code:

A = I strongly agree   B = I slightly agree
C = I slightly disagree   D = I strongly disagree

_____ 1. Men are by nature more sexually aggressive than women are and enjoy sex more than women do.

_____ 2. Sex-role definitions and stereotypes get in the way of mutually satisfying sexual relations.

_____ 3. Concern over sexual performance is quite common.

_____ 4. Psychologically healthy people don't experience any guilt over their sexual activities.

_____ 5. If a woman doesn't experience orgasm, it is generally because the man has not been sensitive enough to her needs.

_____ 6. If a man experiences erection problems, it is generally because of the woman's lack of appreciation of his manhood.

_____ 7. In a sexual relationship, it is the job of each partner to make the other feel like a woman or a man.

_____ 8. Getting in touch with our sexual attractions and feelings toward others generally leads to overt sexual behavior.

_____ 9. The quality of a sexual relationship is usually parallel to the quality of the partners' relationship in general.

_____ 10. Sexual freedom implies doing whatever consenting adults agree to.

_____ 11. If we want to, we can reeducate ourselves so that we can experience sexual relationships with numerous partners without feeling guilty.

_____ 12. Sexual freedom ought to be counterbalanced by sexual responsibility.

_____ 13. We will probably be no more sexually attractive to others than we are to ourselves.

_____ 14. Discussing sexual wants and needs generally leads to mechanical and unspontaneous sex.

_____ 15. Extramarital sex inevitably causes dissatisfaction in the marital relationships.

_____ 16. Today's generation is really unconcerned about being sexually inadequate.

_____ 17. Most people who are intimate with each other find it relatively easy to talk openly and honestly about the intimate details of sexuality.

_____ 18. The key to improving sexual satisfaction is to master sexual techniques and skills.

_____ 19. Sex without love is unsatisfying.

8.4 My Relationship Wants and Needs

Directions

1. What are your wants and needs in a love relationship? Choose the three most important items from the list below.

   _____

   _____

   _____

2. Consider the list again and choose the singlemost important item.

   _____

3. Write your choices and the reasons for choosing them.

   _____

   _____

   _____

4. Optional: Which items does your partner choose?

   _____

   I want someone to…

   Love me

   Confide in me

   Show me affection

   Respect my needs

   Appreciate what I wish to achieve

   Understand my moods

   Help me make important decisions

   Stimulate my ambition

   Look up to

   Give me self-confidence

   Stand by me in difficulty

   Appreciate me as I am

   Admire my ability

   Make me feel that I count for something

   Relieve my loneliness

   Support me and our children

   Accept my need to be self-sufficient and independent

8.5 My Relationship Values

What are your priorities in a love relationship? Rate the items in the list below with a number from 1 to 10, using 1 to indicate least importance to you and 10 most importance to you.

Write a one-page essay in which you describe the three items you feel most strongly about and why.

_____ Being able to talk comfortably to my partner about my innermost feelings

_____ Having my partner share with me his/her innermost feelings

_____ Sharing with my partner nearly all of my leisure time

_____ Both of us having similar political beliefs

_____ Each of us having our own careers

_____ Being able to express anger to my partner

_____ Having my partner express his/her anger to me

_____ Being able to have sexual relations with other people

_____ Having good relations with my parents and family

_____ Enjoying what we have now without concern for a lifelong relationship

_____ Having mutual close friends

_____ Having similar religious beliefs

_____ Having major interests and friendships of my own outside the relationship

_____ Wanting the same material possessions (house, car, etc.)

_____ Being able to tell my partner when I feel jealous

_____ Having the most influence over how we as a couple spend money

_____ Trying with my partner new sexual experiences and techniques

_____ Working together on tasks rather than dividing them between us

_____ Having children

9.1 Parenthood and Me

Directions

In the list below, indicate how strongly you agree with each motivation for becoming a parent. Can you add any motivations to the list?

Motivation	Strongly agree	Agree	Disagree
To have a child who looks like me			
To have child who will carry on the family name			
To have a child who will be successful			
To have someone to inherit my money or property			
To have someone who will regard me highly			
To have someone who will return my love			
To do something I know I can do well			
To feel pride in creating another human being			
To keep me young at heart			
To help me feel fulfilled			
To make my marriage happier			
To make me feel masculine/feminine			
To please my family and society			
To teach someone about the beauty of life			
To help someone grow and develop			
Other			
Other			

CHAPTER 10

10.1 Choosing a Contraceptive

Directions

Indicate the suitability <u>for you</u> of the fertility control methods in the list below and give reasons for your choices.

Method	Very suitable	Suitable	Not suitable	Reasons
Abstinence	_____	_____	_____	_____
Condom (female)	_____	_____	_____	_____
Condom (male)	_____	_____	_____	_____
Diaphragm	_____	_____	_____	_____
Fertility awareness	_____	_____	_____	_____
Hormonal pill	_____	_____	_____	_____
Hormonal patch	_____	_____	_____	_____
Hormonal ring	_____	_____	_____	_____
Intrauterine device (IUD)	_____	_____	_____	_____
Progestin-only method	_____	_____	_____	_____
Spermicidal foam/gel	_____	_____	_____	_____
Tubal ligation	_____	_____	_____	_____
Vasectomy	_____	_____	_____	_____

11.1 AIDS and Me

How has HIV/AIDS touched your life? Write a response to this question considering the following aspects:

1. Personal experience with someone with HIV/AIDS
2. Whether HIV/AIDS has affected your personal behaviors
3. The ways HIV/AIDS has affected your community and society
4. The ways the worldwide HIV/AIDS epidemic affects your life

11.2 AIDS in Film

1. Watch the HBO film "*And the Band Played On*," a dramatization of the beginnings of the AIDS epidemic in the 1980s.

2. After viewing the film, write a reaction paper in which you respond to these questions:
   - What was your overall impression of the film?
   - What were the two most interesting things about HIV/AIDS that you learned?
   - What is your opinion of the scientists who do HIV/AIDS research?
   - What effect did the video have on your attitude about HIV/AIDS?
   - Would you recommend that others watch this film? Why or why not?

Note: The 2008 Nobel Prize in Medicine was awarded to two of the scientists portrayed in the film, Luc Montagnier and Françoise Barre-Sinoussi (see the Nobel Foundation website: http://nobelprize.org/nobel_prizes/).

CHAPTER 12

12.1 My Vaccination Record

Directions

Make a record of your vaccinations using the chart below.

Vaccine	Year initial series completed	Years revaccinated					
Diphtheria							
Hepatitis A							
Hepatitis B							
Influenza							
Measles							
Mumps							
Pertussis (whooping cough)							
Polio							
German measles (rubella)							
Tetanus							
Tuberculosis							
Other							

13.1 My Cancer Risks

Directions

1. Go to the online assessment tool Your Disease Risk (http://www.yourdiseaserisk.wustl.edu/).
2. Click on "What Is Your Cancer Risk?"
3. Assess your risks for any three of the cancers listed here:

   Bladder

   Breast

   Cervix

   Colon

   Kidney

   Lung

   Skin

   Ovary

   Pancreas

   Prostate

   Stomach

   Uterus

13.2 My Environmental Cancer Risks

Many environmental factors are linked to cancer, including those in the list below.

Directions

1. Estimate your exposure to each potential carcinogen listed in the chart below.
2. Write down some ideas about how you could reduce your exposure to some of them.

Potential Carcinogen	Exposure			
	High	Moderate	Low	None
Personal cigarette smoking	_____	_____	_____	_____
Secondhand smoke	_____	_____	_____	_____
Smokeless tobacco	_____	_____	_____	_____
Asbestos (in old buildings, including schools)	_____	_____	_____	_____
Radon (a radioactive gas in soil)	_____	_____	_____	_____
Indoor solid fuel (wood, coal) burning	_____	_____	_____	_____
Photochemical smog (from cars)	_____	_____	_____	_____
Human papillomavirus	_____	_____	_____	_____
Human immunodeficiency virus	_____	_____	_____	_____
Hepatitis B virus	_____	_____	_____	_____
Epstein-Barr virus	_____	_____	_____	_____
Helicobacter pylori infection	_____	_____	_____	_____
Sun exposure (or artificial tanning)	_____	_____	_____	_____
Well-done cooked meats	_____	_____	_____	_____
Postmenopausal estrogen therapy	_____	_____	_____	_____
Diethylstilbestrol (DES)	_____	_____	_____	_____
Benzene	_____	_____	_____	_____
Formaldehyde	_____	_____	_____	_____
Nickle-containing materials	_____	_____	_____	_____
Gamma irradiation	_____	_____	_____	_____
X-rays	_____	_____	_____	_____
Radioactive chemicals	_____	_____	_____	_____
Dioxin	_____	_____	_____	_____
Vinyl chloride	_____	_____	_____	_____
Coal tars	_____	_____	_____	_____
Soot	_____	_____	_____	_____
Wood dust	_____	_____	_____	_____

14.1 My Risk for Heart Disease

Directions

1. Go to the online assessment tool Your Disease Risk (http://www.yourdiseaserisk.wustl.edu/).
2. Click on "What Is Your Heart Disease Risk?"
3. Complete the Questionnaire.
4. List any risk factors that you could/should lower, and for each, identify one health behavior you could change that would help reduce that risk.

15.1 My Family Medical History

Directions

1. In the chart below, mark an "X" in a column to indicate the occurrence of a particular disease in a family member.

	Disease						If deceased, age at death	Cause of death
	Cancer	Diabetes	Heart disease	Hypertension	Stroke	Other		
Father								
Mother								
Brother								
Brother								
Sister								
Sister								
Father's father								
Father's mother								
Father's brother or sister								
Mother's father								
Mother's mother								
Mother's brother or sister								

2. For any "X" in your chart, research any possibility that the disease has some degree of inherited component.

16.1 Being Knowledgeable About Drugs

What do you know about the drugs and medicines that you consume?

Directions

1. Go to one of the websites listed on this page (or an authoritative alternative) to learn about any medications or dietary supplements you are taking or have taken or a particular "recreational" or social drug you currently use or once used.

2. Describe something of interest that you learned.

_____

_____

_____

_____

Medicines

MedlinePlus Drug Information, http://www.nlm.nih.gov/medlineplus/druginformation.html

Dietary Supplements

National Center for Complementary and Alternative Medicine, http://nccam.nih.gov/health/supplements

Nonmedical Drug Use

National Institute on Drug Abuse, http://www.nida.nih.gov/

Alcohol Use and Abuse

National Institute on Alcohol Abuse and Alcoholism, http://www.niaaa.nih.gov/

16.2 Medicines I Take

Directions

1. In the chart below, list any medicines you are taking. Consult the product packaging, your doctor, the pharmacist, authoritative books (e.g., *Physician's Desk Reference*), or the U.S. National Library of Medicine's MedlinePlus website (https://medlineplus.gov/druginformation.html) for information about side effects and reasons not to take the medicine (*contraindications*).

2. Assess the risks of taking a medicine in relation to its therapeutic benefits.

   _____

   _____

3. Search for nondrug alternatives to the drugs on your list.

   _____

   _____

Drug	Side effects	Contraindications

16.3 Nonessential Drugs I Consume

Americans consume too many drugs, in part because of the belief (promoted by drug manufacturers) that health and well-being are enhanced by chemicals. Whereas many drugs, when used appropriately, can promote wellness and relieve illness, too often people consume drugs unnecessarily.

Directions

1. For 1 week, make a list of the nonessential drugs you ingest. Be sure to include coffee, tea, and cola and "energy" drinks, all of which contain caffeine; alcohol; nicotine; and pain relievers.

2. After recording your nonessential drug consumption during Week 1, for another week try to eliminate one of the nonessential drugs you ingest and make notes about how you feel.

Week 1	Sun	Mon	Tues	Wed	Thurs	Fri	Sat
Caffeine (How many cups of coffee or 12-oz. servings of cola drinks per day?)							
Alcohol (How many 12-oz. beers, glasses of wine, or mixed drinks per day?)							
Nicotine (How many cigarettes, cigars, pipes, or dips of snuff or chewing tobacco per day?)							
Pain relievers (How many tablets per day?)							
Other:							
Other:							

Week 2	Sun	Mon	Tues	Wed	Thurs	Fri	Sat
Caffeine (How many cups of coffee or 12-oz. servings of cola drinks per day?)							
Alcohol (How many 12-oz. beers, glasses of wine, or mixed drinks per day?)							
Nicotine (How many cigarettes, cigars, pipes, or dips of snuff or chewing tobacco per day?)							
Pain relievers (How many tablets per day?)							
Other:							
Other:							

16.4 Drugs in Media and Advertising

Directions

Find two examples of advertising in magazines, newspapers, radio, film, TV, or the Web that promote or facilitate the use of alcohol, tobacco, or prescription and nonprescription drugs. For each example, write an analysis in which you do the following:

1. Describe the images in the advertisement (e.g., the ages, appearance, and activities of the models; if a story is being depicted).

   _____

   _____

2. Identify the means by which the advertiser links the images in the ad to the product being sold.

   _____

   _____

3. Identify the audience to which the ad is directed and how the imagery is used to "grab" that audience.

   _____

   _____

4. Offer your opinion of the commercial effectiveness of the ad (i.e., does it sell?).

   _____

   _____

   _____

   _____

5. Offer your opinion of the effect of the ad on society.

   _____

   _____

   _____

17.1 Why Do I Smoke?

Smoking can provide a variety of rewards. Knowing the reasons you smoke can help you quit and stay smoke-free.

Directions

1. Answer the questions below by entering one of the following numbers for each:

   1 = Never
   2 = Seldom
   3 = Occasionally
   4 = Frequently
   5 = Always

2. Use the scoring section to calculate your score for each of the smoking categories.

3. Consult the scoring interpretation page to find out what your score means.

		Score
A.	I smoke cigarettes to keep myself from slowing down.	_____
B.	Handling a cigarette is part of the enjoyment of smoking it.	_____
C.	Smoking cigarettes is pleasant and relaxing.	_____
D.	I light up a cigarette when I feel angry about something.	_____
E.	When I have run out of cigarettes I find it almost unbearable until I can get them.	_____
F.	I smoke cigarettes automatically without even being aware of it.	_____
G.	I smoke cigarettes to stimulate me, to perk myself up.	_____
H.	Part of the enjoyment of smoking a cigarette comes from the steps I take to light up.	_____
I.	I find cigarettes pleasurable.	_____
J.	When I feel uncomfortable or upset about something, I light up a cigarette.	_____
K.	I am very much aware of the fact when I am not smoking a cigarette.	_____
L.	I light up a cigarette without realizing I still have one burning in the ashtray.	_____
M.	I smoke cigarettes to give me a "lift."	_____
N.	When I smoke a cigarette, part of the enjoyment is watching the smoke as I exhale it.	_____
O.	I want a cigarette most when I am comfortable and relaxed.	_____
P.	When I feel "blue" or want to take my mind off cares and worries, I smoke cigarettes.	_____
Q.	I get a real gnawing hunger for a cigarette when I haven't smoked for a while.	_____
R.	I've found a cigarette in my mouth and didn't remember putting it there.	_____

Adapted from Horn, D. (1969). *Smoker's Self-Testing Kit*. U.S. National Clearinghouse for Smoking and Health, U.S. Public Health Service, Health Services and Mental Health Administration, Regional Medical Programs Service, Division of Chronic Disease Programs.

How to Score

1. Insert the numbers you have entered in the spaces below, putting the number you have entered to question A over line A, to question B over line B, etc.

2. Add the three scores on each line to get your totals. For example, the sum of your scores over lines A, G, and M gives you your score on Stimulation, lines B, H, and N give the score on Handling, and so on.

Totals

_____	+	_____	+	_____	=	_____	
A		G		M		Stimulation	
_____	+	_____	+	_____	=	_____	
B		H		N		Handling	
_____	+	_____	+	_____	=	_____	
C		I		O		Pleasurable relaxation	
_____	+	_____	+	_____	=	_____	
D		J		P		Crutch: tension reduction	
_____	+	_____	+	_____	=	_____	
E		K		Q		Craving: psychological addiction	
_____	+	_____	+	_____	=	_____	
F		L		R		Habit	

Scores of 11 or above indicate that this factor is an important source of satisfaction for the smoker. Scores of 7 or less are low and probably indicate that this factor does not apply to you. Scores in between are marginal. A description of what your scores mean can be found below.

What My Scores Mean

Scores can vary from 3 to 15 in each category. A score of 11 or above is high; a score of 7 or less is low.

Stimulation

Smoking stimulates/energizes you. You believe smoking helps you wake up, concentrate, organize your energies, and keep going. If you scored more than 11 in this category, you need to find other ways to feel energized, such as the following:

- Avoid fatigue: get sufficient sleep so you won't feel tired.
- Take a walk (or do other exercise) to get yourself moving.
- Meditate to clear your mind and prepare yourself for a day's activities.
- Do some yoga or stretching exercises to balance your energy.
- Use a journal to plan your day's activities.
- Talk to someone or log on to a chat room.
- Chew cinnamon gum (or another strong flavor) to stimulate your sense of taste.

Handling

You like to handle cigarettes, a lighter, or matches. If you scored more than 11 in this category, you need to find other ways to satisfy your desire to handle things, such as the following:

- Hold a special object that has healing significance for you (a stone, beads, etc.).
- Hold a pen or pencil (or plastic cigarette).
- Doodle.
- Play with a coin, a piece of jewelry, or some other harmless object.
- Clean and polish your nails.

Pleasure

Smoking gives you pleasure (or reduces unpleasant feelings). If you scored more than 11 in this category, you need to find alternative ways to feel pleasure, such as the following:

- Meditate.
- Do a pleasurable activity.
- Remind yourself of the harmful effects of smoking.
- Chew a flavored gum that you like.
- Talk to someone or log on to a chat room.

Reduction of negative feelings or crutch

Smoking helps you cope with uncomfortable feelings and stress. If you scored more than 11 in this category, you need to find alternative ways to deal with unpleasant feelings, such as the following:

- Meditate.
- Write your thoughts and feelings in a journal.
- Talk to someone about your feelings.
- Take a walk or exercise.
- Listen to music.
- Identify common stressful situations in your life and experiment with nonsmoking coping methods to find ones that work best.

Craving

You experience cravings for cigarettes. If you scored more than 11 in this category, you need to find other ways to cope with cravings, such as the following:

- Become mindful of—and avoid—situations and circumstances that "trigger" smoking.
- Use deep breathing or meditation to help you let cravings pass.
- Use nicotine replacement products (patch or gum).
- Use craving-reducing medications (e.g., buproprion).
- Take soothing baths or showers.

Habit

For you, smoking is virtually automatic. You do it without thinking. If you scored more than 11 in this category, you need to replace smoking-related habits with nonsmoking ones, such as the following:

- Remove ash trays, cigarettes, and other smoking-related paraphernalia from your house, office, and car so they won't trigger automatic/mindless smoking.
- Designate smoke-free places in your home and office; make your car smoke-free.
- Sit in nonsmoking sections of restaurants.
- Don't go to bars and other locales that permit (and encourage) smoking.
- Make a pact with friends and coworkers who smoke not to smoke around you.

17.2 Am I Addicted to Nicotine?

Nicotine addiction (also called physical dependence) is a major reason for habitual tobacco use. Without nicotine, a tobacco-addicted person experiences withdrawal syndrome consisting of being grouchy and irritable, having headaches, having trouble sleeping, feeling depressed, and having intense cravings for cigarettes.

Directions

- For questions 1–6, choose the answer that best represents you.
- Add your points in column 3.
- Refer to the scoring section below to determine your level of nicotine addiction.

Questions	Answers	Points
1. How soon after you wake do you smoke your first cigarette?	Within 5 minutes	3
	6 to 30 minutes	2
2. Do you find it difficult to refrain from smoking in places where it is forbidden (e.g., in church, at the library, at the movies)?	Yes	1
	No	0
3. Which cigarette would you most hate to give up?	The first one in the morning	1
	All others	0
4. How many cigarettes per day do you smoke?	10 or less	0
	11 to 20	1
	21 to 30	2
	31 or more	3
5. Do you smoke more frequently during the first hours after waking than during the rest of the day?	Yes	1
	No	0
6. Do you smoke if you are so ill that you are in bed most of the day?	Yes	1
	No	0

Scoring

0 to 2—very low dependence

3 to 4—low dependence

5—medium dependence

6 to 7—high dependence

8 to 10—very high dependence

Adapted from Fagerström, K. O., Heatherton, T. F., & Kozlowski, L. T. (1991). Nicotine addiction and its assessment. *Ear, Nose, and Throat Journal, 1990, 69*, 763–765.

17.3 If You Want to Quit

Cigarette smoking is the worst thing one can do to one's health, worse than all other unhealthy behaviors (not exercising, eating too much fat, etc.) combined.

- Cigarette smoke contains over 4,000 chemicals, about 40 of which cause cancer.
- Cigarette smoking increases the risk of heart disease, emphysema (a fatal lung disease), and all types of cancer.
- About 1,000 people die each day as a long-term consequence of their smoking habit.
- 40 million Americans have quit smoking, and most of them are glad they did, so you know it can be done.
- Quitting can be difficult, so the quitter's motto should be "If at first you don't succeed, try, try again."

Why People Start Smoking

- Smoking almost always begins in late childhood or adolescence because of peer pressure, modeling after family members and media personalities, and the influence of advertising.

Why People Continue to Smoke

- Nicotine is highly addicting.
- Cigarettes are easy to get.
- Smoking becomes linked to a wide variety of emotional states, social situations, and activities.
- Nicotine is used to change one's mental state
  - to arouse ("a wake me up")
  - to sedate ("a calm me down")
  - to change a mood (dampen unpleasant emotions)
- Smokers often deny that their health is at risk.

How to Quit

Step 1: Understand the Quitting Process

- The smoker must be ready to stop. When the mind is ready to stop smoking, steps can be taken to bring the body along.
- There is no single method for quitting successfully.
- Many people try several times before achieving permanent success. Relapse can be seen as a step to a final goal rather than a defeat.

Step 2: Precontemplation

- Understanding why you smoke cigarettes (see Exercise 17.1)
- Accepting that smoking is harmful to one's own health and the health of others
- Believing that one can quit successfully
- Having social support during the quitting and maintenance phases of quitting

Step 3: Understanding Withdrawal and Urges

- The first few days are the toughest; withdrawal symptoms peak in two to four days.
- After withdrawal, ex-smokers may continue to experience the urge to smoke in situations in which they smoked in the past (e.g., stress, anger, after a meal, talking on the phone, etc.).
- An urge to smoke rarely lasts for more than a few seconds…so have a way to chill while it passes.
- During the quitting process, consider using nicotine-containing gum, the nicotine patch, and any of a variety of medications that lessen the urge to smoke. Be aware of the *denial trap*, which

is believing that by choosing pharmacological help you are substituting one habituating drug for another. Stop-smoking medications are used only during the few weeks of the quitting process. And they work!

Step 4: Set a Quit Date—the Day You Will Stop Smoking Forever

- Put it on your calendar.
- Announce it to your family and friends.

Step 5: Prepare for the Quit Date

- Cut back on the number of cigarettes smoked (see Exercise 17.4).
- Find alternatives to smoking in the usual smoking situations.
- Come up with strategies for dealing with the urge to smoke after you've quit.
- Stop smoking in your car; clean your car and clothes of cigarette smell.

Step 6: On the Quit Date and for the Next 14 Days

- Discard all cigarettes and smoking paraphernalia (lighters, ashtrays).
- Limit time spent with smokers and in smoking situations.
- Employ alternative behaviors to smoking.
- Employ your strategies for dealing with urges to smoke.

Step 7: Preparing for Possible Relapse

- Be aware that nearly all ex-smokers are tempted to smoke again during the first few months after quitting.
- Never delude yourself into thinking "I'll have only this one."
- Relapse tends to occur during negative emotional states, so quitters should develop alternatives to smoking (e.g., meditating, walking, journal-writing, etc.) for the times of difficult emotions.
- Relapse should be seen as a normal step in the quitting process and not a sign of failure (which can trigger negative, punishing inner self-talk, the soothing of which can be to smoke).

Online Resources for Help with Quitting:

- QuitNet
- SmokeFree.gov…Quitting info from the National Cancer Institute
- You Can Quit Smoking Now…a guide from the National Institutes of Health
- Quit Smoking Program…from the Canadian Lung Association
- The Quit Smoking Company…information and products to help smokers quit including learning how to set a quit date, quit and avoid weight gain, and making quitting easier…lots of resources

17.4 The Cut-Back Method for Quitting Smoking

Prepare for Quit Day (see Exercise 17.3) by cutting back on the number of cigarettes smoked.

- Buy only ONE pack of cigarettes at a time (no more cartons!).
- Change to a less desirable brand of cigarettes.
- Cut cigarettes in half before smoking them.
- Don't carry cigarettes with you so you will have to "bum" them from others.
- Don't smoke on breaks at work, prior to a class, at clubs, or in your car.

Keep a smoking diary to help cutting back on smoking.

Step 1: For 2 days that are representative of your usual smoking pattern, keep a list of all the cigarettes you smoke. For each cigarette record:

- the time of day it was smoked
- how much you wanted/needed the cigarette—1 = not much, 2 = medium, 3 = a lot
- your feelings at the time it was smoked (happy, sad, neutral, depressed, angry, bored, etc.)
- what you were doing when it was smoked (eating, watching TV, driving, etc.)
- whom you were with when it was smoked (alone, with friends or family, etc.)

Step 2: Refer to your smoking diary and identify the cigarettes that you need the least (score of "1" or "2") and cut back on one cigarette a day for as many cigarettes as you can. When you are ready, come up with a plan for eliminating them from your life.

18.1 My Alcohol Use

The CRAFFT and AUDIT (Alcohol Use Disorders Identification Test) questionnaires were developed to identify persons whose alcohol consumption may be hazardous to their health.

Directions:

- Visit the websites listed below and do the online questionnaires.
- If your scores indicate a drinking problem, talk with your doctor or a counselor.

CRAFFT:

http://www.ceasar-boston.org/CRAFFT/

AUDIT:

https://www.drugabuse.gov/sites/default/files/files/AUDIT.pdf

CAGE:

https://pubs.niaaa.nih.gov/publications/inscage.htm

18.2 Cutting Down on Drinking

Directions

1. Respond to these questions:

   - Do you drink alone when you feel angry or sad?

     _____

     _____

   - Does your drinking ever make you late for work?

     _____

     _____

   - Does your drinking worry your family?

     _____

     _____

   - Do you ever drink after telling yourself you won't?

     _____

     _____

   - Do you ever forget what you did while you were drinking?

     _____

     _____

   - Do you get headaches or have a hangover after you have been drinking?

     _____

     _____

If you answered yes to any of the questions, you may have a drinking problem. If you want to cut down on your drinking, follow these steps:

1. Write your reasons for cutting down or stopping.

   _____

   _____

2. Set a drinking goal.

   Choose a limit for how much you will drink. You may choose to cut down or not to drink at all. If you are cutting down, keep below these limits:
   - Women: No more than one drink a day
   - Men: No more than two drinks a day

   Now write your drinking goal on a piece of paper. Put it where you can see it, such as on your refrigerator or bathroom mirror. Your paper might look like this:

   My drinking goal

       I will start on this day _____.

       I will not drink more than _____ drinks in one day.

       I will not drink more than _____ drinks in one week.

       or

       I will stop drinking alcohol.

3. Keep a diary of your drinking. Write down every time you have a drink for 3 to 4 weeks.

Week:

	No. of drinks	Type of drinks	Place consumed
Mon			
Tues			
Wed			
Thurs			
Fri			
Sat			
Sun			

Now you know why you want to drink less and you have a goal. There are many ways you can help yourself to cut down. Try the tips.

4. Watch it at home.

Keep a small amount or no alcohol at home. Don't keep temptations around.

5. Drink slowly.

When you drink, sip your drink slowly. Take a break of one hour between drinks. Drink soda, water, or juice after a drink with alcohol. Do not drink on an empty stomach! Eat food when you are drinking.

6. Take a break from alcohol.

Pick a day or two each week when you will not drink at all. Then, try to stop drinking for one week. Think about how you feel physically and emotionally on these days. When you succeed and feel better, you may find it easier to cut down for good.

7. Learn how to say *NO*.

You do not have to drink when other people drink. You do not have to take a drink that is given to you. Practice ways to say no politely. For example, you can tell people you feel better when you drink less. Stay away from people who give you a hard time about not drinking.

8. Stay active.

9. Get support.

Cutting down on your drinking may be difficult at times. Ask your family and friends for support to help you reach your goal. Talk to your doctor if you are having trouble cutting down. Get the help you need to reach your goal.

10. Watch out for temptations.

Watch out for people, places, or times that make you drink when you do not want to. Stay away from people who drink a lot or bars where you used to go. Plan ahead of time what you will do to avoid drinking when you are tempted.

Do not drink when you are angry or upset or have a bad day. These are habits you need to break if you want to drink less.

11. Do not give up!

Most people do not cut down or give up drinking all at once. Just like a diet, it is not easy to change. That is okay. If you do not reach your goal the first time, try again. Remember, get support from people who care about you and want to help.

Adapted from National Institutes of Health, National Institute on Alcohol Abuse and Alcoholism. (1996). How to cut down on your drinking. http://pubs.niaaa.nih.gov/publications/handout.htm

19.1 My Medical History

As you are likely to have more than one healthcare provider in your life (thus increasing the risk of record-keeping errors), use the charts below to keep (and update regularly) your own medical records.

Illness History

Illness	No	Yes	When	Treatment	Special problems
German measles					
Mumps					
Chicken pox					
Scarlet fever					
Diphtheria					
Pneumonia, bronchitis, asthma					
Arthritis					
Rheumatic fever					
Heart disease or heart murmur					
Anemia					
Bleeding problem					
Ulcer, colitis					
Epilepsy					
Severe headaches					
Mononucleosis					
Jaundice or hepatitis					
Eye injury					
Ear disease or injury					
Skin disease					
Varicose veins					
Kidney or bladder problem					

Surgical History

What	When	Where	Physician

19.2 Using the Internet for Health Research

Your tax dollars are definitely at work at the National Library of Medicine (part of the U.S. Department of Health and Human Services), the most comprehensive medical library in the world. One of the library's services is providing consumers with accurate, up-to-date, authoritative health and medical information through its MedlinePlus website: http://www.medlineplus.gov.

Directions

1. Visit the MedlinePlus website and click any links that interest you.
2. Describe your experience.

_____

_____

_____

_____

_____

20.1 Exploring Complementary and Alternative Medicine

Directions

1. Visit the website of the National Center for Complementary and Alternative Medicine (http://nccam.nih.gov/), a division of the National Institutes of Health (NIH).

2. On the home page, click the link What Is CAM? and write a paragraph summary on what you find.

3. Browse the website and write a paragraph describing something of interest that you discover.

20.2 Evaluating Complementary and Alternative Websites

Several thousand websites offer information about complementary and alternative medicine. Many online health resources are useful, but others may present information that is inaccurate or misleading, so it is prudent to know how to evaluate their content. Be cautious if a website is selling something, does not identify and give the professional credentials of contributors who are providing information, includes outdated or undated information, makes excessive claims for what a product can do, or is sponsored by an organization whose goals differ from yours.

Directions:

Visit, evaluate, and write a review of three websites that discuss/present a complementary or alternative approach to health. Address these questions for each website.

1. What is the name and URL of the website?
2. What is the purpose of the website?
3. What information does the website contain?
4. What is the source of information on the website? Are references cited?
5. Is the information on the pages of the website current?
6. Who is responsible for the content of the website?
7. How do you know that the information provider(s) is an authority in the field?
8. How is the website funded and does sponsorship influence the content of the website?
9. Does the website ask for personal information, and if so, for what purpose?

21.1 Preventing Intentional Injury

Directions

Answer the questions in number 1 below and then respond to 2 and 3.

1. Answer yes or no to the following questions.

1. I have guns in my home.	_____
If yes, are they stored safely?	_____
When used, are they always used safely?	_____
2. I am involved in an abusive relationship.	_____
3. I live in a heavy-crime area.	_____
4. I abuse alcohol or other drugs.	_____
5. I work in a high-risk job.	_____
6. I clearly communicate my intentions and boundaries in a dating situation.	_____
7. I know, and have immediate access to, emergency phone numbers.	_____
8. I have sources of personal support.	_____
9. I know the warning signs of suicide.	_____
10. I know resources for mental health counseling in my community.	_____

2. Based on your responses to the questions in number 1, are there behaviors or situations in your life that need to be addressed? If so, what are they?

   _____

   _____

   _____

   _____

   _____

3. What concerns do you have, both as an individual and a member of your community, related to intentional injury and death?

   _____

   _____

   _____

   _____

   _____

21.2 Preventing Unintentional Injury

Directions
Answer the questions in number 1 below and then respond to 2 and 3.

1. Circle yes or no to the following questions.

1.	I abuse alcohol or other drugs.	Y	N
2.	I wear seat belts when driving or riding in a car.	Y	N
3.	I have a car with front air bags.	Y	N
4.	I drive defensively rather than competitively.	Y	N
5.	I drive appropriately for weather conditions.	Y	N
6.	I maintain my car's tires, wipers, brakes, and lights.	Y	N
7.	I wear a helmet when riding on a bicycle, motorcycle, or roller blades.	Y	N
8.	I follow safety rules when riding a bicycle.	Y	N
9.	I keep gasoline, paint, oily rags, newspapers, plastics, and other flammable materials away from sources of heat.	Y	N
10.	I avoid overloading electrical circuits.	Y	N
11.	I use only safe sources of heat in my living quarters.	Y	N
12.	I avoid smoking in bed.	Y	N
13.	I have a smoke detector on each floor of my house.	Y	N
14.	I have a fire extinguisher in my house.	Y	N
15.	I keep a first-aid kit at home and in my car.	Y	N
16.	I post local emergency numbers and the poison control center number.	Y	N
17.	I follow safety procedures when involved in recreational activities.	Y	N

2. Based on your responses to the questions in number 1, are there behaviors or situations in your life that need to be addressed?

_____

_____

_____

3. What concerns do you have, both as an individual and a member of the community, related to unintentional injury and death?

_____

_____

22.1 Healthy Aging

The health habits you observe as a young and middle-aged adult will greatly determine your health as an older person.

Directions

1. Indicate how frequently you practice each of the health behaviors listed below.
2. Among the health behaviors you do not practice regularly, choose one that you could work on this year to make it a regular part of your life.

Health behavior	Frequency		
	Regularly	Once in a while	Rarely
Do not smoke	_____	_____	_____
Consume recommended amount of fiber	_____	_____	_____
Consume recommended amount of calcium	_____	_____	_____
Consume five servings of fruits and vegetables per day	_____	_____	_____
Limit consumption of well-done meat	_____	_____	_____
Maintain normal body weight	_____	_____	_____
Practice physical activity 3–4 times a week	_____	_____	_____
Have social relationships and ties	_____	_____	_____
Have daily quiet time	_____	_____	_____
Consume minimal or no alcohol	_____	_____	_____
Consume minimal or no fast food	_____	_____	_____
Brush teeth twice a day	_____	_____	_____
Floss teeth once a day	_____	_____	_____
Obtain flu shots	_____	_____	_____
Obtain mammograms (if over age 40)	_____	_____	_____
Obtain Pap smear	_____	_____	_____
Practice human papillomavirus prevention	_____	_____	_____
Practice AIDS prevention	_____	_____	_____
Obtain colorectal screening (if over age 50)	_____	_____	_____
Obtain blood pressure screening	_____	_____	_____
Obtain cholesterol check screening	_____	_____	_____

23.1 Do I Protect Myself from Crime?

Crime Protection

Rate yourself on a scale of 1 to 5 to show how often you follow these crime prevention methods.

    1 = always

    2 = frequently

    3 = sometimes

    4 = rarely

    5 = never

_____	1. I walk in well-lit areas.
_____	2. I watch where I am going and what is happening to me.
_____	3. I try to avoid walking alone at night.
_____	4. I carry a whistle in my hand when walking alone.
_____	5. I lock my car doors and do not leave valuables in sight.
_____	6. I get out my car keys before I reach my car.
_____	7. I park in well-lit and well-traveled areas of the parking lot.
_____	8. I know the location of campus pay phones and call boxes.
_____	9. I always carry cash in case of an emergency.
_____	10. I avoid working or studying in buildings alone.
_____	11. I take the safest, not the fastest, route when walking on campus.
_____	12. I use shuttle buses or a campus escort service after dark.
_____	13. I have memorized the phone number of the campus police.
_____	14. When jogging or biking, I go with a friend and exercise on well-traveled routes.
_____	15. If strangers harassed me, I would leave the scene and go to an open store, gas station, or anywhere people are present.
_____	16. If I were held up, I would give the perpetrator my possessions and not fight.
_____	17. If I were assaulted, I would try not to panic and look at the attacker carefully in order to give a good description to police.

Adapted from Ball State University Campus Safety Tips. (2017). http://cms.bsu.edu/About/AdministrativeOffices/StudentAffairs/ HealthSafety/CampusSafetyHandbook/safetytips. Columbus, Ohio Police Crime Prevention Tips. (2015). http://www.columbuspolice.org/Units/srb/crimeprevention.hml

24.1 Environmental Awareness Questionnaire

Directions

Check the response that is most appropriate for each question. Do you use pesticides in the house to kill insects such as ants, roaches, or flies?

❏ Frequently (1)

❏ Occasionally (2)

❏ Almost never (3)

Do you use pesticides or herbicides around the garden and yard to kill insects and weeds?

❏ Frequently (1)

❏ Occasionally (2)

❏ Almost never (3)

Do you recycle newspapers or other kinds of paper?

❏ Almost never (1)

❏ Sometimes (2)

❏ Regularly (3)

Do you recycle bottles, cans, or plastics?

❏ Hardly ever recycle these items (1)

❏ Some of these items sometimes (2)

❏ Most of the items regularly (3)

When you go on a picnic or hike do you pack up and dispose of all trash in proper trash receptacles?

❏ Very infrequently (1)

❏ Sometimes (2)

❏ All the time (3)

If you need to run an errand that is less than a half mile away, do you walk or bike instead of drive?

❏ Almost never (1)

❏ Occasionally (2)

❏ Most of the time (3)

Do you conserve electricity by turning off unneeded lights and by not running appliances when you don't really need to (like the air conditioner)?

❏ Hardly ever (1)

❏ Some of the time (2)

❏ Almost always (3)

Do you make an effort to conserve water when showering, flushing, washing the car, etc.?

❏ Almost never (1)

❏ Sometimes (2)

❏ Almost always (3)

Do you pour dangerous chemicals such as gasoline or paint solvents down the drain or into sewer systems instead of arranging for proper disposal?

❑ Often (1)

❑ Sometimes (2)

❑ Almost never (3)

Have you thrown an empty can or bottle into the environment?

❑ Within the past week (1)

❑ Within the past month (2)

❑ Not within the past year that you can remember (3)

If you smoke, do you throw your butts into the environment when smoking outside?

❑ Usually (1)

❑ Occasionally (2)

❑ Never (3)

What kind of mileage does your automobile average?

❑ Less than 20 miles per gallon (1)

❑ 20 to 30 miles per gallon (2)

❑ More than 30 miles per gallon (3)

If you play a radio outdoors, how loud do you play it?

❑ About as loud as it will go (1)

❑ Just loud enough for me to hear (2)

❑ Never play a radio outdoors where it might disturb others (3)

When shopping for needed products, do you look for environmentally safe ones?

❑ Never, just look for the cheapest and best product (1)

❑ Sometimes, depends on what is needed (2)

❑ Almost always, if I can find one (3)

How many motor vehicles do you own, including cars, motorcycles, motorboats, jet skis, and others?

❑ More than four (1)

❑ Two to four (2)

❑ Only one (3)

Add up the point values indicated in parenthesis after each answer you checked. A perfect score on these specific environmental questions is 45, but remember that no one is perfect. Perhaps by reviewing your answers you can find ways to improve your environmental awareness—and also contribute to your own health.

24.2 How Environmentally Friendly Is My Car?

Directions

1. Go to the U.S. Department of Energy's Fuel Economy Guide (https://www.fueleconomy.gov/feg/findacar.shtml).

2. In the "Browse By Model" boxes enter the data for your or any other car. Click **GO**.

3. Scroll to find your model and note the MPG.

4. Click on the "Energy and Environment" tab. Scroll to find your model and note the Energy Impact score and the Tailpipe Emissions value. Multiply the tailpipe emission value by the number of miles you drive in a year.

24.3 How Healthy Is My Drinking Water?

The Environmental Protection Agency sets health standards for drinking water. Obtain a report from your local water supplier's most recent report on the quality of the water distributed to you. The easiest way to do this is to contact your local water system (phone or email) and ask. An alternative is to use the EPA website: http://www.epa.gov/ccr/ccr-information-consumers.